Children
with
Disabilities
Seventh Edition

Children
with
Disabilities
Seventh Edition

edited by

Mark L. Batshaw, M.D.
Children's National Medical Center
The George Washington University
School of Medicine and Health Sciences
Washington, D.C.

Nancy J. Roizen, M.D.
University Hospital's Rainbow Babies and Children's Hospital
Division of Developmental-Behavioral Pediatrics and Psychology
Cleveland, Ohio

Gaetano R. Lotrecchiano, Ed.D., Ph.D.
Department of Clinical Research and Leadership
The George Washington University
School of Medicine and Health Sciences
Washington, D.C.

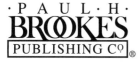
·P·A·U·L·H·
BROOKES
PUBLISHING Co ®

Baltimore • London • Sydney

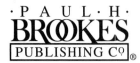

Paul H. Brookes Publishing Co.
Post Office Box 10624
Baltimore, Maryland 21285-0624

www.brookespublishing.com

Typeset by BLPS Content Connections, Chilton, Wisconsin.
Manufactured in the United States of America by
Sheridan Books, Inc., Chelsea, Michigan.

Illustrations, as listed, copyright © 2013 by Mark L. Batshaw. All rights reserved. Figures 1.1–1.3, 1.5–1.13, 1.15, 2.2–2.6, 4.2, 6.1, 6.2, 7.3, 7.4, 7.6, 9.1–9.3, 9.6, 9.9, 9.10, 10.1–10.5, 10.7, 10.8, 10.11, 10.12, 11.1–11.6, 11.9, 12.1a, 12.1c, 12.2–12.5, 12.8–12.10, 15.1–15.4, 16.1, 18.1, 19.1–19.3, 24.6 (drawings only), 24.7, 24.11, 24.12, 24.14, 24.16, 24.17, 24.18 (drawing only), 25.2–25.8, 27.1–27.3, and 35.1.

Illustrations, as listed, copyright © by Lynn Reynolds. All rights reserved. Figures 4.3, 4.5, 9.5, 9.8, 9.11, 11.8, 13.1, 32.3, and 32.5.

Appendix C, Commonly Used Medications, which appears on pages 803–818, provides information about numerous drugs frequently used to treat children with disabilities. This appendix is in no way meant to substitute for a physician's advice or expert opinion; readers should consult a medical practitioner if they are interested in more information.

The publisher and the authors have made every effort to ensure that all of the information and instructions given in this book are accurate and safe, but they cannot accept liability for any resulting injury, damage, or loss to either person or property, whether direct or consequential and however it occurs. Medical advice should only be provided under the direction of a qualified health care professional.

The vignettes presented in this book are composite accounts that do not represent the lives or experiences of specific individuals, and no implications should be inferred. In all instances, names and identifying details have been changed to protect confidentiality.

Library of Congress Cataloging-in-Publication Data

Children with disabilities / edited by Mark L. Batshaw, Nancy J. Roizen, and Gaetano R. Lotrecchiano.—7th ed.
  p.   cm.
  Includes bibliographical references and index.
  ISBN 978-1-59857-194-3 (case)—ISBN 1-59857-194-X (case)
  I. Batshaw, Mark L., 1945– II. Roizen, Nancy J. III. Lotrecchiano, Gaetano R.
[DNLM: 1. Disabled Children. WS 368]
618.92—dc23   2012012739

British Library Cataloguing in Publication data are available from the British Library.

2016

10   9   8   7   6   5   4   3

Contents

I   As Life Begins

1   Genetics and Developmental Disabilities
   Mark L. Batshaw, Andrea Gropman, and Brendan Lanpher 3
   Genetic Disorders
   Chromosomes
   Cell Division and Its Disorders
   Genes and Their Disorders
   Epigenetics
   Genetic Testing
   Environmental Influences on Heredity

2   Fetal Development
   Adré J. du Plessis 25
   Structural Development of the Brain
   Functional Development of the Fetal Nervous System

3   Environmental Toxicants and Neurocognitive Development
   Jerome Paulson 37
   Scope of the Issue
   Susceptible Periods of Development
   Specific Toxicants
   Public Policy Implications

4   Birth Defects and Prenatal Diagnosis
   Rhonda L. Schonberg 47
   Screening Evaluations During Pregnancy
   Prevention and Alternative Reproductive Choices
   Psychosocial Implications

5   Newborn Screening: Opportunities for
      Prevention of Developmental Disabilities
   Joan E. Pellegrino 61
   What Is a Screening Test?
   Why Screen Newborns?
   How Is Newborn Screening Done?
   What Should Be Done When a Child Has a Positive Newborn Screen?
   What Happens to Children with Confirmed Disease?
   What Is the Risk of Developmental Disability in Children with Confirmed Disease?

About the Online Companion Materials

Attention Instructors! Online companion materials are available to help you teach a course using *Children with Disabilities, Seventh Edition.*

Please visit www.brookespublishing.com/batshaw to access

- Customizable PowerPoint presentations for every chapter, totaling over 450 slides
- All original illustrations from the book downloadable for easy use in your PowerPoint presentations, tests, handouts, and other course purposes
- Study questions for every chapter to help students check their knowledge of key concepts
- Extension activities for class use, group projects, and homework to help students apply the information from the text
- Extended case studies to enrich discussions of how concepts are interconnected
- Sample syllabi from various fields to help you determine what chapters and sequence best suits the needs of your course
- Resource listings with functional links for easy access

About the Editors

Mark L. Batshaw, M.D., is the "Fight for Children" Chair of Academic Medicine and Chief Academic Officer at the Children's National Medical Center (CNMC) in Washington, D.C., and Professor and Chairman of Pediatrics and Associate Dean for Academic Affairs at The George Washington University School of Medicine and Health Sciences in Washington, D.C.

Dr. Batshaw is a board-certified neurodevelopmental pediatrician who has treated children with developmental disabilities for more than 35 years. In 2006, Dr. Batshaw received both the Capute Award for notable contributions to the field of children with disabilities by the American Academy of Pediatrics and the Distinguished Research Award from The Arc.

Before moving to Washington in 1998, he was Physician-in-Chief of Children's Seashore House, the child development and rehabilitation institute of The Children's Hospital of Philadelphia. Dr. Batshaw is a graduate of the University of Pennsylvania and of the University of Chicago Pritzker School of Medicine. Following pediatric residency at the Hospital for Sick Children in Toronto, he completed a fellowship in developmental pediatrics at the Kennedy Krieger Institute at The Johns Hopkins Medical Institutions.

Dr. Batshaw continues to pursue his research on innovative treatments for inborn errors of metabolism, including gene therapy. He has published more than 150 articles, chapters, and reviews on his research interests and on the medical aspects of the care of children with disabilities. Dr. Batshaw was the founding editor-in-chief (1995–2001) of the journal *Mental Retardation and Developmental Disabilities Research Reviews*.

Dr. Batshaw lives in Washington, D.C. He and his wife Karen have three children and six grandchildren.

Nancy J. Roizen, M.D., is Director of the Division of Developmental-Behavioral Pediatrics and Psychology at University Hospital's Rainbow Babies and Children's Hospital in Cleveland. She is certified in neurodevelopmental disabilities and in developmental behavioral pediatrics.

Dr. Roizen received her B.S. and M.D. degrees from Tufts University. After completing an internship in pediatrics at Massachusetts General Hospital, she did a residency in pediatrics at The Johns Hopkins Hospital. Her fellowships were in neurodevelopmental disabilities at the Kennedy Krieger Institute and in developmental and behavioral pediatrics at University of California, San Francisco. She then was a staff physician at the Child Development Center at Oakland Children's Hospital for 8 years, followed by 16 years as Chief of the Section of Developmental Pediatrics at the University of Chicago. Then, at SUNY Upstate Medical University, she was Vice Chair of Pediatrics, Professor of Pediatrics, and Chief of the Division of Neurosciences for 4 years. Next stop was the Cleveland Clinic, where she was the Chief of the Department of Developmental Pediatrics and Physiatry for 2 years.

Dr. Roizen has published more than 100 articles, chapters, and reviews on her clinical and research interests in Down syndrome and hearing loss, and on collaborations in congenital toxoplasmosis and velocardiofacial syndrome. She lives in Shaker Heights, Ohio, with her husband. They have a daughter who is working on a postdoctorate fellowship in organic chemistry at Stanford University and a son who is a fellow in pediatric endocrinology at Children's Hospital of Philadelphia.

Gaetano R. Lotrecchiano, Ed.D., Ph.D., is a former Leadership Education in Neurodevelopmental Disabilities Program Director and is presently Academic Director of Translational Science Programs as Assistant Professor of Clinical Research and Leadership and of Pediatrics at The George Washington University School of Medicine and Health Sciences, Washington, D.C.

Dr. Lotrecchiano received a Ph.D. in ethnomusicology in 2005 from the University of Maryland and an Ed.D. in human and organizational learning in 2012 from The George Washington University Graduate School of Education and Human Development. He is a member of the Center for Neuroscience Research at Children's National Medical Center and the Center for the Study of Learning at The George Washington University. He has served in a number of positions administering disabilities and rare disease programs throughout his career, including the Intellectual and Developmental Disabilities Research Center (IDDRC), the Rare Diseases Clinical Research Center (RCDRC), and the Child Health Research Center (CHRC). Presently, he is the Director of Education for the Khalifa Bin Zayed al Nehyan Foundation initiative to create a sustainable rehabilitation center and professional education in the Eastern United Arab Emirates. Dr. Lotrecchiano focuses on professional development through his dedication to those who care for children with special needs. As a result, his scholarly interests have focused on complexity leadership, transdisciplinarity team science, and blended-learning models in professional development, which he feels are key aspects of contemporary professional health care. Recently recognized as a Morton A. Bender Teaching Scholar, Dr. Lotrecchiano has dedicated his entire career to excellence in teaching and instruction. His recent published material is in the *International Journal of Transdisciplinary Research* and *VINE: The Journal of Information and Knowledge Management Systems and Integral Leadership Review*. Dr. Lotrecchiano and his partner Paul live in Beltsville, Maryland, with a historic home in Snow Hill, in the lower Delmarva Peninsula.

Contributors

Kruti Acharya, M.D.
Assistant Professor of Pediatrics and
Medicine
University of Chicago
950 East 61st Street, SSC Suite 207
Chicago, IL 60637

George Acs, D.M.D, M.P.H
ACS Consulting and Publishing
7120 Chilton Court
Clarksville, MD 21029

Laura Gutermuth Anthony, Ph.D.
Assistant Professor
The George Washington University School
of Medicine and Health Sciences
Children's National Medical Center
111 Michigan Avenue, NW
Washington, D.C. 20010

Donna Bernhardt Bainbridge, B.S., M.S.,
Ed.D.
Special Olympics Global Advisor for
FUNfitness & Fitness Programming,
Faculty, MPH Program, University of
Montana
Adjunct Faculty, University of Indianapolis
Special Olympics, Universities of Montana
and Indianapolis
1133 19th Street, NW
Washington, D.C. 20036

Stephen Baumgart, M.D., FAAP
Senior Staff Physician
Professor of Pediatrics
Department of Neonatology, Children's
Hospital National Medical Center
The George Washington University
111 Michigan Avenue, NW
Washington, D.C. 20010

Michelle Bestic, Pharm.D.
Clinical Pharmacologist/Toxicologist
Akron Children's Hospital
1 Perkins Square
Akron, OH 44308

Michael J. Bina, Ed.D.
President
The Maryland School for the Blind
3501 Taylor Avenue
Baltimore, MD 21236

Pamela Buethe, Ph.D.
Director of Audiology
Children's National Medical Center
Children's Hearing and Speech Center
111 Michigan Avenue, NW
Washington, D.C. 20010

Philippa H. Campbell, Ph.D.
Professor
Thomas Jefferson University
6th Floor Edison, Suite 663
130 South 9th Street
Philadelphia, PA 19107

Marilyn Cataldo, M.A.
Director of Behavioral Services in Education
Case Manager (Educational Manager &
Clinical Instructor)
Kennedy Krieger Institute
707 North Broadway
Baltimore, MD 21205

Michael F. Cataldo, Ph.D.
Director of Behavioral Psychology
Kennedy Krieger Institute
707 North Broadway
Baltimore, MD 21205

Taeun Chang, M.D.
Director, Neonatal Neurology
Children's National Medical Center
111 Michigan Avenue, NW
Washington, D.C. 20010

Robin P. Church, Ed.D.
Senior Vice President for Education
Associate Professor of Education
Kennedy Krieger Institute
Johns Hopkins University
3825 Greenspring Avenue
Baltimore, MD 21211

Elissa Batshaw Clair, Ed.S., M.Ed.
School Psychologist
Special School District
12110 Clayton Road
St. Louis, MO 63131

Iser DeLeon, Ph.D.
Associate Professor
Kennedy Krieger Institute
Johns Hopkins University School of
  Medicine
3825 Greenspring Avenue
Baltimore, MD 21211

Dewi Frances T. Depositario-Cabacar, M.D.
Assistant Professor, Neurology and
  Pediatrics
The George Washington University Medical
  Center
Children's National Medical Center
111 Michigan Avenue, NW
Washington, D.C. 20010

Larry W. Desch, M.D.
Clinical Associate Professor of Pediatrics,
Director of Developmental Pediatrics
Chicago Medical School, Rosalind Franklin
  University
Advocate Hope Children's Hospital
4440 West 95th Street
Oak Lawn, IL 60453

Nienke P. Dosa, M.D., M.P.H.
Associate Professor of Pediatrics
Center for Development, Behavior and
  Genetics
Department of Pediatrics
SUNY Upstate Medical University
750 East Adams Street
Syracuse, New York 13210

Adré du Plessis, M.D., MBChB, M.P.H.
Chief of Fetal and Transitional Medicine,
Children's National Medical Center,
Professor of Pediatrics and Neurology
The George Washington University School
  of Medicine
111 Michigan Avenue, NW
Washington, D.C. 20010

Peggy S. Eicher, M.D.
Medical Director, Center for Pediatric
  Feeding and Swallowing Disorders
St. Joseph's Children's Hospital
DePaul Ambulatory Care Center
11 Getty Avenue
Paterson, NJ 07503

Patrick C. Friman, Ph.D., ABPP
Director of the Boys Town Center for
  Behavioral Health
Boys Town
Youth Care Building
13603 Flanagan Boulevard
Boys Town, NE 68010

William Davis Gaillard, M.D.
Professor, Neurology and Pediatrics
Chief Division Neurophysiology, Epilepsy,
  Critical Care Neurology
The George Washington University Medical
  Center
Children's National Medical Center
111 Michigan Avenue, NW
Washington, D.C. 20010

Chrysanthe Gaitatzes, M.D., Ph.D.
Neonatology Attending Physician
Holy Cross Hospital
1500 Forest Glen Road
Silver Spring, MD 20910

Brooke E. Geddie, D.O.
Pediatric Ophthalmologist
Helen DeVos Children's Hospital
330 Barclay, Suite 104, MC 183
Grand Rapids, MI 49503

Arlene Gendron
Project Lead
Children's National Medical Center
111 Michigan Avenue, NW
Washington, D.C. 20010

Angelo P. Giardino, M.D., Ph.D., M.P.H.
Chief Medical Officer/Clinical Professor
Texas Children's Health Plan/Baylor College
  of Medicine
2450 Holcombe Boulevard, Suite 34L
Houston, TX 77021

Marianne M. Glanzman, M.D.
Clinical Associate Professor of Pediatrics
Division of Child Development
  Rehabilitations and Metabolism
The Children's Hospital of Philadelphia
The University of Pennsylvania School of
  Medicine
3550 Market Street, 3rd Floor
Phildelphia, PA 19104

James Gleason, PT, M.S.
Associate Director, University Centers for
    Excellence in Developmental Disabilities
Eunice Kennedy Shriver Center
University of Massachusetts Medical School
200 Trapelo Road
Waltham, MA 02452

Andrea Gropman, M.D.
Associate Professor
The George Washington University of the
    Health Sciences
Children's National Medical Center
Department of Neurology
111 Michigan Avenue, NW
Washington, D.C. 20010

Rebecca M. Haesler, M.S., RD, LD
Clinical Dietitian
Texas Children's Hospital
6621 Fannin St.
Houston, TX 77030

Gilbert R. Herer, Ph.D., CCC-A/SLP
Director Emeritus, Children's Hearing and
    Speech Center
Children's National Medical Center,
Professor Emeritus of Pediatrics
The George Washington University
111 Michigan Avenue, NW
Washington, D.C. 20010

Alexander H. Hoon, Jr., M.D., M.P.H.
Director, Phelps Center for Cerebral Palsy
    and Neurodevelopmental Medicine
Kennedy Krieger Institute
3825 Greenspring Avenue
Baltimore, MD 21211

Susan L. Hyman, M.D.
Associate Professor of Pediatrics
University of Rochester School of Medicine
Division of Neurodevelopmental and
    Behavioral Pediatrics
Box 671
601 Elmswood Avenue
Rochester, NY 14642

SungWoo Kahng, Ph.D.
Senior Behavior Analyst
Kennedy Krieger Institute
3825 Greenspring Avenue
Baltimore, MD 21211

Peter B. Kang, M.D.
Director, EMG Laboratory
Assistant Professor of Neurology
Children's Hospital Boston
Harvard Medical School
Department of Neurology
300 Longwood Avenue
Boston, MA 02115

Robert F. Keating, M.D.
Professor and Chief
Children's National Medical Center
The George Washington University School
    of Medicine
111 Michigan Avenue, NW
Washington, D.C. 20010

Lauren Kenworthy, Ph.D.
Pediatric Neuropsychologist
Director, Center for Autism Spectrum
    Disorders
Associate Professor Pediatrics, Neurology,
    Psychiatry
Children's National Medical Center
The George Washington University Medical
    School
111 Michigan Avenue, NW
Washington, D.C. 20010

Brendan Lanpher, M.D.
Assistant Professor of Pediatrics
Division of Genetics and Metabolism
The George Washington University
Children's National Medical Center
111 Michigan Avenue, NW
Washington, D.C. 20010

Susan E. Levy, M.D.
Associate Professor of Pediatrics
The Children's Hospital of Philadelphia
The University of Pennsylvania School of
    Medicine
3550 Market Street, 3rd Floor
Philadelphia, PA 19104

M.E.B. Lewis, Ed.D.
Director, Education Projects
Kennedy Krieger Institute
3825 Greenspring Avenue
Baltimore, MD 21211

Michelle Huckaby Lewis, M.D., J.D.
Research Scholar
Genetics and Public Policy Center, Berman
    Institute of Bioethics
Johns Hopkins University
1717 Massachusetts Avenue, NW
Washington, D.C. 20036

Gregory S. Liptak, M.D., M.P.H.
Upstate Foundation Professor of Pediatrics
SUNY Upstate Medical University
Syracuse, NY

Toby M. Long, Ph.D.
Associate Professor
Director of Training
Director of Physical Therapy
Georgetown University
Department of Pediatrics
Center for Child and Human Development
Box 571485
Washington, D.C. 20057-1485

Brian K. Martens, Ph.D.
Professor of Psychology
Syracuse University
Department of Psychology
430 Huntington Hall
Syracuse, NY 13244-2340

Marijean Miller, M.D.
Associate Professor
Ophthamology and Pediatrics
Children's National Medical Center
The George Washington University
111 Michigan Avenue, NW
Washington, D.C. 20010

Jocelyn Mills, RD, CSP, LD
Senior Pediatric Clinical Dietitian
Texas Children's Hospital
6621 Fannin Street
Houston, TX 77030

Scott M. Myers, M.D.
Neurodevelopmental Pediatrician
Geisinger Health System
Clinical Assistant Professor of Pediatrics
Temple University School of Medicine
100 North Academy Avenue
Danville, PA 17822

Jerome A. Paulson, M.D.
Director, Mid-Atlantic Center for Children's
    Health & the Environment
Children's National Medical Center
The George Washington University Schools
    of Medicine and Public Health
2233 Wisconsin Avenue, NW, Suite #317
Washington, D.C. 20007

Joan E. Pellegrino, M.D.
Associate Professor of Pediatrics
SUNY Upstate Medical University
750 East Adams Street
Syracuse, NY 13210

Louis Pellegrino, M.D.
Assistant Professor of Pediatrics
SUNY Upstate Medical University
Department of Pediatrics
750 East Adams Street
Syracuse, NY 13210

Steven Perlman, D.D.S., M.Sc.D., D.H.L
    (Hon.)
Professor of Pediatric Dentistry
Boston University School of Dentistry
Global Clinical Advisor and Founder
Special Olympics Special Smiles
77 Broad Street
Lynn, MA 01902

Khodayar Rais-Bahrami, M.D.
Director, Neonatal-Perinatal Medicine
    Fellowship Program
Children's National Medical Center
The George Washington University School
    of Medicine
111 Michigan Avenue, NW
Washington, D.C. 20010

Adelaide Robb, M.D.
Associate Professor Psychiatry and Pediatrics
Children's National Medical Center
The George Washington University
111 Michigan Avenue, NW
Washington, D.C. 20010

Rhonda L. Schonberg, M.S.
Clinical Instructor
The George Washington University School
    of Medicine and Health Sciences
Genetic Counselor and Coordinator
Division of Fetal and Transitional Medicine
Division of Genetics and Metabolism
Children's National Medical Center
111 Michigan Avenue, NW
Washington, D.C. 20010

Scott C. Schultz, M.D.
Instructor
Kennedy Krieger Institute
John Hopkins School of Medicine
707 North Broadway
Baltimore, MD 21205

Vincent Schuyler, B.S., FABDA
Director, Quality & Community
    Partnerships
Goldberg Center for Community Pediatric
    Health,
Children's National Medical Center
Director
District of Columbia Partnership to Improve
    Children's Health Care Quality
111 Michigan Avenue, NW
Washington, D.C. 20010

Neelam Sell, M.D.
Fellow, Developmental-Behavioral Pediatrics
The Children's Hospital of Philadelphia
3350 Market Street, 3rd Floor
Phildelphia, PA 19104

Bruce K. Shapiro, M.D.
The Arnold J. Capute, M.D., M.P.H.
    Chair in Neurodevelopmental Disabilities
Professor of Pediatrics
The Johns Hopkins University School of
    Medicine
Vice President, Training
Kennedy Krieger Institute
707 North Broadway
Baltimore, MD 21205

Billie Lou Short, M.D.
Chief, Division of Neonatology
Professor of Pediatrics
Children's National Medical Center
The George Washington School of Medicine
111 Michigan Avenue, NW
Washington, D.C. 20010

Kara L. Simpson, M.S., CGC
Certified Genetic Counselor
Children's National Medical Center
111 Michigan Avenue, NW, #1950
Washington, D.C. 20010

Peter J. Smith, M.D., M.A.
Assistant Professor of Pediatrics
University of Chicago
950 East 61st Street
SSC Suite 207
Chicago, IL 60637

Sheela L. Stuart, Ph.D., CCC-SLP
Director, Children's Hearing and Speech
    Center
Children's National Medical Center
The George Washington University
111 Michigan Avenue, NW
Washington, D.C. 20010

Adrienne S. Tedeschi, M.D.
Fellow, Developmental-Behavioral Pediatrics
Division of Developmental-Behavioral
    Pediatrics and Psychology
Rainbow Babies and Children's Hospital
11100 Euclid Avenue, Walker Building,
    Suite 3150
Cleveland, OH 44106

Frances Tolley, R.N., B.S.N.
Nurse Clinician, Phelps Center for Cerebral
    Palsy and Neurodevelopmental Medicine
Kennedy Krieger Institute
801 North Broadway
Baltimore, MD 21205

Melissa K. Trovato, M.D.
Assistant Profeesor
Kennedy Krieger Institute
John Hopkins School of Medicine
707 North Broadway
Baltimore, MD 21205

Renee M. Turchi, M.D., M.P.H.
Associate Professor of Pediatrics and
    Community Health and Prevention
St. Christopher's Hospital for Children
Drexel University School of Public Health
3601 A Street
Philadelphia, PA 19134

Betty Vohr, M.D.
Director of Neonatal Follow-up
Professor of Pediatrics
Women & Infants Hospital
Alpert Medical School of Brown University
Division of Neonatology
101 Dudley Street
Providence, RI 02905

H. Barry Waldman, D.D.S., M.P.H., Ph.D.
Distinguished Teaching Professor
Stony Brook University School of Dental
    Medicine
Stony Brook, NY 11794

Patience H. White, M.D., M.A.
Vice President, Public Health
Arthritis Foundation
Professor of Medicine and Pediatrics
The George Washington University School
  of Medicine and Health Sciences
1615 L Street, NW Suite 320
Washington, D.C. 20006

Amanda L. Yaun, M.D.
Assistant Professor, Neurosurgery
Children's National Medical Center
111 Michigan Avenue, NW
Washington, D.C. 20010

Michaela L. Zajicek-Farber, M.S.W., Ph.D.
Associate Professor
The Catholic University of America,
  National Catholic School of Social Service
Shahan Hall #112
620 Michigan Avenue, NE
Washington, D.C. 20064

Tesfaye Getaneh Zelleke, M.D.
Assistant Professor of Pediatrics and
  Neurology
The George Washington University
Children's National Medical Center
111 Michigan Avenue, NW
Washington, D.C. 20010

Michelle H. Zimmer, M.D.
Assistant Professor of Pediatrics
Cincinnati Children's Medical Center
3430 Burnet Avenue MLC 4002
Cincinnati, OH 45229

A Personal Note to the Reader

As it enters its seventh edition, *Children with Disabilities* has continued to evolve. The first edition was derived from lectures I gave for a special education course I taught at The Johns Hopkins University in Baltimore. The book contained 23 chapters, and I authored or co-authored virtually all of them. When I started writing the first edition I was 3 years out of my neurodevelopmental disabilities fellowship training program, and I thought I knew everything about developmental disabilities! I also considered myself an expert in my own children's development, having just welcomed into our family our third child, Andrew.

With this edition of the book the number of chapters and pages has basically doubled since its inception, and I have authored but a few chapters. I have recognized the need for additional help and counsel and have brought on two valued colleagues, Dr. Gaetano R. Lotrecchiano and Dr. Nancy J. Roizen, to coedit the book with me. Guy directed our Leadership Education in Neurodevelopmental Disabilities (LEND) program at Children's National, and my friendship with Nancy dates back to our training at Hopkins. Based on our areas of expertise, we divided the book up. I took the sections As Life Begins and The Developing Child, Nancy focused on Developmental Disabilities, and Guy edited the chapters in the section Interventions, Families, and Outcomes.

The book has also become somewhat of a family affair. My daughter Elissa, a special education teacher and school psychologist, authored the chapter "Special Education Services." And Drew has continued his autobiographical letters concerning the effect of attention-deficit/hyperactivity disorder on his life.

It has been both personally and professionally very rewarding to develop this book over the past 30 years. Many of those rewards have come from the students, colleagues, and parents who have shared with me their thoughts and advice about the book. It is my hope that *Children with Disabilities* will continue to fill the needs of its diverse users for many years to come.

Mark L. Batshaw

Preface

One of the first questions asked about a subsequent edition of a textbook is "What's new?" The challenge of determining what to revise, what to add, and, in some cases, what to delete is always significant in preparing a new edition in a field changing as rapidly as developmental disabilities. Since the publication of the sixth edition in 2007, advances in the fields of neuroscience and genetics have greatly enhanced our understanding of the brain and inheritance. This brings forth opportunities for treatments previously not thought possible for children with developmental disabilities. The human genome has been mapped and the brain probed by functional imaging techniques. The need to examine and explain this increased knowledge and its significance for children with disabilities has necessitated an increase in the depth and breadth of the subjects covered in the book. Yet, while the book is now more expansive and has several new chapters, we have worked hard to ensure that it retains its clarity and cohesion. Its mission continues to be to provide the individual working with and caring for children with disabilities the necessary background to understand different disabilities and their treatments, thereby enabling affected children to reach their full potential.

THE AUDIENCE

Since it was originally published, *Children with Disabilities* has been used by students in a wide range of disciplines as a medical textbook addressing the impact of disabilities on child development and function. It has also served as a professional reference for special educators, general educators, physical therapists, occupational therapists, speech-language pathologists, psychologists, child-life specialists, social workers, nurses, physicians, advocates, and others who provide care for children with disabilities. Finally, as a family resource, parents, grandparents, siblings, and other family members and friends have used the book. They have found useful information on the medical and rehabilitative aspects of care for the child with developmental disabilities.

FEATURES FOR THE READER

We have been told that the strengths of previous editions of this book have been the accessible writing style, the clear illustrations, and the up-to-date information and references. We have dedicated our efforts to retaining these strengths. Some of the features you will find include the following:

- *Teaching goals*—Each chapter begins with learning objectives to orient you to the content of that particular chapter.

- *Situational examples*—Most chapters include one or more stories, or case studies, to help bring alive the conditions and issues discussed in the chapter.

- *Key terms*—As medical terms are introduced in the text, they appear in boldface type at their first use; definitions for these terms appear in the Glossary (Appendix A).

- *Illustrations and tables*—More than 200 drawings, photographs, x rays, imaging scans, and tables reinforce the points of the text and provide ways for you to more easily understand and remember the material you are reading.

- *Summary*—Each chapter closes with a final section that reviews its key elements and provides you with an abstract of the covered material.

- *References*—The reference list accompanying each chapter can be thought of as more than just a list of the literature cited in the chapter. These citations include review articles, reports of study findings, research discoveries, and other key references that can help you find additional information.

- *Appendixes*—In addition to the Glossary, there are three other helpful appendices 1) Syndromes and Inborn Errors of Metabolism, a mini-reference of pertinent information on inherited disorders causing developmental disabilities; 2) Commonly Used Medications, to describe indications and side effects of medications often prescribed for children with disabilities; and 3) Childhood Disabilities Resources, Services, and Organizations, a directory of a wide range of national organizations, federal agencies, information sources, self-advocacy and accessibility programs, and support groups that can provide assistance to families and professionals.

CONTENT

In developing this seventh edition, we have aimed for a balance between consistency with the text that many of you have come to know so well in its previous editions and innovation in exploring the new topics that demand our attention. All chapters have been substantially revised and many have been rewritten to include an expanded focus on psychosocial, rehabilitative, and educational interventions as well as to provide information discovered through educational, medical, and scientific advances since 2007. In addition, four new chapters have been added to address the following topics: 1) the new face of developmental disabilities (long-term outcomes of previously fatal disorders), 2) novel therapies and treatment efficacy (alternative medicine), 3) understanding and using neurocognitive assessment, and 4) diagnosing a child with developmental disabilities. They focus on recently gained knowledge that is transforming our understanding of the causes of developmental disabilities.

The chapters are grouped into sections and have been organized to help guide readers through the breadth of content. The book starts with a section titled As Life Begins, which addresses what happens before, during, or shortly after birth to cause a child to be at increased risk to manifest a developmental disability. The concepts and consequences of genetics, embryology, infections and fetal development, the birth process, and prematurity are explained. The next section of the book, The Developing Child, covers environmental causes of developmental disabilities and examines the various organ systems—how they develop and work and what can go wrong. Nutrition, vision, hearing, language, patterns of development, and the brain and musculoskeletal systems are discussed in individual chapters. As its title implies, the third section, Developmental Disabilities, provides comprehensive descriptions of various developmental disabilities and genetic syndromes causing disabilities and includes chapters on intellectual disability, Down syndrome, inborn errors of metabolism, psychiatric disorders in developmental disabilities, autism spectrum disorders, attention-deficit/hyperactivity disorder, specific learning disabilities, cerebral palsy, neural tube defects, epilepsy, and traumatic brain injury. The final section, Interventions, Families, and Outcomes, contains chapters that focus on various interventions, including early intervention and special education services, feeding, dental care, behavioral assessment and support, assistive technology, and physical and occupational therapy. This section also concentrates on the ethical, legal, emotional, and transition-to-adulthood issues that are common to most families of children with disabilities and to professionals who work with them. The book closes with a discussion of the prospects for providing health care in the 21st century.

THE AUTHORS AND EDITORS

Nancy J. Roizen joined me as an editor for the sixth edition of the text. Like me, she is a neurodevelopmental pediatrician. Gaetano R. Lotrecchiano, an educator for interdisciplinary training in developmental disabilities, joined as an editor on this edition. We have chosen physicians, psychologists, social workers, therapists, and other health care professionals who are experts in the areas they write about as authors of *Children with Disabilities*. Many are colleagues from Children's National Medical Center in Washington, D.C. Each chapter in the book has undergone editing at Paul H. Brookes Publishing Co. to ensure consistency in style and accessibility of content. Once the initial drafts were completed, each chapter was sent for peer review by major clinical and academic leaders in the field and was revised according to their input.

A FEW NOTES ABOUT TERMINOLOGY AND STYLE

As is the case with any book of this scope, the editor or author faces decisions about the use of particular words or the presentation style of information. We would like to share with you some of the decisions we have made for this book.

- *Categories of intellectual disability*—This book uses the American Psychiatric Association's categories according to the term *mental retardation* (i.e., mild, moderate, severe, profound) when discussing medical diagnosis and treatment and uses the categories that the American Association on Intellectual and Developmental Disabilities (formerly the American Association on Mental Retardation) established in 1992 (i.e., requiring limited, intermittent, extensive, or pervasive support) when discussing educational and other interventions, thus emphasizing the capabilities rather than the impairments of individuals with intellectual disability.

- *"Typical" and "normal"*—Recognizing diversity and the fact that no one type of person or lifestyle is inherently "normal," we have chosen to refer to the general population of children as "typical" or "typically developing," meaning that they follow the natural continuum of development.

- *Person-first language*—We have tried to preserve the dignity and personhood of all individuals with disabilities by consistently using person-first language, speaking, for example, of "a child with autism," instead of "an autistic child." In this way, we are able to emphasize the person, not define him or her by the condition.

As you read this seventh edition of *Children with Disabilities*, we hope you will find that the text continues to address the frequently asked question "Why this child?" and to provide the medical background you need to care for children with developmental disabilities.

Acknowledgments

We would like to thank our colleagues at Paul H. Brookes Publishing Co. for their great help. Steve Plocher served as Associate Editor for the text and Johanna Cantler as Acquisitions Editor, and both provided developmental oversight of the project; Danica Crittenden assisted with the review process. A book such as *Children with Disabilities* is best understood with illustrations that help to explain medical concepts. An expert medical illustrator is crucial in this effort. Lynn Reynolds has contributed to this endeavor in both past editions and with new additions in this volume. We deeply acknowledge her important contribution. We also gratefully acknowledge Arlene Gendron, who helped organize the project as well as contributed to the book's appendixes. We thank previous contributors whose work on the sixth edition laid an excellent foundation for this text: Terry Adirim, Karen Batshaw, Michael Batshaw, Michael J. Bell, Nathan J. Blum, Jill E. Brown, W. Bryan Burnette, Seth Canion, Charles J. Conlon, Philip W. Davidson, Carolyn Drews-Botsch, Ann-Christine Duhaime, Diana M. Escolar, Sara Helen Evans, Erynn S. Gordon, Karl F. Gumpper, Michael J. Guralnick, William H.J. Haffner, Mark L. Helpin, Janet S. Isaacs, Dorothy O. Jones, Annie Kennedy, Carol A. Knightly, Alan E. Kohrt , Lisa A. Kurtz, Mary F. Lazar, Sheryl J. Menacker, Gretchen A. Meyer, Linda J. Michaud, Gary J. Myers, Man Wai Ng, Jeffrey P. Rabin, Mark Reber, Howard M. Rosenberg, Andrew J. Satin, Tomas Jose Silber, Harvey S. Singer, Annie G. Steinberg, Ana Carolina Tesi Rocha, Cynthia J. Tifft, Laura L. Tosi, Kenneth E. Towbin, Symme Wilson Trachtenberg, Mendel Tuchman, Kim Van Naarden Braun, Shari L. Wade, Steven L. Weinstein, and Marshalyn Yeargin-Allsopp. Finally, many of our colleagues reviewed and edited the manuscript for content and accuracy, and we would like to acknowledge their efforts.

Why me?
Why me?
Why do I have to do so much more than others?
Why am I so forgetful?
Why am I so hyperactive?
And why can't I spell?
Why me? O'why me?

I remember when I almost failed first grade because I couldn't read. I would cry hour after hour because my mother would try to make me read. Now I love to read. I couldn't write in cursive but my mother helped me and now I can. I don't have as bad a learning disability as others. At lest I can go to a normal school. I am trying as hard as I can (I just hope it is enough). My worst nightmare is to go to a special school because I don't want to be treated differently.

I am getting to like working. I guess since my dad is so successful and has a learning disability, it helps make me not want to give up. Many people say that I am smart, but sometimes I doubt it. I am very good at math, but sometimes I read a number like 169 as 196, so that messes things up. I also hear things incorrectly, for instants entrepreneur as horse manure (that really happened). I guess the reason why a lot of people don't like me is because I say the wrong answer a lot of times.

I had to take medication, but then I got off the medication and did well. Then in 7th grade I wasn't doing well but I didn't tell my parents because I thought they would just scream at me. My dad talked to the guidance counselor and found out. It wasn't till a week ago that I started on the medication again; I have been doing fine since than. As I have been getting more organized, I have had more free time. I guess I feel good when I succeed in things that take hard work.

This is my true story. . .

Andrew Batshaw

Andrew Batshaw
1989

In applying to colleges during my senior year of high school, I found that most had as an essay topic, "Tell us something about yourself." I decided to write about my ADHD and learning disability as it is a big part of who I am. I wrote "I have found that while a disability inherently leaves you with a weakness, adapting to that disability can provide rewards. I feel that from coping with my disability, I have gained pride, determination, and a strength that will be with me all of my life." I guess Vassar College agreed; they admitted me.

When it came time for high school graduation, we had a problem. My sister was graduating from the University of Chicago on the same day that I graduated from high school in Philadelphia. The only solution was for one parent to attend my graduation while the other one was with my sister in Chicago. The decision as to who would go to which graduation was easy. My mother insisted that she attend my graduation because it was a product of her hard work as well as my own. I remember she said to me that day, "When I think of the boy who cried himself to sleep because he could not remember how to spell the word 'who,' it makes me so happy to see you now."

My parents expressed themselves in different ways about my leaving for college. My mother and I found ourselves getting into many arguments over simple things (the old severing of the umbilical cord; I am the baby of the family). My father, however, made sure to remind me to start my stimulant medication 2 weeks before classes began!

The first semester I took four courses: Poetry, Linear Algebra, Computer Science, and Music Theory. As the semester continued, I developed an increasing interest in computer science, until finally I decided to become a computer science major. I was very flattered, however, when during a meeting with my English professor, she asked if I planned to be an English major. To think that someone who could not read until the end of second grade would become a member of the Vassar English department seemed almost unbelievable. Well, I might have been proud but not that proud. I stuck with computer science.

On the whole, I would say that my freshman year was a good one. I learned a great deal, both inside and outside of classes, about myself and others. What will I do after college? What will I end up doing with my life? These are questions that continually run through my mind. I have no clear answers, but there is one thing of which I am sure: My disability will not keep me from doing anything. I will not let it.

andrew Batshaw

Andrew Batshaw
1996

As a college graduate, I find that my ADHD and learning disabilities are much less of an issue; however, that was not the case during my early college years. In my second year of college, I took a year-long introductory German class that fulfilled my language requirement. Forgetting that languages don't come easily to me, I chose the intensive German class that met an extra day a week and moved faster than the regular class. I watched my exam grades slowly slide into the C range during the first semester and decided to switch to the regular class for the rest of the year. While this was happening, some medical warnings were issued concerning the stimulant medication I was taking, so I decided to discontinue its use.

In the new German class, we had exams every other week, so I received regular feedback on how I was doing. Unfortunately, it was not positive feedback. After receiving an F on the first quiz, I decided that I needed to work harder in the class. I started studying more and was less than relieved when on my next exam my grade rose to a D! Again, I studied even more and still received a D on the test that followed. At this point, I began to doubt myself. I felt like I was doing everything I could, and still I wasn't improving. I said to myself, "I know you have always told yourself that you could do anything you really gave your all to, but maybe there are just some things you can't do." I was disheartened, but felt that I had no choice but to just keep working. I received a C and then a C+ on my next two exams, but my overall class grade was still very low. My professor spoke to me and said that as long as I received at least a C+ on the final exam, he would pass me. I did all I could to prepare for the test and took the exam without reservation, simply willing to accept the results, whatever they might be. I ran into my professor a week after the final exam and was told that not only had I passed the final exam, but that I had received an A, one of the highest grades in the class. As you might expect, I was ecstatic. I looked back on the day when I had thought, "Maybe there really are things that I just can't do," and smiled, because I proved myself wrong. On top of that, I had accomplished it without the help of medication. That was when I truly felt that I had overcome my ADHD and learning disabilities.

In fact, some of the most important activities in my life are things that at first glance you wouldn't think someone with ADHD would find attractive. I meditate every day, which involves sitting in one place and not moving for long periods of time. When I meditate, I am actually watching how my mind works. I see how easily I am distracted from simply sitting by thinking about all kinds of things, like what I did yesterday or what I am going to do later. Nevertheless, I keep bringing myself back, over and over again, and sometimes my mind becomes very quiet and clear. I find that this has had a positive impact on all aspects of my life. I was talking with my older brother, Michael, after attending my first 3-day meditation retreat, and he told me how proud he was of me. He said that after seeing me bounce off the walls and have such difficulty concentrating while growing up, he was amazed that I could sit still and meditate for 3 days.

After 4 years, including 6 months at the University of York in England, I graduated from Vassar College with a B.A. in Computer Science in May 1999. After graduation, I worked for a year as a software engineer and then started my own company with my brother and a friend. Unfortunately, after developing the company for a year, we became one of the many casualties of the dot-com collapse. Naturally, I was very disappointed, but it was an incredible experience that I will always value. It sparked in me a passion for entrepreneurship that led to my decision to attend business school.

Throughout the process of applying to business school, it became clear to me how my learning disability had been transformed from a hindrance to an asset. The work habits I had developed to overcome my disability allowed me to stick to a rigorous preparation program for my business school entrance exams. As a result, I scored in the 98th percentile. In addition, when preparing my applications, I chose to include an essay about how overcoming a disability had taught me to treat failure as a natural and necessary part of important accomplishments. Furthermore, it instilled in me a drive to achieve and to take calculated risks that are essential to being successful in business. I will be attending the University of Southern California Business School with a full scholarship.

Drew Batshaw
2002

Five eventful years have passed since I wrote my foreword to the fifth edition of this text. I graduated from business school, fell in love and married an amazing woman, and have been pursuing a career in business. Through all of these experiences, my ADHD and learning disability continue to impact my life in both subtle and not-so-subtle ways.

At the end of my last letter, I spoke about pursuing an MBA at the University of Southern California. My experience in business school was positive, both academically and socially. I'd come a long way from my childhood struggles; my ADHD and learning deficits had little effect on my performance. I excelled, my teachers respected me, and other students regularly sought me out to work on projects with them.

For me, business school was easier than college for a number of reasons. The subject matter was generally more engaging and played to my strengths: thinking on my feet, presenting ideas orally, and using analytical reasoning. In addition, much of the learning took place in an interactive and experiential environment that kept my interest and attention. For example, we discussed real situations that companies have had in the past and how we would have managed them, and we role-played as consultants with 90 minutes to prepare a thorough presentation for the class. Another significant factor was that writing (which historically has been my most challenging form of communication) is different and easier for me in a business setting than an academic one. In business writing, lengthy discourse is discouraged and traditional writing rules are far less important than presenting information in a clear and concise way; plus, of course, I'd had many years to hone my writing skills since I entered Vassar. Finally, I'd learned to manage my disability and identify environments like business school where I would be most successful.

After graduating with my MBA, I launched a company that provided coaching services for young executives and business owners. My job as a coach was to assist clients in their effectively working through problems, as opposed to the traditional consultant model of doing the work for them. After about 18 months, I realized that my heart was no longer in building the business; I missed managing tangible projects and found coaching to be lonely. I had many clients but no peers to interact with on a daily basis. I then moved to my current job, where I run the operations and technology of an education technology company that helps low-income children improve their reading skills. It is very satisfying to be involved in a business that helps children who have reading difficulties like I had. In contrast to the coaching work, this job allows me to manage many different projects and work with a great team.

I have also found that I reap unexpected benefits from my ADHD. Professionally, I am known for my ability to effectively problem-solve with limited information. Unlike others who are intimidated by their lack of knowledge or information, I delight in jumping right into the problem and figuring it out as I go (much like how I used to raise my hand all the time in grade school even though I didn't know the answer). In addition, I juggle many different projects and priorities with finesse. I thrive in environments that offer variety, allow me to wear many different hats, and require the use of a broad set of skills throughout the course of each day. Perhaps because of this I have changed jobs every 1 to 2 years since graduating from college (7 years ago): I have been a software developer, a dot-com founder, a business school student, and an executive coach, and now I am a manager of technology and finance. When I first start a job, I'm very excited and engaged in the work, but after I become proficient, I start to itch to do something different. Does my ADHD cause me to need a certain kind of sustained and varied stimulation that I have not yet found? I'm not sure, but I do know that I require a high level of change and stimulation to stay engaged and productive.

My ADHD impacted my early adulthood in other ways. For many years, no matter how much I achieved or how well I succeeded, I was still left with the shame of not being good enough during my formative years. As a child, my disability affected my self-image as well as my academic performance. Despite my mother telling me, "You are intelligent. It's just your learning disability that affects how you do in school," I still measured my worth in comparison to everyone else—for example, how far I got in a spelling bee, how long it took me to read a book, or what grade I received on a writing assignment. Through much of my twenties, when something didn't go well in my life—professionally, personally, or sometimes even when I was just sick—I would feel like that little boy again who just couldn't do anything right. I can see now that no amount of achievement would have transformed those feelings of inadequacy.

What has helped me most in dealing with this legacy is counseling and rewarding intimate relationships. Counseling has helped me to recognize when this old shame is triggered and how to notice it and move on. Through intimate relationships, I've come to understand and own my worth in a greater sense— how I offer so much more than just what I can achieve. For example, I have a positive impact on others by just being in their lives, and I can move people with my emotions and words. These things are all effortless. I don't have to try or work hard to make them happen. They simply occur as a natural result of who I am inherently.

My greatest teacher in this has been my wife, Amy. We were married in August 2005 after dating for 2 years. Her capacity for love, joy, and compassion amazes me. While preparing this letter, I asked her how my disability impacts our relationship. She smiled and said, "Well, you don't like to wash the dishes or go clothes shopping with me!" Much as I'd like to blame that on ADHD, I'm not sure that would be fair. What I *have* noticed are some of Amy's qualities that make her an especially good match for someone like me with ADHD. Professionally, she is a coach and organizing consultant, and, as a result, naturally provides structure and organization to our lives. In addition, she gives me a lot of space and honors the transition time I need between being by myself and being with her. Finally, she is very accepting and offers me constant appreciation and encouragement. I am a lucky man!

In sum, I lead an extraordinarily blissful life. I have a wonderful wife, my current work is stimulating and meaningful, and my relationships with family and friends are warm and fulfilling. I am immensely grateful for all I have been given and all I have been able to accomplish—in spite of and *because of* my disability.

Andrew Batshaw
2007

Reflecting on the impact of my learning disability and ADHD on my current life, I am struck by how little impact I still feel. At the age of 33, I appreciate the fact that my learning disability and ADHD are not at the heart of any of my current struggles: My lack of sleep, lack of free time and lack of time with my wife can all be attributed to having two small children (Gia, 3½ and Mika, 18 months). I did not anticipate all the challenges that having children would create. For example, when my wife, Amy, and I are both exhausted and sleep deprived, it is really difficult to find energy for the activities that nourish our relationship. We have to work hard to find the energy and make the time for these activities. It has been worth the effort and I am delighted that as Gia and Mika get older it's getting easier and easier. There is something satisfying about being challenged not by my disability, but by things that are difficult for most parents with young kids.

I can confidently say that I no longer need to manage my disability. I have overcome most of it and view any remnants as the same challenges everyone faces. Some challenges include: I prefer to be able to structure my own work; I get stressed at work when I have multiple items with close deadlines that aren't movable; When I am with my kids, I need to work hard to stay present and not think about other things. I could build a case for how each of these challenges are rooted in my disability but I don't because in the end, they are like any other factors I work with to create the best life that I can. So, I choose jobs where I will be able to structure my work. Also, I set up processes to minimize deadlines being set without my consideration. When I notice I am not being present with my kids, I change what I am doing so I won't be as distracted. Doing these things happens naturally. For example, I am simply more attracted to work environments where I can structure my work. When I start a new job, I don't methodically create processes to minimize deadlines without my consideration; it just happens in the way I establish working relationships. I believe that managing my disability shaped the ways I now automatically manage myself, my work environment and my personal life. As a result, I can go months without even thinking about the fact that I have a disability (in fact, I am tempted to say "had" a disability instead of "have").

The one trigger that reconnects me to the emotions of growing up with a disability is witnessing others with disabilities. A few years ago, I happened across a Craigslist ad written by an older brother. He wanted to buy an inexpensive video game system to play with his little brother who had (I believe physical) disabilities. He didn't need the latest generation system; he just wanted to find a way to connect and play because things were so challenging for his brother. His thoughtfulness and commitment to creating joy for his brother still move me today.

Four years ago in my last letter, I mentioned my concern about changing jobs frequently and needing a lot of varied stimulation. I am happy to report that my current job has the potential for me to remain sufficiently challenged and satisfied for many years. As the Director of Product Development for a small technology company, I have just the right mix of activities: I spend about 50% of my time writing software (coding) and the other 50% managing people and projects. In addition, my job desires have shifted a little since having children. Work stability and predictability have become more important financially, and also provide a balance to all of the constant change and stimulation at home.

As I think back to the writing of my previous letters, I see a reassuring arc in my relationship with my disability. At first my identity was inextricably tied to being someone with learning disabilities. As I began to achieve success in spite of them, I saw myself as someone who was overcoming disabilities. Further into adulthood, I was someone minimally impacted by disabilities. And today, I don't even think of myself as having disabilities. It has been quite a ride, and I look forward to what comes next.

Andrew Batshaw
2011

This book is dedicated to all of the families we have been honored to serve and to the health care professionals we have taught so they could care for children with disabilities.

We would also like to dedicate this book to Greg Liptak, M.D., a developmental pediatrician and an author in this text who made major contributions to the field of children with disabilities. His recent death has been a major loss to the field and to the children and families he served.

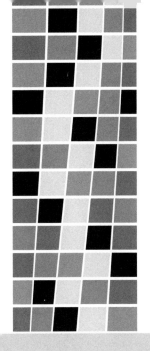

I

As Life Begins

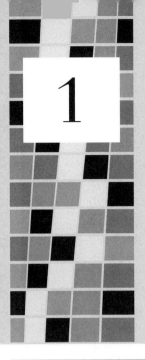

1

Genetics and Developmental Disabilities

Mark L. Batshaw, Andrea Gropman, and Brendan Lanpher

Upon completion of this chapter, the reader will

- Know about the human genome and its implication for the origins of developmental disabilities

- Be able to explain errors in mitosis and meiosis, including nondisjunction, translocation, and deletion

- Know the differences and similarities among autosomal recessive, autosomal dominant, and X-linked genetic disorders

- Understand epigenetics and the related concepts of genomic imprinting and copy number variation

- Understand the ways that genes can be affected by the environment in which they reside

Whether we have brown or blue eyes is determined by genes passed on to us from our parents. Other traits, such as height and weight, are affected by genes and by our environment both before and after birth. In a similar manner, genes alone or in combination with environmental factors can place children at increased risk for many developmental disorders, including birth defects such as meningomyelocoele or spina bifida (see Chapter 4). The spectrum of disorders that leads to developmental disabilities has a range of genetic and environmental causes. Some disorders are purely genetic, such as Rett syndrome and certain forms of muscular dystrophy (see Chapter 19), which result from a **single-gene defect**, and Down syndrome (see Chapter 18), which results from an extra chromosome (aneuploidy). At the other end of the

spectrum are disorders that are almost purely environmentally induced, including infectious diseases such as cytomegalovirus and those caused by teratogens like alcohol (see Chapter 3). Then there are conditions in which genes are affected by their environment leading to epigenetic disorders such as fragile X and Angelman syndrome. As an introduction to the discussion in the chapters that follow, this chapter describes the human cell and explains what chromosomes and genes are. It also reviews and provides some illustrations and examples of the errors that can occur in the processes of **meiosis** (cell division) and **mitosis** (cell reproduction), discusses inheritance patterns of single-gene disorders, and presents the new concept of epigenetics. As you progress through this book, bear in mind that the purpose of this discussion is to focus on the abnormalities that can occur in human development. These disorders are typically rare, however, genetic mechanisms underlie a large proportion of childhood disease and disability.

■ ■ ■ KATY

Katy was developing typically until she was 2 years old, when she started to have episodes of vomiting and lethargy after high-protein meals. Her parents became very concerned because their older son, Andrew, had died in infancy after lethargy and seizures were followed by coma, although no specific diagnosis had been made. With extensive testing by a genetic metabolic specialist, Katy was discovered to have an error (mutation) in the gene that codes for ornithine transcarbamylase (OTC), an enzyme that prevents the accumulation of ammonia in body and brain that can lead to coma. The OTC gene is located on the X chromosome so its deficiency is inherited as an X-linked disorder. Because girls have two X chromosomes, one with the mutation and one normal copy, they are therefore less likely to be affected than boys and, when affected, they generally have less severe manifestations. It turns out that Andrew also carried this mutation. Katy was placed on a low-protein diet and given medication to provide an alternate pathway to rid the body of ammonia, and she has done well. Now age 7, it looks like she may have a mild nonverbal learning disability; if Katy had been left untreated, she would probably not be alive.

GENETIC DISORDERS

The human body is composed of approximately 100 trillion cells. There are many cell types, including nerve cells, muscle cells, white blood cells, and skin cells, to name a few. All cells except for the red blood cell are divided into two compartments: 1) a central, enclosed core—the nucleus; and 2) an outer area—the **cytoplasm** (Figure 1.1). The red blood cell differs insofar as it does not have a nucleus. The nucleus houses **chromosomes,** structures that contain the genetic code (**deoxyribonucleic acid;** DNA), which is organized into hundreds of units of heredity (**genes**) in each chromosome. These genes are responsible for physical attributes and biological functioning. Under the direction of the genes, the products that are needed for the organism's development and functions, such as waste disposal and the release of energy, are made in the cytoplasm. The nucleus, then, contains the blueprint for the organism's growth and development, and the cytoplasm manufactures the products needed to complete the task.

When there is a defect within this system, the result may be a genetic disorder. These disorders take many forms. They include the addition of an entire chromosome in each cell (e.g., Down syndrome), the loss of an entire chromosome in each cell (e.g., Turner syndrome; aneuploidy), and the loss or deletion of a significant portion of a chromosome (e.g., Cri-du-chat syndrome). There can also be a **microdeletion** of a number of closely spaced or contiguous genes within a chromosome (e.g., chromosome 22q11.2 deletion syndrome or velocardiofacial

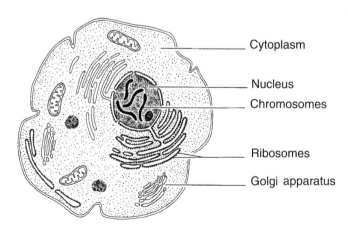

Figure 1.1. An idealized cell. The genes within chromosomes direct the creation of a product on the ribosomes. The product is then packaged in the Golgi apparatus and released from the cell.

syndrome [VCFS]), which may have varied expression depending on environmental influences (Gothelf, Schaer, & Eliez, 2008). Finally, there can be a defect within a single gene (e.g., phenylketonuria) or altered expression of the gene (e.g., Rett syndrome). This chapter discusses each of these types of genetic defects, beginning with a discussion of chromosomes and problems in their division.

CHROMOSOMES

Each organism has a fixed number of chromosomes that direct the cell's activities. In each human cell, there are 46 chromosomes. Generally speaking, each chromosome contains hundreds of genes, but some chromosomes have more (e.g., 500–800 gene loci in chromosomes 1, 19, and X) and others have fewer (50–120 in chromosomes 13, 18, 21, and Y). The 46 chromosomes are organized into 23 pairs. Normally, one chromosome in each pair comes from the mother and the other chromosome comes from the father. Egg and sperm cells, unlike all other human cells, each contain only 23 chromosomes. During conception, these **germ cells** fuse to produce a fertilized egg with the full complement of 46 chromosomes.

Among the 23 pairs of chromosomes, 22 are termed **autosomes.** The 23rd pair consists of the X and Y chromosomes, or the **sex chromosomes.** The Y chromosome, which determines "maleness," is one third to one half the size of the X chromosome, has a different shape, and has far fewer genes. Two X chromosomes determine the child to be female; an X and a Y chromosome determine the child to be male.

CELL DIVISION AND ITS DISORDERS

Cells have the ability to divide into daughter cells that contain genetic information that is identical to the information from the parent cell. The prenatal development of a human being is accomplished through cell division, differentiation into different cell types, and movement of cells to different locations in the body. There are two kinds of cell division: mitosis and meiosis. In mitosis, or nonreductive division, two daughter cells, each containing 46 chromosomes, are formed from one parent cell. In meiosis, or reductive division, four daughter cells, each containing only 23 chromosomes, are formed from one parent cell. Although mitosis occurs in all cells, meiosis takes place

only in the germ cells in order to create sperm and eggs.

The ability of cells to continue to undergo mitosis throughout the life span is essential for proper bodily functioning. Cells divide at different rates, however, ranging from once every 10 hours for skin cells to once a year for liver cells. This is why a skin abrasion heals in a few days, but the liver may take a year to recover from hepatitis. By adulthood, some cells, including neurons and muscle cells, appear to have a significantly decreased ability to divide. This limits the body's capacity to recover after medical events such as strokes or from injuries.

One of the primary differences between mitosis and meiosis can be seen during the first of the two meiotic divisions. During this cell division, the corresponding chromosomes line up beside each other in pairs (e.g., both copies of chromosome 1 line up together). Unlike in mitosis, however, they intertwine and may "cross over," exchanging genetic material, which adds variability (Figure 1.2). Although this crossing over (or recombination) of the chromosomes may result in disorders (e.g., deletions), it also allows for the mutual transfer of genetic information, reducing the chance that siblings end up as exact copies (clones) of each other. Some of the variability among siblings can also be attributed to the random assortment of maternal and paternal chromosomes during the first of two meiotic divisions.

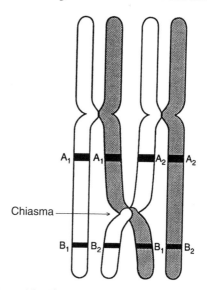

Figure 1.2. The process of crossing over (i.e., recombination) at a chiasma permits exchange of genetic material among chromosomes and accounts for much of the genetic variability of human traits. In this illustration, there is an exchange between two chromosomes at the banding area labeled B. (*Source:* Jorde, Carey, & Bamshad, 2001.)

Throughout the life span of the male, meiosis of the immature sperm produces **spermatocytes** with 23 chromosomes each. These cells will lose most of their cytoplasm, sprout tails, and become mature sperm. This process is termed spermatogenesis. In the female, meiosis forms oocytes that will ultimately become mature eggs, in a process called oogenesis. By the time a girl is born, her body has produced all of the approximately 2 million eggs she will ever have. A number of events that adversely affect a child's development can occur during meiosis (Hassold, Hall, & Hunt, 2007). When chromosomes divide unequally, a process known as **nondisjunction** occurs: One daughter egg or sperm contains 24 chromosomes and the other 22 chromosomes. Usually, these cells do not survive, but occasionally they do and can lead to the child being born with too many chromosomes (e.g., Down syndrome) or too few chromosomes (e.g., Turner syndrome). It is interesting to note that the most commonly found **trisomy** in miscarriages is trisomy 16, but embryos with trisomy 16 are never carried to term (Brown, 2008). The chromosome 16 contains so many genes important to development that its disruption is incompatible with life. Conversely, trisomies 13, 18, and 21 are the most commonly observed chromosomal

disorders at birth, probably because these chromosomes contain a relatively small number of gene loci and their disruption does not cause death, even though it does cause severe developmental disabilities (Parker et al., 2003).

The majority of fetuses carrying chromosomal abnormalities are spontaneously aborted. Among those children who survive these genetic missteps, **intellectual disability,** unusual (dysmorphic) facial appearances, and various **congenital organ** malformations are common. In the general population, chromosomal errors causing disorders occur in 6–9 per 1,000 of all live births. In children who have intellectual disability, however, the prevalence of chromosomal abnormality increases 10- to 40-fold (Flint et al., 1995).

Chromosomal Gain: Down Syndrome

The most frequent chromosomal abnormality is nondisjunction of autosomes, and the most common clinical consequence is trisomy 21, or Down syndrome (Wiseman, Alford, Tybulewicz, & Fisher, 2009; see Chapter 18). Nondisjunction can occur during either mitosis or meiosis but is more common in meiosis (Figure 1.3). When nondisjunction occurs during the first meiotic division, both copies of

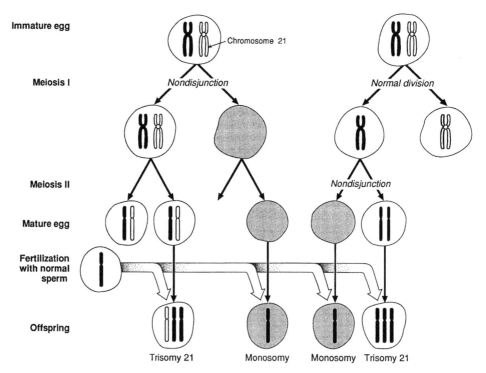

Figure 1.3. Nondisjunction of chromosome 21 in meiosis. Unequal division during meiosis I or meiosis II can result in trisomy or monosomy.

chromosome 21 end up in one cell. Instead of an equal distribution of chromosomes among cells (23 each), one daughter cell receives 24 chromosomes and the other receives only 22. The cell containing 22 chromosomes is unable to survive. However, the egg (or sperm) with 24 chromosomes occasionally can survive. After fertilization with a sperm (or egg) containing 23 chromosomes, the resulting embryo contains three copies of chromosome 21, or trisomy 21. The child will be born with 47 rather than 46 chromsomes in each cell and have Down syndrome (Figure 1.4).

A majority of individuals with Down syndrome (approximately 90%) acquire it as a result of a nondisjunction during meiosis in oogenesis; about 5% acquire Down syndrome from nondisjunction during spermatogenesis (Soares, Templado, & Blanco, 2001). This disparity is partially due to the increased rate of autosomal nondisjunction in egg production, but also to the lack of viability of sperm with an extra chromosome 21. Another 3%–4% of individuals acquire Down syndrome as a result of **translocation** (discussed later) and 1%–2% acquire it from **mosaicism** (some cells being affected and others not; this is also discussed later).

Chromosomal Loss: Turner Syndrome

Turner syndrome (sometimes called 45,X, which describes its genetic construction), affects girls. It is the only disorder in which a fetus can survive despite the loss of an entire chromosome. Even so, more than 99% of the 45,X conceptions appear to be miscarried (Morgan, 2007). Females with Turner syndrome (1 in every 5,000 live births) have a single X chromosome and no second X or Y chromosome, for a total of 45, rather than 46, chromosomes. In contrast to Down syndrome, 80% of individuals with **monosomy** X conditions are affected by meiotic errors in sperm production; these children usually receive an X chromosome from their mothers but no sex chromosome from their fathers.

Girls with Turner syndrome have short stature, a webbed neck, a broad "shield-like" chest with widely spaced nipples, and nonfunctional ovaries. Twenty percent have obstruction of the left side of the heart, most commonly caused by a **coarctation** of the **aorta.** Unlike children with Down syndrome, most girls with Turner syndrome have typical intelligence. They do, however, have visual–perceptual impairments that predispose them to develop nonverbal learning disabilities (Hong, Scaletta Kent, & Kesler, 2009). Human growth hormone injections have been effective in increasing height in girls with Turner syndrome, and **estrogen** supplementation can lead to the emergence of secondary sexual characteristics; however, these girls remain infertile.

Mosaicism

In mosaicism, different cells have a different genetic makeup (Conlin et al., 2010). For example, a child with the mosaic form of Down syndrome may have trisomy 21 in blood cells

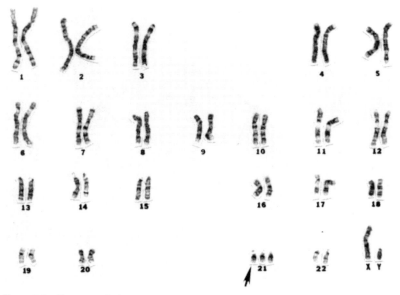

Figure 1.4. Karyotype of a boy with Down syndrome (47, XY). Note that the child has 47 chromosomes; the extra one is a chromosome 21.

but not in skin cells; or the individual may have trisomy 21 in some, but not all, brain cells. Children with mosaicism often appear as though they have a particular condition (in this example, Down syndrome); however, the physical abnormalities and cognitive impairments may be less severe. Usually mosaicism occurs when some cells in a trisomy conception lose the extra chromosome via nondisjunction during mitosis. Mosaicism also can occur if some cells lose a chromosome after a normal conception (e.g., some cells lose an X chromosome in mosaic Turner syndrome). Mosaicism is rare and present in only 5%–10% of all children with chromosomal abnormalities.

Translocations

A relatively common dysfunction in cell division, translocation can occur during mitosis and meiosis when the chromosomes break and then exchange parts with other chromosomes. Translocation involves the transfer of a portion of one chromosome to a completely different chromosome. For example, a portion of chromosome 21 might attach itself to chromosome 14 (Figure 1.5). If this occurs during meiosis, one daughter cell will then have 23 chromosomes but will have both a chromosome 21 and a chromosome 14/21 translocation. Fertilization of this egg, by a sperm with a cell containing the normal complement of 23 chromosomes, will result in a child with 46 chromosomes. This includes two copies of chromosome 21, one chromosome 14/21, and one chromosome 14. This child will have Down syndrome because of the functional trisomy 21 caused by the translocation.

Deletions

Another somewhat common dysfunction in cell division is deletion. Here, part, but not all of a chromosome is lost. Chromosomal deletions occur in two forms, visible deletions and microdeletions. Those that are large enough to be seen through the microscope are called visible deletions. Those that are so small that they can only be detected at the molecular level are called microdeletions.

Cri-du-chat ("cat cry") syndrome is an example of a visible chromosomal deletion in which a portion of the short arm of chromosome 5 is lost. Cri-du-chat syndrome affects approximately 1 in 50,000 children, causing microcephaly and an unusual facial appearance with a round face, widely spaced eyes, **epicanthal folds,** and low-set ears. Individuals with the syndrome have a high-pitched cry and intellectual disability (Cerruti Mainardi, 2006).

Examples of **microdeletion syndromes** include Williams syndrome and VCFS (Gothelf, Schaer, & Eliez, 2008; Mervis & John, 2010). The former is due to a deletion in the long arm of chromosome 7, and the latter is due to a deletion in the long arm of chromosome 22. Children with Williams syndrome have intellectual disability with a distinctive facial appearance, cardiac defects, and a unique cognitive profile with apparent expressive language skills beyond what would be expected based on their cognitive abilities. Children with VCFS syndrome may have a cleft palate, a congenital heart defect, a characteristic facial appearance, and/or a nonverbal learning disability. Cognitive problems are present in the majority of individuals with VCFS, and many

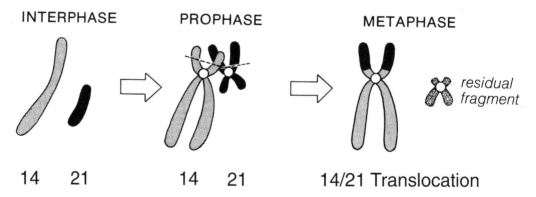

Figure 1.5. Translocation. During **prophase** of meiosis in a parent, there may be a transfer of a portion of one chromosome to another. In this figure, the long arm of chromosome 21 is translocated to chromosome 14, and the residual fragments are lost.

affected children satisfy the criteria for the diagnosis of autism.

Microdeletion syndromes are also called **contiguous gene syndromes** because they involve the deletion of a number of adjacent genes. A number of microdeletion syndromes can be diagnosed using **fluorescent *in situ* hybridization** (FISH) technology. These include Miller-Dieker syndrome, Williams syndrome, VCFS, and Smith-Magenis syndrome. FISH employs a fluorescently labeled compound that binds with and identifies a specific gene sequence on the chromosome. FISH and karyotype analysis are now being largely replaced by targeted genomic microarray analysis (Li & Andersson, 2009). These diagnostic tools are discussed later in the chapter.

Frequency of Chromosomal Abnormalities

In total, approximately 25% of eggs and 3%–4% of sperm have an extra or missing chromosome, and an additional 1% and 5%, respectively, have a structural chromosomal abnormality (Hassold, Hall, & Hunt, 2007). As a result, 10%–15% of all conceptions have a chromosomal abnormality. Somewhat more than 50% of these abnormalities are trisomies, 20% are monosomies, and 15% are **triploidies** (69 chromosomes). The remaining chromosomal abnormalities are composed of structural abnormalities and **tetraploidies** (92 chromosomes). It may therefore seem surprising that more children are not born with chromosomal abnormalities. The explanation is that more than 95% of fetuses with chromosomal abnormalities do not survive to term. In fact, many are lost very early in gestation, before a pregnancy may be recognized.

GENES AND THEIR DISORDERS

The underlying problem with the previously mentioned chromosomal disorders is the presence of too many or too few genes, resulting from extra or missing chromosomal material. Genetic disorders can also result from an abnormality in a single gene. The Human Genome Project, a public–private partnership developed to unravel the genetic makeup of mankind, established that the human **genome** contains 20,000–25,000 genes (http://www.ncbi.nlm.nih.gov/genome/guide/human). This is quite remarkable given that the fruit fly has approximately 13,000 genes, the round worm 19,000 genes, and a simple plant

26,000 genes. Before the project started it was projected that humans would have more than 100,000 genes. How is it possible that human beings have fewer than 25,000 genes, given that genes are responsible for producing specific protein products (e.g., hormones, enzymes, blood-type proteins) as well as regulating the development and function of the body? It was previously thought that each gene regulated the production of a single protein. Now it is known that the situation is much more complicated than this; single genes in humans code for multiple proteins, giving humans the combinational diversity that lower organisms lack. Humans can produce approximately 100,000 proteins from one quarter of that many genes. However, it must be acknowledged that the chimp shares 99% of the human genome. Having now examined the genome of innumerable organisms, the minimum number of genes necessary for life appears to be approximately 300, and all living organisms share these same 300 genes.

The mechanism by which genes act as blueprints for producing specific proteins needed for body functions is as follows. Genes are composed of various lengths of DNA that, together with intervening DNA sequences, form chromosomes. DNA is formed as a **double helix,** a structure that resembles a twisted ladder (Figure 1.6). The sides of the ladder are composed of sugar and phosphate molecules, whereas the "rungs" are made up of four chemicals called **nucleotide bases: cytosine** (C), **guanine** (G), **adenine** (A), and **thymine** (T). Pairs of nucleotide bases interlock to form each rung: cytosine bonds with guanine, and adenine bonds with thymine. The sequence of nucleotide bases on a segment of DNA (spelled out by the 4–letter alphabet C, G, A, T) make up an individual's genetic code. Genes range in size, containing from 1,500 to more than 2 million nucleotide-base pairs. Overall there are approximately 3.3 billion base pairs in the human genome, but less than 3% encode genes that serve as a blueprint for protein production. It should also be noted that all genes are not "turned on" or expressed at all times. Some are only active during fetal life (e.g., the fetal hemoglobin gene), and it is hoped that some never are expressed (e.g., oncogenes, which have the potential to cause cancer). The turning on and off of genes may follow a carefully developmentally regulated process. Regulation of gene expression plays a particularly important role during fetal development; as a result, problems involving gene expression during fetal development can be

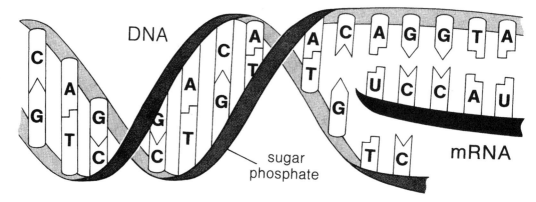

Figure 1.6. Deoxyribonucleic acid (DNA). Four nucleotides (C, cytosine; G, guanine; A, adenosine; T, thymine) form the genetic code. On the mRNA molecule, uracil (U) substitutes for thymine. The DNA unzips to transcribe its message as mRNA.

particularly devastating. The way gene expression is regulated involves a number of structural changes to the DNA and its architecture without altering the actual nucleotide sequence of the DNA. This process is termed *epigenetics* and is a cause of a number of genetic syndromes that are associated with developmental disabilities.

Transcription

The production of a specific protein begins when the DNA comprising that gene unwinds, and the two strands (the sides of the ladder) unzip to expose the code (Jorde, Carey, & Bamshad, 2009). The exposed DNA sequence then serves as a template for the formation, or **transcription,** of a similar nucleotide sequence called **messenger ribonucleic acid** (mRNA; Figure 1.7). In all RNA, the nucleotides are the same as in DNA except that uracil (U) substitutes for thymine (T). As might be expected, errors or mutations may occur during transcription; however, a proofreading enzyme generally catches and repairs these errors. If not corrected, transcription errors can lead to the production of a disordered protein and a disease state.

Translation

Once transcribed, the single-stranded mRNA detaches, and the double-stranded DNA zips back together. The mRNA then moves out of the nucleus into the cytoplasm, where it provides instructions for the production of a protein, a process termed **translation** (Figure 1.8). Once the mRNA is in the cytoplasm, the process of translation begins. The mRNA attaches itself to a **ribosome.** The ribosome moves along the mRNA strand, reading the message in three-letter "words," or **codons,** such as GCU, CUA, and UAG. Most of these triplets code for specific **amino acids,** the building blocks of proteins. As these triplets are read, another type of RNA, transfer RNA (tRNA), carries the requisite amino acids to the ribosome, where they are linked to form a protein. Certain triplets, termed *stop codons*, instruct the ribosome to terminate the sequence by indicating that all of the correct amino acids are in place to form the complete protein.

Once the protein is complete, the mRNA, ribosome, and protein separate. The protein is released into the cytoplasm and is either used by the cytoplasm or prepared for secretion into the bloodstream. If the protein is to be secreted, it is transferred to the **Golgi apparatus** (Figure 1.1), which packages it in a form that can be released through the cell membrane and carried throughout the body.

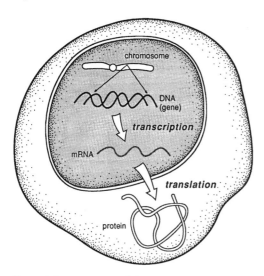

Figure 1.7. A summary of the steps leading from gene to protein formation. Transcription of the DNA (gene) onto mRNA occurs in the cell nucleus. The mRNA is then transported to the cytoplasm, where translation into protein occurs.

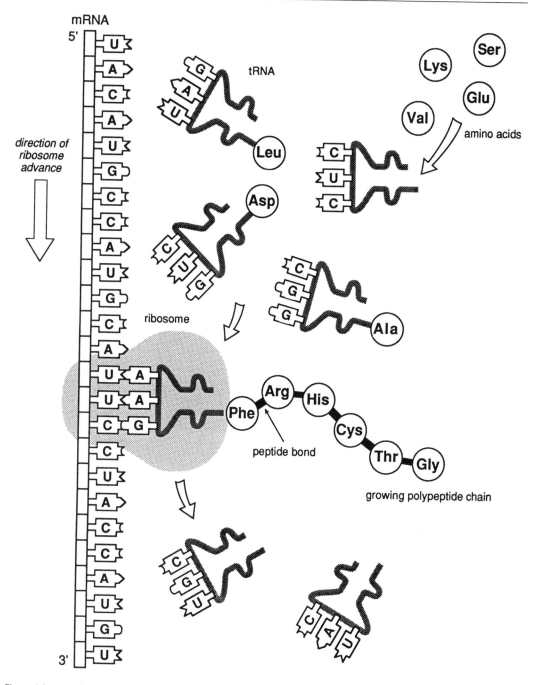

Figure 1.8. Translation of mRNA into protein. The ribosome moves along the mRNA strand assembling a growing polypeptide chain using tRNA–amino acid complexes. In this example, it has already assembled six amino acids (phenylalanine [Phe], arginine [Arg], histidine [His], cystine [Cys], threonine [Thr], and glycine [Gly]) into a polypeptide chain that will become a protein.

Mutations

An abnormality at any step in this translation process can cause the body to produce: 1) a structurally abnormal protein, 2) reduced amounts of a protein, or 3) no protein at all. When the error occurs in the gene itself, thus disrupting the subsequent steps, that mistake is termed a *mutation*. The likelihood of mutations occurring increases with the size of the gene. In sperm cells, the point mutation rate also increases with paternal age. Although most mutations occur spontaneously, they can be induced by radiation, toxins, and viruses. Once they occur, mutations become part of a person's genetic code. If they are present in the germline, they can be passed on from one generation to the next.

Point Mutations

The most common type of mutation is a single base pair substitution (Jorde, Carey, & Bamshad, 2009), also called a **point mutation.** Because there is redundancy in human DNA, many point mutations have no adverse consequences. Depending on where in the gene they occur, point mutations are capable of causing a **missense mutation** or a **nonsense mutation** (Figure 1.9). A missense mutation results in a change in the triplet code that substitutes a different amino acid in the protein chain. For example, in most cases of the inborn error of metabolism, **phenylketonuria** (PKU), a single base substitution causes an error in the production of phenylalanine hydroxylase, the enzyme necessary to metabolize the amino acid **phenylalanine.** The result is an accumulation of phenylalanine in blood and brain that can cause brain damage (see Chapter 19). In a nonsense mutation, the single base pair substitution produces a stop codon that prematurely terminates the protein formation. In this case, no useful protein is formed. Neurofibromatosis-1 (NF1) is an example of a disorder commonly caused by a nonsense mutation. In NF1 a tumor suppressor, neurofibromin, is not formed. As a result, multiple benign neurofibroma tumors form on the body and in the brain. Children with NF1 also have a high incidence of attention-deficit/hyperactivity disorder (Ferner, 2010).

Insertions and Deletions

Mutations can also involve the insertion or deletion of one or more nucleotide bases. The most common mutation in individuals with spinal muscular atrophy (associated with severe muscle loss and weakness throughout the body) involves an insertion in the survival motor neuron gene, rendering it defective (Farrar, Johnston, Grattan-Smith, & Turner, 2009). In contrast, a common mutation in another inherited muscle disease, Duchenne muscular dystrophy, usually involves a deletion in the dystrophin gene (see Chapter 13).

Base additions or subtractions may also lead to a **frame shift** in which the three base pair reading frame is shifted. All subsequent triplets are misread, often leading to the production of a stop codon and a nonfunctional protein. Certain children with Tay-Sachs disease (see later in the chapter; Appendix B) have this type of mutation. Other mutations can affect regions of the gene that regulate transcription but that do not actually code for an amino acid. These areas are called promoter and enhancer areas. They help turn other genes on and off and are very important in the normal development of the fetus. A mutation in a transcription gene leads to Rubinstein-Taybi syndrome, which is associated with multiple congenital malformations and severe intellectual disability

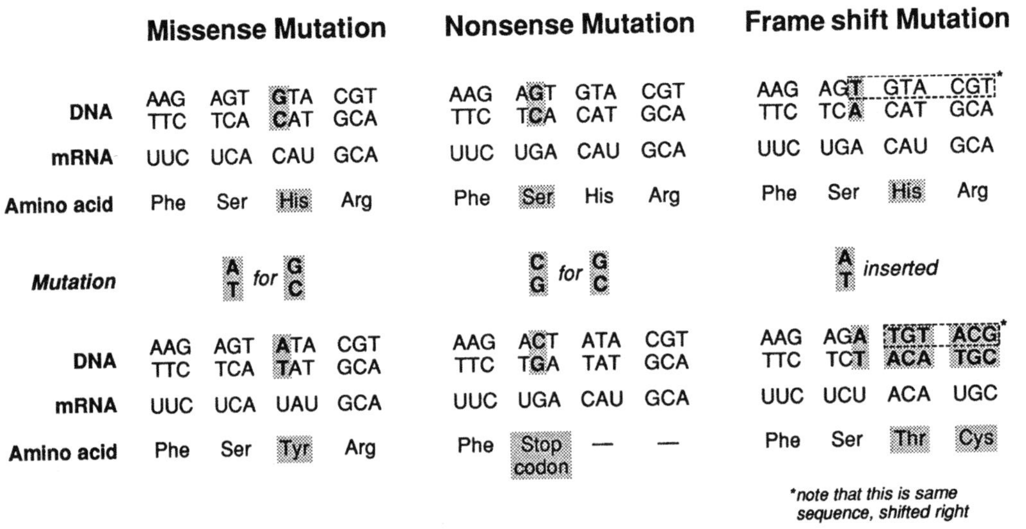

Figure 1.9. Examples of point mutations: Missense mutation, nonsense mutation, and frame shift mutation. The shaded areas mark the point of mutation.

(Roelfsema & Peters, 2007). Mutations in a transcription gene also may result in a normal protein being formed but at a much slower rate than usual, leading to an enzyme or other protein deficiency.

Selective Advantage

The **incidence** of a genetic disease in a population depends on the difference between the rate of mutation production and that of mutation removal. Typically, genetic diseases enter populations through mutation errors. Natural selection, the process by which individuals with a selective advantage survive and pass on their genes, works to remove these errors. For instance, because individuals with sickle cell disease (an **autosomal recessive** inherited blood disorder) historically have had a decreased life span, the gene that causes this disorder would have been expected to be removed from the gene pool over time. Sometimes natural selection, however, favors the individual who is a carrier of one copy of a mutated recessive gene. In the case of sickle cell disease, unaffected carriers (called heterozygotes), who appear clinically healthy, actually have minor differences in their hemoglobin structure that make it more resistant to a malarial parasite (López, Saravia, Gomez, Hoebeke, & Patarroyo, 2010). In Africa, where malaria is endemic, carriers of this disorder have a selective advantage. This selection has maintained the sickle cell trait among Africans. Northern Europeans, for whom malaria is not an issue, rarely carry the sickle cell gene at all; this mutation has presumably died out via natural selection (Jorde, Carey, & Bamshad, 2009).

Single Nucleotide Polymorphisms (SNPs)

Of the more than 3 billion base pair genetic code, people of all races and geography share 99.9% genetic identity (Ridley, 2006). Although this is quite remarkable, that 0.1% difference means there are about 3 million DNA sequence variations, also called **single nucleotide polymorphisms** (SNPs). This genetic variation is the basis of evolution, but it can also contribute to health, unique traits, or disease. One SNP involved in muscle formation, if present, makes individuals much more likely to become "buff" if they weight lift; another SNP is associated with perfect musical pitch. There is a SNP that makes individuals more susceptible to adverse effects from certain medications, because it leads to slower metabolism of drugs by the liver. There also are SNPs that place people at greater risk for developing Alzheimer's disease and Crohn's disease (an inflammatory bowel disease; Amre et al., 2010; Seshadri et al., 2010). It is likely that at some time in the not too distant future, doctors will take blood samples to test for various SNPs associated with health and disease in order to practice individualized (personalized) medicine (McCabe, 2010).

Single Gene (Mendelian) Disorders

Gregor Mendel (1822–1884), an Austrian monk, pioneered our understanding of single-gene defects. While cultivating pea plants, he noted that when he bred two differently colored plants—yellow and green—the **hybrid** offspring all were green, rather than mixed in color. Mendel concluded that the green trait was **dominant,** whereas the yellow trait was **recessive** (from the Latin word for "hidden"). However, the yellow trait sometimes appeared in subsequent generations. Later, scientists determined that many human traits, including some birth defects, are also inherited in this fashion. They are referred to as **Mendelian traits.**

Table 1.1 indicates the prevalence of some common genetic disorders associated with developmental disabilities. Approximately 1% of the population has a known single-gene disorder. These disorders can be transmitted to offspring on the autosomes or on the X chromosome. Mendelian traits may be either dominant or recessive. Thus, Mendelian disorders are characterized as being **autosomal recessive, autosomal dominant,** or X-linked.

Autosomal Recessive Disorders

Among the currently recognized Mendelian disorders, approximately 1,000 are inherited as autosomal recessive traits (McKusick-Nathans Institute of Genetic Medicine & National Center for Biotechnology Information, 2010). For a child to have a disorder that is autosomal recessive, he or she must carry an abnormal gene on both copies of the relevant chromosome. In the vast majority of cases, this means that the child receives an abnormal copy from both parents. The one exception is uniparental dysomy (see the following section).

Tay-Sachs disease is an example of an autosomal recessive, progressive neurological disorder. It is caused by the absence of an enzyme, hexosaminidase A, which normally metabolizes a potentially toxic product of nerve cells (Kaback, 2006). In individuals with Tay-Sachs disease, this product cannot be broken down

Table 1.1. Prevalence of genetic disorders

Disease	Appropriate prevalence
Chromosomal disorders	
Down syndrome	1/700–1/1,000
Klinefelter syndrome	1/1,000 males
Trisomy 13	1/10,000
Trisomy 18	1/6,000
Turner syndrome	1/2,500–1/10,000 females
Single-gene disorders	
Duchenne muscular dystrophy	1/3,500 males
Fragile X syndrome	1/4,000 males; 1/8,000 females
Neurofibromatosis Type I	1/3,000–1/5,000
Phenylketonuria	1/10,000 to 1/15,000
Tay-Sachs disease	1/3,000 Ashkenazi Jews
Mitochondrial inheritance	
Leber hereditary optic neuropathy	Rare
MELAS and MERRF	Rare
Mitochondrial encephalopathy	Rare

Source: Jorde, Carey, and Bamshad (2001).

Key: MELAS, mitochondrial encephalomyelopathy, lactic acidosis, and stroke-like episodes; MERRF, myoclonic epilepsy and ragged red fibers.

and is stored in the brain, leading to progressive brain damage and early death.

Alternate forms of the gene for hexosaminidase A are known to exist. The different forms of a gene, called **alleles,** include the normal gene, which can be symbolized by a capital "A" because it is dominant, and the mutated allele (in this example, carrying Tay-Sachs disease), which can be symbolized by the lowercase "a" because it is recessive (Figure 1.10). Upon fertilization, the embryo receives two genes for hexosaminidase A, one from the father and one from the mother. The following combinations of alleles are possible: **homozygous** (carrying the same allele) combinations, AA or aa; and **heterozygous** (carrying alternate alleles) combinations, aA or Aa. Because Tay-Sachs disease is a recessive disorder, two abnormal recessive genes (aa) are needed to produce a child who has the disease. Therefore, a child with aa would be homozygous for the Tay-Sachs gene (i.e., have two copies of the mutated gene and manifest the disease), a child with aA or Aa would be heterozygous and a healthy carrier of the Tay-Sachs gene, and a child with AA would be a healthy noncarrier.

If two heterozygotes (carrying alternate alleles) were to have children (aA × Aa or Aa × aA), the following combinations could occur: AA, aA or Aa, or aa (Figure 1.10). According to the law of probability, each pregnancy would carry a 1 in 4 chance of the child being a noncarrier (AA), a 1 in 2 chance of the child being a carrier (aA or Aa), and a 1 in 4 risk of the child having Tay-Sachs disease (aa). If a carrier has children with a noncarrier (aA × AA), each pregnancy carries a 1 in 2 chance of the child being a carrier (aA, Aa), a 1 in 2 chance of the child being a noncarrier (AA), and virtually no chance of the child having the disease (Figure 1.10). Siblings of affected children, even if they are carriers, are unlikely to produce children with the disease because this can only occur if they have children with another carrier, which is an unlikely occurrence in these rare diseases, except in cases of intermarriage.

The 1 in 4 risk when two carriers have children is a probability risk. This does not mean that if a family has one affected child, the next three will be unaffected. Each new pregnancy carries the same 1 in 4 risk; the parents could, by chance, have three affected children in a row or five unaffected children. In the case of Tay-Sachs disease, carrier screening is used to identify at-risk couples and prenatal diagnosis to provide information about whether the fetus is affected (see Chapter 5).

Because it is unlikely for a carrier of a rare condition to have children with another carrier of the same disease, autosomal recessive disorders are quite rare in the general population, ranging from 1 in 2,000 to 1 in 200,000 births (McKusick-Nathans Institute of Genetic Medicine & National Center for Biotechnology Information, 2010). When intermarriage occurs within an extended family (e.g., cousin marriage; Figure 1.11) or when marriages among ethnically, religiously, or geographically isolated populations occur (founder effect), the incidence of these disorders increases markedly.

Like Tay-Sachs disease, certain other autosomal recessive disorders are caused by mutations that lead to an enzyme deficiency of some kind. In most cases, there are a number of different mutations within the gene that can produce the same disease. Because these enzyme deficiencies generally lead to biochemical abnormalities involving either the insufficient production of a needed product or the buildup of toxic materials, **developmental disabilities** or early death may result (see

Chapter 19). Autosomal recessive disorders affect males and females equally, and there tends to be clustering in families within sibships (i.e., more than one affected child per family). However, a history of the disease in past generations rarely exists unless there has been intermarriage.

Autosomal Dominant Disorders

Approximately 950 autosomal dominant disorders have been identified, the most common ones having a frequency of 1 in 500 births (McKusick-Nathans Institute of Genetic Medicine & National Center for Biotechnology Information, 2010). Autosomal dominant disorders are quite different from autosomal recessive disorders in mechanism, incidence, and clinical characteristics (Table 1.2). Because autosomal dominant disorders are caused by a single

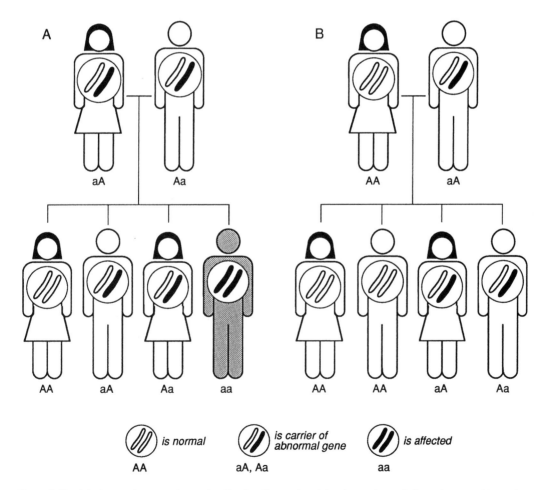

Figure 1.10. Inheritance of autosomal recessive disorders. Two copies of the abnormal gene (aa) must be present to produce the disease state: A) Two carriers mating will result, on average, in 25% of the children being affected, 50% being carriers, and 25% not being affected; B) A carrier and a noncarrier mating will result in 50% noncarriers and 50% carriers, no children will be affected.

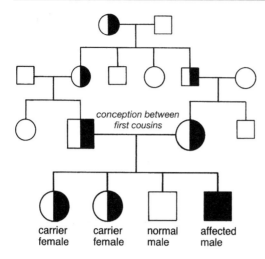

conception between
first cousins

carrier	carrier	normal	affected
female	female	male	male

Figure 1.11. A family tree illustrating the effect of consanguinity (in this case, a marriage between first cousins) on the risk of inheriting an autosomal recessive disorder. The chance of both parents being carriers is usually less than 1 in 300. When first cousins conceive a child, however, the chance of both parents being carriers rises to 1 in 8. The risk, then, of having an affected child increases almost fortyfold.

abnormal allele, individuals with the **genotypes** Aa or aA are both affected to some degree.

To better understand this, consider NF1, the neurological disorder discussed previously. Suppose *a* represents the normal recessive gene and *A* indicates the mutated dominant gene for NF1. If a person with NF1 (aA or Aa) has a child with an unaffected individual (aa) there is a 1 in 2 risk, statistically speaking, that the child will have the disorder (aA or Aa), and a 1 in 2 chance he or she will be unaffected (aa; Figure 1.12). An unaffected child will not carry the abnormal allele and, therefore, cannot pass it on to his or her children.

Autosomal dominant disorders affect men and women with equal frequency. They tend to involve structural (physical) abnormalities rather than enzymatic defects. In affected individuals, there is often a family history of the disease; however, approximately half of affected individuals represent a new mutation. Although

individuals with a new mutation will risk passing the mutated gene to their offspring, their parents are unaffected and at no greater risk than the general population of having a second affected child. There can also be partial penetrance of the gene, which produces a less severe disorder (e.g., in NF1 or tuberous sclerosis), or delayed onset form of the disease (e.g., in Huntington disease).

X-Linked Disorders

Unlike autosomal recessive and autosomal dominant disorders, which involve genes located on the 22 nonsex chromosomes, X-linked (previously called sex-linked) disorders involve mutant genes located on the X chromosome. X-linked disorders primarily affect males (Stevenson & Schwartz, 2009). The reason for this is that males have only one X chromosome; therefore, a single dose of the abnormal gene causes disease. Because females have two X chromosomes, a single recessive allele usually does not cause disease, provided there is a normal allele on the second X chromosome. Approximately 1,100 X-linked disorders have been described, including Duchenne muscular dystrophy and hemophilia (McKusick-Nathans Institute of Genetic Medicine & National Center for Biotechnology Information, 2010; Figure 1.13). Carrier mothers in two thirds of the cases pass on these disorders from one generation to the next; one third of these cases represent new mutations. It is becoming increasingly recognized that the distinction between X-linked recessive and X-linked dominant is often cloudy and may not be clinically useful.

As an example, children with Duchenne muscular dystrophy develop a progressive muscle weakness (Bushby et al., 2010a, 2010b). The disease results from a mutation in the dystrophin gene (located on the X chromosome), the function of which is to ensure stability of the muscle cell membrane. Because the disease affects all muscles, eventually the heart muscle and the diaphragmatic muscles needed for

Table 1.2. Comparison of autosomal recessive, autosomal dominant, and X-linked inheritance patterns

	Autosomal recessive	Autosomal dominant	X-linked
Type of disorder	Enzyme deficiency	Structural abnormalities	Mixed
Examples of disorder	Tay-Sachs disease Phenylketonuria (PKU)	Achondroplasia Neurofibromatosis	Fragile X syndrome Muscular dystrophy
Carrier expresses disorder	No	Yes	Sometimes
Increased risk in other family members from intermarriage	Yes	No	No

circulation and breathing are impaired. Dystrophin is also required for typical brain development and function; so affected boys may have cognitive impairments.

In fact, approximately 10% of males with intellectual disability and l0% of females with learning disabilities are affected by X-linked conditions (Inlow & Restifo, 2004). The finding that males are more than twice as likely to have intellectual disability than females is attributable to a combination of factors: first, X-linked disorders affect males disproportionately more than females; second, there is an unusually large number of genes residing on the X chromosome that are critical for normal brain development, nerve cell function, learning, and memory. Up to 10% of all known genetic errors causing intellectual disability are on the X chromosome,

despite the X chromosome containing only 4% of the **genome** (i.e., all the genes contained in the 46 chromosomes).

The mechanism for passing an X-linked recessive trait to the next generation is as follows: Women who have a recessive mutation (Xa) on one of their X chromosomes and a normal allele on the other (X) are carriers of the gene (XaX). Although these women are usually clinically unaffected, they can pass on the abnormal gene to their children. Assuming the father is unaffected, each female child born to a carrier mother has a 1 in 2 chance of being a carrier (i.e., inheriting the mutant Xa allele from her mother and the normal X allele from her father; Figure 1.13). A male child (who has only one X chromosome), however, has a 1 in 2 risk of having the disorder. This occurs

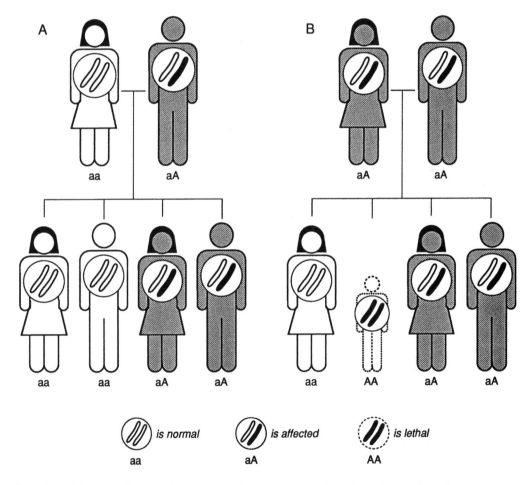

Figure 1.12. Inheritance of autosomal dominant disorders. Only one copy of the abnormal gene (A) must be present to produce the disease state: A) If an affected person conceives a child with an unaffected person, statistically speaking, 50% of the children will be affected and 50% will be unaffected; B) If two affected people have children, 25% of the children will be unaffected, 50% will have the disorder, and 25% will have a severe, often fatal, form of the disorder as a result of a double dose of the abnormal gene.

if he inherits the X chromosome containing the mutated gene (XaY) instead of the normal one (XY). A family tree frequently reveals that some maternal uncles and male siblings have the disease.

Occasionally, females are affected by X-linked diseases. This can occur if the woman has adverse **lyonization** (inactivation of one of the X chromosomes) or if the disorder is X-linked dominant. Regarding the former mechanism, geneticist Mary Lyon questioned why women have the same amount of X-chromosome directed gene product as men instead of twice as much, as would be predicted from their genetic makeup. Dr. Lyon postulated that early in embryogenesis, one of the two X chromosomes in each cell was inactivated, making every female fetus a mosaic. This implied that some cells would contain an active X

chromosome derived from the father, whereas others would contain an active X chromosome derived from the mother. This lyonization hypothesis was later proven to be correct. In most instances, the cells in a woman's body have a fairly equal division between maternally and paternally derived active X chromosomes. In a small fraction of women, however, the distribution is very unequal. If the normal X chromosome is inactivated preferentially in cells of a carrier of an X-linked disorder, the woman will manifest the disease, although usually in a less severe form than the male. An example is ornithine transcarbamylase (OTC) deficiency, the disorder Katy had in this chapter's opening case study (see also Chapter 19).

The second mechanism for a female to manifest an X-linked disorder is if the disorder is transmitted as X-linked dominant.

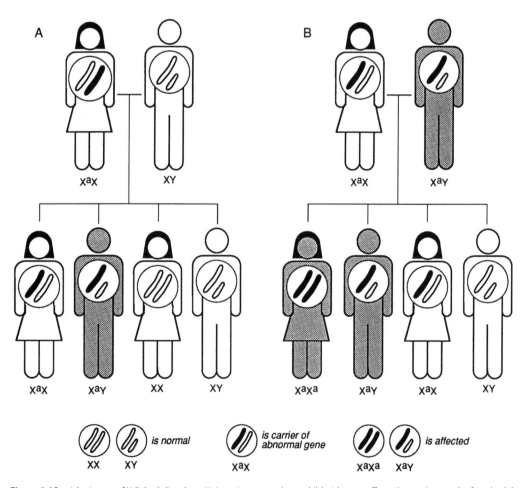

Figure 1.13. Inheritance of X-linked disorders: A) A carrier woman has a child with an unaffected man. Among the female children, statistically speaking, 50% will be carriers and 50% will be unaffected. Among the male children, 50% will be affected and 50% will be unaffected; B) A carrier woman has a child with an affected man. Of the female children, 50% will be carriers and 50% will be affected. Of the male children, statistically speaking, 50% will be unaffected and 50% will be affected.

Although most X-linked disorders are recessive, a few appear to be dominant. One example is Rett syndrome (Chahrour & Zoghbi, 2007; Matijevic, Knezevic, Slavica, & Pavelic, 2009; Percy, 2008). It appears that in this disorder, the presence of the mutated transcription gene, *MECP2*, on the X chromosome of a male embryo nearly always leads to lethality. When it occurs in one of the X chromosomes of the female, however, it is compatible with survival but results in a syndrome marked by microcephaly, intellectual disability, and autism-like behaviors.

Mitochondrial Inheritance

Each cell contains several hundred mitochondria in its cytoplasm (Figure 1.1). Mitochondria produce the energy needed for cellular function through a complex process termed **oxidative phosphorylation.** It has been proposed that mitochondria were originally independent microorganisms that invaded our bodies during the process of human evolution and then developed a symbiotic relationship with the cells in the human body. They are unique among cellular organelles (the specialized parts of a cell) in that they possess their own DNA, which is in a double stranded circular pattern rather than the double-helical pattern of nuclear DNA and contains genes that are different from those contained in nuclear DNA (Figure 1.14). Most of the proteins necessary for mitochondrial function are coded by nuclear genes, and disorders caused by abnormalities in these genes are most often inherited in an autosomal recessive manner. Certain mitochondrial functions, however, are dependent on genes encoded on the mitochondrial DNA. A mutation in a mitochondrial gene can result in defective energy production and a disease state (Calvo & Mootha, 2010). An example of a disorder with mitochondrial inheritance is mitochondrial encephalomyelopathy, lactic acidosis, and stroke-like episodes (MELAS), a progressive neurological disorder marked by episodes of stroke and dementia. Other disorders with mitochondrial inheritance can lead to blindness, deafness, or muscle weakness. Sixty-five mitochondrial disorders have been described thus far (McKusick-Nathans Institute of Genetic Medicine & National Center for Biotechnology Information, 2010). Every cell contains many mitochondria, but not every mitochondrion may carry a given mutation. In many disorders that are inherited through the mitochondrial genome, there is great clinical variability based on the "heteroplasmy," or the

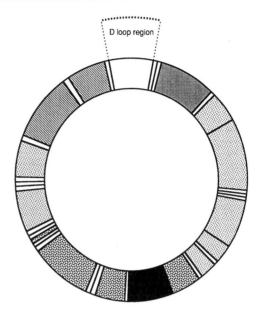

Figure 1.14. Mitochondrial DNA genome. The genes code for various enzyme complexes involved in energy production in the cell. The displacement loop (D loop) is not involved in energy production. (This figure was published in Medical genetics, revised 2nd edition, by Jorde, L.B., Carey, J.C., & Bamshad, M.J., et al., p. 105, Copyright C.V. Mosby [2001]; adapted by permission.) (*Key:* ▨ Complex I genes [NADH dehydrogenase], ▩ Complex III genes [ubiquinol: cytochrome c oxidoreductase], □ tRNA genes, ▨ Complex IV genes [cytochrome c oxidase], ■ Complex V genes [ATP synthase], ▨ ribosomal RNA genes.)

mix of different mitochondrial genomes within a single individual. There may be significant variability amongst specific tissues in an individual so that some organs or tissues may be affected by the mitochondrial disorder and others may not be.

Because eggs, but not sperm, contain cytoplasm, mitochondria are inherited from one's mother. As a result, mitochondrial DNA disorders are passed on from generally unaffected mothers to their children, both male and female. Men affected by a mitochondrial disorder cannot pass the trait to their children. In some cases, a mother with significant heteroplasmy may have only mild effects of a disease but may pass on only mutated mitochondrial genomes to a child. In that case, a child would have a homoplasmic mitochondrial mutation and would have a much more severe clinical course (Figure 1.15).

Trinucleotide Repeat Expansion Disorders

There has been an increased recognition that **copy number variability** accounts for several developmental disabilities (Stranger, 2007). This discovery has been made possible by

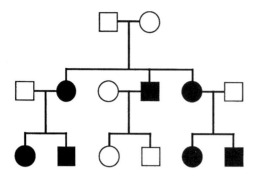

Figure 1.15. Mitochondrial inheritance. Because mitochondria are inherited exclusively from the mother, defects in mitochondrial disease will be passed on from the mother to her children, as illustrated in this pedigree. (*Key:* Shading indicates affected individuals, squares are males, circles are females.)

advances in molecular cytogenetics, specifically microarray based technologies that allow for high-resolution, simultaneous screening of the entire human genome (Li & Andersson, 2009; Stankiewicz & Beaudet, 2007).

One particular type of copy number variation is the trinucleotide repeat expansion (triplet repeat disorder), which has been linked to a number of disorders that do not follow typical Mendelian inheritance. Trinucleotide repeat disorders result from problems in recombination and replication during meiosis. Certain genes have highly repetitive sequences of trinucleotides. These repetitive sequences may expand (or contract) in size during meiosis. Once the repetitive sequence reaches a certain size threshold, it may interfere with the function of the gene and lead to a clinically apparent disorder. The expansion length is linked to the phenotype, with the longer expansions often presenting with earlier and more severe clinical signs and symptoms.

The first triplet repeat disorder discovered was fragile X syndrome. Fragile X syndrome is the most common inherited cause of intellectual disability. Boys and girls with fragile X syndrome have a phenotype that includes a characteristic physical appearance, cognitive skills deficits, and impaired adaptive behaviors (Chonchaiya, Schneider, & Hagerman, 2009; Schneider, Hagerman, & Hessl, 2009). Many affected children satisfy the criteria for the diagnosis of autism. The prevalence of fragile X syndrome (the full mutation) for males is about 1:3,600. The prevalence of the full mutation in females is estimated to be at least 1:4,000 to 1:6,000. Fragile X syndrome arises from an expansion of the number of cytosine-guanine-guanine (CGG) trinucleotide repeats occurring

within the fragile X mental retardation protein gene (*FMR1*). Inheritance of the instability in CGG regions leads to expansion from the normal number of repeats (6–40) to a premutation state (50–200 repeats) or from a premutation state to full mutation (>200 repeats). The stability of the CGG repeat depends upon the length of the repeat as well as the sex of the individual passing on the mutation. The increased risk of CGG expansion from one generation to another is a phenomenon termed *anticipation*. Anticipation leads to a worsening clinical phenotype in successive generations. When a child is suspected of having fragile X syndrome the diagnosis can be confirmed by detecting the number of trinucleotide repeats in FMR1 using a clinically available molecular genetic blood test (Collins et al., 2010). There is a correlation between the number of trinucleotide repeats and the severity of disease.

EPIGENETICS

The diagnostic evaluation of children with intellectual disability and other developmental disabilities has become increasingly complex in recent years owing to a number of newly recognized genetic mechanisms and sophisticated methods to diagnosis them. It has been appreciated that changes in gene expression can occur by mechanisms that do not permanently alter the DNA sequence (Urdinguio, Sanchez-Mut, & Esteller, 2009), a phenomenon termed **epigenetics.** Epigenetic mechanisms are important regulators of biological processes because they include genome reprogramming during embryogenesis (Gropman & Batshaw, 2010; Gräff & Mansuy, 2009; Kumar, 2008). Epigenetic modification, which is important in developmental processes, may have long-term effects on learning and memory formation. Epigenetic abnormalities may result from dysfunction of certain enzymes, genomic imprinting, and triplet repeat copy number variation. A number of conditions causing developmental disabilities, including fragile X syndrome, Rett syndrome, Rubinstein-Taybi syndrome, Prader-Willi syndrome, and VCFS, can be attributed to disruptions in epigenetic function. It is interesting to note that virtually all epigenetic disorders have been found to have a high incidence of symptoms consistent with autism spectrum disorders (Moss & Howlin, 2009). In addition, the risk of epigenetic disorders has been found to be increased in pregnancies assisted by in vitro fertilization (IVF; Owen & Segars, 2009).

Rubinstein-Taybi syndrome is an example of epigenetic dysfunction caused by the dysfunction of a histone acetyltransferase, an enzyme that regulates gene expression (Roelfsema & Peters, 2007). An autosomal dominant disorder, Rubinstein-Taybi syndrome is characterized by intellectual disability and physical anomalies, including broad thumbs, growth deficiency that is later followed by excessive weight gain, characteristic facial appearance, and an increased risk for developing tumors. This syndrome is caused by mutations in the cAMP response element-binding (CREB) protein gene. As a coactivator of transcription, CREB has dual functions in mediating both gene activation and epigenetic modification.

According to Mendelian genetics, the **phenotype,** or appearance, of an individual should be the same whether the given gene is inherited from the mother or the father. This is not always the case, however, because of **genomic imprinting.** This is an epigenetic phenomenon in which the activity of the gene is modified depending upon the sex of the transmitting parent (Butler, 2009). Most autosomal genes are expressed in both maternal and paternal alleles. However, imprinted genes show expression from only one allele (the other is silenced or used differently), and this is determined during production of the egg or sperm. Imprinting implies that the gene carries a "tag" placed on it during spermatogenesis or oogenesis. This is most often accomplished by adding methyl groups to the DNA, affecting the expression of the methylated genes. Imprinted genes are important in development and differentiation, and if expression from both alleles is not maintained, disturbances in development can result (Wilkins & Ubeda, 2011). The first human imprinting disorder discovered was Prader-Willi syndrome. It is caused by a paternal deletion in chromosome 15 or by maternal uniparental disomy in which both chromosome 15s come from the mother. It can also result if both copies of chromosome 15 are imprinted as if they came from the mother, regardless of the actual parent of origin (Conlin et al., 2010). Prader-Willi syndrome is characterized by severe hypotonia and feeding difficulties in early childhood, followed by an insatiable appetite and obesity by school age. It features significant motor and language delays in the first 2 years of life, borderline to moderate intellectual disability, and severe behavioral problems, including compulsive and hording behaviors. Many affected children satisfy the criteria for the diagnosis of autism (Goldstone, Holland, Hauffa, Hokken-Koelega, & Tauber, 2008). Other examples of imprinted neurogenetic disorders include Angelman syndrome and Beckwith-Wiedemann syndrome (Dan, 2009; Gurrieri & Accadia, 2009).

GENETIC TESTING

Over the past few decades, the availability of tests for specific genetic disorders has increased exponentially. The term *genetic testing* is broad and may encompass many different kinds of tests and technologies.

Perhaps the most well-known genetic test is a karyotype. A karyotype is essentially a photograph of all of the chromosomes from a single cell, arranged in numbered pairs so the banding pattern is visible. This is an ideal test for aneuploidies (irregularities in the number of chromosomes, such as Down syndrome) or for translocations (see preceding discussion). Some relatively large deletions and duplications also may be visible on karyotype. Smaller deletions and duplications may be detected by FISH. With FISH, the presence or absence of specific chromosome regions is assessed. DNA probes specific to the target region are given a fluorescent signal tag and are attached to the patient's DNA. The presence or absence of the fluorescent signal then indicates the presence or absence of the corresponding region in the patient's sample.

In many ways, karyotype and FISH techniques have been largely supplanted by chromosome microarray analysis, also called comparative genomic hybridization (CGH) (Koleen et al., 2009). Much like a karyotype or FISH, CGH requires about a teaspoon of blood. A comparison is performed between the patient's blood and a reference sample; differences in the DNA of the two samples allows detection of chromosomal imbalances. Both the patient DNA sample and the control DNA sample are labeled with fluorescent dyes, and differences in the relative fluorescence intensities on the microarray are indicative of the differences in copy number between the two genomes (Sebat et al., 2007). Newer-generation arrays also involve the use of single-nucleotide polymorphisms (SNPs) to detect very small copy number variations in DNA sequences (Friedman et al., 2006).

One of the limitations of chromosomal microarray technology is that it is not able to detect balanced rearrangements of chromosomal material. Additionally, chromosomal microarrays do not detect point mutations (single nucleotide changes) and therefore would not be an appropriate test to screen for diseases such as Rett syndrome (which is caused by a point mutation in *MECP2* gene).

To assess for point mutations or very small deletions or duplications within a specific gene, DNA sequencing is typically used. There are a number of different technologies available for this, but they all essentially deliver the patient's sequence for a given gene that can then be compared with a reference sequence. This can be very useful when, based on clinical evaluation, a genetic disorder relatable to a known gene is suspected.

There are many other types of genetic tests available for specific disorders. For example, some inborn errors of metabolism may be identified by detecting specific metabolites in blood, urine, or other types of samples. Testing for methylation patterns on DNA samples may detect certain epigenetic disorders. Other genetic disorders may be detected radiologically. The decision about which tests are most appropriate for a specific patient is complex, and physicians with expertise in medical genetics may help guide testing and interpret results. Over the coming years, technological advances will allow for much more comprehensive and in-depth genetic analysis. Sequence analysis of an entire human genome was completely unfathomable just a few years ago, but may become clinically available in the near future. It is very challenging for clinicians to keep up with the changing understanding and availability of genetic tests. One extremely valuable resource for clinicians is http://www.genetests.org, which is a NIH-supported web site that catalogues the most up-to-date and authoritative information about currently available genetic tests and their uses.

ENVIRONMENTAL INFLUENCES ON HEREDITY

The particular genes that a person possesses determine his or her genotype, and the expression of the genes results in the physical appearance of traits—that is, the phenotype of the individual. For some traits and clinical disorders, however, the same genotype can produce quite different phenotypes, depending on environmental influences. In terms of traits, bright parents tend to have bright children and tall parents tend to have tall children; however, the interaction of genetics with the pre- and postnatal environments allows for many possible outcomes. For example, it has been found that as a result of an increased protein intake

during childhood, Asian Americans who grow up in the United States are significantly taller than their parents who grew up in Asia. Diabetes, meningomyelocele, cleft palate, and pyloric stenosis are examples of disorders that have both genetic and environmental influences (Au, Ashley-Koch, & Northrup, 2010). Taking the example of PKU, an affected child will develop intellectual disability if the PKU is not treated early but will have typical development if it is treated with a diet low in phenylalanine from infancy (Feillet et al., 2010; see Chapter 19).

SUMMARY

Each human cell contains a full complement of genetic information encoded in genes contained in 46 chromosomes. Not only does this genetic code determine our physical appearance and biological makeup, it is also the legacy we pass on to our children. The unequal division of the reproductive cells, the deletion of a part of a chromosome, the mutation in a single gene, or the modification of gene expression can each have significant consequences. Yet, despite these and other potential problems that can occur during the development of the embryo and fetus, approximately 97% of infants are born without birth defects.

REFERENCES

Amre, D.K., Mack, D.R., Morgan, K., Israel, D., Deslandres, C., Seidman, E.G., … Levy, E. (2010). Association between genome-wide association studies reported SNPs and pediatric-onset Crohn's disease in Canadian children. *Human Genetics, 128*(2), 31–35.

Au, K.S., Ashley-Koch, A., & Northrup, H. (2010). Epidemiologic and genetic aspects of spina bifida and other neural tube defects. *Developmental Disabilities Research Reviews, 16*(1), 6–15.

Brown, S. (2008). Miscarriage and its associations. *Seminars in Reproductive Medicine, 26*(5), 391–400.

Bushby, K., Finkel, R., Birnkrant, D.J., Case, L.E., Clemens, P.R., Cripe, L., … Constantin, C., DMD Care Considerations Working Group. (2010a). Diagnosis and management of Duchenne muscular dystrophy, Part 1: Diagnosis, and pharmacological and psychosocial management. *Lancet Neurology, 9*(1), 77–93.

Bushby, K., Finkel, R., Birnkrant, D.J., Case, L.E., Clemens, P.R., Cripe, L., … Constantin, C., DMD Care Considerations Working Group. (2010b). Diagnosis and management of Duchenne muscular dystrophy, Part 2: Implementation of multidisciplinary care. *Lancet Neurology, 9*(2), 177–189.

Butler, M.G. (2009). Genomic imprinting disorders in humans: A mini-review. *Journal of Assisted Reproduction and Genetics, 26*(9–10), 477–486.

Calvo, S.E., & Mootha, V.K. (2010). The mitochondrial proteome and human disease. *Annual Review of Genomics and Human Genetics, 11*, 25–44.

Cerruti Mainardi, P. (2006). Cri du chat syndrome. *Orphanet Journal of Rare Disease, 5*(1), 33.

Chahrour, M., & Zoghbi, H.Y. (2007). The story of Rett syndrome: From clinic to neurobiology. *Neuron 56*(3), 422–437.

Chonchaiya, W., Schneider, A., & Hagerman, R.J. (2009). Fragile X: A family of disorders. *Advances in Pediatrics, 56*, 165–186.

Collins, S.C., Coffee, B., Benke, P.J., Berry-Kravis, E., Gilbert, F., Oostra, B., ...Warren, S.T. (2010). Array-based FMR1 sequencing and deletion analysis in patients with a fragile X syndrome-like phenotype. *Public Library of Science, 5*(3), e9476.

Conlin, L.K., Thiel, B.D., Bonnemann, C.G., Medne, L., Ernst, L.M., Zackai, E.H., ... Spinner, N.B. (2010). Mechanisms of mosaicism, chimerism, and uniparental disomy identified by single nucleotide polymorphism array analysis. *Human Molecular Genetics, 19*(7), 1263–1275.

Dan, B. (2009). Angelman syndrome: Current understanding and research prospects. *Epilepsia, 50*(11), 2331–2339.

Farrar, M.A., Johnston, H.M., Grattan-Smith, P., Turner, A., & Kiernan, M.C. (2009). Spinal muscular atrophy: Molecular mechanisms. *Current Molecular Medicine, 9*(7), 851–862.

Feillet, F., van Spronsen, F.J., MacDonald, A., Trefz, F.K., Demirkol, M., Giovannini, M., ... Blau, N. (2010). Challenges and pitfalls in the management of phenylketonuria. *Pediatrics, 126*(2), 333–341.

Ferner, R.E. (2010). The neurofibromatoses. *Nature Clinical Practice Neurology, 10*(2), 82–93.

Flint, J., Wilkie, A.O., Buckle, V.J., Winter, R.M., Holland, A.J., & McDermid, H.E. (1995). The detection of subtelomeric chromosomal rearrangements in idiopathic intellectual disability. *Nature Genetics, 9*, 132–140.

Friedman, J.M., Baross, A., Delaney, A.D., Ally, A., Arbour, L., Armstrong, L., ... Marra, M.A. (2006). Oligonucleotide microarray analysis of genomic imbalance in children with mental retardation. *The American Journal of Human Genetics, 79*, 500–513.

Goldstone, A.P., Holland, A.J., Hauffa, B.P., Hokken-Koelega, A.C., & Tauber, M. (2008). Recommendations for the diagnosis and management of Prader-Willi syndrome. *Journal of Clinical Endocrinology and Metabolism, 93*(11), 4183–4197.

Gothelf, D., Schaer, M., & Eliez, S. (2008). Genes, brain development and psychiatric phenotypes in velo-cardio-facial syndrome. *Developmental Disabilities Research Reviews, 14*(1), 59–68.

Gräff, J., & Mansuy, I.M. (2009). Epigenetic dysregulation in cognitive disorders. *European Journal of Neuroscience, 30*(1), 1–8.

Gropman, A., & Batshaw, M.L. (2010). Epigenetics, copy number variation, and other molecular mechanisms underlying NDD: New insights and diagnostic approaches. *Journal of Developmental and Behavioral Pediatric, 31*(7), 582–591.

Gurrieri, F., & Accadia, M. (2009). Genetic imprinting: The paradigm of Prader-Willi and Angelman syndromes. *Endocrine Development, 14*, 20–28.

Hassold, T., Hall, H., & Hunt, P. (2007). The origin of human aneuploidy: Where we have been, where we are going. *Human Molecular Genetics, 16*(2), R203–R208.

Hong, D., Scaletta Kent, J., & Kesler, S. (2009). Cognitive profile of Turner syndrome. *Developmental Disabilities Research Reviews, 15*(4), 270–278.

Inlow J.K., & Restifo, L.L. (2004). Molecular and comparative genetics of mental retardation. *Genetics 166*(2), 835-81.

Jorde, L.B., Carey, J.C., & Bamshad, M.D. (2001). *Medical Genetics* (4th ed.). Philadelphia, PA: Mosby Elsevier.

Kaback, M.M., & Hexosaminidase, A. (2006). Deficiency. In: R.A. Pagon, T.C. Bird, C.R. Dolan, & K. Stephens (Eds.), *Gene Reviews*. Seattle, WA: University of Washington. Retrieved from http://www.ncbi.nlm.nih.gov/bookshelf/br.fcgi?book=gene&part=tay-sachs

Koleen, D.A., Pfundt, R., de Leeuw, N., Hehir-Kwa, J.Y., Nillesen, W.M., ... de Vries, B.B. (2009). Genomic microarrays in mental retardation: A practical workflow for diagnostic applications. *Human Mutation, 30*, 283–292.

Kumar, D. (2008). Disorders of the genome architecture: A review. *Genome Medicine, 2*(3–4), 69–76.

Li, M.M., & Andersson, H.C. (2009). Clinical application of microarray-based molecular cytogenetics: An emerging new era of genomic medicine. *Journal of Pediatrics, 155*(3), 311–317.

López, C., Saravia, C., Gomez, A., Hoebeke, J., & Patarroyo, M.A. (2010). Mechanisms of genetically-based resistance to malaria. *Gene, 467*(1–2), 1–12.

Matijevic, T., Knezevic, J., Slavica, M., & Pavelic, J. (2009). Rett syndrome: From the gene to the disease. *European Neurology, 61*(1), 3–10.

McCabe, E.R. (2010). Nanopediatrics: Enabling personalized medicine for children. *Pediatric Research 67*(5), 453–457.

McKusick-Nathans Institute of Genetic Medicine & The National Center for Biotechnology Information. (2010). *Online Mendelian Inheritance in Man* (OMIM). Retrieved from http://www.ncbi.nlm.nih.gov/omim/

Mervis, C.B., & John, A.E. (2010). Cognitive and behavioral characteristics of children with Williams syndrome: Implications for intervention approaches. *American Journal of Medical Genetics, 154C*(2), 229–248.

Morgan, T. (2007). Turner syndrome: Diagnosis and management. *American Family Physician, 76*(3), 405–410.

Moss, J., & Howlin, P. (2009). Autism spectrum disorders in genetic syndromes: Implications for diagnosis, intervention, and understanding the wider autism spectrum disorder population. *Journal of Intellectual Disability Research, 53*(10), 852–873.

National Center for Biotechnology Information. (2011). *Human genome resources*. Retrieved from http://www.ncbi.nlm.nih.gov/genome/guide/human

Owen, C.M., & Segars, Jr., J.H. (2009). Imprinting disorders and assisted reproductive technology. *Seminars in Reproductive Medicine, 27*(5), 417–428.

Parker, M.J., Budd, J.L., Draper, E.S., & Young, I.D. (2003). Trisomy 13 and trisomy 18 in a defined population: Epidemiological, genetic and prenatal observations. *Prenatal Diagnosis, 23*(10), 856-860.

Percy, A.K. (2008). Rett syndrome: Recent research progress. *Journal of Child Neurology, 23*(5), 543–549.

Ridley, M. (2006). *Genome: The autobiography of a species in 23 chapters*. New York, NY: HarperCollins.

Roelfsema, J.H., & Peters, D.J. (2007). Rubinstein-Taybi syndrome: Clinical and molecular overview. *Expert Reviews in Molecular Medicine, 9*(23), 1–16.

Schneider, A., Hagerman, R.J., & Hessl, D. (2009). Fragile X syndrome: From genes to cognition. *Developmental Disabilities Research Reviews, 15*(4), 333–342.

Sebat, J., Lakshmi, B., Malhotra, D., Troge, J., Lese-Martin, C., Walsh, T., ...Wigler, M. (2007). Strong association of de novo copy number mutations with autism. *Science 316*, 445–449.

Seshadri, S., Fitzpatrick, A.L., Ikram, M.A., DeStefano, A.L., Gudnason, V., Boada, M., ... Breteler, M.M. (2010). CHARGE Consortium; GERAD1 Consortium; EADI1 Consortium. Genome-wide analysis of genetic loci associated with Alzheimer disease. *Journal of the American Medical Association, 303*(18), 1832–1840.

Soares, S.R., Templado, C., Blanco, J., Egozcue, J., & Vidal, F. (2001). Numerical chromosome abnormalities in the spermatozoa of the fathers of children with trisomy 21 of paternal origin: Generalised tendency to meiotic non-disjunction. *Human Genetics, 108*(2), 134–139.

Stankiewicz, P., & Beaudet, A.L. (2007). Use of array CGH in the evaluation of dysmorphology, malformations, developmental delay, and idiopathic mental retardation. *Current Opinion in Genetics & Development, 17*(3), 182–192.

Stevenson, R.E., & Schwartz, C.E. (2009). X-linked intellectual disability: Unique vulnerability of the male genome. *Developmental Disabilities Research Reviews 15*(4), 361–368.

Stranger, B.E., Forrest, M.S., Dunning, M., Ingle, C.E., Beasley, C., ... Dermitzakis, E.T. (2007). Relative impact of nucleotide and copy number variation on gene expression phenotypes. *Science, 315*, 848–853.

Urdinguio, R.G., Sanchez-Mut, J.V., & Esteller, M. (2009). Epigenetic mechanisms in neurological diseases: Genes, syndromes, and therapies. *Lancet Neurology, 8*(11), 1056–1072.

Vogel, F., & Rathenberg, R. (1975). Spontaneous mutation in man. *Advances in Human Genetics, 5*, 267.

Wilkins, J.F., & Úbeda, F. (2011). Diseases associated with genomic imprinting. *Progress in Molecular Biology and Translational Science, 101*, 401–45.

Wiseman, F.K., Alford, K.A., Tybulewicz, V.L., & Fisher, E.M. (2009). Down syndrome—recent progress and future prospects. *Human Molecular Genetics, 18*(R1), R75–83.

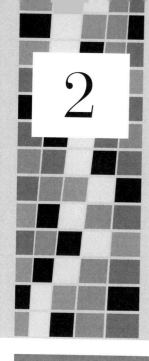

2

Fetal Development

Adre J. du Plessis

Upon completion of this chapter the reader will

- Understand the fundamental principles of structural brain development from conception to birth

- Be able to explain the complex interplay between development of brain structure and brain function across fetal life

- Know the mechanisms by which environmental factors and their timing disrupt the normal process of fetal brain development

- Understand how the development of neural pathways that ultimately connect the rest of the body to the deep brain structures, and then to the developing cortex, relate to the emergence of sensory experience and consciousness

Neurologic integrity at birth is a major determinant of quality of life across a person's lifespan. This chapter will discuss fundamental aspects of normal brain development in the fetus. Although development of the peripheral neuromotor and sensorineural systems is important for postnatal function (see Chapters 12 and 13), this chapter will focus only on the development of the central nervous system.

A mature brain possesses more than one billion neurons, each with many connections to other cells. Precise differentiation (specialization), localization, and connectivity of these cells are critical for normal neurologic function. Most of these processes are complete prior to birth, and any disruption may lead to irreversible structural and functional brain impairment. Even though many such problems are

detectable soon after birth, research increasingly suggests that many neurobehavioral conditions presenting later in life, such as attention deficit disorder, autism spectrum disorders, and schizophrenia, originate in fetal life.

Until relatively recently, understanding of fetal brain development was based solely on animal studies and human autopsy tissue. Advances in two major areas, neurogenetics and neuroimaging, have markedly accelerated understanding of fetal brain development (Bystron, Blakemore, & Rakic, 2008; Prayer et al., 2006; Rados, Judas, & Kostovic, 2006; Ten Donkelaar & Lammens, 2009). Along with recent insights into the genetic determinants of normal brain development, recognition has been rapidly growing of the impact of environmental influences on neural development, either directly or through epigenetic mechanisms (see Chapter 1). In fact, advances in both these areas have blurred the traditional distinction between viewing influences on development as one of either genetic or environmental.

Any discussion of events during fetal brain development requires a consistent starting point reference. Embryologists use postconceptional age (PCA), which dates the onset of development from the presumed date of ovulation, as a metric for development. Within this context intrauterine development is divided into two major phases, the embryonic period, over the first 8 postconceptional weeks and the fetal period, from 9 weeks until birth (Figure 2.1). Clinicians use gestational age (GA) in weeks referenced to start on the first day of the last menstrual period (i.e., 2 weeks earlier than postconceptional age); this divides the intrauterine period into three trimesters. The first trimester extends over the first 12 weeks, the second from 13 to 28 weeks, and the third trimester from 29 weeks until term (40 weeks). In this chapter we will primarily use GA to describe developmental events.

STRUCTURAL DEVELOPMENT OF THE BRAIN

Brain development proceeds along a highly programmed series of overlapping phases, each of which has a period of peak growth that moves across the different brain regions in a tightly regulated schedule. Each of these maturational phases has a "critical period" during which disruption of development may have irreversible and far-reaching consequences. In this sense the timing of a disruption is as important as its nature, i.e., "when" is as important as "what." Paradoxically, these periods of accelerated maturation are also periods of particular vulnerability to injury since the precise mechanisms that promote development normally may increase disruption under adverse conditions.

There are a number of classification schemes that have been used to outline the major events in neural development. Table 2.1 lists one such approach that defines the various overlapping developmental phases and their peak periods of activity. These phases include neurulation, neural proliferation,

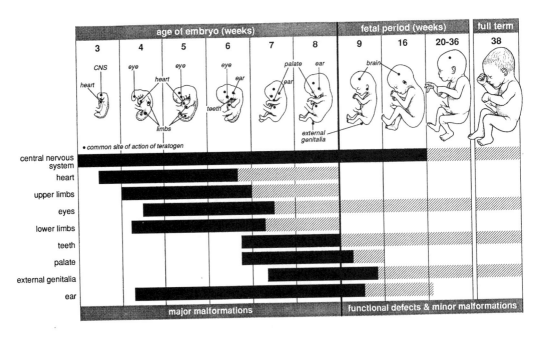

Figure 2.1. Embryogenesis and fetal development. The changes that take place during embryogenesis, between 3 and 8 weeks after fertilization, are enormous. All body systems are formed, and the embryo takes on a human form. Length increases 20-fold during this time. The fetal period lasts from 9 weeks to birth. Teratogens cause malformations if acting during the time a specific organ or group of organs are being formed. Damage to an organ during the time represented by a solid bar will lead to a major malformation, and damage during the time represented by the hatched bar will lead to functional defects or minor morphological abnormalities. (From Moore, K.L., & Persaud, T.V.N. [1993]. *Before we are born: Essentials of embryology and birth defects* [4th ed., inside back cover]. Philadelphia, PA: W.B. Saunders; adapted by permission.)

neuronal migration, and myelination; and each is described in the following sections (Volpe, 2008).

Neurulation

The first major phase of nervous system development in the embryo is neural tube formation, or **neurulation** (Figures 2.2 and 2.3). Between 2 and 4 weeks' GA, the **rostral** (anterior) and **caudal** (posterior) poles of the developing embryo are established. Along this axis arises a region of tissue (the primitive streak) which becomes the neural plate. Structures appear adjacent to both ends of the neural plate, the rostral prechordal plate and the caudal eminence. There are two stages of neurulation, primary and secondary. *Primary neurulation* is the process by which the neural plate develops a midline groove, the edges of which fold over, converge, and close to form the neural tube. The openings (**neuropores**) of the neural tube close around 6 weeks' GA. Defects in primary neurulation and neural tube

formation result in congenital malformations such as spina bifida/meningomyelocoele, and encephaloceles (see Chapter 25).

Secondary neurulation is a series of events at the neural tube's lower edge in which the caudal eminence develops into the bottom-most spine segments and elements of the lower intestine. Defects in secondary neurulation result in the **caudal regression syndrome** and can result in major malformations of the lower vertebrae, pelvis, and spine. Around the time of neural tube closure a ridge develops along its **dorsolateral** (backside) aspects. This tissue forms the neural crest, which in turn develops into a variety of structures including spinal and brainstem **ganglia** (masses of nerve cell bodies), **melanocytes** (pigment-forming skin cells), certain endocrine structures (e.g., thymus, adrenal medulla), elements of the heart, and the **enteric nervous system** (the subdivision of the autonomic nervous system that controls the gastrointestinal system). By 6 weeks' GA, the rostral end of the

Table 2.1. Time table of major developmental events in fetal brain development

Developmental event	Period of peak activity (GA)	Abnormalities (*etiologies*)
Dorsal induction		
Neural tube formation (primary neurulation)	3–4 weeks	Spina bifida (*folate deficiency; anti-epileptic drugs; maternal diabetes; excess vitamin A; trisomies 13 and 18*); encephaloceles
Caudal eminence development (secondary neurulation)	4–7 weeks	Caudal regression syndromes (*maternal diabetes*)
Ventral induction		
Prosencephalic development	2–3 months	
Cleavage		Holoprosencephaly (*Smith-Lemli-Opitz syndrome; fetal alcohol exposure; maternal diabetes; retinoic acid*)
Midline formation		Agenesis of the corpus callosum (*Aicardi syndrome; pyruvate dehydrogenase deficiency; glycemic encephalopathy*); septo-optic dysplasia
Neural proliferation	3–4 months	Microcephaly (*alcohol, phenytoin, Accutane; radiation; congenital infections; maternal PKU*)
Neuronal migration	3–5 months	Schizencephaly (*EMX2 gene mutation, fetal stroke*), heterotopias, lissencephaly (*Miller-Dieker syndrome; Fukuyama congenital muscular dystrophy*)
Cortical organization	5 months to years postnatal	Polymicrogyria (*fetal growth restriction; congenital infections; metabolic disorders*)
Myelination	Birth to years postnatal	Hypomyelination (*metabolic disorders, congenital infection; prematurity, hypothyroidism*)
Cerebellar-brainstem development	2 months to postnatal	(Ponto) cerebellar hypoplasia (*congenital defects in glycosylation; congenital infections*); Joubert syndrome; Dandy-Walker malformation

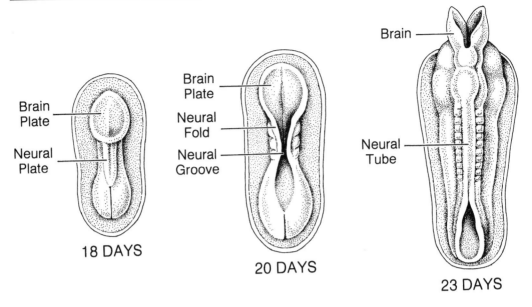

Figure 2.2. Development of the central nervous system (CNS) during the first month of the embryonic period. This is a longitudinal view showing the gradual closure of the neural tube to form the spinal column and the rounding up of the head region to form the primitive brain.

neural tube begins to differentiate into three primary sections, which go on to form the major components the brain: the forebrain, midbrain, hindbrain, and cerebellum (Figure 2.4). In summary, by 6 weeks' GA the basic parts of the brain and spinal cord have been established.

Subsequent events in neural tube development proceed by specialization in which regional genetic organizing centers generate molecular products that stimulate and/or inhibit growth differentially. *Ventral induction* describes the development of the precursor of

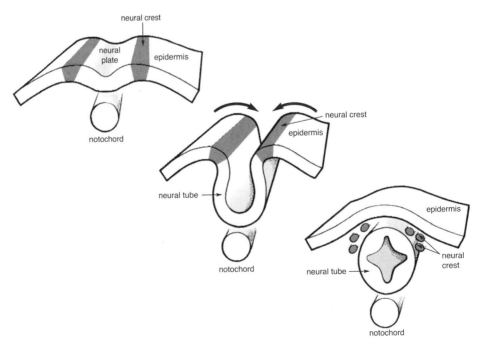

Figure 2.3. Stages in dorsal induction with formation of the neural tube, neural crest, and overlying skin and soft tissue.

the forebrain, and its cleavage into two cerebral hemispheres (Figure 2.4). This is followed by development of the midline structures including the corpus callosum, optic and olfactory vesicles, pituitary gland, and parts of the face (see Figure 2.4). This process is regulated by certain genetic pathways, and mutations in these genes can result in a spectrum of brain anomalies, including agenesis (absence) of the corpus callosum, and **holoprosencephaly,** which involves impaired cleavage of the cerebral hemispheres and associated facial malformations (Edison & Muenke, 2003). Such disturbances in brain development may be seen after early alcohol exposure (fetal alcohol syndrome) or retinoic acid exposure (high-dose vitamin A given for treatment of severe acne), as well as in certain genetic disorders such as the Smith-Lemli-Opitz syndrome (see Appendix B).

Each cerebral hemisphere forms a dorsal region which generates major parts of the cerebral cortex. These phenomena are discussed below. Subsequent phases of cerebral hemispheric development can be summarized as 1) neural proliferation, 2) neuronal migration, 3) cortical organization and synapse formation, and 4) myelination.

Neural Proliferation

Neural proliferation occurs during a sustained period of vigorous cellular division which peaks between 6 and 22 weeks' GA, giving rise to precursors of the future neuronal (grey matter)

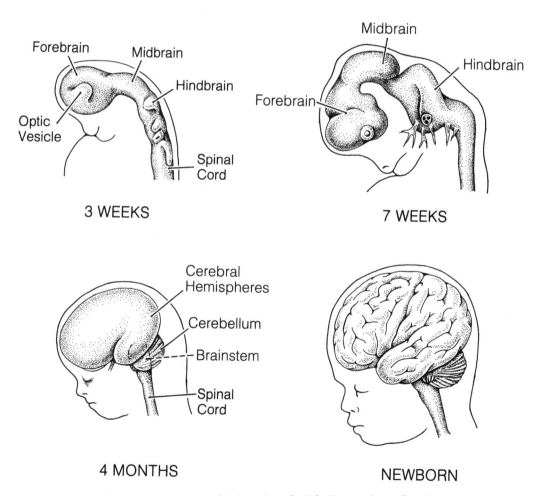

Figure 2.4. Development of the brain during fetal life. This is a side view illustrating the increasing complexity of the brain over time. The forebrain, or prosencephalon, develops into the cerebral hemispheres; the midbrain, or mesencephalon, develops into the brainstem; and the hindbrain, or rhombencephalon, develops into the cerebellum. Although all brain structures are formed by 4 months, the brain grows greatly in size and complexity during the final months of prenatal development.

and **glial** (white matter) cell populations of the brain. **Neurogenesis** (the birth of neurons) starts in the spinal cord and brainstem, but by the early fetal period involves the entire **periventricular region** (the area surrounding the ventricles which contain cerebrospinal fluid). The cerebral ventricular zone is divided into the dorsal and ventral neuroepithelium. The dorsal neuroepithelium goes on to form the excitatory neuron population (with glutamate as its primary neurotransmitter) and the future projection pathways. These pathways are important for cognition, motivation, and memory. The ventral neuroepithelium gives rise to the future interneuronal population, which produces the neurotransmitter gamma aminobutyric acid (GABA). During early brain development GABA exerts an excitatory function but later switches to become the principal inhibitory neurotransmitter (see Chapter 12).

The rapidly growing periventricular regions are particularly susceptible to certain viruses (such as cytomegalovirus) and other injurious agents such as radiation and alcohol. Not surprisingly, agents that impair neural proliferation result most commonly in **microcephaly** (abnormally small head), amongst other developmental disturbances.

Neuronal Migration

After multiple divisions resulting in the proliferation of neurons, they start to migrate out toward the surface of the brain in successive waves beginning at 12 weeks' GA and ending by 20 weeks' GA (Bystron et al., 2008). The excitatory pyramidal neurons migrate along radial glia, which are specialized cells that act as guide "wires" from the ventricular surface to the brain periphery (Figure 2.5). The pyramidal neurons are destined to play a critical role in future projection neuronal networks in the brain which are involved in cognition. Radial migration occurs in an inside-out manner, with successive waves of migration passing through earlier layers to occupy a more superficial location until a mature six-layered cerebral cortex is established. The outermost layer contains specialized cells that produce reelin, a chemical signal responsible for arresting the migration of cells once they reach their appropriate destination layer (Zhao et al., 2006). A genetic lack of reelin causes **lissencephaly,** a "smooth" brain with a lack of development of folds (gyri) and grooves (sulci). Disturbances in reelin production may also play a role in complex partial seizures and autism.

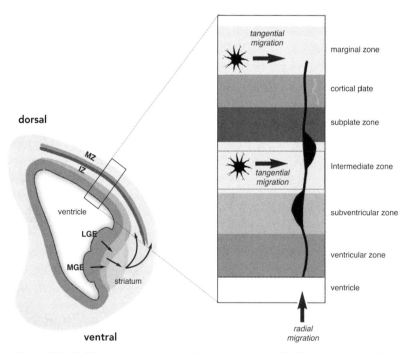

Figure 2.5. Radial and tangential neuronal migration between 12–20 weeks' gestation. Radial migration emanates from the ventricular zone of the dorsal part of the brain, while tangential migration emanates from the lateral (LGE) and medial (MGE) ganglionic eminences and course in the intermediate (IZ) and marginal (MZ) zones of the developing brain.

The subplate zone just under the developing cortex is a transient architectonic zone that plays a critical role in development of the thalamocortical pathways and their ultimate cortical connectivity in the neocortex. The major events in organizing the subplate and thalamocortical systems occur between 22 and 40 weeks' GA. Between 26 and 28 weeks' GA, the thalamocortical projections begin to penetrate the cortical plate and form synapses (Kostovic & Judas). By 29 weeks' GA, evoked potentials triggered in extremities can be detected over the cortex, suggesting functional connectivity between peripheral sensory fibers and the cerebral cortex, setting the stage for a host of functions such as the conscious experience of sensation and other functions coordinating movements of the extremities. Once the thalamocortical connectivity is established the subplate begins to recede.

Tangential migration, the other major form of neural migration, follows a more circuitous and prolonged path than radial migration (Figure 2.5). These neurons migrate parallel to the surface of the brain and perpendicular to the radial glia. As these tangentially migrating neurons approach their destination, they switch to a brief radial phase of migration. These cells are precursors of the inhibitory (GABAergic) interneuronal system of the mature brain, which enhances regulation and discrete control of excitatory systems in the cortex. Abnormalities here place the child at greater risk for seizures.

Neural Proliferation and Migration in the Developing Cerebellum

The cerebellum has a particularly protracted development starting in the embryonic period and extending across even the first few years of postnatal life (Ten Donkelaar & Lammens, 2009). This in turn constitutes a prolonged period of vulnerability to injury and potential disruption of its developmental program. The cerebellum originates at the midbrain-hindbrain junction between 6 and 8 weeks' GA, and its development combines regional growth and inhibition. The developing cerebellum has two growth regions (Figure 2.6). A primary proliferative zone adjacent to the ventricle sends cells to form the cerebellar nuclei and Purkinje cells (which are the only cerebellar output pathway for motor coordination). A second wave of neural progenitors migrates to the lateral aspects of the future cerebellum, where a further wave of migration occurs tangentially across the surface of the cerebellum to form the rapidly growing external granular cell layer. After a series of cell divisions, these granular cells migrate inwards across the Purkinje cell layer to form the internal granular layer, a process that extends into postnatal life (Ten Donkelaar & Lammens, 2009). The sustained growth in the developing cerebellum exposes it to a prolonged period of being at risk for injury and developmental disruption from viruses (e.g., cytomegalovirus), and toxins (e.g., alcohol) that stunt the cerebellum's growth. In addition, cerebellar hypoplasia has been associated with certain genetic disorders including Dandy-Walker syndrome, Werdnig-Hoffman syndrome, and Walker-Warburg syndrome.

The relevance of cerebellar development to developmental disabilities is demonstrated by the significant deficits described after fetal or neonatal cerebellar injury. The traditional view of the cerebellum as a purely motor relay center responsible for maintaining balance and coordinated movements has been challenged by a growing body of evidence suggesting a far more diverse and pervasive role in neurologic function. A cerebellar cognitive affective syndrome, with nonmotor deficits in cognition, language, and behavioral regulation, has been described in adults after cerebellar injury. This syndrome includes impairment of executive functions such as planning, set-shifting, verbal fluency, abstract reasoning and working memory; difficulties with spatial cognition including visual-spatial organization and memory; and personality change with blunting of affect or disinhibited and inappropriate behaviour (Schmahmann & Sherman, 1998). More recently, a **developmental cerebellar cognitive affective syndrome** has been described in children who survive prematurity-related cerebellar injury (Limperopoulos et al, 2007). Here deficits range from impaired executive function to severe behavioral disturbances that fall into the autism spectrum.

Cortical Organization and Synapse formation

Neuronal activation (i.e., firing of electical impulses) is critical for brain development. Normal cortical organization and connectivity requires appropriate regional neuronal activation in order to maintain local growth factor levels and to activate local genetic programs. This is the basis for the dictum that *Neurons that fire together, wire together; those that don't,*

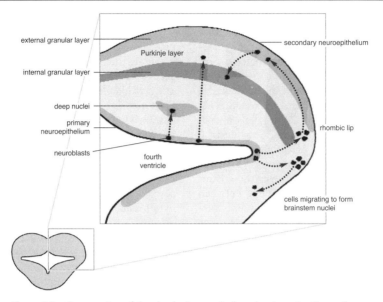

Figure 2.6. Cross section of the developing cerebellum showing migration pathways from the primary and secondary neuroepithelial layers.

won't. The interplay between neuronal activation and structural development occurs in the immature brain in two major ways: nonsynaptic communication, and development of synaptic communication During early brain development, *nonsynaptic communication* occurs with neurons and neural networks being driven by a rudimentary excitability. Neurons are coupled by electrical "synapses" that facilitate rapid co-firing of neuronal populations. During this phase the neurotransmitter GABA has an excitatory action, and the re-uptake system that removes GABA is poorly developed (Ben-Ari, 2006). This results in elevated GABA levels surrounding the cells which keep neuronal circuits in a partially depolarized, and thus excitable, state (Akerman & Cline, 2007). This, in turn, facilitates the generation of a primitive neural activity presenting as spontaneous and recurrent bursts of high-voltage activity, called giant depolarizing potentials (GDP). Although these GDP are not related to environmental stimulation and contain little information, they are fundamental to constructing early functional neural networks and to forming basic cortical maps (Khazipov et al., 2004). Although this neural activation is itself independent of chemical synapses, it is an important trigger for subsequent synapse formation through gene activation and growth factor support. In fact, this activity results in major overproduction of synapses, which require "pruning back" during subsequent phases or reorganization (see Chapter 12). This pruning activity is affected

negatively in Down syndrome and fragile X syndrome and has also been implicated in ADHD and learning disabilities.

At this point in development, pathways from the periphery have not yet established effective connectivity with the cerebral circuitry and are confined, for the most part, to loops of activity between the spine and brainstem, the so-called primitive reflexes. The next phase is marked by the *development of synaptic communication* and synapse-driven networks. The abundant chemical synapses generated earlier are unstable and require a threshold of activation to become stabilized synapses; if not activated, they recede. This switch to a cortical receptor-mediated synaptic network is critical for establishing the level of complexity required for the behaviorally relevant actions essential for postnatal life. Synapses are concentrated on spine-like processes of the neuronal dendrites (branched projections that conduct electrochemical stimulation received from another neuron to the cell body). During this critical period, refinement of cortical maps becomes experience-driven, which only becomes possible when: 1) GABA's action shifts from excitation to inhibition (Jelitai & Madarasz, 2005); 2) sufficient density of the excitatory neurotransmitter glutamate synapses is achieved; and 3) information transfer across synapses becomes more discrete, with rapid clearance of neurotransmitters from the synaptic cleft. In summary, although complex genetic mechanisms drive the organization and connectivity of the developing cerebral cortex, both spontaneous and experience-driven activity plays a critical role in establishing and consolidating neural networks. When this does not occur, the risk for various developmental disabilities increases. For example, in Rett syndrome (see Appendix B) there is a decrease in dendritic spines and resultant abnormal synaptic function.

As fundamental as the progressive acquisition of neural elements described above is to normal neurodevelopment, so too are subsequent events that actively prune and reorganize the brain structure. Failure of such events may cause impaired neurologic function. During fetal brain development, an excess of neural structures is created, ranging from whole cells to cellular elements such as synapses. Significant reorganization then takes place involving the regression of redundant synapses, withdrawal of axons from crowded areas, and changes in the profile of neurotransmitters. In addition, redundant neurons are culled by the active energy-dependent process called **apoptosis** (programmed cell death; Narayanan, 1997).

Myelination

The efficacy of neural connectivity depends not only on successful conduction of electrical impulses to target sites, but on the speed and coordination of their transmission. Connectivity is driven by axonal growth cones, which respond to attractant and repellant signals that guide them to their destination. Conduction along axons is accelerated by the process of myelination. In this process a group of oligodendrocytes (a type of glial cell) that attach along the length of an axon wrap the axon in a lipid-rich myelin sheath, interrupted by minute nodes of exposed axonal membrane. By allowing action potentials to "hop" from one node to the next, neural transmission is markedly accelerated. During fetal development myelination starts in the spinal cord and brainstem, then proceeds upward into the cerebrum. However, by the time of birth at term myelination has only advanced into the brainstem, cerebellum, and internal capsule (white matter near the thalamus). Myelination of the cerebral white matter is relatively late, reaching its peak during the first year of postnatal life (Kinney, Brody, Kloman, & Gilles, 1988). During the fetal period oligodendrocytes go through several stages of development before becoming capable of forming myelin. During this period of maturation the immature oligodendrocyte

is particularly vulnerable to injury, such as that generated by infection-inflammation and hypoxia-ischemia (lack of adequate oxygenation or circulation). This is a particular risk for premature infants. Such injury of immature oligodendrocytes typically has a delayed presentation, only becoming evident when the expected myelination fails to occur. One manifestation of this injury is a form of cerebral palsy termed spastic diplegia (see Chapter 24).

FUNCTIONAL DEVELOPMENT OF THE FETAL NERVOUS SYSTEM

For obvious reasons the study of functional brain development in the fetus has been based primarily on observations of fetal motor behavior. The earliest description of fetal movements was by Erbkam in 1837 who reported on the behaviors of spontaneous miscarriages. It was not until the advent of fetal ultrasound in the early 1970s that visualization of the fetus's active behavior became possible (de Vries, Visser, & Prechtl, 1985). Since then rapid advances in ultrasound technology, such as 3D ultrasound in the early 1990's and more recently 4D ultrasound (showing fetal activity), have provided increasingly detailed observations of fetal behavior. This approach provides a potential window on the functional development of the fetal nervous system, complementing the insights into structural brain development provided by advanced fetal imaging. Under adverse conditions neurologic function becomes impaired before the development of permanent structural brain injury. Consequently, a greater understanding of fetal behavior and its relationship to brain development may provide important indicators of failing intrauterine support prior to the development of irreversible brain injury, opening the possibility of intervention during fetal life to prevent or ameliorate brain injury.

Specific fetal movements start very early in development, well before development of the fundamental structural apparatus of the central nervous system. Studies in primates confirmed that these early fetal movements are expressions of spontaneous neural discharges (discussed above). The earliest fetal movements are seen between 10 and 12 weeks' GA and consist of brief flexion/extension movements of the trunk. These are followed one week later by isolated movements of the head and extremities. Thereafter a broad repertoire of fetal movement patterns accumulates, although many of the earliest movement patterns are retained through fetal life and into early neonatal life. Certain early patterns of stereotypic movements reflect activation in the spinal cord and brainstem. Initially the activation of these movement patterns is spontaneous, but later they may be triggered by sensory stimuli. Sensorimotor spinal reflex loops generating primitive reflex responses may be present as early as 10 weeks' GA as evidenced by, for example, fetal motor responses to tactile stimulation from a co-twin.

Early reflex responses are shock-like and massive, suggesting a paucity of synapses and little modulating influence from the brain centers down onto the spinal nerves. With maturation, descending cerebral influences act upon intervening synapses in these spinal and brainstem reflex loops, resulting in more discrete and localized reflex movements. This cerebral modulation of spinal-brainstem activity is mainly inhibitory, as evidenced by the diminution of reflexes to repeated stimulation. For example, ringing a loud bell will lead to startle-like fetal movements, but repeated close-interval ringing will cause the startle to dampen and then disappear. This is an early example of learning.

From 17 to 22 weeks' GA a variety of facial movements emerge including mouthing, swallowing, yawning, and hiccuping. Facial responses to peripheral stimulation develop early in gestation, and are probably mediated by subcortical systems. More complex facial movements resembling emotional expressions emerge during the third trimester, at a time when connections between the thalamus and cortex are being formed. Fetal eye movements start at 18 weeks, become rapid at 21 weeks, and become consolidated into active and nonactive periods between 26 and 28 weeks' GA (Nijhuis, Prechtl, Martin, & Bots, 1982).

Development of the autonomic nervous system is reflected in changing heart rate and breathing patterns with advancing gestation. These various aspects of fetal activity (gross motor, facial and eye movement, heart rate and breathing) become clustered together and stabilize into recognizable coordinated behavioral states around 36 weeks' GA. In summary, these patterns of fetal motility and behavioral state have a well-characterized development in the normal fetus which can now be followed by advanced fetal ultrasound techniques.

A number of external influences on fetal movements have been reported, including maternal steroid administration, cigarette smoking, maternal stress, fetal growth restriction, and maternal diabetes mellitus (Visser, Laurini, de Vries, Bekedam, & Prechtl, 1985). Although lacking in sensitivity and specificity, fetal movements in the growth-restricted fetus are described as slow, monotonous, and erratic, with decreased variability in strength and amplitude, while those in diabetic pregnancies appear monotonous, rigid or chaotic. In the anencephalic fetus which has no cerebral hemispheres (see Appendix B), jerky, forceful, large-amplitude movements probably reflect the lack of modulation as a result of absence of the cerebral hemispheres.

SUMMARY

Assembly of the basic neural apparatus required for a newborn infant to engage in postnatal life requires the successful unfolding of a highly complex series of events during fetal life. Fundamental to the development of a structurally and functionally integrated nervous system is the emergence of nerve cell activation, at first resulting from spontaneous discharges in crude regional circuits. Toward the end of gestation and into postnatal life discrete synaptic connectivity becomes established and modified by sensory stimuli from the internal and external environment. Conversely, other underutilized neural structures are pruned back. A host of blood-borne influences may act through the placenta to disrupt this complex interaction between brain activation and development. Understanding of the critical *in vivo* events of normal brain development has been accelerated by increasingly sophisticated fetal imaging of brain structure and function. These advances promise to lead to the earlier detection of abnormalities and the enhancement of interventions to minimize the often catastrophic repercussions of abnormal fetal brain development.

REFERENCES

Akerman, C.J., & Cline, H.T. (2007). Refining the roles of GABAergic signaling during neural circuit formation. *Trends in Neuroscience, 30*(8), 382–389.

Ben-Ari, Y. (2006). Basic developmental rules and their implications for epilepsy in the immature brain. *Epileptic Disorders, 8*(2), 91–102.

Bystron, I., Blakemore, C., & Rakic, P. (2008). Development of the human cerebral cortex: Boulder Committee revisited. *Nature Reviews Neuroscience 9*, (2), 110–122.

de Vries, J.I., Visser, G.H., & Prechtl, H.F. (1985). The emergence of fetal behaviour. II. Quantitative aspects. *Early Human Development, 12*(2), 99–120.

Edison, R., & Muenke, M. (2003). The interplay of genetic and environmental factors in craniofacial morphogenesis: Holoprosencephaly and the role of cholesterol. *Congenital Anomalies (Kyoto), 43*(1), 1–21.

Jelitai, M., & Madarasz, E. (2005). The role of GABA in the early neuronal development. *International Review of Neurobiology, 71*, 27–62.

Khazipov, R., Sirota, A., Leinekugel, X., Holmes, G.L., Ben-Ari, Y., & Buzsaki, G. (2004). Early motor activity drives spindle bursts in the developing somatosensory cortex. *Nature, 432*(7018), 758–761.

Kinney, H.C., Brody, B.A., Kloman, A.S., & Gilles, F.H. (1988). Sequence of central nervous system myelination in human infancy. II. Patterns of myelination in autopsied infants. *Journal of Neuropathology and Experimental Neurology, 47*(3), 217–234.

Kostovic, I., & Judas, M. (2010). The development of the subplate and thalamocortical connections in the human foetal brain. *Acta Paediatrica, 99*(8), 1119–1127.

Limperopoulos, C., Bassan, H., Gauvreau, K., Robertson, R.L. Jr, Sullivan, N.R., Benson, C.B., … du Plessis, A.J. (2007). Does cerebellar injury in premature infants contribute to the high prevalence of long-term cognitive, learning, and behavioral disability in survivors? *Pediatrics, 120*(3), 584–93.

Narayanan, V. (1997). Apoptosis in development and disease of the nervous system: Naturally occuring cell death in the developing nervous sytem. *Pediatric Neurology, 16*(1), 9–13.

Nijhuis, J.G., Prechtl, H.F., Martin, C.B., Jr., & Bots, R.S. (1982). Are there behavioural states in the human fetus? *Early Human Development, 6*(2), 177–195.

Prayer, D., Kasprian, G., Krampl, E., Ulm, B., Witzani, L., Prayer, L., & Brugger, P.C. (2006). MRI of normal fetal brain development. *European Journal of Radiology, 57*(2), 199–216.

Rados, M., Judas, M., & Kostovic, I. (2006). In vitro MRI of brain development. *European Journal of Radiology, 57*(2), 187–198.

Schmahmann, J.D., & Sherman, J.C. (1998). The cerebellar cognitive affective syndrome. *Brain, 121*(4), 561–579

Ten Donkelaar, H.J., & Lammens, M. (2009). Development of the human cerebellum and its disorders. *Clinics in Perinatology, 36*(3), 513–530.

Visser, G.H., Laurini, R.N., de Vries, J.I., Bekedam, D.J., & Prechtl, H.F. (1985). Abnormal motor behaviour in anencephalic fetuses. *Early Human Development, 12*(2), 173–182.

Volpe, J.J. (2008). Human brain development *Neurology of the Newborn* (5th ed.). Philadelphia, PA: Saunders.

Zhao, H., Wong, R.J., Nguyen, X., Kalish, F., Mizobuchi, M., Vreman, H.J., … Contag, C.H. (2006). Expression and regulation of heme oxygenase isozymes in the developing mouse cortex. *Pediatric Research, 60*(5), 518–523.

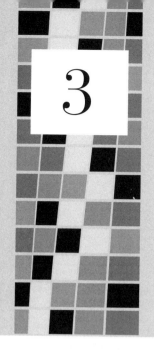

3

Environmental Toxicants and Neurocognitive Development

Jerome Paulson

Upon completion of this chapter, the reader will be able to

■ Describe vulnerable periods in the neurocognitive development of children

■ List and discuss several known neurotoxicants

■ Describe possible mechanisms of action of neurotoxicants

■ Discuss current limitations on protecting children from neurotoxins and other hazardous chemicals

A pregnant woman, 4 weeks after conception, ingests a chemical called glutarimide (N-phthalimido) and subsequently delivers a term infant with severely malformed and shortened arms and legs (phocomelia). A woman at 30 weeks' gestation ingests the same chemical and delivers a term infant with no visible congenital anomalies. This chemical is also known as thalidomide. It was widely marketed over the counter in Europe, Canada, and Japan in the 1950s and early 1960s, specifically recommended for the control of morning sickness in pregnant women. Neither premarket testing nor postmarket follow-up of the effects of the chemical exposure were required at the time. It is estimated that about 10,000 infants were born worldwide with various birth defects resulting from first trimester thalidomide exposure (Franks, Macpherson, & Figg, 2004; Silverman, 2002). The widely diverse consequences of thalidomide exposure underscore the importance of specific windows of vulnerability *in utero*. Windows of vulnerability, both before and after

birth, are discussed in the following sections. The experience with thalidomide also underscores the importance of premarket testing and postmarket surveillance, not only of chemicals that are intended for ingestion by humans (i.e., drugs), but of all chemicals that enter the human body. These issues are the focus of this chapter.

Via animal and human studies, over 1,000 chemicals have been identified as potential neurotoxicants (causes of neurologic injury; Grandjean & Landrigan, 2006). The range of outcomes from exposure to these chemicals includes: 1) fetal death; 2) death at an older age related to early or recent exposure; 3) malformations related to *in utero* exposure; 4) growth retardation related to *in utero* or later exposure; 5) developmental disabilities including intellectual disability, learning disabilities, and cerebral palsy; and 6) so-called "subclinical outcomes," such as statistically significant decrements in IQ, executive functioning, and/or adaptive skills (Faustman, Silbernagel & Fenske, et al.,

2000; Gilbert, 2008; Grandjean et al., 2008; Grandjean & Landrigan, 2006; Selevan, Kimmel, & Mendola, 2000; Weiss, 2000).

Many chemicals have been shown to have similar detrimental effects in animals and humans. For example, learning deficits have been associated with exposure to metals including cadmium, lead, mercury, and manganese; solvents including toluene, xylene, and ethanol; and other chemicals including polychlorinated biphenyls (PCBs), nicotine, and dioxins (Koger, Schettler, & Weiss, 2005). These observations suggest that different toxicants—acting on specific developmental processes that occur at a given time in development—can have the same or similar outcomes.

Conversely, individual chemicals have been associated with a range of outcomes. For example, exposure to PCBs in children has been associated with learning disabilities, attention-deficit/hyperactivity disorder (ADHD), and memory impairments. Exposure to lead has been associated with learning disabilities, decreased IQ, ADHD, violent behaviors, and aggression. This suggests that exposure to the same toxicant during different developmental time periods can lead to different adverse effects. Beyond chemicals, toxicants such as radiation can also adversely affect neurodevelopment.

Only a small fraction of the thousands of known chemicals have been proven to cause developmental neurotoxicity in humans (see Figure 3.1). This does not necessarily mean that other chemicals do not cause neurotoxicity, only that this association remains untested or unproven.

SCOPE OF THE ISSUE

In 2000, an expert panel, convened by the U.S. National Academy of Sciences (NAS), estimated that 3% of all neurobehavioral disorders in children are directly caused by exposure to environmental contaminants and that another 25% are caused by interactions among environmental factors, including "infection, nutritional deficiencies and excesses, life-style factors (e.g., alcohol), hyperthermia, ultraviolet radiation, X-rays, and…the myriad of manufactured and natural agents encountered by humans" (National Academy of Sciences Committee on Developmental Toxicology, 2000). In 2006, the World Health Organization estimated that environmental causes, including metals, pesticides, stress, and so forth, account for about 13% of all neuropsychiatric diseases (Prüss-Üstün & Corvalán, 2006). Landrigan et al. (2002) have estimated that in the United States the annual cost for lead poisoning is $43.4 billion and the annual cost for neurobehavioral disorders is $9.2 billion.

SUSCEPTIBLE PERIODS OF DEVELOPMENT

The environment can affect development before conception by influencing the sperm or ova. Once conception takes place, the embryo and (later) the fetus are susceptible to a number of factors including drugs, chemical toxicants, infections, and physical factors, such as radiation, that influence developmental outcomes. Even after a child is born, infection, chemical, and physical factors can influence

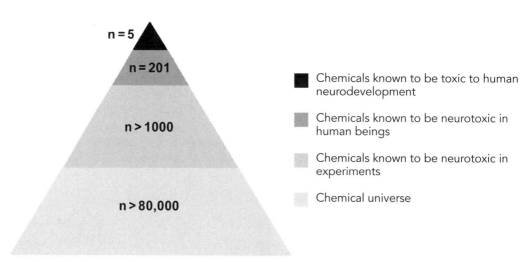

Figure 3.1. Diagram of the extent of knowledge of neurotoxic chemicals. (From Grandjean, P. and Landrigan, P.J. Developmental neurotoxicity of industrial chemicals. Reprinted with permission from Elsevier [*The Lancet*, 2006, Vol. 368, pp. 2167–2178]).

developmental outcomes. Because brain maturation continues into early adulthood, with completion of myelination of the frontal lobes, it can theoretically be influenced by environmental factors for two decades (Brent, Tanski, & Weitzman, 2004; Faustman, Silbernagel, Fenske, & Burbacher, 2000; Mendola, Selevan, Gutter, & Rice, 2002; Rice & Barone, 2000; Selevan et al., 2000).

SPECIFIC TOXICANTS

While it is impossible to discuss each of the over 1,000 chemicals that have been identified as potential neurotoxicants, this section will focus on several chemicals that are common causes of neurotoxicity. These are examples of neurotoxicants that are better understood than others or they represent emerging concerns.

■ ■ ■ MP

MP is a 22-year-old African American male. He was the product of an uncomplicated pregnancy, labor, delivery, and neonatal course. From 12–36 months of age, he lived in an apartment with deteriorating lead paint. His venous blood lead levels were: 18 mcg/dL at 18 months, 24 mcg/dL at 20 months, 26 mcg/dL at 24 months, and 16 mcg/dL at 48 months. There is no history of head trauma, meningitis, or other central nervous system (CNS) pathology. He dropped out of high school in the 11th grade after failing all academic subjects for 2 years, and he has been incarcerated twice for illicit drug use. Neuropsychological testing at age 22 shows a Full-scale IQ of 95, evidence of attention deficit disorder on trail-making and other tests, and evidence of executive function disorder. MP's lead poisoning is a contributing factor in his neurocognitive and behavioral problems.

Lead

ı is one of the most studied neurotoxicants, h the Greeks and Romans first describing the ɔxicity of lead in adults. In 1904, J. Lockhart Gibson, an Australian pediatrician, recognized lead poisoning in children related to exposure to paint. Gibson recommended that lead-based paint be banned in environments where children live and play. Bans on lead paint were put in place in many European and Latin American countries by the 1930s. As a result of industrial lobbying, lead paint was not banned for interior use in the United States until 1978 and was not removed from gasoline until the late 1990s. Because of these bans, the median blood lead level among children 1–6 years of age in the United States has decreased from 14.9 mcg/dL in the late 1970s to less than 2 mcg/dL today (America's Children and the Environment, 2010).

Despite these improvements, lead poisoning remains a significant problem, primarily because of lead dust in the home (United States Environmental Protection Agency, 2010a). Lead-containing paint flakes off surfaces in microscopic or macroscopic particles, and these settle to the floor. Young children are frequently on the floor, and these particles stick to their hands. The lead is then ingested as the children engage in normal hand-to-mouth activity. Children younger than 2 years of age absorb about half of the lead that they ingest, much more than adults, who absorb only 10% (Agency for Toxic Substances and Disease Registry, 2007). The lead enters the bloodstream and can damage many organ systems, including the brain.

The degree and type of damage from lead is a function of the timing of exposure. For example, lead exposure causes **peripheral neuropathy** (damage to nerves in the arms and legs) in adults, whereas it results in damage to the CNS in young children. The degree and type of damage from lead is also a function of dose. It is not clear, however, whether the best measure of dose is the maximum blood lead level, a lifetime average blood lead level, or some other measure. The duration of exposure also influences degree and type of damage to the CNS (Canfield et al., 2003; Canfield et al., 2004; Lanphear et al., 2005).

More is known about the specific neuropathology and functional neurological defects related to lead exposure than other toxicants. Low levels of lead interfere with the structure of the CNS and with neurotransmitter function. CNS support cells, oligodendrocytes, and astrocytes are damaged by lead. This results in abnormal myelination and disruption of the movement of nerve cells from one place to another in the developing CNS (**neuronal migration**). In animal research models, exposure to low levels of lead reduces the number of neural stem cells that are transformed into neurons and oligodendrocytes, and increases the number that are transformed into astrocytes (Lidsky & Schneider, 2003). This means there are fewer cells involved in cognition and motor function and more support cells. Low levels of lead also alter the function of the dopamine system in animals. This may explain the association between lead exposure, attention deficits, and executive-function deficits in children. Structural and functional neuroimaging studies in humans document that early exposure to lead decreases adult gray matter, alters white matter microstructure (which is associated with decreased brain volume), and affects language function.

In terms of treatment, chelation therapy (i.e., administration of medication that binds to lead and increases its excretion in the urine) for children with extremely high blood lead levels (≥ 70 mcg/dL; level of concern is ≥10 mcg/dL) can prevent seizures, coma, and death. Unfortunately, chelation has not been found to prevent or reverse the neurocognitive damage (Dietrich et al., 2004)..

Mercury

Mercury is neurotoxic in the form of elemental mercury (primarily when it enters the body via inhalation of mercury vapor) and as inorganic or organic compounds, particularly methyl mercury (MeHg; Agency for Toxic Substances and Disease Registry, 2001). There is no evidence to support the concern that ethyl mercury, when used as a preservative in vaccines, is neurotoxic. More specifically, extensive review by the U.S. National Academies of Sciences and other groups have found no evidence that ethyl mercury in the form of Thimerosal is a cause of autism (Andrews et al., 2004; Institute of Medicine, Immunization Safety Review Committee, 2004).

Mercury vapor exposure can occur through breakage of mercury containing devices such as thermometers, barometers, and fluorescent light fixtures. The amount of mercury vapor in an individual compact fluorescent light bulb is not sufficient to be toxic. However, disposing of millions of such light bulbs is a pending environmental health challenge.

The release of mercury vapor into the air through coal combustion is not likely to cause toxicity because concentrations are low. However, when that mercury deposits on the land or in aquatic environments, bacteria in the soil or water convert mercury to methylmercury (MeHg). In aquatic environments, the MeHg is bioaccumulated in small organisms and then biomagnified up the food chain as larger organisms eat many smaller ones. Humans are exposed to the MeHg when they eat contaminated fish or shellfish. Although fish are the most likely source of MeHg, they are also an important source of omega-3 fatty acids, which are important for normal brain growth and development. At this point, the benefits of eating fish outweigh the risks (Budtz-Jorgensen, Grandjean, & Weihe, 2007). However, young children as well as women who may become pregnant, who are pregnant, or who are nursing should avoid high-mercury fish: shark, swordfish, king mackerel, and tilefish. They should preferentially consume lower-mercury fish and seafood: shrimp, canned light tuna, salmon, pollock, and catfish (Environmental Protection Agency and the Food and Drug Administration, 2004).

Prenatal exposure to extremely high doses of MeHg results in severe brain damage with microcephaly, seizures, and severe cognitive and motor deficits (Bakir et al., 1973). These effects were first recognized in 1956 in Minamata, Japan, where MeHg was released into the wastewater by a chemical plant (Ekino, Susa, Ninomiya, Imamura, & Kitamura, 2007). Childhood exposure to acute doses of MeHg (as occurred in Minamata) is associated with cognitive and motor deficits; however, adults similarly exposed may have only minimal effects (Elhassani, 1982; Pierce et al., 1972).

Research on low-dose MeHg exposure in the Faeroe and Seychelle Islands, where fish containing MeHg is consumed as a primary food, has yielded variable results. Some studies showed evidence of dose-responsive decrements in IQ and impairments in memory, attention, language, and visuospatial perception (Grandjean et al., 1999; Grandjean et al., 2003; Yorifuji, Debes, Weihe, & Grandjean, 2011). Other studies did not find a relationship between prenatal exposure to MeHg and subsequent neurocognitive deficits in the children (Davidson, Myers, Weiss, Shamlaye, & Cox, 2006; Myers et al., 2009).

In the years 2005–2008, about 3% of women of childbearing age in the United States were found to have blood mercury levels about 5.8 parts per billion, levels indicated by the EPA that put children at some risk of adverse health effects (United States Environmental Protection Agency, 2010b). In a review of all data on prenatal exposure to MeHg, the National Academy of Sciences Committee on Developmental Toxicology (2000) concluded that there is a strong association between MeHg exposure *in utero* and neurocognitive deficits, including small decreases in IQ and abnormalities in neuropsychological tests of memory, attention, language, and visuospatial perception.

The mechanism of MeHg toxicity is not as well known as that of lead, but it is probably similar. Like the damage caused by lead, the damage caused by MeHg is dependent on the timing and the amount of the exposure. High doses adversely affect mitosis, cellular migration, and organization of neurons in the cortex. MeHg is associated with oxidative damage to neurons and alteration of calcium metabolism. At low doses, MeHg is associated with alterations in neurotransmitters (Meyers et al., 2009).

Arsenic

Arsenic in high doses can be fatal, and chronic arsenic exposure can lead to neurotoxicity and cancer (Grandjean & Murata, 2007; Tofail et al., 2009; Vahidnia et al., 2007; Vahter et al., 2008). Exposure of children usually occurs through ingestion of naturally contaminated drinking water or through contact with contaminated industrial sites. Over 100 million people worldwide are exposed to elevated levels of arsenic in drinking water. Arsenic can cross the placenta and enter breast milk when mothers are exposed through water or land/industrial contamination. Manifestations of central neurotoxicity are similar to other toxicants: problems with learning, short-term memory, decreased IQ, and concentration. Peripheral neurotoxicity, with delayed nerve conduction velocities, is also common. Mechanisms of action are thought to be DNA hypomethylation leading to abnormal gene expression and interactions with the endocrine system.

Alcohol

Maternal ingestion of alcoholic beverages during pregnancy can lead to fetal alcohol spectrum disorder (FASD), a wide range of physical, behavioral, and cognitive problems in the child; damage depends on the amount, timing, and duration of the consumption (American Academy of Pediatrics Committee on Substance Abuse and Committee on Children with Disabilities, 2000). Moderating factors include maternal nutrition, stress, and tobacco consumption (Guerrini, Thomson, & Gurling, 2007; Riley & McGee, 2005). There is no known safe level of alcohol consumption during pregnancy. More severe manifestations of FASD are termed fetal alcohol syndrome (FAS), and more subtle manifestations are termed **partial fetal alcohol syndrome** (pFAS). Another term used to describe FASD manifestation is **alcohol-related neurodevelopmental disorder** (ARND; Chasnoff, Wells, Telford, Schmidt, & Messer, 2010).

Guidelines for diagnosing FAS are available (National Center on Birth Defects and Developmental Disabilities, the Centers for Disease Control and Prevention & the Department of Health and Human Services, 2004). Developmentally and behaviorally, *in utero* ethanol exposure can manifest itself as microcephaly, behavior problems, ADHD, executive function deficits, and learning problems. Imaging studies document decreased brain volume and abnormalities of the corpus callosum, basal ganglia, and other brain structures (Guerri, Bazinet, & Riley, 2009).

Polychlorinated Biphenyls

Polychlorinated biphenyls (PCBs) are a group of industrial chemicals that share a similar molecular structure; they were used in the electronics, plastics, paint, and pesticide industries from the 1930s to 1970s. PCBs are fat-soluble; therefore, they bioaccumulate and persist for extremely long periods of time in the environment. This accounts for why they remain a concern 40 years after being banned. PCBs can cross the placenta and are also found in breast milk. Postnatal human exposure is generally through food but can also occur through exposure to contaminated waste sites. Fish are the most likely source of PCBs, however, because fish are an important source of the omega-3 fatty acids, the benefits of children eating fish outweigh the risks (Budtz-Jorgenson et al., 2007). While low in MeHg, farm-raised salmon, whether sold fresh or canned, may be high in PCBs and should be avoided by young children and by women who might become pregnant, who are pregnant, and who are nursing.

PCBs have been shown to be neurotoxic in animals, and high-dose human intake through food contamination has been associated with cognitive delays, behavior disorders, growth retardation, and other findings. Outcomes associated with low-dose exposure to PCBs *in utero* and after birth indicate small deficits in neuromotor development and IQ, along with problems with attention and impulse control (Eubig, Aguiar, & Schantz, 2010; Faroon, Keith, Jones, & De Rosa, 2001; Schantz, Widholm, & Rice, 2003).

Pesticides

There are over 1,300 chemicals registered as pesticides in the United States. These range from elements such as sulfur to complex organic molecules. In 2001, over 1.2 billion pounds of pesticides (e.g., herbicides, insecticides, fungicides) were used in the United States. Most insecticides kill pests by disrupting their nervous systems. About three quarters of households in the United States use pesticides (either inside the home or outside), and exposure also occurs through consumption of food that has been contaminated in agricultural settings. Pesticides (as sold) are mixtures of an active ingredient plus so-called "inert ingredients" (i.e., those components which do not kill pests). However, inert ingredients actually may be harmful to animals and humans.

Dichlorodiphenyltrichloroethane (DDT), an organochlorine insecticide, was banned in the United States in the 1970s, but it is still used elsewhere in the world. DDT and its breakdown product dichlorodiphenyldichloroethylene (DDE) are still present in the environment, can cross the placenta, and can be transferred from mother to child via breast milk. Higher levels are present in the blood and breast milk of individuals living in countries still using DDT; however, nearly 100% of Americans have some DDE in their bodies. Although animal studies show a clear connection between early life exposure and adverse neurodevelopmental outcomes, studies in humans (particularly those examining DDE exposure) show variable effects, perhaps related to the dose of the exposure, whether the exposure is bolus or continuous low dose, the timing of the exposure during development, and co-factors, such as stress and nutrition.

Prenatal exposure to the organophosphate chlorpyrifos has been associated with an increased risk of developmental delay, ADHD, and autism at 3 years of age (Eskenazi et al., 2008; Rauh et al., 2000) and deficits in Working Memory Index and Full-Scale IQ at 7 years of age (Rauh et al., 2011). Based on findings in animal models these abnormalities may be related to alterations in neurotransmitters, and in axonal growth and development (Ahlbom, Fredriksson, & Eriksson, 1994; Ahlbom et al., 1995; Nasuti et al., 2007). Chlorpyrifos and diazinon were banned for residential use in the early 2000s, but other organophosphates are still on the market for home use.

Endocrine Disrupting Chemicals

In 2009, the Endocrine Society published a comprehensive review of the literature regarding endocrine disrupting chemicals (EDCs; Diamanti-Kandarakis et al., 2009). The U.S. Environmental Protection Agency (EPA) defines an EDC as "an exogenous agent that interferes with synthesis, secretion, transport, metabolism, binding action, or elimination of natural blood-borne hormones that are present in the body and are responsible for homeostasis, reproduction, and developmental process" (United States Environmental Protection Agency, 2009). A very diverse group of chemicals have endocrine disrupting properties including phthalates, PCBs, polychlorinated dibenzodioxins, brominated flame retardants, dioxins, DDT, perfluorinated compounds (PFCs), organochlorine pesticides, bisphenol A, and some metals. EDCs can have estrogenic, antiestrogenic, antiandrogenic, antithyroid, or antiprogestin effects.

Exposure to phthalates, some of the pesticides, PCBs, and other EDCs have been shown to be associated with decreased IQ and other neurodevelopmental abnormalities. Perchlorate is a compound that has been the object of much concern. Perchlorate is a component of rocket fuel, and it has been found to contaminate the water systems of over 11 million people in the United States at concentrations of at least 4 parts per billion. It has also been found in vegetables and in milk. One concern is that perchlorate might induce a relative hypothyroid state in pregnant women or young children, thus causing developmental deficits. However, in a review of all available data prior to 2005, the National Academy of Sciences (Committee to Assess the Health Implications of Perchlorate Ingestion, 2005) found no evidence of an association between perchlorate exposure and congenital hypothyroidism or changes in thyroid function of newborns. The NAS cautioned that, "epidemiologic evidence is inadequate to determine whether or not there is a causal association between perchlorate exposure and adverse neurodevelopmental outcomes" (Committee to Assess the Health Implications of Perchlorate Ingestion, 2005).

Mixed Toxicants

In laboratory settings, animals can be exposed to single toxicants. In the real world, children are usually exposed to multiple toxicants. Discerning which toxicant is related to which outcome and whether the various toxicants act synergistically (i.e., additively or protectively) is very difficult. For example, children eating large amounts of seafood can be exposed to both MeHg and PCBs. Children living near hazardous waste sites may be exposed to any of the contaminants present. In areas where there are metal smelters, children can be exposed to lead, arsenic, and other metals that are being recovered for commercial purposes or which co-occur in the raw ore.

Environmental Tobacco Smoke

Environmental tobacco smoke is a mixture of over 4,000 chemicals (California Air Resources Board, 2005). Prenatal exposure can occur if the mother smokes or if she is exposed to environmental tobacco smoke. In animal studies, prenatal exposure to tobacco smoke via the mother leads to reductions in cortical gray matter and alteration in the development of white matter. Studies of children exposed prenatally to tobacco smoke revealed deficits in speech and language skills, visual/spatial abilities, behavior, and IQ (Best et al., 2009; Rauh et al., 2004).

Dietary Exposures and Attention-Deficit/Hyperactivity Disorder

Since Feingold (1973) first introduced the idea of an association between ADHD and dietary components, there have been hundreds of individual articles and several extensive reviews on the subject (Schab & Trinh, 2004; Stevens, Kuczek, Burgess, Hurt, & Arnold, 2011). The following dietary components have been considered: artificial food colorings (AFC), sugar, wheat, eggs, monosodium glutamate (MSG), and other artificial or naturally occurring dietary components. In 2008, the Food and Drug Administration (FDA) was petitioned to ban certain food additives from the diets of all children, not just those with ADHD (Center for Science in the Public Interest, 2008).

The literature reviews generally indicate that there is a small subset of children with ADHD who do have a worsening of their behavior when exposed to certain food constituents; however, there is a debate regarding whether this is an allergic or a pharmacologic mediated behavior change. Only through a carefully constructed elimination diet can a practitioner determine if a given child with ADHD is a member of this subset, and it is not recommended that all children with ADHD be subjected to an elimination diet. Rather, the elimination diet should be reserved for children whose families suspect a link between dietary constituents and the child's behavior.

The FDA has concluded that there is insufficient evidence of an association between food additives and behavioral change to ban those additives from food for all children (U.S. Department of Health and Human Services and the Food and Drug Administration, 2011).

On the other hand, the European Food Standards Agency has decided that foods containing the colors Tartrazine (E102), Quinoline Yellow (E104), Sunset Yellow (E110), Carmoisine (E122), Ponceau 4R (E124), and Allura Red (E129) must carry a warning label stating that the color "may have effects on activity and attention in children" (Foods Standards Agency, 2010).

PUBLIC POLICY IMPLICATIONS

Over the past several years, concerns over children's exposure to neurotoxicant chemicals have included (among others) bisphenol-A in baby bottles (Grady, 2010), phthalates in soft toys (Eilperin, 2009), and perfluorinated chemicals in cookware (Adams, 2010). From this author's perspective, the United States' primary federal law that controls exposure to toxic chemicals—the Toxic Substances Control Act (TSCA) of 1976 (PL 94-469)—does not sufficiently protect the health of children and pregnant women (United States Government Accountability Office, 2005). Unlike pharmaceuticals and pesticides, chemicals intended for any other use do not have to be tested prior to marketing; furthermore, they do not have to be monitored (postmarket) for problems. In other words, when a new drug is proposed, the FDA requires testing for both safety and efficacy, but no such process takes place when new chemicals are developed for use in the environment. In fact, TSCA (again, the primary law that addresses these issues) creates a disincentive with regard to toxicity testing. The law states that if a company knows of problems with a chemical, the company must reveal those problems; however, if the company does not know of problems (e.g., if they have not tested for problems), they have nothing to report.

A number of organizations have called for the reform of TSCA, and legislation has been introduced in several Congresses but has not passed. Some states are now trying to pass state chemical management laws. In some other places, laws (Canada) and regulations (European Union) that regulate chemicals are more protective of children than TSCA. Moving forward, this author believes that the United States should adopt legislation that requires premarket testing of new chemicals and the timely evaluation of existing chemicals. These evaluations should include tests that are sensitive to neurodevelopmental endpoints. (See Paulson, 2011, for a more expansive discussion.)

SUMMARY

Based on animal and human studies, over 1,000 chemicals have been identified as potential neurotoxicants. Exposures to different types of chemicals have been documented to result in similar outcomes both in animal models and in humans. These observations suggest that different toxicants can have the same or similar effects on developmental processes when exposure occurs at the same time in development. Conversely, exposure to the same toxicant at different developmental time periods can lead to different adverse effects. In most cases any damage to the CNS by environmental hazards is irreversible. For that reason, the focus must be on prevention of exposure. This author provides the argument that the current legislative framework, the Toxic Substances Control Act, is inadequate and needs to be revised.

REFERENCES

Adams, J.U. (2010, October 11). Trying to understand our chemical exposure. Los Angeles, CA: Los Angeles Times. Retrieved from http://www.latimes.com/health/la-he-biomonitoring-20101011,0,6430509

Agency for Toxic Substances and Disease Registry. (2001, March). ToxFAQs for metallic mercury. Retrieved from http://www.atsdr.cdc.gov/toxfaqs/TF.asp?id=1195&tid=24

Agency for Toxic Substances and Disease Registry. (2007, August). Toxicological profile for lead. Retrieved from http://www.atsdr.cdc.gov/ToxProfiles/tp13.pdf

Ahlbom, J., Fredriksson, A., & Eriksson, P. (1994). Neonatal exposure to a type-I pyrethroid (bioallethrin) induces dose-response changes in brain muscarinic receptors and behaviour in neonatal and adult mice. Brain Research, 645, 318–324.

Ahlbom, J., Fredriksson, A., & Eriksson, P. (1995). Exposure to an organophosphate (DFP) during a defined period in neonatal life induces permanent changes in brain muscarinic receptors and behaviour in adult mice. Brain Research, 677, 13–19.

American Academy of Pediatrics, Committee on Substance Abuse and Committee on Children with Disabilities. (2000). Fetal alcohol syndrome and alcohol–related neurodevelopmental disorders. Pediatrics, 106, 358–361.

America's Children and the Environment. (2010, November 19). Measure B1: Lead in the blood of children. Retrieved from http://www.epa.gov/ace/body_burdens/b1-graph.html

Andrews, N., Miller, E., Grant, A., Stowe, J., Osborne, V., & Taylor, B. (2004). Thimerosal exposure in infants and developmental disorders: A retrospective cohort study in the United Kingdom does not support a causal association. Pediatrics, 114, 584–591.

Bakir, F., Damluji, S.F., Amin-Zaki, L., Murtadha, M., Khalidi, A., al-Rawi, N.Y., ... Doherty, R.A. (1973). Methylmercury poisoning in Iraq. Science, 181, 230–241.

Brent, R.L., Tanski, S., & Weitzman, M. (2004). A pediatric perspective on the unique vulnerability and resilience of the embryo and the child to environmental toxicants: The importance of rigorous research concerning age and agent. Pediatrics, 113, 935–944

Budtz-Jorgensen, E., Grandjean, P., & Weihe, P. (2007). Separation of risks and benefits of seafood intake. Environmental Health Perspectives, 115, 323–327.

Canfield, R.L., Henderson, C.R., Cory-Slechta, D.A., Cox, C., Jusko, T.A., & Lanphear, B.P. (2003). Intellectual impairment in children with blood lead concentrations below 10 µg per deciliter. New England Journal of Medicine, 348, 1517–26.

Center for Science in the Public Interest. (2008). Petition to ban the use of Yellow 5 and other food dyes, in the interim to require a warning on foods containing these dyes, to correct the information the food and drug administration gives to consumers on the impact of these dyes on the behavior of some children, and to require neurotoxicity testing of new food additives and food colors. Washington, DC: Center for Science in the Public Interest. Retrieved from http://cspinet.org/new/pdf/petition-food-dyes.pdf

Canfield, R.L., Gendle, M.H., & Cory-Slechta, D.A. (2004). Impaired neuropsychological functioning in lead-exposed children. Developmental Neuropsychology, 26, 513–540.

Chasnoff, I.J., Wells, A.M., Telford, E., Schmidt C., & Messer, G. (2010). Neurodevelopmental functioning in children with FAS, pFAS, and ARND. Journal of Developmental and Behavioral Pediatrics, 31, 192–201.

Committee to Assess the Health Implications of Perchlorate Ingestion. (2005). Health implications of perchlorate ingestion. Washington, DC: National Academy of Sciences. Retrieved from http://www.nap.edu/openbook.php?isbn=0309095689

Davidson, P.W., Myers, G.J., Weiss, B., Shamlaye, C.F., & Cox, C. (2006). Prenatal methyl mercury exposure from fish consumption and child development: A review of evidence and perspectives from the Seychelles Child Development Study. Neurotoxicology, 27, 1106–1109.

Diamanti-Kandarakis, E., Bourguignon, J.P., Giudice, L.C., Hauser, R., Prins, G.S., Soto, A.M., ... Gore, A.C. (2009). Endocrine-disrupting chemicals: An Endocrine Society scientific statement. Endocrine Reviews, 30, 293–342.

Dietrich, K.N., Ware, J.H., Salganik, M., Radcliffe, J., Rogan, W.J., Rhoads, G.G., ... Jones, R.L. (for the Treatment of Lead-Exposed Children Clinical Trial Group). (2004). Effect of chelation therapy on the neuropsychological and behavioral development of lead-exposed children after school entry. Pediatrics, 114, 19–26.

Eilperin, J. (2009, November 24). Mothers' exposure to chemicals may affect boys. The Washington Post. Retrieved from http://www.washingtonpost.com/wp-dyn/content/article/2009/11/20/AR2009112003698.html

Ekino, S., Susa, M., Ninomiya, T., Imamura, K., & Kitamura, T. (2007). Minamata disease revisited: An update on the acute and chronic manifestations of methyl mercury poisoning. Journal of the Neurological Sciences, 262, 131–144.

Elhassani, S.B. (1982). The many faces of methylmercury poisoning. Journal of Toxicology—Clinical Toxicology, 19, 875–906.

Environmental Protection Agency and the Food and Drug Administration. (2004, March). What you need to know about mercury in fish and shellfish: Advice for: Women who might become pregnant, women who are pregnant, nursing mothers, young children (EPA-823-R-04-005). Retrieved from http://www.fda.gov/Food/FoodSafety/Product-SpecificInformation/Seafood/FoodbornePathogensContaminants/Methylmercury/ucm115662.htm

Eskenazi, B., Rosas, L.G., Marks, A.R., Bradman, A., Harley, K., Holland, N., ... Barr, D.B. (2008). Pesticide toxicity and the developing brain. *Basic and Clinical Pharmacology and Toxicology, 102*, 228–236.

Eubig, P.A., Aguiar, A., & Schantz, S.L. (2010). Lead and PCBs as risk factors for attention-deficit/hyperactivity disorder. *Environmental Health Perspectives, 118*(12), 1654–1667. doi: 10.1289/ehp.0901852

Faroon, O.M., Keith, S., Jones, D., & De Rosa, C. (2001). Effects of polychlorinated biphenyls on development and reproduction. *Toxicology and Industrial Health, 17*, 63–93.

Faustman, E.M., Silbernagel, S.M., Fenske, R.A., Burbacher, T.M., & Ponce, R.A. (2000). Mechanisms underlying children's susceptibility to environmental toxicants. *Environmental Health Perspectives, 108*, 13–21.

Feingold, B.F., (1973). Adverse reactions to food additives. Paper presented at the meeting of the American Medical Association, Chicago, IL.

Food Standards Agency. (2010, July 22). Compulsory warnings on colours in food and drink. London, England: Author. Retrieved from http://www.food.gov.uk/news/newsarchive/2010/jul/eucolourswarn

Franks, M.E., Macpherson, G.R., & Figg, W.D. (2004). Thalidomide. *The Lancet, 363*(9423), 1802–1811.

Gilbert, S.G. (2008). Scientific consensus statement on environmental agents associated with neurodevelopmental disorders. Retrieved November 30, 2010 from http://www.iceh.org/pdfs/LDDI/LDDIStatement.pdf

Gibson, J.L. (1904). A plea for painted railings and painted rooms as the source of lead poisoning amongst Queensland children. *Australasian Medical Gazette, 23*, 149–153.

Grady, D. (2010, September 6). In feast of data on bpa plastic, no final answer. *New York Times.* Retrieved from http://www.nytimes.com/2010/09/07/science/07bpa.html?_r=1&ref=bisphenol_a

Grandjean, P., Bellinger, D., Bergman, A., Cordier, S., Davey-Smith, G., Eskenazi, B., ... Weihe, P., (2008). The faroes statement: Human health effects of developmental exposure to chemicals in our environment. *Basic & Clinical Pharmacology & Toxicology, 102*, 73–5.

Grandjean, P., Budtz-Jorgensen, E., White, R.F., Jorgensen, P.J., Weihe, P., Debes, F., & Keiding, N. (1999). Methylmercury exposure biomarkers as indicators of neurotoxicity in children aged 7 years. *American Journal of Epidemiology, 150*, 301–305.

Grandjean, P., & Landrigan, P.J. (2006). Developmental neurotoxicity of industrial chemicals. *The Lancet, 368*, 2167–2178.

Grandjean, P., & Murata, K. (2007). Developmental arsenic neurotoxicity in retrospect. *Epidemiology, 18*, 25–26.

Grandjean, P., White, R.F., Weihe, P., & Jørgense, P.J. (2003). Neurotoxic risk caused by stable and variable exposure to methylmercury from seafood. *Ambulatory Pediatrics, 3*, 18–23.

Guerri, C., Bazinet, A., & Riley, E.P. (2009). Fetal alcohol spectrum disorders and alterations in brain and behaviour. *Alcohol and Alcoholism, 44*, 108–114.

Guerrini, I., Thomson, A.D., & Gurling, H.D. (2007). The importance of alcohol misuse, malnutrition and genetic susceptibility on brain growth and plasticity. *Neuroscience and Biobehavioral Reviews, 31*, 212–220.

Institute of Medicine, Immunization Safety Review Committee. (2004). *Immunization safety review: Vaccines and autism.* Washington, DC: National Academies Press.

Koger, S.M., Schettler, T., & Weiss, B. (2005). Environmental toxicants and developmental disabilities a challenge for psychologists. *American Psychologist, 60*, 243–255.

Landrigan, P.J., Schechter, C.B., Lipton, J.M., Fahs, M.C., Schwartz, J., (2002). Environmental pollutants and disease in American children: Estimates of morbidity, mortality, and costs for lead poisoning, asthma, cancer, and developmental disabilities. *Environmental Health Perspectives, 110*, 721-728

Lanphear, B.P., Hornung, R., Khoury, J., Yolton, K., Baghurst, P., Bellinger, D.C. ... Roberts, R. (2005). Low-level environmental lead exposure and children's intellectual function: An international pooled analysis. *Environmental Health Perspectives, 113*, 894–899.

Lidsky, T.I. & Schneider, J.S. (2003). Lead neurotoxicity in children: Basic mechanisms and clinical correlates. *Brain, 126*, 5–19.

Mendola, P., Selevan, S.G., Gutter, S., & Rice, D. (2002). Environmental factors associated with a spectrum of neurodevelopmental deficits. *Mental Retardation and Developmental Disabilities Research Reviews, 8*, 188–197.

Myers, G.J., Thurston, S.W., Pearson, A.T., Davidson, P.W., Cox, C., Shamlaye, C.F. ... Clarkson, T.W. (2009). Postnatal exposure to methyl mercury from fish consumption: A review and new data from the Seychelles Child Development Study. *Neurotoxicology, 30*, 338–349.

National Academy of Sciences Committee on Developmental Toxicology. (2000). *Scientific frontiers in developmental toxicology and risk assessment.* Washington, DC: National Academy Press.

National Academy of Sciences. (2000). Toxicological effects of methylmercury. Washington, DC: National Academy Press. Retrieved from http://books.nap.edu/catalog/9899.html?onpi_newsdoc071100

National Center on Birth Defects and Developmental Disabilities, Centers for Disease Control and Prevention, & Department of Health and Human Services (with National Task Force on Fetal Alcohol Syndrome and Fetal Alcohol Effect, American Academy of Pediatrics, American College of Obstetricians and Gynecologists, March of Dimes, & National Organization on Fetal Alcohol Syndrome). (2004). Fetal alcohol syndrome: Guidelines for referral and diagnosis. Retrieved from http://www.cdc.gov/ncbddd/fasd/documents/FAS_guidelines_accessible.pdf

Nasuti, C., Gabbianelli, R., Falcioni, M.L., Di Stefano, A., Sozio, P., & Cantalamessa, F. (2007). Dopaminergic system modulation, behavioral changes, and oxidative stress after neonatal administration of pyrethroids. *Toxicology, 229*, 194–205.

Paulson, J.A., & the American Academy of Pediatrics Council on Environmental Health. (2011). Chemical management policy: Prioritizing children's health. *Pediatrics, 127,* 983–990.

Pierce, P.E., Thompson, J.F., Likosky, W.H., Nickey, L.N., Barthel, W.F., & Hinman, A.R. (1972). Alkyl mercury poisoning in humans: Report of an outbreak. *Journal of the American Medical Association, 220,* 1439–1442.

Prüss-Üstün, A., & Corvalán, C. (2006). *Preventing disease through healthy environments: Towards an estimate of the environmental burden of disease. World Health Organization.* Retrieved from https://www.who.int/quantifying_ehimpacts/publications/preventingdiseasebegin.pdf

Rauh, V.A., Whyatt, R.M., Garfinkel, R., Andrews, H., Hoepner, L., Reyes, A., ... Perera, F.P. (2004). Developmental effects of exposure to environmental tobacco smoke and material hardship among inner city children. *Neurotoxicology and Teratology, 26,* 373–385.

Rice, D., & Barone, S., Jr. (2000). Critical periods of vulnerability for the developing nervous system: Evidence from humans and animal models. *Environmental Health Perspectives, 108*(3), 511–533.

Riley, E.P., & McGee, C.L. (2005). Fetal alcohol spectrum disorders: An overview with emphasis on changes in brain and behavior. *Experimental Biology and Medicine, 230,* 357–365.

Schab, D.W., & Trinh, N.T. (2004). Do artificial food colors promote hyperactivity in children with hyperactive syndromes? A meta-analysis of double-blind placebo-controlled trials. *Journal of Developmental and Behavioral Pediatrics, 25,* 423–434.

Schantz, S.L., Widholm, J.J., & Rice, D.C. (2003). Effects of PCB exposure on neuropsychological function in children. *Environmental Health Perspectives, 111,* 357–376.

Selevan, S.G., Kimmel, C.A., & Mendola, P. (2000). Identifying critical windows of exposure for children's health. *Environmental Health Perspectives, 108*(3) 451–455.

Silverman, W.A. (2002). The schizophrenic career of a "monster drug." *Pediatrics, 110*(2), 404–406.

State of California Air Resources Board. (2005). *Proposed identification of environmental tobacco smoke as a toxic air contaminant.* Sacramento, CA: California Environmental Protection Agency.

Stevens, L.J., Kuczek, T., Burgess, J.R., Hurt, E., & Arnold, L.E. (2011). Dietary sensitivities and ADHD

symptoms: Thirty-five years of research. *Clinical Pediatrics, 50,* 279–293.

Tofail, F., Vahter, M., Hamadani, J.D., Nermell, B., Huda, S.N., Yunus, M., ... Grantham-McGregor, S.M. (2009). Effect of arsenic exposure during pregnancy on infant development at 7 months in rural Matlab, Bangladesh. *Environmental Health Perspectives, 117,* 288–293

U.S. Department of Health & Human Services, Food and Drug Administration. (2011, March 30–31). Food Advisory Committee meeting minutes: *Certified color additives in food and possible association with attention deficit hyperactivity disorder in children.* Retrieved from http://www.fda.gov/advisorycommittees/committeesmeetingmaterials/foodadvisorycommittee/ucm250901.htm

U.S. EPA 2009 Endocrine Disruptors Research available at http://www.epa.gov/endocrine/#eds, accessed 6 December 2010

United States Environmental Protection Agency (2010a). America's children and the environment measure B1: Lead in the blood of children. Retrieved from http://www.epa.gov/economics/children/body_burdens/b1-graph.html

United States Environmental Protection Agency (2010b) *America's children and the environment measure B4: Distribution of concentration of mercury in blood of women of child-bearing age* Retrieved from http://www.epa.gov/economics/children/body_burdens/b4-graph.html

United States Government Accountability Office (2005, June). *Chemical regulation: Options exist to improve EPA's ability to assess health risks and manage its chemical review program.* Washington, DC: Author. Publication No. GAO-05-458. Retrieved from http://www.gao.gov/new.items/d05458.pdf

Vahidnia, A., van der Voet, G.B., & de Wolff, F.A. (2007). Arsenic neurotoxicity—a review. *Human Experimental Toxicology, 26,* 823-832.

Vahter, M. (2008) Health effects of early life exposure to arsenic. *Basic & Clinical Pharmacology & Toxicology 102,* 204–211

Yorifuji, T., Debes, F., Weihe, P., & Grandjean, P. (2011). Prenatal exposure to lead and cognitive deficit in 7- and 14-year-old children in the presence of concomitant exposure to similar molar concentration of methylmercury. *Neurotoxicology and Teratology, 33,* 205–211.

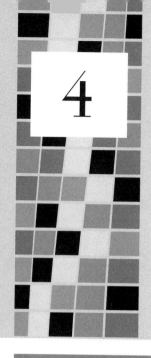

4

Birth Defects and Prenatal Diagnosis

Rhonda L. Schonberg

Upon completion of this chapter, the reader will

- Understand the uses and limitations of noninvasive prenatal maternal blood screening for birth defects

- Be knowledgeable regarding the indications for, and limitations of, first- and second-trimester evaluation of birth defects using the techniques of ultrasonography, fetal magnetic resonance imaging, and echocardiography

- Be aware of the techniques of amniocentesis and chorionic villus sampling to be able to determine when these invasive diagnostic tests may be indicated

- Be familiar with alternative reproductive techniques, including in vitro fertilization, and understand under what circumstances couples might benefit from such technologies

- Learn about new noninvasive prenatal diagnosis technologies currently being explored

- Understand the psychosocial needs of families who are at increased risk for having children with genetic disorders or birth defects

The birth of a child with a developmental disability or a genetic disorder can have a devastating impact on parents, siblings, and extended family members. As couples grieve the loss of their expected "normal" child and work to accept the child they have been given, they try to understand what happened to them and why. Although most infants are born without complications, in the United States 3% of births result in a child with a birth defect or a genetic disorder (Centers for Disease Control and Prevention, 2006). These events can affect any pregnant woman regardless of age, socioeconomic status, or ethnicity. Although we know of circumstances that can increase the risk of having a child with a birth defect, some of which are discussed in this chapter, most affected newborns will be born to couples who are unaware they are at risk and who have no family history of similarly affected children. When this occurs, genetic evaluation (discussed in Chapter 1) can help determine a diagnosis and/or mode of inheritance. Advances in prenatal diagnosis and prenatal screening have provided couples with the opportunity to gain information about their fetus (e.g., the presence of, or increased risk for a birth defect or genetic disorder) and to examine a range of family planning options.

This chapter discusses genetic screening that is available prior to and during pregnancy, diagnostic testing available for fetuses who have been determined to be at an increased risk for specific genetic disorders, and alternative reproductive choices.

■ ■ ■ CHELSEA

Susan, a 31-year-old woman who had previously miscarried, was enjoying an uneventful second pregnancy. Her fears were raised in the second trimester, however, when a maternal serum screening test revealed an elevated **alpha-fetoprotein** (AFP) level. Her obstetrician recommended a detailed fetal ultrasound, which showed a fetal abdominal wall defect (**gastroschisis**). Susan and her husband Rick met with the genetics staff, who explained that gastroschisis is usually an isolated malformation. It is not associated with a chromosomal abnormality, additional medical problems, or intellectual disability. After considering the information provided and weighing their risks, the couple decided not to undergo amniocentesis. They met with a pediatric surgeon to discuss the management of a newborn with gastroschisis and visited the high-risk nursery where their baby would be treated. On the basis of the information they received, Susan and Rick decided to continue the pregnancy, and they prepared for the birth of their child. Susan had ultrasound studies every 3–4 weeks throughout the remainder of the pregnancy to monitor fetal growth and **amniotic fluid** volume. When delivery came, the family and the surgical team were prepared. Surgery was performed on baby Chelsea's first day of life with an uneventful recovery. At 1 year of age, Chelsea is a growing, thriving, healthy child.

GENETIC ASSESSMENT

Assessing reproductive risk generally involves reviewing an individual's medical and pregnancy history and obtaining an extended family history, including the presence of birth defects,

genetic disorders, unexplained infant deaths, and recurrent pregnancy losses. Information about maternal medication use and occupational or other exposures can also provide clues to possible reproductive risks. Throughout the United States, many centers offer the skills of a genetic counselor (http://www.nsgc.org) combined with the medical expertise of physicians trained in genetics to perform this genetic assessment (An updated listing of these centers can be found at http://www.GeneClinics.org).

Knowing an individual's ethnic background can be one of the initial steps in assessing reproductive risk. Individuals from specific ethnic backgrounds have a higher chance of carrying certain gene mutations known to be associated with a particular genetic disorder (see Table 4.1). Most of the disorders amenable to carrier screening are inherited in an autosomal recessive pattern and often have high morbidity and mortality (e.g., Tay Sachs disease in the Ashkenazi Jewish population). Both parents would have to be carriers for there to be an increased risk (25% with each pregnancy) of having an affected child (see Chapter 1). Advanced knowledge of this risk provides couples with the opportunity to consider alternative reproductive options or to undergo prenatal diagnostic testing.

A couple may also be at increased risk for having a child with a genetic disorder if a previous child or other family member has been diagnosed with the disorder. In these situations, a detailed review of the family history, pregnancy history, and medical records (if available) is performed as well as examination of the affected individual to verify or establish the diagnosis. This process can be extremely helpful in discussing reproductive risks and prenatal testing options.

As of January 2011, more than 20,000 genetic disorders have been identified (Online Mendelian Inheritance in Man, 2011). Specific genetic testing is clinically available for over 2,000 of these disorders, and the number continues to grow (http://GeneTests.org). Information about these genetic disorders is available to the lay public through the Genetics Home Reference, a National Library of Medicine supported database (http://ghr.nlm.nih.gov); the Genetic Alliance, a clearinghouse for information and support groups for genetic disorders (http://www.geneticalliance.org); and the National Organization for Rare Disorders (http://www.rarediseases.org).

Table 4.1. Disorders with increased carrier frequencies in particular ethnic groups

Ethnic group	Disorder at risk	Estimated carrier frequency
European and North American (Caucasian)	Cystic fibrosis	1 in 25
Ashkenazi Jewish (Eastern European Jewish)	Tay-Sachs disease	1 in 27
	Canavan disease	1 in 40
	Cystic fibrosis	1 in 25
	Gaucher disease (type 1)	1 in 15
	Bloom syndrome	1 in 100
	Niemann Pick disease (type A)	1 in 90
	Fanconi anemia	1 in 90
	Glycogen storage disease (type 1A)	1 in 71
	Maple syrup urine disease (MSUD)	1 in 81
	Mucolipidosis IV (ML IV)	1 in 125
	Familial dysautonomia	1 in 36
African American or Western African	Sickle cell anemia	1 in 12
	Beta thalassemia	1 in 50
	Cystic fibrosis	1 in 61
Mediterranean	Beta thalassemia	1 in 15 to 1 in 20
Asian	Alpha thalassemia	1 in 8 to1 in 20
French Canadian	Tay-Sachs disease	1 in 27
Southeast Asian	Beta thalassemia	1 in 4 to 1 in 150

This table was published in *Medical complications during pregnancy* (5th ed.), B.N. Burrow & T.P. Duffy, in the chapter Clinical Genetics, by Seashore, M.R., p. 216. Copyright W.B. Saunders, 1999; adapted by permission.

SCREENING EVALUATIONS DURING PREGNANCY

First- and second-trimester screening tests, offered to all pregnant women, can modify the risk for having a child affected with Down syndrome, trisomy 18, or trisomy 13. Screening also helps reduce the risk of pregnancy loss, which can result from invasive diagnostic testing that may not be needed. It is well known that women who will be 35 years old or older at the birth of their child have an increased risk to have a baby with trisomy 21 (Down syndrome) or other chromosomal abnormalities (Hook, 1981; Morris, Wald, & Mutton, 2003; see Figure 4.1). It has been recommended for many years that women in this age group have routine screening. More recently, the American College of Obstetrics and Gynecology (ACOG) has recommended that prenatal screening be offered to all women, regardless of age (American College of Obstetricians and Gynecologists, 2007).

The standard of care for prenatal service providers in developed countries is to offer screening evaluations and genetic diagnostic testing during pregnancy. The following sections describe the options available during the first and second trimesters (Anderson & Brown, 2009; Benn, 2002).

First Trimester

Screening in the first trimester of pregnancy allows for earlier assessment, diagnosis, genetic counseling, and discussion of follow-up testing. Such evaluations can take the form of first-trimester ultrasonography, maternal serum (blood) screening, and screening for disorders that may be common in specific ethnic groups (e.g., mutations associated with cystic fibrosis, sickle cell disease, Tay Sachs; see Table 4.1). Although there have been continued advances in first-trimester screening, ACOG continues to recommend that all women age 35 or older also be offered diagnostic testing for chromosome abnormalities using **chorionic villus sampling** (CVS) performed in the first trimester or **amniocentesis** performed in the second trimester (American College of Obstetricians and Gynecologists, 2007; see Table 4.2).

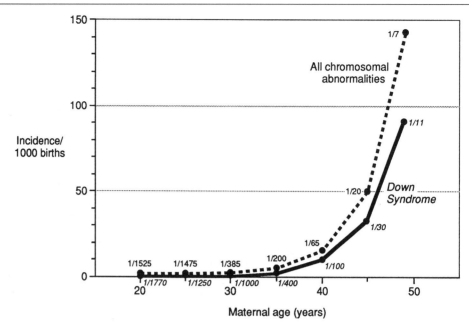

Figure 4.1. Risk of trisomy 21 and all chromosome abnormalities in pregnant women of various ages. Risk increases markedly after 35 years of age (*Source:* Hook, 1981).

First-Trimester Ultrasound

Early ultrasound can establish fetal viability, determine the number of fetuses (especially useful in cases involving assisted reproductive technology), and confirm placental position. It improves gestational dating, which can result in fewer inductions of labor for suspected post maturity (Whitworth, Bricker, Neilson, & Dowswell, 2010). Early ultrasound (11–14 weeks' gestation) can also measure the nuchal translucency (the transparency of the fluid-filled cavity at the nape of the fetus's neck; Sheppard & Platt, 2007; Sonek & Nicolaides, 2010). Increased nuchal translucency, even in the absence of a chromosomal abnormality, is associated with adverse outcomes including a greater incidence of congenital heart disease, other fetal anomalies, and fetal death (Hafner, Schuller, Metzenbauer, Schuchter, & Philipp, 2003; Souka, von Kaisenberg, Hyett, Sonek, & Nicolaides, 2005). Therefore, increased nuchal translucency warrants a recommendation for further ultrasound studies and a fetal echocardiogram later in the pregnancy. Other first-trimester ultrasound findings that may help detect Down syndrome include abnormal Doppler flow in the ductus venosus and tricuspid regurgitation; these are signs of congenital heart disease commonly found with this disorder. With improved technology, including three-dimensional ultrasound studies, other

birth defects can also be identified in the first trimester, allowing for decisions about follow-up testing (Nyberg, Hyett, Johnson, & Souter, 2006).

First-Trimester Maternal Serum Screening

Testing of maternal serum free beta human chorionic gonadotropin (free beta hCG) and pregnancy-associated plasma protein A (PAPP-A) at 10–14 weeks' gestation, when used in combination with the first-trimester ultrasound, further informs the risk assessment. This combined screening has been found to correctly identify approximately 87% of fetuses with Down syndrome and has a less than 5% false-positive rate (Anderson & Brown, 2009; Nicolaides, 2004). In addition to identifying a fetus with Down syndrome, extreme variations in the maternal serum free beta-hCG or PAPP-A can indicate an adverse pregnancy outcome, including low birth weight, stillbirth, fetal loss, and early delivery (Anderson & Brown, 2009).

The finding of cell-free fetal DNA in the plasma of pregnant women has opened up new possibilities for noninvasive prenatal diagnosis. Fetal DNA can be detected in a large background of maternal DNA (i.e., in maternal plasma) based on fetal-specific DNA methylation patterns (see Chapter 1). Using these fetal epigenetic markers permits noninvasive prenatal assessment of fetal chromosomal

Table 4.2. Common indications for amniocentesis and chorionic villus sampling (CVS)

Indication	CVS	Amniocentesis
Maternal age 35 or older	X	X
Previous offspring with a chromosome abnormality	X	X
Increased risk to have a child with a genetic disorder (e.g., previous affected child, positive carrier testing, carrier of X-linked disorder)	X	X
Previous offspring with a neural tube defect (e.g., spina bifida, anencephaly)		X
Increased nuchal trans-lucency and screen, positive first-trimester maternal serum screening	X	X
Increased risk for having a child with a chromo-some abnormality or neural tube defect based on a second trimester maternal serum screening test		X
Anatomic abnormality identified via ultrasound	X	X

abnormalities such as Down syndrome and certain pregnancy-associated disorders such as Rh incompatability and single nucleotide variations (see Chapter 1). Initial research studies are promising, but further work needs to be done before this technique becomes widely available for clinical use (Chiu & Lo, 2010; Hung, Chiu, & Lo, 2009).

Chorionic Villus Sampling

Chorionic villus sampling (CVS) involves obtaining a minute biopsy of the **chorion,** the outermost membrane surrounding the embryo. Chorionic **villi,** consisting of rapidly dividing cells of fetal origin, can be analyzed directly or grown in culture prior to testing (Blakemore, 1988). CVS can be used for chromosome analysis, enzyme assay (for inborn errors of metabolism; see Chapter 19), or molecular DNA analysis (identifying specific mutations that cause genetic diseases). It is not, however, diagnostic for neural tube defects such as spina bifida.

CVS is performed at approximately 10–12 weeks' gestation, usually before a woman appears pregnant and prior to **"quickening"**

(the detection of fetal movement by the mother). Using ultrasound guidance, a chorionic villus biopsy is performed either by suction through a small catheter passed through the cervix or by aspiration via a needle inserted through the abdominal wall and uterus (Figure 4.2). CVS is considered the safest invasive prenatal diagnostic procedure prior to the 14th week of gestation. There is less than a 1% risk of procedure-related pregnancy loss when CVS is performed by skilled practitioners. Provided CVS is performed after 10 weeks' gestation, there is no increased risk of causing a fetal anomaly (Wapner, 2005).

Second Trimester

Maternal serum screening and ultrasonography are also offered in the second trimester. Magnetic resonance imaging (MRI) and fetal echocardiography can add important information in select circumstances at this point in the pregnancy.

Second-Trimester Maternal Serum Screening

Approximately 70% of women in the United States currently have a maternal serum screening test and/or detailed ultrasound study performed in the second semester to detect or indicate an increased risk for common birth defects. Screening tests are designed to maximize the number of affected fetuses correctly identified while limiting the number of false-positive results. Women 35 years of age and older are also offered diagnostic testing for chromosome disorders. Although screening sensitivity is improving, it is still not diagnostic. If screening results are abnormal, additional studies are needed to confirm the diagnosis.

Typically a maternal blood specimen can be drawn at approximately 16 weeks' gestation and analyzed for AFP, hCG, and unconjugated serum estriol (uE3). A fourth marker, Inhibin A, has been added to improve the detection rate for Down syndrome in the second trimester to 80%, with a 5% false-positive rate (Canick & Macrae, 2005). In combination with first-trimester screening results, fully integrated screening and stepwise sequential screening can increase the detection rate for Down syndrome to about 95%, with a 5% false-positive rate (Anderson & Brown, 2009; Malone et al., 2005). Because not all women present themselves for prenatal care in the first trimester, second-trimester screening is useful (Shamshirsaz, Benn, & Egan, 2010). The level of these serum

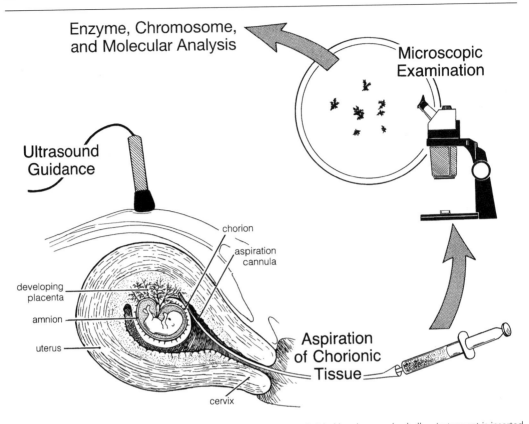

Enzyme, Chromosome, and Molecular Analysis

Microscopic Examination

Ultrasound Guidance

chorion

aspiration cannula

developing placenta

amnion

uterus

Aspiration of Chorionic Tissue

cervix

Figure 4.2. Transcervical CVS is performed at 10–12 weeks' gestation. Guided by ultrasound, a hollow instrument is inserted through the vagina and passed into the uterus. A small amount of chorionic tissue is removed by suction. The tissue is then examined under a microscope to make sure it is sufficient. Karyotype, enzyme, and/or DNA analyses can be performed without first growing the cells, although cell culture is needed for most analyses. Results are available in a few days in select situations; more often they are ready in 10–14 days.

markers, combined with other indicators including maternal age, weight, race, diabetes status, and number of fetuses, can also be used to assess the risk for neural tube defects (e.g., **spina bifida, anencephaly**; see Chapter 25), abdominal wall defects (e.g., **gastroschisis, omphalocele**), and trisomy 18 syndrome (see Appendix B). As an example, increased levels of AFP suggest a fetus at risk for a neural tube defect, an abdominal wall defect, or a rare kidney disorder. High AFP levels can also be associated with a multiple gestation; gestational age greater than anticipated; or a pregnancy at a higher risk for preterm delivery, stillbirth, or intrauterine loss. Adverse pregnancy outcome has also been associated with extreme variations of the other first- and second-trimester serum biochemical markers (Dugoff et al., 2004; Gagnon et al., 2008).

If the maternal serum screen in the second trimester suggests an increased risk for the presence of a fetus with Down syndrome, trisomy 18, or trisomy 13, diagnostic testing by amniocentesis and a detailed ultrasound evaluation

are recommended. It should be noted that correct gestational age is important for an accurate interpretation of the screening results. Second-trimester screening, with appropriate follow-up, can lead to a diagnosis of an abnormal (or normal) outcome by 18–20 weeks' gestation. Sequential screening using first- and second-trimester serum results is improving accuracy and influencing decisions about invasive testing.

Second-Trimester Ultrasonography

Approximately two thirds of pregnant women undergo **real-time ultrasonography** during their pregnancy. Prenatal ultrasound studies at 18–20 weeks' gestation can identify more than 60% of fetuses with major structural anomalies. Once an abnormality is identified, other technology, such as a fetal echocardiogram or MRI, may be suggested to further delineate the diagnosis and contribute to management (Filkins & Koos, 2005; Gagnon et al., 2009; Stewart, 2004). The absence of any abnormal marker on a second-trimester scan can imply a 50%–80% reduction in the prior risk that was based on maternal age or serum screen results (Benac-erraf, 2005). Not only can imaging be used to diagnose neural tube defects and abdominal wall defects (screened for by second-trimester serum testing), it also can be used to diagnose facial clefts, renal anomalies, skeletal anomalies, hydrocephalus, heart defects, and other malformations. Although the identification of structural abnormalities by ultrasound is improving, it cannot replace definitive diagnostic testing for chromosomal abnormalities, genetic mutations, and biochemical analyses that are possible using amniocentesis or CVS. Often ultrasound

and other diagnostic testing complement each other in making a diagnosis.

Amniocentesis

Amniocentesis is traditionally performed at approximately 15–18 weeks' gestation. Under ultrasound guidance in a sterile field, a needle is inserted just below the mother's umbilicus and through the abdominal and uterine walls. It enters the amniotic sac, and 1–2 ounces of amniotic fluid are aspirated (Figure 4.3). Through natural processes (mostly fetal urination), the fluid is replaced within 24 hours. The risk of

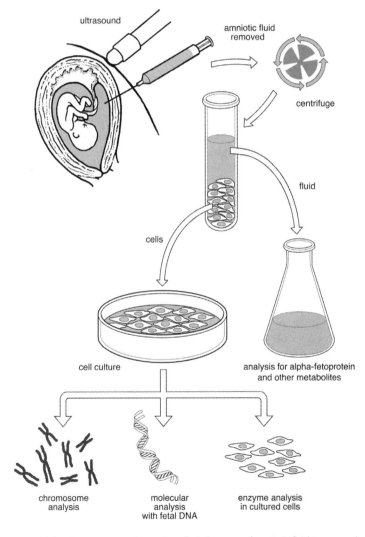

Figure 4.3. Amniocentesis. Approximately 1–2 ounces of amniotic fluid is removed at 16–18 weeks' gestation. The sample is spun in a centrifuge to separate the fluid from the fetal cells. The alpha-fetoprotein (AFP) in the fluid is measured to test for a neural tube defect. When indicated, the fluid can also be used to check for metabolites associated with inborn errors of metabolism. The cells are grown for a week, and then a karyotype, enzyme, or DNA analyses can be performed. Most results are available in 10–14 days (*Source:* Rose & Mennuti, 1993).

pregnancy loss following a genetic amniocentesis at 15+ weeks ranges from 0.5%–1.0% (Wilson, 2000). Early amniocentesis, performed before 14 weeks' gestation, has been found to cause an increased risk of pregnancy loss, a higher incidence of musculoskeletal deformities (most often clubfoot), and a greater chance of amniotic fluid leakage. For this reason, CVS (not amniocentesis) continues to be the preferred procedure for first-trimester diagnosis (Wapner, 2005).

One advantage of amniocentesis is the ability to assay the amniotic fluid directly for abnormal levels of biochemical compounds, such as AFP. Although ultrasound evaluations have improved in specificity and accuracy, they do not detect all cases of neural tube defects. However, when combined with an elevated amniotic fluid AFP level and a positive acetylcholinesterase test, an abnormal ultrasound identifies virtually all neural tube defects (Rose & Mennutti, 1993).

Magnetic Resonance Imaging (MRI)

High-resolution ultrasound has revolutionized the identification of fetal anatomic abnormalities, but this technology has limitations. In selected circumstances, MRI can add to the clinical understanding of an ultrasound variation when used at approximately 17 weeks' gestation or later (Bulas, 2007; Reddy, Filly, & Copel, 2008). Because MRI uses ultrafast imaging sequences, neither mother nor fetus requires sedation for a detailed study. Although there have been no known risks associated with the use of MRI to date, the long-term effects

are unknown (De Wilde, Rivers, & Price 2005). MRI of the central nervous system can demonstrate the presence (Figure 4.4A) or absence (Figure 4.4B) of the corpus callosum (i.e., the band of tissue connecting the two cerebral hemispheres), **Chiari malformations** of the brain (the downward displacement of the cerebellum through the opening at the base of the skull, which is seen in spina bifida), and the cause of enlarged ventricles (**hydrocephalus** Glenn & Berkovich, 2006). Alternatively, MRI can also confirm normal anatomy (as demonstrated by the images of the corpus callosum in Figure 4.4A) when ultrasound has identified an increased risk of abnormality. Fetal MRI interpretation requires special training, and centers that focus on fetal care and management often have the most experienced radiologists available to perform this task. Because it is not considered standard care, special authorization from insurance companies may be needed for this costly study.

Fetal Echocardiography

Congenital heart disease (CHD) is the most common anatomical abnormality, contributing to greater than one third of congenital anomaly deaths in childhood (Reddy et al., 2008). Echocardiography has become a valuable tool in the assessment of a fetus with CHD. This targeted ultrasound is performed at 18–22 weeks' gestation, when the fetal heart is approximately the size of an adult's thumbnail. With fetal echocardiography, it is possible to evaluate the structure and function of the fetal heart and monitor fetal blood flow. Three- and four-dimensional

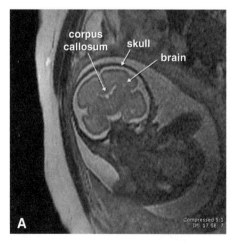 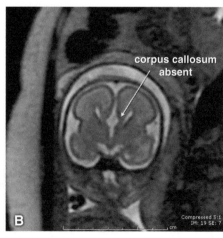

Figure 4.4. A) Magnetic resonance imaging (MRI) of a fetal brain with a corpus callosum. B) MRI images of a fetal brain with agenesis of the corpus callosum. (Courtesy of Dorothy I. Bulas, M.D., Department of Diagnostic Imaging, Children's National Medical Center, Washington, D.C.)

studies offer the opportunity for multiple views of normal and complex anatomy (Devore, 2005). A family history of CHD, increased nuchal translucency in the first trimester (Hafner et al., 2003; Souka et al., 2005), maternal diabetes or lupus, a fetal diagnosis of Down syndrome or velocardiofacial syndrome (VCFS; see Appendix B), or other birth defects noted by ultrasound increase the likelihood that a congenital heart defect will be identified. Because fetal circulation differs from that of the newborn, coarctation (severe narrowing) of the aorta, interrupted aortic arch, and small atrial or ventricular septal defects (ASD or VSD) may not be accurately diagnosed using fetal echocardiography. A careful cardiac evaluation should also be performed postnatally in infants known to be at increased risk for a CHD. Prenatal diagnosis of a CHD can result in earlier postnatal diagnosis and earlier intervention (Mohan, Kleinman, & Kern, 2005; Reddy et al., 2008).

When CHD is identified *in utero*, a detailed ultrasound study is indicated to screen for other malformations. Approximately 10%–15% of infants with CHD have an underlying chromosomal abnormality and will often have additional anomalies, developmental delay, or intellectual disability (Table 4.3; Brown, 2000). When a fetus is identified with CHD, genetic

counseling and diagnostic testing via amniocentesis are warranted because the long-term outcome for a child with an isolated CHD can be much different than the expected outcome for a child with a chromosomal abnormality.

Diagnostic Testing of Fetal Cells

Both CVS and amniocentesis are well-established techniques for obtaining fetal cells. The most common test requested is chromosomal analysis; however, biochemical analysis for inborn errors of metabolism or DNA analysis for disorders such as fragile X syndrome or cystic fibrosis also can be performed (Thompson, McInnes, & Willard, 2004). Indeed, any genetic disorder for which a familial DNA mutation has been identified can be assessed using DNA isolated from the fetal cells. Studies other than traditional chromosome analysis are generally only considered when a pregnancy is thought to be at increased risk for a particular condition.

Fluorescent in situ hybridization (FISH) is a technique that utilizes short pieces of DNA of known sequence (called a DNA probe) that can hybridize, or attach to, a unique region on a chromosome. The probe contains a fluorescent tag, making it visible under a fluorescent microscope. FISH is used to identify specific chromosomes or to indicate small deletions of a defined region of a specific chromosome. When a rapid result is required for prenatal diagnosis, this technique can be used to test for trisomies 13, 18, and 21 and variations in the number of X or Y chromosomes (Ward et al., 1993). In addition, FISH can be used to diagnose some genetic syndromes caused by chromosome microdeletions or variations that are too small to be detected by conventional analysis. For example, the discovery of certain CHDs by fetal ultrasound or echocardiography should prompt consideration of FISH analysis to detect the 22q11.2 deletion that occurs in 1 in 4,000 live births and is associated with VCFS/ DiGeorge Syndrome (see Appendix B). Array comparative genomic hybridization (CGH) is a newer technology allowing the evaluation of small, submicroscopic genomic deletions and duplications that are responsible for approximately 15% of unknown genetic disorders (see Chapter 1; Vissers, Veltman, van Kessel, & Brunner, 2005). Advances in this technology have enabled high-resolution examination of genetic alterations that are not otherwise identifiable by traditional chromosome analysis. As the technology improves, its application to prenatal diagnosis and assisted reproductive technology (ART)

Table 4.3. Ultrasound findings in certain chromosomal abnormalities

Syndrome	Findings
Trisomy 13	Cleft lip and palate
	Congenital heart defect
	Cystic kidneys
	Polydactyly
	Midline facial defect
	Brain abnormalities (holoprosencephaly
Trisomy 18	Clenched hands with overlapping fingers
	Congenital heart defect
	Polyhydramnios
	Growth retardation
	Rocker-bottom feet
	Omphalocele
Trisomy 21	Gastrointestinal malformations (duodenal atresia)
	Congenital heart defect
	Excess neck skin/ increased nuchal translucency
	Absent nasal bone

Sources: D'Alton & DeCherney, 1993; Nicolaides, 2005; and Viora et al., 2005.

will expand. CGH should be considered when multiple anomalies are identified via ultrasound and conventional chromosomal analysis is normal (American College of Obstetricians and Gynecologists, 2009b; Kleeman et al., 2009).

As technology improves, the indications for prenatal diagnosis will increase and detection may be improved. Unfortunately, even the most sophisticated prenatal diagnostic technology cannot guarantee the birth of a "normal" child. Most of the disorders that cause developmental disabilities in the absence of structural malformations are not currently amenable to prenatal diagnosis. Prenatal testing, however, has offered some parents at high risk for having a child with a severe genetic disorder the opportunity to have healthy children. For other families, it provides time to prepare for immediate surgical or medical intervention following a timed delivery, or it provides time to plan for end-of-life care for a child who may not survive because of the severity of the birth defect.

PREVENTION AND ALTERNATIVE REPRODUCTIVE CHOICES

Although birth defects cannot be prevented, attention to a number of factors can contribute to a decreased risk for certain fetal abnormalities. Recommendations such as receiving early prenatal care, avoiding alcoholic beverages and tobacco, and minimizing unnecessary medication are familiar to most women. In addition, women should try to avoid exposure to infection, excess vitamin A, and frequent consumption of fish that are known to have elevated mercury content (American College of Obstetricians and Gynecologists, 2009a).

In addition, ingestion of 0.4 mg of folic acid (found in most multivitamins) by all women of childbearing age starting 3 months before attempted conception is now recommended in order to reduce the risk of neural tube defects. If a neural tube defect is detected, *in utero* repair of a myelomeningocele should be considered based on results of a randomized trial that demonstrated a reduced risk of the child developing hydrocephalus and an increased likelihood of future independent ambulation. Because there can be maternal morbidity from this procedure, the benefits versus risks must be carefully evaluated (Adzick et al., 2011).

If not treated appropriately, a number of maternal conditions can predispose an infant to birth defects or developmental delay. For example, a woman with phenylketonuria (PKU) is at risk of having a child with microcephaly and intellectual disability if she does not maintain a phenylalanine-restricted diet during pregnancy (see Chapter 19). If not under good control, other maternal disorders, including diabetes and lupus, increase the risk to the fetus. In addition, certain medications taken to control illness, such as anti-epileptic drugs, can increase the risk of birth defects. Ideally, the risks versus benefits of chronic medication use during pregnancy will be discussed between the patient and her care provider prior to conception.

Assisted Reproduction Technology

When a couple has an increased risk of having a child with a serious genetic disorder and they prefer not to face the possibility of terminating an affected pregnancy, other reproductive options may be available utilizing assisted reproductive technology (ART). Mendelian genetic disorders may be inherited as autosomal recessive (with two carrier parents), X-linked recessive (with a carrier mother), or autosomal dominant (with one parent being affected; see Chapter 1). A parent may also be known to be a carrier of a balanced chromosome translocation and be at risk to have a child with an unbalanced amount of genetic material. Options such as artificial insemination using donor sperm or **in vitro fertilization (IVF)** with a donor egg may be appropriate considerations under these circumstances. Couples considering these options should assess how donors are chosen: what carrier testing is performed to make sure the donor is not a carrier for an identifiable genetic disease, the ethnic/racial background of the donor, and the donor's family history. When considering ART, families should also inquire about the rate of successful pregnancies, the risk for multiple gestation (e.g., twins, triplets), and the increased risk of birth defects (Hansen, Bower, Milne, de Klerk, & Kurinczuk, 2005; Shiota & Yamada, 2009; Wen et al., 2010). The use of proteomics (methodology for measuring proteins) may assist in identifying embryos with the highest implantation potential, thus avoiding further complications from multiple gestation. Evaluating the secretome, the proteins the embryo produces and secretes into the environment, may provide these clues (Katz-Jaffe, McReynolds, Gardner, & Schoolcraft, 2009).

Another ART approach is intracytoplasmic sperm injection (ICSI), a technology available to infertile males who have low sperm count or poor sperm motility (Palermo et al., 1998). Sperm from the prospective father are harvested, and the cytoplasmic portions of the sperm are removed. The nucleus of the sperm is then introduced into a harvested egg by microinjection, and the developing blastocyst (early embryo) is subsequently transferred into the uterus. Genetic causes of male infertility, including microdeletion within fertility-associated regions of the Y chromosome, carriers for certain cystic fibrosis mutations, and Klinefelter syndrome, may be indications for ICSI. For approximately 1% of conceptions accomplished through ICSI, sex chromosome aneuploidy (e.g., an extra X or Y chromosome) has been reported. In addition there is a 6.5% malformation rate secondary to the procedure; therefore, genetic counseling is recommended prior to initiating ICSI (Hindryckx et al., 2010).

Preimplantation Genetic Diagnosis

Preimplantation genetic diagnosis (PGD) is available for couples who are at high risk of having a child with a known genetic disorder, who wish to conceive an unaffected child that is biologically their own, and who want to avoid the risk of pregnancy termination. Originally introduced in 1990 for couples at risk of having a child with an X-linked disorder, PGD has expanded with the development of FISH technology to identify common trisomies (13, 18, and 21) in women of advanced age (Kuliev & Verlinsky, 2004) and with the development of molecular technology to identify DNA sequence differences (i.e., single gene mutations).

There are two approaches to PGD, as illustrated in Figure 4.5. The first involves **polar body testing** of the woman's eggs to establish the presence or absence of the mutation in question (e.g., looking for the Tay Sachs gene in a couple who are both carriers of this disorder). Only embryos from fertilized eggs determined to contain the normal gene are transferred to the mother's uterus to establish a pregnancy. The second approach is to perform in vitro fertilization on harvested eggs and allow them to develop in culture to the blastomere, or eight-cell stage. A single cell is then microdissected from each blastomere and analyzed for the presence of mutations or aneuploidy (abnormal chromosome number). Only unaffected embryos are subsequently transferred to the uterus. Approximately 20% of implanted embryos will survive to birth.

Pregnancies utilizing these methods have been successful for couples at high risk for bearing a child with a number of genetic disorders or common trisomies (Verlinsky et al., 2004). However, diagnosis from a single cell remains a technical challenge and the risk of misdiagnosis cannot be eliminated (Wilton, Thornhill, Traeger-Synodinos, Sermon, & Harper, 2009). Therefore, prenatal diagnosis via CVS or amniocentesis is recommended after PGD is done to confirm the diagnosis.

ARTs are costly in terms of physical, emotional, and financial resources; at present these services are rarely covered by health insurance plans. The risk of multiple gestations is also a concern, particularly if fetal reduction (i.e., abortion of one or more fetuses) is not an option the parents are willing to consider. Publications from Europe, the United States, and Australia have suggested an association between ART and imprinting (epigenetic) disorders such as Beckwith Weidemann Syndrome (Chapter 1; Appendix B). However, because the absolute incidence is small, routine screening for these imprinting disorders in children conceived by ART is not recommended at this time (Manipalviratn, DeCherney, & Segars, 2009). As with IVF, couples should request detailed information regarding techniques that are used, risk of error in diagnosis, risk of other anomalies of birth defects, cost per attempt, rate of successful pregnancies, and risk of multiple gestations.

PSYCHOSOCIAL IMPLICATIONS

With advances in prenatal screening technology and testing, choices can be overwhelming for a family. Health care professionals and patients often avoid difficult preliminary discussions about how a couple would respond to the diagnosis of an abnormality or (if they already have a child with special needs) how they would respond to a recurrence of the problem in their next child. For some couples, having advanced knowledge allows for preparation prior to birth; for others, it may mean ending a pregnancy.

Many of these issues are best addressed prior to attempting pregnancy so that prenatal diagnostic techniques, genetic screening, and other specialized tests can be investigated in advance. Exploring each individual's reproductive choices and available options is time consuming, but necessary. It is imperative that health care professionals focus on the family's psychosocial needs as well as the clinical information the couple is requesting.

When a woman gives birth to a child with special needs or a child who does not survive, the experience can be devastating for

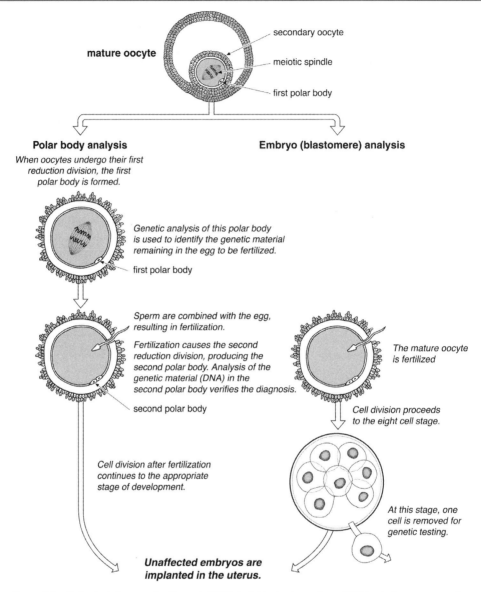

Figure 4.5. Preimplantation genetic diagnosis (PGD). Individuals who undergo PGD begin the process as they would for in vitro fertilization. The ovary is stimulated to produce mature oocytes, which are then harvested for fertilization outside of the woman's body. These mature oocytes can be used for polar body analysis or they can be fertilized and processed for a blastomere biopsy. This figure describes the path toward the preimplantation diagnosis using both methods. Polar body analysis is limited to those disorders or variations that would be present in the maternal genetic material whereas an embryo biopsy can analyze both maternal and paternal genetic contributions. As with in vitro fertilization, not all pregnancies will progress to term. Prenatal diagnosis at a later stage of gestation via chorionic villus sampling (CVS) or amniocentesis is recommended to confirm the preimplantation diagnosis.

the family. Each family is unique, and assumptions by health care providers as to what a family should or should not do in a given situation must be avoided. Genetic counselors and medical geneticists, who are trained in nondirective counseling, can help families understand their options and choose a course of action that is consistent with the family's own values and resources. Often, support groups or individual counseling can be beneficial.

SUMMARY

A wealth of information exists for couples considering a pregnancy. This is particularly true for couples who have an increased risk for conceiving a child with a specific genetic disorder or who have previously conceived a child with a birth defect, special needs, or genetic disorder. The array of screening and diagnostic tests can be both overwhelming and reassuring. Health care providers, working together with genetics professionals, are in a unique position to help families carefully consider and understand their reproductive options and the effects that prenatal diagnosis or genetic screening will have on them physically, emotionally, and financially.

REFERENCES

American College of Obstetricians and Gynecologists. (2007, January 11). Screening for Fetal Chromosomal Abnormalities: ACOG Practice Bulletin; No. 77. *Obstetrics and Gynecology, 109*, 217–227.

American College of Obstetricians and Gynecologists. (2009a). Reducing Your Risk of Birth Defects: ACOG Education pamphlet AP146. Washington, DC: Author.

American College of Obstetricians and Gynecologists. (2009b). Array comparative genomic hybridization in prenatal diagnosis: ACOG Committee Opinion No. 446. 09. *Obstetrics and Gynecology, 114*(5), 1161–1163.

Adzick, N.S., Thom, E.A., Spong, C.Y., Brock, J.W., Burrows, P.K., Johnson, M.P., ... Farmer, D.L. (2011). A randomized trial of prenatal versus postnatal repair of myelomeningocele. *New England Journal of Medicine, 364*(11), 993–1004.

Anderson, D.L., & Brown, C.E.L. (2009). Fetal chromosome abnormalities: Antenatal screening and diagnosis. *American Family Physicians, 79*(2), 117–123.

Benacerraf, B. (2005). The role of second-trimester genetic sonogram in screening for Down syndrome. *Seminars in Perinatolology, 29*(6), 386–394.

Benn, P.A. (2002). Advances in prenatal screening for Down syndrome: II. First trimester testing, integrated testing, and future directions. *Clinica Chimica Acta, 324*(1–2), 1–11.

Blakemore, K.J. (1988). Prenatal diagnosis by chorionic villus sampling. *Obstetrics and Gynecology Clinics of North America, 15*, 179–213.

Brown, D.L. (2000). Family history of congenital heart disease. In C.B. Benson, P.H. Arger, & E.I. Bluth (Eds.), *Ultrasonography in obstetrics and gynecology: A practical approach* (pp. 155–166). New York, NY: Thieme Medical.

Bulas, D. (2007). Fetal magnetic resonance imaging as a complement to fetal ultrasonography. *Ultrasound Q, 23*(1), 3–22.

Canick, J., & Macrae, A. (2005). Second trimester serum markers. *Seminars in Perinatology, 29*(4), 203–208.

Centers for Disease Control and Prevention. (2006). Improved national prevalence estimates for 18 selected major birth defects—United States, 1999–2001. *Morbidity and Mortality Weekly Report, 54*(51–52), 1301–1305.

Chiu, R.W., & Lo, Y.M. (2010). Non-invasive prenatal diagnosis by fetal nucleic acid analysis inmaternal plasma: The coming of age. *Seminars in Fetal and Neonatal Medicine, 16*, 88–93.

D'Alton, M.E., & DeCherney, A.H. (1993). Prenatal diagnosis. *The New England Journal of Medicine, 328*, 114–119.

Devore, G. (2005). Three-dimensional and four-dimensional fetal echocardiography: A new frontier. *Current Opinion Pediatrics, 17*(5), 592–604.

De Wilde, J.P., Rivers, A.W., & Price, D.L. (2005). A review of the current use of magnetic resonance imaging in pregnancy and safety implications for the fetus. *Progress in Biophysics and Molecular Biology, 87*, 335–353.

Dugoff, L., Hobbins, J., Malone, F., Porter, T.F., Luthy, D., Comstock, C.H., ... D'Alton, M.E. (2004). First-trimester maternal serum papp-a and free-beta sub-unit human chorionic gonadotropin concentrations and nuchal translucency are associated with obstetric complications: A population-based screening study (the faster trial). *American Journal of Obstetrics and Gynecology, 191*, 1446–1451.

Filkins, K., & Koos, B.J. (2005). Ultrasound and fetal diagnosis. *Current Opinion in Obstetrics and Gynecology, 17*, 185–195.

Gagnon, A., Wilson, R.D., Allen, V.M., Audibert, F., Blight, C., Brock, J.A., ... Wyatt, P. (2009). Evaluation of prenatally diagnosed structural congenital anomalies. *American Journal of Obstetrics & Gynecology Canada, 31*(9), 875–881.

Gagnon, A., Wilson, R.D., Audibert, F., Allen, V.M., Blight, C., Brock, J.A., ... Wyatt, P. (2008). Obstetric complications associated with abnormal maternal serum marker analytes. *American Journal of Obstetrics & Gynecology Canada, 30*(10), 918–949.

GeneTests. (2011). Retrieved from http://www.ncbi.nlm.nih.gov/sites/genetests?db=genetests=Limits

Genetics Home Reference. (2012). Retrieved from http://ghr.nlm.nih.gov

Glenn, O.A. & Barkovich, J. (2006). Magnetic resonance imaging of the fetal brain and spine: An increasingly important role in prenatal diagnosis: Part 2. *American Journal of Neuroradiology, 27*, 1807–1814.

Hafner, E., Schuller, T., Metzenbauer, M., Schuchter, K., & Philipp, K. (2003). Increased nuchal translucency and congenital heart defects in a low-risk population. *Prenatal Diagnosis, 23*, 985–989.

Hansen, M., Bower, C., Milne, E., de Klerk, N., & Kurinczuk, J. (2005). Assisted reproductive technologies and the risk of birth defects: A systematic review. *Human Reproduction, 20*, 328–338.

Hindryckx, A., Peeraer, K., Debrock, S., Legius, E., deZegher, F., Francois, I., ... D'Hooghe, T. (2010). Has the prevalence of congenital abnormalities after intracytoplasmic sperm injection increased? The Leuven data 1994–2000 and a review of the literature. *Gynecological and Obstetric Investigation, 70*(1), 11–22.

Hook, E.B. (1981). Rates of chromosomal abnormalities at different maternal ages. *Obstetrics and Gynecology, 58*, 282–285.

Hung, E.C., Chiu, R.W., & Lo, Y.M. (2009). Detection of circulating fetal nucleic acids: A review of methods and applications. *Journal of Clinical Pathology, 62*(4), 308–313.

Katz-Jaffe, M.G., McReynolds, S., Gardner, D.K., & Schoolcraft, W.B. (2009). The role of proteomics in defining the human embryonic secretome. *Molecular Human Reproduction, 15*(5), 271–277.

Kleeman, L, Bianchi, D.W., Sharrrer, L.G., Rorem, E., Cowan, J., Craigo, S.D., ... Wilkins-Haug, L.E. (2009). Use of array comparative genomic hybridization for prenatal diagnosis of fetuses with sonographic anomalies and normal metaphase karyotype. *Prenatal Diagnosis, 29*(13), 1213–1217.

Kuliev, A., & Verlinsky, Y. (2004). Meiotic and mitotic nondisjunction: Lessons from preimplantation genetic diagnosis. *Human Reproduction Update, 10*, 401–407.

Malone, F.D., Canick, J.A., Ball, R.H., Nyberg, D.A., Comstock, C.H., Bukowski, R., ... D'Alton, M.E.

(for the First- and Second-Trimester Evaluation of Risk [FASTER] Research Consortium). (2005). First-trimester or second trimester screening, or both, for Down's syndrome. *New England Journal of Medicine, 353*(19), 2001–2011.

Manipalviratn, S., DeCherney, A., & Segars, J. (2009). Imprinting disorders and assisted reproductive technology. *Fertility and Sterility, 91*(2), 305–315.

Mohan, U., Kleinman, C., & Kern, J. (2005). Fetal echo-cardiography and its evolving impact 1992–2002. *American Journal of Cardiology, 96*(1), 134–136.

Morris, J.K., Wald, N.J., Mutton, D.E., & Alberman, E. (2003). Comparison models of maternal age-specific risk for Down syndrome live births. *Prenatal Diagnosis, 23,* 252–258.

National Society of Genetic Counselors. (1983). *Genetic counseling as a profession.* http://www.nsgc.org

Nicolaides, K.H. (2004). Nuchal translucency and other first-trimester sonographic markers of chromosomal abnormalities. *American Journal of Obstetrics and Gynecology, 191,* 45–67.

Nyberg, D.A., Hyett, J., Johnson, J., & Souter, V. (2006). First trimester screening. *Radiologic Clinics of North America, 44,* 837–861.

On Line Mendelian Inheritance in Man. (2011). Retrieved from http://www.ncbi.nlm.nih.gov/sites/entrez?db=omim&TabCmd=Limits

Palermo, G.D., Schlegel, P.N., Sills, E.S., Veeck, L., Zaninovic, M., Menendez, S., & Rosenwaks, Z. (1998). Births after intracytoplasmic injection of sperm obtained by testicular extraction from men with nonmosaic Klinefelter's syndrome. *The New England Journal of Medicine, 338,* 588–590.

Reddy, U.M., Filly, R.A., & Copel, J.A. (2008). Prenatal imaging: Ultrasonography and magnetic resonance imaging. *Obstetrics and Genecology, 112*(1), 145–157

Rose, N.C., & Mennutti, M.T. (1993). Alpha-fetoprotein and neural tube defects. In J.J. Sciarra & P.V. Dilts, Jr. (Eds.), *Gynecology and Obstetrics* (Rev. ed., pp. 1–14). New York, NY: HarperCollins.

Seashore, M.R. (1999). Clinical genetics. In B.N. Burrow & T.P. Duffy (Eds.), *Medical Complications During Pregnancy* (5th ed., pp. 197–223). Philadelphia, PA: W.B. Saunders.

Shamshirsaz, A.A., Benn, P., & Egan, J.F. (2010). The role of second-trimester screening in the post-first-trimester screening era. *Clinics in Laboratory Medicine, 30*(3), 667–676.

Sheppard, C., & Platt, L.D. (2007). Nuchal translucency and first trimester risk assessment: A systematic review. *Ultrasound Q, 23*(2), 107–116.

Shiota, K. & Yamada, S. (2009). Intrauterine environment-genome interaction and children's development (3): Assisted reproductive technologies and developmental disorders. *Journal of Toxicological Sciences, 34*(Suppl 2), SP287–SP291.

Sonek, J., & Nicolaides, K. (2010). Additional first-trimester ultrasound markers. *Clinics in Laboratory Medicine, 30*(3), 573–592.

Souka, A., von Kaisenberg, C., Hyett, J., Sonek, J.D., & Nicolaides, K.H. (2005). Increased nuchal translucency with normal karyotype. *American Journal of Obstetrics and Gynecology, 192*(4), 1005–1021.

Stewart, T.L. (2004). Screening for aneuploidy: The genetic sonogram. *Obstetrics and Gynecology Clinic of North America, 31,* 21–33.

Thompson, M.W., McInnes, R.R., & Willard, H.F. (Eds.). (2004). *Thompson & Thompson Genetics in Medicine* (6th ed.). Philadelphia, PA: W.B. Saunders.

Van den Veyver, I.B., & Beaudet, A.L. (2006). Comparative genomic hybridization and prenatal diagnosis. *Current Opinion in Obstetrics and Gynecology, 18,* 185–191.

Verlinsky, Y., Cohen, J., Munne, S., Gianaroli, L., Simpson, J.L., Ferraretti, A.P., & Kuliev, A. (2004). Over a decade of experience with preimplantation genetic diagnosis: A multicenter report. *Fertility and Sterility, 82,* 292–294.

Viora, E., Errante, G., Sciarrone, A., Bastonero, S., Masturzo, G., Martiny, G., & Campogrande, M. (2005). Fetal nasal bone and trisomy 21 in the second trimester. *Prenatal Diagnosis, 25*(6), 511–515.

Vissers, L.E., Veltman, J.A., van Kessel, A.G., & Brunner, H.G. (2005). Identification of disease genes by whole genome CGH arrays. *Human Molecular Genetics, 14* (Suppl. 2), R215–R223.

Wapner, R.J. (2005). Invasive prenatal diagnostic techniques. *Seminars in Perinatology, 29*(6), 401–404.

Ward, B.E., Gersen, S.L., Carelli, M.P., McGuire, N.M., Dackowski, W.R., Weinstein, M., ... Klinger, K.W. (1993). Rapid prenatal diagnosis of chromosomal aneuploidies by fluorescence in situ hybridization: Clinical experience with 4,500 specimens. *American Journal of Medical Genetics, 52,* 854–865.

Weisz, B., Pandya, P.P., David, A.L., Huttly, W., Jones, P., Rodeck, C.H. (2007). Ultrasound findings after screening for Down syndrome using the integrated test. *Obstetrics and Genecology, 109*(5), 1046–1052.

Wen, S.W., Leader, A., White, R.R., Léveillé, M.C., Wilkie, V., Zhou, J., & Walker, M.C. (2010). A comprehensive assessment of outcomes in pregnancies conceived by in vitro fertilization/intracytoplasmic sperm injection. *European Journal of Obstetrics & Gynecology and Reproductive Biology, 150*(2), 160–165.

Whitworth, M., Bricker, L., Neilson, J.P., & Dowswell, T. (2010). Ultrasound for fetal assessment in early pregnancy. *Cochrane Database System Review, 14*(4): CD007058.

Wilson, R.D. (2000). Amniocentesis and chorionic villus sampling. *Current Opinion in Obstetrics and Gynecology, 12,* 81–86.

Wilton, L., Thornhill, A., Traeger-Synodinos, J., Sermon, K.D., & Harper, J.C. (2009). The causes of misdiagnosis and adverse outcomes in PGD. *Human Reproduction, 24*(5), 1221–1228.

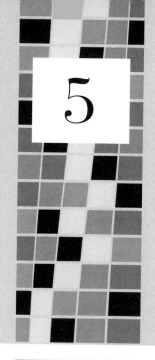

5 Newborn Screening

Opportunities for Prevention of Developmental Disabilities

Joan E. Pellegrino

Upon completion of the chapter the reader will

- Understand the rationale for newborn screening
- Understand the difference between a screening test and diagnostic test
- Be familiar with the types of screening tests available
- Understand the limitations and pitfalls of screening

The birth of a new baby is a joyous time, but for some families, a shadow is cast on their first hopes by the worrisome results of a newborn screening test. The baby's mother will have undergone a number of screening procedures during the pregnancy (see Chapter 4), but she may be unaware that her newborn infant will also have several screening tests performed. This chapter describes the rationale for newborn screening, summarizes the types of disorders for which screening is conducted, and reviews the methods for assuring proper follow up on the results of newborn screening.

■ ■ ■ ASHLEY

Denise, a 32-year-old healthy woman, was pregnant with her second child. The pregnancy was uncomplicated. She had a normal maternal serum screening test in the second trimester and normal prenatal ultrasounds. The delivery was uncomplicated, and she and her daughter, Ashley, were discharged home from the hospital when Ashley was 3 days old. Ashley's parents were therefore upset and confused to receive

a telephone call four days later that Ashley had screened positive for medium chain acyl-CoA-dehydrogenase deficiency (MCAD). They did not know what this disease was, and they did not understand why Ashley should screen positive for an "inherited" condition when they already had a healthy 2-year-old daughter at home. Denise did recall reading that her state had expanded newborn screening, but she was unsure what this meant. Ashley was seen by her pediatrician and underwent diagnostic testing for MCAD. The diagnosis was confirmed, and Ashley was treated with a frequent, regular feeding schedule. Her sister had not been tested for MCAD, as this test was not part of the newborn screen in her state at the time of her birth. She was subsequently tested and found to be affected as well.

WHAT IS A SCREENING TEST?

A **screening test,** as the name implies, is a test designed to screen for, but not definitively diagnose, a particular condition. When applied to a group of individuals, a screening test separates those who are at risk for a condition from those who are not. The ideal screening test would perform this operation with perfect accuracy; but in reality, all screening tests produce false-positive results (unaffected individuals identified as being at risk), and some screening tests produce false-negative results (affected individuals identified as not being at risk). Because the goal of newborn screening is to identify *all* truly affected individuals, interpretive methods and screening algorithms are devised to eliminate false-negative results while still trying to minimize false positives. In some cases, this is accomplished by setting a numerical cut-off for a test that favors the identification of truly affected individuals, at the expense of over-identifying some unaffected individuals as being at risk for the tested condition (Figure 5.1). Because any particular condition tested for by newborn screening is relatively rare, the number of individuals affected by that condition will be much smaller than the number of unaffected individuals. Depending on the technology used, this means that the majority of positive screens may turn out to be false positives. For some conditions, retesting a child using the same or alternative screening tests will improve the screening process; but ultimately, a final group of individuals with positive-screening results

must undergo diagnostic testing. A **diagnostic test** is designed to definitively confirm or exclude the presence of a disease or condition in a particular individual. Diagnostic tests, in theory, should produce no false-positive or false-negative results, so they would actually represent the ideal "screening test." In practice, diagnostic tests are generally either too cumbersome or too expensive to perform on large numbers of individuals, hence the need for screening tests.

WHY SCREEN NEWBORNS?

Of the hundreds of diseases and conditions that may potentially affect infants and young children, a limited number are appropriate for inclusion in a newborn screening program. In the United States, the number of conditions tested for varies widely among the individual states. Due to this variability, the American College of Medical Genetics completed a report commissioned by the Health Resources and Services Administration (HRSA) that recommended universal screening for 29 specific core conditions (the uniform panel) and 25 specific secondary conditions (Newborn Screening Expert Group, 2005). In general terms, the conditions screened for are serious, identifiable, and treatable. In this context, being "treatable"

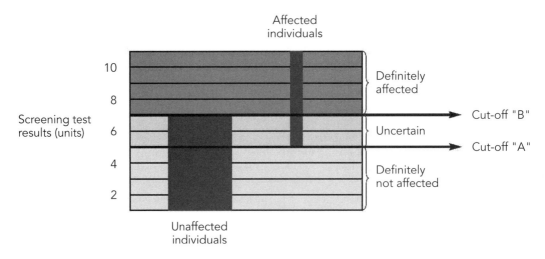

Figure 5.1. Setting a cut-off level for a screening test. In this example, a hypothetical screening test is applied with the ultimate goal of identifying individuals who are affected by a particular disease or condition. Individuals who ultimately prove to be unaffected show test results from 0 to 7 units; individuals who prove to be affected show test results ranging from 5 to 11 units. Individuals with test results above 7 or below 5 will be definitely identified by the screen as affected or unaffected; individuals testing between 5 and 7 may or may not be affected. If cut-off "A" is selected, all affected individuals will be correctly identified, but some unaffected individuals will be incorrectly identified as having disease (false positives). Because the number of unaffected individuals is so much larger than the number with disease, the majority of individuals testing positive will turn out to be unaffected. If cut-off "B" is selected, all unaffected individuals will be correctly identified, but some individuals with disease will be missed (false negatives). Selecting a cut-off level between "A" and "B" will result in a mix of false positives and false negatives.

does not necessarily mean that the condition is curable; it means that interventions should result in significant amelioration of the expected consequences of that condition. The types of diseases and disorders usually screened for fall into the following categories: endocrine disorders, lung disorders, blood disorders, infectious diseases, immune disorders, and metabolic disorders. In addition, hearing loss is screened for in the newborn period (Choo & Meinzen-Derr, 2010; Wolff et al., 2010; see Chapter 10).

This chapter focuses on medical conditions that can be identified by newborn screening and that place the child at significant risk for developmental disabilities. It should be noted, however, that screenings are conducted in the newborn period for additional conditions that carry significant medical and related emotional issues (i.e., congenital adrenal hyperplasia; White, 2009), cystic fibrosis (Southern, Mérelle, Dankert-Roelse, & Nagelkerke, 2009), and sickle cell anemia/hemoglobinopathies (Benson & Therrell, 2010). Screening also occurs prenatally based on family history, ethnicity, and routine maternal serum screening with ultrasound (see Chapter 4).

Endocrine Disorders

The endocrine system produces and regulates a variety of hormones that are critical to maintaining the body in a normal and balanced physiological state, called **homeostasis**. Several specific hormones are critical to the early growth and development of the central nervous system. Congenital hypothyroidism is a condition in which the newborn produces inadequate thyroid hormone; 1 in 3,000 infants is born with the condition, making it relatively common compared with other disorders screened for in the newborn period. Early identification of this condition allows for early treatment with thyroid hormone replacement. Untreated infants have severe growth problems and abnormal brain development, resulting in serious lifelong cognitive disability (Fingerhut & Olgemöller, 2009; Pass, 2009).

Infectious Diseases

Currently, three states screen for human immunodeficiency virus (HIV), and another two screen for **Toxoplasmosis gondii**. These are potentially serious infections in newborns. A positive screen for either of these organisms would require consultation with an infectious disease specialist for confirmation and treatment. A positive HIV screen in the newborn indicates that the mother is infected, and the newborn needs to be followed for the increased risk of disease. The goal of treatment for affected newborns with HIV is long-term suppression of viral replication in order to prevent clinical symptoms of acquired immunodeficiency virus (AIDS) and preserve the immune system. Guidelines for treatment are available (see http://www.hivatis.org). All pregnant women are offered HIV screening prenatally so that they can start treatment and reduce the risk of transmission to the fetus. Untreated congenital toxoplasmosis results in multisystem disease including neurologic complications such as seizures, visual impairments, and intellectual disability. The incidence of congenital toxoplasmosis ranges from 1 in 1,000 to 1 in 8,000 live births. Newborns identified through newborn screening require treatment with medication to reduce the incidence of the sequelae (Röser, Nielsen, Petersen, Saugmann-Jensen, & Nørgaard-Pedersen, 2010).

Immune Disorders

Severe Combined Immunodeficiency (SCID) is a group of disorders that leads to early childhood death as a result of severe infections (Puck, 2007). SCID is known as the "bubble boy" disease because affected children used to be placed in a protected environment to reduce the risk of infection. The Secretary's Advisory Committee on Heritable Disorders in Newborns and Children recently recommended adding this group of diseases to the 29 others in the core panel (see http://www.hrsa.gov/heritabledisorderscommittee). Currently, three states have added this to their newborn screening panels. Children receiving early diagnosis can benefit from stem cell transplants (Lipstein, Vorono, et al., 2010).

Metabolic Disorders

Metabolic disorders, also known as inborn errors of metabolism, represent a diverse group of genetic conditions that manifest as abnormalities of body chemistry at the cellular level (see Chapter 19). These conditions are often associated with the accumulation of abnormal substances, or metabolites, in body fluids and tissues as a consequence of abnormal functioning of proteins known as enzymes. Phenylketonuria (PKU) is a classic example of a screenable metabolic condition. In the United States, the incidence of PKU is 1 in 10,000, with an increased incidence in Caucasians of European decent. The disorder belongs to a group of metabolic conditions known as **amino**

acid disorders. In PKU, a genetic mutation results in the deficiency of an enzyme needed to process phenylalanine, an amino acid common to most protein-laden foods, including meat and dairy products. Early identification of PKU by newborn screening allows implementation of a protein-restricted diet. The lack of treatment results in accumulation of phenylalanine in blood and body tissues, with particularly severe consequences for the developing central nervous system.

Another relatively common metabolic disorder (with an incidence of 1 in 15,000) is MCAD, the disorder that Ashley, our case study in the beginning of the chapter, has. This disorder is the most common example of a group

Table 5.1. Metabolic disorders detectable in newborns by tandem mass spectroscopy

Type of disorder	Specific disorder
Amino acid disorders	5-oxoprolinuria
	Argininemia
	Argininosuccinate lyase deficiency (ASL)
	Citrullinemia
	Citrullinemia II
	Defects of biopterin cofactor biosynthesis
	Defects of biopterin cofactor regeneration
	Homocystinuria
	Hyperammonemia, hyperornithinemia, homocitrullinemia (HHH)
	Hypermethioninemia
	Maple syrup urine disease (MSUD)
	Nonketotic hyperglycinemia
	Phenylketonuria (PKU)
	Tyrosinemia type I, II, and III
Organic acid disorders	2-methyl-3-hydroxybutyryl CoA dehydrogenase (2M3HBA)
	2-methylbutyrl CoA dehydrogenase deficiency (2MBG)
	3-hydroxy-3-methylglutaryl-CoA lyase deficiency (HMG)
	3-methylcrotonyl-CoA carboxylase deficiency (3-MCC)
	3-methylglutaconyl-CoA hydratase deficiency (3MGA)
	Beta-ketothiolase deficiency (BKT)
	Glutaric acidemia type 1 (GA1)
	Isobutyryl-CoA dehydrogenase deficiency (IBG)
	Isovaleric acidemia (IVA)
	Malonic aciduria (MAL)
	Methylmalonic acidemia–Cbl A, B
	Methylmalonic acidemia–Cbl C, D
	Methylmalonic acidemia–mutase deficiency (MUT)
	Multiple carboxylase deficiency (MCD)
	Propionic acidemia (PA)
Fatty acid oxidation disorders	2,4, dienoyl-CoA reductase deficiency (DE RED)
	3-hydroxy long chain acyl-CoA dehydrogenase deficiency (LCHAD)
	Carnitine palmitoyltransferase I and II (CPT I and II)
	Carnitine uptake defects (CUD)
	Carnitine/acylcarnitine translocase deficiency (CACT)
	Medium chain acyl-CoA dehydrogenase deficiency (MCAD)
	Medium chain ketoacyl-CoA thiolase deficiency (MCKAT)
	Medium/short chain hydroxy Acyl-CoA dehydrogenase deficiency (M/SCHAD)
	Multiple acyl-CoA dehydrogenase deficiency (glutaric acidemia Type II)
	Short chain Acyl-CoA dehydrogenase deficiency (SCAD)
	Trifunctional protein deficiency (TFP)
	Very long chain acyl-CoA dehydrogenase deficiency (VLCAD)

of metabolic conditions called **fatty acid oxidation disorders** (Kompare & Rizzo, 2008; Leonard & Dezateux, 2009). Normally, the body processes fat in order to release energy through oxidation. This is especially important during periods of fasting, when fat becomes the main source of energy for the body. Children with MCAD may become seriously ill after a period of fasting and may suffer permanent brain damage as a consequence. Careful monitoring and frequent feedings are essential, especially during infancy. Several other categories of metabolic disease, including organic acid disorders (e.g., **organic acidemias**), disorders of carbohydrate metabolism (e.g., **galactosemia**), and several miscellaneous enzyme deficiencies (e.g., **biotinidase deficiency**) are amenable to dietary intervention or to specific medical treatments. As a group, the metabolic disorders now represent the largest number of potentially treatable conditions that can be identified through newborn screening and are the primary targets of the newest screening technologies.

HOW IS NEWBORN SCREENING DONE?

Most newborn screening tests rely on blood samples obtained during the first few days after birth (Fernhoff, 2009; Hiraki & Green, 2010; Levy, 2010). Testing begins by collecting a blood sample from a heel prick and blotting this onto a special filter-paper collection device. The sample is collected before the newborn is discharged from the birthing facility but after the infant has had an opportunity to feed, ideally at least 24 hours after birth. The infant must eat first because certain metabolic disorders cannot be detected until the body is challenged to metabolize the substances present in breast milk or formula. The filter paper is dried and sent to a newborn screening laboratory. The specimen is then divided into multiple samples for use in a variety of tests looking for specific diseases. In the past, a different test was required for each disease. With the advent of **tandem mass spectroscopy,** the number of tests that can be run on one sample has increased exponentially.

The mass spectrometer is a device that separates and quantifies ions based on their mass-to-charge ratio (American College of Medical Genetics & American Society of Human Genetics, 2000). The **tandem mass spectrometer** (MS/MS) consists of two of these devices separated by a reaction chamber such that accurate measurements of many different types of metabolites can be obtained at once (Chace, DiPerna, & Naylor, 1999). This is a very rapid and sensitive method for mass screening because a single sample can be screened in 1–2 minutes for numerous disorders (Table 5.1; Chace, Kalas, & Naylor, 2003). This technology can also improve the detection rate (lower the number of false positives) for other diseases such as PKU (Chace, Sherwin, Hillman, Lorey, & Cunningham, 1998; Marsden, Larson, & Levy, 2006). It is important to note that not all of the currently mandated disorders can be screened in this way, so other methods will continue to be needed (Table 5.2).

The use of tandem mass spectroscopy has increased the number of diagnoses of inborn errors of metabolism. In one study, the detection rate using this method to screen for 12 diseases (excluding PKU) was 10.6 in 100,000 (Waisbren et al., 2003). Among this group, 40% of infants had MCAD. In another study the detection rate was increased from the previous rate of 9 in 100,000 births to 15.7 in 100,000 births over a 4-year period when 31 diseases (again excluding PKU) were screened for using MS/MS (Wilcken, Wiley, Hammond, & Carpenter, 2003). In this study, the most commonly diagnosed disorder was again MCAD.

Many states have second-tier testing once the initial biochemical test is abnormal. This typically involves genetic testing (testing of the DNA of the infant). Second-tier testing is usually performed by the same laboratory that performed the initial screen and occurs automatically as part of the screening algorithm. Under this method, a sample is tested and flagged as abnormal relative to an expected range for the test. The sample is then sent for a second-tier test that aids in the interpretation

Table 5.2. Disorders detected in newborns by technologies other than tandem mass spectroscopy

Arginase deficiency

Biotinidase deficiency

Congenital adrenal hyperplasia

Congenital hypothyroidism

Congenital toxoplasmosis

Cystic fibrosis

Galactokinase deficiency

Galactose epimerase deficiency

Galactose-1-phosphate uridyltransferase deficiency

Glucose-6-phosphate dehydrogenase deficiency

Hemoglobinopathies: S/S; S/C; S/ßTh variants

Human immunodeficiency virus (HIV)

Hearing loss

of the initial screening result. Only abnormal samples have second-tier tests. For example, a specimen might be abnormal for immunoreactive trypsinogen (IRT), a test for cystic fibrosis. That sample is then tested for some of the more common DNA mutations associated with cystic fibrosis. If two mutations are found, the sample may be coded as positive. If no mutation, or only one mutation, is found then the sample may be coded as negative or positive depending on the level of IRT. By adding second-tier DNA testing for multiple mutations, the sensitivity of the test is increased, but an increased number of carriers (individuals with a single copy of the mutated gene who do not have cystic fibrosis) are also identified, creating another layer of complexity from a genetic counseling perspective (Comeau et al., 2004).

WHAT SHOULD BE DONE WHEN A CHILD HAS A POSITIVE NEWBORN SCREEN?

In practice, each state decides how to handle positive screening results and how to follow up. In general, there should be prompt notification of the physician of record (usually the primary care pediatrician or family practitioner) and the infant's family. Treatment should be initiated if appropriate, and the infant should be evaluated further. Definitive testing should confirm the diagnosis. If the diagnosis is confirmed, a treatment plan specific to that disorder should be initiated. The family is typically referred to a specialty consultant or program, and genetic counseling is offered. Some of the conditions screened require urgent evaluation, such as the organic acidemias, carbohydrate and urea cycle disorders, and the immune and endocrine diseases. All interventions require close collaboration with the specialist, primary care physician, public health department, and the families.

Even when follow-up on a positive newborn screen operates efficiently and effectively, families may still experience significant stress related to the process. As previously mentioned, many positive screens turn out to be false positives. In many conditions, for every 10 infants with a positive screen, only 1 will be found to have the disease. Even though these other 9 children will ultimately prove to be without disease, the process leading to this conclusion can be difficult for families. Mothers of false-positive infants have been found to have significantly increased stress level scores compared to mothers of screen-negative infants, and they score higher on measures of parent–child dysfunction. Having the child seen through a specialty center (e.g., a metabolic disorders clinic at an academic medical center) or communicating repeat screening results in person seems to improve this situation (Waisbren et al., 2003). On the one hand, it is important for families to understand that a positive newborn screen does not automatically mean that their infant has a problem. On the other hand, it is obviously important that appropriate follow-up is pursued in a timely fashion to allow identification of truly affected infants.

When a child screens positive for a particular disorder, follow-up testing methods and algorithms will differ depending on the characteristics of the specific disorder and the methods used for the initial screen. The American College of Medical Genetics has developed ACT SHEETS and confirmatory algorithms for the 29 core conditions and many of the secondary targets as well. These are available on their web site (http://www.acmg.net).

WHAT HAPPENS TO CHILDREN WITH CONFIRMED DISEASE?

Infants with a positive newborn screen are often referred to a center where they can be seen by a physician who has expertise in the condition for which positive screening occurred (James & Levy, 2006). This may be a hematologist, a pulmonologist, an endocrinologist, or a geneticist. In some states, families may have access to multidisciplinary programs that include nurses, genetic counselors, social workers, and nutritionists in addition to specialty physicians. Additional testing is then obtained to confirm the specific diagnosis or to aid in genetic counseling. Once the diagnosis is established, the child will require ongoing (and often lifelong) care for that condition. The specific interventions employed will depend on the diagnosis obtained (e.g., see Chapter 19). In general, the goal is to provide long-term therapy for the child and ongoing counseling to the family, with the ultimate goal of improving medical, neurodevelopmental, and psychosocial outcomes. Some disorders are relatively easy to manage with medications or supplements (e.g., thyroid hormone replacement therapy for congenital hypothyroidism, or biotin therapy [a B vitamin] for biotinidase deficiency). Other disorders are more complex and may require a combination of medications, supplements, and dietary changes. For example, the treatment of PKU requires protein restriction and replacement of normal food items with synthetic, non-phenylalanine-containing substitutes. This is usually achieved using special formulas in children or supplemental nutrition bars in adults. Although this sounds quite simple, it is for most individuals and families a very burdensome diet and is complicated by the fact that these specialized foods are costly and may not be covered by medical insurance.

Because most of these disorders are genetic, genetic testing may be recommended to confirm the diagnosis or to provide additional prognostic information. Once a specific mutation is identified, prenatal diagnosis may be available in the next pregnancy, if the family chooses to pursue this. Recurrence risk (risk that another child will be born with the same condition in the future) is an appropriate concern. Because most metabolic disorders are inherited as an autosomal recessive trait (see Chapter 1), the statistical risk of recurrence is 25%. By comparison, an individual actually diagnosed with a metabolic disorder is at much lower risk for having a child with the same condition. There are additional issues to consider, however, when a woman with a metabolic disorder becomes pregnant: Her disease may have an impact on the developing fetus, even though the fetus does not have the disease (e.g., see description of maternal PKU in Chapter 19). Although the teratogenic effects of phenylalanine on the fetus have been well described, this is not the case for many other metabolic disorders. With increasing numbers of individuals being identified with severe metabolic disorders earlier and treated sooner, it is expected that more affected women will survive into childbearing age and the effects of these disorders on the developing fetus will be further elucidated.

WHAT IS THE RISK OF DEVELOPMENTAL DISABILITY IN CHILDREN WITH CONFIRMED DISEASE?

The neurodevelopmental and functional sequelae of a particular disorder identified through newborn screening is specific to that disorder. A few studies have addressed the issue of developmental outcomes in children who have an underlying metabolic disorder. A population-based surveillance study of children with severe developmental disabilities (intellectual disability, cerebral palsy, hearing loss, and vision impairment) who had a true-positive newborn screen revealed that only 3 of 147 infants showed signs of these disorders (Van Naarden Braun, Yeargin-Allsopp, Schendel, & Fernhoff, 2003). Two of the infants had maple syrup urine disease (MSUD) and one had galactosemia. All three children had intellectual disability that was attributable to their metabolic disorder. However, when this study was expanded to look for children with positive newborn screen who were receiving special education services, there were 9 children out of 216 who had a less severe form of developmental disability (developmental delay, speech-language impairment, learning disability). Seven children had a form of galactosemia, and two had congenital hypothyroidism. One child with classic galactosemia had developmental delays, another child had a specific learning disability, and the remaining seven had speech-language impairments. In the Waisbren study (2003), the children identified by newborn screening had fewer developmental and health problems and functioned better (as evidenced by developmental testing) compared with those children diagnosed at a later age based on clinical symptoms. The children identified through screening had fewer hospitalizations, shorter hospital stays, and 60% fewer medical problems, and they scored significantly higher on developmental testing. Despite the positive outlook in these studies, many of these diseases are still associated with severe developmental disabilities (Dhondt, 2010).

HOW CAN SCREENING FAIL?

There are a number of steps during which newborn screening can fail. It is important to keep in mind that a newborn may not have been screened at the hospital. Many states allow for exemptions from newborn screening based on religious or other reasons. Other possibilities are that the newborn may have been born at home, the newborn may have been transferred to another hospital, or the specimen could have been lost or misidentified. There are also reasons why an infant could screen negative but still have a disease (i.e., a false-negative result). For example, it is possible that the specimen was obtained at the wrong time. As previously noted, for some of the metabolic disorders, the infant needs to be at least 24 hours old and must have been fed an adequate amount of formula or breast milk before a screening test can be valid. If the infant has not eaten, then the metabolites for some of the diseases will not accumulate and the test will yield a false-negative result. For some disorders, the test is not accurate if the infant has had a blood transfusion. Things as simple as how much blood is collected, how long the sample is dried, how long it took to get to the lab, and even the weather conditions during shipment can result in inaccurate test results. In addition, infants are sometimes "lost" to follow-up. It may be difficult to actually locate a specific infant due to a name change for the baby, family relocations, inadequate information provided with the sample (e.g., wrong address or telephone number), or a new physician of record.

Newborn screening can be particularly challenging in infants who are born prematurely. False-positive rates (FPRs) increase with decreasing birth weight and gestation age and are significantly increased in very low birth weight neonates (<1000g) and infants <32 weeks gestational age. The majority of false-positive screens in this population are for endocrine disorders. Strategies to decrease the FPRs may include waiting for >48 hours to obtain the first sample in infants <32 weeks gestation (Slaughter et al., 2010).

The purpose of newborn screening is to identify affected infants, but as previously noted, a certain number of unaffected infants will be identified as being at risk. For some conditions, these false-positive cases turn out to represent individuals who are carriers for the condition. With the advent of DNA testing, an increasing number of carrier infants have been identified. These infants do not have the disease but are carrying one DNA mutation for the screened disease. In many cases, the families of these newborns will be referred to a specialty center for further testing and counseling. If it is determined that the infant is a carrier, then genetic counseling will be offered to the parents so that they can better understand the risk of recurrence for themselves, for their child (and his or her future children), and for the child's siblings (who may also be carriers for the condition).

THE PAST, PRESENT, AND FUTURE OF NEWBORN SCREENING

The first successful newborn screening program was started in Massachusetts in 1962 with screening for PKU (MacCready, 1963). Preventive screening was mandated by the state and subsequently adopted by other states over a period of several years. Expansion of newborn screening began in earnest in 1975 when a test

was developed to screen for congenital hypothyroidism (Dussault et al., 1975; LaFranchi 2010). The success of newborn screening for this disorder led to the addition of testing for an increasing number of disorders. Each year more than 4 million babies are screened in the United States for a variety of disorders, and approximately 6,000 infants are diagnosed with a detectable and treatable disorder (National Newborn Screening and Genetics Resource Center, 2010; for more information see http://HRSA.gov/heritabledisorderscommittee). Each state decides which disorders will be screened for, but the majority of states are providing universal screening for the 29 core conditions (see Table 5.3). While the majority of states have mandatory screening (i.e., all infants must be screened), some have voluntary screening (i.e., parents may choose whether their child is screened). Some states require written informed consent; others have an implied consent, but require written informed dissent (i.e. the parents must sign if they choose not to participate). Some states have a single designated laboratory that performs all screening testing others contract with regional centers, university laboratories, or private laboratories. Each state must decide how the screening process is to be conducted, how to notify the parents and professionals of the results, and how to follow up on abnormal results. Each state may make a different decision depending on a number of factors including its resources, population mix, and birth rate. However, with the passage of The Newborn Screening Saves Lives Act of 2008 most states began to follow a uniform practice for performing and following up on newborn screening (National Newborn Screening and Genetics Resource Center, 2010).

Further expansion of screening programs has been driven by consumer activism and new technologies (especially tandem mass spectroscopy). The HHS Secretary's Advisory Committee on Heritable Disorders in Newborns and Children has developed an evidence review process to consider additional conditions for universal screening. As of February 2010 they have evaluated nine conditions and recommended the addition of one (SCID) to the uniform panel. The advisory committee looks at the scientific evidence to make recommendations for inclusion in the screening panel by reviewing the condition, diagnosis, and treatment and screening methods. They look at the natural history of the disease, at how early and by what method the disease is diagnosed, and at the clinical variability and burden of disease

They also review information on the methods available for newborn screening, including the validity, sensitivity, positive-predictive value, cost, and whether or not it can be multiplexed (more than one disease identified from the same run). Then they review the diagnosis and treatment options to see if confirmation of the diagnosis is available and if early identification and treatment can improve the outcome (Calonge et al., 2010; Watson, 2006).

A state can also add diseases to their newborn screening panel through their own legislative acts. Therefore some conditions that were not accepted by the advisory committee are, in fact, being tested for in a few specific states. The lysosomal storage disorders are a good example of this. Many people feel that this group of diseases is a good candidate for newborn screening. However, they were not recommended by the advisory committee.

Lysosomal storage disorders are a group of about 40 diseases in which there is progressive accumulation of a substance in the lysosome that is normally broken down. In lysosomal

Table 5.3. Recommended newborn screening core panel

Disorder	Number of states mandated[a]
Amino acid disorders	
Argininosuccinate lyase deficiency (ASA)	51
Citrullinemia	51
Homocystinuria	51
Maple syrup urine disease (MSUD)	51
Phenylketonuria (PKU)	51
Tyrosinemia type I	47
Organic acid disorders	
3-hydroxy-3-methylglutaryl-CoA lyase deficiency (HMG)	51
Glutaric acidemia type 1 (GA1)	51
Isovaleric acidemia (IVA)	51
3-methylcrotonyl-CoA carboxylase deficiency (3-MCC)	49
Multiple carboxylase deficiency	50
Methylmalonic acidemia (Cbl A,B)	51
Methylmalonic acidemia (mutase deficiency)	51
Beta-ketothiolase deficiency	51
Propionic acidemia (PA)	51
Fatty acid oxidation disorders	
Carnitine uptake defect	50
3-hydroxy long chain acyl-CoA dehydrogenase deficiency (LCHAD)	51
Medium chain acyl-CoA dehydrogenase deficiency (MCAD)	51
Trifunctional protein deficiency (TFP)	50
Very long chain acyl-CoA dehydrogenase deficiency (VLCAD)	51
Hemoglobinopathies	
Hb S/S; Hb S/ßTh; Hb S/C	51
Other	
Congenital adrenal hyperplasia	51
Biotinidase deficiency	50
Congenital hypothyroidism	51
Cystic fibrosis	51
Galactose-1-phosphate uridyltransferase deficiency (Galactosemia)	51
Hearing loss	36[b]

Based on data from National Newborn Screening and Genetics Resource Center (NNSGRC). Data retrieved November 15, 2010, from http://genes-r-us.uthscsa.edu, from material updated by NNSGRC as of August 8, 2010. Please see http://genes-r-us.uthscsa.edu/nbsdisorder5s.htm for most updated list.

[a]Only states that universally require a screening by law are counted (other states have universally offered screening but do not require it universally or for selected populations); Washington, D.C., is counted for "51 states."

[b]Additional states universally offer but do not universally require hearing screening.

storage disorders, the substance is unable to be metabolized due to a defect in an enzyme. Some of these disorders are treatable by either enzyme replacement therapy or stem cell transplant. However, in order to optimize treatment it should begin as soon as possible, making early identification critical. New York State added one lysosomal storage disorder, Krabbe disease, to its screening panel in 2006 (Duffner et al. 2009). Several other states have recommended screening for some of these disorders as well. Screening methods have been reported for Krabbe, Gaucher, Fabry, Sandhoff, Niemann Pick, Tay Sachs, Maroteaux-Lamy, Adrenoleukodystrophy, and Pompe (Duffey, Sadilek, Scott, Turecek, & Gelb, 2010; Kemper, 2007; Marsden & Levy, 2010; Matern, 2008; Raymond, Jones, & Moser, 2007). It is likely that some of these disorders will be added to newborn screening panels in the future.

As new technologies are developed and therapeutic advances are made, the list of conditions recommended for newborn screening is likely to expand. As an example, with the completion of the Human Genome Project, the discovery of hundreds of mutations causing disorders being screened for opens the possibility of using expression microarray technology to screen for these mutations in the newborn period rather than to screen for metabolic abnormalities resulting from the mutations (the MS/MS method). Chromosomal microarray has become the first-tier test for individuals with developmental disabilities or congenital anomalies (Miller et al, 2010). This technology could be used for newborn screening as well.

There is no doubt that newborn screening will expand in the future. The challenge will be to balance the legal, ethical, and social concerns that can be raised by expanded screening (Bailey, Skinner, Davis, Whitmarsh, & Powell, 2008). There is clinical variation in many of the screenable diseases, making it difficult to know who to treat and when to institute therapy. DNA-based technology can detect carriers and can also detect sequence variations and polymorphisms for which we have little information, making it difficult to know the clinical significance (Fleischman, Lin, & Howse, 2009). There may also be a paradigm shift from the newborn as the patient, to the family as the patient. In this view the family receives the information on carrier status and its implication for prenatal diagnoses in future pregnancies (McCabe & McCabe, 2008).

PRENATAL SCREENING

Complementary to newborn screening is **prenatal screening** (screening during pregnancy to identify conditions that affect the fetus). As with newborn screening, numerous prenatal screening tests are now available (see Chapter 4). One can choose first-trimester screening tests, consisting of a blood test combined with a fetal ultrasound examination, or a second-trimester maternal serum screening. In addition, screening can be done before pregnancies in certain at-risk populations (e.g., carrier detection for Tay-Sachs disease in the Ashkenazi Jewish population or mutation analysis for fragile X syndrome in an extended family in which one family member has been previously identified as having the disorder). Population-based screening of pregnant women is also available for cystic fibrosis, spinal muscular atrophy, and fragile X syndrome. Prenatal screening tests are particularly relevant in instances where increased risk is recognized on the basis of advanced maternal age, ethnicity, or a positive family history for a particular inherited disorder. Positive results from screening tests may prompt more involved diagnostic testing, including high-resolution fetal imaging, amniocentesis, chorionic villus sampling, and even percutaneous umbilical blood sampling. These are considered diagnostic tests because they are performed to look for a specific disorder. Chromosomal analysis, enzymatic assays, and molecular testing can all be done on fetal tissue that is obtained through diagnostic testing in order to confirm a diagnosis or to rule it out.

SUMMARY

Screening tests are important tools used to help define increased risk for significant medical and genetic conditions. These tests can be used for mass screening of newborns, and they are also useful for prenatal screening and targeted screening of specific at-risk populations and ethnic groups. Newborn screening is one of the most important and effective public health measures. Many infants have been identified through this early screening and have been successfully treated with resultant improved outcomes. However, some of the metabolic disorders can have lifelong complications despite therapy. The number of diseases and disorders screened for has grown over time and will likely continue to increase. Parents have been the greatest advocates for expanding newborn screening and will continue to play a major role as we move forward (Lipstein, Nabi, et al., 2010). As more infants are identified with more diseases and disorders, future research will be aimed at developing innovative therapies to further improve outcomes.

REFERENCES

American College of Medical Genetics/American Society of Human Genetics Test and Technology Transfer Committee Working Group. (2000). Tandem mass spectroscopy in newborn screening. *Genetics in Medicine, 2,* 267–269.

Bailey, D.B., Skinner, D., Davis, A.M., Whitmarsh, I., & Powell, C. (2008). Ethical, legal, and social concerns about expanded newborn screening: Fragile X syndrome as a prototype for emerging issues. *Pediatrics, 121,* e693–704.

Benson, J.M., Therrell, B.L., Jr. (2010). History and current status of newborn screening for hemoglobinopathies. *Seminars in Perinatology, 34*(2), 134–44.

Calonge, N., Green, N.S., Rinaldo, P., Llyod-Puryear, M., Dougherty, D., Boyle, C., ... The Advisory Committee on Heritable Disorders in Newborns and Children. (2010). Committee report: Method for evaluating conditions nominated for population-based screening of newborns and children. *Genetics in Medicine, 12*(3), 153–159.

Chace, D.H., DiPerna, J.C., & Naylor, E.W. (1999). Laboratory integration and utilization of tandem mass spectroscopy in neonatal screening: A model for clinical mass spectroscopy in the next millennium. *Acta Paediatric Supplement, 88,* 45–47.

Chace, D.H., Kalas, T.A., & Naylor, E.W. (2003). Use of tandem mass spectrometry for multianalyte screening of dried blood specimens from newborns. *Clinical Chemistry, 49,* 1797–1817.

Chace, D.H., Sherwin, J.E., Hillman, S.L., Lorey, F., & Cunningham, G.C. (1998). Use of phenylalanine-to-tyrosine ratio determined by tandem mass spectroscopy to improve newborn screening for phenylketonuria of early discharge specimens in the first 24 hours. *Clinical Chemistry, 44,* 2405–2409.

Choo, D., & Meinzen-Derr, J. (2010). Universal newborn hearing screening in 2010. *Current Opinion in Otolaryngology & Head and Neck Surgery, 18*(5), 399–404.

Comeau, A.M., Parad, R.B., Dorkin, H.L., Dovey, M., Gerstle, R., Haver, K., ... Eaton, R.B. (2004). Population-based newborn screening for genetic disorders when multiple mutation DNA testing is incorporated: A cystic fibrosis newborn screening model demonstrating increased sensitivity but more carrier detections. *Pediatrics, 113,* 1573–1581.

Dhondt, J.L. (2010). Expanded newborn screening: Social and ethical issues. *Journal of Inherited Metabolic Disease, 33*(Suppl 2), S211–7.

Duffey, T.A., Sadilek, M., Scott, C.R., Turecek, F., & Gelb, M.H. (2010). Tandem mass spectrometry for the direct assay of lysosomal enzymes in dried blood spots: Application to screening newborns for Mucopolysaccharidosis VI (Maroteaux-Lamy syndrome). *Analytical Chemistry, 82*(22), 9587–9591.

Duffner, P.K., Caggana, M., Orsini, J.J., Wenger, D.A., Patterson, M.C., Crosley, C.J., ... Wasserstein, M.P.

(2009). Newborn screening for Krabbe disease: The New York State model. *Pediatric Neurology, 40*(4), 245–252.

Dussault, J.H., Coulombe, P., Laberge, C., Letarte, J., Guyda, H., & Khoury, K. (1975). Preliminary report on a mass screening program for neonatal hypothyroidism. *Journal of Pediatrics, 86,* 670–674.

Fernhoff, P.M. (2009). Newborn screening for genetic disorders. *Pediatric Clinics of North America, 56*(3), 505–513.

Fingerhut, R., & Olgemöller, B. (2009). Newborn screening for inborn errors of metabolism and endocrinopathies: An update. *Analytical and Bioanalytical Chemistry, 393*(5), 1481–1497.

Fleischman, A.R., Lin, B.K., & Howse, J.L. (2009). A commentary on the President's Council on Bioethics report: The changing moral focus of newborn screening. *Genetics in Medicine, 11*(7), 507–509.

Hiraki, S., & Green, N.S. (2010). Newborn screening for treatable genetic conditions: Past, present, and future. *Obstetrics & Gynecology Clinics of North America, 37*(1), 11–21.

James, P.M., & Levy, H.L. (2006). The clinical aspects of newborn screening: Importance of newborn screening follow-up. *Mental Retardation and Developmental Disabilities Research Reviews, 12*(4), 246–254.

Kemper, A.R., Hwu, W.L., Lloyd-Puryear, M., & Kishnani, P.S. (2007). Newborn screening for Pompe disease: Synthesis of the evidence and development of screening recommendations. *Pediatrics, 120*(5), e1327–1334.

Kompare, M., & Rizzo, W.B. (2008). Mitochondrial fatty-acid oxidation disorders. *Seminars in Pediatric Neurology, 15*(3), 140–149.

LaFranchi, S.H. (2010). Newborn screening strategies for congenital hypothyroidism: An update. *Journal of Inherited Metabolic Disease, 33*(Suppl 2), S225–233.

Leonard, J.V., & Dezateux, C. (2009). Newborn screening for medium chain acyl CoA dehydrogenase deficiency. *Archives of Disease in Childhood, 94*(3), 235–238.

Levy, P.A. (2010). An overview of newborn screening. *Journal of Developmental & Behavioral Pediatrics, 31*(7), 622–631.

Lipstein, E.A., Nabi, E., Perrin, J.M., Luff, D., Browning, M.F., & Kuhlthau, K.A. (2010). Parents' decision-making in newborn screening: Options, choices, and information needs. *Pediatrics, 126,* 696–704.

Lipstein, E.A., Vorono, S., Browning, M.F., Green, N.S., Kemper, A.R., Knapp, A.A., ... Perrin, J.M. (2010). Systematic evidence review of newborn screening and treatment of severe combined immunodeficiency. *Pediatrics, 125*(5), e1226–1235.

MacCready, R. (1963). Phenylketonuria screening program. *The New England Journal of Medicine, 269,* 52–56.

Marsden, D., Larson, C., & Levy, H.L. (2006). Newborn screening for metabolic disorders. *Journal of Pediatrics, 148,* 577–584.

Marsden, D., & Levy, H. (2010). Newborn screening of lysosomal storage disorders. *Clinical Chemistry, 56*(7), 1071–1079.

Matern, D. (2008). Newborn screening for lysosomal storage disorders. *Acta Paediatrica Supplement, 97*(457), 33–37.

Miller, D.T., Adam, M.P., Aradhya, S., Biesecker, L.G., Brothman, A.R., Carter, N.P., ... Ledbetter, D.H. (2010). Consensus statement: Chromosomal microarray is a first tier clinical diagnostic test for individuals with developmental disabilities or congenital anomalies. *The American Journal of Human Genetics,* *86,* 749–764.

McCabe, L.L., & McCabe, E.R.B. (2008). Expanded newborn screening: Implications for genomic medicine. *Annual Review of Medicine, 59,* 163–175.

National Newborn Screening and Genetics Resource Center. (2010). National newborn screening status report. Retrieved from http://genes-r-us .uthscsa.edu /nbsdisorders.htm

Newborn Screening Expert Group. (2005). Newborn screening: Towards a uniform screening panel and system. *Federal Register, 70,* 44. Retrieved from http://mchb.hrsa.gov/screening

Pass, K.A., & Neto, E.C. (2009). Update: Newborn screening for endocrinopathies. *Endocrinology Metabolism Clinics of North America, 38*(4), 827–737.

Puck, J.M. (2007). Neonatal screening for severe combined immune deficiency. *Current Opinion in Allergy and Clinical Immunology,* 7(6), 522–527.

Raymond, G.V., Jones, R.O., & Moser, A.B. (2007). Newborn screening for adrenoleukodystrophy: Implications for therapy. *Molecular Diagnosis and Therapy,* 11(6), 381–384.

Röser, D., Nielsen, H.V., Petersen, E., Saugmann-Jensen, P., & Nørgaard-Pedersen, P.B. (2010). Congenital toxoplasmosis: A report on the Danish neonatal screening programme 1999–2007. *Journal of Inherited Metabolic Disease, 33*(Suppl 2), S241–247.

Slaughter, J.L., Meinzen-Derr, J., Rose, S.R., Leslie, N.D., Chandraesekar, R., Linard, S.M., & Akinbi, H.T. (2010). The effects of gestational age and birth weight on false positive newborn screening rates. *Pediatrics, 126*(5), 910–916.

Southern, K.W., Mérelle, M.M., Dankert-Roelse, J.E., & Nagelkerke, A.D. (2009). Newborn screening for cystic fibrosis. *Cochrane Database Systematic Review,* *21*(1), CD001402.

Van Naarden Braun, K., Yeargin-Allsopp, M., Schendel, D., & Fernhoff, P. (2003). Long-term developmental outcomes of children identified through a newborn screening program with a metabolic or endocrine disorder: A population-based approach. *Journal of Pediatrics, 143*(2), 236–242.

Waggoner, D.J., & Pagon, R.A. (2009). Internet resources in medical genetics. *Current Protocols in Human Genetics,* Unit 9.12. doi:10.1002/0471142905. hg0912s62

Waisbren, S.E., Albers, S., Amato, S., Ampola, M., Brewster, T.G., Demmer, L., ... Levy, H.L. (2003). Effect of expanded newborn screening for biochemical genetic disorders on child outcomes and parental stress. *Journal of the American Medical Association,* *290*(19), 2564–2572.

Watson, M.S. (2006). Current status of newborn screening: Decision-making about the conditions to include in screening programs. *Mental Retardation and Developmental Disabilities Research Review,* 12(4), 230–235.

White, P.C., & Medscape. (2009). Neonatal screening for congenital adrenal hyperplasia. *Nature Reviews Endocrinology,* 5(9), 490–498.

Wilcken, B., Wiley, V., Hammond, J., & Carpenter, K. (2003). Screening newborns for inborn errors of metabolism by tandem mass spectroscopy. *The New England Journal of Medicine,* 348, 2304–2312.

Wolff, R., Hommerich, J., Riemsma, R., Antes, G., Lange, S., & Kleijnen, J. (2010). Hearing screening in newborns: Systematic review of accuracy, effectiveness, and effects of interventions after screening. *Archives of Disease in Childhood,* 95(2), 130–135.

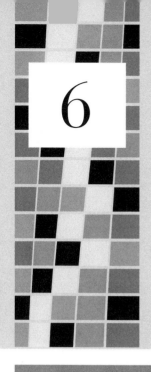

6

The First Weeks of Life

Chrysanthe Gaitatzes, Taeun Chang, and Stephen Baumgart

Upon completion of this chapter the reader will have

- A basic understanding of the events taking place during the transition from fetal to extrauterine life

- A basic understanding of neonatal problems that may be associated with developmental disabilities, including:

    - persistent pulmonary hypertension

    - hypoxic ischemic encephalopathy

    - neonatal seizures

    - hypoglycemia and other metabolic disturbances

    - neonatal stroke

    - neonatal infection

Given that most infants are born into the world without any special difficulty, it is easy to take for granted the astonishing complexity of the birth process. A number of events must take place in a precise and well-timed sequence for the newborn to have a healthy beginning. Understanding the basic principles of normal fetal physiology is key to understanding the normal transition to the extrauterine environment that occurs at the time of birth. In the sections that follow, the typical fetal-to-neonatal transition process is described for a full-term infant. Some of the most commonly encountered early-life problems that may be associated with future physiological and developmental impairments are highlighted.

■ ■ ■ JUSTIN

Justin was born at 39 weeks' gestation to a 26-year-old mother. This was her third pregnancy; she had previously delivered two healthy full-term infants. Justin's mother developed insulin-dependent diabetes during her pregnancy (gestational diabetes). Other prenatal laboratory screening tests were unremarkable. She presented to the hospital in active labor. **Fetal heart rate monitoring** by ultrasound revealed fetal distress, with long periods of abnormally low heart rate during and between labor contractions. This indicated that inadequate oxygen was being supplied to the infant's heart muscle and other vital organs. Justin was therefore delivered by emergency **Cesarean section** within 20 minutes. The obstetrician noted that Justin had passed thick **meconium** (the first bowel movement, usually passed after birth) into the amniotic fluid before his delivery. Because of his mother's diabetes, he was large for gestational age, weighing more than 4 kilograms, or over 9 pounds. This made his delivery difficult through the small Cesarean incision. His further hospital course is described throughout the chapter.

THE FETUS BEFORE BIRTH

The condition of the fetus before birth depends primarily on three things. First, fetal circulation must be adequate to support oxygenation and nutrition of the fetus. Second, the amniotic fluid must be of adequate volume to permit fetal breathing movements, and thus support normal lung development. And third, the fetal digestive system must be functioning well to perform amniotic fluid swallowing and thus support development of the stomach, intestines, and other digestive organs.

Fetal Circulation

The fetal heart begins to develop during the third week of gestation and starts to beat during the fourth week; soon thereafter blood circulation is established. Blood carrying oxygen and

nutrients circulates from the placenta through the umbilical cord via a single umbilical vein (Figure 6.1). The blood in the umbilical vein then passes through the **ductus venosus** (a major blood channel that develops through the embryonic liver) into the **inferior vena cava** (the main vein feeding into the infant's heart). The vena cava blood flows into the right atrium and then the **right ventricle** of the heart. In adult circulation, blood exits the right ventricle via the pulmonary artery into the lungs, but in the fetus only about 10% of this blood volume passes into the lungs. The rest is shunted away from the right and into the left side of the fetal heart through the **foramen ovale** (a tiny window between the right atrium and the left atrium) and the **ductus arteriosus** (a fetal blood vessel that bypasses the main pulmonary artery and lungs). In this way oxygenated blood from the placenta flows into the **aorta**, the major artery supplying oxygenated blood to the body and brain. After the vital organs extract oxygen and nutrients from the arterial blood circulation, deoxygenated venous blood returns to the placenta via two umbilical arteries that pass out of the umbilical cord. Here it is replenished with oxygen and nutrients that are derived from the mother's circulation, and carbon dioxide, heat, and other metabolic waste products (e.g., acids) are removed. The fetal lungs play no role in oxygenation or ventilation (removal of carbon dioxide from the infant) prior to birth.

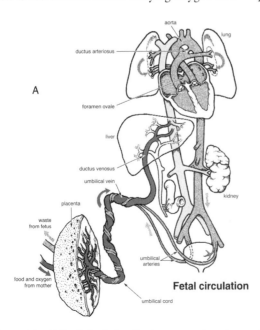

Fetal circulation

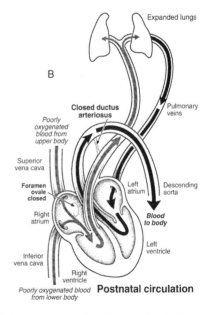

Postnatal circulation

Figure 6.1. A) **Fetal circulation.** The foramen ovale and patent (open) ductus arteriosus allow the blood flow to bypass the unexpanded lungs. B) **Postnatal circulation.** The fetal bypasses close off with expansion of the lungs.

Amniotic Fluid

The fetal lungs are filled with a clear fluid secreted by the lung cells, which act like a gland during prenatal life. Some of this fluid, in combination with the fetus' urine, comprises the amniotic fluid, which is essential for: 1) cushioning the fetus within the mother's uterus, 2) allowing free movement of the fetal limbs and muscles, and 3) promoting symmetric unrestricted body growth. Amniotic fluid is also essential for normal lung development as the fetus practices breathing movements before birth. The presence of too little fluid (**oligohydramnios**) can be associated with **hypoplastic** (small, underdeveloped) lungs, limb abnormalities, poor fetal growth, and prematurity or stillbirth. Oligohydramnios can occur for a number of reasons (Smith, 1976); for example, this occurs in genetic syndromes associated with absent or malfunctioning kidneys, such as Potter syndrome. **Polyhydramnios**, the presence of too much amniotic fluid, also has a number of causes, including maternal causes (e.g., maternal infections, diabetes) and fetal causes. Polyhydramnios may be associated with certain malformations that obstruct the amniotic fluid circulation through the gastrointestinal system, kidneys, and the fetal heart (i.e., duodenal atresia in a fetus with Down syndrome).

The gastrointestinal tract is very active during fetal development. The fetus swallows and absorbs amniotic fluid regularly. **Meconium** (fetal stool) consists mostly of swallowed amniotic fluid debris, gastrointestinal mucous, green bile secretions from the liver, and sloughed off gastrointestinal lining cells. It begins to form during the first trimester of pregnancy. Under normal nonstress conditions the fetus does not pass meconium *in utero*. Meconium-stained amniotic fluid results from an early bowel movement and is a sign of intrauterine fetal distress, usually caused by lack of oxygen from the placenta. Meconium is thick, tar-like, and can irritate or damage the infant's lungs if aspirated at the time of delivery (March of Dimes, 2010).

THE NERVOUS SYSTEM

Normal fetal brain development requires a complex sequence of events, and disruptions can lead to a range of brain malformations (see Chapter 2). The fetal brain has been shown to be active prenatally. Many fetal neurologic reflexes have been identified, including swallowing and sucking. These provide a crucial foundation of skills needed for the infant to feed during the early days and weeks of postnatal life (Health Grades Inc., 2011).

THE BIRTH PROCESS

■ ■ ■ JUSTIN (CONTINUED)

After the obstetrician delivered Justin's head but before delivering his body, she suctioned his nostrils and throat with a bulb syringe. This was done to clear as much of the meconium out of his airways as possible prior to his first breath. After Justin was delivered, he was quickly placed under a radiant heating lamp to maintain his temperature. He was **apneic** (not breathing on his own) and limp. The pediatrician in attendance for this high-risk delivery placed a plastic tube into his airway (**tracheal intubation**) and suction was applied. She aspirated thick, tar-like meconium out of the trachea. The pediatrician repeated the procedure three times, until no more meconium was cleared. By then Justin was 80 seconds old and had not yet taken his first breath. His heart rate was about 60 beats per minute (normal is over 100 beats per minute). At this point a first minute Apgar score (see Table 6.1; Apgar score section) was assigned, giving him only 1 point out of 10 (for the presence of a heart rate under 100 beats per minute).

Justin was vigorously stimulated by rubbing his chest and abdomen with a warm, dry towel. Positive pressure ventilation (PPV; artificial breathing) was provided with a rubber facemask and bag, connected to 100% oxygen. Despite 30 seconds of PPV, Justin still showed no respiratory efforts, and his heart rate was now less than 60 beats per minute. The pediatrician started chest compressions of the sternum over the infant's heart while the nurse continued PPV. After 30 more seconds, Justin's heart began to beat at a normal rate. The medical team continued to stimulate Justin, but his breathing effort remained erratic. A tube was once again placed into his trachea, but this time it was taped into place to allow Justin to receive mechanical ventilation. His Apgar score at 5 minutes was 3 (2 points were awarded for heart rate above 100 per minute, and 1 point for attempted but poor respirations). He remained completely flaccid, with no muscle tone or spontaneous movement.

The First Breath

In a typical birth, the process of clearing the fluid from the lung **alveoli** (the tiny air sacs where gases are exchanged) is stimulated by the initiation of labor (Bland, 1992; Welty, Hansen, & Corbet, 2005). The mechanical compression of the infant's chest as it passes through the narrow birth canal further contributes to the fluid's evacuation from the alveoli. After the first few breaths, the majority of the fluid has been pushed out of the alveoli and absorbed into the pulmonary capillaries and lymphatic vessels. Thereafter, breathing becomes much easier, and normal gas exchange (oxygen for carbon dioxide) takes place. The effort required to breathe is also reduced when the first breath stimulates the secretion of **surfactant** from gland-like cells in the lung. Surfactant is a lipoprotein that acts like a soap bubble, allowing for a significant decrease in the alveolar membrane's surface tension, making breathing much easier and the lungs more flexible.

Aeration improves the amount of oxygen in the infant's blood and the pH (blood acidity), and it decreases the amount of carbon dioxide, a waste by-product of the infant's metabolism. These changes enhance pulmonary **vasodilation** (relaxation and dilation of blood vessels within the lung) in response to gas entry, allowing blood to circulate more freely through the lungs. The flow of blood thru the lungs stimulates the closure of the ductus arteriosus (mostly closed within 6 hours, completely closed by 3 days) and the foramen ovale, completing the transition from fetal circulation to the postnatal "adult" circulation.

The Apgar Score

Virginia Apgar (1909–1974) was a physician and humanitarian who is best known for the scoring system she devised in 1952 for systematically assessing the well-being of newborns. This scoring system remains in routine use today and consists of a total of 10 points that are given for the infant's color/appearance, heart rate, respirations, reflex irritability when stimulated, and muscle tone at rest (see Table 6.1). The Apgar score is usually assigned at 1 minute and again at 5 minutes following birth. When resuscitation is required, as for baby Justin, a 10-minute Apgar score is added. The 1-minute Apgar score primarily reflects the infant's condition resulting from the intrauterine experience immediately prior to birth; the 5- and 10-minute scores reflect the infant's condition in the immediate postnatal period. Apgar scores are most helpful in allowing health care professionals to communicate their impression of a newborn's condition with other health care professionals. Apgar scores are not intended to determine decisions regarding resuscitation and are generally not predictive of long-term developmental outcomes (Behnke et al., 1988).

▓ ▓ ▓ JUSTIN (CONTINUED)

While Justin was still in the delivery room and after the umbilical cord was cut by the obstetrician, a central (deep vein) intravenous catheter was placed via Justin's umbilical cord. The umbilical vein enters the abdominal wall and then runs through the liver and into the inferior vena cava near the heart. As a result, fluid infused through an umbilical catheter is rapidly carried throughout the body. Justin received an infusion of **normal saline** (a salt solution used to improve circulatory perfusion and to correct low blood pressure). Initial measurement of his serum glucose level showed significant **hypoglycemia** (a dangerously low blood sugar level), probably due to the mother's poor blood sugar regulation with her gestational diabetes

Table 6.1. Apgar scoring system

	Sign	0 Points	1 Point	2 Points
A	Activity (muscle tone)	Absent, flaccid	Arms and legs flexed	Vigorous movements
P	Pulse	Absent	< 100 bpm	> 100 bpm
G	Grimace (reflex irritability)	No response	Grimaces only	Sneeze, cough, cry
A	Appearance (skin color)	Blue-gray, pale despite oxygen administration	Normally pink, except for extremities, may require oxygen to become pink	Normally pink over entire body without giving extra oxygen
R	Respiration	Absent (apnea)	Slow, irregular, or gasping	Good, vigorous, crying

Note: The Apgar scoring system evaluates the newborn's transition to normal breathing and activity during the first 5 minutes of life after birth.

(March of Dimes, 2010). Justin was then given intravenous **dextrose** (a simple sugar similar to glucose) through the umbilical vein catheter to correct his blood sugar. Then he was transferred to the neonatal intensive care unit (NICU) for further management.

In the NICU, Justin's endotracheal tube was connected to a mechanical ventilator to assist his breathing. He was started on a continuous infusion of **dopamine** (an adrenaline-like drug) to increase his falling blood pressure and to promote circulation to his brain. He continued to require 100% oxygen to stay pink (instead of ambient 21% oxygen). That high oxygen requirement, in combination with the history of meconium aspiration in the delivery room, suggested the possibility that Justin had developed a condition known as **persistent pulmonary hypertension of the newborn** (PPHN).

Persistent Pulmonary Hypertension of the Newborn

In the fetus, the pulmonary blood vessels offer high resistance to blood flow from the heart, allowing blood that has been oxygenated in the placenta to bypass the nonfunctioning fetal lungs and flow to the rest of the body. At birth, the pulmonary vascular resistance must drop (i.e., the blood vessels of the lungs must dilate) to allow the lungs to take over the function of delivering oxygen to the blood. For reasons that are not fully understood, this drop in pulmonary vascular resistance does not occur in a timely manner in some infants, causing persistent pulmonary hypertension (PPHN; also called persistent fetal circulation). The first spontaneous breath facilitates vasodilation by causing alterations in the blood (i.e., the improved pH, oxygen, and carbon dioxide content previously noted), so the absence of a first breath may hamper the changeover process. Persistent pulmonary blood vessel constriction causes decreased circulation through the lungs. As a result, deoxygenated blood is shunted from the right side to the left side of the heart through the patent ductus arteriosus (PDA) and/or the foramen ovale (that failed to close as in normal transition described above), without first going through the lungs to get oxygenated and to be rid of carbon dioxide (Figure 6.2). This causes a significant strain to the heart from both hypoxia and high blood pressure in the lungs and can cause heart failure.

In addition to meconium aspiration, there are other causes of PPHN including **pneumonia**, **sepsis** (bacterial infections of the lungs or blood), and lung **hypoplasia**. Most infants with PPHN respond to mechanical ventilation or inhaled nitric oxide (iNO), a therapeutic gas that is added to the infant's oxygen supply. For infants who do not respond to mechanical ventilation or iNO, a life-saving procedure known as extracorporeal membrane oxygenation (ECMO) is used. The infant's

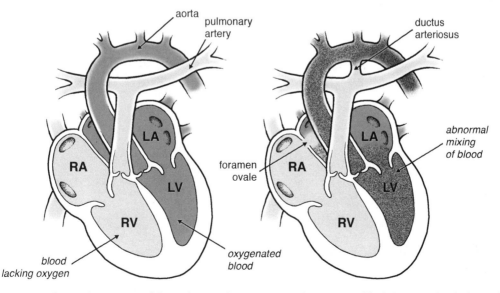

Figure 6.2. Pulmonary hypertension of the newborn resulting in a postnatal persistence of fetal shunting within the heart of blue blood across the ductus arteriosus and the foramen ovale (fetal channels). This results in hypoxia throughout the systemic circulation; red color indicates oxygenated blood, blue indicates blood lacking oxygen, and purple indicates abnormal mixing of blue with red blood, resulting in poor oxygen delivery out of the heart into systemic circulation (especially to the brain).

circulating blood is redirected by a mechanical pump through an artificial lung oxygenator, thus bypassing the infant's lungs and/or heart. ECMO is, in effect, a heart–lung bypass machine. It is used until the infant's lung blood vessels are no longer under increased pressure.

■ ■ ■ JUSTIN (CONTINUED)

Justin responded well to iNO. Within a few days his oxygen level was weaned from 100% back to room air, and by 2 weeks after birth, he was able to breathe on his own. Unfortunately, a head CT brain scan obtained when he was 4 days old revealed evidence of diffuse hypoxic injury (Figure 6.3). Just before going home, Justin had a magnetic resonance imaging (MRI) scan of the brain, which confirmed global, severe cerebral injury involving multiple cortical and subcortical areas of the brain (see HIE in the next section).

By his third week of life, Justin was taken off intravenous nutrition. He was able to tolerate formula provided through a feeding tube, but he showed no evidence of a suck or a protective gag reflex. At the time of his discharge from the NICU, Justin was receiving his feedings through a nasogastric tube, with the understanding that

if he was unable to recover oral feeding skills, he might require placement of a permanent gastrostomy feeding tube (see Chapter 31). Justin's parents also understood that he was at a high risk for developing cerebral palsy as well as hearing and vision problems. Therefore medical follow-ups were scheduled, and he was referred to an early intervention therapy program (see Chapter 10).

Hypoxic Ischemic Encephalopathy

Justin developed his brain injury as a result of **hypoxic ischemic encephalopathy (HIE)**. This is a condition involving both inadequate oxygen and inadequate blood circulation to the brain, leading to dysfunction. The principal prenatal cause of HIE is compromise of the placental blood supply to the fetus (placental insufficiency). This can occur with maternal diabetes (as in Justin's case) or maternal hypertension (**preeclampsia** or toxemia of pregnancy), **placental abruption** (early separation of the placenta from the uterine wall), maternal shock, umbilical cord prolapse (delivery of the cord prior to the infant, with compression of cord and blood supply as the infant is delivered), and intrauterine growth restriction (often resulting from abnormal

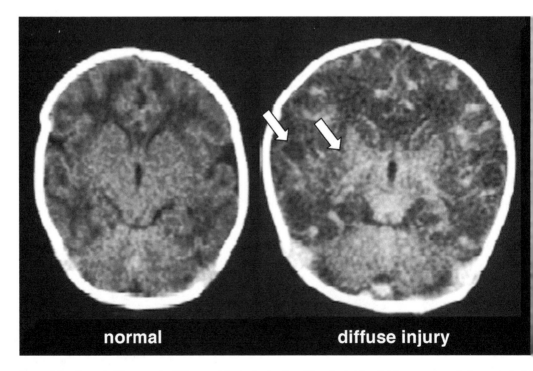

Figure 6.3. Computed tomography (CT) scan of the brain showing diffuse brain injury (white areas, arrows). Arrows indicate absence of normal cortex rim, which is noted throughout the cortex with beginnings of cystic formations in the cortex and edematous basal ganglia.

placental development). When HIE develops, the infant's body responds by redistributing blood away from "nonvital organs" (e.g., kidneys, liver, lungs, intestines, skeletal muscles) and towards perfusion of the "vital organs" (e.g., heart, brain, adrenal glands). This is why kidney and liver failure often occur concurrently with severe HIE. Neonates with HIE have symptoms of abnormal neurological function including decreased activity level, poor suck and feeding, respiratory difficulty, temperature instability (hypothermia, and/or fevers in early infancy), and seizures.

The most popular system for grading the severity of HIE in neonates is known as the Sarnat Neurological Score and includes several clinical findings as well as EEG testing (Sarnat & Sarnat, 1976). HIE is graded into three stages, with Stage 3 being the most severe (Table 6.2). Unlike the Apgar score, the Sarnat neurological score is more useful in prediction of subsequent delayed neurological development. An infant with a Sarnat score of 1 may be hyper-alert and jittery for a day after birth but is likely to recover completely, breathing and feeding normally before going home in a few days. These infants are at low risk for developing cerebral palsy or intellectual disability. An infant with a Sarnat score of 3 (like Justin) has a 70% risk of either dying shortly after birth or going on to have physical and cognitive impairments by 1–2 years of age. An infant with a Sarnat score of 2 has an outcome between those described for Sarnat scores of 1 and 3 (de Vries & Jongmans, 2010).

Neuroimaging is very helpful in assessing the extent of the hypoxic-ischemic injury (Figures 6.4 and 6.6). A magnetic resonance imaging (MRI) scan obtained shortly after birth showing abnormalities in both cerebral hemispheres and deep structural abnormalities (indicated in the figure by arrows), as in Justin's case, is strongly correlated with a poor neurodevelopmental outcome (Bianioni et al., 2001; Rutherford et al., 2004; Massaro, Nadja Kadom, Chang, & Baumgart, 2010). An MRI technique known as **diffusion-weighted imaging** (DWI) is currently the gold-standard for identifying early ischemic injury in specific regions of the brain (Figure 6.4).

The medical management of infants with HIE focuses on correcting physiological abnormalities that are life threatening. These include hypoxemia (low blood oxygen content), hypercarbia (high blood carbon-dioxide content), acidosis, hypotension (low blood pressure/shock), hypoglycemia, and seizures. These disturbances are corrected with the use of oxygen, mechanical ventilation, intravenous medications, seizure medications, and thermoregulation (temperature support). Drugs and nonpharmacologic interventions that may be neuroprotective during HIE are also being studied (Whitelaw & Thoresen, 2002). The major nonpharmacologic intervention involves therapeutic hypothermia (whole body cooling) and results in a decrease in brain temperature and therefore a decrease of metabolic activity, inflammation, and later neuronal death (Gluckman et al., 2005; Gunn & Gunn, 1998; Hoehn et al., 2008; Jacobs, 2010; Shankaran et al., 2005; Simbruner, Mittal, Rohlmann, Muche, & nEURO.network Trual Participants, 2010).

Long-term follow-up with neurologists and developmental specialists is imperative for

Table 6.2. Sarnat examination for scoring neonatal encephalopathy

Factor	Stage 1[a]	Stage 2[b]	Stage 3[c]
Level of consciousness	Hyper-alert	Obtunded/lethargic	Stuporous/coma
Neuromuscular tone	Normal, vigorous	Hypotonia, looseness	Flaccid or fixed stiffness (decerebrate posturing)
Reflexes	Hyperactive Moro reflex	Weak primitive reflexes	Absent reflexes
Autonomic (vital signs)	Fast heart rate (tachycardia)	Slow heart rate (bradycardia) Pupils constricted	Slower heart rate Pupils dilated/unreactive
Seizures	None	Multifocal	Brainstem reflex only
Electroencephalogram (EEG)	Normal, organized rhythms Sleep cycles present	Epileptic threshold (delta waves seen)	Depressed or absent Voltages flat EEG/Electrographic seizures present

Source: Sarnat and Sarnat (1976).

Note: [a]Stage 1: **Mild encephalopathy** <24hr likely to have normal developmental outcome.
[b]Stage 2: **Moderate encephalopathy** <5days normal, >7days likely to have poor outcome.
[c]Stage 3: **Severe encephalopathy** severe impairment, or death 70% likely.

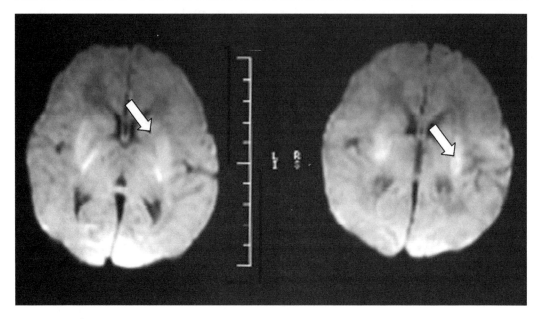

Figure 6.4. Diffusion-weighted imaging/magnetic resonance imaging scans highlighting severe global cerebral injury involving the cerebral cortex, the underlying white matter (corticospinal tracts; arrow on the left scan), and the centrally located basal ganglia (arrow on the right scan) on both sides of the brain.

infants like Justin. Long-term deficits range from mild to severe and include learning disabilities (Chapter 23), visual and hearing impairment (Chapters 10 and 11), intellectual disability (Chapter 17), and cerebral palsy (Chapter 24). According to the National Collaborative Perinatal Project (NCPP; Hardy, 2003), factors that were found to be associated with increased morbidity included ongoing neonatal seizures, decreased activity after the first day of life, temperature instability past the first 3 days of life, and ongoing problems with feeding and breathing.

Neonatal Seizures

Neonatal seizures can present clinically or as EEG abnormalities (see Chapter 27). Clinical seizures often manifest as stiffening (tonic) or jerking (clonic) movements of the arms or legs, or as rhythmic bicycling or rowing movements of the extremities. They can also be very subtle, such as oral–lingual movements (spasmodic lip smacking or tongue thrusting), ocular movements (excessive blinking or prolonged eye opening/staring), or as apneas associated with bradycardia (brief respiratory arrests associated with low heart rate).

There are many possible causes of neonatal seizures. They may be a consequence of HIE,

metabolic disturbances such as hypoglycemia, hypocalcemia (low blood calcium), hyper-, or hyponatremia (high or low blood sodium concentration), and other electrolyte imbalances. They may also result from traumatic brain injury (from forceps/vacuum-assisted deliveries or prenatal maternal trauma), thrombosis (clot) or brain hemorrhage, infections (e.g., meningitis), inborn errors of metabolism (see Chapter 19), and maternal substance abuse (withdrawal symptoms).

EEG is the standard tool for assessing clinically observed seizures (Figure 6.5). An abnormal EEG announces the presence of a central nervous system injury. The underlying cause of the seizure (e.g., inborn errors of metabolism, HIE, congenital infections) is independently important to prognosis for disability. Poor background organization or reactivity to stimuli suggests a diffuse insult to the brain, whereas focal areas of irritability or seizures suggest an acute localized brain injury. Subtle seizures or electrographic seizures (seizures that are not clinically evident) can also be distinguished using EEG and monitored for response to medical treatment. The prognostic value of the EEG is increased if performed within the first 48 hours of life, and if repeated every 24–48 hours to evaluate recovery during the acute episode. An EEG pattern that fails to improve or becomes progressively more abnormal during the first few days of life is associated with long-term neurological sequelae.

The use of antiepileptic drugs (AEDs) for control of seizures in neonates is an area of active debate. The most commonly used AEDs in newborns are phenobarbital and phenytoin (Dilantin). Traditionally, AEDs were prescribed for infants up to 2 years of age to prevent seizure recurrence. The current approach, however, attempts to avoid the potentially adverse effects of long-term AEDs on the developing neonatal brain by a trial period off medications before hospital discharge (Kim, Kondratyev, Tomita, & Gale, 2007). If there is no recurrence of seizure activity, the infant is discharged home, without AEDs and with a plan for close neurological follow-up and monitoring.

Hypoglycemia

Newborns are vulnerable to hypoglycemia (low blood sugar) because their ability to access liver glycogen stores (the main form of glucose energy storage present at the time of birth) is poorly regulated and immature. When it is severe or prolonged, hypoglycemia is just as harmful as lack of oxygen because the neonatal brain is completely dependent on glucose for generating energy. The level of hypoglycemia that is considered abnormal depends on the age of the infant. During their first day of life, newborns normally have lower levels of circulating glucose than older newborns. Neonatal hypoglycemia can be completely asymptomatic but may result in seizures or nonspecific symptoms such as jitteriness, tremors, apneic spells, a weak or high-pitched cry, limpness, lethargy, or difficulty feeding.

Hypoglycemia is common in infants of diabetic mothers (as in Justin's case) and necessitates monitoring of blood glucose testing every 30 minutes to 2 hours during the first few days of life. The hypoglycemia is the result of the infant continuing to produce excessive insulin for a few days after birth (as it did *in utero* in response to the mother's gestational diabetes).

Other full-term neonates who are at high risk for developing hypoglycemia include infants who are small for gestational age or who have intrauterine growth restriction, asphyxia, hypoxia, or sepsis. Prevention of hypoglycemic

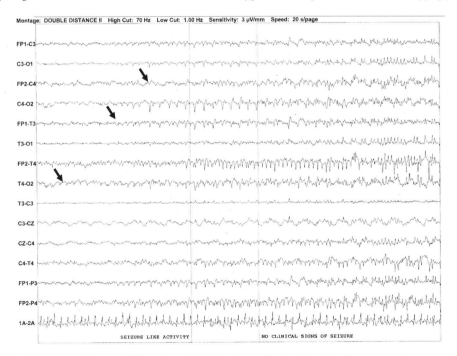

Figure 6.5. Electroencephalogram (EEG) polygraph showing increased electrical activity (bumpy waves) corresponding to electrographic seizures recorded from wires taped to the scalp over the right side of the brain and resulting in left-sided seizure movements clinically as noted at the bottom. First arrow indicates seizure activity beginning in the right frontal-temporal region. Seizures quickly spread to involve the entire right hemisphere by the second arrow and then the entire brain by the third arrow. Note that clinical seizure activity is not noted until the first vertical event marker at the bottom of this figure and that clinical seizure activity is no longer seen after the second vertical event marker, despite the fact that there is generalized electrographic seizures on the EEG, which continues on for another 20–30 seconds beyond what is shown here. Cortical seizures may be present even in the absence of abnormal movements in a brain-injured baby.

encephalopathy requires the continuous intravenous infusion of dextrose for a few days until the infant is feeding and the blood glucose levels become consistently normal.

Neonatal Stroke

Neonatal stroke occurs in 2–9 per 10,000 live births and can cause cerebral palsy (Boardman et al., 2005; Mercuri et al., 2004) and other associated developmental disabilities. The stroke is most often arterial in origin (Figure 6.6), although sinus vein thrombosis (clotted vein) is also an important cause (Ferriero, 2004; de Veber et al., 2001). The most common clinical presenting sign of a neonatal stroke is seizures in the first few days of life. However, other neonates with stroke may present with later onset of seizures (in the first weeks of life as opposed to the first days) or develop a motor deficit. Risk factors implicated in neonatal stroke include inherited or acquired **thrombophilia** (the tendency for one's blood to clot more rapidly than normal) or a structural vascular abnormality in the brain (e.g., arterial–venous malformation or AVM). Preeclampsia and intrauterine growth restriction also have been associated with an increased occurrence of neonatal stroke (Wu et al., 2004). It should be noted that the risk

of recurrence for neonatal stroke is minimal, except for infants with congenital heart disease who develop clots emanating from abnormal cardiac structures. There is no specific medical treatment for neonatal stroke except when a clotting disorder is identified, in which case antiplatelet or anticoagulation medications (aspirin or heparin) may be used. Early institution of physical therapy after a stroke is important for improving functional outcome and helping avoid muscle weakness and joint contractures. Other developmental specialties may be required to address additional, motor, cognitive, and neurobehavioral abnormalities.

Neonatal Sepsis

At birth, the newborn's immunity to bacteria and viruses is immature. Newborns have fewer white blood cells than older infants, and the white blood cells that are present are less immunologically active. This condition, combined with lower concentrations of specific immunoglobulin antibodies, makes the newborn vulnerable to infection. The newborn infant's white blood cells, which are responsible for primary defense against bacteria, exhibit poor **chemotaxis** (the ability to migrate toward areas of infection). The **T-cell lymphocyte** population

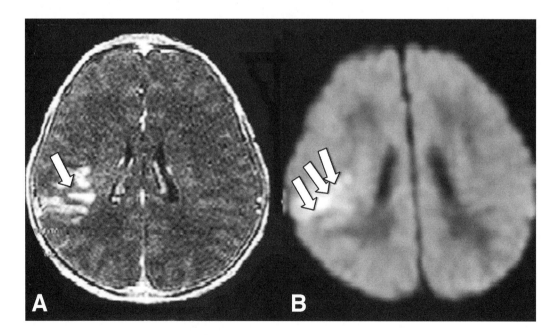

Figure 6.6. A) Magnetic resonance imaging (MRI) showing a right-side middle cerebral artery (MCA) infarction (white areas, arrow). B) Diffusion-weighted MRI showing an area of restricted diffusion of water in the same region on the infarction as in A (arrows).

(white blood cells responsible for recognizing and chemically encoding into immunologic memory any foreign bacterial substances) is also not as effective in infants under 6 months of age. In addition, the presentation of bacterial **antigen** to a newborn does not stimulate an **antibody** formation response as quickly as it does in older children. Also, the neonate's physical barriers to infection (i.e., the skin and the mucous membranes lining the upper respiratory passages, lungs, intestines, and urinary tract) are not as robust a defense barrier, as they will become later in childhood. These deficits in immune defenses are particularly egregious in premature infants, where bacterial infections are generally more common and more devastating.

Neonatal sepsis can be divided into two time periods: 1) early onset, presenting within the first 7 days of life; and 2) late onset, presenting after 7 days. Early onset sepsis is caused by maternal microorganisms that infect the newborn either during passage through the colonized vaginal canal or transplacentally. The most common bacteria that cause early onset neonatal sepsis are *Group B Streptococcus* (GBS), *Escherichia coli, Haemophilus influenza*, and *Listeria monocytogenes*. In some cases, GBS infection results from direct aspiration into the infant's mouth, throat, and lungs during the birth process, with subsequent passage of the bacteria directly into the bloodstream. GBS can also cause late onset sepsis. Late onset sepsis is most often due to bacteria acquired from the environment (onto the skin) or from the infant's own gastrointestinal tract. Most common late onset pathogens in addition to GBS are **Staphylococcus aureus** (now becoming disturbingly resistant to the usual first-line antibiotics), *Escherichia coli, Klebsiella pneumoniae, Pseudomonas, Enterobacter*, and *Candida*. Pneumonia is the most common presentation for early onset sepsis, whereas meningitis is the most common infection in late onset sepsis. Viruses such as adenovirus, enterovirus, Coxsackie virus and Herpes virus can also be the causative agents of neonatal sepsis, and can cause **meningoencephalitis** (a generalized and often devastating infection of the brain and central nervous system).

The mortality of neonatal sepsis can be greater than 50% among untreated or late-treated infants. As a result, physicians need to be suspicious of sepsis in the neonate and aggressive in starting appropriate intravenous antibiotics with suspected sepsis. As one approach to early detection of neonatal sepsis, the American College of Obstetrics and Gynecology (ACOG; Barclay, 2010) recommends screening of all pregnant women for the presence of GBS colonization at 35–37 weeks' gestation.

The clinical presentation of sepsis in the neonate can be vague and nonspecific; the infant may even appear to be well until the sepsis becomes overwhelming. The most common clinical features are 1) poor feeding, probably the first and most sensitive sign of an ill infant; 2) excessive sleepiness or irritability; 3) hypothermia or hyperthermia; 4) increased respiratory rate; and/or 5) hypoglycemia. Any fever above 37.4 °C or 99.3 °F is considered a medical emergency in a neonate. Blood, cerebrospinal fluid, and urine must be sent for microscopic analysis and cultures for the most likely organisms. Neuroimaging with brain CT or MRI can be useful in identifying focal areas of infection, and repeat scans can be useful in assessing response to therapy and delineating injury to determine prognosis.

Outcomes of neonatal sepsis and meningitis vary and depend on the organ systems most severely involved. Meningitis and meningoencephalitis can be devastating, with cognitive impairment and hearing loss being among the most common complications. Up to 25% of newborns with bacterial or viral meningitis will have some degree of serious, lifelong neurological deficit (Grimwood et al., 1995); behavioral audiometry and vision testing should also be planned, since the risk for sensorineural hearing loss is particularly high following meningitis.

■ ■ ■ JUSTIN (CONTINUED)

Justin did not feed orally during his initial hospital stay and required surgical placement of a permanent feeding (gastrostomy) tube. Justin went home with his parents on tube feedings and was seen by a pediatric neurologist and developmental psychologist in a specialized infant development clinic (high risk clinic) at 6, 12, 18, and 24 months of age. By 6 months he demonstrated hypertonic extensor posturing with neck and back arching. The State's Infants and Toddlers Program was already involved, and referral was made specifically for physical therapy to assist his parents in providing exercises for increasing range of motion for his limbs. He was fitted for splints. Additionally, a referral to an audiologist was made because he had failed his neonatal and early infant hearing screens.

At 12 months of age Justin was clearly developmentally delayed. He could not sit without support, feed orally, or move and position his limbs without adult assistance. He had been fitted for glasses and hearing aids. By 18 months of age, the neurologist had diagnosed cerebral palsy affecting all limbs (spastic quadriplegia) and made a referral to the March of Dimes to support intervention. He was chronically medicated for epilepsy. By school age, he was in special placement for comprehensive care and was considered to have severe intellectual disability.

SUMMARY

Although the vast majority of infants make the transition from intrauterine to extrauterine life without difficulty, for some infants prenatal injuries, genetic disorders, malformations, environmental factors, including the birth process and subsequent hazards in the weeks immediately following birth, present challenges. Persistent pulmonary hypertension, hypoxic–ischemic encephalopathy, neonatal seizures, metabolic disturbances, neonatal stroke, and neonatal infection can result in neurodevelopmental disabilities and require aggressive medical intervention. Advances in perinatal and neonatal care provide hope that progress will continue to reduce the incidence of adverse outcomes.

REFERENCES

Barclay, L. (2011, March). ACOG endorses CDC guidelines for newborn group B strep prevention. *Medscape Medical News.* Retrieved from http://www.medscape.com/viewarticle/739334

Behnke, M., Eyler, F.D., Carter, R.L., Hardt, N., Cruz, A.C., & Resnick, M.B. (1988). The predictive value of Apgar scores for developmental outcome in low-birthweight infants. *American Journal of Perinatology, 6,* 18–21.

Bianioni, E., Mercuri, E., Rutherford, M.A., Cowan, F., Azzopardi, D., Frisone, M.F., ... Dubowitz, L. (2001). Combined use of EEG and MRI in full-term neonates with acute encephalopathy. *Pediatrics, 107*(3), 461–468.

Bland, R.D. (1992). Developmental changes in lung epithelial ion transport and liquid movement. *Annual Review of Physiology, 54,* 373.

Boardman, J.P., Ganesan, V., Rutherford, M.A., Saunders, D.E., Mercuri, E., & Cowan, F. (2005). Magnetic resonance image correlates of hemiparesis after neonatal and childhood middle cerebral artery stroke. *Pediatrics, 115,* 321–326.

Bruno, V.M.G., Goldberg, M.P., Dugan, L.L., Giffard, R.G., & Choi, D.W. (1994). Neuroprotective effect of hypothermia in cortical cultures exposed to oxygen-glucose deprivation or excitatory amino acids. *Journal of Neurochemistry, 63,* 1398–1406.

Connell, J., Oozeer, R., de Vries, L., Dubowitz, L.M.S., Dubowitz, V. (1989). Continuous EEG monitoring of neonatal seizures: Diagnostic and prognostic considerations. *Archives of Disease in Childhood, 64,* 452–458.

de Veber, G., Andrew, M., Adams, C., Bjornson, B., Booth, F., Buckley, D.J., ... Gillet, J. (for the Canadian Pediatric Ischemic Stroke Study Group). (2001). Cerebral sinovenous thrombosis in children. *New England Journal of Medicine, 345,* 417–423.

de Vries, L.S., & Jongmans, M.J. (2010). Long-term outcome after neonatal hypoxic-ischaemic encephalopathy. *Archives of Disease in Childhood, 95,* F220–F224. doi:10.1136/adc.2008.148205

Ferriero, D.M. (2004). Medical progress: Neonatal brain injury. *New England Journal of Medicine, 351,* 1985–1995.

Gluckman, P.D., Wyatt, J.S., Azzopardi, D., Ballard, R., Edwards, A.D., Ferriero, ... Gunn, A.J. (on behalf of the Cool Cap Study Group). (2005). Selective head cooling with mild systemic hypothermia after neonatal encephalopathy: Multicentre randomized trial. *Lancet, 365,* 663–70.

Grimwood, K., Anderson, V.A., Bond, L., Catroppa, C., Hore, R.L., Kier, E.H., ... Roberton, D.M. (1995). Adverse outcomes of bacterial meningitis in school-age survivors. *Pediatrics, 95,* 646–656.

Gunn, A.J., & Gunn, T.R. (1998). The 'pharmacology' of neuronal rescue with cerebral hypothermia. *Early Human Development, 53,* 19–35.

Hardy, J.B. (2003). The collaborative perinatal project: Lessons and legacy. *Annals of Epidemiology, 13*(5), 303–311.

Health Grades Inc. (2011). *Feeding problems in newborn.* Retrieved from http://www.rightdiagnosis.com/medical/feeding_problems_in_newborn.htm

Hoehn, T., Hansmann, G.B., Uhrer, C., Simbruner, G., Gunn, A.J., Yager, J., ... Thoresen, M. (2008). Therapeutic hypothermia in neonates: Review of current clinical data, ILCOR recommendations, and suggestions for implementation in neonatal intensive care units. *Resuscitation, 78,* 7–12. doi:10.1016/j.resuscitation.2008.04.027.

Jacobs, S. (2010, May). *ICE Trial Australia Through 2010.* Paper presented at Society for Pediatric Research, Vancouver, Canada.

Kim, J.S., Kondratyev, A., Tomita, Y., & Gale, K. (2007). Neurodevelopmental impact of antiepileptic drugs and seizures in the immature brain. *Epilepsia, 48*(Suppl 5), 19–26.

March of Dimes. (2010). *Amniotic fluid.* White Plains, NY: Author. Retrieved from http://www.marchofdimes.com/pregnancy/complications_amniotic.html

Massaro, A.N., Nadja Kadom, N., Chang, T., & Baumgart, S. (2010). MRI quantitative assessment in patients with neonatal encephalopathy (NE) treated with whole body hypothermia. *Journal of Perinatology, 30,* 596-603.

Mercuri, E., Barnett, A., Rutherford, M., Guzzetta, A., Haataja, L., Cioni, G., ... Dubowitz, L. (2004). Neonatal cerebral infarction and neuromotor outcome at school age. *Pediatrics, 113,* 95–100.

Rutherford, M., Counsell, S., Allsop, J., Boardman, J., Kapellou, O., Larkman, D., ... Cowan, F. (2004). Diffusion-weighted magnetic resonance imaging in term perinatal brain injury: A comparison with site of lesion and time from birth. *Pediatrics, 114,* 1004–1014.

Sarnat, H.B., & Sarnat, M.S. (1976). Neonatal encephalopathy following fetal distress. *Archives of Neurology, 33,* 696–705.

Shankaran, S., Laptook, A.R., Ehrenkranz, R.A., Tyson, J.E., McDonald, S.A., Donovan, E.F. ... Jobe, A.H. (for the National Institute of Child Health and Human Development Neonatal Research Network). (2005). Whole body hypothermia for neonates with hypoxic-ischemic encephalopathy. *New England Journal of Medicine, 353,* 1574–1584.

Simbruner, G., Mittal, R.A., Rohlmann, F., Muche, R., & neo.nEURO.network Trial Participants. (2010). Systemic hypothermia after neonatal encephalopathy: Outcomes of neo.nEURO.network, RCT. *Pediatrics, 126,* e771–e778.

Smith, D.W. (1976). Oligohydramnios sequence (Potter syndrome). In *Recognizable patterns of human malformation,* (3rd ed., pp. 484-485). pp. 484–485. Philadelphia, PA: Saunders.

Welty, S., Hansen, T.N., & Corbet, A. (2005). Respiratory distress in the preterm infant. In H.W. Taeusch, R.A. Ballard, & C.A. Gleason (Eds.), *Avery's diseases of the newborn* (8th ed.). Philadelphia, PA: Saunders/ Elsevier.

Whitelaw, A., & Thoresen, M. (2002). Clinical trials of treatments after perinatal asphyxia. *Current Opinion in Pediatrics, 14,* 664–668.

Wu, Y.W., March, W.M., Croen, L.A., Grether, J.K., Excobar, G.J., & Newman, T.B. (2004). Perinatal stroke in children with motor impairment: A population-based study. *Pediatrics, 114,* 612–619.

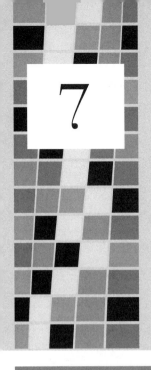

7

Premature and Small-for-Dates Infants

Khodayar Rais-Bahrami and Billie Lou Short

Upon completion of this chapter, the reader will

■ Recognize some of the causes of prematurity and being small for gestational age

■ Be able to identify physical characteristics of the premature infant

■ Understand the complications and illnesses associated with preterm birth

■ Be aware of the methods used to care for low birth weight infants

■ Know the results of outcome studies

The preterm infant is at an immediate disadvantage compared with the full-term infant. In addition to facing all of the usual challenges of making the transition from intrauterine to extrauterine life (see Chapter 6), the preterm infant must make these changes using organs that are not yet ready to perform the task. Almost every organ is immature (Hyman, Novoa, & Holzman, 2009). Decreased production of a substance called surfactant in the lungs can lead to respiratory distress syndrome (RDS); immaturity of the central nervous system places the preterm infant at increased risk for an **intraventricular hemorrhage** (IVH), **periventricular leukomalacia** (PVL), and **hydrocephalus;** and inadequate kidney function makes fluid and metabolic management difficult. An immature gastrointestinal tract impairs the infant's ability to digest and absorb certain nutrients and places the gut at risk for developing a life-threatening disorder called **necrotizing enterocolitis** (NEC), that results from inadequate blood supply. Finally, the preterm infant's eyes are more susceptible to the damaging effects of the oxygen that is used to treat respiratory distress. This may result in **retinopathy of prematurity** (ROP) and potential for subsequent vision loss (see Chapter 11). Given these risks, it is remarkable that most preterm infants overcome these acute problems with little residual effects. A minority, however, do sustain long-term medical and neurodevelopmental complications. A discussion of these complications and their prevention is the focus of this chapter.

■ ■ ■ ERIN

Erin was born prematurely, at 23 weeks' gestation, and weighed less than 500 grams (about 1 pound). During Erin's first day of life, she needed artificial ventilation and surfactant therapy to keep the air passages in her lungs open. By 2 months of age, she was doing well

87

enough to receive a pressurized oxygen–air mixture through a high flow **nasal cannula** (HFNC-Vapotherm), but she had brief breathing arrests (**apnea**) associated with a slowed heart rate (**bradycardia**). These problems were treated successfully with caffeine and frequent physical stimulation. In addition, she developed NEC, leading to bowel perforation that required two major abdominal surgeries 10 weeks apart.

Meeting Erin's nutritional requirements was also a problem. Initially, she needed intravenous nutrition. Gradually, she was able to tolerate increasing amounts of elemental infant formula by a nasogastric tube, and by 3 months, she was strong enough to receive some of her feedings by bottle. At her 168th day of life (i.e., postconceptional age of 45 weeks), weighing 3,760 grams (8 pounds, 4½ ounces), Erin went home on oxygen and caffeine and was hooked up to an apnea monitor while taking all feedings by mouth. Her parents had been instructed how to administer oxygen therapy, how to use the monitor, and how to administer cardiopulmonary resuscitation (CPR) in an emergency. Although her overall prognosis is good, Erin will need continued medical and neurodevelopmental monitoring until she is school age.

DEFINITIONS OF PREMATURITY AND LOW BIRTH WEIGHT

A preterm or premature infant is one born at 36 weeks gestation or before. Although there is no universal system for birth-weight classification, it is commonly accepted that an infant with a birth weight less than 2,500 grams (5½ pounds) is **low birth weight** (LBW); an infant born weighing less than 1,500 grams (3⅓ pounds) is **very low birth weight** (VLBW); and an infant with a birth weight lower than 1,000 grams (2¼ pounds) is **extremely low birth weight** (ELBW). An infant weighing less than 800 grams (1¾ pounds) is sometimes called a **micro-preemie** (Dani, Poggi, Romangnoli, & Bertini, 2009). Assessment of gestational age is also important, because infants of low birth weight may represent prematurely born infants or those who are **small for gestational age** (SGA).

Small for Gestational Age Infants

Infants can be either full term or premature. In either case, they have a birth weight below the 10th percentile for a graph of population-specific birth weight verses gestational age (Figure 7.1). SGA infants are also referred to as dysmature or small for dates. In addition to being small, these infants also appear malnourished, usually because

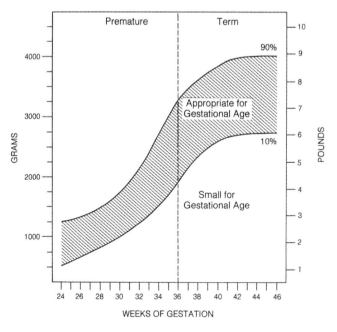

Figure 7.1. Newborn weight by gestational age. The shaded area between the 10th and 90th percentiles represents infants who are appropriate for gestational age. Weight below the 10th percentile makes an infant small for gestational age (SGA). Prematurity is defined as being born before 36 weeks' gestation. (From Lubchenco, L.O. [1976]. *The high risk infant.* Philadelphia: W.B. Saunders; reprinted by permission.)

of **intrauterine growth restriction** (IUGR). About one half of SGA births are attributable to maternal illness, smoking, or malnutrition (Grivell, Dodd, & Robinson, 2009). These infants tend to be underweight but have normal length and head circumference; they are said to have asymmetric SGA because of this discrepancy in growth pattern. The other half of SGA births are said to have symmetric SGA (equally deviant in length, weight, and head circumference). These infants may have been exposed *in utero* to alcohol or to infections such as cytomegalovirus. Infants with certain chromosomal and other genetic disorders also present as symmetrical SGA infants (Suresh, Horbar, Kenny, Carpenter, & Vermont Oxford Network, 2001). SGA infants, whether full term or preterm, are recognized as having an increased risk for many complications in the newborn period (e.g., hypoxia, hypothermia, hypoglycemia), increased perinatal and neonatal mortality, long-term growth impairments, and developmental disabilities (Argente, Mehls, & Barrios, 2010; Bottino, Cowett, & Sinclair, 2009; Casey, 2008; de Bie, Oostrom, & Delemarre-van de Wall, 2010; McCall, Alderdice, Halliday, Jenins, & Vohra, 2010; McCowan & Horgan, 2009; Sinclair, Bottino, & Cowett, 2009).

Assessment of Gestational Age

Assessment of gestational age helps distinguish an appropriate-for-gestational-age infant from an SGA infant. In addition, it influences treatment approaches, neurodevelopmental assessment, and outcome. The gestational age is calculated from the projected birth date, or estimated date of confinement (EDC). This can be obtained using the Nägele rule: Add 7 days and subtract 3 months from the date of the last menstrual period. The accuracy of menstrual dating, however, is quite variable, especially in anticipated preterm deliveries. In most cases, uterine size is an accurate predictor of gestational age and can be measured by clinical and ultrasound examination. Another way of estimating gestational age is by noting when fetal activity first develops. **Quickening** is first felt by the mother at approximately 16–18 weeks' gestation. Fetal heart sounds can be first detected at approximately 10–12 weeks by ultrasound and at 20 weeks by fetoscope (similar to a stethoscope). Following birth, gestational age can be assessed using a clinical scoring system called the modified Dubowitz examination (discussed next). Another technique allows for estimating the degree of prematurity by examining the maturity of the lens of the eye in the first 24–48 hours of life (Nagpal, Kumar, & Ramji,

2004). Using a combination of these methods increases the accuracy of gestational age assessment.

Physical and Behavioral Characteristics of the Premature Infant

Several physical and developmental characteristics distinguish the premature infant from the full-term infant. A scoring system developed by Dubowitz, Dubowitz, and Goldberg (1970) and updated by Ballard et al. (1991; Figure 7.2), takes these characteristics into account and enables the physician to estimate the infant's gestational age with some accuracy. The limitation of this scoring system is the postnatal age of the infant. If the scoring is not performed within the first 24 hours of birth, neurological and some physical features (e.g., skin texture) can change, making the infant appear more mature. Also, any severely ill infant can be difficult to evaluate due to altered neurological status.

The main physical characteristics that distinguish a premature infant from a full-term infant are the presence in the premature infant of fine body hair (**lanugo**) and smooth, reddish skin, along with the absence of skin creases, ear cartilage, and breast buds (Figure 7.3). In addition to the physical appearance, premature infants display distinctive neurological and behavioral characteristics, including reduced muscle tone and activity and increased joint mobility (Constantine et al., 1987). Low muscle tone is particularly evident in the infant born before 28 weeks' gestation; it gradually improves with advancing gestational age, starting with the legs and moving up to the arms by 32 weeks' gestational age. Thus, although the premature infant lies in a floppy, extended position, the full-term infant rests in a semi-flexed position. As flexion tone improves over the weeks after birth, increased joint mobility disappears. Finally, as compared with the full-term infant, the premature infant may appear behaviorally passive and disorganized in the first weeks of life (Mandrich, Simons, Ritchie, Schmidt, & Mullet, 1994).

INCIDENCE OF PRETERM BIRTHS

Preterm birth occurs in about 13% of all pregnancies worldwide. While this represents a minority of pregnancies, it is responsible for the majority of neonatal deaths and nearly one half of all cases of neonatal-onset neurodevelopmental disabilities, including cerebral palsy

(Nelson, 2008). The risk is highest in infants born before 32 weeks' gestation, representing 2% of all births. The incidence of preterm births has declined by 1% since 2006, but overall has risen 16% since 1990; furthermore, preterm births occur twice as frequently in African Americans as in Caucasians. Of LBW infants weighing less than 2,500 grams, 70% are preterm and 30% are full-term infants who are SGA (Heron et al., 2010).

CAUSES OF PREMATURE BIRTH

The rise in reported rates of preterm delivery is certainly a cause for concern and has been attributed to many co-factors including: increased obstetric intervention (e.g., Cesarean sections), use of assisted reproduction techniques (e.g., in vitro fertilizations), high number of multiple pregnancies from fertility drugs, increased prevalence of substance abuse

Neuromuscular Maturity

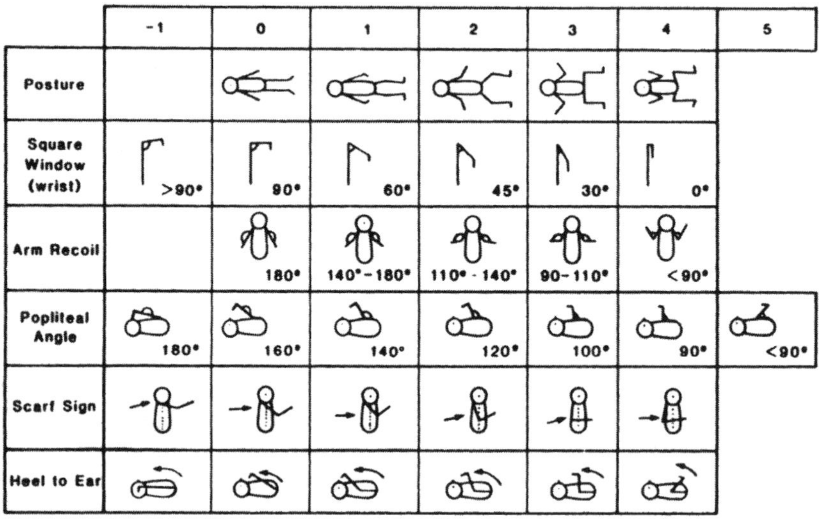

Physical Maturity

Skin	sticky friable transparent	gelatinous red, translucent	smooth pink, visible veins	superficial peeling &/or rash. few veins	cracking pale areas rare veins	parchment deep cracking no vessels	leathery cracked wrinkled
Lanugo	none	sparse	abundant	thinning	bald areas	mostly bald	
Plantar Surface	heel-toe 40-50 mm: -1 <40 mm: -2	>50mm no crease	faint red marks	anterior transverse crease only	creases ant. 2/3	creases over entire sole	
Breast	imperceptible	barely perceptible	flat areola no bud	stippled areola 1-2mm bud	raised areola 3-4mm bud	full areola 5-10mm bud	
Eye/Ear	lids fused loosely: -1 tightly: -2	lids open pinna flat stays folded	sl. curved pinna; soft; slow recoil	well-curved pinna; soft but ready recoil	formed &firm instant recoil	thick cartilage ear stiff	
Genitals male	scrotum flat, smooth	scrotum empty faint rugae	testes in upper canal rare rugae	testes descending few rugae	testes down good rugae	testes pendulous deep rugae	
Genitals female	clitoris prominent labia flat	prominent clitoris small labia minora	prominent clitoris enlarging minora	majora & minora equally prominent	majora large minora small	majora cover clitoris & minora	

Maturity Rating

score	weeks
-10	20
-5	22
0	24
5	26
10	28
15	30
20	32
25	34
30	36
35	38
40	40
45	42
50	44

Figure 7.2. Scoring system to assess newborn infants. The score for each of the neuromuscular and physical signs is added together to obtain a score called the "total maturity score." Gestational age is determined from this score. (This figure was published in *Journal of Pediatrics*, *119*, 418, Ballard, J.L., Khoury, J.C., Wedig, K., et al. New Ballard score, expanded to include extremely premature infants, Copyright Elsevier, 1991; reprinted by permission.)

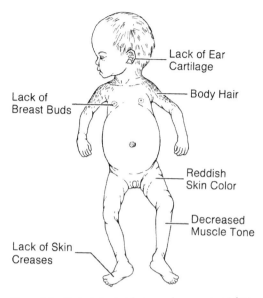

Figure 7.3. Typical physical features of a premature infant.

in urban areas, a rise in idiopathic preterm delivery rates due to the adverse effect of low socioeconomic factors, and maternal educational level (Morgen, Bjork, & Andersen, 2008; Shah, 2010). Other common causes of preterm delivery are maternal infections and adolescent pregnancies, conditions that often co-occur. Although less than 3% of all pregnancies occur in adolescents, these pregnancies account for 14%–18% of all preterm births. Maternal age under 18 years is a major risk factor for complications in both mothers and neonates, especially in mothers aged younger than 15 years (Najati & Gojazadeh 2010). In addition, up to 80% of early preterm births (births before 30 weeks' gestation) are associated with an intrauterine infection that precedes the rupture of membranes (Klein & Gibbs, 2005). Other risk factors include inadequate prenatal care, poverty, acute and chronic maternal illness, multiple-gestation births, history of previous premature pregnancies, placental bleeding, preeclampsia, smoking, and substance abuse (Morgen et al., 2008). Congenital anomalies or injuries to the fetus may also lead to premature birth. Certain fetal conditions such as **Rh incompatibility** and poor fetal growth may require early delivery.

COMPLICATIONS OF PREMATURITY

The premature infant must undergo the same physiologic transitions to extrauterine life as the full-term infant (see Chapter 6). The preterm infant, however, must accomplish this difficult task using immature body organs. The result is a significant risk of complications in virtually every organ system in the body. This risk increases with the degree of prematurity.

Respiratory Problems

Respiratory problems are one of the most common and potentially life threatening problems for premature infants born before 34 weeks. These problems result from the immaturity of the fetal lungs and the lack of production of surfactin. We will discuss the acute respiratory issue of hyaline membrane disease as well as the potential long-term consequences leading to bronchoplulmonary dysplasia.

Hyaline Membrane Disease

Hyaline membrane disease (HMD), also called respiratory distress syndrome (RDS), is a disorder characterized by respiratory distress in the newborn period. The underlying abnormality is decreased production of surfactant that normally keeps the alveoli (the terminal airway passages) stable, permitting the exchange of oxygen and carbon dioxide (Figure 7.4). A chest x ray can clinically confirm HMD, showing a "ground glass" appearance of the lungs. This results from the collapsed alveoli appearing dense and hazy in comparison with the air-filled lung of a typical full-term newborn, which appears translucent and black (Figure 7.5). The clinical course of HMD involves peak severity between 24 and 48 hours after birth, followed by improvement over the next 24–48 hours. In uncomplicated cases, HMD will resolve within 72–96 hours after birth. This classical course of HMD has fortunately been modified by the administration of exogenous surfactant replacement (Wirbelauer & Speer, 2009). Improvement in pulmonary function usually begins within minutes after the first dose of surfactant is injected through the trachea, and after one or two doses of surfactant, effective gas exchange can be achieved with a significantly lower level of oxygen and ventilatory support. Except in severe cases of HMD, it is unusual for an infant to require more than two doses of surfactant.

Infants with mild HMD generally do well with supplemental oxygen alone or in combination with **continuous positive airway pressure** (CPAP). CPAP involves providing a mixture of oxygen and air under continuous pressure; this prevents the alveoli from collapsing between breaths. More severely affected infants may require the placement of an endotracheal tube for mechanical ventilatory support as well as administration of exogenous

Inflated Alveolus in Full-term Infant

Collapsed Alveolus in Premature with RDS

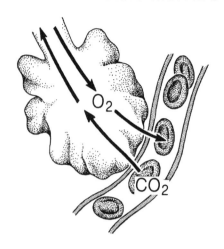

Figure 7.4. Schematic drawing of alveoli in a normal newborn and in a premature infant with respiratory distress syndrome (RDS). Note that the inflated alveolus is kept open by surfactant. Oxygen (O_2) moves from the alveolus to the red blood cells in the pulmonary capillary. Carbon dioxide (CO_2) moves in the opposite direction. This exchange is much less efficient when the alveolus is collapsed; the result is hypoxia.

surfactant. Although surfactant therapy has significantly reduced mortality in ELBW premature infants, there has been no appreciable change in long-term pulmonary and neurodevelopmental complications in these infants (Patrianakos-Hoobler et al., 2010). Therefore, close follow up to school entry is important.

A related approach to treating surfactant deficiency is to stimulate its production. There is evidence that administration of steroids to mothers 24–36 hours before delivery stimulates surfactant production and pulmonary maturation in the fetus. This lessens the likelihood and/or severity of HMD. The effect of antenatal steroids is additive to postnatal surfactant replacement therapy in reducing respiratory distress and mortality. It is therefore recommended that **steroids** be given prior to birth for potential preterm delivery of fetuses between 24 and 34 weeks' gestational age (NIH Consensus Development Panel on the Effect of Corticosteroids for Fetal Maturation on Perinatal Outcomes, 1995).

Bronchopulmonary Dysplasia

The improved survival of ELBW newborns has increased the number of infants at risk for various forms of respiratory morbidity associated with mechanical ventilation, including **bronchopulmonary dysplasia** (BPD). This term is generally used to describe infants who require supplemental oxygen and/or mechanical ventilation beyond

28 days postnatal age and/or corrected gestational age of 36 weeks and who have persistently abnormal chest x rays and respiratory examinations (e.g., rapid breathing, wheezing). BPD primarily occurs in infants who are born at less than 32 weeks' gestation and require mechanical ventilation during the first week of life for treatment of HMD. Although the frequency of BPD in VLBW neonates is high, in the majority of cases the disease is mild. Severe BPD is more common in neonates with associated comorbidities such as late-onset sepsis or advanced intraventricular hemorrhage (Walsh et al., 2005; Woynarowska, Rutkowska, & Szamotulska, 2008).

The development of BPD has been attributed to lung injury from a combination of barotrauma (pressure damage from prolonged mechanical ventilation), oxygen toxicity, infection, and inflammation; the exact mechanism of BPD remains poorly understood. Since the 1970s, newer methods of respiratory support, including high-frequency ventilation and surfactant therapy, have increased the survival rate of smaller and less mature infants, but the total number of infants who develop BPD has not decreased. BPD remains the most common chronic lung disease of infancy in the United States, with some 7,000 new cases being diagnosed each year. Long-term studies of pulmonary function in this population indicate that as these infants grow, there is clinical improvement. Children with mild BPD exhibit impairments in respiratory mechanics and lung

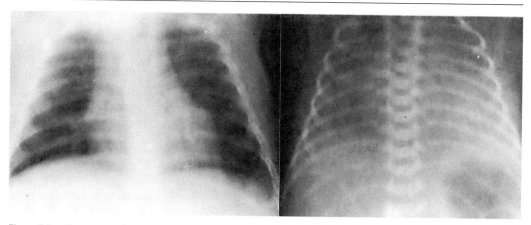

Figure 7.5. Chest x rays of a normal newborn (left) and of a premature infant with respiratory distress syndrome (RDS; right), which shows a "white out" of the lungs due to surfactant deficiency.

structure. The widespread involvement of the peripheral airways suggests that all children diagnosed with BPD are potentially at risk of developing chronic obstructive pulmonary disease later in life. As a result, abnormalities in airway resistance and pulmonary compliance persist into adulthood, resulting in a high risk of reactive airway disease (RAD) or asthma (Broström et al., 2010).

Approaches to postnatal prevention and treatment of BPD have included steroid therapy, supplemental vitamin A, high-frequency ventilation, use of bronchodilators (asthma medication), and administration of diuretics to increase urinary excretion of excessive lung fluids. The use of postnatal steroid medication such as dexamethasone (Decadron) for prevention and treatment of BPD has been a matter of controversy. Although early postnatal corticosteroid treatment facilitates extubation and reduces the risk of BPD, it can cause short-term adverse effects including gastrointestinal bleeding, intestinal perforation, hyperglycemia, hypertension, hypertrophic cardiomyopathy, and growth failure. There is also the potential for steroids having long-term effects on physical growth and neurodevelopment. Long-term follow-up studies report an increased risk of abnormal neurological examination and cerebral palsy (Halliday, Ehrenkranz, & Doyle, 2009).

It is not unusual for infants with BPD to require prolonged support with supplemental oxygen, diuretics, and bronchodilators after discharge from the hospital. Even with supportive care and treatment, infants with BPD may continue to have long-term problems, including limited tolerance of physical activity, feeding difficulties that contribute to poor physical growth, excessive caloric requirement, and an increased risk of developmental disabilities (Valleur-Masson et al., 1993).

Neurologic Problems

Premature infants are also at increased risk for neurologic problems that are often linked to their respiratory problems. These problems include bleeding into the brain (intraventricular hemorrhage), damage to the white matter of the brain (periventricular leukomalicia), damage to hearing from antibiotic use, and periods of respiratory arrest and heart slowing (apnea and bradycardia).

Intraventricular Hemorrhage

Intraventricular hemorrhage (IVH), defined as bleeding into the ventricular space within the brain hemispheres, is an important neurological complication of extremely premature infants. The risk of IVH correlates directly with the degree of prematurity. Fortunately, its incidence appears to be declining. About half of IVH cases occur during the first day of life, and 90% occur by the third day of life (Bassan, 2009; Owens, 2005). Ultrasound of the head is the most reliable and safest technique for diagnosis of IVH. The American Academy of Neurology Practice Parameter for "Neuroimaging of the Neonate" suggests that an initial screening ultrasound shortly after birth be performed on all preterm neonates of <30 weeks' gestation to detect signs of IVH. In addition, they recommend a follow-up ultrasound at 36–40 weeks postmenstrual age in order to detect CNS lesions such as periventricular leukomalacia and ventriculomegaly, which will affect long-term outcomes (Ment et al., 2002; Vassilyadi, Tataryn, Shamji, & Ventureyra, 2009). Magnetic resonance imaging (MRI) is better than ultrasound at detecting white matter abnormalities, hemorrhagic lesions, and cysts. Emerging data are providing evidence for the importance of this imaging modality at term-equivalent as a predictor of neurological outcome in VLBW preterm infants (El-Dib, Massaro, Buas, & Aly, 2010).

IVH is commonly graded by severity into four levels (Volpe, 2008). Grade I is defined by bleeding into the germinal matrix, a network of blood vessels in the roof of the lateral ventricles. If the hemorrhage expands beyond the germinal matrix into the ventricular system, it is Grade II. Grades I and II account for the majority of IVH cases, and significant neurological impairment is fortunately rare with these types. About 20% of hemorrhages, however, are severe enough to dilate the ventricle (Grade III) or invade the brain substance (Grade IV). Grade IV is often called *periventricular hemorrhagic infarction*. These hemorrhages can lead to periventricular leukomalacia (PVL), or damage of the white matter surrounding the ventricles (Volpe, 2008). The long-term neurological outcome for infants with IVH is related to the severity of the hemorrhage. Cerebral palsy (with or without intellectual disability) is seen in 30% of patients with Grade III hemorrhages and in 75% of those with Grade IV hemorrhages (Pleacher, Vohr, Katz, Ment, & Allan, 2004; Sarkar, Bhagat, Dechert, Schumacher, & Donn, 2009).

Avoidance of hypoxic–ischemic events that lead to fluctuations in cerebral blood pressure, expert delivery room stabilization, effective resuscitation and ventilation, gentle handling, and use of muscle relaxants during mechanical ventilation have all been associated with a reduction in the incidence and severity of IVH (Volpe, 2008). A number of medications have been studied for preventing or treating IVH, with varied results. These include antenatal use of steroids and postnatal use of phenobarbital, vitamin K, vitamin E, indomethacin, ethamsylate, ibuprofen, and recombinant activated factor VIIa (McCrea & Ment 2008).

Periventricular Leukomalacia

The periventricular white matter is the region of the brain closest to the ventricles. PVL results when this area sustains damage either due to low oxygen or low blood flow. This area is especially vulnerable to injury in the premature infant. This is because the glial cells, a major constituent of white matter, undergo rapid growth by the end of the second trimester and are more susceptible to injury caused by

fluctuations in cerebral blood pressure during this period. There is also evidence that maternal infection involving the membranes surrounding the fetus (chorioamnionitis) increases the risk of PVL. (Blumenthal, 2004; Volpe, 2001).

PVL has been reported to occur in 4%–15% of premature infants (Perlman, Risser, & Broyles, 1996). It may occur in association with IVH or independently (Figure 7.6). The diagnosis of PVL is best made by serial cranial (head) ultrasounds that may show the development of cystic lesions in the white matter. Serial cranial ultrasounds or an MRI at near term gestation or at term-equivalent gestation in VLBW neonates also have been shown to be important predictors of the subsequent development of **spastic diplegia** (a form of cerebral palsy that impairs lower extremity function) and **hemiplegia** (a form of cerebral palsy that affects one side of the body; Mirmiran et al., 2004; see Chapter 24). Large cysts (greater than 3 millimeters in diameter) place the neonate at increased risk of developing **spastic quadriplegia** (a form of cerebral palsy that affects all four limbs), visual impairment, intellectual disability, and seizures in early childhood (Okumura et al., 2003).

Auditory Toxicity

ELBW infants are at increased risk for hearing loss because of multisystem illness and the frequent use of medications, such as aminoglycoside antibiotics and diuretics, that can be toxic to the auditory system. The overall prevalence of sensorineural hearing impairment is about 4 per 10,000 in full-term infants. This increases to 13 per 10,000 in LBW infants and to 51 per 10,000 among VLBW infants (Robertson, Howarth, Bork, & Dinu, 2009; Van Naarden & Decoufle, 1999). In 1995, the Joint Committee on Infant Hearing recommended that all VLBW infants undergo auditory screening. The committee further expanded this statement in 2000 to advocate testing for all newborns. The most commonly performed tests are brainstem auditory evoked response (BAER) and **otoacoustic emission** (OAE; Ohl, Dornier, Czajka, Chobaut, & Tavernier, 2009).

Apnea and Bradycardia

Apnea is clinically defined as a respiratory pause lasting 15–20 seconds, associated with a decrease in heart rate to below 80–100 beats per minute. It is the most common disorder of respiratory control found in the neonatal intensive care unit (NICU) and is related to immaturity of the central nervous system. About

10% of all LBW infants and more than 40% of VLBW infants experience clinically significant apnea (Baird, 2004).

Apnea of prematurity (AOP) remains a major clinical problem and requires the neonatologist to make treatment choices, which are sometimes difficult. AOP occurs in most infants of gestational age less than 33 weeks (Abu-Shaweesh & Martin, 2008). It is a developmental disorder that usually reflects a physiological immaturity of brain control of respiration. However, neonatal diseases may be associated with AOP and play an additive role, resulting in an increased incidence of apnea. Careful screening should therefore be performed in order to make sure that no factor other than immaturity is involved in the occurrence of apnea. Short apnea (less than 10 seconds, without bradycardia and/or desaturation) is not clinically relevant. Prolonged apnea is defined as lasting for more than 15 or 20 seconds and/or is associated with bradycardia or oxygen desaturation. Prolonged apnea results in short-term disturbances of cerebral hemodynamics and oxygenation, which may negatively affect neurodevelopmental outcome. Treatment involves the administration of caffeine, which has been shown to reduce the

incidence of apnea and decrease the risk of bronchopulmonary dysplasia, patent ductus arteriosus, and subsequent development of cerebral palsy (Moriette, Lescure, El Ayoubi, & Lopez, 2010; Pillekamp, Hermann, von Gontard, Kribs, & Roth, 2007).

Sudden Infant Death Syndrome

Sudden infant death syndrome (SIDS) occurs more than twice as frequently in premature infants as in full-term infants, usually between 2 and 5 months of life (Kinney & Thach, 2009; Mitchell, 2009; Ostfeld, Esposito, Perl, & Hegyi, 2010). Contrary to earlier beliefs, apnea of prematurity is not a major predisposing factor for SIDS. However, because of the increased incidence of SIDS among this population, extremely premature infants who are having significant apneic spells in the 2 weeks before discharge may be sent home with an apnea monitor (Committee on Fetus and Newborn, American Academy of Pediatrics, 2003). Although these monitors emit an alarm if the infant stops breathing and alerts the parents to intervene, studies on their use have not shown effectiveness in reducing the occurrence of SIDS. The monitors do, however, provide

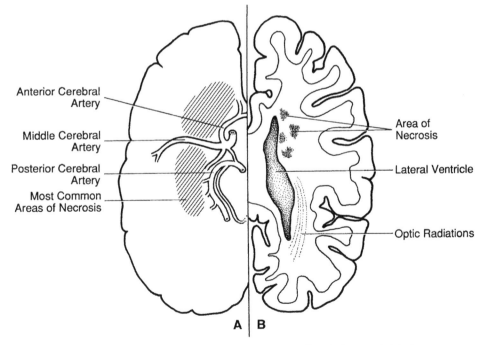

Figure 7.6. Periventricular leukomalacia (PVL). A) The blood vessel supply to the brain, and B) the brain structures. The area of the white matter surrounding the lateral ventricle (particularly the top part) is especially susceptible to hypoxic-ischemic damage because it is not well supplied by blood vessels. It lies in a watershed area between the anterior, middle, and posterior cerebral arteries. In premature infants, poor oxygenation and decreased blood flow associated with respiratory distress syndrome (RDS) may lead to necrosis of this brain tissue, a condition termed *periventricular leukomalacia*. When the posterior portion is affected, the optic radiations may be damaged, resulting in cortical blindness.

reassurance to parents and physicians about the status of the infant. Parents of such high-risk infants should be trained in neonatal CPR prior to taking their infant home on an apnea monitor. The monitor is generally not required for more than a few months.

In 1992, in an effort to prevent SIDS, the American Academy of Pediatrics' Task Force on Infant Position and SIDS, began recommending that infants be placed on their back for sleep. In addition, the Task Force recommended that fluffy blankets and toys not be placed in an infant's crib during sleep times and that the home environment be smoke free. These changes have resulted in a 40% reduction in the incidence of SIDS (Gibson, Dembofsky, Rubin, & Greenspan, 2000).

Cardiovascular Problems

The most common cardiovascular problem in LBW infants is a **patent ductus arteriosus (PDA)**. The ductus arteriosus is the fetal vessel that diverts blood flow from the lungs. It normally closes at birth, allowing blood to flow to the lungs and be oxygenated. About 30% of all premature infants, and more than 50% of those born weighing less than 1,000 grams, will have a patent (open) ductus arteriosus diagnosed during the first few days of life (Hamrick & Hansmann, 2010). This is especially true in premature infants who have RDS. In these children, a PDA will divert blood from the lungs and further decrease oxygenation to the body and brain, increasing the work of the heart. This can lead to hypoxia, decreased blood flow to specific organs, and heart failure. The presence of a PDA can be detected by echocardiography, a form of ultrasound of the heart. Its management involves medical and supportive measures, including fluid restriction, diuresis (stimulation of urination), and the use of CPAP. If these measures fail, closure is possible using medications such as indomethacin or ibuprofen. In a small percentage of infants, surgical closure is required (Noori, 2010; Ohlsson, Walia, & Shah, 2010).

Gastrointestinal Problems

Although premature infants may be born with a suck-and-swallow response, it is immature and poorly coordinated until approximately 32 to 34 weeks' gestation. Thus, most premature infants require nasogastric or nasojejunal tube feedings until they can make the transition to oral feeds (Premji & Chessell, 2001). The nutritional needs of the premature infant are also different from those of the full-term infant and thus require the use of specialty formulas. In addition to physiological problems, premature infants are at increased risk for two major gastrointestinal disorders—necrotizing enterocolitis (NEC) and **gastroesophageal reflux disease (GERD)**—that can inhibit growth and be life threatening.

Necrotizing Enterocolitis

NEC is the most commonly acquired life-threatening intestinal disease in premature infants (Bradshaw, 2009; Henry & Moss, 2009; Thompson & Bizzarro, 2008). It involves severe injury to a portion of the bowel wall. The exact cause of NEC is unknown, but prematurity appears to be the most common predisposing factor. Approximately 80% of infants with NEC are born at less than 38 weeks' gestation and weigh less than 2,500 grams at birth. Other predisposing factors include fetal distress, premature rupture of membranes, low Apgar scores, and exchange transfusion (where blood is gradually removed from the newborn and replaced with matched adult blood to treat Rh incompatibility). The incidence of NEC is 1–2 per 1,000 live births, and the overall mortality rate for infants with NEC is 20%. The mortality rate of ELBW infants with NEC, however, is greater than 40% (Snyder et al., 1997).

Medical management of NEC involves withholding feedings, applying nasogastric suction to decrease pressure on the bowel wall, administering antibiotics to fight the suspected underlying infection, and providing intravenous fluids and nutrition to prevent dehydration and weight loss. Although medical treatment can be successful in many infants with NEC, approximately half require surgery to remove the diseased section of the bowel (Chandler & Hebra, 2000). Survivors of NEC may experience a variety of postoperative complications related to the disease, the operation, or treatment measures. For example, surgery for NEC is the leading cause of short bowel syndrome in infancy (Horwitz et al., 1995). The removal of a large portion of the bowel leads to decreased absorption of nutrients. This occurs in up to 11% of postsurgical NEC survivors and results in chronic diarrhea, malabsorption, nutritional deficiencies, impaired growth, and the long-term need for intravenous nutrition (e.g., fats, carbohydrates, amino acids).

Gastroesophageal Reflux Disease

The immaturity of gastric sphincter muscular control and delayed stomach emptying in premature infants may result in GERD, a syndrome in which the contents of the stomach are regurgitated back into the **esophagus** (Birch & Newell, 2009). Infants with severe GERD are at increased risk for vomiting and **aspiration pneumonia** (a lung infection precipitated by the **aspiration** of food into the lung), which may be worsened by nasogastric tube feedings. Signs of GERD include refusal of oral feeding, apnea, irritability, and back arching. Treatment is targeted toward special positioning techniques and medications (see Chapter 9).

Ophthalmologic Problems

Abnormalities in retinal vascular development after preterm birth lead to retinopathy of prematurity (ROP), formerly called retrolental fibroplasia. ELBW infants are at the greatest risk for developing ROP (Askin &Diehl-Jones 2009; Sylvester, 2008). A pediatric ophthalmologist should perform an examination for early detection of ROP at 4–6 weeks after birth or at 32–33 weeks' gestation (whichever comes first). Follow-up examinations should be done until retinal vascularization is complete, around term gestation (see Chapter 11). Preventive therapy with early human milk feeding and vitamins A and E supplements may decrease the severity of ROP in susceptible infants (Porcelli & Weaver, 2010). Severe ROP is treated by laser to prevent permanent retinal detachment.

Immunologic Problems

The premature infant is born with an immature immune system. As a result, the infant is at increased risk for infection in the first months of life (Klein & Gibbs, 2005). Generalized bacterial and fungal infections, occurring in approximately 30% of extremely premature infants, are major life-threatening illnesses and can lead to a poor neurodevelopmental outcome (Wheater & Renie, 2000). Premature infants who remain in the hospital for prolonged periods should receive routine immunizations based on their chronological age.

Other Physiologic Abnormalities

Premature infants are at increased risk for many of the same transient physiological abnormalities that occur in full-term infants (see Chapter 6). These include hyperbilirubinemia, anemia, hypoglycemia, hyperglycemia, hypocalcemia, and hypothermia. These problems place the premature infant at increased risk for brain damage.

Acidosis and hypoxia, resulting from inadequate respiration, can increase the permeability of the blood–brain barrier to bilirubin, making preterm infants more susceptible to kernicterus. Thus, the bilirubin level that is used to determine whether phototherapy or an exchange transfusion should be performed is lower for the preterm infant than for the full-term infant (Watchko & Maisels, 2010). **Glucose** and **electrolyte** instability are also common in premature infants, especially the micropreemie.

Anemia is also more of a problem for the premature infant than for the full-term infant because it decreases the oxygen-carrying capacity of the red blood cells and can lead to hypoxic–ischemic brain damage. Preterm infants, especially ELBW infants, are exposed to frequent blood draws as part of their care in the NICU. ELBW infants develop anemia of prematurity due to inadequate production of erythropoietin. In severe cases (based on indications and guidelines that are relatively nonspecific: hematocrit/hemoglobin levels, ventilation and oxygen need, apneas, bradycardias, and poor weight gain), anemia of prematurity is corrected with blood transfusion and/or treatment with erythropoietin to stimulate the bone marrow to produce red blood cells (Bishara & Ohls, 2009). In recent years, studies evaluating transfusion guidelines have shown that changes in transfusion practices have significantly reduced the need for transfusion in the LBW premature infant and reduced the need for erythropoietin (which is very costly and does not affect the transfusion requirement) in ELBW infants (Bishara & Ohls, 2009).

Finally, premature infants often have a transient deficiency of thyroid hormone production. In severe cases, this condition may be associated with neurodevelopmental impairments. However, in most cases, the transient hypothyroidism resolves without the need for thyroid hormone replacement therapy and does not negatively impact long-term outcomes (Fisher, 2008).

MEDICAL AND DEVELOPMENTAL CARE OF LOW BIRTH WEIGHT INFANTS

The best treatment for LBW infants is prevention of preterm births. This starts with identifying women at risk and providing them with education and prenatal health care. In addition, detecting preterm labor early and using labor-arresting agents and antenatal steroid therapy are very effective methods for preventing neonatal mortality and morbidity (Mwansa-Kambafwile, Cousens, Hansen, & Lawn, 2010). Prenatal care has improved appreciably since the 1970s, but the incidence of preterm delivery remains high and might even be rising (Heron et al., 2010). Preterm and SGA infants are best managed and cared for in high-risk obstetrical centers with NICUs.

Unfortunately increased survival rate of preterm infants has been associated with an increased risk of significant neurodevelopmental impairment (Wilson-Costello, Friedman, Minich, Fanaroff, & Hack, 2005). As survival rates of preterm infants have improved, the focus of care is now including a consideration of the optimal environment within the NICU for the premature infant to develop. Traditional NICU care has focused on medical protocols and procedures. A newer approach uses a more relationship-based, individualized, developmentally supportive model. This approach recognizes that the usual NICU setting is not optimal for the premature infant's developmental progress. Typical NICU care has involved the infant experiencing prolonged diffuse sleep states, unattended crying, a high ambient noise level, bright ambient light, a lack of opportunity for sucking, and poorly timed social and caregiving interactions.

The newer approach seeks to observe the infant's behavior and respond to it appropriately by providing individualized neurodevelopmental care and actively involving the parents in their infant's care (Als et al., 2005). It involves documenting infant behavior, including breathing pattern, color fluctuations, startles, posture, and sleep state. This then leads to caregiving suggestions and environmental modifications. One of the techniques involving the parent is termed "kangaroo care." Once the premature infant has reached physiologic stability and does not require major respiratory support, he or she is placed on the parent's chest. Kangaroo care (parent–infant skin-to-skin contact) improves preterm growth, decreases hospital-acquired infections, and may shorten hospital length of stay (Aucott, Donohue, Atkins, & Allen, 2002).

These developmental approaches have been associated with improved functioning in the NICU, including a reduced number of apnea events, faster weight gain, improved oxygenation, motor maturity, and state organization.

Research is ongoing to determine whether this approach carries long-term benefits.

In addition to environmental modifications that support development, early intervention services can be provided even before the child is discharged from the NICU. Once the infant is medically stable, a team consisting of a physical and/or occupational therapist, speech pathologist, developmental psychologist, and/or developmental pediatrician should evaluate the child. Care plans should be developed to provide parents with training regarding the ongoing developmental needs of the child after discharge. This may also include referral to an early intervention program (see Chapter 30).

SURVIVAL OF LOW BIRTH WEIGHT INFANTS

Advances in the technology of newborn intensive care and their application to the premature infant have been very successful in reducing mortality. Since 1960, survival of LBW infants has increased from 50% to more than 90% (Table 7.1). This improvement has been even more remarkable in ELBW and micropremie infants; in one study comparing the 1980s with the 1990s, the survival among preterm infants born with birth weight of 500 to 999 grams has increased from 49% to 67% (Wilson-Costello et al., 2005). A more recent study has shown that ELBW infants who survive the first few days have by far a much better chance of long-term survival. Although the overall survival for infants with birth weight <500 g was only 8%, those who lived through the first three days of life had up to a 50% chance of survival. Infants in the 500- to 749-g birth weight category had an overall survival rate of 50%. That increased to 70% if they survived through the third day, and 80% by the end of the first week of life (Mohamed, Nada, & Aly, 2010).

Table 7.1.   Improvement in survival rates of premature infants

	Survival (%)		
Birth weight (g)	1960	1990	2004
500–750	10	30	50
750–1,000	20	70	85
1000–1,500	30	90	98
1500–2,000	50	90	>98

Sources: Emsley et al. (1998); O'Shea et al. (1997); O'Shea et al. (1998); and Mohamed et al. (2010).

CARE AFTER DISCHARGE FROM THE HOSPITAL

The medical cost of the hospitalization and care of preterm infants who require prolonged NICU stays is extraordinarily high, often measured in hundreds of thousands of dollars. Length of stay is a major factor in this cost; as a result, many centers are developing care pathways that allow the medical team to consider earlier discharge than previously practiced for stable premature infants. This new approach needs to be monitored closely to ensure that earlier discharge does not compromise the health of infants and result in an increased risk of readmission to the hospital for treatment of medical complications.

Clinical criteria for discharging preterm LBW infants are based on the achievement of sufficient weight and maturity of body organ function to ensure medical stability and continued growth in a home environment. This generally involves the infant being able to feed well by mouth, continue to gain weight, maintain a stable body temperature outside of an isolette, and no longer experience episodes of apnea and bradycardia. Most preterm LBW infants meet these eligibility criteria at a postconceptional age of 35–37 weeks. For ELBW infants, discharge at a postconceptional age of 37–42 weeks is a more realistic goal (Rawlings & Scott, 1996). At the time of discharge, most infants weigh between 1,800 and 2,000 grams (4–4½ pounds).

When premature infants are discharged, parents may be faced with the stress and difficulty of caring for an infant with many special needs. The prolonged duration of hospitalization and separation from parents also may have interfered with the usual parent–infant bonding. Premature infants may be more irritable, cry more often, and have poorer sleep–wake cycles compared with full-term infants. Because of an immature sucking pattern, premature infants often require more frequent feedings. Specialized formula and/or breast milk supplementation with a human milk fortifier are now available to meet the caloric needs of premature infants post discharge.

As a result of these stresses, it is important to provide adequate support for the family after discharge, including close medical supervision and home care visits by nursing and/or social work staff (Broedsgaard & Wagner, 2005). Parental education regarding the needs of a growing preterm infant is extremely important. Ideally the infant should be discharged to a home environment that is free of smoke and any other potential respiratory irritants such as kerosene heaters, fresh paint, and people with respiratory-related viral illness; each of these factors plays a crucial role in causing subsequent respiratory illnesses or in exacerbating the underlying lung disease.

To prepare premature infants and their parents for the infant's discharge, most centers provide rooming-in services for the parents. This allows the parents to take over the care of their infant under the supervision of the NICU staff members who determine whether there are unforeseen problems. The parents also learn about the care of their infant, thereby reducing the stress and anxiety of taking a preterm infant home.

EARLY INTERVENTION PROGRAMS

Early intervention programs have been shown to benefit the neurodevelopment of most premature infants through 3–5 years of age, although longer-term effects are still debated (Koldewijn et al., 2009; Koldewijn et al., 2010; Spittle, Orton, Doyle, & Boyd, 2007). In a recent study of children with birth weight less than 2 kilograms, there was no significant difference in Mental Developmental Index scores at 3 years of age (after adjustment for maternal education) between children who receive early intervention services and those who do not; however, there was a statistically significant benefit shown via full-scale IQ scores at 5 years. With respect to motor outcomes, there were no differences between the groups receiving services and those not receiving services (Nordhov et al., 2010).

These programs should start for many premature infants prior to discharge from the hospital and continue until the child reaches 3 years corrected age. Corrected age is calculated by first determining how premature the child was in weeks (subtract the child's gestational age at birth from 40 weeks); then that number is subtracted from the child's current chronological age. For example, a child born at 28 weeks was 12 weeks early. To get the corrected age, 12 weeks (i.e., 3 months) should be subtracted from the child's age. The corrected age of an 8-month-old born at 28 weeks' gestation is 5 months. This correction is generally done until 12–24 months chronological age.

The intervention strategy incorporates group meetings for parents, home visits, and after 24 months chronological age, attendance at a multidisciplinary child development center with a low teacher–infant ratio (1:3–1:4; see

Chapter 30). It is important to recognize that even after completion of the early intervention program, many of these children continue to need special education services, including speech-language therapy, physical and/or occupational therapy, special education, behavior therapy, and treatment of emotional problems. If these children do not receive these services, the benefits of early intervention may be lost over time (Guralnick, 2005).

NEURODEVELOPMENTAL OUTCOME

Most infants born prematurely can be viewed during infancy as developing at a typical rate when their corrected or adjusted age is determined from their expected date of birth rather than from their actual birth date. There are, however, differences between full-term and preterm infants, even when gestational age is taken into account. Although few premature infants develop cerebral palsy, in terms of motor skills, they often lack the smooth, rhythmic movement patterns of full-term infants. Devices such as walkers and jumpers should be avoided because they encourage the infant to stand on tiptoe and walk in an abnormal pattern. In later infancy, visual-motor tasks that require the planned use of arms and hands are also more difficult. Coordinating reach and grasp, scooping with a spoon, managing a standard cup, copying block constructions, and completing crayon/paper tasks can be more difficult (Atkinson & Braddick, 2007).

By school age, the developmental status of preterm children who had birth weights above 1,500 grams is not very different from full-term infants (Gurka, LoCasale-Crouch, & Blackman, 2010). Children with birth weights below 1,500 grams, however, have an increased risk for developmental disabilities. School-age children who were born very preterm or had ELBW are at greater risk of developing executive function deficits (seen in ADHD, learning disabilities, and autism) and at greater risk of requiring ongoing neuropsychological follow-up through middle childhood (Aarnoudse-Moens, Smidts, Oosterlaan, Duivenvoorden, & Weisglas-Kuperus, 2009; Aarnoudse-Moens, Weisglas-Kuperus, van Goudoever, & Oosterlaan, 2009; Adams-Allan, 2008; Anderson & Doyle, 2008; Delobel-Ayoub et al., 2009; Johnson et al., 2010; Spittle et al., 2009; Stephens & Vohr, 2009; Wilson-Costello et al., 2007). In terms of behavior issues, children born prematurely are at risk for lower levels of social competence, and they are less adaptable, less regular in their habits, less persistent, and more withdrawn. ADHD is also more common in this group (Hack et al., 2004). Signs of ADHD may appear as early as 2 years of age with hyperactivity and difficulty following verbal directions and listening to a story. In addition, there may be behavior differences such as sleep disturbances, feeding difficulties, tantrums, or resistance to limit setting (Gray, Indurkhya, & McCormick, 2004). Learning differences may be anticipated in children whose language is delayed and who demonstrate poor visual–motor coordination (Breslau, Paneth, & Lucia, 2004). Family factors have also been found to be strong predictors of future school performance (Gross, Mettelman, Dye, & Slagle, 2001). Optimal school outcome has been significantly associated with increased parental education, child rearing by two parents, and stability in family composition and geographic residence.

Major developmental disabilities have been found in about one quarter of children with birth weight less than 1,000 grams (ELBW and micropreemies). This includes cerebral palsy (15%), hearing impairment (9%–11%), and visual impairment (1%– 9%; Hack et al., 2000). At 18–22 months corrected age, the mean Bayley Mental Developmental Index (Bayley, 1993) was 75, and 29% of the children had a score less than 70. Although cerebral palsy, especially spastic diplegia, is not uncommon in children who were VLBW, many "outgrow" this diagnosis by school age and simply appear to be less coordinated or have motor-associated learning difficulties.

In terms of predicting future neurodevelopmental disabilities, in one study, nearly 30% of ELBW infants with a normal cranial ultrasound were later found to have either cerebral palsy or intellectual disability (Laptook, O'Shea, Shankaran, Bhaskar, & the NICHD Neonatal Network, 2005). Neonatal brain MRI at corrected term gestation and/or before discharge appears to be a better predictor of severe neurodevelopmental disorders (El-Dib et al., 2010). Sensorineural hearing impairments were correlated with neonatal sepsis and jaundice. Neurological, developmental, neurosensory, and functional morbidities increased with decreasing birth weight, and overall, males were more at risk for disabilities than were females. Infants born SGA are at increased risk for lower cognitive performance as young adults. However, this lower capacity is not considered sufficiently severe to affect their educational level or social adjustment (Paz et al., 1995; Viggedal, Lundalv, Carlsson, & Kjellmer, 2004).

SUMMARY

When compared with full-term infants, LBW infants—in particular, VLBW infants/micro-premies—are at greater risk in the newborn period for many problems that may lead to long-term complications. Physiologic immaturity of organ systems often leads to RDS, hyperbilirubinemia, hypoglycemia, and hypocalcemia. Fortunately, most of these infants recover from these transient complications without major long-term sequelae. Other problems, however, such as IVH, PVL, sepsis, and persistent apnea and bradycardia are associated with poor neurodevelopmental outcome. With increased public awareness, improved prenatal care, advanced neonatal intensive care, increased parent involvement in the NICU, and access to early intervention services, the outcome of premature and SGA infants is likely to continue to improve.

REFERENCES

Aarnoudse-Moens, C.S., Smidts, D.P., Oosterlaan, J., Duivenvoorden, H.J., & Weisglas-Kuperus, N. (2009). Executive function in very preterm children at early school age. *Journal of Abnormal Child Psychology, 37*(7), 981–993.

Aarnoudse-Moens, C.S., Weisglas-Kuperus, N., van Goudoever, J.B., & Oosterlaan, J. (2009). Meta-analysis of neurobehavioral outcomes in very preterm and/or very low birth weight children. *Pediatrics, 124*(2), 717–728.

Abu-Shaweesh, J.M., & Martin, R.J. (2008). Neonatal apnea: What's new? *Pediatric Pulmonology, 43*(10), 937–944.

Als, H., Duffy, F.H., McAnulty, G.B., Rivkin, M.J., Vajapeyam, S., Mulkern, R.V., ... Eichenwald, E.C. (2005). Early experience alters brain function and structure. *Pediatrics, 113*, 846–857.

American Academy of Pediatrics Task Force on Infant Position and SIDS. (1992). Position and SIDS. *Pediatrics, 89*, 1120–1126.

Anderson, P.J., & Doyle, L.W. (2008). Cognitive and educational deficits in children born extremely preterm. *Seminars in Perinatology, 32*(1), 51–58.

Argente, J., Mehls, O., & Barrios, V. (2010). Growth and body composition in very young SGA children. *Pediatric Nephrology, 25*(4), 679–85.

Askin, D.F., & Diehl-Jones, W. (2009). Retinopathy of prematurity. *Critical Care Nursing Clinics of North America, 21*(2), 213–233.

Atkinson, J., & Braddick, O. (2007). Visual and visuo-cognitive development in children born very prematurely. *Progress in Brain Research, 164*, 123–49.

Aucott, S., Donohue, P.K., Atkins, E., & Allen, M.C. (2002). Neurodevelopmental care in the NICU. *Mental Retardation and Developmental Disabilities Research Review, 3*, 298–308.

Baird, T.M. (2004). Clinical correlates, natural history and outcome of neonatal apnoea. *Seminars in Neonatology, 9*, 205–211.

Ballard, J.L., Khoury, J.C., Wedig, K., Wang, L., Eilers-Walsman, B.L., & Lipp, R. (1991). New Ballard score, expanded to include extremely premature infants. *The Journal of Pediatrics, 119*, 417–423.

Bassan, H. (2009). Intracranial hemorrhage in the preterm infant: Understanding it, preventing it. *Clinics in Perinatology, 36*(4), 737–62.

Bayley, N. (1993). *Bayley Scales of Infant Development—Second Edition*. San Antonio, TX: Harcourt Assessment.

Birch, J.L., & Newell, S.J. (2009). Gastrooesophageal reflux disease in preterm infants: Current management and diagnostic dilemmas. *Archives of Disease in Childhood: Fetal and Neonatal Edition, 94*(5), F379–F383.

Bishara, N., & Ohls, R.K. (2009). Current controversies in the management of the anemia of prematurity. *Seminars in Perinatology, 33*, 29–34.

Blumenthal, I. (2004). Periventricular leucomalacia: A review. *European Journal of Pediatrics, 163*, 435–442.

Bottino, M., Cowett, R.M., & Sinclair, J.C. (2009). Interventions for treatment of neonatal hyperglycemia in very low birth weight infants. *Cochrane Database System Review, 21*(1), CD007453.

Bradshaw, W.T. (2009). Necrotizing enterocolitis: Etiology, presentation, management, and outcomes. *Journal of Perinatal and Neonatal Nursing, 23*(1), 87–94.

Breslau, N., Paneth, N.S., & Lucia, V.C. (2004). *Pediatrics, 114*, 1035–1040.

Broedsgaard, A., & Wagner, L. (2005). How to facilitate parents and their premature infant for the transition home. *International Nursing Review, 52*, 196–203.

Broström, E.B., Thunqvist, P., Adenfelt, G., Borling, E., & Katz-Salamon, M. (2010). Obstructive lung disease in children with mild to severe BPD. *Respiratory Medicine, 104*, 362–70.

Casey, P.H. (2008). Growth of low birth weight preterm children. *Seminars in Perinatology, 32*(1), 20–27.

Chandler, J.C., & Hebra, A. (2000). Necrotizing enterocolitis in infants with very low birth weight. *Seminars in Pediatric Surgery, 9*, 63–72.

Committee on Fetus and Newborn, American Academy of Pediatrics. (2003). Apnea, sudden infant death syndrome, and home monitoring. *Pediatrics, 111*(4), 914–917.

Constantine, N.A., Kraemer, H.C., Kendall-Tackett, K.A., Bennett, G.C., Tyson, J.E., & Gross, R.T. (1987). Use of physical and neurologic observations in assessment of gestational age in low-birth-weight infants. *The Journal of Pediatrics, 110*, 921–928.

Dani, C., Poggi, C., Romagnoli, C., & Bertini, G. (2009). Survival and major disability rate in infants born at 22–25 weeks of gestation. *Journal of Perinatal Medicine, 37*(6), 599–608.

de Bie, H.M., Oostrom, K.J., & Delemarre-van de Waal, H.A. (2010). Brain development, intelligence and cognitive outcome in children born small for gestational age. *Hormone Research in Paediatrics, 73*(1), 6–14.

Delobel-Ayoub, M., Arnaud, C., White-Koning, M., Casper, C., Pierrat, V., Garel, M., & EPIPAGE Study Group. (2009). Behavioral problems and cognitive performance at 5 years of age after very preterm birth: The EPIPAGE Study. *Pediatrics, 123*(6), 1485–1492.

Dubowitz, L.M., Dubowitz, V., & Goldberg, C. (1970). Clinical assessment of gestational age in the newborn infant. *The Journal of Pediatrics, 77,* 1–10.

El-Dib, M., Massaro, A.N., Bulas, D., & Aly, H. (2010). Neuroimaging and neurodevelopmental outcome of premature infants. *American Journal of Perinatology, 27*(10), 803–818.

Emsley, H.C.A., Wardle, S.P., Sims, D.G., Chiswick, M.L., & D'Souza, S.W. (1998). Increased survival and deteriorating developmental outcome in 23 to 25 week old gestation infants, 1990–4 compared with 1984–9. *Archives of Disease in Childhood, Fetal and Neonatal Edition, 78,* F99–F104.

Fisher, D.A. (2008). Thyroid system immaturities in very low birth weight premature infants. *Seminars in Perinatology, 32*(6), 387–397.

Gibson, E., Dembofsky, C.A., Rubin, S., & Greenspan, J.S. (2000). Infant sleep position practices 2 years into the "Back to Sleep" campaign. *Clinical Pediatrics, 39,* 285–289.

Gray, R.F., Indurkhya, A., & McCormick, M.C. (2004). Prevalence, stability, and predictors of clinically significant behavior problems in low birth weight children at 3, 5, and 8 years of age. *Pediatrics, 114,* 736–743.

Grivell, R., Dodd, J., & Robinson, J. (2009). The prevention and treatment of intrauterine growth restriction. *Best Practice & Research Clinical Obstetrics and Gynaecology, 23*(6), 795–807.

Gross, S.J., Mettelman, B.B., Dye, T.D., & Slagle, T.A. (2001). Impact of family structure and stability on academic outcome in preterm children at 10 years of age. *The Journal of Pediatrics, 138,* 16–75.

Guralnick, M.J. (Ed.). (2005). *The developmental systems approach to early intervention.* Baltimore, MD: Paul H. Brookes Publishing Co.

Gurka, M.J., LoCasale-Crouch, J., & Blackman, J.A. (2010). Long-term cognition, achievement, socioemotional, and behavioral development of healthy late-preterm infants. *Archives of Pediatrics and Adolescent Medicine, 164*(6), 525–532.

Hack, M., Wilson-Costello, D., Friedman, H., Taylor, G.H., Schuchter, M., & Fanaroff, A.A. (2000). Neurodevelopment and predictors of outcomes of children with birth weights of less than 1000g: 1992–1995. *Archives of Pediatric and Adolescent Medicine, 154,* 725–731.

Hack, M., Youngstrom, E.A., Cartar, L., Schluchter, M., Gerry Taylor, H., Flannery, D., ... Borawski, E. (2004). Behavioral outcomes and evidence of psychopathology among very low birth weight infants at age 20 years. *Pediatrics, 114*(4), 932–940.

Halliday, HL., Ehrenkranz, RA., & Doyle, LW. (2009). Early (< 8 days) postnatal corticosteroids for preventing chronic lung disease in preterm infants. *Archives of Pediatrics & Adolescent Medicine, 16,* 999–1004.

Hamrick, S.E., & Hansmann, G. (2010). Patent ductus arteriosus of the preterm infant. *Pediatrics, 125*(5), 1020–1030.

Henry, M.C., & Moss, R.L. (2009). Necrotizing enterocolitis. *Annual Review of Medicine, 60,* 111–124.

Heron, M, Sutton, P.D., Xu, J, Ventura, S.J., Strobino, D.M., & Guyer, B. (2010). Annual summary of vital statistics: 2007. *Pediatrics, 125,* 4–15.

Horwitz, J.R., Lally, K.P., Cheu, H.W., Vasquez, W.D., Grosfeld, J.L., & Ziegler, M.M. (1995).

Complications after surgical intervention for necrotizing enterocolitis: A multicenter review. *Journal of Pediatric Surgery, 30,* 994–998.

Hyman, S.J., Novoa, Y., & Holzman, I. (2009). Perinatal endocrinology: Common endocrine disorders in the sick and premature newborn. *Endocrinology Metabolism Clinics of North America, 38*(3), 509–524.

Johnson, S., Hollis, C., Kochhar, P., Hennessy, E., Wolke, D., & Marlow, N. (2010). Autism spectrum disorders in extremely preterm children. *Journal of Pediatrics, 156*(4), 525–531.

Joint Committee on Infant Hearing. (1995). Joint Committee on Infant Hearing 1994 Position Statement. *Pediatrics, 95*(1), 152–156.

Joint Committee on Infant Hearing. (2000). Year 2000 position statement: Principles and guidelines for early hearing detection and intervention programs. *Pediatrics, 106*(4), 798–817.

Kinney, H.C., & Thach, B.T. (2009). The sudden infant death syndrome. *New England Journal of Medicine, 361*(8), 795–805.

Klein, L.L., & Gibbs, R.S. (2005). Infection and preterm birth. *Obstetrics and Gynecology Clinics of North America, 32,* 397–410.

Koldewijn, K., van Wassenaer, A., Wolf, M.J., Meijssen, D., Houtzager, B., Beelen, A., ... Nollet, F. (2010). A neurobehavioral intervention and assessment program in very low birth weight infants: Outcome at 24 months. *Journal of Pediatrics, 156*(3), 359–365.

Koldewijn, K., Wolf, M.J., van Wassenaer, A., Meijssen, D., van Sonderen, L., van Baar, A., ... Kok, J. (2009). The Infant Behavioral Assessment and Intervention Program for very low birth weight infants at 6 months corrected age. *Journal of Pediatrics, 154*(1), 33–38.

Laptook, A.R., O'Shea, T.M., Shankaran, S., Bhaskar, B., & the NICHD Neonatal Network. (2005). Adverse neurodevelopmental outcomes among extremely low birth weight infants with a normal head ultrasound: Prevalence and antecedents. *Pediatrics, 115*(3), 673–680.

Lubchenco, L.O. (1976). *The high risk infant.* Philadelphia, PA: Saunders.

Mandrich, M., Simons, C.J., Ritchie, S., Schmidt, D., & Mullett, M. (1994). Motor development, infantile reactions and postural responses of preterm, at-risk infants. *Developmental Medicine and Child Neurology, 36,* 397–405.

McCall, E.M., Alderdice, F., Halliday, H.L., Jenkins, J.G., & Vohra, S. (2010). Interventions to prevent hypothermia at birth in preterm and/or low birthweight infants. *Cochrane Database System Review, 17*(3), CD004210.

McCowan, L., & Horgan, R.P. (2009). Risk factors for small for gestational age infants. *Best Practice & Research Clinical Obstetrics & Gynaecology, 23*(6), 779–793.

McCrea, H.J., & Ment, L.R. (2008). The diagnosis, management and postnatal prevention of intraventricular hemorrhage in the preterm neonate. *Clinics in Perinatology, 35,* 777.

Ment, L.R., Bada, H.S., Barnes, P.D., Grant, P.E., Hirtz, D., Papile, L.A., ... Slovis, T.L. (2002). Practice parameter: Neuroimaging of the neonate. *Neurology, 58,* 1726–1738.

Mitchell, E.A. (2009). SIDS: Past, present and future. *Acta Paediatrica, 98*(11), 1712–1719.

Mirmiran, M., Barnes, P.D., Keller, K., Constantinou, J.C., Fleisher, B.E., Hintz, S.R., & Arigno, R.L.

(2004). Neonatal brain magnetic resonance imaging before discharge is better than serial cranial ultrasound in predicting cerebral palsy in very low birth weight preterm infants. *Pediatrics, 114*(4), 992–998.

Mohamed, M.A., Nada, A., & Aly, H. (2010). Day-by-day postnatal survival in very low birth weight infants. *Pediatrics, 126*(2), e360–e366.

Morgen, C.S., Bjork, C., & Andersen, P.K. (2008). Socioeconomic position and the risk of preterm birth: A study within the Danish National Birth Cohort. *International Journal of Epidemiology, 37*, 1109–1120.

Moriette, G., Lescure, S., El Ayoubi, M., & Lopez, E. (2010). Apnea of prematurity: What's new? *Archives of Pediatrics & Adolescent Medicine, 16*, 186–190.

Mwansa-Kambafwile, J., Cousens, S., Hansen, T., & Lawn, J. (2010). Antenatal steroids in preterm labour for the prevention of neonatal deaths due to complications of preterm birth. *International Journal of Epidemiology 39*, i122–i133.

Nagpal, J., Kumar, A., & Ramji, S. (2004). Anterior lens capsule vascularity in evaluating gestation in small for gestation neonates. *Indian Pediatrics, 41*, 817–821.

Najati, N., & Gojazadeh, M. (2010). Maternal and neonatal complications in mothers aged under 18 years. *Journal of Patient Preference and Adherence, 4*, 219–222.

Nelson, K.B. (2008). Causative factors in cerebral palsy. *Clinical Obstetrics and Gynecology, 51*(4), 749–762.

NIH Consensus Development Panel on the Effect of Corticosteroids for Fetal Maturation on Perinatal Outcomes. (1995). Effect of corticosteroids for fetal maturation on perinatal outcomes. *Journal of the American Medical Association, 273*(5), 413–418.

Noori, S. (2010). Patent ductus arteriosus in the preterm infant: To treat or not to treat? *Journal of Perinatology, 30*, S31–S37.

Nordhov, S.M., Rønning, J.A., Dahl, L.B., Ulvund, S.E., Tunby, J., & Kaaresen, P.I. (2010). Early intervention improves cognitive outcomes for preterm infants: Randomized controlled trial. *Pediatrics, 126*(5), e1088–e1094. Advance online publication. doi: 10.1542/peds.2010-0778

Ohl, C., Dornier, L., Czajka, C., Chobaut, J.C., & Tavernier, L. (2009). Newborn hearing screening on infants at risk. *International Journal of Pediatrics Otorhinolaryngol, 73*(12), 1691–1695.

Ohlsson, A., Walia, R., & Shah, S. (2008). Ibuprofen for the treatment of patent ductus arteriosus in preterm and/or low birth weight infants. *Cochrane Database System Review, 4*(1), CD003481.

Okumura, A., Hayakawa, F., Kato, T., Maruyama, K., Kubota, T., Suzuki, M., ... Watanabe, K. (2003). Abnormal sharp transients on electroencephalograms in preterm infants with periventricular leukomalacia. *Journal of Pediatrics, 143*(1), 26–30.

O'Shea, T.M., Klinepeter, K.L., Goldstein, D.J., Jackson, B.W., & Dillard, R.G. (1997). Survival and developmental disability in infants with birth weights of 501 to 800 grams, born between 1979 and 1994. *Pediatrics, 100*(6), 982–986.

O'Shea, T.M., Preisser, J.S., Klinepeter, K.L., & Dillard, R.G. (1998). Trends in mortality and cerebral palsy in a geographically based cohort of very low birth weight neonates born between 1982 and 1994. *Pediatrics, 101*(4) 642–647.

Ostfeld, B.M., Esposito, L., Perl, H., & Hegyi, T. (2010). Concurrent risks in sudden infant death syndrome. *Pediatrics, 125*(3), 447–453.

Owens, R. (2005). Intraventricular hemorrhage in the premature neonate. *Neonatal Network, 24*, 55–71.

Paz, I., Gale R., Laor, A., Danon, Y.L., Stevenson, D.K., & Seidman, D.S. (1995). The cognitive outcome of full-term small for gestational age infants at late adolescence. *Obstetrics & Gynecology, 85*, 452–456.

Patrianakos-Hoobler, A.I, Msall, M.E., Huo, D., Marks, J.D., Plesha-Troyke, S., & Schreiber, M.D. (2010). Predicting school readiness from neurodevelopmental assessments at age 2 years after respiratory distress syndrome in infants born preterm. *Developmental Medicine & Child Neurology, 52*(4), 379–85.

Perlman, J.M., Risser, R., & Broyles, R.S. (1996). Bilateral cystic periventricular leukomalacia in premature infants: Associated risk factors. *Pediatrics, 97*, 822–827.

Pillekamp, F., Hermann, C., Keller, T., von Gontard, A., Kribs, A., & Roth, B. (2007). Factors influencing apnea and bradycardia of prematurity: Implications for neurodevelopment. *Neonatology, 91*(3), 155–161.

Pleacher, M.D., Vohr, B.R., Katz, K.H., Ment, L.R., & Allan, W.C. (2004). An evidence-based approach to predicting low IQ in very preterm infants from the neurological examination: Outcome data from the Indomethacin intraventricular hemorrhage prevention trial. *Pediatrics, 113*, 416–419.

Porcelli, P.J., & Weaver, R.G., Jr. (2010). The influence of early postnatal nutrition on retinopathy of prematurity in extremely low birth weight infants. *Early Human Development, 86*, 391–396.

Premji, S., & Chessell, L. (2001). Continuous nasogastric milk feeding versus intermittent bolus milk feeding for premature infants less than 1500 grams. *Cochrane Database of Systematic Reviews*, CD001819.

Rawlings, J.S., & Scott, J.S. (1996). Postconceptional age of surviving preterm low-birth-weight infants at hospital discharge. *Archives of Pediatrics and Adolescent Medicine, 150*, 260–262.

Robertson, C.M., Howarth, T.M., Bork, D.L., & Dinu, I.A. (2009). Permanent bilateral sensory and neural hearing loss of children after neonatal intensive care because of extreme prematurity: A thirty-year study. *Pediatrics, 123*(5), e797–e807.

Sarkar, S., Bhagat, I., Dechert, R., Schumacher, R.E., & Donn, S.M. (2009). Severe intraventricular hemorrhage in preterm infants: Comparison of risk factors and short-term neonatal morbidities between grade 3 and grade 4 intraventricular hemorrhage. *American Journal of Perinatology, 26*(6), 419–424.

Shah, P.S., & Knowledge Synthesis Group on Determinants of LBW/PT Births. (2010). Parity and low birth weight and preterm birth: A systematic review and meta-analyses. *Acta Obstetrica et Gynecologica Scandinavica, 89*(7), 862–875.

Sinclair, J.C., Bottino, M., & Cowett, R.M. (2009). Interventions for prevention of neonatal hyperglycemia in very low birth weight infants. *Cochrane Database System Review, 8*(3), CD007615.

Snyder, C.L., Gittes, G.K., Murphy, J.P., Sharp, R.J., Ashcraft, K.W., & Amoury, R.A. (1997). Survival after necrotizing enterocolitis in infants weighing less than 1000 g: 25 years' experience at a single institution. *Journal of Pediatric Surgery, 32*, 434–437.

Spittle, A.J., Orton, J., Doyle, L.W., & Boyd, R. (2007). Early developmental intervention programs post hospital discharge to prevent motor and cognitive impairments in preterm infants. *Cochrane Database System Review, 18*(2), CD005495.

Spittle, A.J., Treyvaud, K., Doyle, L.W., Roberts, G., Lee, K.J., Inder, T.E., ... Anderson, P.J. (2009). Early emergence of behavior and social-emotional problems in very preterm infants. *Journal of the American Academy of Child and Adolescent Psychiatry*, *48*(9), 909–918.

Stephens, B.E., & Vohr, B.R. (2009). Neurodevelopmental outcome of the premature infant. *Pediatric Clinics of North America, 56*(3), 631–646.

Suresh, G.K., Horbar, J.D., Kenny, M., Carpenter, J.H., & Vermont Oxford Network. (2001). Major birth defects in very low birth weight infants in the Vermont Oxford Network. *The Journal of Pediatrics, 139*(3), 366–373.

Sylvester, C.L. (2008). Retinopathy of prematurity. *Seminars in Ophthalmology, 23*(5), 318–323.

Thompson, A.M., & Bizzarro, M.J. (2008). Necrotizing enterocolitis in newborns: Pathogenesis, prevention and management. *Drugs, 68*(9), 1227–1238.

Valleur-Masson, D., Vodovar, M., Zeller, J., Laudat, F., Masson, Y., Kassis, M., ... Voyer, M. (1993). Bronchopulmonary dysplasia: Course over 3 years in 88 children born between 1984 and 1988. *Archives Francaises de Pediatrie, 50*(7), 553–559.

Van Naarden, K., & Decoufle, P. (1999). Relative and attributable risks for moderate to profound bilateral sensorineural hearing impairment associated with lower birth weight in children 3 to 10 years old. *Pediatrics, 104*, 905–910.

Vassilyadi, M., Tataryn, Z., Shamji, M.F., & Ventureyra, E.C. (2009). Functional outcomes among premature infants with intraventricular hemorrhage. *Pediatric Neurosurgery, 45*(4), 247–255.

Viggedal, G., Lundalv, E., Carlsson, G., & Kjellmer, I. (2004). Neuropsychological follow-up into young adulthood of term infants born small for gestational age. *Medical Science Monitor, 10*, 8–16.

Volpe, J.J. (2008). *Neurology of the newborn* (5th ed.). Philadelphia, PA: Saunders.

Walsh, M.C., Morris, B.H., Wrage, L.A., Vohr, B.R., Poole, W.K., Tyson, J.E., ... Fanaroff, A.A. (2005). Extremely low birthweight neonates with protracted ventilation: Mortality and 18-month neurodevelopmental outcomes. *The Journal of Pediatrics, 146*, 798–804.

Watchko, J.F., & Maisels, J.M. (2010). Enduring controversies in the management of hyperbilirubinemia in preterm neonates, *Seminars in Fetal and Neonatal Medicine, 15*, 136–140.

Wheater, M., & Renie, J.M. (2000). Perinatal infection is an important risk factor for cerebral palsy in very-lowbirth-weight infants. *Developmental Medicine and Child Neurology, 42*, 364–367.

Wilson-Costello, D., Friedman H., Minich N., Fanaroff, A.A., & Hack, M. (2005). Improved survival with increased neurodevelopmental disability for extremely low birth weight infants in the 1990s. *Pediatrics, 115*, 997–1003.

Wilson-Costello, D., Friedman, H., Minich, N., Siner, B., Taylor, G., Schluchter, M., & Hack, M. (2007). Improved neurodevelopmental outcomes for extremely low birth weight infants in 2000–2002. *Pediatrics, 119*, 37–45.

Wirbelauer, J., & Speer, C.P. (2009). The role of surfactant treatment in preterm infants and term newborns with acute respiratory distress syndrome. *Journal of Perinatology, 29*(Suppl 2), S18–S22.

Woynarowska, M., Rutkowska, M., & Szamotulska, K. (2008). Risk factors, frequency and severity of bronchopulmonary dysplasia (BPD) diagnosed according to the new disease definition in preterm neonates. *Medycyna Wieku Rozwojowego, 12*, 933–941.

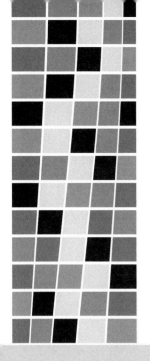

II

The Developing Child

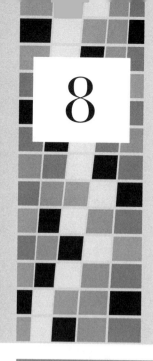

8

Nutrition and Children with Disabilities

Rebecca M. Haesler and Jocelyn J. Mills

Upon completion of this chapter, the reader will

- Understand nutritional requirements and their assessment in children
- Identify how developmental disabilities modify nutritional requirements
- Understand the fundamental role of nutrition in the growth and development of children
- Understand how nutritional interventions are included in children's care plans

Nutrition is the study of foods, their nutrients, and other components of the diet that affect biological processes and health (Brown, 2007). Human requirements for protein, fats, carbohydrates, vitamins, and minerals vary with age, activity level, medical diagnosis, genetic heritage, and physiological state (Institute of Medicine, 2005). A typical diet provides all of the nutrients, minerals, and vitamins needed for typical growth and development. In children with developmental disabilities, however, a typical diet may present challenges. As a result of motor impairments, a child with cerebral palsy may have difficulty ingesting sufficient food. A child with an autism spectrum disorder (ASD) may have food selectivity that results in nutritional deficiencies (see Chapter 21). Conversely, a child with Prader-Willi syndrome often engages in **hyperphagia** (pathological overeating), and a child with **meningomyelocoele** may become obese through inactivity. Typically, the impact of nutrition is greatest during infancy and childhood when the body is actively growing. For children with developmental disabilities, however, the need for medical nutritional therapy may be lifelong. *Medical nutrition therapy* is defined as the manipulation of nutrients and dietary components to affect a disease or condition (American Dietetic Association, 2010). This therapy also takes into account the psychosocial environment in which the child lives. Food selection and preparation are major cultural characteristics of all societies, and within the context of home and family, providing and preparing food for children expresses parental love and concern. This chapter focuses on the nutritional needs of children with developmental disabilities and emphasizes medical nutrition therapy as part of a comprehensive care plan.

◼◼◼ ALYSSA

Alyssa's parents were notified at 7 days of age that she had an abnormal blood test, specifically an abnormal newborn screening test. She was examined in the metabolism clinic of the local children's hospital, where studies confirmed the diagnosis of **phenylketonuria** (PKU), and her parents met with a geneticist and dietitian. The geneticist explained PKU, its genetics, and laboratory test results (see Chapter 19). The parents came to understand that the basic problem in PKU was the inability to metabolize a specific essential amino acid, phenylalanine, one of the building blocks of protein. The dietitian explained that Alyssa would have a lifelong need to be on a special diet restricted in natural protein and supplemented with a phenylalanine-free formula, which would allow her to meet her protein requirements. The parents learned how to measure the phenylalanine content in various foods. Each time Alyssa and her parents came into the metabolism clinic they would meet with the dietitian who would measure her growth, review her diet, provide educational material, answer their questions, and adjust her formula and food intake as needed. As Alyssa began eating more solid foods, the dietitian educated the family on ways to vary the diet by incorporating low-protein versions of common food items that could be ordered on the Internet. These specialty foods were initially developed for adults with kidney failure who also require low-protein diets. By age 7, Alyssa was selecting most of her foods and was able to make her formula without assistance. She was learning to "own" the responsibility for her disorder.

At age 9, her blood phenylalanine test results showed Alyssa was eating too much "regular" food. She rebelled sometimes about finishing her phenylalanine-free formula. The dietitian recommended a lower-volume formula so that Alyssa's formula was more age-appropriate and easier to consume. It was also emphasized that low-protein food substitutes provide greater variety and allow for a diet closely resembling that of her peers. Routine blood phenylalanine test results were used by the dietitian to adjust the diet, along with growth measurements, Alyssa's likes and dislikes, and her parent's concerns. Alyssa wanted to be just like everyone else, and the geneticist, dietitian, and family worked together to find solutions to Alyssa's life on a strict diet. Her parents were

encouraged to let Alyssa attend a PKU camp the following summer when she was to be 10 years old so she could interact with peers challenged by the same issues.

TYPICAL GROWTH DURING CHILDHOOD

Nutritional requirements for infants and children are determined by what is needed to produce optimal growth and development. The average full-term infant weighs 3.4 kilograms (about 7½ pounds) at birth, and gains 20–30 grams (about 1 ounce) each day for several months. By 4–6 months of age, the infant's birth weight has doubled, and by 12 months, it has tripled (National Center for Health Statistics, 2000; National Center for Health Statistics, 2008a). As the child becomes more active, weight gain slows to about 5 pounds per year until approximately 9–10 years of age, when the adolescent growth spurt begins. Length advances at a slower pace than weight, increasing by 50% during the first year of life (from an average of 50 centimeters or about 19½ inches at birth), doubling by 4 years of age, and tripling by 13 years of age. Increase in head circumference parallels brain growth. Head circumference increases by 3 inches during the first year of life, and brain weight doubles by 2 years of age (National Center for Health Statistics, 2000; National Center for Health Statistics, 2008a).

In addition to the basic measures of growth (i.e., weight, length, head circumference), a number of useful growth indices have been developed that provide a more nuanced and clinically relevant way of measuring a child's nutritional status. Among these, the index used most often is the **body mass index (BMI)**, a measure of the relationship between weight and stature (length) across ages that was developed by the Centers for Disease Control and Prevention (CDC; National Center for Health Statistics, 2010; Speiser et al., 2005; see Table 8.1). By placing weight into the context of a child's overall size and body habitus, the BMI can be a useful screening tool to assess whether a child is over- or underweight. Direct measures of body fat utilizing specialized equipment and techniques are not as widely available but offer an even more accurate way of assessing this critical aspect of a child's nutritional status.

NUTRITIONAL GUIDELINES

Research-based nutrition guidelines published by the National Academies of Sciences estimate daily intake of specific vitamins and minerals based on age and gender (Institute of Medicine, 1997, 2001). Energy and protein intake recommendations were updated in 2005 (Institute of Medicine, 2005) and have been incorporated into the nutrients included in food labels. They are also reflected in the standard growth charts commonly used by health care professionals (National Centers for Health Statistics, 2000). The concept of a "balanced diet" derives from standard nutritional guidelines, and is based on the notion that typical children will require specific amounts and proportions of certain nutrients. Although these guidelines are a good starting point for determining the nutrition requirements for children with disabilities, adjustments are often required. In some cases an apparently "unbalanced" diet is appropriate for a child with a specific condition. For example, a typical 10-year-old girl who is active needs about 2,000 calories daily. In contrast, a 10-year-old girl with meningomyelocoele may need fewer calories daily due to a below typical activity level, whereas a child with **choreoathetoid** cerebral palsy may be more active and thus require more calories (Bell & Davies, 2010; Liusuwan, Widman, Abresch, Styne, & McDonald, 2007; see Chapter 24). An all-liquid diet or a diet of only a few different foods may be recommended for a child with limited oral-motor skills. For a child like Alyssa with a special metabolic condition, it is critically important that certain elements of

the diet be reduced, eliminated, or enhanced to avoid the build-up of toxic metabolites. Table 8.2 provides other examples of how specific dietary components and calorie content can be manipulated to address the special needs of specific medical conditions and disabilities (Isaacs & Zand, 2007).

NUTRITIONAL ISSUES IN CHILDREN WITH DEVELOPMENTAL DISABILITIES

Children with developmental disabilities have many of the same nutrition problems as typically developing children. These include being over- or underweight, refusing to eat or drink a variety of foods and beverages, and fighting for control with parents at mealtimes. Children with disabilities, however, are prone to more serious and varied problems that are especially related to impaired oral motor skills (e.g., swallowing incoordination among children with cerebral palsy), medical problems (e.g., chronic gastroesophageal reflux [GER] among children who were premature infants), and food refusal (e.g., dislike of certain food textures among children with autism specrum disorders [ASDs]; Bandini et al., 2010; Marchand, Motil, & the North American Society for Pediatric Gastroenterology, Hepatology, and Nutrition [NASPGHAN] Committee on Nutrition, 2006). As a result, common nutritional advice for typically developing children may not be appropriate for children with disabilities (see Table 8.3). Instead, diets must be targeted to specific conditions and developmental disabilities, as illustrated in Table 8.2.

Table 8.1. Growth parameters and nutrition assessment

Growth parameter	Utility in nutrition assessment
Weight for age (pounds or kilograms)	Provides direct comparison to established norms for age; key parameter for monitoring short- and long-term changes in nutritional status
Length for age (inches or centimeters)	Provides direct comparison to established norms for age; key measure of linear growth
Head circumference for age (inches or centimeters)	Provides direct comparison to established norms for age; key proxy for brain growth
Weight-to-height proportionality	Provides a rough estimate of nutritional status by relating weight to stature; birth to 36 months of age
Body mass index (weight in pounds x 703 / height in inches x height in inches)	Provides an estimate of body fat relative to weight and height; >2 years of age
Rate of weight and length accretion (change in weight or length over a given time interval)	Precise method of tracking patterns and rates of growth
Body fat indices	Direct measures of body fat using reliable, specialized equipment and techniques

Obesity

Intake of food energy, or kilocalories (more commonly referred to simply as *calories*), is a critical aspect of nutrition, and disorders involving excess or insufficient energy intake are common among children with disabilities (Bandini et al., 2005). Obesity is caused by excessive energy intake relative to energy expenditure and is typically defined, using the CDC growth chart, by a BMI greater than the 95th percentile BMI for age. Obesity and overweight are increasing worldwide, but controversy continues about how to best assess the risks of obesity in children and adolescents (Speiser et al., 2005). BMI includes assumptions about stature and body composition that may not apply to children with disabilities. For example, **scoliosis** may interfere with accurate height measurements, which in turn can affect the calculation of the BMI. Other disorders that may not be well described by the BMI criteria are Prader-Willi syndrome, meningomyelocoele, and Down syndrome (Bandini et al., 2005).

Undernutrition

Concern about the adequacy of energy intake is more common in children with disabilities than in typically developing children. Needs for increased energy and protein are commonly observed in children with such conditions as prematurity (Agostoni et al., 2010), cystic fibrosis (Munck, 2010), choreoathetoid cerebral palsy (Bell & Davies, 2010), and Rett syndrome (Oddy et al., 2007). In these cases, the goal of medical nutrition therapy is to provide extra calories and protein as food or nutritional supplements.

When Disabilities Affect Stature

Extra calories and nutrients may not normalize growth in many disabilities that are known to be associated with short stature, such as translocation chromosomal disorders, Turner syndrome, Down syndrome, Williams syndrome, chromosome 22q11 microdeletion syndromes (e.g., Velocardiofacial syndrome, DiGeorge syndrome), meningomyelocoele (Liusuwan, et al., 2007), chronic kidney disease (Mahan & Warady, 2006), and fetal alcohol syndrome (FAS; Chudley et al., 2005). These short-stature syndromes are discussed in Appendix B. Providing extra calories in these conditions may simply result in obesity. To increase linear growth, could be treated with growth hormone therapy in some of these conditions (Cohen et al., 2008). Diagnosis-specific growth

Table 8.2.   Dietary adjustments for specific medical conditions and disabilities

Dietary element	Condition	Specific adjustment required
Fats	Smith-Lemli-Opitz syndrome	Cholesterol (purified form) increased
	Long chain fatty acid oxidation disorders	Fat decreased, greater than 75% of nutrition from fat-free foods
	Uncontrollable seizures	Ketogenic diet, fat increased
Proteins	Phenylketonuria, Maple syrup urine disease	Natural protein decreased by more than 80%, addition of protein substitutes, vitamins and minerals
Carbohydrates	Glycogen storage disease Type 1	Specific types of sugar (e.g., sucrose, fructose, galactose, lactose) decreased
	Galactosemia, lactose intolerance	Specific types of sugar (e.g., galactose, lactose) decreased
	Hereditary fructose intolerance	Specific types of sugar (e.g., fructose) decreased
Vitamins and minerals	Vitamin B_{12} disorders	Vitamin B12 increased, often protein content decreased
	Iron-deficiency anemia	Foods rich in iron increased or supplemental iron added
	Rickets	Foods rich in calcium and vitamin D increased or supplements added
Energy (calorie)	Obesity and overweight	Calories decreased 10%–30% (fats, proteins, and carbohydrates), activity level increased
	Hypotonia in Down syndrome or Prader-Willi syndrome	Calories decreased 30%–40% (fats, proteins, and carbohydrates)

reports are based on smaller population groups than the standard growth charts for typical children (Arvay et al., 2005). They help set realistic expectations for growth after the diagnosis. Conditions in which excess growth is unrelated to nutritional intake also are known, including genetic conditions such as **Sotos syndrome, Marfan syndrome,** and types of gigantism that result from an overproduction of growth hormone. Typically, an important measure of sufficient nutrition is adequate growth. Yet, many developmental disabilities are associated with these atypical growth patterns. As a result, it may be difficult to determine whether a child with a developmental disability who has apparent inadequate growth is truly undernourished (Marchand et al., 2006).

When Disabilities Limit Eating

Children with developmental disabilities may lack an appetite or have physical difficulties in eating. Mealtime, rather than being a pleasure, becomes aversive for both the child and parents. It is thus imperative to identify the root causes of the feeding disorder and to design an appropriate therapy program. A child unable to eat because of fatigue and weakness resulting from a neuromuscular disability merits a different approach than a child who refuses to eat due to behavioral or cognitive issues. Children with dyskinetic cerebral palsy may have such

severe difficulty chewing and swallowing that they may risk aspiration pneumonia as well as undernutrition. In this case, nutritional therapy might be directed at providing alternative routes for nutrition, such as **gastrostomy** tube formula feedings (Bell et al., 2010).

Children with ASDs may have severe and persistent restricted food preferences. However, a study by Emond, Emmet, Steer, and Golding in 2010, shows that while children with ASDs may have decreased variability in their diets, adequate energy intake is maintained, resulting in typical growth. Behavior management techniques may be utilized to gradually add new food items to the ASD child's menu (see Chapter 21). Such techniques may involve rewards for trying new foods or encouraging the child to participate in food preparation.

Recognizing undernutrition and malnutrition may also be difficult because nutrient needs and activity levels of children with disabilities may be higher or lower than typical (Taylor & Rogers, 2005). For example, short stature is usually not a sign of limited nutrition in children with Turner syndrome (Cohen et al., 2008), but it can reflect long-term inadequate nutrition in PKU (Williams, Mamotte, & Burnett, 2008). Thin appearance is common in spastic quadriplegia (a severe form of cerebral palsy; Motil 2010; see Chapter 24). Also, although short stature can result from **undernutrition**, it

Table 8.3. Common nutrition advice that may not apply to children with disabilities

Common nutrition advice	How this advice may not apply to children with disabilities
"If she won't eat now, don't worry; she will eat when she is hungry."	The child may not respond to hunger cues. Hunger may be masked by fatigue, medications, or specific medical conditions.
"Don't worry. Others in the family are small."	Genetic and hereditary factors are important to identify, but many "small" children with disabilities are often undernourished due to lack of sufficient intake.
"He's just picky."	Behaviorally based feeding problems are common in children with disabilities. Some food refusals are key symptoms of an underlying medical problem.
"He's failing to thrive."	Many disabilities are associated with atypical growth patterns (disability-specific growth charts allow for more accurate interpretation of growth patterns).
"He eats the same foods all the time. He should eat a variety of foods."	Monotonous self-restricted eating patterns are common in children with developmental disabilities, especially those who have autism spectrum disorders. Some medical conditions (especially metabolic disorders) require a limited range of food types to prevent complications.

may instead result from muscle atrophy due to central nervous system damage. With undernutrition, nutritional intake should be increased; with muscle atrophy, added nutrition will add fat but not improve muscle bulk and may contribute to obesity.

MEDICAL NUTRITIONAL THERAPY

The overall goal of medical nutrition therapy (MNT) is to improve a child's health and nutritional status while promoting a family's enjoyment of their child at mealtimes. Examples of positive outcomes include encouraging success with self-feeding, meeting general nutritional needs, and correcting energy imbalances.

Nutrition Assessment and Nutrition Care Plan

The tools of MNT are the nutritional assessment and the nutritional care plan that is customized to the needs of each child. A nutritional assessment usually answers the following three questions (Riddick-Grisham, 2004, p. 328):

1. Is the child being fed a diet that meets his or her nutritional requirements?

2. Is the child growing as expected for his or her age, gender, and condition?

3. Is there a feeding or eating problem interfering with growth or with meeting nutritional requirements?

The nutrition assessment is the first step in the process of documenting a child's nutritional status. This involves the steps outlined in Table 8.4; the measurement and interpretation of growth parameters are defined in Table 8.1. If a child's nutritional status is not optimal, recommendations are made to improve the diet and feeding or eating practices.

The nutrition care plan articulates these recommendations and spells out monitoring and follow-up needs. Table 8.5 shows common interventions in a nutrition care plan. In addition to offering general dietary and feeding recommendations, a well-developed nutrition care plan addresses the role of food in the family and in the family's culture, including meal and snack patterns, food choices, and food preparation. Take the example of a child with Down syndrome who is significantly overweight. If obesity is a family problem, the weight loss plan should involve changing the entire family's eating patterns. If the family culture involves ingesting fatty and fried foods, a plan should be developed with the family to incorporate different cooking patterns. When providing food is

equated by the parents to providing love, emotional needs may be interfering with nutritional requirements. If food is used as a behavioral reinforcer, another equally effective reinforcer may need to be identified.

Nutrition Support for Children Who Cannot Eat

Nutrition support provides nutrients at high enough levels to meet nutrition requirements when the child is unable to ingest food and drink in the usual manner. It separates the delivery of nutrients from the act of eating by providing complete nutritional supplements and nutrients enterally—that is, directly to the gastrointestinal (GI) tract—or parenterally—that is, directly into the blood stream. **Enteral feeding** involves a gastric tube or **gastrostomy** placement surgery, resulting in feeding directly into the stomach. Successful placement not only improves nutrition but may also decrease the family's psychological stress around feeding issues. When it is important for feeding to bypass the GI tract, **parenteral feeding** is used. Usually parenteral feeding is administered in a hospital setting on a short-term basis (Carney, 2010).

The most common developmental disabilities that require nutrition support include cerebral palsy (spastic quadriplegia), progressive neurologic disorders (e.g., Tay-Sachs disease), uncontrolled seizures (e.g., Lennox-Gastaut syndrome), and certain inborn errors of metabolism (Carney, 2010). Table 8.6 illustrates a sample dietary intake for a child with spastic quadriplegia. Although nutritional support can correct the signs and symptoms of

---

Table 8.4. Elements of a nutrition assessment

Review the child's medical history (including diagnosis, laboratory findings, medications used, and developmental levels).

Assess and interpret the child's growth parameters (see Table 8.1).

Obtain the child's dietary history from caregivers (including intake patterns for food and drink, portion sizes, meal duration, and use of supplements).

Analyze and interpret the dietary intake information, based on the child's age and gender, for macronutrients (protein, fats, and carbohydrates), micronutrients (vitamins and minerals), fluids, and other dietary components (e.g., dietary fiber); computer dietary analysis programs can be used.

Summarize impressions of the child's nutritional status and the adequacy of his or her diet; make recommendations and referrals.

undernourishment, no special nutritional interventions have been identified to correct the short stature and low weight that is typical in severe cerebral palsy (Krick et al., 1996). These issues are discussed further in Chapter 24.

Nutrition Support Formulas

A wide range of formulas are available as food replacements, food supplements, and nutrition support as described in Table 8.7. These differ from infant formulas in terms of energy content, **osmolarity**, and the level of supplemented vitamins and minerals. Nutrition-support formulas differ further from one another in specific nutrients, caloric density, intended use, and mode of administration. Infants older than 1 year of age who require nutritional supplementation may be transitioned to pediatric formulas (intended for children up to 10 years old) that provide 30 calories per fluid ounce (as compared with regular infant formulas that provide 20 calories per fluid ounce). Children older than age 10 may use a formula intended

for adults (Joeckel & Phillips, 2009). Protein-free or carbohydrate-free formulas employed in inborn errors of metabolism entail additional arrangements (see Chapter 19). They are not used alone, as they create a nutritional deficiency if not mixed with other formulas or foods (Isaacs & Zand, 2007). The goals of maintaining regular foods in the diet and minimizing reliance on complete nutritional supplements are common for children with oral-motor feeding problems such as Rett syndrome and certain forms of cerebral palsy (Marchand et al., 2006).

SPECIAL NUTRITIONAL CONCERNS IN CHILDREN WITH DISABILITIES

Some of the nutritional concerns associated with specific developmental disabilities are listed in Table 8.8. In most cases, families of children with specialized diets benefit from the involvement of a registered dietitian, who can help monitor the diets and provide consultative support to schools and other agencies. Such support assures appropriate implementation of dietary recommendations.

Therapeutic Diets

Diets for inborn errors of metabolism, such as PKU, and the **ketogenic diet** used in some children with intractable epilepsy provide examples of customized diets that differ in composition and goals. Both types of diet are similar in requiring close monitoring and in causing behavior problems around food at home, in school, and at restaurants. Table 8.9 shows a sample daily nutritional intake for a 10 year old

Table 8.5. Sample interventions found in a nutrition care plan

Recommend meal and snack schedules or timing.

Counter side effects from medications (e.g., increased appetite, effect on taste).

Prevent overweight or underweight.

Monitor planned weight gain, weight loss, or catch-up growth.

Apply specialty (disease-specific) growth charts for growth assessment.

Estimate fat stores and body composition for in-depth growth assessment.

Analyze and interpret home intake diet record.

Modify diets for specific nutrients, such as low protein, high calorie, or low fat.

Reinforce breast feeding, infant formula, or formula preparation steps.

Select foods to address food texture problems or avoid choking.

Manage food refusals, food jags, or other food behaviors.

Demonstrate how to determine portion sizes and measure foods.

Order special formulas or supplements.

Reinforce signs of hunger, fullness, and right pace of eating or feeding.

Document food insecurity and refer the family to community nutrition programs.

Coordinate with other health care providers and educators.

Complete referrals for WIC (Special Supplemental Nutrition Program for Women, Infants and Children), early intervention services, or other providers.

Table 8.6. Sample intake and feeding schedule for a child with a limited ability to eat by mouth and supplemented feedings via gastrostomy tube

6:30 A.M.	Stop night feeding pump
9:30 A.M.	Oral snack at school: milk in a cup and spoon-fed applesauce
11:45 A.M.	School lunch: modified soft texture, 30% self-feeding
1:00 P.M.	Gastrostomy feeding of 8 fluid ounces of complete nutritional supplement
3:30 P.M.	After-school snack at home: self-fed cookie and milk in a cup
6:00 P.M.	Supper with family: mashed potato with gravy on a spoon and juice in a cup
8:30 P.M.	Start night feeding of 50 milliliters per hour complete nutritional supplement, providing 40% of daily calories and 60% of daily protein intake

Table 8.7. Selected formulas for children with disabilities

Formulas and their components	Use based on diagnosis or condition
Standard infant formulas; 20 calories per fluid ounce*	Full-term newborns up to 1 year
Premature transitional formula; 22 calories per fluid ounce*	Discharge formula for infants with birth weight of <1800 grams, on limited volume intake or history of osteoporosis or poor growth
Complete nutritional supplements (e.g., Pediasure, Boost); 30 calories per fluid ounce*	Meal or snack substitutes Increase calories Ensure intake of specific nutrients (e.g., protein)
Formulas modified in the balance of nutrients; these are not used alone	Protein free: protein-restricted diets Carbohydrate restricted: ketogenic diet Fat altered: diets for gastrointestinal disorders or long chain fatty acid oxidation disorders Specific amino acids removed: phenylketonuria

*Calories per fluid ounce can be adjusted based on a child's needs

with PKU who is complying well with a low-protein diet.

With the rapid expansion of screening of newborns for a variety of genetic and metabolic conditions (Chapter 19), a parallel expansion will be necessary to address the special nutritional requirements of children having such disorders (Longo, 2006). As a result of the effectiveness of early dietary treatment for PKU, the list of inborn errors of metabolism treated early in life through diet has increased markedly (American College of Medical Genetics, 2006; Longo, 2006). Treatment and follow-up of these rare genetic conditions has provided a model of customized nutrition therapy that may have broader applications in creating nutritional interventions tailored to the genetic characteristics of adult individuals as well (American College of Medical Genetics, 2006).

Table 8.10 shows a sample dietary intake for an older child on a ketogenic diet. A ketogenic diet is deliberately designed to be very high in fat content and very low in carbohydrates while providing adequate calories and protein for growth. This diet results in the accumulation of ketones in the body; ketones are thought to be the mechanism of improved seizure control (see Chapter 27). The sample diet shown is for an older child who eats regular foods; however some children on the ketogenic diet are not able to consume food by mouth and rely on specific fat-modified formulas that are administered through a gastrostomy tube (Zupec-Kania & Spellman, 2008).

Food Allergies

The public is increasingly concerned about links between various types of food allergies and chronic illnesses. A food allergy is an adverse reaction to food caused by an immune response. The most common food allergens in the United States are milk, soy, egg, wheat, peanut, tree nut, fish, and seafood. Poor nutritional outcomes may occur in children with food allergies as a consequence of diet restrictions that may severely impact nutrient intake. Nutrition education should focus on foods that should be avoided. Nutritionally complete hypoallergenic formulas are available to supplement a child's intake and ensure adequate growth (Feuling, Levy, & Goday, 2010).

Constipation

Gastrointestinal dysfunction is another frequent concern for children with developmental disabilities. Substituting whole wheat bread for white bread, and fresh unpeeled apples for apple juice, are typically suggested to families dealing with a toddler who has meningomyelocoele or Down syndrome. For tube-fed children, providing a fiber-containing formula and additional fluid may alleviate constipation. However, constipation that is refractory to routine dietary interventions (i.e., increasing fiber in the diet) can be treated using medications. A variety of laxatives at small daily doses have shown effectiveness in preventing impaction, discomfort, and constipation-caused **anorexia** (Sullivan, 2008).

Celiac Disease

Celiac disease involves a permanent sensitivity to gluten, the protein portion of wheat and rye. Some children with celiac disease also have to avoid oats. Children with a number of conditions associated with developmental disabilities have a higher incidence of celiac disease than children in the typically developing population; these conditions include Down syndrome, Turner syndrome, and Williams syndrome (Hill et al., 2005). Emerging evidence and case reports suggest a higher incidence of celiac disease in autism spectrum disorders; however evidence remains inconclusive (Genuis, & Bouchard, 2010). In affected children, a gluten-free diet has to be followed strictly, even when children are asymptomatic. Many processed foods, from both grocery stores and restaurants, must be avoided because they contain wheat and other flours for fillers and binding agents. Potato-, soy-, and rice-based products can be substitutes for regular breads and pastas, although these specialized foods may be prohibitively expensive for many families.

Dietary Self-Restriction

Dietary self-restriction is a common problem in children with developmental disabilities, manifesting itself in food refusal, selectivity by type of food or food texture, oral-motor delay, and **dysphagia** (Levy et al., 2009; see also Chapter 9). Autism spectrum disorders (see Chapter 21) are particularly associated with a selective eating pattern resulting from a resistance to change (Emond et al., 2010). Sensitivities to the food colors, textures, and temperature are often reported, in which case a child refuses to eat many foods and rigidly insists on what he or she will eat. When not given preferred foods, the child completely refuses to eat and may have temper tantrums. The child may also prefer to drink rather than to eat foods, so a

Table 8.8. Common nutrition concerns of particular developmental disabilities

Prematurity-related nutrition problems likely in the first 3 years	Formula changes to accommodate medical problems Delayed self-feeding Rate of growth corrected for preterm birth Difficulty with setting feeding schedules Variable appetite, especially with illness Gastrointestinal problems (constipation, gastroesophageal reflux, reduced appetite)
Neuromuscular disorders (e.g. cerebral palsy)	Difficulty gaining weight, particularly with frequent illness Underweight with small muscle mass Short stature Constipation which may or may not be alleviated with dietary fiber Feeding problems/swallowing incoordination limiting food types Need to consider supplementation or gastrostomy
Developmental delays/intellectual disability (e.g., Down syndrome, Prader-Willi syndrome)	Unusual growth patterns Underweight or overweight Unusual level of activity, either higher or lower Delayed self-feeding skills Self-restricted diet Difficulty identifying hunger and fullness Constipation which may or may not be alleviated with dietary fiber
Attention-deficit/hyperactivity disorder	Inability to sit long enough to eat a meal Distractibility interfering with eating and meals Lack of structured meal and snack patterns Possible decreased appetite as a medication side effect Difficulty with socializing at meals
Epilepsy	A growth plateau is likely, even if eating well Possible changes in appetite as medication side effect A postseizure state is likely to interfere with meals and energy intake Unusual growth patterns in children with poorly controlled seizures

Table 8.9.   Sample diet for a 10-year-old with phenylketonuria (PKU)

Breakfast	½ cup Froot Loops 6 fluid ounces rice milk 1 low-protein blueberry muffin 8 fluid ounces PKU formula
Lunch	Medium garden salad with 2 tablespoons of ranch dressing Small order of fast food french fries 12 fluid ounces Sprite
After-school snack	Baked apple slices with brown sugar and cinnamon 8 fluid ounces PKU formula
Dinner	Hot dog bun with 1 slice low-protein cheese, mustard, ketchup, and pickles 1-ounce bag Wise Onion Rings Pear 8 fluid ounces PKU formula

high proportion of total calories comes from one type of drink. Interventions to improve the child's diet might include providing a complete vitamin and mineral supplement and adding new foods one at a time by offering them many times (15–20 times) over 1–2 months, paired with positive reinforcers (i.e., foods the child likes; see Chapter 32). Usually children with ASDs have typical growth and caloric intake despite their unusual eating habits.

Issues Specific to Premature Infants

Nutritional interventions for preterm infants represent the frontier of nutrition science. Premature infants may have behaviorally based feeding problems complicated by medical and growth concerns. In one study, children born before 26 weeks of gestation age and assessed at 6 years of age were shown to have continued feeding difficulties (Samara, Johnson, Lamberts, Marlow, & Wolke, 2010). Immaturity of the gastrointestinal system is one of the limiting factors in meeting nutrition requirements in premature infants, resulting in the need to supplement human breast milk with increased calories, specific fats, protein, vitamins, and minerals (O'Connor et al., 2008). Recommendations about specific vitamin and mineral requirements and long-chain fatty acid supplements after preterm birth are evolving, but findings show that increased intake of energy and protein result in greater lean-body mass accretion as opposed to fat mass (Agostoni et al., 2010). As one example, 400 international units of vitamin D per day from food or supplements is now recommended for all infants and children because of an increased risk of **rickets** (Wagner, & Greer, 2008).

Table 8.10.   Sample ketogenic diet: Intake for an older child on a 4:1 (fat:protein + carbohydrate) ratio

Breakfast	Omelet made with: 35 grams egg, 35 grams butter, 20 grams mushroom
Lunch	55 grams beef bologna 15 grams black olives 30 grams mayonnaise 20 grams tomato
After-school snack	Carbohydrate-free multivitamin and mineral pill 20 grams strawberries 55 grams heavy whipping cream
Dinner	25 grams chicken breast cooked in 25 grams butter 25 grams avocado 25 grams green beans cooked in 20 grams butter
Snack	50 grams carrot sticks 25 grams mayonnaise

NUTRITION WITHIN COMPLEMENTARY AND ALTERNATIVE MEDICAL CARE

In response to the large number of children with developmental disabilities, many products, treatments, and medicines have been created to improve nutrition. Products claiming to boost energy or correct nutritional deficiencies are attractive to parents of children with developmental disabilities. Data from the 2007 National Health Interview Survey (NHIS) shows that one in nine children used complementary and alternative medicine (CAM) in the previous year (National Center for Health Statistics, 2008b). CAM is most commonly used by children with asthma, attention-deficit/hyperactivity disorder, autism, cancer, cerebral palsy, cystic fibrosis, inflammatory bowel disease, and/or juvenile rheumatoid arthritis. CAM approaches that are promoted to improve nutrition include **megavitamin therapy**, amino acid and mineral supplements, and herbal remedies. Although CAM approaches are often presumed to be harmless, the safety of these approaches has not been well-documented, and no CAM nutritional therapy has been proven effective by scientific methods (Kemper, Vohr, & Wells, 2008). Furthermore, some CAM is clearly unsafe—for example, some CAM therapies targeted for pediatric oncology patients may negatively interact with chemotherapy and radiation therapy (Roth, Lin, Kim, & Moody, 2009). CAM in the form of nutritional supplements can also lead to increased risk for or new side effects of medication received to control the underlying disability (e.g., antiepileptic medication). Thus, a child's medical and nutrition history should include a comprehensive list of supplements (Kemper, Vohr, & Wells, 2008). CAM is further discussed in Chapter 38.

SUMMARY

Underweight, overweight, constipation, food allergies, feeding difficulties, and other GI disturbances that interfere with appetite are more common in children with developmental disabilities than in typically developing children. Dietary guidelines for Americans (U.S. Department of Agriculture, 2010) and the MyPlate Plan (U.S. Department of Agriculture, n.d.) are not sufficient resources for customizing nutrition recommendations for many children with developmental disabilities. Thus, medical nutrition therapy that includes a nutrition

assessment and care plan should be part of the comprehensive care for children with developmental disabilities. Pediatric nutrition experts work in a variety of care settings (e.g., schools, clinics, hospitals) to ensure that children with disabilities receive good nutrition services and that the children's parents are supported in their efforts to make feeding and nutrition a positive aspect of parenting and family life.

REFERENCES

Agostoni, C., Buonocore, G., Carnielli, V.P., De Curtis, M., Darmaun, D. Decsi, T., ... ESPGHAN Committee on Nutrition. (2010). Enteral nutrient supply for preterm infants: Commentary from the European Society for Paediatric Gastroenterology, Hepatology, and Nutrition Committee on Nutrition. *Journal of Pediatric Gastroenterology and Nutrition, 50*, 85–91.

American College of Medical Genetics. (2006). Newborn screening: Toward a uniform screening panel and system: Final report. *ACMG Medical Geneticist 8,* (5, Suppl.), 12–252.

American Dietetic Association. (2002). Position of the American Dietetic Association: Ethical and legal issues in nutrition, hydration and feeding. *Journal of the American Dietetic Association, 102*, 716–725.

American Dietetic Association. (2010). Position of the American Dietetic Association: Integration of medical nutrition therapy and pharmacotherapy. *Journal of the American Dietetic Association, 110*, 950–956.

Arvay, J., Zemel, B.S., Gallagher, P.R., Rovner A.J., Mulberg, A.E., Stallings, V.A., & Haber, B.A. (2005). Body composition of children aged 1 to 12 years with biliary atresia or Alagille syndrome. *Journal of Pediatric Gastroenterology and Nutrition, 40*, 146–150.

Bandini, L.G., Anderson, S.E., Curtin, C., Cermak, S., Evans, E.W., Scampini, R., ... Must, A. (2010). Food selectivity in children with autism spectrum disorders and typically developing children. *Pediatrics, 157*, 259–264.

Bandini, L.G., Curtin, C., Hamad, C., Tybor, D.J., & Must, A. (2005). Prevalence of overweight in children with developmental disorders in the continuous national health and nutrition examination survey (NHANES) 1999–2002. *Pediatrics, 146*(6), 738–743.

Bell, K.L., Boyd, R.N., Tweedy, S.M., Weir, K.A., Stevenson, R.D., & Davies, P.S. (2010). A prospective, longitudinal study of growth, nutrition and sedentary behavior in young children with cerebral palsy. *Biomedical Central Public Health, 10*, 1–12.

Bell, K.L., & Davies, S.W. (2010). Energy expenditure and physical activity of ambulatory children with cerebral palsy and of typically developing children. *American Journal of Clinical Nutrition, 92*, 313–319.

Brown, J.E. (Ed.). (2007). *Nutrition through the life cycle* (3rd ed.). Belmont, CA: Wadsworth.

Carney, L.N., Nepa, A., Cohen, S.S., Dean, A., Yanni, C., & Markowitz, G. (2010). Parenteral and enteral nutrition support: Determining the best way to feed. In M. Corkins (Ed.), *The A.S.P.E.N. pediatric nutrition support core curriculum*. Silver Springs, MD: American Society for Parenteral and Enteral Nutrition.

Chudley, A.E., Conry, J., Cook, J.L., Loock, C., Rosales, T., & LeBlanc, N. (2005). Fetal alcohol spectrum disorder: Canadian guidelines for diagnosis. *Canadian Medical Association Journal, 172*(5, Suppl.), S1–S21.

Cohen, P., Rogol, A.D., Deal, C.L., Saenger, P., Reiter, E.O., Ross, J.L., ... Wit, J.M. (2008). Consensus statement on the diagnosis and treatment of children with idiopathic short stature: A summary of the growth hormone research society, the Lawson Wilkins Pediatric Endocrine Society, and the European Society for Paediatric Endocrinology Workshop. *The Journal of Clinical Endocrinology and Metabolism, 93,* 4210–4217.

Emond, A., Emmett, P., Steer, C., & Golding, J. (2010). Feeding symptoms, dietary patterns, and growth in young children with autism spectrum disorders. *Pediatrics, 126,* e337–e342.

Feuling, M.B., Levy, M.B., & Goday, P.S. (2010). Food allergies. In M. Corkins (Ed.), *The A.S.P.E.N. pediatric nutrition support core curriculum.* Silver Springs, MD: American Society for Parenteral and Enteral Nutrition.

Genuis, S.J., & Bouchard, T.P. (2010). Celiac disease presenting as autism. *Journal of Child Neurology, 25,* 114–119.

Hill, I.D., Dirks, M.H., Liptak, G.S., Colletti, R.B., Fasano, A., Guandalini, S., ... Seidman, E.G. (2005). Guideline for the diagnosis and treatment of celiac disease in children: Recommendations of the North American Society for Pediatric Gastroenterology, Hepatology and Nutrition. *Journal of Pediatric Gastoenterology and Nutrition, 40,* 1–19.

Institute of Medicine, Food and Nutrition Board. (1997). *Dietary reference intakes for calcium, phosphorus, magnesium, vitamin D, and fluoride.* Washington, DC: National Academies Press.

Institute of Medicine, Food and Nutrition Board. (2001). *Dietary reference intakes for vitamin A, vitamin K, arsenic, boron, chromium, copper, iodine, iron. molybdenum, nickel, silicon, vanadium, and zinc.* Washington, DC: National Academies Press.

Institute of Medicine, Food and Nutrition Board. (2005). *Dietary reference intakes for energy, carbohydrate, fiber, fat, fatty acids, cholesterol, protein, and amino acids.* Retrieved August 3, 2010, from http://www.nap.edu

Isaacs, J.S., & Zand, D.J. (2007). Single-gene autosomal recessive disorders and Prader-Willi syndrome: An update for food and nutrition professionals. *Journal of the American Dietetic Association, 107,* 466–478.

Joeckel, R.J., & Phillips, S.K. (2009). Overview of infant and pediatric formulas. *Nutrition in Clinical Practice, 24,* 356–362.

Kemper, K.J., Vohra, S., Walls, R., & the Task Force of Complementary and Alternative Medicine and the Provisional Section on Complementary, Holistic, and Integrative Medicine. (2008). The use of complementary and alternative medicine in pediatrics. *Pediatrics, 122,* 1374–1386.

Krick, J., Murphy-Miller, P., Zeger, S., & Wright, E. (1996). Patterns of growth in children with cerebral palsy. *Journal of the American Dietetic Association, 96,* 680–685.

Levy, Y., Levy, A., Zangen, T., Kornfield, L., Dalal, I., Samuel, E., ... Levine, A. (2009). Diagnostic clues for identification of nonorganic vs organic causes of food refusal and poor feeding. *Journal of Pediatric Gastroenterology and Nutrition, 48,* 355–362.

Lewith, G.T., & Chan, J. (2002). An exploratory qualitative study to investigate how patients evaluate complementary and conventional medicine. *Complementary Therapies in Medicine, 10,* 69–77.

Liusuwan, R.A., Widman, L.M., Abresch, R.T., Styne, D.M., & McDonald, C.M. (2007). Body composition and resting energy expenditure in patients aged 11 to 21 years with spinal cord dysfunction compared to controls: Comparisons and relationships among groups. *The Journal of Spinal Cord Medicine, 30,* S105–S111.

Longo, N. (2006). Inborn errors of metabolism: New challenges with expanded newborn screening programs. *American Journal of Medical Genetics, 142C,* 61–63.

Mahan, J.D., & Warady, B.A. (2006). Assessment and treatment of short stature in pediatric patients with chronic kidney disease: A consensus statement. *Pediatric Nephrology, 21,* 917–930.

Marchand, V., Motil, K.J., & the North American Society for Pediatric Gastroenterology, Hepatology, and Nutrition [NASPGHAN] Committee on Nutrition. (2006). Nutrition support for neurologically impaired children: A clinical report of the North American Society for Pediatric Gastroenterology, Hepatology, and Nutrition. *Journal of Pediatric Gastroenterology and Nutrition, 43,* 123–135.

Meyer, C. (2004). Scientists probe role of vitamin D: Deficiency a significant problem. *Journal of the American Medical Association, 292,* 1416–1418.

Motil, K.J. (2010). Developmental delay. In M. Corkins, (Ed.), *The A.S.P.E.N. pediatric nutrition support core curriculum.* Silver Springs, MD: American Society for Parenteral and Enteral Nutrition.

Munck, A. (2010). Nutritional considerations in patients with cystic fibrosis. *Expert Reviews of Respiratory Medicine, 4,* 47–56.

National Center for Health Statistics. (2000). *NCHS growth curves for children 0–19 years.* Washington, DC: U.S. Government Printing Office.

National Center for Health Statistics. (2008a). *Anthropometric reference data for children and adults: United States, 2003–2006.* Washington, DC: U.S. Government Printing Office.

National Center for Health Statistics. (2008b). *Complementary and alternative medicine use among adults and children: United States, 2007.* Washington, DC: U.S. Government Printing Office.

National Center for Health Statistics. (2010). *Changes in terminology for childhood overweight and obesity.* Washington, DC: U.S. Government Printing Office.

O'Connor, D.L., Khan, S., Weishuhn, K., Vaughan, J., Jefferies, A., Campbell, D.M., ...Whyte, H. (2008). Growth and nutrient intakes of human milk fed preterm infants provided with extra energy and nutrients after hospital discharge. *Pediatrics, 121,* 766–776.

Oddy, W.H., Webb, K.G., Baikie, G., Thompson, S.M., Reilly, S., Fyfe, S.D., ... Leonard, H. (2007). Feeding experiences and growth status in a Rett syndrome population. *Journal of Pediatric Gastroenterology and Nutrition, 45,* 582–590.

Riddick-Grisham, S. (Ed.). (2004). *Pediatric life care planning and case management.* Boca Raton, FL: CRC Press.

Roth, M., Lin, J., Kim, M., & Moody, K. (2009). Pediatric oncologists' views towards the use of complementary and alternative medicine in children with cancer. *Journal of Pediatric Hematology and Oncology, 31,* 177–182.

Samara, M., Johnson, S., Lamberts, K., Marlow, N., & Wolke, D. (2010). Eating problems at age 6 years in a whole population sample of extremely preterm children. *Developmental Medicine and Child Neurology, 52,* e16–22.

Speiser, P.W., Rudolf, M.C.J., Anhalt, H., Camancho-Hubner, C., Chiarelli, F., Eliakim, A., ... Hochberg, Z. (2005). Consensus statement: Childhood obesity. *Journal of Clinical Endocrinology & Metabolism, 90,* 1871–1887.

Sullivan, P.B. (2008). Gastrointestinal disorders in children with neurodevelopmental disabilities. *Developmental Disabilities Research Review, 14,* 128–136.

U.S. Department of Agriculture. (n.d.). *ChooseMyPlate.* Retrieved August 1, 2011, from http://www.choosemyplate.gov

U.S. Department of Agriculture. (2010). *Dietary guidelines for Americans.* Retrieved November 12, 2010, from http://www.cnpp.usda.gov/DGAs2010-DGACReport.htm

Wagner, C.L., Greer, F.R., American Academy of Pediatrics Section on Breastfeeding, & American Academy of Pediatrics Committee on Nutrition. (2008). Prevention of rickets and vitamin D deficiency in infants, children, and adolescents. *Pediatrics, 122,* 1142–1152.

Williams, R.A., Mamotte, C.D., & Burnett, J.R. (2008). Phenylketonuria: An inborn error of phenylalanine metabolism. *Clinical Biochemical Review, 29,* 31–41.

Zupec-Kania, B.A., & Spellman, E. (2008). An overview of the ketogenic diet for pediatric epilepsy. *Nutrition in Clinical Practice, 23,* 589–596.

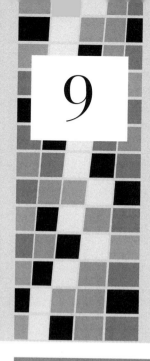

9

Feeding and Its Disorders

Peggy S. Eicher

Upon completion of this chapter, the reader will

■ Be able to describe the feeding-swallowing process and how it changes as an infant grows and develops

■ Understand how medical, motor, and interactional problems influence a child's feeding function

■ Recognize some of the common feeding problems that occur in children with developmental disabilities

■ Identify the basic components of a treatment approach to feeding problems

---

Children with developmental disabilities commonly experience problems feeding; some studies estimate 33%–80% of children with developmental disabilities have such problems (Linscheid, 2006). Although the exact rate is unknown, consensus has emerged that the incidence of swallowing dysfunction in children is increasing (Lefton-Greif, 2008). Feeding problems may vary in manifestation from difficulty chewing to difficulty swallowing (**dysphagia**), severe food selectivity, inadequate intake, or total food refusal. Feeding problems result from a combination of several factors: anatomical abnormality, motor or sensory dysfunction, medical or psychological conditions, growth abnormality, learning difficulties, or social interaction difficulties (Piazza, 2008). Multiple medical causes are present in almost 50% of children with feeding problems. About 90% have at least one medical diagnosis (Lefton-Greif, 2008). There are certain patterns

of clinical presentation associated with specific underlying diagnostic conditions. For example, oral motor dysfunctions or delays are common in children with global developmental delays, cerebral palsy, and Down syndrome, while children diagnosed on the autism spectrum more likely exhibit food selectivity (Lefton-Greif, 2008). The challenge in treating feeding problems for children with developmental disabilities is not only identifying all of the factors interfering with the child's feeding function but also understanding how they interrelate.

This chapter first reviews the normal swallowing process and the changes that occur in that process during growth and development. Next, the chapter traces how various medical and developmental conditions influence the feeding process and how such conditions frequently cause feeding problems in children with developmental disabilities. A case history is presented to illustrate the interaction of the different influences and their impact on feeding function. Examples of common feeding and digestive disorders are discussed, along with approaches to therapy.

▩ ▩ ▩ ANGELINA

Angelina is a 27-month-old girl referred for evaluation because she "doesn't want to eat." She was born prematurely at 25 weeks' gestation, weighing 1 pound. As a complication of her premature birth, Angelina has cerebral palsy and was slow to accept oral feeding for the first 3 months of life.

By the time she was discharged home at 4 months, Angelina had come to accept bottle feeding, although she drank only 2 ounces at a time and needed frequent breaks. Spoon-feeding proved so difficult for Angelina that her mother resorted to putting baby food in the bottle. Angelina transitioned to whole milk at 15 months of age. Her mother reported Angelina's stools became harder and less frequent on whole milk. A 30-calorie per ounce nutritionally complete formula was recommended at 20 months of age because of poor weight gain and to provide more balanced nutrition. Angelina refused to sit in a high chair to eat, so her mother fed Angelina on her lap. Oral-motor problems included minimal mouth-opening for spoon-feeding, and frequent expelling of the few bites of solid foods that she would feed herself.

With baby foods, Angelina didn't open her mouth and pushed the food off the back of the spoon, never letting the food pass through her lips. For bottle feeding, Angelina sat in her mother's lap in a very reclined position. Her extensor tone increased during the bottle feeding. She frequently arched and broke away from the nipple. Stooling was effortful, with one hard stool produced every 3–4 days. Angelina's mother often had to help her evacuate the stools.

On physical examination, Angelina's weight was well below the 3rd percentile for her age (i.e., she weighed less than 97 out of 100 children her age). Her height was at the 10th percentile for age. Angelina's muscle tone was increased throughout, legs more than arms, but with a variable quality. Angelina had developed good head control, but shoulder strength was weak. When sitting upright while supported through the hips, she tended to throw herself backward. Lungs were clear to auscultation with no areas of rhonchi or wheezing. Her stool was palpable on abdominal exam. During a feeding observation, Angelina sat in a high chair. She self-fed a few pieces of dry cereal, placing them near her lateral incisors, and munched them adequately. Her mother attempted to spoon-feed her baby food. Angelina never opened her mouth as her mother tried to push the spoon through her lips repeatedly, resulting in minimal intake despite a prolonged mealtime. With the bottle, her mother reclined Angelina in her lap about 60 degrees. Angelina bit on the nipple without suction. As the feeding progressed, lower extremity extension increased, throwing her into an arched position through her upper body and making it more difficult to control the position of Angelina's head and neck.

Angelina definitely needs intervention. Calorie intake is inadequate, resulting in poor weight gain. Effective intervention must identify what factors are preventing her from eating more successfully. Identifying those factors correctly requires familiarity with the normal feeding process and how it changes over the first few years of life.

THE FEEDING PROCESS

Swallowing

Swallowing is one of the most complex motor activities that humans perform. It entails the coordinated function of striated and smooth muscles of the head and neck, plus the respiratory and gastrointestinal tracts. Swallowing also requires input from the central, peripheral, and autonomic nervous systems (Leopold & Daniels, 2010; Miller, 1986). Swallowing can be divided into four phases (Figure 9.1). The **oral preparatory** (Phase I) and **oral transport phases** (Phase II) are primarily volitional. During these oral phases, food is broken up, forming a bolus by the tongue; the tongue then transports the bolus to the back of the throat. The **pharyngeal transfer phase** (Phase III) begins when the bolus passes the faucial arches (near the tonsils) and triggers the start of the swallowing cascade. The swallowing cascade is the involuntary sequence of highly coordinated movements of the **pharyngeal** (throat) and **esophageal** (tube-to-stomach) muscles. With

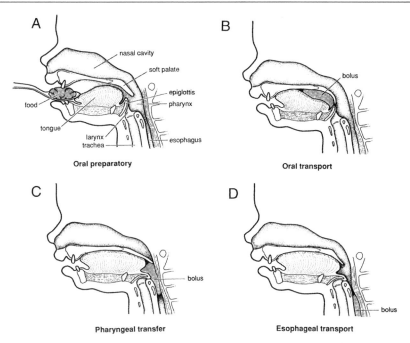

Figure 9.1. The four phases of swallowing. A) Phase I, oral preparatory: Food is taken into the mouth, processed to a manageable consistency, and then collected into a small parcel, or bolus. B) Phase II, oral transport: The bolus is then pushed backward by the tongue toward the pharynx. C) Phase III, pharyngeal transfer: As swallowing begins, the epiglottis normally folds over the opening of the trachea to direct food down the esophagus and not into the lungs. D) Phase IV, esophageal transport: The peristaltic wave moves the bolus down the esophagus toward the stomach.

each swallow, respiration ceases as the soft palate elevates to close off the nasopharynx (entrance to the nasal airway at the back of the mouth). At the same time forward movement and elevation of the hyoid bone results in: 1) tipping of the epiglottis (a projecting piece of cartilage) to cover the trachea (entrance to the lungs) so that food does not slip into the airway, and 2) opening the **upper esophageal sphincter** (UES, or entrance to the esophagus). A wave-like motion (**peristalsis**) originating in the back wall of the throat propels the bolus past the closed airway, through the open UES, and into the esophagus, marking the start of the **esophageal transport phase** (Phase IV). During esophageal transport, the bolus is pushed down the esophagus by continuation of the peristaltic wave, which signals the relaxation, or opening, of the **lower esophageal sphincter** (LES, entrance to the stomach), allowing the bolus to pass into the stomach. Entrance of the bolus into the stomach and subsequent closure of the LES marks the end of the esophageal transport phase.

Developmental Changes in Oral Motor Skills

The process of swallowing evolves as the nervous system matures. Phase I of swallowing (oral preparatory) is most influenced by growth and development. Reflexive oral-motor patterns in the infant are integrated into more complex oral-motor patterns that are learned through practice. Cortical maturation enables more independent and finely graded tongue and jaw movements to develop under increasing volitional control (Leopold & Daniels, 2010). Acquisition of oral motor skills occurs in a sequential, stepwise progression. Mastery of skills at each level provides the foundation for skills at the next level. Thus, no stage can be skipped without interfering with the foundation skills for the next stage.

Suckling

Suckling is the earliest oral pattern. The tongue moves in and out while riding up and down with the jaw, creating a wave-like motion. Suckling motions and swallowing activity have been reported in fetuses as early as 12–14 weeks' gestation (Popescu, Popescu, Wang, Barlow, & Gustafson, 2008). Suckling and swallowing are gradually coupled over the course of gestation so that the fetus can swallow half an ounce at 20 weeks' gestation and up to 15 ounces at 38–40 weeks' gestation. Only following delivery and with some practice, however, does the baby develop the rhythmical suck-swallow bursts coordinated with breathing to allow functional feeding. This stepwise coupling of suck-swallow and then suck-swallow-breath is one reason that even healthy premature infants usually require tube feedings during the first weeks of life (Amaizu, Shulman, Schanler, & Lau, 2008; Gewolb & Vice, 2006; Ross, 2008).

For the first 3–4 months of life, suckling is a reflexively driven activity that occurs involuntarily whenever something enters the infant's mouth. With brain maturation, the reflex is integrated and the infant can control initiation of the suckle pattern. Likewise, the ability to stabilize the jaw increases and the tongue dissociates from the jaw, leading to the next stage, sucking.

Sucking

During sucking, the lips purse, the jaw opening is smaller and more controlled than in suckling, and the tongue is raised and lowered independently of the jaw. When sucking replaces the **anterior/posterior** pattern of suckling, usually around 5 months of age, the child can progress to spoon feeding. Because of the predominant up-and-down pattern of sucking, food can be transported to the back of the mouth without first riding out of the mouth on the tongue.

Munching and Chewing

With munching, small pieces of food are broken off, flattened, and then collected for swallowing. Munching consists of a rhythmical bite-and-release pattern with a series of well-graded jaw openings and closings. More important, however, the emergence of tongue lateralization at this stage enables the child to move food from side-to-side and then regather it in the mid-line. Actual chewing and grinding food into smaller pieces does not occur until the child acquires a rotary component jaw movement, a capacity that emerges around 9 months of age and is gradually modified via repetition until, by around 2 years of age, it approximates the adult pattern (Gisel, 2008).

The Influence of Growth on Oral-Motor Structures

Typically, the attainment of new oral-motor skills coincides with the change in oral-motor structures occurring with growth. The infant, for example, is perfectly equipped for nipple-feeding. The cheek fat pads confine the oral cavity while the tongue, soft palate, and epiglottis fill much of the mouth, easing the formation of the vacuum necessary to draw fluids out of the nipple. The larynx (voice box at the entryway to the lungs) is almost tucked under the tongue, necessitating less throat control to guide the liquid past the airway and into the esophagus (Bosma, 1986).

With growth, jaw and palate enlarge in relation to the soft tissue structures, allowing room for teeth (Figure 9.2). The larger oral cavity is not as efficient for nipple-feeding but facilitates spoon entry and lateralization. The larynx descends and moves backward as the neck lengthens. This elongation necessitates increased postural control of the head and neck to enable safe swallowing. This is achieved as the child develops gross motor control for righting the head and sitting independently. Meanwhile, the changes occurring in the child's oral-motor pattern afford the tongue increasing control of collection and propulsion of the food in the mouth and **pharynx**, enhancing the child's ability to guide the food safely past the airway.

The integration of growth and enlarging structures with increasing neurologic control over posture and oral-motor pattern is so important that delay in gross motor or oral-motor development can decrease feeding efficiency and foster swallowing incompetency (Manno, Fox, Eicher, & Kerwin, 2005). Similarly, feeding difficulties may be the first sign of an anatomical defect involving the oral or nasal cavities, pharynx, or esophagus that can adversely affect swallowing. **Clefts** such as those in the lip or palate interfere with sealing off the oral cavity, decreasing the child's efficiency at generating negative pressure and collecting the food in preparation for swallowing. A change in size or shape of an oral structure that affects coordination of the swallowing process can also be a significant problem; for example, enlarged tonsils and adenoids may render the child dependent on his or her mouth as an airway, influencing suck-swallow-breath timing and even coordination, if the flow of the food bolus is disrupted by the tonsils. Normal esophageal **peristalsis** (the involuntary constriction and relaxation of the muscles of the esophagus and intestine, creating wavelike movements that push food forward) is interrupted in children with **esophageal atresia** or **tracheoesophageal fistulae**, which are abnormal connections of the esophagus to the respiratory tract. Even after repair of these abnormal connections, the child's swallow will be influenced by the degree

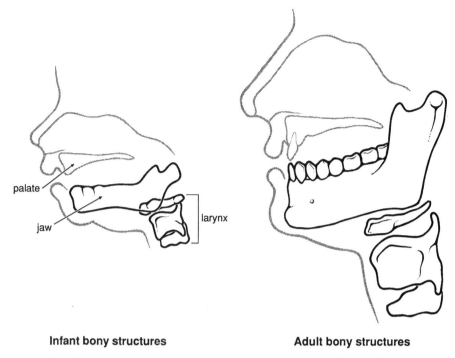

Infant bony structures   **Adult bony structures**

Figure 9.2. The influence of growth on the bony structures of the oropharynx. The mandible (jaw) enlarges, enabling room for teeth and a larger oral cavity. The larynx descends and moves posteriorly, necessitating increased control of bolus propulsion to guide it past the airway.

of abnormal peristalsis remaining in the esophageal phase of the swallow.

Referring back to the case study and Angelina, the development of her feeding problems can now be understood. She was an ineffective bottle feeder. As she was a 25-week preterm baby, suck-swallow-breath coordination would have been absent at birth and would have had to develop while she was intubated and supported with a **nasogastric (NG)** tube running through her nose down to her stomach. Moreover, the lack of buccal fat pads in the so-called micropremi impedes the generation of sucking pressures. In fact, Angelina continues to use more nipple compression than suction to bottle-feed. Because she was not successful at spoon feeding, she did not acquire the foundational skill of sucking, with its jaw stability and independent tongue movement. This prevented her from progressing to lateral movement of the tongue. She is not accustomed to using her tongue as a platform to transport food. Although she can move small pieces of food with the edge of her tongue over to her teeth to flatten them, she does not use her tongue to re-gather the pieces and, thus, she only eats single, small pieces of food that dissolve in the mouth or are very soft. Despite some interest in self-feeding, it is very hard for Angelina to efficiently transport food

to swallow, which explains why she eats only a few bites. However, Angelina's oral-motor function is only partly responsible for her feeding problems. There are medical, motor, and interactional factors that contribute to Angelina's poor feeding function, too.

FEEDING AND THE INFLUENCE OF MEDICAL CONDITIONS

Successful feeding is dependent not only on the anatomy and function of the oral and pharyngeal structures involved in swallowing but also on the child's medical status, especially with regard to respiration and digestion (Manno et al., 2005). Sensory information from the lungs, heart, and **gastrointestinal (GI) tract** goes directly to the swallowing center in the brain. Through this input, a child with breathing difficulty (e.g., wheezing) may start to drool because swallowing frequency slows as a result of the need for increased respiratory rate (Gewolb & Vice, 2006; Khoshoo & Edell, 1999). Current research suggests that the feeding difficulties of preterm infants may relate more to inappropriate swallow–respiration interaction than to the suck–swallow interaction (Lefton-Greif & McGrath-Morrow, 2007).

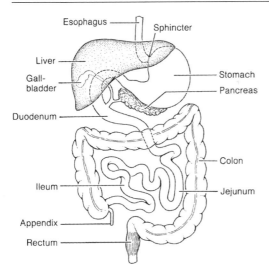

Figure 9.3. After food enters the stomach, it is mixed with acid and is partially digested. Then it passes through the three segments of the small intestine (duodenum, jejunum, and ileum). There, digestive juices are added, and nutrients are removed. The remaining water and electrolytes pass through the colon, where water is removed. Voluntary stooling is controlled by the rectal sphincter muscles.

Esophagus to Stomach: Gastroesophageal Reflux, Dumping, and Delayed Emptying

Input from the GI tract (one long tube, from mouth to anus) also has significant impact on the feeding process (Figure 9.3). Gastroesophageal reflux disease (GERD) is commonly associated with feeding problems in children with developmental disabilities (Williams et al., 2010). The **lower esophageal sphincter (LES)** functions as a one-way valve to prevent the backward flow or reflux of food up into the esophagus (termed *gastroesophageal reflux* [GER]; Figure 9.4). GER can result in vomiting, and if the stomach's contents enter the airway, the reflux can cause coughing, wheezing, and even pneumonia (Gold, 2005). In addition, repeated entry of stomach acid into the esophagus can cause inflammation (esophagitis) that makes eating painful. The child may respond to GER by vomiting, refusing to eat, or taking frequent breaks in the meal. GER can result from a number of abnormalities, and some forms can be inherited (Hu et al., 2004). The most common problem is transient relaxation of the LES, or lowered LES resting tone, that allows reflux of gastric contents (Gold, 2004). LES function can be influenced by meal volume and composition (Fox et al., 2007). Reflux also can result from increased abdominal pressure caused by straining or constipation (Borowitz & Sutphen, 2004).

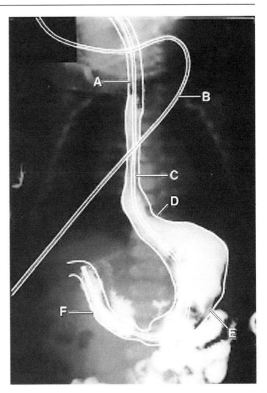

Figure 9.4. Gastroesophageal reflux (GER). Food passes down the esophagus (A), through the lower esophageal sphincter (D), and into the stomach (E) and duodenum (F). If the sphincter does not remain closed after the passage of food, reflux (C) occurs, as shown in this barium study in a child with a nasogastric tube (B) in place.

Vomiting is not the only effect that GER can have on the feeding process. A child with GER who feels uncomfortable all the time may lose interest in eating or may accept only a few favorite foods (Hassall, 2005). GER can also affect the movement of the tongue, throat, and esophagus, causing the child to choose foods that need less oral preparation and are therefore easier to swallow. The resulting lack of practice with more difficult textures can lead to delayed oral–motor development. The most common conditions associated with GER are cerebral palsy and prematurity.

Vomiting, feeding problems, poor weight gain, and irritability are also characteristics of adverse food reactions, including food allergy and food intolerance. The incidence of food allergy has dramatically increased over the last 20 years (Shaker & Woodmansee, 2009). The most common allergenic foods are cow's milk, hen's egg, soy, wheat, fish, peanuts, and shellfish (Berni Canani, Ruotolo, Discepolo, & Troncone, 2008). Eosinophilic gastroenteropathies are a heterogeneous group of non-IgE-mediated food allergies characterized by feeding intolerance and GER symptoms. Biopsies taken from the lining of the involved area of the GI tract demonstrate increased accumulation of eosinophils, the allergy-reactive white blood cells (at least 15 eosinophils per high-powered field; Shaker & Woodmansee, 2009). The affected children also frequently have food sensitivity, shown through skin testing, as well as clinical evidence of other allergic disease (Mukkada et al., 2010).

Nausea, vomiting and bloating may signal delayed stomach emptying (Gariepy & Mousa, 2009). Normally, stomach wall contractions mix and push the stomach contents into the **duodenum**, the upper part of the small intestine. Delayed stomach emptying can be caused by abnormal stomach contractions, a blockage in the **pylorus** (the sphincter at the junction of the stomach and the duodenum), poor intestinal motility, or a meal heavy in fat or protein.

Dumping occurs when the stomach empties too rapidly. Symptoms of dumping include nausea, vomiting, diarrhea, heart palpitations, and weakness (Gariepy & Mousa, 2009). Children receiving carbohydrate-based high-calorie supplements or formulas can have symptoms of dumping. Children who have had a surgical procedure to weaken the pylorus are particularly at risk. Avoidance of dumping requires slowing the rate of stomach emptying or decreasing the concentration of food delivered to the duodenum. This can be accomplished by 1) slowing the feeding rate using continuous feeding, 2) using fat-based instead of carbohydrate-based caloric supplements, or 3) changing to a formula with a lower caloric concentration (Gariepy & Mousa, 2009).

The Small Bowel: Lactase Deficiency

Enzymes and other substances from the pancreas and bile ducts are released into the duodenum and aid in the breakdown of food particles into sugars, fatty acids, amino acids, vitamins, and minerals. Approximately 70% of the world population has an inherited deficiency of the enzyme lactase, which normally breaks down milk sugar (lactose) to allow its absorption (Lomer, Parkes, & Sanderson, 2008). With lactase deficiency, unabsorbed lactose irritates the intestinal wall and causes abdominal discomfort, vomiting, and diarrhea after ingesting milk products. Yet dairy products are an important, if not the main, source of calcium, vitamin D, and protein for many, rendering their potential elimination challenging. Symptoms of lactose-caused GI irritation can be minimized by staggering milk intake throughout the day, taking lactase pills before ingesting a milk product, or using lactase-containing or lactose-free dairy products such as yogurt and cheese (Guandalini, Frye, Rivera, & Borowitz, 2010).

The Colon: Diarrhea and Constipation

The jejunum and ileum, the middle and lower portions of the small intestine, absorb digested nutrients. The nonabsorbable nutrients, called bulk or fiber, pass to the large intestine, or colon. Although movement from the stomach to the end of the ileum may take only 30–90 minutes, passage through the colon may require 1–7 days.

Rapid movement through the colon leads to diarrhea; slower movement causes more water to be absorbed, resulting in hard stools and constipation. Proper bowel evacuation requires adequate fluid, fiber, and coordinated propulsive muscle activity (Walia, Mahajan, & Steffen, 2009). Overly loose stools may be caused by lactase deficiency, inadequate dietary fiber, dumping, overaggressive use of laxatives or enemas, passage of loose stool around an impaction, disruption in the balance of gut flora, or dietary imbalance via over-ingestion of fruit juices.

Constipation is a major problem for many children with developmental disabilities. Constipation is defined as hard stools, or a delay or difficulty in defecation, present for 2 or more weeks, and sufficient to cause significant distress (Loening-Baucke, 2005). In addition to aggravating the risk of reflux by increasing intra-abdominal pressure, constipation can be associated with cramping and discomfort that interferes with appetite, positioning, and sleep (Chao et al, 2008). This can be significant enough to slow growth (Chao et al., 2008). Some evidence indicates a direct relationship between reduction of stool in the rectum (the lowest part of the colon) and decreased abdominal pain with increased appetite, suggesting a communication between rectal fullness and rate of gastric emptying (Boccia et al., 2008; Dupont et al., 2006).

Influence of Other Medical Conditions

Any medical condition that impairs the function of the respiratory tract or GI tract can influence the feeding and swallowing process. For example, asthma, kidney disease, and inborn errors of metabolism (see Chapter 19) can contribute to the development of a feeding problem (Cooper-Brown et al., 2008). Moreover, these disorders can influence one another. An increase in the effort to breathe can influence GI function by changing pressure relationships between the chest and abdomen (Issac, 2009). During an asthma attack, the child generates increased negative lung pressure to breathe; therefore, abdominal pressure is increased relative to chest pressure, increasing the probability of GER. Likewise, GER can contribute to reactive airway narrowing, wheezing, and increased effort to breathe (Gold, 2005). Thus, a vicious cycle can start fairly easily. Unfortunately, if oral feeding is interrupted for prolonged periods of time for any reason, the child may need to restart feeding at an easier texture, especially if the child has cerebral palsy.

FEEDING AND THE INFLUENCE OF TONE, POSTURE, AND DEVELOPMENT

The sensory and motor systems provide both the structural foundation and the sensory information that enable a child to practice and master oral-motor skills. Because the feeding process involves internal activities such as breathing, digestion, and elimination, structural alignment, control, and sensory input affect the feeding process and are in turn affected by it. Abnormal muscle tone, whether high or low,

and/or persistent primitive reflex activity (as seen in cerebral palsy; see Chapter 24) interfere with trunk support as well as the appropriate trunk-, neck-, and head-alignment necessary for successful feeding. Likewise, medical conditions can significantly influence posture and alignment. GI discomfort, whether from irritation (as with esophagitis) or **distension** (as with constipation), compels the child into postures that lessen abdominal pressure. Respiratory conditions that increase the child's effort to breathe compel the child to assume postures that increase the size of the airway. These tend to be extensor positions that interfere with control and alignment through the hips, back, head, and neck. Lack of adequate trunk support and improper alignment greatly hinder rib cage expansion, which ultimately interferes with respiration and increases pressure on the stomach and abdominal cavity. Due to inadequate support and restricted respiration, the shoulders typically elevate, reducing the stability of the base of support for the head and neck. Improper head and neck alignment makes guiding a bolus past the airway more difficult, increasing the risk of aspirating food into the lungs (Larnert & Ekberg, 1995; Sheppard & Fletcher, 2007). Improper alignment also limits tongue movement and interferes with oral-motor patterns (Figures 9.5A and 9.5B).

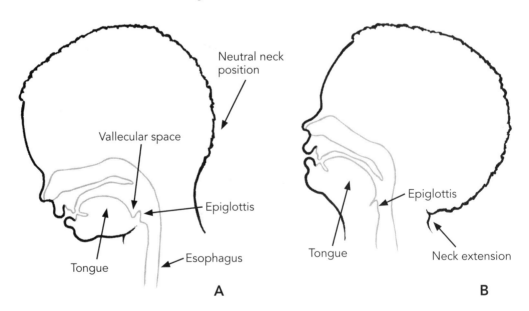

Figure 9.5. A) The child is in a neutral head position with a slight chin tuck. The neutral position allows for open airway while allowing the epiglottis to fall away from the tongue base, opening the vallecular space. This position gives the tongue a strong base of support off of which to move effectively with increased range and control. Widening the vallecular space acts as a "safety net" to catch any early leak of the food bolus from the oral cavity before the swallow. B) The child is in a position of head and neck extension. With neck extension, the tongue base retracts apposing the epiglottis and eliminating the vallecular space. Tongue retraction decreases control of posterior tongue transport. Moreover, by minimizing the vallecular space, this position decreases the possibility of the vallecular "safety net."

For all of these reasons, a child should be seated during feedings with a firm base of support to control positioning of the hips and provided with adequate trunk support to allow neutral positioning of the head and neck. Moreover, the ears and shoulders should be aligned in the same vertical plane as the hips. This may require a slightly reclined position if the child cannot yet sit independently. Some children, in fact, prefer to drink while lying down. Such reclining, if the child has gastrointestinal problems, may start as a way to stretch out and decrease the pressure on the abdomen, or to support the rib cage to facilitate breathing. However, the child then may become dependent on gravity, rather than on active tongue transport, to move the bolus. As a result, spoon feeding or drinking in an upright position, which requires active oral transport, is not successful.

Frequently children will avoid certain sensory experiences that cause them discomfort because a sensation is associated with past or current painful, negative stimuli. In regards to feeding, this may involve refusing certain textures, avoiding oral stimulation, or even a hypersensitivity to the smells or visualization of nonpreferred foods. This hypersensitivity may result from an abnormal response of the child's sensory system, but also it can be seen as part of the sensory feedback from a medical condition. For example, a child with GI discomfort may refuse new textures or feel nauseated and anxious in response to certain smells or even at the sight of a spoon. In fact, GER can contribute to aspiration by desensitizing the larynx and weakening the laryngeal protective responses (Miller, 2009). With treatment of the medical condition, the sensory problems can resolve (Suskind et al., 2006).

The child's fine motor and adaptive skills influence the choice of utensils and level of independence at mealtime, and cognitive abilities help to shape how the child interacts with the mealtime environment. Because children are dependent on their caregivers for feeding, and thus for nutrition, effective caregiver–child communication during mealtime is crucial. An understanding of the child's cognitive level and sensitivity to nonverbal cues prepare the caregiver to effectively communicate with the child. The absence of effective communication increases at mealtime the likelihood of maladaptive behaviors such as expelling, refusal, or tantrums. If the feeder responds to these maladaptive behaviors by removing the disliked food or ending the meal, the child may repeat the maladaptive behavior the next time a meal is served. If this happens repeatedly the maladaptive behavior becomes a learned response.

Many feeding transitions occur in the first 3 years of life, and a child with a developmental disability may have more difficulty during this period in adjusting to changes in textures, utensils, and settings. This heightens the importance of a stable mealtime environment and consistent interactions between the caregiver and child (Manno et al., 2005). Consistency imparts a sense of familiarity that enables children to be comfortable and more tolerant of mealtimes.

FEEDING PROBLEMS IN CHILDREN WITH DISABILITIES

Oral motor problems in children may have a number of causes including 1) abnormalities in muscle tone; 2) compensatory posture and breathing patterns resulting from various medical issues, especially respiratory and gastrointestinal problems; and 3) limited practice of more mature oral-motor patterns. Because children with developmental disabilities have a higher frequency of medical, motor, and learning problems, their risk for feeding problems is greater. A feeding interruption may result from structural or neurological abnormalities that affect the mouth, nose, respiratory system, or GI tract and interfere with safe feeding. A feeding problem may also develop if a medical or developmental condition chronically prevents the child from intaking an appropriate amount without stress. The child then starts to associate discomfort and pain with feeding and learns to avoid feeding situations. This food avoidance or aversion can continue even after the medical condition has resolved, especially in children who have difficulty interpreting or integrating sensory input from elsewhere in the body. An explanation of some of the more common feeding problems follows.

Increased Oral Losses

Loss of food from the mouth, or "messy eating," signals an oral-motor problem, whether related primarily to the **oral pharyngeal musculature** or the impact of medical or postural conditions on oropharyngeal function. The child may have poor lip closure or jaw instability caused by abnormal tone in the facial muscles. As a consequence, once in the mouth, food may 1) be carried out on the tongue as a result of a persistent suckle pattern or exaggerated tongue thrust; 2) fall out of the mouth if the child has not practiced an active transport pattern; or 3) be expelled in an attempt to control bolus size, as when there is swallowing difficulty related to GER or throat infection (Bhatia & Parish, 2009). Sometimes food may be exhaled from the mouth if the oral cavity also serves as the primary airway.

Prolonged Feeding Time

Prolonged feeding time (greater than 30 minutes) usually results from a combination of factors. Oral transport may be slowed by difficulty in collecting food in the mouth or by weakened tongue movements. The suckling pattern of infants with a history of prematurity or cleft palate may utilize more compression than suction, as in Angelina's case. This limits the negative pressure they can generate with which to extract liquid from a nipple, and slows the rate of feeding. If pharyngeal transfer is weak or uncoordinated, the child may need more swallows between bites to clear the food bolus from the pharynx. The child may also slow the meal to allow more time for breathing between bites or to complete transport through the esophagus. The child may appear at times to take breaks, or dawdle, during a meal to allow time for gastric emptying. Prolonged feeding time is a difficult problem for both the child and caregiver and signals the need for an evaluation (Arvedson, 2008).

Food Pocketing

Food pocketing (holding food in the cheeks or the front of the mouth for prolonged periods) suggests either problematic oral transport or food refusal. Children with difficulty moving their tongue from side-to-side or those who use an immature central transport pattern often have trouble transporting food back to the midline before a swallow. As a result, mashed food or chunks migrate toward the cheeks. Alternatively, if a child does not want to swallow the food because of its texture or taste, he or she may trap it in the cheeks in this case, too, and may also trap it under the tongue. Some children with a persistent suckle pattern will move each food bolus to the front of the mouth just behind the front teeth before trying to swallow it. Often this will lead to build up of residue, and pooling under the tongue.

Coughing, Gagging, and Choking

Coughing and gagging indicate difficulty with swallowing. Both are normal defense mechanisms to prevent aspiration. Coughing and gagging during the meal may indicate troublesome food textures. For example, if a child gags on lumpy foods but not on purées, it indicates difficulty adequately chewing or transporting the more highly textured food. The child who coughs while drinking may have a problem controlling flow through the pharynx and past the airway. If the child coughs or gags at the end of or after a meal but not during the meal, GER should be considered. Coughing or gagging during meals that persists for several weeks is a serious warning sign and requires evaluation as soon as possible (Lefton-Greif, 2008).

Choking occurs when food becomes stuck in the pharynx. This happens most commonly when large pieces of soft solids are given to a child whose munching pattern or suckle transport is inadequate, or if the child tends to stuff his or her mouth before swallowing. Cutting foods up into smaller pieces or offering only a couple of pieces at a time may decrease choking. After some practice and with positive reinforcement, the child may be able to gradually increase the size and/or number of chunks accepted. Choking can also occur when there is dysfunction in the upper esophageal sphincter, as with GER, or when using the mouth as an airway while eating (Manno et al., 2005). A full evaluation can help to ascertain the etiology quickly and limit anxiety.

Aspiration

Aspiration refers to food or a foreign substance entering into the airway (Figures 9.6A, 9.6B, and 9.6C). It may occur before, during, or after a swallow or as a result of reflux. Everyone aspirates small amounts of food occasionally, but our protective responses—gagging and coughing—help to clear them from the airway. Children with developmental disabilities that affect sensory or motor coordination of the **oropharynx**, larynx, or **trachea**, however, are at increased risk for recurrent aspiration (Giambra & Meinzen-Derr, 2010). Furthermore, these children often have impaired protective responses that limit their ability to clear their airway once aspiration occurs. Signs of aspiration are influenced by the age of the child. In infants, it may be present as **apnea** and **bradycardia** (slowed heart rate)

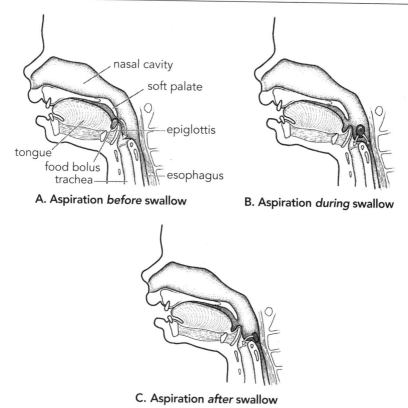

A. Aspiration *before* swallow

B. Aspiration *during* swallow

C. Aspiration *after* swallow

Figure 9.6. Aspiration. A) If a part of the bolus leaks past the soft palate before a swallow is triggered, it can flow past the open epiglottis and into the trachea. B) If the epiglottis is not completely closed as the bolus passes, aspiration can also occur. C) Food residua in the pharynx after a swallow can be carried into the airway with the next breath, resulting in aspiration after the swallow.

during meals, whereas in older infants and children, it may appear as coughing, congestion, or wheezing. Some children aspirate without a protective response from the body; this is called *silent aspiration* and is particularly dangerous because it often goes undetected. Recurrent aspiration and resultant accumulation of foodstuffs in the airway causes irritation and inflammation that can lead to pneumonia, bronchitis, or tracheitis (Lefton-Greif, 2008). If aspiration is suspected, a multidisciplinary feeding team should see the child to evaluate if aspiration is occurring, and, if so, why (Cass, Wallis, Ryan, Reilly, & McHugh, 2005; Cooper-Brown et al., 2008).

Food Refusal

Food refusal can be total, in which case the child does not accept and swallow any food, or partial, in which the child eats some food but not enough to sustain adequate growth and nutritional health. Food refusal is most often associated with an ongoing medical problem such as

asthma or GER. Because of the resulting lack of practice eating, these children's oral-motor skills are also commonly immature or dysfunctional, which further complicates matters. Food refusal requires a coordinated approach among the child's medical provider, an oral-motor therapist, and a behavioral therapist (Williams et al., 2010).

Food Selectivity

Food selectivity implies that the child will accept only a small number of foods, although he or she may eat large quantities of them. Children with autism spectrum disorders often display selectivity of foods (see Chapter 21). Texture-focused selectivity is most commonly seen in children with cerebral palsy who have oral-motor problems. Selectivity may initially stem from an underlying medical condition, but then becomes a learned response perpetuated by environmental or interactional factors, even after the instigating factor has been resolved (Manno et al., 2005; Williams et al., 2010).

Food selectivity is a difficult problem that, like food refusal discussed above, also requires the coordinated efforts of a medical care provider, oral-motor specialist, and behavioral therapist.

Vomiting

GI issues including vomiting and constipation are a major problem for children with developmental disabilities (Sullivan, 2008). Not all vomiting is a consequence of GER. Other medical conditions that produce vomiting and gastric intolerance that mimic reflux are increased intracranial pressure, obstruction of the stomach's outflow tract as with **pyloric stenosis** or intestinal malrotation, kidney disease, and food allergies (Mullen, 2009). Therefore, an appropriate medical evaluation is important. Sometimes the pattern or content of emesis can suggest a cause (e.g., bilious vomiting suggests obstruction; emesis immediately after ingesting a certain food suggests an allergy).

Poor Weight Gain

Poor or inadequate weight gain describes growth that is falling away from the typical growth curve or the individual child's own established growth curve for weight. Historically, the term used was "failure to thrive" (Kessler, 1999), although "poor weight gain" has gained currency recently. Poor weight gain can result from inadequate caloric intake, excessive caloric expenditures, or an inability to use the calories that have been ingested. Nutritionists can be very helpful in determining the caloric intake and nutritional balance of a child's diet as well as providing an estimate of the child's daily caloric and protein needs (Cowin & Emmett, 2007; Sneve, Kattelmann, Ren, & Stevens, 2008). This information then guides further evaluation for the underlying cause of the inadequate weight gain. Children with developmental disabilities are at increased risk of poor growth for both nutritional and nonnutritional reasons (see Chapter 8).

Angelina's story illustrates several topics discussed in this section. Her feeding problems can be described as prolonged feeding time, food selectivity by texture (in her case, refusal of purées), partial food refusal (volume limitation) in that she stops eating after only a few bites, and inadequate intake or poor weight gain. Due to her lack of experience with spoon feeding, she cannot manipulate her tongue effectively to transport food, and tongue lateralization is also weak.

In light of her cerebral palsy and its connection to persistent primitive reflexes, it would be easy to assume that cerebral palsy is the cause of Angelina's oral motor dysfunction. However, if cerebral palsy was actually the cause, she would more likely demonstrate an immature suckle (thrusting) pattern and not have the ability to even weakly lateralize. It would also be easy to attribute her preference for neck extension in feeding and her refusal to sit in the high chair to her cerebral palsy. However, because she possesses the motor control to reciprocally crawl, it is less likely that she would be dominated by extension related to her cerebral palsy. Moreover, cerebral palsy does not explain her limiting the volume of liquids or her refusing purées. Volume limitation and refusal are more commonly associated with GI tract discomfort, as with GER and/or constipation. Angelina's difficulty with the introduction of spoon feeding is consistent with avoidance of spoon pressure on her tongue. Children commonly avoid tongue pressure because of an increased gag response related to GI discomfort, as with GER. The constipation and arching reported by her mother also suggest that Angelina has GI **dysmotility** manifested as constipation and GER. Angelina's constipation slows her GI motility and increases intra-abdominal pressure and the possibility of GER, which makes her less motivated to increase food-intake volume or practice new oral motor patterns.

Angelina's mother has also contributed to Angelina's feeding problems. Because Angelina does not like the high chair, her mother continues to feed her in her lap, which does not provide adequate support to increase ease of breathing or to optimize control of oral-motor movements. Because Angelina does not open her mouth for the spoon, her mother has offered her table foods in which she seems more interested. Angelina prefers these foods not only because she may like the taste, but also because she can self-feed them. This carries mixed results. On the one hand, self-feeding increases her independence. However, by keeping her mother away from her mouth and avoiding spoon placement on her tongue, Angelina has too much control over what foods she accepts and where she puts them in her mouth. She thus can avoid any therapeutic benefit that her mother's placement of the spoon in her mouth could provide her. Food and liquid intake is limited for Angelina due to the influence of GI dysmotility, inefficient oral motor pattern for liquid and food pieces, and spoon refusal. Thus her total caloric intake remains inadequate, and she exhibits poor weight gain.

EVALUATION OF A FEEDING PROBLEM

Because of the complexity of the feeding process and the multiple influences on it, evaluation of a feeding problem should employ a multidisciplinary perspective (Manno et al., 2005; Sheppard & Fletcher, 2007). Information is needed regarding how and when the feeding problem started, how it has changed over time, and what interventions have been used. Background information regarding the child's medical, motor, and behavioral history is also important. A thorough evaluation includes the child's medical history and physical examination, neurodevelopmental assessment, oral-pharyngeal evaluation, feeding history, and mealtime observation (Sheppard & Fletcher, 2007). A nutritional analysis of a 3-day record of the child's intake can provide helpful information regarding the total calories ingested, vitamin and mineral content, and nutritional balance of the diet (Cowin & Emmett, 2007). The information gleaned from the evaluation will identify the feeding problem and the medical, motor, and motivational factors contributing to it.

Diagnostic procedures may be needed to provide further information to support or clarify the clinical impression. Films of the airway can aid in detecting upper airway obstruction. If aspiration of oral feedings is suspected, a modified barium swallow with video fluoroscopy is commonly used. In this procedure, the child is positioned in the usual feeding position and offered foods to which barium, a milk-like substance visible on x ray, has been added. The radiologist uses a video fluoroscope to visualize the pharynx and watch how the pharyngeal muscles guide the food bolus past the airway. The texture of the food and liquids can be varied to evaluate whether the child has more difficulty with one texture than another (Lefton-Greif, 2008). Videofluoroscopy can also give information about airway size and the interface of swallowing and respiration. **Flexible endoscopic evaluation of swallowing** (FEES) has become more frequently used in evaluating swallowing dysfunction. With FEES, a small endoscope is inserted into the nose to the back of the throat in order to directly visualize the **hypopharynx** where the larynx, the entrance to the lungs, sits next to the entrance to the esophagus. The endoscopist can see whether some of the bolus has entered the airway before, during, or after the swallow. The drawback is that the area cannot be captured via the camera during a swallow, so the exact mechanism of the aspiration/penetration may not be clear. FEES with sensory testing (FEES-ST) can yield important information about the sensory thresholds of the area, information that is unavailable from the modified barium swallow (MBS; Lefton-Greif, 2008).

If GI dysmotility is suspected, an upper GI series can be done to rule out anatomical problems. For this procedure, too, barium is either ingested by the child or infused into the stomach by a nasogastric (NG) tube. As the fluid moves through the esophagus, stomach, and small intestine, the radiologist can identify structural abnormalities (Figure 9.4; Vandenplas et al., 2009). A second procedure, the milk scan or gastric emptying study, provides information about height and frequency of GER episodes and assesses the rate of gastric emptying (Figures 9.7A and 9.7B; Vandenplas et al., 2009). During the milk scan, the child swallows a formula to which a small amount of a radioactive tracer has been added, enabling the radiologist to track the milk as it moves through the GI tract. In addition, if the radioactive tracer is found in the lungs after several hours, it suggests that aspiration has occurred during a reflux episode.

The final two tests, the **pH probe** and **gastroesophageal duodenoscopy** (endoscopy), are considered the gold standards in the evaluation of GER and esophagitis, respectively (Vandenplas et al., 2009). For the pH probe, an NG-like tube is inserted through the nose and passed down the esophagus to just above the junction of the stomach and esophagus. At the tip of the tube is a small sensor, which detects the pH, or acidity, above the gastroesophageal junction. If acid in the stomach refluxes into the esophagus, the sensor records a sudden drop in the pH level, signaling GER (Figure 9.8). A symptom diary or videotaping of the child's activities and behaviors during the study period enhances the interpretation of the pH changes. A relatively new technology, **multiple intraluminal impedance** (MII), measures the movement of fluids, solids, and air in the esophagus. MII and pH electrodes should be combined on a single catheter. This combination can detect extremely small amounts of refluxed material, whether or not it is acidic (Vandenplas et al., 2009). Endoscopy entails passing a fiber-optic tube through the mouth down the esophagus and into the stomach. The child is sedated during this procedure. The gastroenterologist can then look directly at the esophagus and stomach and take small biopsy specimens to look for signs of

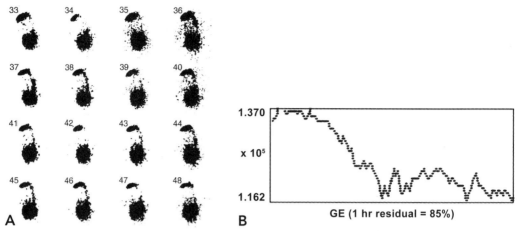

Figure 9.7. Milk scan. In this study, the child is fed a milk formula containing minute amounts of a radioactive label that can be seen on scanning. A) Shown here is a sequence of images taken after the child drinks the milk. The images are generated by a computer from information obtained by the scanner every 120 seconds. The area of radioactivity at the top of each image represents residual formula in the mouth, whereas the lower area of radioactivity is the stomach. Images 34–39 show increased activity in the mouth and esophagus, reflecting a reflux episode to the mouth and descending back to the stomach. In frames 44–48, radioactivity can be seen flowing up from the stomach into the mid-esophagus, indicating another episode of reflux. A repeat scan after the child was placed on antireflux medication would show an absence of stomach reflux. B) In addition to diagnosing reflux, the milk scan can also evaluate whether the stomach is emptying food into the small intestine at a normal rate. Delayed gastric emptying increases stomach pressure and the possibility of reflux or vomiting. In the study shown, residual gastric radioactivity decreased by 15% 1 hour after the labeled milk was ingested (decreasing from 1.370×10^5 counters per minute to 1.162×10^5). This 85% 1-hour residual is high, the normal being 67% or less. Prokinetic agents such as metoclopramide (Reglan) not only decrease gastroesophageal reflux directly but also indirectly by increasing gastric emptying. Following effective medication, the rate of gastric emptying would be expected to increase, potentially to normal levels.

inflammation, allergy, or infection with organisms such as *Candida* or *Helicobacter pylori* (Vandenplas et al., 2009).

MANAGING FEEDING PROBLEMS

Because feeding problems in children with developmental disabilities usually result from the interaction of multiple factors, managing such problems can be difficult, time-consuming, and frustrating. Effective treatment usually requires intervention from more than one therapeutic discipline, and any plan of intervention must be potentially applicable across the child's environments (home, school, and therapist's office) to be truly effective. The treatment team, which should include the child's caregiver, teacher, medical care provider(s), and therapists, needs to prioritize the treatment goals and outline a plan integrating the child's medical, nutritional, and developmental needs (Arvedson, 2008; Ayoob & Barresi, 2007; Cooper-Brown et al., 2008). The primary caregiver, with team input, oversees the plan and

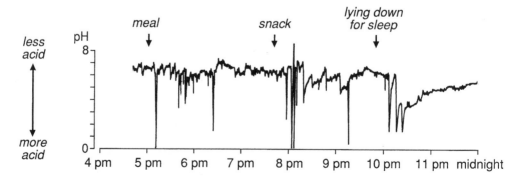

Figure 9.8. A pH probe study is done by passing a tube containing a pH electrode down the esophagus and positioning it just above the stomach. If there is reflux, the pH should drop as the acid contents of the stomach reach the lower esophagus, where the probe is placed. Shown here is an abnormal study with multiple episodes of low pH, occurring about half an hour after feeding and when the child is laid down to sleep. (From Batshaw, M.L. [1991]. *Your child has a disability: A complete sourcebook of daily and medical care* [p. 224]. Baltimore: Paul H. Brookes Publishing Co., Inc.; reprinted by permission. Copyright © 1991 Mark L. Batshaw. Illustration copyright © 1991 by Lynn Reynolds. All rights reserved.)

monitors progress toward the goals, however, open lines of communication among all team members are crucial. Components of a successful treatment strategy include 1) minimizing negative medical influences, 2) ensuring positioning for feeding, 3) facilitating oral-motor function, 4) improving the mealtime environment, 5) promoting appetite, and 6) using alternative methods of feeding (if needed).

All of these components entail constant monitoring of the child's progress. Recognizing the interaction among the medical, motor, and motivational components enables the team to anticipate changes and treat several components at the same time (Manno et al., 2005). Obviously, for a feeding program to be successful, the therapists need to be consistent in and mindful of how the skills they are forging will affect the child's feeding function.

Minimize Negative Medical Influences

Because feeding is a complex skill, a child's feeding function may be very sensitive to even minor medical issues. Thus, parents' and therapists' observations of subtle changes in the child's behaviors, especially during and after feedings, are important and should be shared with medical care providers. Problems with GI irritation and dysmotility can adversely affect respiratory and GI function, as well as the child's level of comfort, and should be treated effectively. For example, Angelina's extensor tone and posturing with meals decreased significantly when she had daily, easily passed stools. This improved her tolerance for sitting in a high chair, as well as her ability to tolerate a larger volume of intake. With better body-positioning, the stimulation from spoon placement on her tongue was more effective in modifying her oral-motor pattern. Constipation can be remediated by 1) establishing regular toileting times to take advantage of the **gastrocolic reflex** that occurs after meals; 2) providing adequate fluids to minimize dry, cakey stools; and 3) encouraging active or passive physical exercise. Dietary fiber in the form of fruits, vegetables, and whole-grain foods can also increase movement through the GI tract (Lee et al., 2008), while more explicitly fiber-intensive products (e.g., Metamucil, Benefiber) may also be helpful (Muller-Lissner et al., 2005).

When constipation is persistent, additional measures may be needed. Laxatives and suppositories can be used, including milk of magnesia, senna concentrate (Senokot), bisacodyl (Dulcolax), lactulose, polyethylene glycol, or glycerin suppositories (Dupont et al., 2006; Loening-Baucke, 2005; Pijpers, Tabbers, Benninga, & Berger, 2009). Enemas, such as Fleet Enema for Children, also may help, but continuous use of enemas can interfere with normal rectal sphincter control and should be avoided. A combination of the discussed approaches may be needed to establish regular bowel movements.

If GI irritation or GER is present, a number of therapeutic modalities are available, including proper positioning, meal modification, medications, and surgery (Vandenplas et al., 2009). The goal is to minimize gastric irritation and protect the esophagus from reflux of stomach acid, either by reducing the amount of gastric contents or by decreasing stomach acid production. Small, frequent meals help to decrease the volume of food in the stomach at any one time. In addition, studies show that whey-based formulas improve stomach-emptying and decrease vomiting in children with certain forms of spastic cerebral palsy (Fried et al., 1992). Similarly, a change in formula to a different protein source or predigested protein may alleviate irritation in those children with milk or soy protein intolerance (Vandenplas et al., 2009). Upright positioning and thickened feedings simply rely on gravity to help keep stomach contents from refluxing into the esophagus. Recent research with premature infants shows that side-lying positions can significantly increase the rate of emptying after a feeding, which then can be used to minimize reflux after the meal. As for medications, H2 antagonists (cimetidine [Tagamet], ranitidine [Zantac], and famotidine [Pepcid]), as well as proton pump inhibitors (omeprazole [Prilosec], lansoprazole [Prevacid], and esomeprazole [Nexium]) decrease stomach acidity and thereby lower the risk of reflux-caused inflammation of the esophagus (Vandenplas et al., 2009). Motility agents such as urecholine (Bethanechol), metoclopramide (Reglan), and erythromycin increase the tone or movement in the esophageal sphincter and stomach, making it harder for reflux to occur (Gariepy & Mousa, 2009).

When GER cannot be controlled by positioning and medication alone, surgery may be needed to prevent problems associated with prolonged reflux. These problems include poor weight gain, recurrent aspiration pneumonia, esophageal stricture, and recurrent apneic episodes (Gariepy & Mousa, 2009; Hassall, 2005). The most common surgical procedure is **fundoplication**, in which the top of the stomach is wrapped around the opening of the esophagus

(Figure 9.9). This decreases reflux while permitting continued oral feeding. An alternative to fundoplication is surgically placing a **gastrojejunal (G-J) tube** that allows access to the stomach as well as the jejunum, permitting some portion of the feeds to bypass the stomach, thereby decreasing the risk of reflux (Figure 9.10; Gariepy & Mousa, 2009).

Ensure Proper Positioning for Feeding

Feeding is a flexor activity that requires good breath support. Appropriate positioning maximizes the child's ability to breathe as well as providing the best alignment to optimize function of the muscles involved in the swallowing process (Larnert & Ekberg, 1995; Sheppard & Fletcher, 2007). The child should be firmly supported though the hips and trunk to provide a stable base. The head and neck should be aligned in a neutral (upright) position, which decreases extension through the oral musculature while maintaining an open airway (Figure 9.11). Such positioning improves coordination and control of the steps in oral-motor preparation and transport. This, in turn, results in more positive feedback to the child and caregiver as a result of good feeding experiences (Kerwin & Eicher, 2004; Manno et al., 2005). If the child does not appear comfortable or appropriately supported for feeding in the currently constructed chair, the child's occupational or physical therapist can make changes to improve the support and alignment.

Facilitate Oral-Motor Function

Any technique that eases the child's practice of an oral motor pattern correctly facilitates oral-motor function. It may consist of oral motor stimulation or desensitization without food, specific placement of food, or manipulation of the food to make it easier for the child to control. Recent research with premature infants has demonstrated that providing patterned **orocutaneous stimulation** that mimics the temporal organization of sucking can enhance the premature infant's acquisition of a functional suckle pattern, and thereby decrease the time needed to establish nipple feedings, and then attain full oral feeding (Miller, 2009; Poore, Zimmerman, Barlow, Wang, & Gu, 2008) In older infants, chin support can often facilitate transition of tongue pattern from a suckle to sucking, and later to tongue lateralization (Gisel, 2008). Chewing can be enhanced

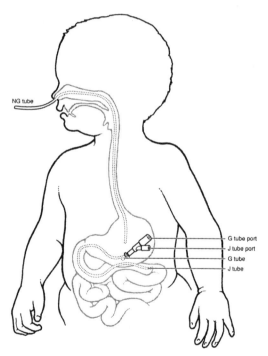

Figure 9.10. Enteral feeding tubes. The nasogastric (NG) tube is placed through the nostril and into the stomach. An NG tube is helpful when problems with the child's oral function are the primary obstacle to adequate nutrition and are temporary. A gastrojejunal (G-J) tube allows access to the stomach as well as directly into the intestine. The G-J tube has 2 openings, or ports, and two parts of tubing. The G port connects with the G tube, which empties the stomach. The J port connects with the J tube, which empties into the intestine. A G-J tube can be helpful when the stomach is unable to tolerate the quantity of nutrients needed for adequate growth.

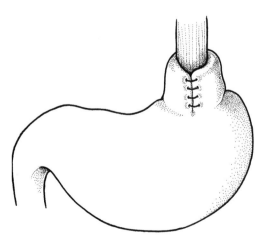

Figure 9.9. In the surgical procedure of fundoplication, the upper stomach is wrapped around the lower esophagus to create a muscular valve that prevents reflux.

by placing food between the upper and lower back teeth. This stimulates crushing movements of the jaw as well as lateral movement of the tongue, both of which are needed to master a munching pattern. Another technique is manipulating food textures to facilitate safe, controlled swallowing (Manno et al., 2005). Thickening of liquids slows their rate of flow, allowing more time for the child to organize and initiate a swallow. **Thickening agents** (e.g., Thick-It, instant pudding powders) can transform any thin liquid into a nectar-, honey-, or milkshake-like consistency. Almost any food can be finely chopped or puréed to a texture that the child can more competently manage.

It is important to remember that the primary goal of eating is to achieve adequate nutrition. Thus, when a child is first learning to accept a higher texture of foods, these foods should be presented during snack time, when volumes are smaller. During this transition period, easier textures should be used at mealtimes to ensure consumption of adequate calories for continued growth. A speech-language pathologist or an occupational therapist can provide information about the child's oral-motor patterns and the appropriate food textures to facilitate improvement in feeding efforts.

Improve the Mealtime Environment

Eating requires more coordination among muscle groups than any other motor activity, including speech. Failure to "perform the work" competently can result in aspiration, which is unpleasant, frightening, and dangerous. Therefore, it is important to make eating as easy as possible (Kerwin & Eicher, 2004). This can be accomplished by increasing the child's focus on the meal and including desirable foods in each meal that are easier to control. Let the child know that mealtime is coming so that he or she can prepare for the "work" to be done. This may entail a premealtime routine of going to a special corner of the room and putting on a bib or napkin or performing relaxation therapy followed by oral stimulation to get the needed muscles ready for eating. Children with feeding difficulties usually eat better in one-to-one situations or in small groups because there are fewer distractions, aiding the ability to focus on the eating process (Williams et al., 2010). Parental provision of undivided attention also makes mealtimes more reinforcing.

When a child is eating well and interested in self-feeding, a number of adaptive devices can promote independence in eating. These include

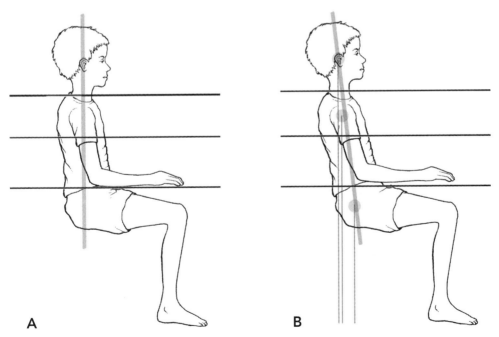

A   **B**

Figure 9.11. A) A child with a neutral pelvis and adequate trunk support to allow neutral positioning of the head and neck. Note how the ears and shoulders align in the same plane as the hips. B) A child is seated with a posterior pelvic tilt, which decreases lordosis, increases kyphosis, and throws him into a head-forward posture. Note how in this position ear, shoulder, and hip are out of alignment.

bowls with high sides, spoons with built-up or curved handles, and cups with rocker bottoms. The satisfaction that children obtain from eating can be increased by social attention during the meal or earning time for a favorite activity after the meal is completed.

Social interaction is an important part of mealtime as well, although it can be distracting. When peer interaction is the focus, it may be helpful to make the meal small (e.g., a snack) and to provide less challenging foods that do not require as much concentration for the child to successfully eat.

Promote Appetite

Some children have little or no appetite regardless of whether they are receiving enough calories to progress along their growth curve. This may be caused by an underlying medical condition, such as a kidney or metabolic disorder or zinc deficiency, or it may be a sign that a chronic medical condition (e.g., diabetes) is inadequately controlled. Alternatively, some children's appetite may be poor as a consequence of being satiated by their tube or supplemental feedings (Linscheid, 2006).

There are differing opinions about whether day versus night, or bolus versus continuous, tube feedings are better for promoting appetite (Dsilna, Christensson, Alfredsson, Lagercrantz, & Blennow, 2005; Dsilna, Christensson, Gustafsson, Lagercrantz, & Alfredsson, 2008). Actually, the important thing is to look at how the child is tolerating the tube feedings. If the child retches, gags, vomits, or needs time to recover after tube feedings, he or she is not tolerating them. Sometimes it takes hours for the child to feel comfortable enough to eat orally again. With this in mind, the best tube-feeding schedule to promote a child's appetite is the one that is tolerated without GI discomfort, even if this involves continuous feedings.

Use Alternative Methods of Feeding

In some cases, oral feeding may not be safe or sufficient to permit adequate nutrition (Mahant, Friedman, Connolly, Goia, & Macarthur, 2009). For these children, NG tube feedings or the placement of a gastrostomy (G) or G-J feeding tube is required (see Figure 9.10). A commercially prepared **enteral formula** (e.g., Nutren Jr., Pediasure) can be used with any of these tubes. Although puréed table food feedings can be given through an NG or a G tube, they are not appropriate for a jejunostomy (J) tube because they will obstruct it. With an NG or a G tube, feedings can be given as single large volumes (boluses) of 3–8 ounces every 3–6 hours or as a continuous drip throughout the day or overnight. J tube feedings must be given continuously, not as a bolus. The advantage of large-volume feedings is that they do not interfere with typical daily activities. The feeding itself takes about 30 minutes. As mentioned previously, however, the large volume may be difficult for the child to tolerate and may lead to vomiting or abdominal discomfort. If this happens, continuous drip feedings can be instituted. A Kangaroo or similar type of automated pump is then used to deliver the formula at a set rate. Sometimes tube feedings are used to supplement oral feedings. In this case, tube feedings generally are used at night so that the child remains hungry for oral feedings during the day. A nutritionist can recommend the appropriate type of enteral formula as well as the amount of supplementation necessary to provide a nutritionally balanced intake that meets the child's daily caloric needs.

SUMMARY

Feeding a child with a developmental disability often requires a number of creative approaches and the involvement of a variety of health care professionals (Manno et al., 2005). When well-integrated, these methods not only allow the child to have optimal oral feeding experiences with their positive social and developmental ramifications but also allow him or her to receive the necessary combination of nutrients and fluids needed to grow and remain healthy.

REFERENCES

Amaizu, N., Shulman, R., Schanler, R., & Lau, C. (2008). Maturation of oral feeding skills in preterm infants. *Acta Paediatrica, 97*, 61–67.

Arvedson, J.C. (2008). Assessment of pediatric dysphagia and feeding disorders: Clinical and instrumental approaches. *Developmental Disabilities Research Review, 14*, 118–27.

Ayoob, K.T., Barrese, I. (2007). Feeding disorders in children: Taking an interdisciplinary approach. *Pediatric Annals, 36*, 478-83.

Batshaw, M.L. (1991). *Your child has a disability: A complete sourcebook of daily and medical care.* Baltimore, MD: Paul H. Brookes Publishing Co.

Berni Canani, R., Ruotolo, S., Discepolo, V., & Troncone, R. (2008). The diagnosis of food allergy in children. *Current Opinion in Pediatrics, 20*, 584–589.

Bhatia, J. & Parish, A. (2009). GERD or not GERD: The fussy infant. *Journal of Perinatology, 29*, S7–S11.

Boccia, G., Buonavolonta, R., Coccorullo, P., Manguso, F., Fuiano, L., & Staino, A. (2008). Dyspeptic symptoms in children: The result of a constipation-induced cologastric brake? *Clinical Gastroenterology and Hepatology, 6,* 556–560.

Borowitz, S.M., & Sutphen, J.L. (2004). Recurrent vomiting and persistent gastroesophageal reflux caused by unrecognized constipation. *Clinical Pediatrics, 43,* 461–466.

Bosma, J.F. (1986). Development of feeding. *Clinical Nutrition, 5,* 210–218.

Cass, H., Wallis, C., Ryan, M., Reilly, S., & McHugh, K. (2005). Assessing pulmonary consequences of dysphagia in children with neurological disabilities: When to intervene? *Developmental Medicine & Child Neurology, 47,* 347–352.

Chao, H., Chen, S., Chen, C., Chang, K., Kong, M., Lai, M., & Chiu, C. (2008). The impact of constipation on growth in children. *Pediatric Research, 64,* 308–311.

Cooper-Brown, L., Copeland, S., Dailey, S., Downey, D., Peterson, M.C., Stimson, C., & Van Dyke, D.C. (2008). Feeding and swallowing dysfunction in genetic syndromes. *Developmental Disabilities Research Reviews, 14,* 147–157.

Cowin, I. & Emmet, P. (2007). Diet in a group of 18 month-old children in South West England, and comparison with the results of a national survey. *Journal of Human Nutrition & Diet, 20,* 254–67.

Dsilna, A., Christensson, K., Alfredsson, L., Lagercrantz, H., & Blennow, M. (2005). Continuous feeding promotes gastrointestinal tolerance and growth in very low birth weight infants. *Journal of Pediatrics, 147,* 43–49.

Dsilna, A., Christensson, K., Gustafsson, A.S., Lagercrantz, H., & Alfredsson, L. (2008). Behavioral stress is affected by the mode of tube feeding in very low birth weight infants. *Clinical Journal of Pain, 24,* 447–55.

Dupont, C., Leluyer, B., Amar, F., Kalach, N., Benhamou, P.H., Mouterde, O., & Vannerom, P.Y. (2006). A dose determination study of polyethylene glycol 4000 in constipated children: Factors influencing the maintenance dose. *Journal of Pediatric Gastroenterology and Nutrition, 42,* 178–185.

Eicher, P.S., McDonald-McGinn, D.M., Fox, C.A., Driscoll, D.A., Emanuel, B.S., & Zackai, E.H. (2000). Dysphagia in children with a 22q11.2 deletion: Unusual pattern found on modified barium swallow. *The Journal of Pediatrics, 137,* 158–164.

Fox, M., Barr, C., Nolan, S., Lomer, M., Anggiansah, A., & Wong, T. (2007). The effects of dietary fat and calorie density on esophageal acid exposure and reflux symptoms. *Clinical Gastroenterology & Hepatology, 5,* 439–44.

Fried, M.D., Khoshoo, V., Secker, D.J., Gilday, D.L., Ash, J.M., & Pencharz, P.B. (1992). Decrease in gastric emptying time and episodes of regurgitation in children with spastic quadriplegia fed a whey-based formula. *The Journal of Pediatrics, 120,* 569–572.

Gariepy, C. E., & Mousa, H. (2009). Clinical management of motility disorders in children. *Seminars in Pediatric Surgery, 18,* 224–238.

Gewolb, I.H., & Vice, F.L. (2006). Maturational changes in the rhythms, patterning, and coordination of respiration and swallow during feeding in preterm and term infants. *Developmental Medicine & Child Neurology, 48,* 589–594.

Giambra, B.K., & Meinzen-Derr, J. (2010). Exploration of the relationships among medical health history variables and aspiration. *International Journal of Pediatric Otorhinolaryngology, 74,* 387–92.

Gisel, E.G. (2008). Interventions and outcomes for children with dysphagia. *Developmental Disabilities Research Review, 14,* 165–173.

Gold, B.D. (2004). Gastroesophageal reflux disease: Could intervention in childhood reduce the risk of later complications? *American Journal of Medicine, 117,* 23S–29S.

Gold, B.D. (2005). Asthma and gastroesophageal reflux disease in children: Exploring the relationship. *The Journal of Pediatrics, 146,* S13–S20.

Guandalini, S., Frye, R.E., Riera, D.M., & Borowitz, S. (2010). *Lactose intolerance.* Retrieved November 29, 2010, from http://www.Emedicine.medscape.com/article/930971, 1–10.

Hassall, E. (2005). Decisions in diagnosing and managing chronic gastroesophageal reflux disease in children. *The Journal of Pediatrics, 146,* S3–S12.

Hu, F.Z., Donfack, J., Ahmed, A., Dopico, R., Johnson, S., Post, J.C., ... Preston, R.A. (2004). Fine mapping a gene for pediatric gastroesophageal reflux on human chromosome 13q14. *Human Genetics, 114,* 562–572.

Issac, K.M. (2009). The relationship between GERD and asthma. *US Pharmacist, 34,* 30-35.

Kerwin, M.L.E., & Eicher, P.S. (2004). Behavioral intervention and prevention of feeding difficulties in infants and toddlers. *Journal of Early and Intensive Behavioral Interventions, 1,* 129–140.

Kessler, D.B. (1999). Failure to thrive and pediatric undernutrition: Historical and theoretical context. In D.B. Kessler & P. Dawson (Eds.), *Failure to Thrive and pediatric undernutrition: A transdisciplinary approach.* Baltimore, MD: Paul H. Brookes Publishing Co.

Khoshoo, V., & Edell, D. (1999). Previously healthy infants may have increased risk of aspiration during respiratory syncytial viral bronchiolitis. *Pediatrics, 104,* 1389–1390.

Larnert, G., & Ekberg, O. (1995). Positioning improves the oral and pharyngeal swallowing function in children with cerebral palsy. *Acta Paediatrica, 84,* 689–692.

Lee, W.T.K., Ip, K.S., Chan, J.S.H., Lui, N.W., & Young, B.W. (2008). Increased prevalence of constipation in preschool children is attributable to underconsumption of plant foods: A community-based study. *Journal of Paediatric Child Health, 44,* 170–175.

Lefton-Greif, M.A. (2008). Pediatric dysphagia. *Physical Medicine and Rehabilitation Clinics of North America, 19,* 837–851.

Lefton-Greif, M.A., & McGrath-Morrow, S.A. (2007). Deglutition and respiration: Development, coordination, and practical implications. *Seminars in Speech and Language, 28,* 166–79.

Leopold, N.A., & Daniels, S.K. (2010). Supranuclear control of swallowing. *Dysphagia, 25,* 250–257.

Linscheid, T.R. (2006). Behavioral treatment for pediatric feeding disorders. *Behavioral Modification, 30,* 6–23.

Loening-Baucke, V. (2005). Prevalence, symptoms and outcome or constipation in infants and toddlers. *The Journal of Pediatrics, 146,* 359–63.

Lomer, M.C., Parkes, G.C., & Sanderson, J.D. (2008). Review article: Lactose intolerance in clinical practice. *Alimentary Pharmacology and Therapeutics, 27,* 93–103.

Mahant, S., Friedman, J.N., Connolly, B., Goia, C., & Macarthur, C. (2009). Tube feeding and quality of life in children with severe neurological impairment. *Archives of Disease in Children, 94,* 668–73.

Manno, C.J., Fox, C.A., Eicher, P.S., & Kerwin, M.L.E. (2005). Early oral-motor interventions for pediatric feeding problems: What, when and how. *The Journal of Early and Intensive Behavior Intervention, 3,* 145–159.

Miller, A.J. (1986). Neurophysiological basis of swallowing. *Dysphagia, 1,* 91–100.

Miller, C.K. (2009) Updates on pediatric feeding and swallowing problems. *Current Opinion in Otolaryngology & Head and Neck Surgery, 17,* 194–199.

Mukkada, V.A., Haas, A., Creskoff Maune, N., Capocelli, K.E., Henry, M., Gilman, N., … Atkins, D. (2010). Feeding dysfunction in children with eosinophilic gastrointestinal diseases. *Pediatrics, 126,* e672–e677.

Mullen, N. (2009). Vomiting in the pediatric age group. *Pediatric Health, 3,* 479–503.

Muller-Lissner, S.A., Kamm, M.A., Scarpignato, C., Wald, A. (2005). Myths and misconception about chronic constipation. *American Journal of Gastroenterology, 100,* 232–242.

Piazza, C. (2008). Feeding disorders and behavior: What have we learned? *Developmental Disabilities Research Reviews, 14,* 174–181.

Pijpers, M.A., Tabbers, M.M., Benninga, M.A., Berger, M.Y. (2009). Currently recommended treatments of childhood constipation are not evidence based: A systematic literature review on the effect of laxative treatment and dietary measures. *Archives of Disease in Children, 94,* 117–131.

Poore, M., Zimmerman, E., Barlow, S.M., Wang, J., & Gu, F. (2008). Patterned orocutaneous therapy improves sucking and oral feeding in preterm infants. *Acta Paediatrica, 97,* 920–927.

Popescu, E.A, Popescu, M., Wang, J., Barlow, S.M., & Gustafson, K.M. (2008). Nonnutritive sucking recorded in utero via fetal magnetography. *Physiologic Measurement, 29,* 127–139.

Ross, E.S. (2008). Feeding in the NICU and issues that influence success. *Perspectives on Swallowing and Swallowing Disorders (Dysphagia), 17,* 94–100.

Salvia, G., DeVizia, B., Manguso, F., De Vizia, B., Manguso, F., Iula, V.D., Terrin, G.,… Cuchiarra, S. (2001). Effect of intragastric volume and osmolality on mechanisms of gastroesophageal reflux in children with gastroesophageal reflux disease. *American Journal of Gastroenterology, 96,* 1725–1732.

Shaker, M., & Woodmansee, D. (2009). An update on food allergy. *Current Opinion in Pediatrics. 21,* 667–674.

Sheppard, J.J., & Fletcher, K.R. (2007). Evidence-based interventions for breast and bottle feeding in the neonatal intensive care unit. *Seminars in Speech and Language, 28,* 204–212.

Sneve, J., Kattelmann, K., Ren, C., & Stevens, D.C. (2008). Implementation of a multidisciplinary team that includes a registered dietitian in a neonatal intensive care unit improved nutrition outcomes. *Nutrition Clinical Practice, 23,* 630–4.

Sullivan, P.B. (2008). Gastrointestinal disorders in children with neurodevelopmental disabilities. *Developmental Disorders Research Reviews, 14,* 128–136.

Suskind, D.L., Thompson, D.M., Gulati, M., Huddleston, P. Liu, D.C., & Baroody, F.M. (2006). Improved infant swallowing after gastroesophageal disease treatment: A function of improved laryngeal sensation? *Laryngoscope, 116,* 1397–1403.

Thompson, D. Laryngopharyngeal sensory testing and assessment of airway protection in pediatric patients. (2003). *American Journal of Medicine, 115,* 166s–168s.

Vandenplas, Y., Rudolph, C.D., Di Lorenzo, C., Hassall, E., Liptak, G., Mazur, L., … European Society for Pediatric Gastroenterology Hepatology and Nutrition. (2009). Pediatric gastroesophageal reflux clinical practice guidelines: Joint recommendations of the North American Society for Pediatric Gastroenterology, Hepatology, and Nutrition (NASPGHAN) and the European Society for Pediatric Gastroenterology, Hepatology, and Nutrition (ESPGHAN). *Journal of Pediatric Gastroenterology and Nutrition, 49,* 498–547.

Walia, R., Mahajan, L., & Steffen, R. (2009). Recent advances in chronic constipation. *Current Opinion in Pediatrics, 21,* 661–666.

Williams, K.E., Field, D.G., & Seiverling, L. (2010). Food refusal in children: A review of the literature. *Research in Developmental Disabilities, 31,* 625–33.

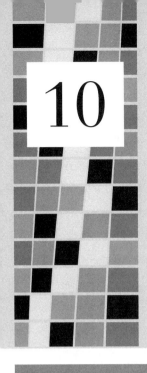

10 Hearing and Deafness

Pamela Buethe, Betty R. Vohr, and Gilbert R. Herer

Upon completion of this chapter, the reader will

- Be able to describe the components of the auditory pathway
- Know the different types of hearing loss, their causes, and their incidence rates
- Gain an understanding of newborn hearing screening
- Know the age-appropriate hearing screen and diagnostic tests
- Understand the importance of family-centered early intervention, communication options, and amplification options for children with hearing loss
- Be able to discuss the educational options and outcomes for children with hearing loss

The sense of hearing is integral to one of the most fundamental of human activities: the use of language for communication. Through hearing children acquire a linguistic system to both transmit and receive information, express thoughts and feelings, learn, and influence the behaviors of their parents and peers. Problems with hearing can negatively affect a child in the areas of language and speech, social-emotional development, literacy, and learning abilities in school; therefore, early identification and intervention are imperative for children with hearing loss and their families. This chapter reviews the human auditory system, hearing loss and its effects on the development of a child's communication skills, and various approaches to treating and educating children with hearing loss.

The following story illustrates the array of opportunities, needs, and circumstances surrounding a child born with a severe hearing loss. These issues are summarized in Table 10.1.

◼◼◼ MATT

Matt, a healthy 7½-pound baby who was born to hearing parents and cared for in a well-infant nursery, failed his newborn hearing screen with otoacoustic emissions (OAE) at 2 days of age and a rescreen at 4 weeks of age. He was referred for a diagnostic **auditory brainstem response** (ABR) test that revealed no measurable responses in his left ear and a moderate to severe **sensorineural** hearing loss in his right ear at 6 weeks of age. Several interventions were initiated immediately, including 1) taking earmold impressions in preparation for hearing aid use, 2) providing Matt's parents with information about hearing loss, 3) a referral to early intervention, and 4) a medical evaluation by his physician. It was explained to his parents that a consultation with an otolaryngologist would be required and that seeking genetic counseling was recommended to explore the origin of his hearing loss. Matt underwent genetic screening for Connexin 26 deafness, which yielded positive results, identifying it as the cause of Matt's hearing loss.

At 3 months of age, Matt was fitted with behind-the-ear hearing aids that included a

Table 10.1. Principles of an effective early hearing detection and intervention (EHDI) system

1. All infants should have access to hearing screening using a physiologic measure at no later than 1 month of age.
2. All infants who do not pass the initial hearing screening and the subsequent rescreening should have appropriate audiological and medical evaluations to confirm the presence of hearing loss at no later than 3 months of age.
3. All infants with confirmed permanent hearing loss should receive early intervention services as soon as possible after diagnosis but at no later than 6 months of age. A simplified, single point of entry into an intervention system that is appropriate for children with hearing loss is optimal.
4. The EHDI system should be family centered with infant and family rights and privacy guaranteed through informed choice, shared decision-making, and parental consent in accordance with state and federal guidelines. Families should have access to information about all intervention and treatment options and counseling regarding hearing loss.
5. The child and family should have immediate access to high-quality technology including hearing aids, cochlear implants, and other assistive devices when appropriate.
6. All infants and children should be monitored for hearing loss in the medical home. Continued assessment of communication development should be provided by appropriate professionals to all children with or without risk indicators for hearing loss.
7. Appropriate interdisciplinary intervention programs for infants with hearing loss and their families should be provided by professionals who are knowledgeable about childhood hearing loss. Intervention programs should recognize and build on strengths, informed choices, traditions, and cultural beliefs of the families.
8. Information systems should be designed and implemented to interface with electronic health charts and should be used to measure outcomes and report the effectiveness of EHDI services at the patient, practice, community, state, and federal levels.

frequency modulation (FM) system and a wireless microphone for his parents' use. The FM system coupled with Matt's hearing aids enabled him to hear his parents' speech message regardless of their location in the room or amount of impeding background noise. Matt, his mother, and his 3-year-old brother (who has normal hearing) were seen for weekly early intervention sessions as part of his individualized family service plan (IFSP), established with the family and their state's early intervention infants and toddlers program in their county of residence. Matt's intervention services were designed to demonstrate auditory and speech-language activities for use at home, share information about hearing and hearing loss, and provide continuing family support. Because Connexin 26 deafness can cause progressive hearing loss, Matt was monitored with audiological evaluations every 3 months.

Matt received weekly home visits from an early intervention professional (e.g., a teacher of the deaf and hard of hearing), who focused on auditory-, speech-, and language-developmental skills until age 3, when he was enrolled in a preschool program with an individualized education program (IEP) to meet his educational needs. At age 3, he lost all hearing in his right ear, due to his Connexin 26 deafness.

Matt was deemed an appropriate candidate for a cochlear implant in the right ear, which he received three months later. Matt entered kindergarten with his same-age, typical-hearing peers and he continued receiving support services in speech-language development. During his first three school-age years, Matt attended general education classes while receiving support services, such as an FM system and speech-language therapy. Presently, Matt's speech is as intelligible and fluent as that of his same-age peers; however, receptive communication difficulties occur for him in group situations, including in his classroom. Matt sometimes misses key words and phrases that provide contextual meaning, and as a result, his responses are sometimes off-topic. Through his parents' advocacy and his school's cooperation, these circumstances are addressed in school through prevention/intervention services of a speech-language pathologist. Matt has experienced the benefit of a proficient and successful early hearing detection and intervention (EHDI) system. This chapter will discuss in depth the characteristics and interventions that contribute to a good outcome.

THE 1-3-6 GUIDELINES FOR SCREENING AND DIAGNOSIS

EHDI systems have been established by federal and state governmental agencies as a part of the public health system that emphasizes the importance of newborn hearing screening, diagnosis of hearing loss, family support, early intervention, and medical home services (Houston, Behl, White, & Forsman, 2010). The Joint Committee on Infant Hearing (JCIH) 2007 recommendations regarding screening and diagnosis of hearing loss are that all infants be screened by 1 month, diagnosed by 3 months, and start intervention by 6 months of age. These goals were accomplished in Matt's case. The 1-3-6 goals are equally important for infants with mild loss, unilateral loss, and severe to profound deafness.

THE HEARING SYSTEM

The anatomical mechanism for hearing represents a complex system (Moller, 2006). It is divided into a peripheral auditory mechanism, which starts at the external ear and ends at the auditory nerve, and a central auditory system, which extends from the auditory nerve to the brain. A disorder in the peripheral system results in a hearing loss, whereas a central auditory problem interferes with the interpretation of what is heard.

The peripheral auditory system is divided into the external, middle, and inner ear. The external ear includes the **auricle** and the ear canal (Figure 10.1). The auricle channels sound into the ear canal and thence to the middle ear. The skin of the ear canal contains glands that produce **cerumen** (earwax). At the end of the ear canal lies the eardrum, or tympanic membrane, which separates the external ear from the middle ear. The tympanic membrane is attached to the first of a series of three small bones of the middle ear—the **malleus, incus,** and **stapes**—which are collectively called the **ossicles.** The end of the ossicular chain, the stapes footplate, is attached by ligaments to the oval window, which serves as the boundary between the middle ear and the bony housing of the inner ear, the **cochlea.**

When sound waves strike the tympanic membrane, the membrane vibrates and thus sets the ossicular chain into motion. Because the tympanic membrane has a larger surface area than the oval window and because the ossicles act as a lever system, the incoming sound pressure is amplified by about 30 **decibels** (dB).

The **eustachian tube** is also part of the middle ear. This tube runs from the anterior wall of the middle-ear space down to the **nasopharynx.** The eustachian tube is usually closed

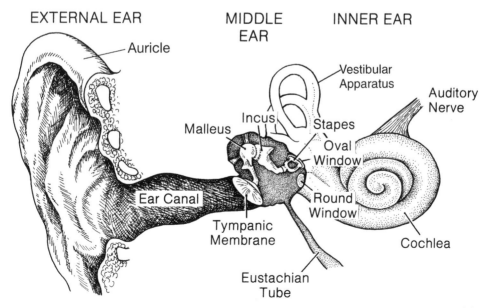

EXTERNAL EAR   MIDDLE EAR   INNER EAR

Figure 10.1. Structure of the ear. The middle ear is composed of the tympanic membrane, or eardrum, and the three ear bones: the malleus, the incus, and the stapes. The stapes footplate lies on the oval window, the gateway to the inner ear. The inner ear contains the cochlea and the vestibular (balance) apparatus, collectively called the **labyrinth**.

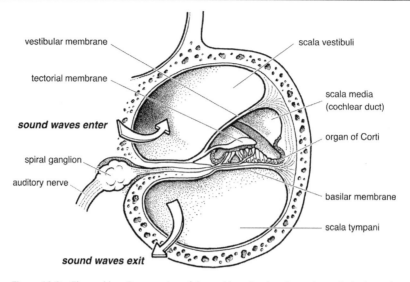

Figure 10.2. The cochlea. Cross-section of the cochlea, showing the scala vestibuli, the scala media, the scala tympani, and the organ of Corti.

but opens during a swallow or yawn, allowing a small amount of air to pass between the naso-pharynx and the middle ear to equalize its air pressure with that in the external canal.

The inner ear is composed of the **vestibular system** and the cochlea. The vestibular system houses the sensory organ of balance, whereas the cochlea houses the sensory organ of hearing (Figure 10.2). The actual end organ of hearing, the **organ of Corti**, consists of multiple rows of delicate hair cells along the organ—three to five rows of outer hair cells and one row of inner—that serve as the receptors for the auditory nerve. The cochlea is arranged **tonotopically**; that is,

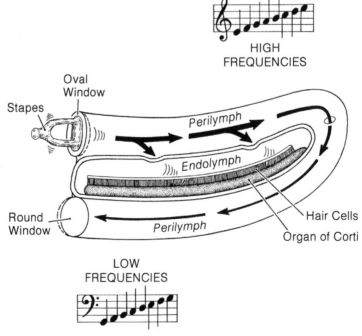

Figure 10.3. The cochlea has been "unfolded" for simplicity. Sound vibrations from the stapes are transmitted as waves in the perilymph. This leads to the displacement of hair cells in the organ of Corti. These hair cells lie above and attach to the auditory nerve, and the impulses generated are fed to the brain. High-frequency sounds stimulate hair cells close to the oval window, whereas low-frequency sounds stimulate the middle and top end of the organ. The sound wave in the perilymph is rapidly dissipated through the round window, and the cochlea is ready to accept a new set of vibrations.

hair cells located at the base of the cochlea, near the **oval window**, respond more specifically to high-frequency sounds (above 2,000 Hz), whereas those in the middle and top respond more to gradually lower-frequency sounds (Figure 10.3). The organ of Corti converts the mechanical energy arriving from the middle ear into electrical energy, or the nerve impulse. As the ossicular chain is activated by the vibrating tympanic membrane, the movement is transmitted through the cochlear chambers and results in release of neurotransmitters from the hair cells. This generates a nerve impulse that is transmitted via the ascending auditory pathway to the brain. Most of the nerve impulses from the right cochlea cross over to ascend the left central auditory pathway to the left portion of the brain, and vice versa for impulses from the left ear (Figure 10.4). When stimulated by an incoming acoustic signal, the outer hair cells produce very soft level sounds called **otoacoustic emissions** that can be measured in the outer ear canal with specialized technology. OAE instrumentation is used in newborn hearing screening programs, in research, and as a diagnostic measurement with pediatric and adult populations.

From the inner ear, sound is carried to the auditory cortex in the temporal lobe of the brain. The route from ear to cortex involves at least four neural relay stations (Figure 10.4). The final (fifth) destination is the auditory cortex, where sound can be associated with other sensory information and memory to permit perception and interpretation. Note that the auditory cortex is not needed to perceive sound, but it is needed to interpret language.

DEFINING SOUND

When we hear a sound, we are actually processing and interpreting a pattern of vibrating air molecules. An initial vibration sets successive rows of air molecules into motion in oscillating concentric circles, or waves. This movement of

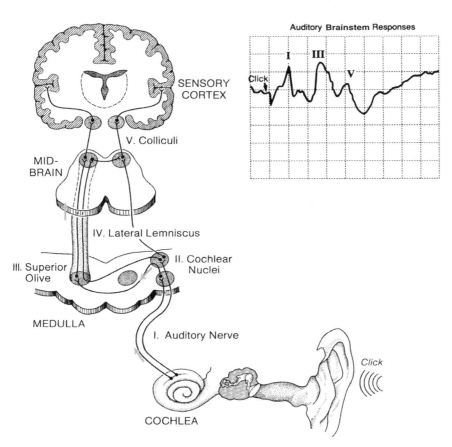

Figure 10.4. The auditory pathway and auditory brainstem responses (ABRs). The auditory nerve carries sounds to the cochlear nuclei in the medullary portion of the brainstem. Here, most impulses cross over to the superior olivary body and then ascend to the opposite inferior colliculus and ultimately the sensory cortex, where the sound is perceived. The function of this pathway can be measured by ABR testing. Each wave corresponds to a higher level of the pathway (denoted by Roman numerals in the pathway and in the reporting of ABRs). (Key: Shaded arrows indicate the direction of travel of the nerve impulse along the pathway.)

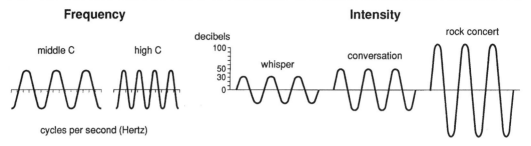

Figure 10.5. Frequency and intensity of sound waves. The frequency of a sound, or its pitch, is expressed as cycles per second, or hertz (Hz). Middle C is 256 Hz; one octave higher (high C) is 512 Hz. Intensity of sound is expressed as decibels (dB) and varies from a whisper at 20 dB to a rock concert at 100 dB or more.

the molecules is described in terms of the frequency with which the oscillations occur and the amplitude of the oscillations from the resting point (Figure 10.5).

The frequency of a sound is perceived as **pitch** and is measured in cycles per second, or **hertz** (Hz). The more cycles that occur per second, the higher the frequency, or pitch, of the sound. Middle C on the musical scale is 256 Hz, whereas the ring of a cellular telephone is approximately 2,000 Hz. The human ear can detect frequencies ranging from 20 Hz to 20,000 Hz, but it is most sensitive to sounds in the 500 Hz to 6,000 Hz range, in which most of the sounds of speech occur (Emanuel & Letowski, 2009).

The amplitude of the molecular oscillation is perceived as the loudness, or intensity, of the sound and is measured in decibels. The softest sound an individual with typical hearing can usually detect is defined as 0 dB hearing level (HL). The intensity of a whisper is about 20 dB HL, typical conversation occurs at about 40 dB HL, and a person's shout registers at about 70 dB HL. A lawn mower or chain saw is measured at about 100 dB HL (Northern & Downs, 2002).

Speech, however, does not occur at a single intensity or frequency. In general, vowel sounds are low frequency in nature and more intense, whereas consonants, particularly the voiceless consonants (e.g., /s/, /sh/, /t/, /th/ as in thin, /k/, /p/, and /h/), are composed of higher frequencies and are the least intense (Figure 10.6). Furthermore, during a conversation, the speaker will change the intensity of speech by talking in a louder or softer voice to express emotion or to emphasize something. This circumstance can adversely affect an individual with a hearing loss, especially if the loss is not consistent at all frequencies. If an individual has a high-frequency hearing loss but normal hearing in the low-frequency region, that individual will be able to hear

speech (because of the relative loudness of vowels) but may not be able to understand it because of the softness of voiceless consonants. The person may hear only parts of words and therefore would find it difficult to follow a conversation.

DEFINING HEARING LOSS

Categories of degree of hearing loss are *minimal, mild, moderate, severe,* and *profound.* Each of these terms is often accompanied by specific threshold levels of loss in the frequency region for speech; that is, the average threshold loss for 500 Hz, 1,000 Hz, and 2,000 Hz (see the section titled Degrees of Hearing Loss for more information). These terms are meant to convey the extent of unilateral loss (for one ear) or bilateral loss (for both ears) and are useful in explaining to parents how much of speech their child can expect to hear.

Hard of hearing is a term frequently used for individuals with losses of 25–70 dB HL for the better ear. Children who are hard of hearing benefit greatly from amplification through hearing aids and communicate primarily through spoken language, as described in Matt's case study at the beginning of the chapter.

Deaf refers to individuals with profound losses, those greater than 70 dB HL. Children with a profound hearing loss may receive limited benefits through the use of hearing aids; they may typically only hear the rhythm of speech, their own voice, and environmental sounds (Boothroyd, 2008); however, with a cochlear implant, they may acquire very effective oral speech-language abilities.

Each child's hearing capacity varies as a consequence of listening circumstances. These descriptive terms, therefore, may only partially explain the listening experiences of a particular child. For example, a child with a mild hearing loss in both ears may encounter as much difficulty in listening as a child with a moderate loss.

PITCH (CYCLES PER SECOND)

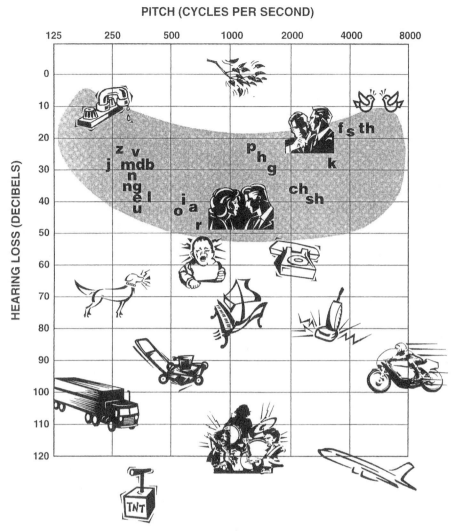

Figure 10.6. Frequency spectrum of familiar sounds plotted on a standard audiogram. The shaded area contains most of the sound elements of speech. (From Northern, J.L., & Downs, M.P. [2002]. *Hearing in children* [5th ed., p. 18]. Philadelphia, PA: Lippincott, Williams & Wilkins. http://www.lww.com Copyright © Lippincott Williams & Wilkins. Reprinted by permission.)

Types of Hearing Loss

Temporary **conductive hearing loss** (CHL) resulting from dysfunction of the external and/or middle ear can be caused by multiple factors, such as a middle ear infection or earwax occluding the ear canal. Other factors are described in the section titled Causes of Hearing Loss.

Permanent hearing loss comprises four types: 1) sensorineural, 2) permanent conductive, 3) mixed loss, and 4) neural hearing disorders. A **sensorineural hearing loss** (SNHL) results from inner ear malfunction of the cochlea. Permanent CHL results from malformations of the outer and/or middle ear that impede the conduction of sound energy to the inner ear. Mixed loss involves the combination of conductive and sensorineural loss as a result of outer and/or middle, and inner ear malfunction. Neural hearing disorders are characterized by normal cochlear outer hair cell function and abnormal inner hair cell function and/or the auditory nerve.

In addition to being classified as sensorineural, conductive, mixed, or neural, permanent hearing loss may be unilateral or bilateral. Unilateral hearing loss affects only one ear, with the other ear having normal hearing; the amount of hearing loss in the affected ear can range from mild to profound. Despite having one ear with normal hearing, children with unilateral hearing loss may experience difficulties understanding speech in noisy environments and localizing to the direction of a sound source. Unilateral hearing loss may also adversely affect a child's speech and language development, interpersonal relationships, and educational achievement (Holstrum, Gaffney, Gravel, Oyler, & Ross, 2008) as a result of receptive communication difficulties.

Hearing losses can also be described as stable or progressive. Progressive hearing losses can be challenging to recognize early and are often associated with genetic factors, intrauterine infections, or syndromes related to hearing loss (Mori, Westerberg, Atashband, & Kozak, 2008; Ravecca et al., 2005).

Degrees of Hearing Loss

In general, defining the degree of hearing loss is meant to predict the difficulty a child will have in understanding speech through hearing alone and, therefore, in acquiring language and information through hearing. Some believe that the more severe the bilateral hearing loss, the more the individual is apt to rely on vision for language acquisition and learning; similarly, the less severe the loss, the more effective amplification with hearing aids is likely to be. These are generalizations, however. Many variables other than the degree of hearing loss affect the way a child can acquire language, learn information, and progress educationally. These include age of onset, the threshold configuration of the hearing loss, supra-threshold speech understanding, general intelligence, and especially family support. Therefore, different language teaching methods, intervention strategies, and educational formats may be required for children with the same degree of hearing loss.

Degree of hearing loss is categorized from minimal to profound using a classification scale. For children, a minimal loss ranges from 15–25 dB HL; a mild loss, from 26–40 dB HL; a moderate loss, from 41–55 dB HL; a moderately severe loss, from 56–70 dB HL; a severe loss, from 71–90 dB HL; and a profound loss, from 91 dB HL and greater (Clark, 1981). As noted, the degree of hearing loss is often determined by measuring and averaging the minimum response levels at three test frequencies (500 Hz, 1,000 Hz, and 2,000 Hz). Generalizations of ranges of hearing levels, albeit convenient, often result in misperceptions of the consequences of the loss. For example, a so-called mild bilateral hearing loss has potentially serious implications for the language and emotional development of a preverbal child, whereas a similar loss in an adolescent may have less of an impact. A description of the functional impact

of the hearing loss is the best measure for a specific child and should accompany any interpretation of audiological testing.

Effects of Hearing Loss on Functional Communication

A minimal loss typically has no significant effect on development, especially if the loss is temporary, such as CHL that occurs with excessive earwax accumulation.

A child with a mild bilateral loss typically has difficulty hearing distant sounds or soft speech, missing 25%–40% of speech at typical conversational loudness. The child has difficulty perceiving the unvoiced consonants /s/, /p/, /t/, /k/, /th/ (as in *thin*), /f/, and /sh/, which are soft, high-frequency sounds. As a result, the child may miss some of the content of class and home discussions and confuse forms of language that depend on these sounds (e.g., plurals or possessives). A hearing aid is often a consideration for a child with a permanent bilateral or unilateral mild loss.

Children with a moderate, moderately severe, or severe bilateral hearing loss may hear conversational level speech as a whisper or simply detect sound when people speak without being able to discern the actual words. These degrees of loss affect the ability to hear even loud conversation without intervention. If the loss is permanent, hearing aid use is essential. Nonetheless, no assumptions can be made about the vocabulary, speech production, or voice quality of children with these degrees of hearing loss. Speech-language evaluations are essential in identifying these behaviors. Learning problems often result, however, from the significantly reduced auditory input associated with a moderate or severe hearing loss. Academic supports, hearing aids, classroom amplification, speech-language therapy, tutoring, and possibly special education services should be considered, based on the needs of the individual child.

A child with a profound bilateral hearing loss may hear very loud environmental sounds nearby without amplification but cannot hear speech of typical conversational volume. Even with amplification, certain consonant sounds are likely to be missed. If the loss occurs before 2 years of age, language and speech may not develop spontaneously, unless identification/intervention begins prior to 6 months of age (Yoshinaga-Itano, 2003).

Children with profound bilateral losses may be helped by powerful hearing aids to stay in contact with the auditory world. They most often benefit from cochlear implantation that provides significant opportunities for spoken-language communication. Spoken language, however, is not the sole language option available to children with a profound hearing loss and their families. Visual communication strategies, the most prominent example of which is sign language, can be very important to a child with profound hearing loss. Many parents who are deaf opt to raise their child in a signing environment to foster the development of the family's language system. The need for visual communication is not limited to children with profound deafness. Some children with severe losses experience enough difficulty in receiving and processing auditory information that they benefit from visual communication as well.

CAUSES OF HEARING LOSS

Genetic, biologic, and environmental risk indicators are associated with hearing loss, as shown in Table 10.2 (JCIH, 2007).

Hearing losses that are present at birth are defined as being "congenital," regardless of their causation, whereas those that develop after birth are described as "acquired."

SNHL in children can be congenital or acquired, occurring as a result of genetic factors, an event or injury *in utero*, perinatal complications, or an occurrence after birth (Smith, Bale, & White, 2005). At least half of SNHL in children is caused by genetic factors, and these are mostly isolated disabilities (Nance, 2003; Norris et al., 2006). For children with SNHL of nongenetic origin, it is estimated that approximately one third have additional developmental disabilities. Nongenetic hearing loss (congenital or acquired) can result from prenatal and postnatal factors related to infections, anoxic brain injury, prematurity, physical trauma, excessively loud noise, or exposure to ototoxic agents (e.g., certain antibiotics).

CHL also can be congenital or acquired. Although CHL can result from malformations of the outer and/or middle ear (e.g., in Down syndrome), it is more often due to middle ear infections (Stach & Ramachandran, 2008).

Congenital external ear (auricle) abnormalities, such as structural deformities, may occur unilaterally or bilaterally, and can be characterized by total or partial failure of auricle development. If the auricle develops only partially, it is called **microtia**; if there is complete absence of development, it is called **anotia** (Artunduaga et al., 2009). **Atresia** often occurs with microtia and refers to the absence of the opening to the external ear canal. When the ear canal opening is present but abnormally narrow it is called **stenosis** (Stach & Ramachandran, 2008). Children with atresia can have significant conductive hearing loss of about 60 dB. Surgical intervention to open the ear canal and remediate the hearing loss may be an option for children with atresia, but not until a child is older and skull growth is complete (Stach & Ramachandran, 2008).

Genetic Causes

In approximately 80% of children with hereditary hearing loss, the hearing loss is inherited as an **autosomal recessive** trait (see Chapter 1)

Table 10.2. Risk indicators associated with permanent congenital, delayed-onset, or progressive hearing loss in childhood

1. Caregiver concern* regarding hearing, speech, language, or developmental delay.
2. Family history* of permanent childhood hearing loss.
3. Neonatal intensive care of more than 5 days or any of the following regardless of length of stay: ECMO,* assisted ventilation, exposure to ototoxic medications (gentamicin and tobramycin) or loop diuretics (furosemide/Lasix), and hyperbilirubinemia that requires exchange transfusion.
4. *In utero* infections, such as CMV,* herpes, rubella, syphilis, and toxoplasmosis.
5. Craniofacial anomalies, including those that involve the pinna, ear canal, ear tags, ear pits, and temporal bone anomalies.
6. Physical findings, such as white forelock, that are associated with a syndrome known to include a sensorineural or permanent conductive hearing loss.
7. Syndromes associated with congenital hearing loss or progressive or late-onset hearing loss,* such as neurofibromatosis, osteopetrosis, and Usher syndrome; other frequently identified syndromes include Waardenburg, Alport, Pendred, and Jervell and Lange-Nielson.
8. Neurodegenerative disorders, such as Hunter syndrome, or sensory motor neuropathies, such as Friedreich's ataxia and Charcot-Marie-Tooth syndrome.
9. Culture-positive postnatal infections associated with sensorineural hearing loss,* including confirmed bacterial and viral (especially herpes viruses and varicella) meningitis.
10. Head trauma, especially basal skull/temporal bone fracture* that requires hospitalization.
11. Chemotherapy.*

Note: Indicators marked with an asterix are more likely to be delayed-onset or progressive.

and is not associated with a syndrome; that is, hearing loss is the child's sole disability. The percentage of deaf or hard of hearing children born to hearing parents is about 92%; only 8% have one or more parents who are deaf or hard of hearing (Mitchell & Karchmer, 2004). About half of all childhood nonsyndromic autosomal recessive hearing losses are caused by mutations in the Connexin 26 (Cx26) gene (*GJB2/DFNB1*; Nance, 2003; Norris et al., 2006). Other hereditary disorders can affect the formation or function of any part of the hearing mechanism (Wolf, 2010). Children with syndromic hearing loss have this loss as part of a genetic condition with broader physical and developmental abnormalities. There are more than 200 documented inherited syndromes associated with deafness, some of which manifest later in life. Table 10.3 describes some of the most common genetic disorders associated with hearing loss.

Cleft palate, in which the roof of the mouth fails to close during embryological development, is a malformation with associated CHL. It has a multifactorial inheritance pattern and may occur alone or together with cleft lip. It may also be part of a genetic syndrome with multiple anomalies (e.g., CHARGE syndrome, caused by a mutation in the *CHD7* gene). According to the Centers for Disease Control and Prevention, the incidence of cleft lip and/or cleft palate is about 1 in 600 live births, making it the most common congenital birth defect (Witt, 2008). Of children with a cleft palate, 50%–90% are susceptible to significant and persistent middle-ear infections with risk of CHL (Sheahan et al., 2003). Because of the absence of closure of the palate, the tensor veli palati muscle does not have a normal midline attachment and functions poorly in opening the eustachian tube, predisposing the child to these infections (Witt, 2008). Close monitoring of hearing in a child with cleft palate is important. Also, surgical **myringotomy** and tympanostomy (pressure equalizing, or PE) tube insertions are often necessary to remediate the middle ear condition and CHL.

Pre-, Peri-, and Postnatal Factors

Environmental exposures to viruses, bacteria, and other toxins such as drugs prior to or following birth can result in SNHL (Roizen, 2003).

Table 10.3. Examples of genetic disorders associated with hearing loss

Syndrome	Inheritance pattern	Type of hearing loss	Other characteristics
Treacher Collins syndrome	Autosomal dominant	Conductive or mixed	Abnormal facial appearance, deformed auricles, defects of ear canal and middle ear
Waardenburg syndrome	Autosomal dominant	Sensorineural, stable	Unusual facial appearance, irises of different colors, white forelock, absent organ of Corti
Bardet-Biedl syndrome	Autosomal recessive	Sensorineural, progressive	Retinitis pigmentosa, intellectual disability, obesity, extra fingers or toes
Usher syndrome	Autosomal recessive	Sensorineural; progressive in type III	Retinitis pigmentosa; central nervous system effects, including vertigo, loss of sense of smell, intellectual disability, epilepsy; half have psychosis
CHARGE association	Autosomal dominant	Mixed, progressive	Eye, gastrointestinal, and other malformations
Down syndrome	Chromosomal	Conductive; occasionally sensorineural	Small auricles, narrow ear canals, high incidence of middle-ear infections
Trisomy 13, trisomy 18	Chromosomal	Sensorineural	Central nervous system malformations
Cleft palate	Multifactorial	Conductive	Cleft lip

Key: CHARGE association, **c**oloboma, congenital **h**eart defect, choanal **a**tresia, **r**etarded growth and development, **g**enital abnormalities, and **e**ar malformations with or without hearing loss.

Neonates with severe respiratory or cardiopulmonary disease requiring extracorporeal membrane oxygenation (ECMO) therapy, treatment with a mechanical device that bypasses the heart and lung, are at risk for developing SNHL as a result of treatment (Fligor et al., 2005).

Very low birth weight infants (born weighing less than 1,500 grams) have an increased risk of perinatal morbidities that predispose them to SNHL, including hyperbilirubinemia (elevated bilirubin level), intracranial hemorrhage, and exposure to systemic antibiotics to treat sepsis (blood poisoning).

Whereas all infants should undergo a newborn hearing screening, infants remaining in a neonatal intensive care unit (NICU) for more than 5 days should undergo an additional audiology diagnostic assessment by 24–30 months of age to detect any SNHL that may be acquired (JCIH, 2007). In addition, parental, health care provider, or education provider concerns regarding a child's hearing abilities should result in a prompt referral for evaluation for any child, at any age.

Infections

Infections during pregnancy, including toxoplasmosis, herpes virus, syphilis, rubella, and **cytomegalovirus** (CMV), may cause severe to profound SNHL. Among these, CMV is the most frequently occurring. It is estimated that congenital CMV is responsible for 15%–20% of cases of moderate to profound bilateral SNHL and is associated with 22%–27% of cases of profound deafness in children (Grosse, Ross, & Dollard, 2008).

Infections during infancy and childhood can also lead to SNHL. Bacterial **meningitis** poses a significant risk for childhood-onset bilateral or unilateral hearing loss from damage to the cochlea, including a risk of profound deafness. Incidence rates reported worldwide vary from 5% to as high as 50%, with *Streptococcus pneumoniae* associated with the largest percentages (Peltola et al., 2010). It is important to recognize severe bilateral SNHL early, as there is only a small window of opportunity to provide a cochlear implant for some losses, such as those resulting from meningitis.

Ototoxic Medications

Specific antibiotics used to treat severe bacterial infections in childhood, particularly aminoglycosides (i.e., kanamycin, gentamicin, vancomycin, and tobramycin), may be **ototoxic** (toxic to the hearing mechanism) and cause irreversible bilateral SNHL due to damage to the sensory cells within the cochlea. The damage is dose-dependent, and the hearing loss is usually in the high frequencies. As we use knowledge of the human genome to develop personalized medicine, we have recognized that an inherited mutation in the mitochondrial 12S ribosomal RNA gene results in an increased risk of ototoxicity from antibiotics (Nance, 2003).

Chemotherapy drugs used to treat cancer, such as cisplatin and carboplatin, also can cause bilateral high-frequency SNHL. In a retrospective study of 134 children, ranged in age by 1.5 weeks to 24 years, the results showed that hearing loss increased in severity based on multiple factors, including the cumulative dose of cisplatin, concurrent treatment with carboplatin, radiation therapy exposure, and the younger age of the child (Chang & Chinosornvatana, 2010).

Children receiving aminoglycosides or undergoing chemotherapy should receive pre-treatment audiological testing to establish baseline auditory test results. They should undergo frequent posttreatment testing and long-term follow-up to monitor the effects of treatment on hearing (Al-Khatib et al., 2010; Bergeron et al., 2005; Berlin et al., 2005).

Middle Ear Disease

*Otitis media with **effusion*** (OME) is the term used to describe a middle ear infection associated with fluid accumulation. It may be treated by antibiotics and pressure equalization (PE) tubes (see Figure 10.7) or left to resolve on its own.

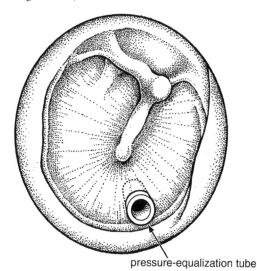

pressure-equalization tube

Figure 10.7. The procedure of myringotomy and pressure equalization tube placement involves the surgical incision of the tympanic membrane. The effusion is withdrawn, and a plastic tube is then inserted through the opening to permit ongoing drainage of fluid and equilibration of air pressure.

Episodic OME, which is acute but not persistent, occurs most commonly in very young children and tends to cause minimal to mild CHL. Such losses often go undiagnosed, are transient, and do not affect communicative development and school achievement.

Persistent OME, defined as more than 6 episodes within a 12-month period, has been shown to increase the risk of CHL, most commonly mild CHL, in young children (Roberts et al., 2004).

Researchers have investigated the link between language and academic skill development in typically developing young children diagnosed with persistent OME. Retrospective studies have found a relationship between a history of persistent OME during early childhood and delays in literacy and language skill development (Nittrouser & Burton, 2005; Shapiro et al., 2008; Winskel, 2006). However, studies performed prospectively have not identified a significant relationship between a history of OME or CHL and children's later academic skills in reading or word recognition (Roberts, Rosenfeld, & Zeisel, 2004); thus, the topic remains controversial. Limitations in study design, small sample sizes, and measurement factors (e.g., home environment contributions, degree of hearing loss) warn against overgeneralizing the results. Furthermore, most study samples have included otherwise healthy children, but impacts of persistent OME with CHL for children with developmental delays, from special populations (e.g., Down syndrome), or with preexisting SNHL and/or speech and language delays, have not been thoroughly investigated (Roberts, Rosenfeld, & Zeisel, 2004).

Collectively, experts support the view that while most children who experience persistent OME during the first years of life manifest no or minor speech, language, and literacy delays, a minority will exhibit persistent deficits throughout primary school grades. Therefore, each child's individuality should be considered when weighing management options for OME. The following reasonable best practices are recommended: 1) evaluate a child's hearing after 3 months of bilateral OME or when a family member or caregiver expresses concern about the child's hearing; 2) screen for OME and hearing loss on a regular basis in special populations of children (including those with intellectual disability, cleft palate, and other conditions that place children at risk for OME); 3) screen a child's language when hearing loss is accompanied by concern about language development; and 4) encourage families of children with OME to provide an enriched language and literacy environment (Roberts et al., 2004).

Trauma

A blow to the skull (traumatic brain injury [TBI]) can cause a longitudinal or transverse skull fracture. In children, this most commonly results from a vehicular accident, but can also be caused by physical abuse and sports injury (Perheentupa et al., 2010; see also Chapter 26). Skull base fractures may lead to 1) a sudden unilateral or bilateral SNHL, as a result of damage to the cochlea; or 2) permanent CHL from trauma to the ossicles of the middle ear (Yetiser, Hidir, & Gonul, 2008).

Noise Exposure

Sudden, explosively loud noises such as firecrackers, fireworks, and firearms may cause SNHL, as can repeated exposure to very loud sounds over time (Fligor, 2009). Examples of the latter include using MP3 players (e.g., iPod) at high-intensity levels, playing in school bands, and attending live rock music concerts and motor sporting events (e.g., NASCAR; Fligor, 2009).

The ubiquitous use of MP3 players among teens has generated concerns regarding risks of gradual but permanent hearing loss due to prolonged listening periods at high-intensity levels (Keith, Michaud, & Chiu, 2008; Torre, 2008). Exposure to levels of 85 dBA of loudness for 8 hours or more per day has been shown to increase the risk of permanent hearing loss. Maximum loudness levels in MP3 players have been measured at 85–107 dBA (Keith et al., 2008). Notably, differences in digital audio players, earphone sensitivity, and the physical fit of earphones (e.g., earbuds, headphones) account for variability in intensity output. Environmental background noise also increases the risk of reaching hazardous listening levels (Keith et al., 2008; Torre, 2008). College students were surveyed regarding their preferred listening levels with their personal devices, and in-ear loudness measurements revealed intensity outputs that ranged from 72–98 dB sound pressure levels (SPL; Torre, 2008). Education and increased public awareness is warranted that long-term use of personal listening devices with earphones may lead to permanent hearing loss.

Syndromes Associated with Intellectual Disability

Children with intellectual disability are at increased risk for hearing loss, especially when a genetic condition is the cause of the disability (see Chapter 17). Children with Down syndrome are particularly prone to developing CHL, with incidence rates as high as 78% reported (Shott, 2006). However, with aggressive medical and surgical interventions for persistent middle ear effusions, incidence rates of CHL have decreased. Normal hearing is achieved for approximately 93% of young children who are treated with pressure equalization tubes for persistent middle ear effusions (Shott, 2006).

Several reports of the results of hearing screenings conducted on adolescent and adult participants in the Special Olympics suggest that many individuals with intellectual disability experience significant undetected hearing loss (Herer, 2012; Neumann et al., 2006). In these studies, 17%–38% of individuals failed screening tests, and a significant proportion of these participants were confirmed as having CHL, SNHL, or mixed hearing loss.

IDENTIFICATION OF HEARING LOSS

Early identification of children with hearing loss in the United States is accomplished through universal newborn hearing screening programs at birthing hospitals (White & Maxon, 2005; JCIH, 2007). As of 2010, all states screen hearing of newborns, and 47 states have legislative mandates to screen hearing before hospital discharge (National Center for Hearing Assessment & Management, 2010).

The importance of identifying hearing loss soon after birth is analogous to the need for early detection of vision loss. The brain pathways for both of these senses are immature at birth and develop normally only when stimulated. Evidence indicates that identifying hearing loss early and implementing family-centered intervention services (including hearing aids) prior to 6 months of age, regardless of the degree of hearing loss, can result in significantly better vocabulary, speech intelligibility, general language abilities, as well as improved parental bonding and social-emotional development for deaf and hard-of-hearing children 1–5 years of age (Moeller, 2000; Yoshinaga-Itano, 2003).

Recent literature confirms the critical function of early intervention on communicative development for deaf and hard-of-hearing infants and toddlers (Vohr et al., 2010; Vohr et al., 2008). Enrollment into early intervention by 3 months of age, compared to enrollment at over 3 months of age, was investigated in young children with minimal or mild to profound SNHL and compared to typically hearing age-mate controls (Vohr et al., 2008; Vohr et al., 2010). Those infants and toddlers with very early enrollment into intervention services were shown to have beneficial effects on their early language development compared to later enrollees.

Nevertheless, children with moderate to profound hearing loss exhibited delayed receptive and expressive language skills in oral and signed English communication modes, compared to peers with either minimal or mild hearing loss or those with typical hearing sensitivity. These outcomes highlight that despite best practices with early detection and management, some children with greater degrees of hearing loss remain at a disadvantage in developing spoken language abilities.

Rates of Hearing Loss and Associated Risk Factors

The prevalence rate for congenital SNHL in babies from the well-infant nursery is approximately 1.2 per 1,000. This rate increases for hospitalized infants admitted to the NICU or specialty-care units to as high as 13.3 per 1,000 (Connolly, Carron, & Roark, 2005). There are risk indicators associated with hearing loss in the neonatal period (see Table 10.2). However, only 50% of the infants with SNHL at birth have identifiable risk-history factors (Connolly et al., 2005). Children with such factors may not demonstrate congenital hearing loss but may acquire hearing loss of a progressive or delayed-onset nature later in childhood. Therefore, it is essential to provide such children with ongoing surveillance. In order to determine the frequency of auditory surveillance, a medical work-up of the infant is performed. This involves a family history of hearing loss, medical history of child and family members, and an examination for findings suggestive of a genetic syndrome associated with hearing loss.

There are usually attributable risk indicators in children who acquire hearing loss; however, hearing loss in adolescents often occurs for reasons that are not well understood (Shargorodsky et al., 2010). According to results from the 2005–2006 National Health and Nutrition Examination Survey (NHANES), one in five adolescents age 12–19 years in the United States exhibited some degree of hearing loss. Compared with data from the 1988–1994 NHANES III, this represents a 33% increase in the prevalence of hearing loss (Shargorodsky et al., 2010). High-frequency hearing loss was more common than low-frequency hearing loss, and females had significantly lower odds of having hearing loss compared to males. Participants reporting income ratios below the poverty threshold had significantly increased odds of having a hearing loss compared to participants above the poverty threshold. Finally, unilateral hearing loss was reported most frequently. Surprisingly, the 2005–2006 NHANES did not find a significant association between hearing loss and adolescents self-reporting noise exposure. The overall worsening of acquired hearing loss in adolescents poses a considerable concern, given that any degree of hearing loss can compromise social development, communication health, and academic achievement.

These data point to the importance of early identification of and education about hearing loss so that hearing loss prevention strategies are taught and practiced.

Factors Indicating Possible Hearing Loss

Parental Concern

Parental concern has been shown to be a sensitive indicator of childhood hearing loss, and providers need to listen to parents' concerns. Since not all children with hearing loss have a risk factor and may pass the screen for newborns, there are new recommendations for ongoing surveillance of language milestones and hearing skills. The JCIH (2007) recommendation is that all infants should undergo an objective standardized screen of global development with a validated tool at 9, 18, and 24–30 months of age. In addition, if a child does not pass a medical home global developmental screen or if there is concern regarding hearing or language, the child should be referred for speech-language evaluation and audiology assessment.

Hearing Milestones for Detecting Hearing Loss

The newborn clearly prefers to listen to speech as opposed to other environmental sounds, just as the infant prefers to fixate visually on a face rather than an object. By 2 months of age, the typically developing infant can distinguish vowel from consonant sounds, and by 4 months, prefers speech patterns that have varied rhythm and stress (Werker & Yeung, 2005). The infant prefers listening to prolonged discourse rather than to repetitive baby talk. During this early period, an infant with typical hearing can be seen orienting his or her body toward a familiar sound source from his or her right or left.

Up to 5 months of age, the speech sounds an infant makes are not influenced by the speech sounds heard. The early vocalizations of infants from different countries sound alike. After 5 months of age, however, the infant's babbling starts to imitate the parents' speech patterns (i.e., native language; Werker & Yeung, 2005). Thus, the babbling of an infant with Spanish-speaking parents becomes different from that of an infant with English-speaking parents.

For all children with normal hearing, listening to spoken language during early life is a critical prerequisite for the typical development of speech. The same can be true for children with hearing loss who, because of detection by newborn hearing screening programs, can access spoken language in early life through early intervention services such as hearing aid amplification.

Signs of Hearing Loss in the Deaf or Hard of Hearing Child

An early sign of severe hearing loss is when the sleeping baby does not awaken to loud noises. Even a deaf infant, however, may react to vibrations, leading family members to assume the infant has actually heard the sound. Between 3 and 4 months of age, infants who are deaf coo and laugh normally. However, their consonant-vowel babbling, which normally occurs around age 6 months, is often reduced, delayed, or absent. Babbling is a sign of prelinguistic and early linguistic development. Children with normal hearing perceive their own babbling from auditory feedback (i.e., self-monitoring stimulation through the hearing sense), whereas infants who are deaf do not perceive this auditory feedback, which is why their babbling is affected (Northern & Downs, 2002).

In children with unaffected hearing, babbling becomes more varied and eventually is attached to meanings (e.g., the babble "dadada-dada" becomes the word *Dada*). The vocalizations of deaf infants show less variety in speech articulation and intonation and are less likely to become meaningful and recognizable words, unless they have benefited from early identification and intervention.

Between the ages of 5–17 months, infants with normal hearing significantly increase their repertoire of consonant sounds. During the same period, their peers who are deaf and hard of hearing, without intervention, demonstrate a reduction in consonant variety resulting in poor speech intelligibility. It is this failure to develop comprehensible speech that leads parents to suspect a hearing loss, if one was not already identified by screening during well-baby visits.

Receptive language also lags in children with hearing loss. By 4 months of age, the child with normal hearing generally orients his or her head or body toward a parent's voice. The child with a hearing loss may or may not exhibit such sound localization behavior, depending on the severity and configuration of the loss. By 8–9 months, a direct head turn (right or left to locate the parent's voice or a familiar sound) can be observed in a baby with typical hearing but not in one with a severe to profound hearing loss. At around 12 months of age, babies respond to verbal instructions accompanied by gestures, such as "Wave bye-bye." At this age, the child who is deaf may seem to understand the message because he or she can figure out the command by following gestures and understanding the context. Similarly, a deaf toddler may get his or her jacket when others do, whether or not he or she understood "Get your coat." By about 16 months of age, the child with normal hearing responds to more complex instructions by words alone. The child with an undiagnosed hearing loss, however, may have great difficulty in doing this and may stop following instructions unless they can be inferred from context or accompanied by gestures. This failure to respond to verbal instructions may lead parents to suspect a hearing loss, but it also can be misperceived as oppositional behavior. Children with normal hearing and with global developmental delays are also delayed in achieving these language milestones. These children, however, are similarly delayed in speech, motor, and cognitive skills. The young child who is deaf or hard of hearing but otherwise typically developing has slow development only in speech and language skills.

Methods of Screening for Hearing Loss

OAE technology and another hearing screening instrument, called screening or ABR, are effective screening tools to detect both SNHL and permanent CHL. Children with neural loss can have a hearing disorder identified as auditory neuropathy/dyssynchrony (auditory neuropathy spectrum disorder, or ANSD) and may have normal OAE results but poor auditory nerve function. Therefore, early detection requires the use of automated ABR technology. Children with ANSD have behavioral hearing test results that reflect substantial loss, as do their interactions with the world of sound. These children often show poor benefit from or dissatisfaction with hearing aid amplification because of the normal outer hair cell function (Berlin et al., 2010; Vlastarakos et al., 2008; Zeng et al., 2005).

Newborn Screening for Hearing Loss

Well Baby Nursery

All babies in the well baby nursery are screened for hearing status before hospital discharge, usually within the first 24 hours of life. The objective, noninvasive physiological procedures of transient-evoked otoacoustic emissions (TEOAE) and distortion product (DPOAE) and/or electrophysiological automated ABR technologies are used. The hearing screening protocols at birthing hospitals can vary with respect to the use of the OAE application and automated ABR. Many hospitals use OAE as a first screen followed by automated ABR for infants failing the OAE screen. Infants who do not pass this discharge screening are followed for postdischarge rescreens within several weeks. For those who do not pass the rescreen, a referral for an audiological diagnostic evaluation is made immediately. The hearing screening protocol can be very efficient, resulting in a 1%–6% referral rate to follow up with postdischarge rescreening or diagnostic audiological testing (Lin et al., 2005; Shulman et al., 2010). However, a longstanding limitation of effectiveness within EHDI systems is that parents of infants who require audiological assessment due to abnormal hearing screening results do not consistently return with their infants for follow-up testing (Mason et al., 2008; Shulman et al., 2010). Data from state-reported hearing screening indicate "lost to follow-up" rates exceeding 40% (CDC, 2011). Health care providers and educators of all specialties are encouraged to stress to families with infants or young children who did not pass their newborn hearing screening the importance of obtaining a hearing assessment regardless of whether a hearing, speech, or language concern exists.

Neonatal Intensive Care Unit

The JCIH (2007) recommended separate newborn hearing screen protocols for NICU infants hospitalized for greater than 5 days. Since NICU infants are considered at increased risk for neural hearing disorders, it was recommended that all NICU infants hospitalized for greater than 5 days be screened with automated ABR.

Hearing Tests

Electrophysiological Methods

In addition to the screening versions being used in EHDI programs, diagnostic OAE and ABR measures are part of the battery of audiological tests for infants, toddlers, and young children (Buz Harlor & Bower, 2009). They are also very useful in assessing children with developmental disabilities who are unable to respond to conventional behavioral audiometric testing (Berlin et al., 2005).

OAE testing is ideal for use in very young children or those with challenging behavior because results are achieved rapidly and do not require the child's cooperation other than sitting quietly. A small probe assembly is placed at the edge of the outer ear canal. The probe contains an earphone and a microphone. The OAE earphone introduces clicks (TEOAE) or tones of various frequencies (DPOAE) into the ear canal that are transmitted to the cochlea. If the cochlea's outer hair cells respond, they transmit low-level sounds called emissions back to the outer ear canal. The OAE probe assembly's microphone receives the emissions from the outer hair cells and transmits them to computer software for analyses. Each ear is tested individually. If there is damage to cochlear structures sufficient to cause a hearing loss of 30 dB or greater, abnormal OAE responses are obtained. OAE responses also may not be recorded due to a middle-ear effusion or malformation. Because OAE testing objectively measures the responses of the cochlear outer hair cells, the outcome data can help differentiate sensory hearing loss from neural components of SNHL. OAEs can also be used to monitor the status of cochlear function that could be affected by use of ototoxic drugs or by exposure to loud sounds, both of which can lead to progressive hearing loss (Lonsbury-Martin, 2005).

Diagnostic ABR testing evaluates both cochlear function and the auditory neural pathway. The ABR method is a highly sensitive test for both hearing loss and neural disruption of the central auditory pathway (Hall, 2006). ABR procedures involve affixing electroencephalogram sensors at various sites on a child's head and presenting sound stimuli through earphones. Click and tone burst stimuli, usually in the 500–4,000 Hz frequency range, are used to assess threshold hearing and neural activity in the brainstem pathway. ABR responses are analyzed using computer software. Either a natural sleeping state or one induced by sedation is required during the procedure. In infants, the ABR waveform is composed of three distinct waves, numbered I, III, and V (Figure 10.4), that represent successively higher levels of the ascending auditory pathway. An absence of waveform at a given intensity suggests a hearing loss, whereas the complete absence of a particular wave suggests an abnormality at a particular location of the brain auditory pathway.

Behavioral Hearing Tests

The outcome of behavioral tests is regarded as the "gold standard" for judging a child's auditory status and function in everyday life. Behavioral hearing testing is performed to 1) determine whether a hearing loss exists, 2) differentiate a CHL from a SNHL, 3) determine each ear's degree of loss across a range of test frequencies, and 4) estimate the clarity with which speech can be understood. The methodology and specific techniques must be modified for the developmental and cognitive age of the child (Madell, 2008).

Testing Infants up to 6 Months Cognitive Age

Both behavioral observation audiometry (BOA) and electrophysiological test methods are used to detect hearing loss in infants up to 6 months of age. BOA relies on subjective observation of a baby's reactions to a variety of sound stimuli in a structured sound environment. Observable responses, such as a change in sucking in response to stimuli, usually occur in response to familiar sounds, such as speech signals and a mother's voice (Madell, 2008). Starting at 4 months of age, infants begin to locate familiar sounds by turning their head toward the sound source, and this is the response sought when using BOA. This head-turning localization behavior becomes quicker and more precise starting at 6 months of age.

Testing Children with Cognitive Ages from 5 Months to 36 Months

As a child's responses to auditory stimuli mature, visual reinforcement audiometry (VRA) can be used to assess hearing sensitivity. VRA pairs sound stimuli produced from a sound source, such as a wall-mounted room speaker (i.e., soundfield speaker) with visual reinforcement stimuli (i.e., a lighted and animated toy) and the child is trained using operant conditioning and control trials to localize with head-turn responses toward the sound source. For most babies and toddlers, a well-defined VRA test protocol can determine reliable hearing responses (although not threshold levels) for tonal and speech stimuli for at least one ear and often both ears. These behavioral data can validate the electrophysiological results of OAE and ABR testing obtained with infants at earlier ages (Madell, 2008; Widen et al., 2005).

Testing Children with Cognitive Ages from 30 Months to 5 Years and Older

Conditioned play audiometry (CPA) can be used for testing children generally between the ages of 2½ and 5 years (Madell, 2008). The child usually wears earphones and is conditioned to perform a play task whenever a pure tone or speech stimulus is heard. For example, the child may stack blocks or put rings on a peg in response to hearing an auditory stimulus. Beginning at 4 years cognitive age for some children, conventional audiometric techniques are employed, with responses consisting of a hand raise in response to the auditory stimulus. If conditioning of the child is successful, audiometric results are as complete as those obtained from an older child or adult (Kemaloglu et al., 2005).

When a child's hearing is assessed via the soundfield room speaker or earphones (i.e., air conduction; Figure 10.8A) and a hearing loss is identified, it is not possible to determine whether the loss is conductive or sensorineural. Therefore, tonal sounds are also presented through a bone conduction vibrator placed on the mastoid bone behind the ear (Figure 10.8B). Air conduction tests the contribution of the external, middle, and inner ear, whereas bone conduction bypasses the external and middle ear and stimulates the inner ear directly. As a result, the child demonstrating a hearing loss by air conduction but normal hearing by bone conduction can be inferred to have a conductive hearing loss. Likewise, if the child evidences hearing loss of equal magnitude by air and bone conduction, the hearing loss is shown to be sensorineural (Figure 10.9; Bess & Humes, 2008).

Speech audiometry is another important method for assessing the auditory function of children 2½ years and older. It complements CPA by determining threshold acuity for speech stimuli, which can validate CPA's tonal threshold results. Speech audiometry methods can also evaluate how well a child understands information at levels above threshold (e.g., comfortable conversational levels), which can provide insight into the effects of a hearing loss on everyday listening/understanding. Test material and methods used in speech audiometry must

be consistent with a child's developmental age (i.e., vocabulary age—e.g., use of pictures of test vocabulary; Mendel, 2008).

Assessing Middle-Ear Function

Measurements of the physiological function of a child's middle-ear system contribute significantly to the differential diagnosis of CHL and SNHL, and they can help monitor the course of middle-ear disease and treatment. To evaluate objectively the function of the middle-ear system, immittance measures (which assess the resistance and compliance of the system) are used. Any significant change to these characteristics of the middle-ear system can affect transmission of sound energy to the cochlea (Lilly, 2005). Immittance tests include **tympanometry** and acoustic reflex measures. Tympanometry examines middle-ear pressure, tympanic membrane compliance, mobility of the ossicles, and eustachian tube function. Acoustic reflex measurements assess the contraction of the muscle tendon attached to the head of the stapes when a very loud sound enters the cochlea.

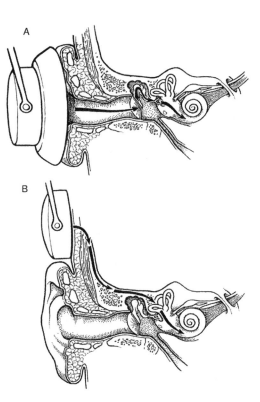

Figure 10.8. Approaches to testing air and mastoid bone conduction of sound. A) In air conduction, the sound comes through the ear canal and middle ear to reach the inner ear. B) In bone conduction, the sound bypasses the external ear and for the most part the middle ear, and then goes directly to the inner ear.

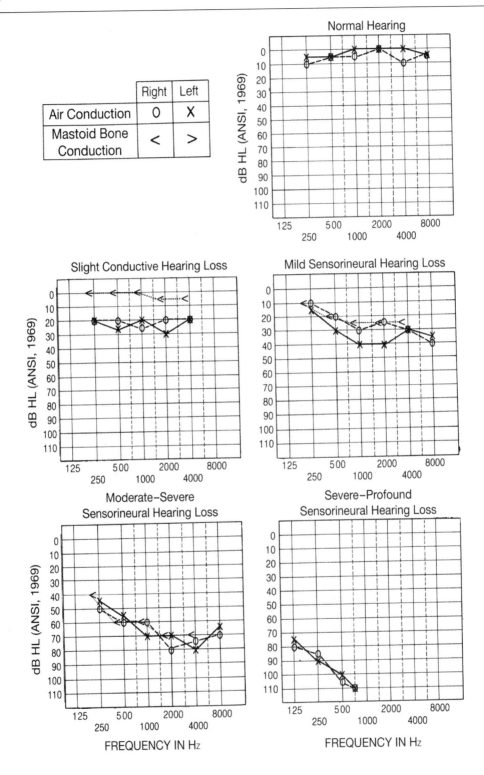

Figure 10.9. Audiograms showing normal hearing and various degrees of hearing loss. Note that in all cases shown, both ears are equally affected. In a conductive hearing loss, bone conduction is found to be better than air conduction because it bypasses the external and the middle ear where the problem exists. In sensorineural hearing loss, bone and air conduction produce similar results because the problem is within the inner ear and/or auditory nerve. (Key: ANSI, American National Standards Institute; Hz, hertz.) (Courtesy of Brad Friedrich, Ph.D.)

In tympanometry, an ear probe that presents a steady-state tone is placed in the ear canal. Varying amounts of air pressure (positive, negative, and atmospheric) are also sent through the probe to the eardrum. A microphone in the probe measures intensity differences of the tone in the ear canal as the air pressure changes. The air pressure–intensity relationships in tympanometry are plotted graphically and can show normal function in the middle-ear system or various problems within it (Figure 10.10). The presence of the acoustic stapedial tendon reflex in a child is strong evidence of a healthy middle-ear system, as well as normal functioning of the inner ear hair cells and eighth nerve (Berlin et al., 2005).

Assessing Central Auditory Function

A child's brain receives, analyzes, identifies, stores, recalls, and relates auditory information in order to make sense of the stimuli/events of the surrounding auditory world. This dynamic process is regarded as among the highest cognitive functions of the human brain. The outcome of this process is readily seen in the rapid evolution of a child's complex speech-language system in early childhood.

For reasons that are currently unclear, some children have auditory processing problems that are attributed to inadequate functioning of sites within the brain's central auditory neurological system. The problems most often emerge as a child approaches school age or enters adolescence, and manifest as difficulties with the following:

- Listening and understanding in noisy conditions
- Paying attention to or remembering spoken information
- Following multistep directions
- Carrying out instructions in a reasonable time frame
- Understanding language
- Developing vocabulary, reading (including comprehension), spelling and vocabulary skills
- Low overall academic performance

Children exhibiting such difficulties are often described as having an auditory processing disorder (APD), but they generally have normal threshold hearing and typical intelligence. APD, however, is also ascribed to coexist with other conditions such as dyslexia, attention-deficit/hyperactivity disorder, autism spectrum disorders, developmental delay, and specific language impairment (Witton, 2010).

Testing for a suspected APD involves presenting special listening tasks that tax the auditory system's ability to understand or integrate auditory information. Most of these behavioral test procedures have normative data only for children 7 years of age and older because of the sophisticated listening–responding tasks.

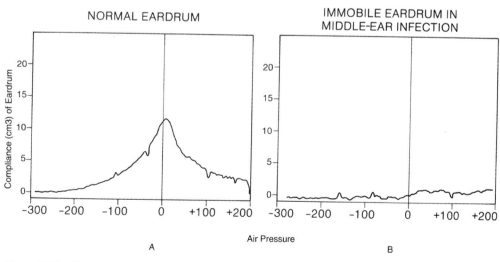

Figure 10.10. Tympanogram. The zero point represents atmospheric air pressure. The positive and negative numbers indicate that positive or negative pressures (relative to atmospheric pressure) have been applied to the eardrum. The compliance values are determined by the intensity of the probe tone at the various pressures and are influenced by the presence or absence of middle-ear pathology. A) A normal tent-shaped tympanogram. B) During otitis media (middle-ear infection), a flattened function may be obtained. (Key: cm³, cubic centimeters.) (Courtesy of Brad Friedrich, Ph.D.)

Electrophysiologic procedures may also be used by audiologists to determine possible clues to APD (Alonso & Schochat, 2009).

INTERVENTION FOR HEARING LOSS

Parents need to make informed decisions for their child about communication methods, hearing aid use, cochlear implantation, and education. They need to be presented with substantial information from professionals with expertise in these important areas, such as physicians, pediatric audiologists, educators of the deaf and hard of hearing, and speech-language pathologists. Other individuals and groups with knowledge about hearing loss also can be helpful to parents, including organizations concerned with hearing loss, other parents of children with hearing loss, and local school systems.

When a child has a hearing loss ranging from mild to severe, the language and speech choices usually focus on a variety of aural/oral intervention methodologies. When a child has a severe or profound loss, the child's family may want to learn about the sign language methods of learning language, as well as aural/oral methods. Parents need immediate access to complete information about the variety of approaches to communication development and education so they can make informed choices (Buz Harlor & Bower, 2009).

Early Intervention

Once a permanent hearing loss has been diagnosed, evidence-based management begins with the child and family's referral to and enrollment in a transdisciplinary, family-centered, comprehensive early intervention program (Mellon et al., 2009). The Individuals with Disabilities Education Improvement Act (IDEA; PL 108–446) ensures services to children with disabilities, including hearing loss. Infants and toddlers aged birth to 2 years who are deaf and hard of hearing receive services under IDEA Part C (see Chapter 31).

The goals for successful intervention include family adaptation to and acceptance of the child's special communication needs and the provision of a linguistically accessible environment at home and school that enhances the child's self-esteem. Optimally, programs should be flexible in their orientation and include family supports and integration with community services. Parent education materials, support groups, and national information centers are now available to assist parents in selecting an appropriate intervention site and a language acquisition strategy.

Methods of Intervention

Language-Learning Options

Various language-learning methods are available to children with severe or profound hearing loss. Auditory oral educational methods emphasize the teaching of listening skills, speech reading, speech articulation, and spoken language. Examples of oral approaches include Cued Speech, which utilizes a limited number of hand shapes next to the face to express phonetic sounds with spoken language, and the auditory-verbal method, which emphasizes the training of residual hearing without reliance on visual stimuli (Lim & Simser, 2005).

Different language-learning options comprise auditory approaches, visual methods, or a combination of both, including the following as noted by Flexer (2008):

- Auditory-oral
- Auditory-verbal
- Cued Speech
- Sign-supported speech and language
- Simultaneous communication
- American Sign Language (ASL)
- Total communication
- Bilingual-bicultural approach

English-oriented sign systems are intended to facilitate the learning of English by combining ASL vocabulary, coined signs, and finger spelling (letter-for-letter spelling of whole words) in an attempt to represent English sentence structure. Proponents of total communication incorporate aural/oral and manual communication modes, such as listening skills, speech reading, English-oriented signing or ASL, gesture/mime, and anything that facilitates the child's comprehension of what is spoken and/or signed. Educators of the deaf who use the bilingual-bicultural approach propose that children must first be immersed in ASL so that they have full access to and can acquire the meaningful use of a language before they can attain a less available (spoken) language. ASL has its own unique grammatical patterns and is structurally different from a spoken language, as it is visually received and spatially expressed. Furthermore, ASL is not English; it is a different language within a distinct culture (Pray & Jordan, 2010).

Amplification

Amplification (i.e., hearing aids, assistive listening devices) is an important part of the services required by the child with hearing loss (Seewald et al., 2005). Hearing aids can be used by children of any age, including young infants. They should be fitted as soon as a persistent or permanent hearing loss has been identified, even if all of the information about the hearing loss is not yet available. Assistive listening devices, such as FM systems, are often used in conjunction with hearing aids in difficult listening environments, such as the classroom, to improve the signal-to-noise ratio of the speech message over impeding ambient room noise (Smaldino & Flexer, 2008).

Audiologists are responsible for the appropriate fitting of amplification devices for children. The selection and utilization of amplification for children, particularly preverbal children, differs significantly from the procedures used in adult fittings (Seewald et al., 2005). First, selection of child-appropriate hearing aids is an ongoing process that extends far beyond identifying hearing loss and the initial fitting of an amplification device. Second, the settings of hearing aids are subject to change as new information regarding the hearing loss and responses to amplification are obtained through frequent audiological evaluations of the child. Finally, the degree of hearing loss is not the only consideration in determining a child's candidacy

for amplification. Profiles of the child's existing speech and language skills, cognitive abilities, commonly encountered listening environments, and school performance are all important factors in determining the appropriateness of hearing aid use and its specific fitting.

Hearing aids have three components: 1) a microphone that changes the acoustic signal into electrical energy, 2) digital amplifiers that increase the intensity of the electrical signal, and 3) a receiver that converts the electrical signal back to an amplified acoustical signal. The amplified sound is channeled into the ear canal through an earmold. A battery powers the hearing aid, and the loudness adjustments are automated by digital sound processing, or, in older children, can be manually adjusted by the user. Children's hearing aids also should permit direct audio input to allow coupling to an FM system and should have tamper-resistant battery compartments to prevent young children from swallowing the batteries.

Hearing aid categories for young children and older youth are behind-the-ear (BTE) aids, in-the-ear (ITE) aids, and bone conduction aids. BTE hearing aids (Figure 10.11) are safer and offer greater flexibility for accommodating the needs of pediatric hearing loss compared to custom ITE hearing aids. This flexibility is especially important if the child's audiometric information is incomplete or if the possibility of progressive hearing loss exists. Also, as the child's

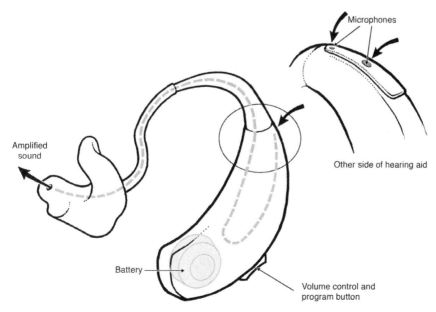

Figure 10.11. The components of a behind-the-ear (BTE) hearing aid. The aid consists of a microphone, a battery power supply, an amplifier, and a receiver that directs the amplified sound through the earmold into the ear canal.

ear canal grows, earmolds can be remade for the BTE aid without having to replace the entire aid as is necessary with the ITE instruments.

Bone conduction hearing aids or bone-anchored hearing aids (e.g., Baha), surgically implanted or worn externally via a soft headband, are most helpful for children who have bilateral malformations of the external and/or middle ear accompanied by conductive hearing loss (e.g, atresia) or who have chronic middle-ear drainage into the external ear canal. The latter condition would prevent use of an earmold with a BTE instrument or an ITE hearing aid (Christensen et al., 2010).

Binaural hearing aids (hearing aids in both ears) are preferred with children, unless there are contraindications to fitting both ears, such as structural abnormalities or the absence of any usable hearing in one ear. Although hearing aids are valuable tools, it is important to understand that they make speech sounds louder but not always clearer. Also, they do not selectively amplify speech versus other sounds. Therefore, when SNHL is present, because of ambient noise, the child may have difficulty understanding what is said even when the hearing aids provide speech sounds that are comfortably loud. The child and family must have realistic

expectations for amplification and recognize the importance of speech and language education and ways to modify the child's listening environment.

Cochlear Implantation for Severe or Profound Sensorineural Hearing Loss

A cochlear implant (CI) is a prosthetic device that electrically stimulates the cochlea via an electrode array surgically implanted in the inner ear. The reasoning behind the use of a CI is that many auditory nerve fibers and the central auditory neurological pathway remain functional even when the sensory hair cells in the cochlea are damaged severely or reduced in number.

The device provides auditory information via five components: 1) a microphone, 2) a signal processor that encodes incoming sounds, 3) a transmitter, 4) a receiver, and 5) the implanted electrodes (Figure 10.12). The sound is received by the microphone and sent to the signal processor, which is a computer that analyzes and digitizes the sound signal into individually programmed electrical information. The electrical information is sent to the transmitter, located

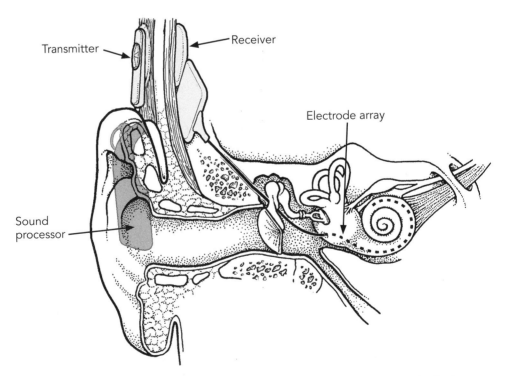

Figure 10.12.   Cochlear implant. The device has five components: a microphone to capture sound, a signal processor that electronically encodes the incoming sounds, a transmitter, a receiver, and the electrodes that have been surgically threaded into the cochlea. The electrodes stimulate nerve fibers along the cochlea, and the child perceives sound.

on the skin surface behind the ear. The transmitter sends the coded signals to an implanted receiver just under the skin. The receiver delivers the coded electrical signals to the array of electrodes that was surgically inserted into the cochlea. These electrodes stimulate auditory nerve fibers at different locations along the cochlea, and sound sensations progress through the central auditory system to the brain.

The primary goal of pediatric cochlear implantation is to provide critical speech information to the auditory system and brain in children who are severely to profoundly deaf, in order to maximize their opportunities for developing spoken language (Geers, 2006). The scientific literature is replete with reports of the positive benefits of multichannel CIs on language, speech, and literacy for children; and early implantation (less than 2 years of age) is a chief variable leading to successful outcomes (Dettman et al., 2007; Holt & Svirsky, 2008; Nicholas & Geers, 2006; Yoshinaga-Itano, Baca, & Sedey, 2010). Additional factors central to children achieving spoken language levels comparable to hearing age-mates include advances in CI technology and clinical practice, enhanced speech coding strategies, extent of preimplantation residual hearing, and effective habilitation/rehabilitation focused on speech and auditory skill development (Geers, 2006).

Cochlear implantation is considered for children in the context of a multidisciplinary team approach that includes an audiologist, speech-language pathologist, an otolaryngologist, the family, and often a psychologist and an educator of the deaf and hard of hearing (Alexiades et al., 2008). Following surgical implantation, the habilitative process begins with the initial activation of the CI and long-term mapping (i.e., programming) of a child's CI by an audiologist. This is critical to the child's successful use of the acoustic features of speech and language. Threshold hearing levels, comfort levels, and the dynamic hearing range change with the CI use throughout life, and this requires remapping (Alexiades et al., 2008).

Current trends in CI surgical methods and device hardware involve simultaneous and sequential bilateral cochlear implantation in children (Peters, Wyss, & Manrique, 2010; Sparreboom, Snik, & Mylanus, 2010; Zeitler et al., 2008). Bilateral CIs have the potential to improve speech perception abilities in the second implanted ear and to provide access to the use of binaural mechanisms, such as improved hearing in noisy environments and enhanced localization abilities.

The families of children using CIs for 4 or more years express a high degree of satisfaction with the results. Parents have a favorable view about the CI's effects on family life and their child's well-being. Their satisfaction with their child's implant, however, is most significantly related to the child's speech-language achievements (Sach & Whynes, 2005). Children with CIs indicate that they are successfully managing the demands of social and educational activities, regardless of post-implant speech-language capabilities (Wheeler, Archbold, Gregory, & Skipp, 2007). There is some evidence, too, that the deaf community is becoming more accepting of cochlear implantation, regarding it as one of a continuum of intervention strategies for parents to consider (National Association of the Deaf, 2000). Deaf parents of some children with CIs have great interest in their children's spoken language development but support the use of signing before and after implantation (Christiansen & Leigh, 2004).

Education and Communication

Education and communication are inextricably linked because educational curricula are language based. Without adequate language skills, a child who is deaf or hard of hearing is at a functional disadvantage in all academic areas. The goal of professionals working with the deaf or hard-of-hearing child should be the facilitation of optimal communication, utilizing whatever tools are most helpful based on the child's cognitive, attentional, and sensory profile and other related variables, including family preferences (Madell & Flexer, 2008). The two factors most predictive of the educational achievement of people who are deaf are language development and educational opportunities (Antia et al., 2009).

To improve communication for a child with hearing loss, education and intervention should focus on developing listening skills and all aspects of language, including syntax and grammar, increasing speech or sign language production, and expanding vocabulary. The educational achievement of students who are deaf or hard of hearing is weakest in the areas of reading and writing (Antia et al., 2009). Good practice specifies that literacy experiences be an intrinsic component of education and intervention, and that preliteracy experiences begin with infants and toddlers (Flexer, 2008).

The roles of interventionists will vary depending on the context of the service provision. Some speech-language pathologists, teachers of students who are deaf or hard of hearing, and educational audiologists, for example, work in the classroom alongside a teacher or special educator. Some work in conjunction with preschool programs for children with hearing loss; still others work as independent contractors either in school-linked consultations or as providers of education/therapy sessions in the homes of infants and toddlers. The variety of available services is highly dependent on the children's ages, their degree of hearing loss and communication problems, the extent of their functional hearing, the local and regional educational philosophy, and other factors such as the family's financial resources and commitment to learning a new communication system. Collaborative interventions are the most supportive for families (Flexer, 2008). Communication approaches reflect speech-language pathology service models and often incorporate a specific type of communication modality, according to the preference of the family, clinician, center, and school.

Infants, toddlers, and preschool children with all degrees of hearing loss may have a variety of possible service delivery systems available to them, ranging from home visits by interventionists, to provision of services in a special preschool, to enrollment in a regular education preschool (with education/therapy services brought to the child in that environment). With the advent of universal newborn hearing screening in birthing hospitals, parents of infants with early identified hearing loss may immediately seek assistance from their school district (Buz Harlor & Bower, 2009).

In general, school-age children with mild and moderate to severe hearing losses will be enrolled in regular education classrooms in community schools. Consultation and collaboration services from speech-language pathologists, educational audiologists, teachers of the deaf and hard of hearing, and other interventionists are brought to the child's classroom. On occasion, the child may leave the general education classroom for individual or small group sessions and may spend part of a day in a special class for intensive small group instruction. Auditory oral language teaching (active listening enhanced with hearing aids, cochlear implants, and assistive listening devices) is usually employed as the mode of communication in these learning environments (Flexer, 2008).

Services for infant and toddler programs under Part C of the IDEA may vary by state (Sorkin, 2008). Table 10.4 lists the services that children who are deaf or hard of hearing and their families may receive under Part C.

School-based services for deaf and hard-of-hearing children begin at 3 years of age and continue through 21 years of age, covered by Part B of the IDEA (Sorkin, 2008). Services for school-age students may vary by school district and are listed in Table 10.5.

The IDEA law requires that children with disabilities have the right to a free and appropriate education (FAPE) and are educated in the least restrictive environment (LRE; U.S. Department of Education, 2006). According to the 2006 regulations, the LRE requirements indicate "a strong preference, not a mandate, for educating children with disabilities alongside their peers without disabilities" (Sorkin, 2008). Educating a child with hearing loss in the LRE is based on the learning needs of the child as the child develops. One goal of early intervention is to provide enough support that education can occur in the LRE. Educational placements are also based on the family's preference, the child's academic and social readiness, and the program options available within the school district (Sorkin, 2008).

An educational placement for young school-age children with a severe or profound degree of hearing loss may include instruction in a special day class taught by an educator of the deaf and hard of hearing, with other service providers coming into the classroom or taking the child or children out for individualized instruction. A special day class placement may mix children with and without hearing loss for some academic subjects or for other school activities. The children who are grouped in a

Table 10.4. Services for children who are deaf or hard of hearing under Part C of the Individuals with Disabilities Education Improvement Act of 2004 (PL 108–446)

- Service coordination by a knowledgeable professional
- Appropriate assessment in all areas of development
- Design of an individual family service plan (see Chapter 30)
- Assistance with parent–child interactions
- Modeling and demonstration of speech and language experiences
- Information that is unbiased to help families decide on communication modes and educational methods
- Emotional support
- Direct instruction to the child (if warranted)
- Caregiver assistance with technology
- Transition services to a preschool program beginning at 2½ years of age

Source: Sorkin (2008).

Table 10.5. Services for school-age children who are deaf or hard of hearing under Part B of the Individuals with Disabilities Education Improvement Act

- Develop and implement individualized education program (IEP)
- Provide hearing assessment
- Supply and maintain assistive listening technology
- Ensure the function of hearing aids, cochlear implant processors, and assistive listening devices
- Management of classroom acoustics
- Provide speech-language therapy
- Provide special education services
- Provide interpreter services (e.g., American Sign Language, Cued Speech, oral transliteration)

Source: Sorkin (2008).

Table 10.6. Specialized curriculum areas and accommodations for students who are deaf or hard of hearing

Specialized curriculum areas
Deaf studies
Use of assistive technology (e.g., telecommunication devices, videophones)
Instruction in manual language (e.g., American Sign Language, Cued Speech)
Speech-language therapy and speech reading
Auditory training
Instruction in social skills
Career and vocational education

Specialized accommodations
Sign language interpreters
Closed captioning
Note-takers
Assistive listening devices
Visual alerts
Communication access real-time translation (CART) system

Source: Sorkin (2008).

special day classroom are usually taught exclusively by a specific language method, such as aural/oral, a sign system, or total communication, depending on the method selected by their parents. As children with all degrees of hearing loss (mild to profound) reach middle-school age, they are often included in general education classes with children who possess typical hearing and receive various types of in-class supports to enable communication access, including interpreters, closed-captioning, and in-service training for teachers and class-mates (Sorkin, 2008).

Other school options for children with severe to profound hearing loss include private schools as well as state schools for students who are deaf. Students who are deaf or hard of hearing in elementary and secondary school programs should be provided instruction in the local school district's adopted core curriculum (IDEA, 2004). It is also important that the students have access to a full range of activities, including after-class and extracurricular options with appropriate accommodations. Modifications and accommodations for each curricular area should be addressed at the IEP plan meetings annually, although parents may request a review of the IEP more frequently if there is a significant change in their child's status (e.g., cochlear implant surgery; Sorkin, 2008). Specialized curriculum areas and accommodations for students who are deaf or hard of hearing are provided in Table 10.6. Facilitating the transition from high school to adult life is also a responsibility of the school system (see Chapters 31 and 40).

For more information and resources regarding the development and education of children who are deaf and hard of hearing, see Laurent Clerc National Deaf Education Center (2011). For information related to families

and their children who are deaf or hard of hearing collaborating in partnership with professionals, see Hands and Voices (2011).

OUTCOME

A wide range of audiological, familial, linguistic, social, and environmental factors can affect speech development, English literacy, language competence, psychosocial function, educational outcomes, and career options for individuals with hearing loss. These factors include age of onset and severity of hearing loss, family response and resources, age of exposure to a language system, psychosocial supports, and the nature of other disabilities or **comorbid** conditions. Formulating a prognosis for the child's ultimate language, educational, and psychosocial development based on any single variable, however, is not possible given the current state of knowledge. Instead, the focus should be on the earliest identification of hearing loss and prompt access to intervention that is individually tailored, family-centered, and carefully monitored.

SUMMARY

Hearing loss can be temporary, persistent, or permanent; conductive, sensorineural, mixed, or neural; unilateral or bilateral; and congenital or acquired. It may exist alone or with other disabilities. Regardless of the degree or the cause of the hearing loss, it is important for professionals working with children with hearing loss and their families to understand the anatomy and physiology of the hearing mechanism and the impact of the hearing loss on the perception and processing of spoken language. Hearing loss in childhood offers a unique opportunity to witness adaptation to perceptual impairment and human resilience in the face of a disruption in communication channels. The child and family's innate strengths, capacities, and vulnerabilities must be viewed within a larger social, linguistic, educational, cultural, and environmental context. Hearing loss does not have to impede typical development, place an individual at a functional disadvantage, or alter ultimate outcomes. Professionals who wish to address the needs of children with hearing loss must recognize, and make recommendations based on, the unique needs of the individual child and family.

REFERENCES

Alexiades, G., De La Asuncion, M., Hoffman, R.A., Kooper, R., Madell, J.R., Markoff, L.B., … Sislian, N. (2008). Cochlear implants for infants and children. In J.R. Madell & C. Flexer (Eds.), *Pediatric audiology: Diagnosis, technology, management*. New York, NY: Thieme Medical Publishers.

Al-Khatib, T., Cohen, N., Carret, A.S., & Daniel, S. (2010). Cisplatin ototoxicity in children, long-term follow up. *International Journal of Pediatric Otorhinolaryngology, 74*, 913–919.

Alonso, R., & Schochat, E. (2009). The efficacy of formal auditory training in children with (central) auditory processing disorder: Behavioral and electrophysiological evaluation. *Brazilian Journal of Otorhinolaryngology, 75*, 726–732.

Antia, S.D., Jones, P.B., Reed, S., & Kreimeyer, K.H. (2009). Academic status and progress of deaf and hard-of-hearing students in general education classrooms. *Journal of Deaf Studies and Deaf Education, 14*, 293–311.

Bergeron, C., Dubourg, L., Chastagner, P., Mechinaud, F., Plouvier, E., Desfachelles, D.F., … Rubie, H. (2005). Long-term renal and hearing toxicity of carboplatin in infants treated for localized and unresectable neuroblastoma: Results of the SFOP NBL90 study. *Pediatric Blood & Cancer, 45*, 32–36.

Berlin, C., Hood, L., Morlet, T., Wilensky, D., Brashears, S., St. John, P., … and Thibodeaux, M. (2005). The battery principle re-visited physiologically, with special attention to auditory neuropathy and Cued Speech. *Perspectives on Hearing and Hearing Disorders in Childhood (ASHA Division 9), 15*, 5–9.

Berlin, C., Hood, L., Morlet, T., Wilensky, D., Li, L., Mattingly, K.R., … Frisch, S. (2010). Multi-site diagnosis and management of 260 patients with auditory neuropathy/dys-syncrony (auditory neuropathy spectrum disorder). *International Journal of Audiology, 49*, 30–43.

Bess, F., & Humes, L. (2008). *Audiology: The fundamentals* (4th ed.). Philadelphia, PA: Lippincott, Williams & Wilkins.

Boothroyd, A. (2008). The acoustic speech signal. In J.R. Madell & C. Flexer (Eds.), *Pediatric audiology: Diagnosis, technology, management*. New York, NY: Thieme Medical Publishers.

Buz Harlor, A.D., Jr., & Bower, C. (2009). Hearing assessment in infants and children: Recommendations beyond neonatal screening. *Pediatrics, 124*, 1252–1263.

Centers for Disease Control and Prevention (CDC). (2011). *Summary of 2008 National CDC EHDI Data* (Version A). Retrieved January 16, 2011 from http://www.cdc.gov/ncbddd/hearingloss/2008-data/2008_EHDI_HSFS_Summary.pdf

Chang, K.W., & Chinosornvatana, N. (2010). Practical grading system for evaluating cisplatin ototoxicity in children. *Journal of Clinical Oncology, 28*, 1788–1795.

Christiansen, J., & Leigh, I. (2004). Children with CIs: Changing parent and deaf community perspectives. *Archives of Otolaryngology—Head and Neck Surgery, 130*, 673–677.

Christensen, L., Smith-Olinde, L., Kimberlain, J., Richter, G.T., & Dornhoffer, J.L. (2010). Comparison of traditional bone-conduction hearing aids with the Baha system. *Journal of the American Academy of Audiology, 21*, 267–273.

Clark, J.G. (1981). Uses and abuses of hearing loss classification. *American Speech Hearing Association, 23*, 493–500.

Connolly, J.L., Carron, J.D., & Roark, S.D. (2005). Universal Newborn Hearing Screening: Are we achieving the Joint Committee on Infant Hearing (JCIH) objectives? *The Laryngoscope, 115*, 232–236.

Emanuel, D.C., & Letowski, T. (2009). Pyschoacoustics. *Hearing science*. Baltimore, MD: Lippincott Williams & Wilkins.

Flexer, C. (2008). Communication approaches for managing hearing loss in infants and children. In J.R. Madell & C. Flexer (Eds.), *Pediatric audiology: Diagnosis, technology, management*. New York, NY: Thieme Medical Publishers.

Fligor, B. (2009). Recreational Noise. In M. Chasin (Ed.), *The consumer handbook on hearing loss and noise*. Sedona, AZ: Auricle Ink Publishers.

Fligor, B.J., Neault, M.W., Mullen, C.H., Feldman, H.A., & Jones, D.T. (2005). Factors associated with sensorineural hearing loss among survivors of extracorporeal membrane oxygenation therapy. *Pediatrics, 115*, 1519–1528.

Geers, A. (2006). Factors influencing spoken language outcomes in children following early cochlear implantation. *Advances in Oto-rhino-laryngology, 64*, 50–65.

Grosse, S.D., Ross, D.S., & Dollard, S.C. (2008). Congenital cytomegalovirus (CMV) infection as a cause of permanent bilateral hearing loss: A quantitative assessment. *Journal of Clinical Virology, 41*, 57–62.

Hall, J.W. (2006). *New handbook of auditory evoked responses*. Boston, MA: Allyn & Bacon.

Hall, J., III, Smith, S., & Popelka, G. (2004). Newborn hearing screening with combined otoacoustic emissions and auditory brainstem responses. *Journal of the American Academy of Audiology, 15*, 414–425.

Hands and Voices. (2011). *What works for your child is what makes the choice right*. Retrieved May 1, 2011 from http://www.handsandvoices.org/index.htm.

Herer, G. (2012). Intellectual Disabilities and Hearing Loss. *Communication Disorders Quarterly*. Accepted for publication March 2012.

Holstrum, W.J., Gaffney, M., Gravel, J.S., Oyler, R.F., & Ross, D.S. (2008). Early intervention for children with unilateral and mild bilateral degrees of hearing loss. *Trends in Amplification, 12*, 35–41.

Holt, R.F., & Svirsky, M.A. (2008). An exploratory look at pediatric cochlear implantation: Is earliest always best? *Ear and Hearing, 29*, 492–511.

Houston, K.T., Behl, D.D., White, K.R., & Forsman, I. (2010). Federal privacy regulations and the provision of Early Hearing Detection and Intervention programs. *Pediatrics, 126*, S28–33.

Individuals with Disabilities Education Improvement Act of 2004, PL 108-446, 20 U.S.C. §§. 1400 et seq.

Joint Committee on Infant Hearing (JCIH). (2007). Year 2007 Position Statement: Principles and guidelines for early hearing detection & intervention programs. *Pediatrics, 120*, 898–921.

Keith, S.E., Michaud, D.S., & Chiu, V. (2008). Evaluating the maximum playback sound levels from portable digital audio players. *Journal of the Acoustical Society of America, 123*, 4227–4237.

Kemaloglu, Y., Gunduz, B., Gokmen, S., & Yilmaz, M. (2005). Pure tone audiometry in children. *International Journal of Pediatric Otorhinolaryngology, 69*, 209–214.

Laurent Clerc National Deaf Education Center. (2011). *Info to go—information and resources on the educational, linguistic, social, and emotional development of deaf and hard of hearing children.* Retrieved May 1, 2011 from http://www.gallaudet.edu/Clerc_Center/Information_and_Resources/Info_to_Go.html

Lilly, D. (2005). The evolution of aural acoustic-immittance measurements. *The ASHA Leader, 6*, 24.

Lim, S., & Simser, J. (2005). Auditory-verbal therapy for children with hearing impairment. *Annals Academy of Medicine Singapore, 34*, 307–312.

Lin, H.C., Shu, M.T., Lee, K.S., Ho, G.M., Fu, T.Y., Bruna, S., & Lin, G. (2005). Comparison of hearing screening programs between one step with transient evoked otoacoustic emissions (TEOAE) and two steps with TEOAE and automated auditory brainstem response. *The Laryngoscope, 115*, 1957–1962.

Lonsbury-Martin, B. (2005). Otoacoustic emissions: Where are we today. *The ASHA Leader, 19*, 6–7.

Madell, J.R., & Flexer, C. (2008). Collaborative team management of children with hearing loss. In J.R. Madell & C. Flexer (Eds.), *Pediatric audiology: Diagnosis, technology, management.* New York, NY: Thieme Medical Publishers.

Madell, J.R., & Flexer, C. (2008). Hearing test protocols for children. In J.R. Madell & C. Flexer (Eds.), *Pediatric audiology: Diagnosis, technology, management.* New York, NY: Thieme Medical Publishers, Inc.

Mason, C., Gaffney, M., Green, D., & Grosse, S. (2008). Measures of follow-up in early hearing detection and intervention programs: A need for standardization. *American Journal of Audiology, 17*, 60–67.

Mendel, L.L. (2008). Current considerations in pediatric speech audiometry. *International Journal of Audiology, 47*, 546–553.

Mitchell, R.E., & Karchmer, M.A. (2004). Chasing the mythical ten percent: Parental hearing status of deaf and hard of hearing students in the United States. *Sign Language Studies, 4*, 138–163.

Moller, A.R. (2006). *Hearing: Anatomy, physiology, and disorders of the auditory system,* (2nd Ed.) Boston, MA: Elsevier.

Mori, T., Westerberg, B.D., Atashband, S., & Kozak, F.K. (2008). Natural history of hearing loss in children with enlarged vestibular aqueduct syndrome. *Journal of Otolaryngology Head Neck Surgery, 37*, 112–118.

Nance, W. (2003). The genetics of deafness. *Mental Retardation and Developmental Disabilities Research Reviews, 9*, 109–119.

National Association of the Deaf (2000). *Position Statement: Cochlear Implants.* Retrieved May 1, 2011 from http://www.nad.org/issues/technology/assistive-listening/cochlear-implants

National Center for Hearing Assessment & Management. (2010). *Early hearing detection and intervention (EHDI) and universal newborn hearing screening (UNHS) programs websites and guidelines.* Retrieved October 25, 2010, from http://www.infanthearing.org/stateguidelines/index.html

Neumann, K., Dettmer, G., Euler, H., Siebel, A., Gross, M., Herer, G., … Montgomery, J. (2006). Auditory status of persons with intellectual disability at the German Special Olympic games. *International Journal of Audiology, 45*, 83–90.

Nicholas, J.G., & Geers, A.E. (2006). Effects of early auditory experience on the spoken language of deaf children at 3 years of age. *Ear and Hearing, 27*, 286–298.

Nittrouer, S., & Burton, L.T., (2005). The role of early language experience in the development of speech perception and phonological processing abilities: Evidence from 5-year-olds with histories of otitis media with effusion and low socio-economic status. *Journal of Communication Disorders, 38*, 29–63.

Norris, V.W., Arnos, K.S., Hanks, W.D., Xia, X., Nance, W.E., & Pandya, A. (2006). Does universal newborn hearing screening identify all children with GJB2 (Connexin 26) deafness? Penetrance of GJB2 deafness. *Ear and Hearing, 27*, 732–741.

Northern, J.L., & Downs, M.P. (2002). *Hearing in children* (5th ed.) Philadelphia, PA: Lippincott, Williams & Wilkins.

Peltola, H., Roine, I., Fernandez, J., Mata, A.G., Zavala, I., & Ayala, S.G. (2010). Hearing impairment in childhood bacterial meningitis is little relieved by dexamethasone or glycerol. *Pediatrics, 125*, e1–8.

Perheentupa, U., Kinnunen, I., Grenman, R., Aitasalo, K., & Makitie, A.A. (2010). Management and outcome of pediatric skull base fractures. *International Journal of Pediatric Otorhinolaryngology, 74*, 1245–1250.

Peters, B.R., Wyss, J., & Manrique, M. (2010). Worldwide trends in bilateral cochlear implantation. *Larngoscope, 120*, S17–44.

Pray, J.L., & Jordan, I.K. (2010). The deaf community and culture at a crossroads: Issues and challenges. *Journal of Social Work in Disability & Rehabilitation, 9*, 168–193.

Ravecca, F., Berrettini, S., Forli, F., Marcaccini, M., Casani, A., Baldinotti, F., … Simi, P. (2005). Cx26 gene mutations in idiopathic progressive hearing loss. *Journal of Otolaryngology, 34*, 126–134.

Roberts, J., Hunter, L., Gravel, J., Rosenfeld, R., Berman, S., Haggard, M., … Wallace, I. (2004). Otitis media, hearing loss, and language learning: Controversies and current research. *Journal of Developmental and Behavioral Pediatrics, 25*, 110–122.

Roberts, J.E., Rosenfeld, R.M., & Zeisel, S.A. (2004). Otitis media and speech and language: A meta-analysis of prospective studies, *Pediatrics, 113*, e238–e248.

Roizen, N. (2003). Nongenetic causes of hearing loss. *Mental Retardation and Developmental Disabilities Research Reviews, 9*, 120–127.

Sach, T.H., & Whynes, D.K. (2005). Paediatric cochlear implantation: The views of parents. *International Journal of Audiology, 44*, 400–407.

Seewald, R., Moodie, S., Scollie, S., & Bagatto, M. (2005). The DSL method for pediatric hearing instrument fitting: Historical perspective and current issues. *Trends in Amplification, 9*, 145–157.

Shapiro, L.R., Hurry, J., Masterson, J., Wydell, T.N., & Doctor, E. (2008). Classroom implication of recent research into literacy development: From predictors to assessment. *Dyslexia, 15*, 1–22.

Shargorodsky, J., Curham, S.G., Curhan, G.C., & Eavey, R. (2010). Change in prevalence of hearing loss in US adolescents. *The Journal of the American Medical Association, 304*, 772–778.

Sheahan, P., Miller, I., Sheahan, J.N., Earley, M.J., & Blayney, A.W. (2003). Incidence and outcome of middle ear disease in cleft lip and/or cleft palate. *International Journal of Pediatric Otorhinolaryngology, 67*, 785–793.

Shott, S.R. (2006). Down syndrome: Common otolaryngologic manifestations. *American Journal of Medical Genetics Part C, Seminars in Medical Genetics, 142C*, 131–140.

Shulman, S., Besculides, M., Saltzman, A., Ires, H., White, K.R., & Forsman, I. (2010). Evaluation of the universal newborn hearing screening and intervention program. *Pediatrics, 126*, s19–s27

Smaldino, J. & Flexer, C. (2008). Classroom acoustics: Personal and soundfield FM and IR systems. In J.R. Madell & C. Flexer (Eds.), *Pediatric audiology: Diagnosis, technology, management*. New York, NY: Thieme Medical Publishers.

Smith, R., Bale, J.J., & White, K. (2005). Sensorineural hearing loss in children. *The Lancet, 365*(9462), 879–890.

Sorkin, D.L. (2008). Education and access laws for children with hearing loss. In J.R. Madell & C. Flexer (Eds.), *Pediatric audiology: Diagnosis, technology, management*. New York, NY: Thieme Medical Publishers.

Sparreboom, M., Snik, A.F., & Mylanus, E.A. (2010). Sequential bilateral cochlear implantation in children: Development of the primary auditory abilities of bilateral stimulation. *Audiology & Neuro-Otology, 16*, 203–213.

Stach, B.A., & Ramachandran, V.S. (2008). Hearing disorders in children. In J.R. Madell & C. Flexer (Eds.), *Pediatric audiology: Diagnosis, technology, management*. New York, NY: Thieme Medical Publishers.

Torre, P., III. (2008). Young adults' use and output level settings of personal music systems. *Ear & Hearing, 29*, 791–799.

U.S. Department of Education. (2006). *Assistance to states for the education of children with disabilities and preschool grants for children with disabilities; final rule.* Retrieved on May 1, 2011, from http://idea.ed.gov/download/finalregulations.pdf

Vlastarakos, P.V., Nikolopoulos, T.P., Tavoulari, E., Papacharalambous, G., & Korres, S. (2008). Auditory neuropathy: Endocochlear lesion or temporal processing impairment? Implications for diagnosis and management. *International Journal of Pediatric Otorhinolaryngology, 72*, 1135–1150.

Vohr, B., Jodoin-Krauzyk, J., Tucker, R., Johnson, M.J., Topol, D., Ahlgren, M. (2008). Early language outcomes of early-identified infants with permanent hearing loss at 12 to 16 months of age. *Pediatrics, 122*, 535-44.

Vohr, B., Jodoin-Krauzyk, J., Tucker, R., Johnson, M.J., Topol, D., Ahlgren, M., et al. (2010). Expressive Vocabulary of Children with Hearing Loss in the First 2 Years of Life: Impact of Early Intervention. *Journal of Perinatology*, 1–7.

Werker, J.F., & Yeung, H.H. (2005). Infant speech perception bootstraps word learning. *Trends in Cognitive Sciences, 9*, 519–527.

Wheeler, A., Archbold, S., Gregory, S., & Skipp, A. (2007). Cochlear implants: The young people's perspective. *Journal of Deaf Studies and Deaf Education, 12*, 303–316.

White, K., & Maxon, A. (2005). *Early identification of hearing loss: Universal newborn hearing screening (an implementation guide).* Retrieved May 29, 2005, http://www.infanthearing.org/impguide/index.html

Widen, J.E., Johnson, J.L., White, K.R., Gravel, J.S., Vohr, B.R., James, M., … Meyer, S. (2005). A multisite study to examine the efficacy of the otoacoustic emission/automated auditory brainstem response newborn hearing screening protocol: Results of visual reinforcement audiometry. *American Journal of Audiology, 14*, S200–S216.

Winskel, H. (2006). The effects of an early history of otitis media on children's language and literacy skill development. *British Journal of Educational Psychology, 76*, 727–744.

Witt, P.D. (2008). *Craniofacial, Cleft Palate.* Retrieved October 29, 2010, from http://emedicine.medscape.com/article/1280866-overview

Witton, C. (2010). Childhood auditory processing disorder as a developmental disorder: The case for a multi-professional approach to diagnosis and management. *International Journal of Audiology, 49*, 83–87.

Wolf, B. (2010). Clinical issues and frequent questions about biotinidase deficiency. *Molecular Genetics and Metabolism, 100*, 6–13.

Yetiser, S., Hidir, Y., & Gonul, E. (2008). Facial nerve problems and hearing loss in patients with temporal bone fractures: Demographic data. *The Journal of Trauma, 65*, 1314–1320.

Yoshinaga-Itano, C. (2003). Early intervention after universal neonatal hearing screening: Impact on outcomes. *Mental Retardation and Developmental Disabilities Research Reviews, 8*, 252–266.

Yoshinaga-Itano, C., Baca, R.L., & Sedey, A.L. (2010). Describing the trajectory of language development in the presence of severe-to-profound hearing loss: A closer look at children with cochlear implants versus hearing aids. *Otology & Neurotology, 31*, 1268–1274.

Zeitler, D.M., Kessler, M.A., Terushkin, V., Roland, T.J., Jr., Svirsky, M.A., Lalwani, A.K., … Waltzman, S.B. (2008). Speech perception benefits of sequential bilateral cochlear implantation in children and adults: A retrospective analysis. *Otology & Neurotology, 29*, 314–325.

Zeng, F., Kong, Y., Michalewski, H., & Starr, A. (2005). Perceptual consequences of disrupted auditory nerve activity. *Journal of Neurophysiology, 93*, 3050–3063.

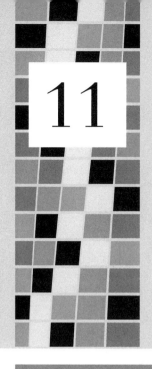

11

Vision and Visual Impairment

Brooke E. Geddie, Michael J. Bina, and Marijean M. Miller

Upon completion of this chapter, the reader will

- Be able to describe the anatomy and function of the eye

- Understand how a child's vision develops

- Be aware of "functional vision assessments" as well as tests used to determine visual acuity and visual fields

- Know about comprehensive ophthalmology and optometric low vision assessments

- Be knowledgeable about ocular abnormalities in children

- Know the definitions and major causes of visual disabilities, including blindness and low vision in children and youth

- Recognize some of the ways in which a young person with visual disabilities develops differently from a child whose vision is within the typical range

- Gain an understanding of some approaches to medical and educational intervention for children with impaired vision

Impaired vision in childhood can have detrimental effects on physical, neurological, cognitive, and emotional development. A severe visual impairment can cause delays in walking, speech and language development, as well as in behavior and socialization if early intervention services are not implemented. Visual impairment can occur as an isolated disability or associated with other developmental disabilities. Once a visual loss has been identified, it is imperative that effective medical and special education interventions be implemented as early as possible. With the goal of early intervention in mind, this chapter explores the *in utero* development of the eye and its normal structure and function. It also examines ocular disorders and common visual problems. Finally, the effects of blindness on a child's development are discussed, and relevant educational resources are introduced.

■ ■ ■ MARY

Mary is a 12-year-old former very low birth weight baby (birth weight 900 g) who has cerebral palsy and poor vision with associated

169

nystagmus. Mary benefits from reading materials with highly contrasted enlarged print. As a consequence of prematurity-caused retinopathy, her retinas have developed myopic degeneration. She requires glasses, with extremely thick lenses (–18.50 right eye and –24.00 left eye) which reduce her visual field. Mary wrote the following essay to describe her disabilities and adaptations at school:

"One thing I don't like about homework is that sometimes I can't see the print. I have a slant board, which brings my work closer so I won't have to bend over. Because of my shyness I don't ask to sit closer to the blackboard even if I can't see the print. Also, I need extended time for assignments and tests. I sometimes use a 'talking' dictionary that has a speech output. My handheld magnifier and distance telescope assist me; however, I often don't always use them when I know they would help. Also, I could do a better job remembering to go back, scan, and check my work."

At the ophthalmologist's office, Mary's binocular visual acuity measures 20/50. However, with her compound visual disabilities of optic atrophy, myopic degeneration, and nystagmus, Mary requires many learning adaptations.

STRUCTURE AND FUNCTION OF THE EYE

General Structure & Function

In many ways, the eye's structure is similar to a camera's (Figure 11.1). The thick, white nontransparent fibrous covering of the eye called the **sclera** functions as the camera body. Like a shutter, the colored region, called the **iris**, responds to changes in light conditions by opening and closing. The **pupil** is the aperture in the center of the iris. Light rays entering the eye through the pupil are refracted by the **cornea** (the clear dome that covers and protects the iris) and by fluids (aqueous and vitreous humor), which fill the globe, before arriving

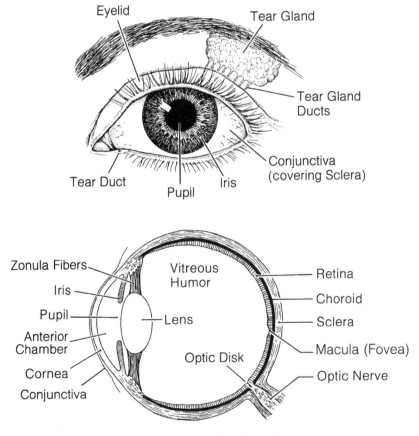

Figure 11.1.   The structure of the eye is similar to that of a camera.

at the retina. When functioning normally, the **lens**, which lies behind the pupil, precisely focuses the light rays on the retina. The cornea is the most important refracting surface of the eye, accounting for approximately two thirds of the refractive power.

When a person looks at a tree, for example, a series of parallel rays of light leave the tree and reach the dome-shaped surface of the cornea, where they are inverted and **refracted**, or bent, toward a focal point. The lens further focuses the light rays through the movement of the attached ciliary muscles. The **ciliary muscles** contract or relax, changing the shape of the lens, accommodating and fine-tuning the focus (Figure 11.2). The image light rays then travel toward the **retina**, the photographic film of the eye, which lines the eye's inner surface.

With conditions such as high myopia (nearsightedness) or hyperopia (farsightedness) the lens cannot focus enough, and the ciliary muscles cannot contract to a degree that reshapes the lens enough to permit normal acuity, necessitating glasses. Likewise, in the case of severe visual impairment, a plus or minus diopter prescription for eyeglasses cannot make up for the degree of impairment and its impact on visual functioning.

Within the retina are two types of **photoreceptor** cells: the **rods** and **cones**. Each retina consists of about 120 million rods and 6 million cones. From a Darwinian perspective, rods were more important than cones for the primal work of our species as hunter-gatherers (i.e., fight or flight, detection of motion, peripheral field). Cones, however, have become more important as humans have evolved to be readers, artists, and artisans.

Both rods and cones respond to light by undergoing a chemical reaction. For detailed vision such as reading, seeing distant objects, and having color vision, cones are needed. They are located primarily in the **fovea centralis** of the **macula**, near the center of the retina. Each cone is sensitive to one of three distinct colors: red, green, or blue. The light from each color of a tree for instance, elicits a different response from each type of cone. In contrast to the macula where cones are mostly found, rods predominate in the more peripheral or outside areas of the retina. Rods function in diminished light and are therefore necessary for night vision.

The retina sends the image via the **optic nerve** to the brain for interpretation. One optic nerve emerges from behind each eye and begins its journey toward the brain. Some of the fibers from each nerve cross over at a point called the **optic chiasm**, which is located just before the nerves enter the brain (Figure 11.3). Each optic nerve (at this point called a *tract*) continues through the cerebral hemisphere to the occipital (back) lobe of the brain. Because some nerve fibers from each eye cross to the opposite side, each eye sends information to both the right

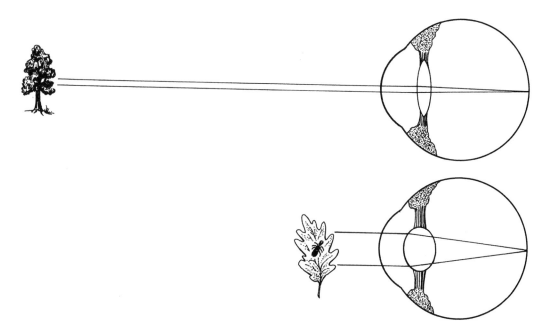

Figure 11.2. Accommodation. The lens changes shape to focus on a near or far object. The lens becomes thin and less refractive for distant objects and thicker and more refractive for near vision.

and left sides of the brain. Therefore, damage to the right or left optic tract at any point after the optic chiasm will cause defects in the visual fields of both eyes (Figure 11.3). By identifying the part of a visual field affected, an ophthalmologist often can determine where the damage has occurred in the brain.

Each structure is important to the eye functioning. If the cornea or lens is cloudy or deformed, images will be indistinct and unclear.

If the retina, optic nerve, or brain is malformed or injured, vision will also be impaired.

Functionally, visual impairment can be divided into disorders affecting 1) transmission of light, 2) central visual field, 3) peripheral visual field, 4) refraction, and 5) a combination of these issues. Categorizing various diagnoses makes it easier to establish common visual needs such as glare reduction, the need for high contrast or print enlargement, the need for high

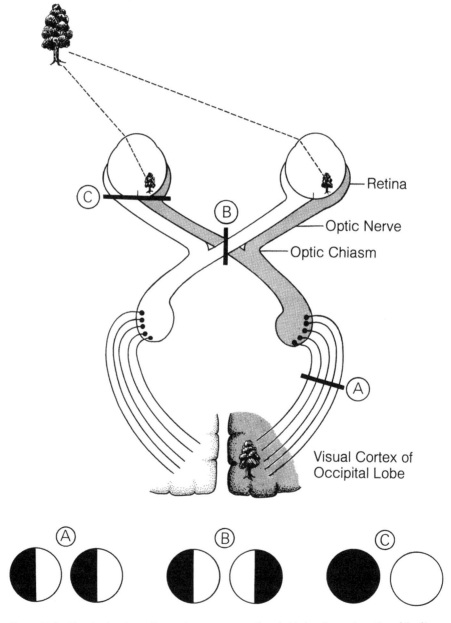

Figure 11.3.   The visual pathway. One optic nerve emerges from behind each eye. A portion of the fibers from each crosses at the optic chiasm. An abnormality at various points along the route (upper figure) will lead to different patterns of visual loss (shown as black areas in the lower figures). These are illustrated A) abnormality at the cortical pathway, B) damage to the optic chiasm, C) retinal damage.

or low illumination, the likelihood for positive benefit from magnifiers or telescopes, and so forth.

Ocular Support

The round shape of the eye is maintained by two substances: the **aqueous humor**, a watery liquid in the **anterior chamber** (the space between the cornea and lens), and the translucent, jelly-like **vitreous humor** that fills the **posterior chamber** (the space between the lens and retina). The anterior chamber is like a water balloon with plumbing to maintain ocular pressure. The aqueous humor is made in the **ciliary body**, located just behind the iris, and drains out of the eye in the angle where the cornea meets the iris through a sponge-like (trabecular) meshwork into **Schlemm's canal** (Figure 11.4). If fluid drainage is obstructed or slowed, the pressure rises. This can result in a condition called **glaucoma**, which can injure the optic nerve and permanently damage vision.

The eye itself sits in a bony socket of the skull (the *recessed orbit*, which provides support and protection) and is surrounded by the protruding forehead, nasal, and cheek bones. This socket also contains blood vessels, muscles that move the eye, a **lacrimal gland** that produces tears, and the optic nerve, which sends images from the eye to the brain. In addition to the recessed orbit, futher protection for the eyeball is provided by the eyelids, eyelashes, and **conjunctiva**. Blinking the eyelids wipes dust and other foreign bodies from the eye surface. Eyelashes help to protect the eye from airborne debris. The **conjunctiva**, a thin, transparent layer covering the sclera, contains tiny nutritive blood vessels supplying the front of the eye. Additional protection includes reflexes that result in the eye turning away and the tough leathery flexible sclera which can sustain insults.

Ocular Motility

Six muscles direct the eye toward an object and maintain **binocular vision** (Figure 11.5). The horizontal recti muscles converge the eyes toward the nose for near activities or diverge the eyes for far ones. The horizontal recti muscles also move the eyes into right and left gaze. The vertical recti muscles serve to move the eye up and down and also have some rotational functions. The oblique muscles lie obliquely above and below the eye; their primary function is to rotate the eyes while their secondary functions handle moving the eyes horizontally and vertically.

Three nerves originating in the brainstem control the movement of these six eye muscles. Two muscles are controlled by their own assigned nerve: the trochlear, or fourth, cranial nerve controls the superior oblique muscle, and the abducens, or sixth, cranial nerve controls

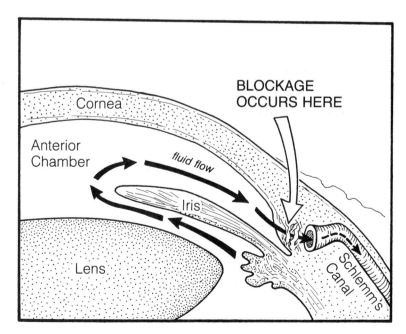

Figure 11.4. Glaucoma. Fluid normally drains from the anterior chamber through Schlemm's canal. A blockage in this passage leads to the accumulation of fluid and, therefore, increased pressure, or glaucoma.

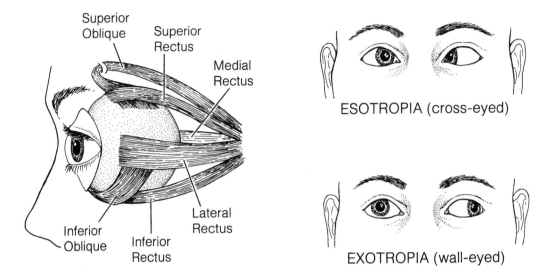

Figure 11.5.   The eye muscles (left). Six muscles move the eyeball. A weakness of one of these muscles causes strabismus. In esotropia, the eye turns in, whereas in exotropia, the eye turns out. Esotropia and exotropia of the left eye are illustrated.

the lateral rectus muscles. The oculomotor, or third, cranial nerve controls the remaining eye muscles. The complex, coordinated movement of these eye muscles allows us to look in all directions without turning our heads and to maintain proper alignment of the eyes. The loss of this coordinated movement leads to **strabismus**, misalignment of the eyes (Figure 11.5).

OCULAR DEVELOPMENT

In the human embryo, the structures that will develop into eyes first appear at 4 weeks' gestation as two spherical bulbs, one on each side of the head (Figure 11.6). They gradually indent to form the optic cups. Three specialized cell layers in these cups subsequently develop into the various parts of the eye. By 7 weeks' gestation, when the embryo is only one inch long, the eyes have already assumed their basic form (Sadler, 2009). As fetal growth continues, the eyes gradually move from the sides of the head to the center of the face.

Deviations from typical development can lead to a wide variety of ocular defects, ranging from **anophthalmia** (lack of eyes), to subtle abnormalities such as irregularly shaped pupils. Ocular malformations can occur as an isolated defect or as part of a syndrome (see Table 11.1; Appendix B). Approximately 15%–30% of children with small eyes and **coloboma**, a cleft-like defect in the eye, have **CHARGE syndrome** (the letters in CHARGE stand for: Coloboma of the eye, Heart defects, Atresia of the choanae, Retardation of growth and/or development,

Genital and/or urinary abnormalities, and Ear abnormalities and deafness; Jongmans et al., 2006; see Appendix B). These children may exhibit a variety of congenital anomalies and in some cases have significant vision and hearing impairments.

Abnormalities occurring later in embryogenesis, when the eyes usually migrate closer together, may lead to abnormal widely spaced eyes, called **hypertelorism**. Finally, intrauterine infections can cause **cataracts**, glaucoma, and/or **chorioretinitis** (an inflammation of the **choroid** and **retina**), depending on when the infection occurs during development and on which tissues are affected.

DEVELOPMENT OF VISUAL SKILLS

As in the acquisition of language and motor skills, vision has developmental milestones. Although infants will fixate briefly on a face soon after birth, steady fixation and tracking of a small target at near range is not expected until 3 months of age in term infants. As visual skills develop, variable eye misalignments can be seen in early infancy. These misalignments should diminish over time with the eyes becoming absolutely straight by 3 months of age.

Visual acuity improves fivefold in the first 6 months after birth and continues to improve over the next 6 years (Braddick & Atkinson, 2011). By age 3–4 years, vision can be objectively measured by identifying a series of pictures at a distance. The test result should be approximately 20/40 or better. (A visual acuity

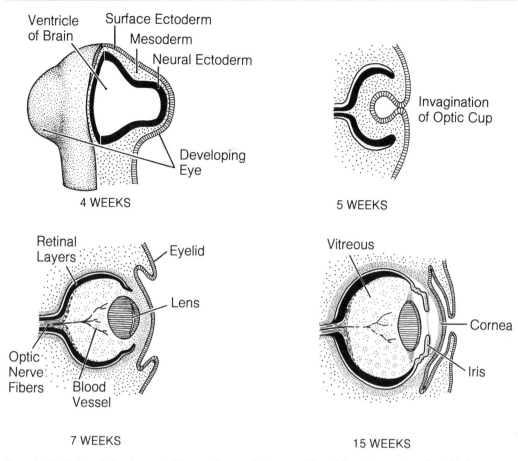

Figure 11.6. Embryonic development of the eye. The eyes first appear at 4 weeks' gestation as two spherical bulges, one on each side of the head. They indent in the next week to form the optic cups. By 7 weeks, the eyes have already assumed their basic form. The eye is completely formed by 15 weeks.

Table 11.1. Selected genetic syndromes associated with eye abnormalities

Syndrome	Eye abnormality
Aicardi syndrome	Retinal abnormalities
CHARGE association	Coloboma, microphthalmia
Galactosemia	Cataracts
Homocystinuria	Dislocated lens, glaucoma
Hurler syndrome	Cloudy cornea
Lowe syndrome	Cataracts, glaucoma
Marfan syndrome	Dislocated lens
Osteogenesis imperfecta	Blue sclera, cataracts
Osteopetrosis	Cranial nerve palsies, optic atrophy
Stickler syndrome	Extreme myopia
Tuberous sclerosis	Retinal defects, iris depigmentation
Tay-Sachs disease	Cherry-red spot in macula, optic nerve atrophy
Trisomy 13, trisomy 18	Microphthalmia, coloboma
Zellweger syndrome	Cataracts, retinitis pigmentosa

Key: CHARGE association: **c**oloboma of the eye, congenital **h**eart defect, choanal **a**tresia, **r**etarded growth and development, **g**enital abnormalities, and **e**ar malformations with or without hearing loss.

result of 20/40 means the child can see clearly at 20 feet an object that a person with typical vision can see at 40 feet.) There also should be minimal vision difference—less than 2 test lines—between eyes. By 6 years of age, visual acuity should be 20/30 or better, and when possible, should be measured with letters rather than pictures (Committee on Practice and Ambulatory Medicine et al., 2003).

Visual Development in Children with Disabilities

Many of the causes of developmental disabilities also influence the visual system (Mervis et al., 2000). In fact, one half to two thirds of individuals with developmental disabilities have a significant ocular disorder. Processes governing eye motions, alignment, visual acuity, and visual perception may mature slowly, partially, or abnormally in these children. Refractive errors, ocular misalignment, and eye movement disorders are especially common. Because of the links between developmental disabilities and vision problems, it is imperative that a pediatric ophthalmologist conduct an examination as part of the overall assessment for a child with a developmental disability.

Amblyopia

Until age 9, the visual system remains immature and susceptible to a unique type of visual regression called **amblyopia**. Amblyopia is most often unilateral, in which a "healthy" eye does not see well because it is "turned off" or ignored by the brain. It is prevalent in 1% to 4% of preschool-aged children (Granet & Khayali, 2011) and can result from deprivation (something obscuring the vision), strabismus, or refractive etiologies such as anisometropia (difference in refractive error between the two eyes). Amblyopia is treated with glasses and/or patching or eye drops to blur the vision of the better seeing eye, encouraging the brain to use and develop the vision of the amblyopic eye (Matta et al., 2010). If left untreated, amblyopia can lead to lifelong visual impairment.

COMMON DISORDERS OF THE EYE IN CHILDREN WITH DISABILITIES

Cataract

Cataract is a defect in lens clarity. Although cataracts primarily occur in adults, they also do so in about 1 in 1000 children ages birth to age 15 years, accounting for about 3% to 39%

of blindness in children (Mickler et al., 2011). A cataract appears as a white spot in the pupil of one or both eyes; if untreated, it will cause amblyopia (Figure 11.7). In the newborn nursery, pediatricians screen for cataracts using an instrument called a direct **ophthalmoscope** and the **red reflex test**. This permits magnification of the pupil and **retroillumination** to look for black spots or irregularities that could indicate a cataract. Any child with a suspected cataract should see a pediatric ophthalmologist promptly. A cataract may be an isolated abnormality or part of a syndrome or disease. For example, children with certain inborn errors of metabolism (e.g., galactosemia; see Appendix B), congenital infections (e.g., rubella), and eye trauma, may develop cataracts.

In the case of a dense congenital cataract (usually larger than 3 mm), surgery is necessary. Studies of children with congenital cataracts indicate that binocular vision develops during the first 3 months after birth. Better visual outcomes for children with severe, unilateral cataracts are found in those who have cataract surgery before 6 weeks of age (Birch & Stager, 1996). Children with dense, bilateral cataracts who have surgery after 2 months of age have poorer vision and unsteady eyes (nystagmus) compared to those having the surgery before 6 weeks (Lambert and Drack, 1996). The surgery involves an outpatient procedure in which the contents of the lens are aspirated, leaving only some of the outer lens capsule intact. These children then require special contact lenses and/or glasses with ongoing care for rehabilitation of vision. Older children requiring cataract surgery may receive a lens implant and will also require glasses and long-term ophthalmologic care.

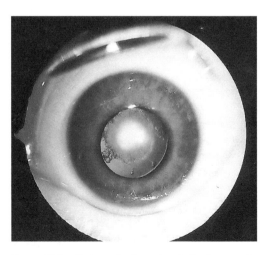

Figure 11.7. Photograph of a cataract, the lens opacity seen through the pupil.

Optic Nerve Hypoplasia

In optic nerve **hypoplasia**, a small, thin optic nerve transmits impaired information to the brain, resulting in decreased vision uncorrectable with glasses. Mid-line structures in the brain can also be underdeveloped, including the pituitary gland. Children with unilateral or bilateral optic nerve hypoplasia have neuroimaging performed, especially when there is poor growth to rule out a growth hormone deficiency from pituitary hypoplasia. Optic nerve hypoplasia is a common cause of visual disability and is often associated with other developmental disabilities.

Retinopathy of Prematurity

In infants, the most common cause of retinal damage is retinopathy of prematurity (ROP), as in the case of Mary. The actual number of affected infants has increased from the mid-2000s (Hameed et al., 2004), which is related partly to increased survival among very low birth weight (VLBW) infants. It is important to identify and treat these infants to preserve their visual function (Chen et al., 2011).

ROP results from vascular damage to the retina. During the fourth month of gestation, retinal blood vessels start growing from the optic nerve root in the back of the eye, and by the ninth month, they have reached the retina's furthest edges (Sylvester, 2008). In premature infants, this blood vessel growth is incomplete. In catching up, some blood vessels can grow into the vitreous instead of along the retinal surface. These abnormal blood vessels cause scar tissue, which can constrict, pulling on the retina. This can cause a retinal detachment and subsequent vision loss in the affected eye (Figure 11.8). All infants weighing less than 1,500 grams at birth or with a gestational age of 30 weeks or less should be screened for ROP by an ophthalmologist until the blood vessels are matured, around 40 to 45 weeks from conception (American Academy of Pediatrics et al., 2006). Additional guidelines have been created for treating "aggressive posterior ROP" which may improve outcomes (International Committee for the Classification of ROP, 2005).

If ROP becomes severe enough to make detachment likely, the affected area of the retina is treated with laser application (Quinn et al., 2011). Despite treatment, children with ROP may have significant visual impairments. Nearly 50% of children born at 27 weeks gestational age or less have been found to have subnormal visual acuity and/or strabismus (Haugen et al., 2010). In addition, extremely low birth weight infants (those weighing less than 1,000 grams) are at increased risk to sustain neurologic insults such as intracerebral hemorrhage and periventricular leukomalacia that further impact vision.

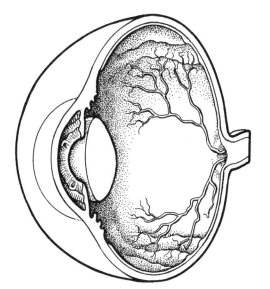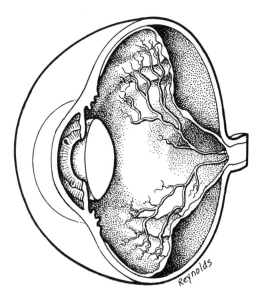

Figure 11.8. Retinopathy of prematurity (ROP). Blood vessels in the retina proliferate (left). Eventually they stop growing, leaving a fibrous scar that contracts in the most severe cases and pulls the retina away from the back of the eye, causing blindness (right). (From Batshaw, M.L., & Schaffer, D.B. [1991]. Vision and its disorders. In M.L. Batshaw, *Your child has a disability: A complete sourcebook of daily and medical care* (p. 165). Baltimore, MD: Paul H. Brookes Publishing Co., Inc.; reprinted by permission. Copyright © 1991 by M.L. Batshaw; illustrations copyright © 1991 by Lynn Reynolds. All rights reserved.)

Infants born at younger gestational ages more commonly have neurodevelopmental disabilities (Leversen et al., 2011) which can be compounded by the effects of ROP on vision.

Other Retinal Disorders

Other disorders that damage the retina include nonaccidental injury (e.g., shaken baby syndrome) that can cause retinal hemorrhages, scarring, and detachment of the retina; toxoplasmosis and other congenital infections; and certain inborn errors of metabolism such as Tay-Sachs disease, in which abnormal cellular storage material is deposited in the retina. Finally, retinal tumors, such as retinoblastoma, can lead to blindness in the affected eye.

DISORDERS OF THE VISUAL CORTEX

The visual cortex is the region of the occipital lobe responsible for receiving and decoding information sent by the eyes. The information is subsequently relayed to the **temporal** and **parietal lobes**. Damage to these areas can result in a type of visual loss called **cortical visual impairment** (CVI; previously called cortical blindness). In children, this condition is most commonly caused by oxygen deprivation (hypoxia), infections of the central nervous system (encephalitis), traumatic brain injury (see Chapter 26), and hydrocephalus (Ospina, 2009).

Cortical Visual Impairment

Cortical visual impairment (CVI) is characterized by visual perceptual deficits in the setting of an ophthalmologic examination that is normal or has only minor abnormalities. CVI is one of the most common causes of visual impairment in children in the developed world (Roman-Lantzy, 2008). Children with CVI present a variety of classic behaviors, and visual attention can range from mildly impaired to absent. Early on, parents note that their infant responds to light and dark but may not look directly at the parents' faces, even at 6 months of age. The parents may be uncertain what the child sees, but they are certain the child has some vision. Later, when the child is more alert, the parents observe intermittent or brief visual tracking behavior. The child may "look over" items but not directly at them. Also, these children can see better peripherally if the object or they are moving. A full ophthalmologic examination must be performed to rule out treatable causes of visual impairment.

Delayed Visual Maturation

In the infant with visual inattention, it is important to differentiate CVI from delayed visual maturation (DVM). Both groups show no response to visual stimuli in early infancy. Children with DVM however, have normal gestational and birth histories, normal eye examinations, no cortical abnormalities, and usually only mild to moderate developmental delays (Mercuri et al., 1997). Nystagmus does not develop as it does in other causes of visual impairment. The cause is still poorly understood. In DVM, visual function improves spontaneously in infancy as the child's overall development progresses. Often, by 6–12 months of age, an infant with DVM can have normal or near normal visual function, with many neurologically normal children reaching a final visual acuity of 20/20 (Nyong'o & Del Monte, 2008). It is therefore important to encourage visual stimulation in all such infants.

STRABISMUS AND OCULAR MOTILITY DISORDERS

Strabismus

Strabismus (misalignment of the eyes) occurs in about 3%–4% of all children. It occurs, however, in 15% of former premature infants and in 40% of children with cerebral palsy (Olitsky & Nelson, 1998). There are three main forms of strabismus: **esotropia** (cross-eyed), in which the eyes turn in, **exotropia** (wall-eyed), in which the eyes turn out (Figure 11.5), or a hyperdeviation, which is a vertical misalignment of the eyes (Granet & Khayali, 2011). Strabismus may be apparent all the time or only intermittently, such as when the child tires. Recall that strabismus is a cause of amblyopia in children younger than 9 years of age. Misalignment of the eyes can result from an abnormality in eye focusing, in the nerves supplying the eye muscles, in the eye muscles themselves, or in the brain regions controlling eye movement (Wright, 2007).

Esotropia can be divided into congenital, accommodative, or other causes (such as secondary to poor vision or acquired from a nerve or brain abnormality). Children with congenital or infantile esotropia have crossed eyes (persisting after 3 months of age) that require surgical correction. With regard to eye focusing, or **accommodation**, the eyes normally converge toward the nose to read a book (near vision). Children who are farsighted must do this same sort of accommodation for both distance and near vision. In some children, this focusing effort leads to esotropia after the age of 2 years, which can be improved with eyeglasses that correct the farsightedness. Neurological problems such as cerebral palsy may alter the brain's signals to the eye muscles and cause strabismus, which would then need to be treated with surgery. This is also true for the child with hydrocephalus who may develop strabismus as a result of nerve palsy caused by increased intracranial pressure. Infants with constant exotropia (after 3 months of age) often have contributing neurologic abnormalities and therefore warrant further evaluation. Intermittent exotropia is more common in the otherwise-healthy child and is often treated with glasses, patching, convergence exercises, or surgery. When necessary, strabismus surgery is done to adjust the position of the eye muscles to achieve better alignment. Approximately 80% of children show good ocular alignment following strabismus surgery, not needing further surgical intervention (Lueder, 2010).

Nystagmus

By 3–4 months of age a child has developed the ability to fixate on objects (Nyong'o & Del Monte, 2008). Interruption of this development results in nystagmus, a rapid jiggling back and forth (most commonly horizontally) of the eyes. A small optic nerve (optic nerve hypoplasia), underdeveloped fovea (foveal hypoplasia), a variety of rod or cone abnormalities, or other causes of visual impairment can result in nystagmus. Some children have idiopathic congenital nystagmus in which there is no anatomic disorder. Nystagmus can be latent (only present with occlusion of one eye) or manifest (constant at all times).

Evaluating children with nystagmus should include a comprehensive pediatric ophthalmologic examination. When the retina appears normal yet the vision is poor, an **electroretinogram** (ERG) may be suggested to test rod and cone function. If there is evidence of neurologic disease or if the nystagmus has atypical features

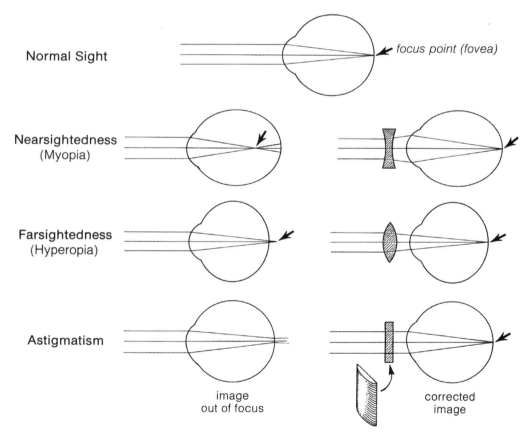

Figure 11.9. Refractive errors. If the eyeball is too long, images are focused in front of the retina (myopia). A concave lens deflects the rays, correcting the problem. If the eyeball is too short, the image focuses behind the retina and is again blurred (hyperopia). A convex lens corrects this. In astigmatism, the eyeball is the correct size, but typically the cornea is misshapen. A cylindrical lens is required to compensate.

such as rotatory or vertical components, then neurologic evaluation with neuroimaging should be considered.

Anomalous Head Posture

Abnormal head postures can be caused by a number of ophthalmologic conditions, including strabismus and nystagmus. Thus, children with tilted or turned heads should see an ophthalmologist as part of their evaluation. Children with nystagmus turn the head so that the eyes are placed where they jiggle the least and vision is most stable (the "null point"). Strabismus surgery can reposition the eyes so that this null point is in the head-straight position. When vertical strabismus is present because of a congenital paralysis of the superior oblique muscle, the head tilts toward the opposite shoulder, to align the eyes. In these children strabismus surgery can be done to correct the **torticollis**.

REFRACTIVE ERRORS IN CHILDREN

As discussed previously, light entering the eye is focused by the cornea and lens. Under optimal conditions, light rays are perfectly refracted onto the retina, resulting in a clearly focused image. If the eye is too long or if the refracting mechanisms of the eye are too strong, the focused image falls in front of the retina, blurring the picture (Figure 11.9). This is called **myopia**, or nearsightedness. If the eye is too short or the refracting mechanisms are too weak, the image is focused behind the retina, also producing a blurred image (Figure 11.9). In this instance, the person has **hyperopia**, or farsightedness. The other common refractive problem is **astigmatism** (Figure 11.9). Astigmatism typically occurs when the surface of the cornea has an elliptical rather than spherical shape. Because of this, light rays entering the eye do not focus on a single point and the image is blurred.

Farsightedness is the most common refractive error of childhood. The important difference between myopia and hyperopia is that with farsightedness, the eye can use its power of accommodation to further focus light rays onto the retina. As a result, most children with mild farsightedness require no correction and have excellent visual acuity. Hyperopia of more than 4 diopters, however, often requires correction with glasses. A diopter is a unit of light-bending power of a lens; it is the reciprocal of the distance in meters to the point where the rays intersect. The accommodative load on the child to maintain sharp focus must be considered, especially in children with disabilities. When farsightedness exceeds 4 diopters, the accommodative load may be so great that the child always has blurred vision except for brief moments when something exceptionally interesting triggers more complete accommodation effort and precise focus. Children with more than 5 diopters of hyperopia can develop both amblyopia and esotropia.

With myopia, the child sees clearly only at a near range. Severe myopia, such as that found in former premature infants who had ROP, may have a clear range of focus of only a few inches from the face. These children need eyeglass correction from infancy to expand their distance vision. Mild refractive errors, conversely, may not necessitate glasses if a child is functioning well. Both severe hyperopia and myopia, however, can impair the development of the visual system, causing amblyopia and affecting the child's interactions with the world.

In children with disabilities, even small refractive errors may be corrected to optimize performance. Furthermore, when there is a significant difference in the refractive error between eyes, glasses must be prescribed to avert amblyopia in the eye with poorer focus. In these cases, glasses ensure that the images focused on the retina of each eye are of equal clarity.

Eyeglasses can be prescribed even for the youngest infant and for the child with multiple disabilities, thanks to a method for assessing refractive errors that relies completely on objective measures rather than on subjective input from the child. After instilling eye-drops, which dilate the pupils and paralyze accommodation, the ophthalmologist views the child's eyes through a **retinoscope** (a magnifying, streaklight source) and can determine, using lenses of varying powers, the refractive error and the required correction. Eyeglasses can then be prescribed.

VISION ASSESSMENT

Primary care providers should follow the American Academy of Pediatrics Policy Statement on eye examination guidelines (Committee on Practice and Ambulatory Medicine et al., 2003). These age-specific screening guidelines include evaluation for the normal and symmetric red reflex from both eyes spontaneously (red reflex test), corneal light reflex or cover test of ocular alignment, and developmentally appropriate visual acuity testing. Any children with a poor visual assessment should be directed to the care of a pediatric ophthalmologist.

Assessing the visual function of children with developmental disabilities is critical in determining the best interventions. It is important to spend time asking the parents from their perspective what the child can see or not see, as the parent observes the child in multiple lighting conditions and in different settings, as well as when the child is rested or tired. Of importance is that parents' "assessment," while not scientific, is more than a one-time snapshot of visual ability. The parents perspective plus the clinical examination can better capture what the child actually sees, doesn't see, what accommodations assist him or her to see better. Blind or low-vision students undergo a formal "functional visual assessment" by their teacher of the visually impaired. The reports of these assessments should be requested by the primary care provider, if available, to provide additional information. This multidisciplinary perspective can be invaluable.

Visual Assessment in Infants and Nonverbal Children

As noted above, regarding infants or children with disabilities, parental report may be the best indicator of visual function. Infants under 3 months of age should blink to a light presented to their eyes, elicit an "eye-popping" reflex when room lights are dimmed, and direct their vision towards faces and high-contrast objects. Red reflex testing is vital for early detection of vision abnormalities such as cataracts, glaucoma, retinal abnormalities, and high refractive errors (American Academy of Pediatrics et al., 2008). Additional steps to assess vision in children 3 months to 3 years of age involve evaluating the child's ability to fixate and follow objects with each eye.

Visual Assessment in Toddlers and Older Children

Various tests are available for measuring visual acuity. Many children beginning at age 3 to 3½ years can identify picture characters or symbols on an eye chart (Chou et al., 2011; US Preventive Services Task Force, 2011). Several symbol tests exist: Allen pictures, LEA symbols, and the HOTV test. For older children, the tumbling E test, Snellen numbers, and Snellen letters are available.

In the nonverbal child, a matching game can be used in which the child points to the figure on a near card to show what he or she sees a distance. Although it is easier to test visual acuity by showing characters one at a time rather than in groups, this tends to underestimate amblyopia, a phenomenon called the crowding effect. This problem is avoided by using a distance chart in which only the letters *H, O, T,* and *V* appear with black bars (crowding bars) around the letters, allowing characters to be shown individually.

Other Techniques for Assessing Visual Function

Several techniques are available for screening or testing visual function without relying on verbal responses or character recognition (Jackson & Saunders, 1999). These techniques include photoscreening, **optokinetic** nystagmus (OKN), preferential looking (PL), visual field, and electrophysiological testing.

Photoscreening

Photoscreeners are computerized devices being more commonly used for visual screening of young children, especially preverbal or children with developmental delays. These devices take images of the red reflexes of the eyes. The data of the images is analyzed for detection of amblyogenic risk factors such as strabismus, significant refractive error, media opacities (such as cataract), and retinal abnormalities. There are a variety of photoscreening devices available with standard detection criteria (Donahue et al., 2003). Photoscreening can be useful for screening large populations of children for potential visual problems, identifying those that need a comprehensive assessment by a pediatric ophthalmologist.

Optokinetic Nystagmus

The OKN response is determined by rotating a black-and-white, vertically striped drum in front of the child's eyes. Similar to the effect of watching a picket fence from a passing car, the child's eyes should jiggle back and forth as they follow the movement of one stripe and then quickly jerk back to fixate on another. OKN is an involuntary response but may not be well-developed until several months of age, even in the normal infant (Nyong'o & Del Monte, 2008). It is estimated that the minimum vision necessary for an OKN response is perception of fingers held in front of the eyes (Brodsky, 2010).

Preferential Looking Techniques

Preferential Looking (PL) testing relies on the fact that an infant or young child will preferentially fixate on a boldly patterned striped target rather than on an equally luminous blank target. In PL testing, the child is shown a series of cards containing a pattern of black-and-white stripes, or gratings, on one side and a blank gray target of equal luminance on the other side (Dobson et al., 1995) while the examiner watches through a peephole. The stripe widths become progressively thinner on successive cards, creating finer gratings that require better visual resolution. The most finely-lined stripes for which the child reliably looks to the patterned side is called the grating visual acuity. Grating visual acuity is an estimate and is not as precise in the low vision setting as is the Snellen vision chart.

Visual Field Testing

The visual field test is a method of measuring an individual's scope of vision. Visual field testing maps the peripheral visual fields of each eye individually. Because it is a subjective examination, requiring the patient to understand the testing instructions, it cannot be accurately performed in young children or individuals with significant cognitive impairment. This testing is important, however, because visual field deficits can functionally interfere with learning. Peripheral vision loss can be an indicator of a progressive degenerative disorder and therefore may worsen over time. These changes may not be appreciated without testing because central vision remains intact. Even though the progressive condition may not be able to be treated medically, identifying it is important as special education services would be highly valuable to an affected student and his or her family.

Electrophysiological Testing

Electrophysiological testing includes electroretinograms (ERGs) and visual evoked potentials (VEPs) to determine whether the vision problem lies primarily in the eyes or the brain (Almoqbel et al., 2008).

Electroretinogram

An ophthalmologist may decide to obtain an ERG when the retina looks normal but vision is absent or very poor. The ERG tests retinal functioning by evaluating the quality of cone and rod response to light stimuli. It is particularly useful in demonstrating diseases of the retina and for assessing poor night vision. In ERG testing, modified contact lenses are placed on the corneas of the child after putting in topical anesthetic drops. Depending on the type of equipment used, one to three electrodes are also affixed to the face and/or body. Lights are momentarily flashed in the child's eyes under different conditions while a computer analyzes the information received from the electrodes and from leads attached to the contact lenses.

Visual Evoked Potential

VEP testing may be considered once an ERG indicates that the retina is functioning normally. Flash VEP testing is used to evaluate the pathway between the eye and the brain in children suspected of having cortical visual impairment. Pattern VEP testing is used to assess visual acuity in infants and children with severe disabilities. Pattern VEP testing for children, however, is available only at a few research centers, and flash VEP provides limited information.

BLINDNESS

The definition of blindness from a legal and federal educational perspective is visual acuity of 20/200 or worse in the better eye with correction, or a visual field that subtends to an angle of not greater than 20 degrees instead of the usual 105 degrees (Individuals with Disabilities Education Improvement Act of 2004, PL 108-446). Individuals with low vision (partially sighted) are defined as having a visual acuity better than 20/200 but worse than 20/70 with correction. Both of these categories of students are considered to have visual impairments. It should be noted that from a functional standpoint, it is not the acuity or field numbers that are all-important. Each person functions differently with the vision they retain. Therefore care providers should guard against making a judgment based on the clinically derived measures alone; talking to parents and getting information from school staff are also important. Most people who are legally blind have considerable useful vision and may be able to distinguish light and dark or to detect objects (20/500 to 20/800) or may read enlarged print or regular print using magnification (20/200 to 20/500). Yet, someone with 20/400 to 20/500 vision is unlikely to read print efficiently enough for it to be a primary learning or information-gathering medium. Other people who are blind, however, cannot perceive the difference between light and dark.

In the educational and rehabilitation field blindness is defined functionally as a degree of vision impairment that is so significant that vision cannot be used as the primary channel for learning. A person with low vision can use their vision as a primary channel for learning, but the individual may also need to use other modalities, such as auditory or tactile, to assist. To provide the best services and treatment to children with multiple disabilities and some degree of visual impairment, it is important to know the extent of limitations from the visual impairment (Holbrook, 2006; Salisbury, 2007).

Causes of Blindness

In childhood, the causes of blindness are many and varied. The three leading causes of visual impairment in the United States are 1) cortical visual impairment, 2) ROP, and 3) optic nerve hypoplasia (Hatton, 2001). Malformations of the visual system range from coloboma of the retina to optic nerve abnormalities and cerebral malformations. Other causes of blindness include traumatic brain injury, severe eye infections, and tumors. Blindness is far more prevalent in developing countries, where nutritional disorders such as vitamin A deficiency and infections such as **trachoma**, measles, and tuberculosis are common.

Identifying the Child with Severe Visual Impairment

Blindness can be an isolated disability or part of a condition involving multiple disabilities. For example, visual impairment caused by an inherited disorder such as albinism (in which there is a reduction in retinal pigment) may be an isolated finding, whereas CVI caused by hypoxia in the newborn period is often associated with cerebral palsy and intellectual disability. About half of all children with severe visual impairments have co-morbid developmental disabilities.

Several clues may indicate that an infant has a severe visual impairment (Brodsky, 2010). The child will not visually fixate on a parent's face or show interest in following brightly colored objects. Parents also may notice abnormalities in the movement of the child's eyes, including wandering eye motions, nystagmus, or eyes that always gaze in one particular direction. In addition, the infant may not blink or react when a threatening gesture is made or a bright light is shined in the eyes. Some children with severe visual impairment habitually press their eyes (known as the oculodigital sign). Any of these findings should lead to a thorough examination by an ophthalmologist.

Developmental Variations in the Child with Severe Visual Impairment

One might expect severe visual impairment to result in lags in early childhood development (Brodsky, 2010). Being unable to establish eye contact with parents could have an impact on the infant's attachment and socialization skills. Preverbal communication, which is dependent on visual observation and imitation, could be delayed. **Hypotonia** and/or fear of movement combined with parental concern about injury might affect the development of motor skills in the child who is blind. Studies that have examined these issues have in fact found developmental delays, but the delays appear to be dependent on the amount of residual vision and the presence or absence of associated developmental disabilities (Hatton et al., 1997).

The early development of children with vision better than 20/500 and with no other severe associated impairments may approximate that of sighted children, whereas that of children with less than 20/500 visual acuity (or 20/800 in some studies) has shown significant lags in early developmental milestones (Figure 11.10). Children with early developmental lags, provided that they have no associated severe developmental disabilities (e.g., cerebral palsy, intellectual disability, hearing impairment), function in the typical range by school age. If there are associated impairments, however, the delays will persist. The origin of the visual loss (eye, optic nerve, brain) does not seem to influence the degree of delay in milestone acquisition.

Children with visual impairments who reach most early developmental milestones at a typical age may show some delays (Dutton & Bax, 2010). Searching for dropped objects, crawling, and walking without support are all acquired later. Decreased motor development in visually impaired children correlates with being less physically fit. There is a higher rate of obesity than in sighted children age 6–12 years, so promoting a healthy and active lifestyle in children with visual impairment is especially important (Houwen, Hartman, & Visscher, 2010). Differences also surface in the use of words and difficulty with pragmatics and pronouns (e.g., saying "you" for "I"; Perez-Pereira & Conti-Ramsden, 1999). In the child who is blind with average intelligence, speech and language reach typical levels by school age. Speech, however, is accompanied by less body and facial "language," and conversation skills may be less developed. In all areas, children with an isolated visual disability will be capable of reaching developmental milestones.

In addition to developmental differences, there may be some atypical behavioral mannerisms. These self-stimulatory actions include pressing the eyes, blinking forcefully, gazing at lights, waving fingers in front of the face, rolling the head, and swaying the body (Fazzi et al., 1999). Pressing the eyes seems to occur only in children with retinal disease, in whom it produces visual stimulation. However, firm pressing or poking the eyes, risks damaging the globe. These mannerisms usually can be extinguished with behavioral intervention.

It is interesting to note that the child with congenital blindness may be unaware of having an impairment until 4–5 years of age. In the school-age child, however, social skills impairments may be related to social isolation and poor self-image. Therefore, including a child in a program with typically developing children should include an agenda to promote socialization (Cochrane et al., 2011).

Most tests of infant development are based primarily on performance of visual skills and may not be optimal in evaluating infants with severe visual impairment. Alternative nonvisually based developmental scales should be used to help in educational planning (Arzubi & Mambrino, 2010).

Early Intervention for the Infant and Young Child with Severe Visual Impairment

The pediatric low-vision population has special needs that require a comprehensive management program, including clinical, rehabilitation, and educational aspects, with an emphasis on early intervention to maximize the child's residual vision (Oldham & Steiner, 2010). As soon as an infant is diagnosed with a severe visual impairment, he or she should be entered into an early intervention program. The early intervention staff should be trained in the effects of visual impairment on a child's early development, and the team should include an orientation and mobility specialist and a teacher certified in the area of visual impairment. The focus should be to increase skills in other senses, to improve body concept and awareness, and to promote locomotion and active exploration of the environment (Roman-Lantzy, 2009).

While awake, infants should be placed on their stomach rather than on the back to strengthen neck and trunk muscles. The young child with a severe visual impairment must explore the world through touch and sound. Brain imaging studies have shown that, in

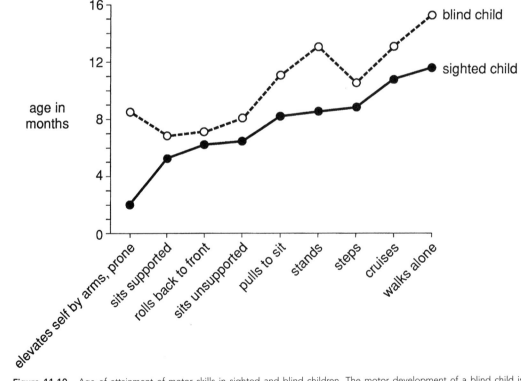

Figure 11.10. Age of attainment of motor skills in sighted and blind children. The motor development of a blind child is delayed. (From *Insights from the blind: Comparative studies of blind and sighted infants* [p. 204], by Selma Fraiberg. Reprinted by permission of Basic Books, member of Perseus Books Group.)

people blind from an early age, the visual cortex can be used for processing tactile and auditory information (Theoret et al., 2004). Therefore, parents and therapists should place or store textured and sound-producing toys at a height the child can reach. If there is any usable vision, the child should be encouraged to take advantage of it; bright colors should be used, and the child's vision and attention directed verbally toward them (Holbrook, 1995). It is very important for the parents, teachers, and therapists to verbally cue the child with information prior to being touched/handled in order to eliminate any resistance to touch (tactile defensiveness; Warren, 1994).

The child's name should be used frequently to encourage inclusion in conversations and to ensure that the child will respond to questions in the absence of verbal cues. There also should be a verbal explanation before, during, and after a task is performed (Ferrell, 1985). While the child is moving from one space to another, the purpose of the move and the orientation of the space should be explained.

Orientation encompasses such skills as laterality and directionality. In terms of orientation and mobility, the child is first taught by an orientation and mobility specialist to locate familiar objects within the home and then progresses to travel outdoors. The child should be urged to walk despite the risks of scrapes and bruises. Poor peripheral vision (tunnel vision) is more of a problem in walking than is the loss of central vision. Any residual vision, however, is better than total absence of vision. The use of mobility aids for walking should be encouraged, including push toys.

The educational placement for the child depends on age, extent of visual impairment, and associated disabilities (see Chapter 31). For the young child, an infant and toddler program usually entails a weekly home-based session in which the early childhood educator visits and works with the parent to set up a stimulating environment. By 2–3 years of age, the child is usually ready for a school-based preschool program. Over the next few years, listening, concept development, conversation, and daily living skills (e.g., dressing, eating, personal hygiene) are emphasized. Literacy modality assessment, called Learning Media Assessments, can also begin at this time so that emergent literacy activities can be part of the child's educational program. Self-dressing can be encouraged by individualized strategies. These include using loose clothing and Velcro straps to fasten shoes, pants, and shirts. Play and

social skills training and strategies to eliminate mannerisms may also be a part of the program. It is important to create an attitude of stimulating all areas of sensory development, including visual skills, in the child who has some residual vision. It is equally important that the parents and other caregivers do not perform too many tasks for the child so that he or she is encouraged to interact with the environment. Otherwise, the child will develop a distorted understanding of how the world works.

Educating the School-Age Child Who is Blind or Has Low Vision

By the time the child reaches school age, the extent of the visual loss is often clear. A child's ability to work efficiently without excessive fatigue, to have an adequate reading rate with a variety of materials, and the possibility of progressive visual loss will all be factors considered by the school. Some children will succeed best with optical aids and devices and larger-print books or electronic readers (e.g., Kindle), whereas others may succeed best with **braille** or learning media or both, referred to as dual media.

Braille is a code formed from a series of raised dots on a page that are read from left to right, as print is read visually (Massof, 2009). Readiness for braille begins in kindergarten (Roth & Fee, 2011). Fine motor skills and tactile sensitivity skills are developed first as these are essential in the learning process. When the child is able to recognize small shapes, differentiate between rough and smooth, and follow a line of small figures across a page, the learning of the braille alphabet can begin.

Children with severe visual impairments should also learn to type on a computer. In addition, a wide variety of books on tape are available from Recording for the Blind & Dyslexic (see http://www.rfbd.org) and from bookstores and libraries. It is critical to make sure that the child has all of the equipment needed for learning and independence and that is appropriate for particular needs. With these tools, children with severe visual impairments should be able to succeed in the general education environment. Other factors in their success are specific and comprehensive instruction in learning braille as early as possible, developing orientation and mobility skills, and utilizing low vision aids. It is imperative that instruction in braille be part of the student's IEP and taught by trained and certified professional special educators.

Assistive Technology

The omnipresence of computers is greatly benefiting individuals with severe visual impairment. Voice recognition software permits individuals to input instructions and dictate to computer applications. Additionally, there are various devices that "talk," including adapted calculators, computers, and other assistive technology devices that provide auditory information. Closed circuit televisions, electronic readers, high-contrast monitors, magnifiers, and telescopes can be very useful in the education and daily living of the school-age child with low vision. There are also computers that convert print into braille and haptic interface technology that makes digital information tactile (Benedict & Baumgardener, 2009).

Communities are also becoming more accessible to individuals with visual impairment by implementing elevators that announce floors, crosswalk indicators that beep when it is safe to cross the street, and ramps. The use of personal global positioning system (GPS) software is also beneficial; however, it provides information as a supplement to a cane but not as a primary orientation aid.

Genetic Advances

Genetic research is advancing with current clinical trials for gene-replacement therapy for genetic forms of visual impairment in which a normal copy of a patient's defective gene is introduced under the retina with a viral carrier (Simonelli et al., 2010). As our knowledge of genetics increases, the possibilities of gene-therapy for visual-impairment conditions may become a reality.

Intervention for Children with Multiple Disabilities

The incidence of blindness in children with multiple developmental disabilities is more than 200 times that found in the general population (Warburg, Frederiksen, & Rattleff, 1979). One third of children with partial sight and two thirds of children with blindness have other developmental disabilities, the most common being intellectual disability, hearing impairments, seizure disorders, and cerebral palsy. The majority of these children have two or more disabilities in addition to visual impairment. Treatment of these children must address all the disabilities and use all the senses and abilities that remain intact. A multidisciplinary approach involving a range of educational and health care professionals is essential.

Outcome for Visually Impaired Child

Visual impairment can be progressive or nonprogressive, dependent on the etiology. Outcome for the child with severe visual impairment depends on the amount of residual vision, the presence of associated disabilities, the motivation of the child and family, and the skills of the child's teachers and therapists. With severe visual impairment, there may be effects on overall health, self-perception, educational attainment, occupational choices, and other social factors (Davidson & Quinn, 2011). In general, less severe visual impairment and absence of associated disabilities predict typical development and good outcomes for independence and occupational success.

SUMMARY

Abnormalities of the visual system are among the many obstacles that children with disabilities may face. These may result from congenital defects or acquired disorders or injuries. The visual challenges encountered may range from minor to severe, transient to permanent, stable to progressive, and ocular to cortical. Children with developmental disabilities, as a group, are at higher risk for visual impairment than children in the general population. Because the visual system is undergoing a process of maturation during childhood, early recognition of visual disorders is essential to ensure prompt treatment and to optimize an outcome of improved vision. Therefore, careful visual assessment is important for all children and can be performed regardless of a child's level of impairment or ability to cooperate. The outcome for children with visual impairments depends on the degree of the visual loss, developmental status, motivation of child and family, and skill of involved teachers and therapists.

REFERENCES

Almoqbel, F., Leat, S.J., & Irving, E. (2008). The technique, validity and clinical use of the sweep VEP. *Ophthalmic and Physiological Optics*, 5, 393–403.

American Academy of Pediatrics, American Academy of Ophthalmology, & American Association for Pediatric Ophthalmology and Strabismus. (2006). Policy statement: Screening examination of the premature infants for retinopathy of prematurity. *Pediatrics*, 117, 572–576.

American Academy of Pediatrics; Section on Ophthalmology, American Association for Pediatric Ophthalmology and Strabismus, American Academy of Ophthalmology, & American Association of Certified Orthoptists. (2008). Red reflex examination in neonates, infants, and children. *Pediatrics, 122*(6), 1401–4.

Arno, P., Capelle, C., Wanet-Defalque, M.C., Catalan-Ahumada, M., & Veraart, C. (1999). Auditory coding of visual patterns for the blind. *Perception, 28,* 1013–1029.

Arzubi, E.F., & Mambrino, E. (2010). *A guide to neuropsychological testing for health care professionals.* New York, NY: Springer.

Batshaw, M.L., & Schaffer, D.B. (1991). Vision and its disorders. In M.L. Batshaw, *Your child has a disability: A complete sourcebook of daily and medical care.* Baltimore, MD: Paul H. Brookes Publishing Co.

Benedict, R.E., & Baumgardner, A.M. (2009). A population approach to understanding children's access to assistive technology. *Disability Rehabilitation, 31*(7), 582–92.

Birch, E.E., & Stager, D.R. (1996). The critical period of surgical treatment of dense congenital unilateral cataract. *Investigative Ophthalmology and Visual Science, 37,* 1532–1538.

Bishop, V.E. (1991). Preschool visually impaired children: A demographic study. *Journal of Visual Impairment and Blindness, 85,* 69–74.

Bitjoka, L., & Pourcelot, L. (1999). New blind mobility aid devices based on the ultrasonic Doppler effect. *International Journal of Rehabilitation Research, 22,* 227–231.

Braddick, O., & Atkinson, J. (2011). Development of human visual function. *Vision Research.* [Epub ahead of print]

Brodsky, M.C. (2010). *Pediatric neuro-ophthalmology.* (2nd ed). New York, NY: Springer Publishing.

Chen, J., Stahl, A., Hellstrom, A., & Smith, L.E. (2011). Current update on retinopathy of prematurity: screening and treatment. *Current Opinions in Pediatrics, 23*(2), 173–8.

Chou, R., Dana, T., & Bougatsos, C. (2011) Screening for visual impairment in children ages 1–5 years: Update for the USPSTF. *Pediatrics, 127*(2), e442–79.

Cochrane, G.M., Marella, M., Keeffe, J.E., & Lamoureux, E.L. (2011). The Impact of Vision Impairment for Children (IVI_C): Validation of a vision-specific pediatric quality-of-life questionnaire using rasch analysis. *Investigative Ophthalmology and Visual Science, 52*(3), 1632–40.

Committee on Practice and Ambulatory Medicine Section on Ophthalmology, American Association of Certified Orthoptists, American Association for Pediatric Ophthalmology and Strabismus, & American Academy of Ophthalmology. (2003). Eye examination in infants, children and young adults by pediatricians. *Pediatrics, 111,* 902–7.

Davidson, S., & Quinn, G.E. (2011). The impact of pediatric vision disorders in adulthood. *Pediatrics, 127*(2), 334–9.

Dekker, R., & Koole, F.D. (1992). Visually impaired children's visual characteristics and intelligence. *Developmental Medicine and Child Neurology, 34,* 123–133.

Dobelle, W.H. (2000). Artificial vision for the blind by connecting a television camera to the visual cortex. *ASAIO Journal, 46,* 3–9.

Dobson, V., Quinn, G.E., Saunders, R.A., Spencer, R., Davis, B.R., Risser, J., & Palmer, E.A. (1995). Grating visual acuity in eyes with retinal residua of retinopathy of prematurity. *Archives of Ophthalmology, 113,* 1172–1177.

Donahue, S.P., Arnold, R.W., Ruben, J.B., & AAPOS Vision Screening Committee. (2003). Preschool vision screening: What should we be detecting and how should we report it? Uniform guidelines for reporting results of preschool vision screening studies. *JAAPOS, 7*(5), 314–6.

Education for All Handicapped Children Act of 1975, PL 94–142, 20 U.S.C. §§ 1400 *et seq.*

Fazzi, E., Lanners, J., Danova, S., Ferrarri-Ginevra, O., Gheza, C., Luparia, A., Balottin, U., & Lanzi, G. (1999). Stereotyped behaviours in blind children. *Brain Development 8,* 522–8.

Fraiberg, S., with the collaboration of Fraiberg, L. (1977). *Insights from the blind: Comparative studies of blind and sighted infants.* New York, NY: Perseus Books Group.

Granet, D.B., & Khayali, S. (2011). Amblyopia and strabismus. *Pediatric Annals, 40*(2), 89–94.

Hameed, B., Shyamanur, K., Kotecha, S., Manktelow, B.N., Woodruff, G., Draper, E.S., & Field, D. (2004). Trends in the incidence of severe retinopathy of prematurity in a geographically defined population over a 10-year period. *Pediatrics, 113,* 1653–1657.

Harding, S., & Nischal, K. (2011). [Review of the book *Visual impairment in children due to damage to the brain: Clinics in developmental medicine,* edited by G. Dutton & M. Bax. New York, NY: Wiley, 2010.] *British Journal of Opthalmology, 95,* 752. doi:10.1136/bjo.2010.199489

Harrison, F. (1993). *Living and learning with blind children: A guide for parents and teachers of visually impaired children.* Toronto, Canada: University of Toronto Press.

Hatton, D.D. (2001). Model registry of early childhood visual impaired collaborative group: First year results. *Journal of Blindness and Visual Impairments, 95,* 418– 433.

Hatton, D.D., Bailey, D.B., Burchinal, J.R., & Ferrell, K.A. (1997). Developmental growth curves of preschool children with vision impairments. *Child Development, 68,* 788–806.

Haugen, O.H., Nepstad. L., Standal, O.A., Elgen, I., Markestad, T. (2010). Visual function in 6 to 7 year-old children born extremely preterm: A population-based study. *Acta Ophthalmology,* doi:10.1111/j.1755-3768.2010.02020.x. [Epub ahead of print].

Hered, R.W. (2011). Effective vision screening of young children in the pediatric office. *Pediatrics, 40*(2), 76–82.

Holbrook, M.C. (2006). *Children with visual impairments: a guide for parents.* Bethesda, MD: Woodbine House.

Houwen, S., Hartman. E., & Visscher, C. (2010) The relationship among motor proficiency, physical fitness, and body composition in children with and without visual impairments. *Research Quarterly Exercise in Sport, 81*(3), 290–9.

Individuals with Disabilities Education Improvement Act of 2004, PL 108–446, 20 U.S.C. §§ 1400 *et seq.*

International Committee for the Classification of Retinopathy of Prematurity. (2005). The international classification of retinopathy of prematurity revisited. *Archives of Ophthalmology, 123,* 991–999.

Jackson, A.J., & Saunders, K.J. (1999). The optometric assessment of the visually impaired infant and child. *Ophthalmic and Physiological Optics, 2,* S49–S62.

Jongmans, M.C., Admiraal, R.J., van der Donk, K.P., Vissers, L.E., Baas, A.F., Kapusta, L., ... van Ravenswaaij, C.M. (2006). CHARGE syndrome: The phenotypic spectrum of mutations in the CHD7 gene. *Journal of Medical Genetics, 43*(4), 306–314.

Lambert, S.R., & Drack, A.V (1996). Infantile cataracts. *Survey of Ophthalmology, 40*, 427–458.

Leversen, K.T., Sommerfelt, K., Rønnestad, A., Kaaresen, P.I., Farstad, T., Skranes, J., Støen, R., … Markestad, T. (2011). Prediction of neurodevelopmental and sensory outcome at 5 years in Norwegian children born extremely preterm. *Pediatrics, 127*(3), e630–8.

Leversen, K.T., Sommerfelt, K., Rønnestad, A., Kaaresen, P.I., Farstad, T., Skranes, J., Støen, R., … Markestad, T. (2010). Predicting neurosensory disabilities at two years of age in a national cohort of extremely premature infants. *Early Human Devevlopment, 86*(9), 581–6.

Lueder, G. (2010). *Pediatric practice ophthalmology.* New York, NY: McGraw-Hill Professional.

Massof, R.W. (2009). The role of Braille in the literacy of blind and visually impaired children. *Archives in Ophthalmology, 127*(11), 1530–1.

Matta, N.S, Singman, E.L., & Silbert., D.I. (2010).Evidenced-based medicine: Treatment for amblyopia. *American Orthopetic Journal, 60*, 17–22.

Mervis, C.A., Yeargin-Allsopp, M., & Winter, S., et al. (2000). Aetiology of childhood vision impairment, Metropolitan Alanta, 1991-93. *Paediatric and Perinatal epidemiology, 14*, 70–77.

Mercuri, E., Atkinson, L., Braddick, O., Anker, S., Cowan, F., Pennock, J., Rutherford, M.A., & Dubowitz, L.M. (1997). The aetiology of delayed visual maturation: Short review and personal findings in relation to magnetic resonance imaging. *European Journal of Pediaetric Neurology, 1*, 31–34.

Mickler, C., Boden, J., Trivedi, R.H., & Wilson, M.E. (2011). Pediatric cataract. *Pediatric Annals, 40*(2), 83–7.

Neitz, M., & Neitz, J. (2000). Molecular genetics of color vision and color vision defects. *Archives of Ophthalmology, 118*, 691–700.

Ng, E.Y., Connolly, B.P., McNamara, J.A., Regillo, C.D., Vander, J.F., & Tasman, W. (2002). A comparison of laser photocoagulation with cryotherapy for threshold retinopathy of prematurity at 10 years: Part 1. Visual function and structural outcome. *Ophthalmology, 109*(5), 928–934.

Nyongo, O., & Del Monte, M. (2008). Childhood visual impairment: Normal and abnormal visual function in the context of developmental disability. *Pediatric Clinics of North America, 55*(6), 1403–15.

Olitsky, S.F., & Nelson, L.B.(1998). Common ophthalmologic concerns in infants and children. *Pediatric Clinics of North America, 45*, 993–1012.

Oldham, J., & Steiner, G.C. (2010). *Being legally blind: observations for parents of visually impaired children.* Anchorage, AK: Shadow Fusion.

Ospina, L.H. (2009). Cortical visual impairment. *Pediatric Review, 11*, e81–90.

Patel, S., Marshall, J., & Fitzke, F.W., 3rd. (1995). Refractive index of the human corneal epithelium and stroma. *Journal of Refractive Surgery, 11*(2), 100–5.

Perez-Pereira, M., & Conti-Ramsden, G. (1999). *Language development and social interaction in blind children.* Philadelphia, PA: Psychology Press.

Quinn, G.E., Dobson, V., Hardy, R.J., Tung, B., Palmer, E.A., Good, W.V., & Early Treatment for Retinopathy of Prematurity Cooperative Group. (2011). Visual field extent at 6 years of age in children who had high-risk prethreshold retinopathy of prematurity. *Arch Ophthalmology, 129*(2), 127–32.

Roman-Lantzy, C. (2008). *Cortical visual impairment: An approach to assessment and intervention.* New York, NY: American Foundation for the Blind Press.

Roth, G.A., & Fee, E. (2011). The invention of Braille. *American Journal of Public Health, 101*(3), 454.

Sadler, T.W. (2009). *Langman's medial embryology* (11th ed.). Baltimore, MD: Lippincott, Williams, & Wilkins.

Salisbury, R. (2007). *Teaching pupils with visual impairment: A guide to making the school curriculum accessible.* New York, NY: Routledge.

Shoval, S., Borenstein, J., & Koren, Y. (1998). The Nav-Belt: A computerized travel aid for the blind based on mobile robotics technology. *IEEE Transactions on Biomedical Engineering, 45*, 1376–1386.

Simonelli, F., Maguire, A.M., Testa, F., Pierce, E.A., Mingozzi, F., Bennicelli, J.L., … Auricchio, A. (2010). Gene therapy for Leber's congenital amaurosis is safe and effective through 1.5 years after vector administration. *Molecular Therapy, 18*(3), 643–50.

Steinkuller, P.G., Du, L., Gilbert, C., Foster, A., Coats, M.L., & Collins, D.K. (1999). Childhood blindness. *Journal of the American Association for Pediatric Opthalmology and Strabismus, 3*, 26–32.

Sylvester, C.L. (2008). Retinopathy of prematurity. *Seminars in Ophthalmology, 23*(5), 318–23.

Theoret, H., Merabet, L., & Pascual-Leone, A. (2004). Behavioral and neuroplastic changes in the blind: Evidence for functionally relevant cross-modal interactions. *Journal of Physiology, 98*, 221–233.

US Preventive Services Task Force. (2011). Vision screening for children 1 to 5 years of age: US Preventive Services Task Force recommendation statement. *Pediatrics, 127*(2), 340–346.

Velazquez R., Hernandez, H., & Preza, E. (2010). A portable eBook reader for the blind. *Conference Proceedings of IEEE English Medical Biology Society, 2010*, 2107–10.

Warburg, M., Frederiksen, P., & Rattleff, J. (1979). Blindness among 7,720 mentally retarded children in Denmark. *Clinics in Developmental Medicine, 73*, 56–67.

Wright, K.W. (2007). *Pediatric ophthalmology for primary care.* (3rd ed.). Elk Grove Village, IL: American Academy of Pediatrics.

Zell Sacks, S., Kekelis, L.S., & Gaylord-Ross, R.J. (Eds.). (1992). *The development of social skills by blind and visually impaired students: Exploratory studies and strategies.* New York, NY: American Foundation for the Blind.

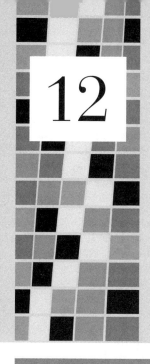

12

The Brain and Nervous System

Amanda Yaun, Robert Keating, and Andrea Gropman

Upon completion of this chapter, the reader will

- Understand the anatomy of the brain and the interaction of its parts

- Be knowledgeable about the roles of the peripheral nervous system and the autonomic nervous system

- Comprehend the structure and importance of the neuron, the functional unit of the central nervous system

- Be able to describe the origin and function of cerebrospinal fluid and its associated blockage in hydrocephalus

- Have knowledge of current and future trends for evaluating the nervous system

- Understand the current imaging technologies used to evaluate the central and peripheral nervous system

---

Long viewed as an incredibly complex computer, the central nervous system (CNS) is considerably more complicated than any machine made to date (Tanaka & Gleeson, 2000). Each component of the nervous system controls some aspect of behavior and affects interaction with the surrounding world. An impairment of any part of this system reduces the ability to adapt to the environment and can lead to disorders as diverse as learning disabilities, **autism spectrum disorders** (ASD), **cerebral palsy**, and **epilepsy**. This chapter provides an overview of the interrelationships between the individual elements of the CNS. It also describes examples of CNS dysfunction and their effects on the child.

THE BRAIN AND SPINAL CORD

The brain and the spinal cord comprise the mature CNS and have six main structures: 1) the cerebral hemispheres, 2) basal ganglia, 3) thalamus, 4) brainstem, 5) cerebellum, and 6) spinal cord (Crossman & Neary, 2010; Goldberg, 2010).

The Cerebral Hemispheres

During embryonic development the neural tube, the primitive precursor to the CNS, develops three bulges that form the main brain components (see Chapter 2). The forward-most bulge, called the **prosencephalon**, develops and becomes the left and right cerebral hemispheres. Each hemisphere consists of an outer cerebral cortex (where most neurons, or brain cells, are located), subcortical white matter (where the "wiring" of the brain is found), and deep masses of gray matter collectively called the **basal ganglia** (containing specialized groupings of neurons). Within each hemisphere there is a fluid-filled cavity called the lateral **ventricle**. The hemispheres are joined together by a band of fibers called the **corpus callosum** that permits the exchange of information between the two hemispheres (Figure 12.1A and 12.1B). There are genetic and environmental factors that may interfere with the normal formation of the corpus callosum and, in the most severe cases, result in its complete lack of development (**agenesis** of the corpus callosum). The importance of this exchange

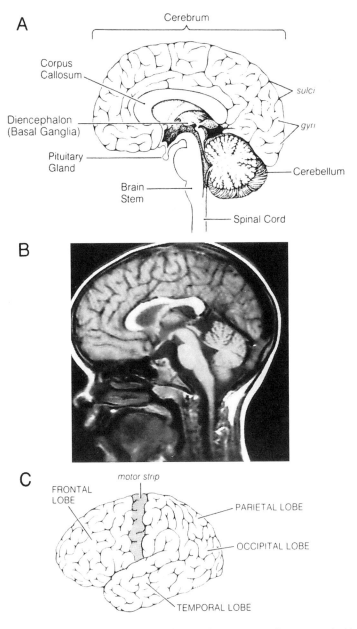

Figure 12.1. A) Lateral view of the brain showing the component elements: cerebral hemispheres, diencephalon, cerebellum, brainstem, and spinal cord. B) Lateral view of brain by magnetic resonance imaging (MRI) scan. Note the excellent reproduction of the structures of the brain. C) Side view of the left hemisphere. The cortex is divided into four lobes: frontal, parietal, temporal, and occipital. The motor strip, lying at the back of the frontal lobe, is highlighted. It initiates voluntary movement and is damaged in **spastic** cerebral palsy.

of information is highlighted by the results of a surgical procedure called a **corpus callosotomy**. In this operation, a portion of the corpus callosum is cut in an attempt to control a severe seizure disorder (Sunaga et al., 2009). It has proven quite effective in decreasing the spread of seizure activity, but in some adults it has resulted in declines in language, visual-perceptual skills, and manual dexterity (Jea et al., 2008; Lin et al., 2011).

In early fetal life, the surface of the cerebral hemisphere is smooth. As the brain's complexity increases during the third trimester, involutions called **fissures** and **sulci** appear. Fissures, which are deeper than sulci, are first visible during fetal development and divide each hemisphere into four functional areas or lobes. The frontal lobe occupies the anterior third of the hemisphere; the parietal lobe sits in the middle-upper part of the hemisphere; the temporal lobe is in the middle-lower region; and the occipital lobe takes up the posterior quarter of each hemisphere (Figure 12.1C). The sulci are smaller involutions within each lobe, and the regions between the sulci are called convolutions or **gyri**. Some gyri vary little in location and contour from one person to another, whereas others vary considerably.

The surface of the cerebral hemisphere is called the **cortex**, consists of gray matter, and is composed principally of **neurons** (nerve cell bodies) and **glia** (supporting cells). Below this gray matter lie the nerve fibers (**axons**) or white matter. The function of the cerebral cortex is to initiate motion and thought processes, and to process sensory input. The cortex of each lobe is responsible for specific activities or functions, outlined in more detail below.

The Frontal Lobe

The frontal lobe controls both voluntary motor activity and important aspects of cognition (Brodal, 2010). It also plays an important role in attention and emotion and may be impaired in intellectual disability (ID) and attention-deficit/hyperactivity disorder (ADHD) as well as in certain genetic disorders (e.g., frontal lobe epilepsy and Pick's disease). The anterior cingulate cortex and frontoinsular cortex, in particular, are connected to processing information across a variety of domains, including those related to attention and emotion (Bush et al., 2000; Carter et al., 1998; Craig, 2009; Critchley et al., 2004; Devinsky et al., 1995).

Within the frontal lobe the different areas of the body are represented topographically along a strip called the primary motor cortex. The tongue and **larynx**, or voice box, are controlled from the lowest point followed in an upward sequence by the face, hand, arm, trunk, thigh, and foot (Figure 12.2). The tongue, larynx, and hand occupy a particularly large area along this strip due to the complexity of speech and fine motor activity.

A nerve impulse initiated in the motor strip passes down the **pyramidal** or **corticospinal** tract that connects the cortex with the spinal cord. Reaching the spinal cord, the impulse passes across a **synapse** (junction between two nerve cells) to an anterior horn cell in the gray matter

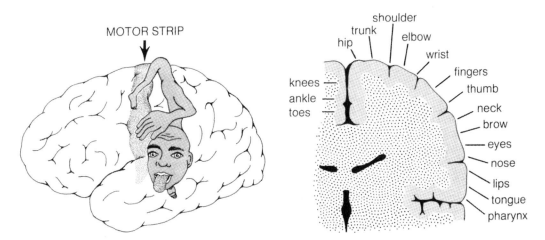

Figure 12.2.   The motor strip. The cartoon figure represents body parts at various points on the strip. Note that the areas representing facial and hand muscles are very large. This is because of the intricate control necessary for speech and fine motor coordination. A cross-section of the motor strip is shown to the right.

section of the spinal cord. This neuron relays the transmission via its axon to a peripheral nerve that connects to an appropriate muscle. The muscle subsequently contracts in response to the original signal from the motor strip in the cortex. In **spinal muscular atrophy** (Werknig-Hoffmann disease), the motor neuron dies during childhood, resulting in **hypotonia** (low muscle tone or "looseness" of the muscle) and weakness (Lorson et al., 2010; Wee et al., 2010; see Chapter 13).

Conversely, if the motor cortex or the pyramidal tract is damaged, increased tone in the form of spasticity results. In spasticity, the underlying involuntary muscle contractions controlled by the brainstem and spinal cord are no longer inhibited by pyramidal tract activity. As a result, voluntary movement becomes less fluid, as seen in cerebral palsy and other movement disorders (see Chapter 24). Therapeutic approaches to spasticity focus on manipulating neurotransmitters to reduce tone. For example, the drug baclofen, which decreases spasticity by increasing the activity of gamma-amino butyric acid (GABA), an inhibitory neurotransmitter, has been administered into the spinal fluid using an implantable pump in individuals with cerebral palsy (Tasseel Ponche et al., 2010; Tilton, 2009; see Chapter 24). Damage to the motor cortex can also lead to seizures that begin as focal twitching and spread to involve large muscle groups (Jacksonian epilepsy; see Chapter 27).

The frontal lobe is also important in abstract thinking. Via functional imaging techniques, the frontal lobe has been identified as the origin of executive function (Arnsten, 2009; Brocki et al., 2008; Green et al., 2008). This high-level abstract thinking is the planner and organizer for future activities. Children with ADHD, learning disabilities, and autism show deficiencies in executive function (Rubia et al., 2011; Tripp & Wickens, 2009; see Chapters 21, 22, and 23). Broca's area (Figure 12.3), the center for expressive language, typically resides in the left frontal lobe, anterior to the motor strip (see Chapter 20). The location can vary, particularly in children who are left-handed, have epilepsy, or have prior destructive lesions such as tumors or stroke (Gaillard et al., 2007).

The Parietal Lobe

Touch, pain, vibration, **proprioception** (ability to sense the position, location, orientation and movement of body parts), and temperature sensation are all processed within the parietal lobe. In addition, the parietal lobe contributes to the integration of other stimuli, promoting a "whole" impression from various sensory inputs. The primary sensory cortex, which receives information from the skin and membranes of the body and face, is located in the somatosensory area of the brain. Via the **thalamus**, this area receives fibers that convey

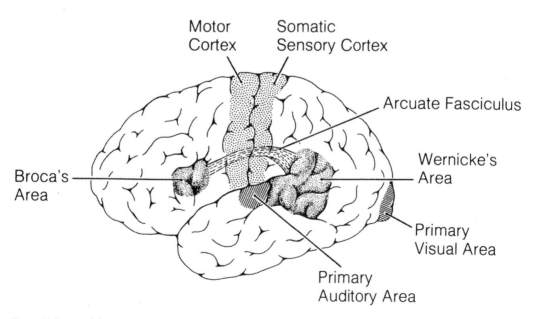

Figure 12.3. An adult neuropathological model of language. Sounds are received in Wernicke's area and passed on to Broca's area via nerve fibers of the arcuate fasciculus. Expressive language is formed here, and the motor cortex is then stimulated to produce speech.

touch and proprioception sensations from the opposite side of the body. Irritation of this area (e.g., by a stroke) may produce **paresthesias** (numbness with a pins-and-needles sensation) of the opposite side of the body. A destructive lesion (e.g., a tumor or hemorrhage) in this area impairs sensation, such as difficulty localizing painful stimuli or measuring their intensity. Although the primary visual cortex is elsewhere (in the occipital lobe), some higher levels of visual processing take place in the parietal lobe. Some evidence indicates that the visual-perceptual problems experienced by children with learning disabilities and the difficulties in performing fine motor tasks found in children with ADHD may be related to parietal region abnormalities (Cubillo et al., 2010; Vaidya & Stollstorff, 2008).

The Temporal Lobe

The temporal lobe is primarily involved in communication and sensation. The dominant hemisphere (the left side in more than 90% of people) is responsible for comprehending speech as well as contributing to the memory of auditory and visual experiences (Gaillard et al., 2011; Vazquez & Mayola, 2008). It receives input from each ear, with point-to-point projection of the **cochlea** (the spiral-shaped cavity of the inner ear that resembles a snail shell and contains nerve endings essential for hearing) upon the acoustic area of the temporal lobe. Wernicke's area, the receptive language center, is found in the superior temporal gyrus. As with Broca's area, it is most commonly found on the left side but its location can vary (Gaillard et al., 2007).

Within the base of each temporal lobe rests two structures, the **hippocampus** and **amygdala**, which serve special cognitive functions. The hippocampus plays an important role in memory and allows for the rapid learning of new information. The amygdala is involved in sensory processing and emotions and is part of the general-purpose "fight or flight" defense-response control system.

Both the amygdala and hippocampus show structural abnormalities in autism, with the degree of abnormality linked to the severity of impairment (Dziobek et al., 2010; Kleinhans et al., 2010). It is unclear if alterations in the hippocampus are a cause or an effect of the disorder's symptomatology. Studies in both animals and humans suggest that the hippocampus can undergo dynamic changes as a result of experience and behavior (Insausti et al., 2010).

In humans, the amygdala is associated with emotional and social functions. Recent use of functional magnetic resonance imaging (fMRI) has demonstrated that the human brain is equipped with specialized circuits for discriminating facial emotions. In particular, the crucial involvement of the amygdala in emotional face processing has been demonstrated by a large number of studies comparing patients with damaged amygdala and normal subjects (Damiano et al., 2011). Amygdala dysfunction has also been strongly implicated in the social deficits of ASD as it is involved in the ability to read and relate to others' emotions.

Recent evidence suggests that several aspects of face processing are impaired in patients with autism (Damiano et al., 2011). The most reproducible features include abnormal patterns of gaze processing, memory for facial identity, and recognition of the emotional content of facial expressions. Research studying face processing in autism focuses on abnormalities in a specific network of brain regions that are implicated in social cognition and face processing. These include the superior temporal sulcus (located in the temporal lobe), which plays a role in processing gaze and facial movements, and the fusiform face area (located on the ventral surface of the temporal lobe). It is not known how alterations in developmental processes and the role of experience interact during normal development and in autism to modify and influence this network.

Temporal lobe dysfunction can contribute to a number of disorders; the two most common are receptive **aphasia** and complex partial seizures (Rosenberger et al., 2009). In receptive aphasia, the temporal lobe may have been damaged by a tumor, vascular insufficiency, or trauma (Siegal & Varley, 2006). The individual is unable to understand spoken words but is able to speak, frequently in an unintelligible fashion (see Chapter 20). Complex partial seizures also arise in the temporal lobe. Before the seizure begins, the individual may experience a déjà vu, or flashback, phenomenon, caused by stimulation of this brain area. The person may also have visual hallucinations, hear bizarre sounds, or smell unpleasant aromas, all of which emanate from the temporal lobe (see Chapter 27).

Treatment of refractory complex partial seizures may involve surgical removal of the seizure focus (McTague & Appleton, 2011). This surgery has been shown in adults to be superior to long-term anti-epileptic drug use in terms of seizure control and quality of life. Although adults who undergo this neurosurgical procedure on the left side of the brain often sustain some language or memory loss, children appear less likely to experience this complication. This suggests that a child's brain is more flexible than an adult's, such that the nondominant hemisphere can take over some of the language functions of the damaged dominant area. In fact, children as old as 6 have undergone total dominant **hemispherectoma** (removal of the left hemisphere for intractable generalized seizures with a left-sided focus) and have been able to recover speech function, presumably by incorporating other cortical locations in a new functional role (Johnston, 2009; Liegeois et al., 2008, 2010; Limbricht et al., 2009). This is known as plasticity (Kuhl & Rivera-Gaxiola, 2008). With hemispherectomy, the degree of language recovery varies according to the underlying cause of the seizure disorder (Mbwana et al., 2009; van Schooneveld et al., 2011).

In the temporal lobe, the primary auditory cortex receives input from both ears by way of the cochlear nerves via multiple synapses in the brainstem. Irritation of this cortex may cause a buzzing or roaring sensation. Because of the bilateral representation, unilateral damage does not result in deafness but may result in mild hearing loss. Bilateral lesions can result in complete hearing loss.

The Occipital Lobe

The primary visual receptive cortex is located in the occipital lobe. The right occipital lobe receives impulses from the right half of each **retina** (the nerve layer that lines the back of the eye, senses light, and creates impulses that travel through the optic nerve to the brain). This creates the left visual field, whereas the left visual cortex receives impulses from the left half of each retina (and creates the right visual field). The upper portion of this cortical area represents the upper half of each retina (the lower visual field), whereas the lower portion represents the lower half (the upper visual field). Irritation of this visual cortex can produce such visual hallucinations as flashes of light, rainbows, brilliant stars, or bright lines. Destructive lesions can cause defects in the visual fields on the opposite side, without loss of central vision.

Visual stimuli are first interpreted in the visual-receptive area, then processed further in an adjacent part of the occipital lobe, before being passed on to the temporal and parietal lobes. Here the identity of a viewed object and its location in space are further determined. In both the temporal and parietal lobes, the image is linked to what is heard and felt so that interpretations can be made. Severe damage to

the occipital region may cause **cortical visual impairment** (cortical blindness; Ospina, 2009). In this condition, despite a normal visual apparatus and pathway, the occipital lobe does not receive the image, and the person is functionally blind (see Chapter 11).

Interconnections

The white matter of the adult cerebral hemispheres contains nerve fibers of many sizes that are **myelinated** (sheathed by an insulating layer that increases the speed at which impulses are conducted). Some of these fibers serve to connect various regions of the brain. The most important of these interconnections is the corpus callosum, noted above (Figure 12.1A).

A second type of interconnection is formed by projection fibers, which connect the cerebral cortex with lower portions of the brain or spinal cord. As an example, the **internal capsule** is a collection of fibers that project from the cortex to the spinal cord; nerve impulses carried by these fibers control distant muscles. Destructive lesions such as tumors or strokes may compress or otherwise compromise the internal capsule and the pyramidal (motor) tract it contains. This will result in **hemiplegia** (spasticity and weakness on the opposite side of the body).

Finally, association fibers connect the various parts of the cerebral hemisphere. Short association fibers, or U fibers, connect adjacent gyri. The fibers which are just beneath the cortex are called *subcortical fibers* while those located in the deeper white matter are called *intracortical fibers*. Long association fibers connect more widely separated areas.

The Basal Ganglia and Thalamus

Deep beneath the cortical surface resides the **diencephalon** (Figure 12.1A), which consists of the **thalamus** and **hypothalamus**. Adjacent to the diencephalon are the **basal ganglia** and related structures. In humans, this primitive part of the brain modulates instructions from the motor cortex in directing voluntary movements (Antonello et al., 2009; Waxman, 2009). In lower vertebrates it directly controls motor activity. Anatomically, the basal ganglia include the **caudate nucleus** and the **putamen** (together called the **corpus striatum**), the **globus pallidus**, and the other gray matter areas at the base of the forebrain. Together, the putamen and the globus pallidus form the **lentiform nucleus**. The caudate nucleus is separated from the lentiform nucleus and thalamus by the **internal capsule**. Functionally, these collections of neurons, together with their connections and neurotransmitters, form an associated motor system.

Damage to the basal ganglia produces various movement disorders. Although voluntary movement is still possible, involuntary jerking or twisting, referred to as **choreoathetosis**, may also occur. Alternatively, individuals may experience rigidity or **dystonic** posturing (involuntary contraction of muscles, forcing limbs into abnormal, sometimes painful postures), manifestations which can be seen in children with **dyskinetic cerebral palsy** (see Chapter 24).

Immediately adjacent to the basal ganglia is the thalamus, through which all sensory input to the cortex must first pass, and which constitutes a gateway or relay station for transmission of information within the brain and across networks and pathways. It also is the seat of normal brain rhythms that are inhibitory and modulate control of movement (Llinás et al., 1999). Damage to the thalamus may cause movement disorders. The thalamus is also thought to be part of a neuronal network concerned with cognitive function, especially language.

Thalamocortical Connectivity

Injury to the thalamocortical pathways (connecting the thalamus to the cortex) have also been found to result in abnormal excitation that may be related to a variety of neuropsychiatric and behavioral disorders (Walsh et al., 2010). Recent neuroimaging studies have demonstrated that injury to thalamic resting state networks correlates with reduced performance on neurocognitive testing (Walsh et al., 2010). A BMRI has already been successfully utilized in detecting alterations in this network in individuals with ADHD, depression, schizophrenia, and autism (Paakkia et al., 2010). Since measures assessing resting-state brain activity can reveal cognitive disorders at an early stage, this is an exciting new area of research. Coupled with genetic analysis, it may reveal insight into earliest manifestations of ID or autism.

The Brainstem

In contrast to the cerebral hemispheres, which control voluntary actions, the brainstem controls more reflexive and involuntary activities. It is comprised of three distinct areas (midbrain, pons, and medulla) and connects the cerebral hemispheres to the spinal cord (Figure 12.4). Within it are the cranial nerves that control functions such as vision, hearing, swallowing, and articulation (Saito, 2009). These cranial nerves also affect facial expression, eye and tongue movement, salivation, and even breathing. In addition to the cranial nerve nuclei, the

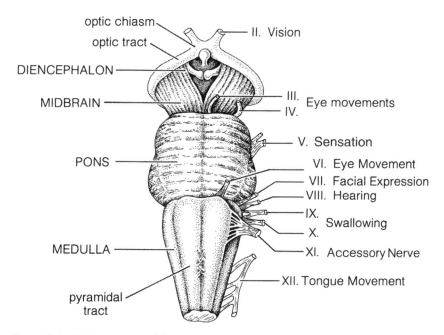

Figure 12.4.   The three regions of the brainstem are shown: midbrain, pons, and medulla. The placement and function of 11 of the 12 cranial nerves are illustrated. (The first cranial nerve [smell] is not shown. It lies in front of the second cranial nerve, below the frontal lobe.) Note that the pyramidal tract runs from the cortex (not shown) into the brainstem. The pyramidal fibers cross over in the medulla. Thus, the right hemisphere controls left-side movement, and the left hemisphere controls right-side movement.

brainstem is composed of a vast array of fiber tracts relaying messages into and out of the brain. The corticospinal tract provides for the passage of neural impulses from the cortex to the spinal cord. Conversely there are tracts bringing sensory information to the cortex via the thalamus. Therefore, any abnormality in this region affects function in distant locations. Children with cerebral palsy may have damage to the brainstem or to pathways that end in the brainstem. This damage might explain the high incidence of excessive salivation, swallowing problems, strabismus, and speech disorders in these children (see Chapter 24).

The Cerebellum

The **cerebellum** (Figure 12.1A) resides in back of the brain stem and immediately below the cerebral hemispheres. It coordinates voluntary motor activity. Its principal role is to dampen skeletal muscular activity, thus enabling smooth transition between activating **agonist** muscles (that work together) while inhibiting their counterpart antagonist muscles. Normal muscle coordination requires that cerebellar functions be integrated with those of the cerebral hemispheres and the basal ganglia. Although voluntary movement can occur without the cerebellum, such movements are ataxic, that is, erratic and uncoordinated. An **ataxic** gait may be seen with cerebellar tumors, progressive neurological disorders (e.g., ataxia telangiectasia), inebriation, or as a side effect of medication (Maria, 2008; Swaiman et al., 2006).

The cerebellum may also influence cognitive function through interconnections with the prefrontal cortex (Bolduc & Limperopoulos, 2009; Ten Donkelaar & Lammens, 2009). It has been implicated in deficits seen in ASD. fMRI reveals cerebellar activation during a variety of cognitive tasks, including those related to language, visual–spatial abilities, and executive function that includes working memory. Furthermore, resting-state functional connectivity data demonstrate that the cerebellum is part of cognitive networks that include the prefrontal and parietal association cortices (Ito et al., 2008; Leiner et al., 1996). The clinical cerebellar cognitive affective syndrome (Schmahmann, et al., 1998) occurring in patients with cerebellar lesions provides further evidence of cerebellar involvement in cognitive functions. The syndrome causes deficits in spatial processing, working memory, language, and emotional ability.

A number of theories have been proposed regarding the specific contribution the cerebellum provides to neural processes, including timing (Ghajar et al., 2009; Ivry et al., 2000), sequencing, and learning associative relationships between elements (Molinari & Leggio, 2007; Timmann et al 2010). This suggests that the cerebellum is important both for extracting relevant information from the environment and also for acquiring procedures related to that information. These ideas support the theory that the cerebellum is crucial to the formation of internal models, which may apply to both movement and cognitive functions (Ito et al., 2008).

The Spinal Cord

The spinal cord transmits motor and sensory messages between the brain and the rest of the body. In addition to permitting voluntary movement, the spinal cord acts to provide protective reflex arcs in both the upper and lower extremities, such as the deep tendon reflex elicited when the knee is tapped. The spinal cord is an elongated, cylindrical mass of nerve tissue that is continuous with the brainstem at its upper end and occupies the upper two thirds of the adult spinal canal within the vertebral column (Figure 12.5). It widens laterally in the neck and the lower back regions. These enlargements correspond to the origins of the nerves of the upper and lower extremities. The nerves of the **brachial plexus** originate at the cervical enlargement of the spinal cord and control arm movement; the nerves of the lumbosacral plexus arise from the lumbar enlargement of the spinal cord and control leg movement. Injury to a newborn's brachial plexus may occur during a difficult vaginal delivery, resulting in weakness of the upper extremity (Abzug & Kozin, 2010).

The spinal cord is divided into approximately 30 segments—8 cervical (neck), 12 thoracic (chest), 5 lumbar (lower back), 5 sacral (pelvic), and a few small coccygeal (tailbone) segments—that correspond to attachments of groups of nerve roots. Individual segments vary in length. They are about twice as long in the mid-thoracic region as in the cervical or upper lumbar area.

There are no sharp boundaries between segments within the cord itself. Each segment contributes four roots: a **ventral** (front) and **dorsal** (back) root arising from the left half and a similar pair of roots arising from the right half. Each root is made up of many individual rootlets. The dorsal nerve roots allow sensory input to ascend to the brainstem, whereas the ventral roots deliver motor input from the brainstem to the appropriate muscle.

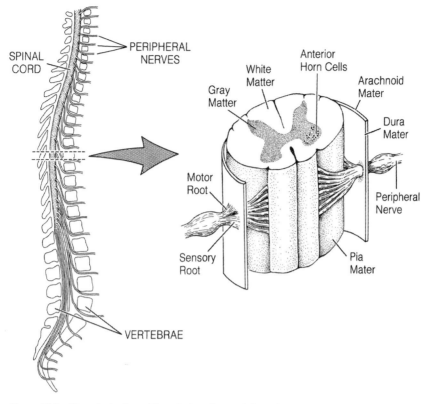

Figure 12.5. The spinal column. The spinal cord extends from the neck to the lower back. It is protected by the bony vertebrae that form the spinal column. The enlargement to the right shows a section of the cord taken from the upper back region. Note the meninges (the dura, arachnoid, and pia mater) surrounding the cord and the peripheral nerve on its way to a muscle. This nerve contains both motor and sensory components (roots). The spinal cord, like the brain, has both gray and white matter. The gray matter consists of various nerve cells, the most important of which are the anterior horn cells. These are destroyed in polio. The white matter contains nerve fibers wrapped in myelin, which gives the cord its glistening appearance.

If the spinal cord is damaged (e.g., due to trauma or a congenital malformation such as a myelomeningocele; see Chapter 25), messages to and from the brain are short-circuited below the area of abnormality. The result is a loss (either partial or complete) of sensation and movement in the affected limbs. The paralysis, which is initially flaccid but ultimately becomes spastic, may involve the legs (**paraplegia**) or all four extremities (**quadriplegia**), depending on the level of damage.

Cerebrospinal Fluid and Hydrodynamic Balance

Long considered simply an aqueous environment for the suspension of the brain, cerebrospinal fluid (CSF) is now known to perform many other functions. In addition to physically supporting the neural elements and serving to buffer the brain and spinal cord from excessive motion, CSF acts to provide nutritional support

as well as to remove excessive hormones and neurotransmitters. CSF may also serve as a "relief valve," adjusting its volume when there is an increase in intracranial pressure. Furthermore, its hydrodynamic properties no doubt influence the physical attributes of the brain.

Approximately a pint of CSF is produced each day by the **choroid plexus**, a collection of blood vessels in the lining of the brain ventricles. This fluid moves throughout the lateral and third ventricles and communicates with the fourth ventricle via the aqueduct of Sylvius (Figure 12.6). At the level of the fourth ventricle, the CSF exits to circulate over the surface of the brain as well as the spinal cord in the subarachnoid space. Absorption of CSF occurs at the arachnoid granulations over the superior surface of the brain. These granulations act as one-way valves to allow CSF to move into the blood stream.

Should an imbalance develop between CSF production and absorption, **hydrocephalus**

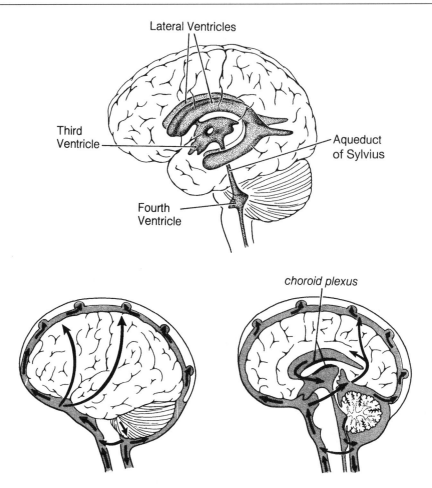

Figure 12.6.   The ventricular system of the brain. The major parts of the ventricular system are shown (top). The flow of cerebrospinal fluid (CSF) is shown (bottom). The fluid is produced by the choroid plexus in the roof of the lateral and third ventricles. Its primary route is through the aqueduct of Sylvius, into the fourth ventricle, and then into the spinal column, where it is absorbed. A secondary route is around the surface of the brain. A blockage, most commonly of the aqueduct of Sylvius, leads to hydrocephalus. (Lower illustrations from Milhorat, T.H. [1972]. *Hydrocephalus and the cerebrospinal fluid.* Philadelphia, PA: Lippincott Williams & Wilkins. http://www.lww.com Copyright © 1972, The Williams & Wilkins Co., Baltimore, MD; adapted by permission.)

may ensue (Figure 12.7). This usually congenital condition involves an abnormal accumulation of fluid in the cerebral ventricles, causing skull enlargement and brain compression. It can be caused by an obstruction of CSF flow within the ventricular system (frequently at the aqueduct of Sylvius) or at the exit of the ventricular system (at the foramina of Luschka and Magendie). This is known as a noncommunicating hydrocephalus. In contrast, a communicating hydrocephalus is caused by malfunction at the level of the arachnoid granulations. In addition to inadequate absorption, it is also possible (though rare) to have an oversupply of CSF, as seen with tumors of the choroid plexus. This excess may overwhelm the ability of the arachnoid granulations to absorb the fluid.

When fluid builds up inside the skull of an infant, the **sutures** (the joints connecting the bones of the skull) expand and dissipate the increased pressure at the expense of an increase in head circumference. This may present as a bulging **anterior fontanelle** ("soft spot"). The same situation in an older child whose sutures have closed, however, may quickly lead to headache, vomiting, lethargy, and focal neurological changes. This buildup of fluid can be life-threatening at any age and is considered a medical emergency.

When hydrocephalus occurs, it is necessary to restore the balance between production and absorption of CSF, a treatment often accomplished via a shunting procedure that results in long-term drainage of CSF. The

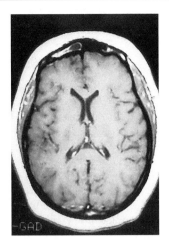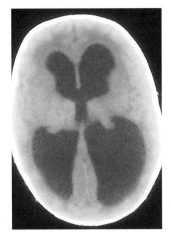

Figure 12.7. Normal magnetic resonance imaging (MRI) scan (left) and computed tomography (CT) scan showing hydrocephalus (right). In the image to the right, note the rounded appearance of the frontal horns (top) as well as the differentially enlarged occipital horns (bottom). This is known as culpocephaly and is frequently seen in individuals with spina bifida.

shunt's objective is to bypass the CSF obstruction, whether at the level of the arachnoid granulations or within the ventricular system. This usually involves diverting CSF from the head to another site, preferably the abdomen. The complication rate for this surgery is low, and the long-term outcome is reasonable good. Once in place, however, numerous obstacles remain in maintaining a working shunt and avoiding infection. Many children require shunt revisions as a result of infection or because obstructions develop within the shunt. Despite present-day imperfections, managing hydrocephalus has been simplified and often allows for a near typical lifestyle.

In children with noncommunicating hydrocephalus, either congenital (e.g., aqueductal stenosis) or acquired (e.g., secondary to a tumor), there is a surgical alternative to shunting. This procedure (endoscopic third ventriculostomy) involves perforating the floor of the third ventricle to create a new outflow route for the CSF, thus bypassing the obstruction completely intracranially (Sandberg, 2008). Endoscopic third ventriculostomy has the benefit of avoiding implants, but is not feasible in all individuals with hydrocephalus. In addition, there is a small but serious risk of injury to nearby vascular and neural structures.

THE PERIPHERAL NERVOUS SYSTEM

The peripheral nerves allow neural impulses to move from the CNS (brain and spinal cord) to distant muscles and sensory organs. These nerves can have both motor and sensory fibers that run in opposite directions. Motor, or **efferent**, fibers transmit impulses from the brain to initiate movement, while sensory, or **afferent**, fibers carry signals from muscles, skin, and joints back to the brain. Sensory fibers convey information related to the position of a joint or the tone of a muscle following movement. Hyperexcitability of sensory neurons in the child with cerebral palsy contributes to spasticity. There are also a number of hereditary neuropathies that interfere with the **peripheral nervous system** (Botez & Herrmann, 2010; Schenone et al., 2011).

The regeneration capacity of the peripheral nervous system differs substantially from that of the CNS. Although the CNS is now considered capable of limited regeneration, the peripheral nervous system can be repaired more easily. This ability to promote the regrowth of peripheral nerves is responsible for the success seen in surgical reconstruction for **brachial plexus** palsy. The brachial plexus is a network of nerves that conducts signals from the spine to the shoulder, arm, and hand. Brachial plexus palsy is caused by damage to those nerves. Symptoms include a limp or paralyzed arm; lack of muscle control in the arm, hand, or wrist; and a lack of feeling or sensation in the arm or hand. Meaningful recovery of neurological function is seen in 60%–90% of young children undergoing these procedures (Abzug & Kozin, 2010).

The **somatic** nervous system (SNS) is the part of the peripheral nervous system that is associated with the voluntary control of body movements via skeletal muscles, and with sensory reception of touch, hearing, and sight. The SNS consists of efferent nerves responsible for stimulating muscle contraction, including all the neurons connected with skeletal muscles, skin, and sense organs. Complex coordination between the motor and sensory system is necessary to ensure normal muscle tone. An imbalance can lead to either increased or decreased tone. Direct injury to the SNS will affect voluntary as well as reflex activities of the involved muscle and will cause flaccid weakness. This is in contrast to a CNS motor injury which results in increased tone in the form of spasticity.

Involuntary activities of the cardiovascular, digestive, endocrine, urinary, respiratory, and reproductive systems are controlled by the **autonomic nervous system**. This control begins in the diencephalon and terminates at the end organ (e.g., stomach, bladder, lungs; Figure 12.8). In contrast to the graded response of voluntary movements, the autonomic nervous system involves an on/off type of control. The best example of this is the "fight or flight"

response. When a person feels threatened, physically or psychologically, several physiological changes take place simultaneously. Digestive system functions are suspended so that blood can be diverted to more important areas for actions involved in "fight or flight," such as the brain and heart. Heart rate and blood pressure increase, and the air passages of the lungs expand in size. All of these changes prepare for a quick reaction to an emergency.

Although the autonomic nervous system works involuntarily in maintaining **homeostasis** (metabolic equilibrium of the body), voluntary adjustments come from the cerebral cortex to modulate these effects. The development of bowel and bladder control is the best example of this. In an infant, when the bladder or rectum fills, the outlet muscles release automatically and the infant urinates or defecates with no conscious control. Between the ages of 12 and 18 months, however, the child gradually gains control over these functions. The cerebral cortex begins to send inhibitory signals to reduce the normal autonomic activity. As any parent knows only too well, this coordination

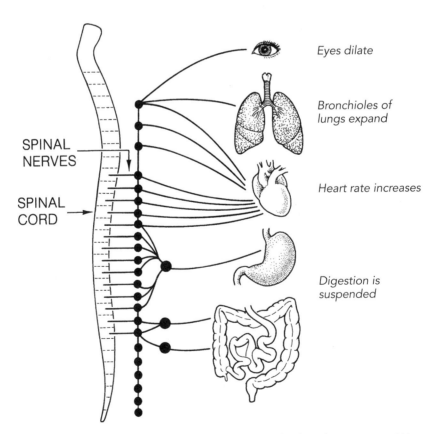

Figure 12.8. Autonomic nervous system. These nerves control such involuntary motor activities as breathing, heart rate, and digestion. This system is involved in "fight or flight" reactions.

requires months of fine-tuning to master consistent control. Individuals who have sustained damage to either the corticospinal tracts or the spinal cord are less able to inhibit the autonomic nervous system in this way. This explains the great difficulty that children with cerebral palsy, myelomeningocele, or traumatic brain injury (see Chapter 26) may have in controlling bowel and bladder function.

THE MICROSCOPIC ARCHITECTURE OF THE BRAIN

The Neuron

Neurons are similar to other cells in that they have a cell body consisting of a nucleus and cytoplasm. Unlike other cells, however, they have a long process called an *axon*, which extends from the cell body, and many short jutting processes called *dendrites* (Figure 12.9). The axon carries impulses away from the nerve cell body, sometimes for a distance greater than a meter. Dendrites receive impulses from other neurons and carry them a short distance toward the cell body. The size and shape of dendrites may change with neuronal activity, suggesting that these changes may represent the anatomical basis for memory.

As the brain begins to organize by 5 weeks' gestation (a process that continues into early childhood) the axons and dendrites grow and differentiate. The major developmental features of this organizational period include 1) the establishment and differentiation of neurons; 2) the attainment of proper alignment, orientation, and layering of cortical neurons; 3) the elaboration of dendrites and axons; 4) the establishment of synaptic contacts; and 5) cell death and selective elimination of neuronal processes and synapses.

Establishment and differentiation

As the neurons develop, growing axons are able to recognize various molecules that are on the surface of other axons and cell bodies. They can use these molecules as cues to navigate the circuitous pathway to their final destination. These axons need to "perceive" this guidance information, distinguishing the correct pathway from the incorrect one. In addition, axons need to move forward (sometimes rapidly), make turns, avoid obstacles, and stop when the target is reached. These guidance functions—sensory, motor, and integrative—are contained within the specialized tip of a growing axon, the growth cone (Squire et al., 2008).

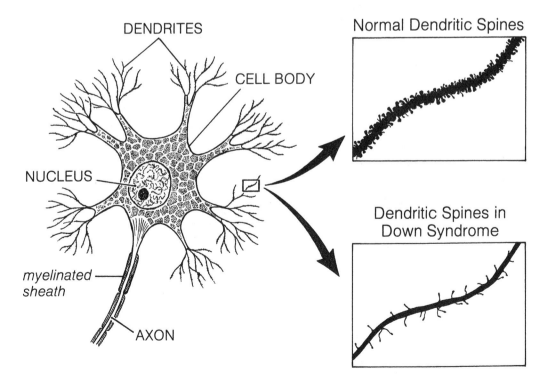

Figure 12.9. Illustration of a nerve cell (neuron), showing its component elements. The enlargements show the minute dendritic spines that increase the number of synapses or junctures among nerve cells. Note the diminished size and number of dendritic spines in a child with Down syndrome.

Alignment, Orientation, and Layering of Cortical Neurons

During neuronal differentiation, the primitive neurons begin to express their distinctive physical and biochemical features. This process, called *arborization*, is much like the growth of a tree from a sapling. It even involves pruning, such that some new connections (synapses) remain established while others disappear. For example, in the visual cortex, synapses form most rapidly between 2 and 4 months after term, a critical time for the development of visual function. Maximum synaptic density is attained at 8 months of age, when the elimination of synapses begins. By 11 months of age, approximately 40% of synapses have been lost (Volpe, 2008).

Dendrites and Axons

As axons grow toward their respective dendritic targets, the dendrites respond by increasing the number of spines, or projections, along their surface (Figure 12.10). The spines increase the surface area of the dendrites, permitting more elaborate communication between the neurons. In fact, increased dendritic outgrowth has been associated with enhanced memory. In contrast, deficient development of dendritic arborization has been observed in individuals with cognitive impairment, most notably in Down syndrome (Huttenlocher, 1991).

Synapses

Proper function of the nervous system requires that two linkages form: 1) the needed connections between an axon from one neuron and the dendrite from a second neuron, and 2) the communication between these two neurons once the connection is established. The point of contact between two neurons is called a **synapse** (Figure 12.10).

Cell Death and Selective Elimination of Neuronal Processes and Synapses

Synapses can be either chemical or electrical, with distinct characteristics for each type.

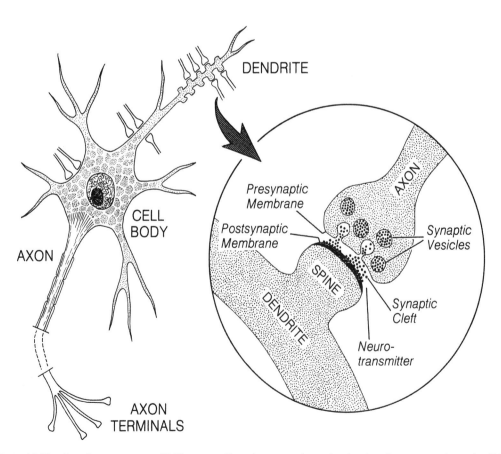

Figure 12.10. Central nervous system (CNS) synapse. The enlargement shows the abutting of an axon against a dendritic spine. The space separating the two is the synaptic cleft. Neurotransmitter bundles are released into the cleft from vesicles in the presynaptic membrane. These permit transmission of an impulse across the juncture.

In electrical synapses, there is a short distance between the two neurons and there is a communication between the cytoplasm of the cells. Because of this, there is very little delay as an electric current passes from one neuron to the next, and the transmission is usually bidirectional.

In contrast, chemical synapses have a larger gap between the two neurons and no direct communication of the cytoplasm. In order to bridge the gap between the two cells, small **vesicles** (small bladder-like cavities) containing specific chemicals (neurotransmitters) are released from the axon of one neuron. These chemicals travel the distance between the cells to reach the receptors for that particular neurotransmitter on the dendrite of the second neuron. The effect on the postsynaptic cell can be either excitatory or inhibitory. Because of the process involved, there is a delay in transmission and the signal is unidirectional. Within a network, the two types of synapses work together to foster synchrony (Brodal, 2010).

Neurotransmitters

Neurotransmitters are chemicals that are released by one cell to cause an effect on a second cell. They differ from hormones in the scale of their action. While hormones are released into the bloodstream and can affect cells distant from the originating cell, neurotransmitters are released within the synapse and only affect cells that are in very close proximity. For a substance to be considered a neurotransmitter, it has to be synthesized within and released from the presynaptic neuron and has to exert a defined effect on the postsynaptic neuron.

With chemical transmission at a synapse, the first step is the synthesis of the neurotransmitter within the presynaptic neuron. Many of these chemicals share a common precursor. For example, dopamine and norepinephrine are both synthesized from the amino acid tyrosine. Each neuron is specialized to use one neurotransmitter. After synthesis, the neurotransmitters are packaged and stored in vesicles within the axon to await release. When a **depolarizing current** (an electrical current causing a change in cell membrane voltage) passes through the axon, the vesicles spill their contents into the synapse. The neurotransmitters then travel the distance between the two neurons. The dendrite of the postsynaptic neuron has receptors that are specific for the released neurotransmitter. When the receptors are activated, there can be an excitatory or inhibitory response. The

excess neurotransmitters within the synapse are then removed either by reuptake or by enzymatic breakdown. The function of the CNS can be altered by manipulating any of the steps in chemical transmission. Many commonly used medications for depression and anxiety belong to a group of prescription drugs known as **selective serotonin reuptake inhibitors** (SSRIs). Examples include fluoxetine (Prozac) and sertraline (Zoloft). These medications block the reuptake of serotonin after its release in the synaptic cleft, thereby increasing the availability and the duration of serotonin action in specific brain regions. Similarly atomoxetine (Strattera) is a selective norepinephrine inhibitor and has been found to be effective in treating ADHD.

Within the central, peripheral, and autonomic nervous system there are a variety of identified neurotransmitters. Table 12.1 provides a simplified summary of the characteristics of some of the major neurotransmitters.

Myelination

The neurons and neuronal processes of the brain and spinal cord form two distinct regions of the CNS, the gray matter and the white matter. The gray matter contains the nerve cell bodies, appearing grayish in color. The white matter is made up of axons sheathed with a protective covering called myelin that promotes the rapid conduction of nerve impulses. During fetal life, most of the axons have no myelin coating. They gradually develop this glistening casing after birth. Effective **myelination** is necessary for the development of voluntary gross and fine motor movement and the suppression of **primitive reflexes** (see Chapter 24). The majority of myelination is completed by 18 months of age, around the time a child can run (Volpe, 2008); however, myelination continues to a lesser degree throughout adolescence and into early adulthood. Deficient myelin formation has been found in a number of conditions including prematurity, congenital hypothyroidism, and malnutrition (van der Voorn et al., 2006).

TECHNIQUES FOR EVALUATING THE CENTRAL NERVOUS SYSTEM

Computed Tomography

In the 1990s, considerable advances in neuroradiology provided more definitive findings regarding the living brain (Barkovich, 2005;

Table 12.1. Characteristics of some of the major neurotransmitters

Neurotransmitter	Location	Function	Associated disorder
Acetylcholine	Nucleus basalis Neuromuscular junction Autonomic nervous system	Stimulates muscle contraction at the neuromuscular junction	Myasthenia gravis (loss of receptors) Botulism (impaired release)
Dopamine	Substantia nigra	Initiates and controls movement	Parkinson's disease (deficiency) Schizophrenia (excess)
Norepinephrine	Locus ceruleus Sympathetic nervous system	Maintains vigilance and responsiveness	Alzheimer's disease
Serotonin	Raphe nuclei	Involved in the sleep–wake cycle, emotions, food intake, thermoregulation, and sexual behavior	Depression (deficiency)
Histamine	Hypothalamus	Regulates hormones	
GABA	Inhibitory interneurons throughout the brain and spinal cord	Principal inhibitory neurotransmitter	Epilepsy (deficiency)
Glycine	Inhibitory interneurons in the spinal cord	Inhibits antagonist muscles	Nonketotic hyperglycinemia (excess)
Glutamate	Excitatory neurons throughout the brain and spinal cord	Principal excitatory neurotransmitter	Huntington disease (excess) Acute brain injury (excess)

Source: Kandel, Schwartz, and Jessell (2000).
Key: GABA, gamma-aminobutyric acid.

Giedd et al., 2010; Lodygensky et al., 2010; Vogel et al., 2010). High-speed computed tomography (CT) scans, which are produced from multiple thin-cut x rays, became a routine part of evaluating the child with hydrocephalus, trauma, craniofacial disorders, new-onset seizures, and brain and skull tumors. The inherent strength of CT resides in its excellent bone definition. Three dimensional CT scans routinely provide sophisticated reconstruction of complex skull-base disorders, and CT angiography offers good resolution of blood vessels or flow abnormalities, with additional information about the adjacent bony structures. Quick and painless acquisition of images means that CT scans can often be obtained without needing to sedate young children, as opposed to magnetic resonance imaging (MRI) scans, which take longer to acquire, making sedation necessary. This also makes CT well-suited for emergency situations, which require rapid acquisition of brain images (e.g., in seeking evidence of intracranial hemorrhage after trauma).

CT can be supplemented with intravenous (IV) contrast, which helps define areas of blood-brain barrier breakdown. Addition of IV contrast is especially helpful in cases of infection or suspected tumor. Most infections and many (but not all) tumors will appear bright with the addition of contrast, aiding in visualization of these lesions. Conversely, IV contrast typically does not aid in clinical scenarios such as closed head injury or hydrocephalus. Caution should be used when administering contrast to any child with dehydration or abnormal renal function.

While CT is a powerful diagnostic tool, the associated radiation exposure is 100 times higher than that from a typical chest x ray (Hall & Brenner, 2008), a level of exposure that is particularly relevant when treating children. Not only are children more sensitive to radiation, and thus at an increased risk from exposure, but they also will have a longer lifetime than adults for any negative effects from exposure to manifest (Bulas et al., 2009). In addition to the risk to the individual, one must consider the potential population risk of increased cancer rates as use of CT becomes more common (Berrington de González et al., 2009). While CT remains a mainstay in evaluating the child's nervous system, one must consider alternative methods of imaging when possible, such as magnetic resonance imaging.

Magnetic Resonance Imagining

MRI scanning has surpassed all other imaging modalities for evaluating brain structure. It is particularly useful in investigating developmental abnormalities of the brain, in assessing the causes of epilepsy (Abdelhalim & Alberico, 2009; Duncan, 2009; Freilich & Gaillard, 2010; Gaillard et al., 2007), in identifying chronic hemorrhage (Kidwell et al., 2004), and in visualizing brain tumors.

Over the last decade, improvements in MRI technology and science have allowed physicians to collect information not only about alterations in structure, but also alteration in function, brain metabolism, and microscopic damage to the brain's gray and white matter. This is done by using special MRI software in the routine MRI scanner. These new sequences have been used clinically, as well as part of research studies to learn more about brain networks that underlie cognition and how different developmental disorders may be similar or different in terms of brain function.

Children with intellectual disability (ID) may have a structural cause for the underlying deficit, which may be qualitative or quantitative, and if so can be measured by MRI. Some findings may be non-specific, but nonetheless may be helpful in identifying a physiologic process (i.e., does it involve the gray matter or

white matter), determining the timing of the insult (i.e., old neonatal stroke versus current stroke in a child with sickle cell disease), assessing the potential for reversibility, or following up to see if a condition is static or progressive. Other findings on MRI may be so specific that they help to identify the definitive cause of ID in a child. An example would be the diagnosis of a major structural brain anomaly such as holoprosencephaly, lissencephaly, or a malformation of the cerebellum (Mochida, 2009; Spalice et al., 2009; Verrotti et al., 2010; see Appendix B). Applying the newer modalities of MRI that probe function, microstructure, and metabolism can be used to assess brain injury at its earliest onset as well as provide a basis for following the course of the disease or gauging the effects of interventions (Giedd et al., 2010; Verbruggen et al., 2009).

New discoveries and applications over the past decades include that of 1) fluid-attenuated inversion recovery (FLAIR; see Figure 12.11) imaging, which allows much better analysis of disorders that affect the white matter (Hoisington et al., 1998); 2) fMRI (see Figure 12.12), which enables one to visualize brain activation patterns while a patient performs a cognitive or motor task in the scanner (Guye et al 2008; O'Shaughnessy et al., 2008); 3) diffusion weighted imaging (DWI) and diffusion tensor

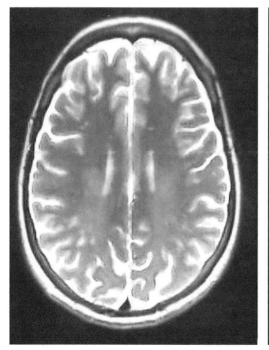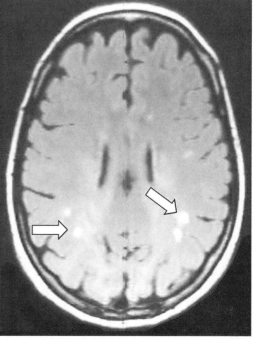

Figure 12.11.   Imaging shows deceivingly normal study on routine T2 (left), but evidence of white matter lesions on FLAIR (right).

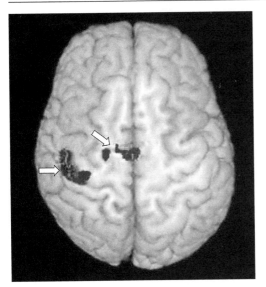

Figure 12.12. Activation map typical of an fMRI. In this figure, the left motor strip is being activated in the area indicated by the arrows. A task that elicits motor response would be expected to produce such a motor response. In an individual who has motor impairment, this area may show less activation and other areas may activate in a compensatory response.

systematic approach based on pattern recognition of brain involvement is particularly useful in the analysis of brain MRI scans in patients with ID due to inborn errors of metabolism (see Chapter 19; Barkovich 2007; van der Knaap et al., 2005).

Over the past two decades, fMRI has emerged as a valuable tool for imaging the time course of activity associated with neurocognitive processes in the brain. This technology has wide-ranging applications for both basic research into brain function and for clinical research into the neurophysiology of neurological and psychiatric illness (Christ et al., 2010). fMRI detects minute changes in regional blood flow and metabolism and can be useful in localizing brain regions involved in such activities as reading, speaking, listening, and moving (Berl et al., 2010; Sun et al., 2010). Differences have been found in individuals with dyslexia versus standard-achievement-level readers. In epilepsy, fMRI is useful in localizing language, memory function, as well as seizure foci (Detre, 2004) and may one day replace more invasive testing of these functions.

imaging (DTI) to look at microscopic damage in white matter (Bennett et al., 2010); and 4) magnetic resonance spectroscopy (MRS), which enables a noninvasive biochemical examination of the brain (Ross et al., 1996; Figure 12.13). A

MRS is a versatile noninvasive technique capable of producing information on a large number of brain chemicals (Pfeuffer et al. 1999). This technology is widely available and can be performed in the same session as

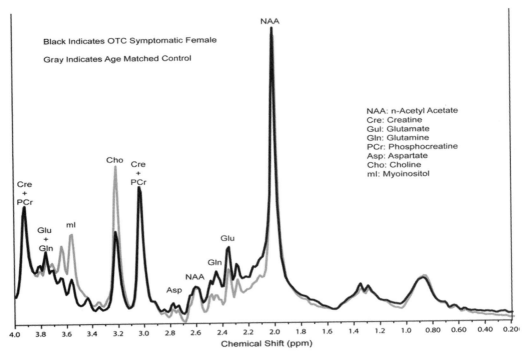

Figure 12.13. 1H MRS comparing a normal subject (gray) with a subject with OTCD (black). Peak difference can be seen, specifically, higher glutamine (GLN) in OTCD, lower choline (CHO) in OTCD, and lower myoinositol (MI) in OTCD. (Key: OTCD, ornithine transcarbamylase deficiency)

conventional MRI (Bizzi et al; 2008; Cecil et al., 2006). MRS techniques complement conventional and advanced imaging and are proving useful in diagnosing, treating, and predicting progression. To date there are no clear guidelines for the use of MRS in childhood neurological diseases, although the literature shows it has contributed to diagnosis and management (Cakmakci et al., 2009; Gropman, 2010; Panigrahy et al., 2010; Xu et al., 2008).

Spectroscopy investigations are performed to study brain chemistry and can measure: 1) N-acetyl aspartate (NAA), a marker of neuronal integrity; 2) creatine, an energy marker; 3) choline, a cell membrane component; 4) myoinositol, a small sugar that is involved in signaling and cell volume; and 5) lactate, which is elevated in conditions affecting energy metabolism. With special software, the neurotransmitters glutamate and glutamine also can be measured. Figure 12.13 demonstrates an MRS comparing a normal subject with one of the inborn errors of metabolism, ornithine transcarbamylase (OCTD).

Single Photon Emission Computer Tomography and Positron Emission Tomography

Like fMRI, single photon emission computer tomography (SPECT) and positron emission tomography (PET) are techniques that demonstrate metabolically active regions in the brain. A radioactive-labeled compound, most commonly glucose, is injected into the bloodstream and SPECT or PET is then used to assess the compound's selective uptake in various brain regions. Both have been used to diagnose strokes, tumors, and brain injury following head trauma (Dubroff & Newberg, 2008; Kou et al., 2010; Lewine et al., 2007; Suskauer & Huisman, 2009), and to predict gross motor development in children with cerebral palsy (Yim et al., 2000). SPECT and PET have also been employed to evaluate seizure disorders prior to surgery (Jafari-Khouzani et al., 2011; Kim et al., 2010; Shore, 2008; Varghese et al., 2009). Table 12.2 summarizes the advantages and disadvantages of each of these different imaging techniques.

As with CT, there is radiation exposure associated with SPECT and PET scans, which must be factored in when weighing the risks and benefits of these diagnostic studies. With regard to radiation the rule is to practice the ALARA principle (As Low As Reasonably Achievable) and only order PET or SPECT in children when there is solid clinical justification. One should always be mindful of a child's cumulative radiation exposure and use pediatric protocols that lower the radiation dosages (Chawla et al., 2010).

Electroencephalography

Whereas CT and MRI show the structure of the brain, and SPECT, PET, and fMRI show its metabolic activity, there are additional tests that can be useful in assessing the function of the brain. Electroencephalography (EEG) utilizes scalp electrodes to measure intracranial electrical activity (see Chapter 27). This is a noninvasive test that detects the summation of neuronal discharges in the superficial layers of the cerebral cortex. In epilepsy, EEG can show a pattern that is indicative of epileptiform ("seizure-like") activity. Coupled with continuous video monitoring, EEG becomes a powerful tool to match seizure type with the location of the seizure focus in the brain (Sullivan et al., 2007). It can detect seizures that may not be evident clinically and can show the effects of various treatments, both medical and surgical, on seizure activity. EEG is also useful in evaluating mental status changes associated with diffuse neurological dysfunction (as might occur in encephalitis or infection of the brain). The background EEG is important as the frequency (Hertz, Hz) of the waveforms is a key characteristic used to define normal or abnormal EEG rhythms. In certain situations, EEG waveforms of a certain frequency for age and/or state of alertness may be viewed as abnormal because they demonstrate irregularities in amplitude or rhythmicity.

Electromyography and Nerve Conduction Studies

To this point, the discussion of techniques for evaluating the nervous system has focused on evaluating the CNS. Although there is limited imaging to assess the peripheral nervous system (e.g., MRI to evaluate the brachial plexus), functional testing is readily available in the form of **electromyography** (EMG) and **nerve conduction studies** (NCS). These studies involve placement of needle electrodes at various points on the body to test motor and sensory function of the peripheral nerves. EMG and NCS can be used to define traumatic injury or peripheral neuropathy and can demonstrate the aftereffects of toxic exposure (Avaria et al., 2004; Pitt; 2011). In addition, these studies can be a helpful aid in surgical cases that involve dissection near either sensory or motor pathways.

Table 12.2. Advantages and disadvantages of each neuroimaging technique

Imaging technique	Advantages	Disadvantages
Computed tomography (CT)	High resolution of bony anatomy; quick and readily available; usually does not require sedation	Lower resolution of brain structures compared to MRI
Magnetic resonance imaging (MRI)	Extremely high resolution of brain structures; images obtained in multiple planes; no radiation exposure	Takes longer to acquire images compared with CT; often requires sedation
Positron emission tomography (PET)/single photon emission computed tomography (SPECT)	Shows brain function in addition to structure by tracking the uptake of radioactive glucose	Limited availability at many centers
Functional MRI (fMRI)	Shows function by detecting variation in regional blood flow; lends better structural resolution than PET/SPECT	Requires significant patient cooperation; not feasible for individuals who are very young or who have severe intellectual disability

SUMMARY

The nervous system is composed of central and peripheral elements. The CNS (the brain and spinal cord) is complex in both its structure and its function. Various techniques allow better assessment of the brain for diagnosis of a broad range of clinical pathology. As our understanding of both normal and abnormal neurological function improves, better therapeutic avenues will be forthcoming.

REFERENCES

Abdelhalim, A.N., & Alberico, R.A. (2009). Pediatric neuroimaging. *Neurologic Clinics, 27*(1), 285–301.

Abzug, J.M., & Kozin, S.H. (2010). Current concepts: Neonatal brachial plexus palsy. *Orthopedics, 33*(6), 430–5. doi: 10.3928/01477447-20100429–25.

Antonello, R.M., Moretti, R., & Toree, P. (2009). *Basal ganglia and thalamus: Their role in cognition and behavior.* Hauppage, NY: Nova Science Publishers. .

Arnsten, A.F. (2009). Toward a new understanding of attention-deficit/hyperactivity disorder pathophysiology: An important role for prefrontal cortex dysfunction. *Central Nervous System Drugs, 23*(1), 33–41. doi: 10.2165/00023210-200923000–00005.

Avaria, M.A., Mills, J.L., Kleinsteuber, K., Aros, S., Conley, M.R., Cox, C., ... Cassorla, F. (2004). Peripheral nerve conduction abnormalities in children exposed to alcohol in utero. *Journal of Pediatrics, 144*(3), 338–343.

Barkovich, A.J. (2005) *Pediatric neuroimaging.* 4th ed. Philadelphia, PA: Lippincott Williams & Wilkins.

Barkovich, A.J. (2007). An approach to MRI of metabolic disorders in children. *Journal of Neuroradiology, 34*, 75–88.

Bennett, I.J., Madden, D.J., Vaidya, C.J., Howard, D.V., & Howard, J.H., Jr. (2010). Age-related differences in multiple measures of white matter integrity: A diffusion tensor imaging study of healthy aging. *Human Brain Mapping, 31*(3), 378–90.

Berl, M.M., Duke, E.S., Mayo, J, Rosenberger, L.R., Moore, E.N., Van Meter, J, ... Gaillard, W.D. (2010). Functional anatomy of listening and reading comprehension during development. *Brain Language, 114*(2), 115–25.

Berrington de González, A., Mahesh, M., Kim, K.P., Bhargavan, M., Lewis, R., Mettler, F., & Land, C. (2009). Projected cancer risks from computed tomographic scans performed in the United States in 2007. *Archives of Internal Medicine, 169*, 2071–2077.

Bizzi, A., Castelli, G., Bugiani, M., Barker, P.B., Herskovits, E.H., Danesi, U., ...Uziel, G. (2008). Classification of childhood white matter disorders using proton MR spectroscopic imaging. *American Journal of Neurological Research, 29*, 1270–1275.

Bolduc, M.E., & Limperopoulos, C. (2009). Neurodevelopmental outcomes in children with cerebellar malformations: A systematic review. *Developmental Medicine and Child Neurology, 51* (4),256–67.

Botez, S.A., & Herrmann, D.N. (2010). Sensory neuropathies, from symptoms to treatment. *Current Opinions in Neurology, 23*(5), 502–8.

Brocki, K., Fan, J., & Fossella, J. (2008). Placing neuroanatomical models of executive function in a developmental context: Imaging and imaging—genetic strategies. *Annals of the New York Academy of Sciences, 1129*, 246–55.

Brodal, P. (2010). *The central nervous system: Structure and function* (4th ed.). New York, NY: Oxford University Press.

Bulas, D.I., Goske, M.J., Applegate, K.E., & Wood, B.P. (2009). Image gently: Why we should talk to parents about CT in children. *American Journal of Roentgenology, 192*, 1176–1178.

Bush, G., Luu, P., & Posner, M.I. (2000). Cognitive and emotional influences in anterior cingulate cortex. *Trends in Cognitive Science, 4*, 215–222.

Cakmakci, H., Pekcevik, Y., Yis, U., Unalp, A., & Kurul, S. (2009). Diagnostic value of proton MR spectroscopy and diffusion–weighted MR imaging in childhood inherited neurometabolic brain diseases and review of the literature. *European Journal of Radiology, 74*(3), e61–71.

Carter, C.S., Braver, T.S., Barch, D.M., Botvinick, M.M., Noll, D., & Cohen, J.D. (1998). Anterior cingulate cortex, error detection, and the online monitoring of performance. *Science, 280*, 747–749.

Cecil, K.M., & Kos, R.S. (2006). Magnetic resonance spectroscopy and metabolic imaging in white matter diseases and pediatric disorders. *Top Magnetic Resonance Imaging, 17*, 293.

Chawla, S.C., Federman, N., Zhang, D., Nagata, K., Nuthakki, S., McNitt–Gray, M., & Boechat, M.I. (2010). Estimated cumulative radiation dose from PET/CT in children with malignancies: A 5–year retrospective review. *Pediatric Radiology*, *40*, 681–686.

Craig, A.D. (2009). How do you feel — now? The anterior insula and human awareness. *Nature Reviews Neuroscience*, *10*, 59–70.

Christ, S.E., Moffitt, A.J., & Peck, D. (2010). Disruption of prefrontal function and connectivity in individuals with phenylketonuria. *Molecular Genetics and Metabolism*, *99* (1), S33–40.

Critchley, H.D., Wiens, S., Rotshtein, P., Ohman, A., & Dolan, R.J. (2004). Neural systems supporting interoceptive awareness. *Nature Reviews Neuroscience*, *7*, 189–195.

Crossman, A.R., & Neary, D. (2010). *Neuroanatomy: An illustrated colour text* (42nd ed.). Philadelphia, PA: Churchill Livingstone.

Cubillo. A., Halari, R., Ecker, C., Giampietro, V., Taylor, E., & Rubia, K. (2010). Reduced activation and inter–regional functional connectivity of fronto–striatal networks in adults with childhood attention–deficit/hyperactivity disorder (ADHD) and persisting symptoms during tasks of motor inhibition and cognitive switching. *Journal of Psychiatric Research*, *44*(10), 629–39.

Damiano, C., Churches, O., Ring, H., & Baron–Cohen, S. (2011) The development of perceptual expertise for faces and objects in autism spectrum conditions. *Autism Research*, *4*(4), 297–301.

Detre, J.A. (2004). FMRI: Applications in epilepsy. *Epilepsia*, *45*(4), 26–31.

Devinsky, O., Morrell, M.J., & Vogt, B.A., (1995). Contributions of anterior cingulate cortex to behaviour. *Brain*, *118*, 279–306.

Dubroff, J.G., & Newberg, A. (2008). Neuroimaging of traumatic brain injury. *Seminars in Neurology*, *28*(4), 548–57.

Duncan, J. (2009). The current status of neuroimaging for epilepsy. *Current Opinions in Neurology*, *22*(2), 179–84.

Dziobek, I., Bahnemann, M., Convit, A., & Heekeren, H.R. (2010). The role of the fusiform–amygdala system in the pathophysiology of autism. *Archives of General Psychiatry*, *67*(4), 397–405.

Freilich, E.R., & Gaillard, W.D. (2010). Utility of functional MRI in pediatric neurology. *Current Neurological Neuroscience Reports*, *10*(1), 40–6.

Gaillard, W.D., Berl, M.M., Duke, E.S., Ritzl, E., Miranda, S., Liew C., ... Theodore, W.H. (2011). fMRI language dominance and FDG–PET hypometabolism. *Neurology*, *76*(15), 1322–9.

Gaillard, W.D., Berl, M.M., Moore, E.N., Ritzl, E.K., Rosenberger, L.R, Weinstein, S.L., ... Theodore, W.H. (2007). Atypical language in lesional and non-lesional complex partial epilepsy. *Neurology*, *69*(18), 1761–71.

Giedd, J.N., & Rapoport, J.L. (2010). Structural MRI of pediatric brain development: What have we learned and where are we going? *Neuron*, *67*(5), 728–734.

Giedd, J.N., Stockman, M., Weddle, C., Liverpool, M., Alexander–Bloch, A., Wallace, G.L., ... Lenroot, R.K. (2010). Anatomic magnetic resonance imaging of the developing child and adolescent brain and effects of genetic variation. *Neuropsychological Review*, *20*(4), 349–61.

Goldberg, S. (2010). *Clinical neuroanatomy made ridiculously simple* (42nd ed.). Miami, FL: Medmaster.

Greene, C.M., Braet, W., Johnson, K.A., & Bellgrove, M.A. (2008). Imaging the genetics of executive function. *Biological Psychology*, *79*(1), 30–42.

Gropman, A. (2010). Brain imaging in urea cycle disorders. *Molecular Genetics and Metabolism*, *100*, S20–S30.

Guye, M., Bartolomei, F., & Ranjeva, J.P. (2008). Imaging structural and functional connectivity: Towards a unified definition of human brain organization? *Current Opinions in Neurology*, *213*, 93–403

Hall, E.J., & Brenner, D.J. (2008). Cancer risks from diagnostic radiology. *British Journal of Radiology*, *81*, 362–378.

Hoisington, L., Miller, R.A., & Vreibel, B. (1998). Fast FLAIR techniques in MR imaging of the brain. *Radiologic Technology*, *69*, 351–357

Huttenlocher, P.R. (1991). Dendritic and synaptic pathology in mental retardation. *Pediatric Neurology*, *7*, 79–85.

Insausti, R., Cebada–Sánchez, S., & Marcos, P. (2010). Postnatal development of the human hippocampal formation. *Advances in Anatomy, Embryology, and Cell Biology*, *206*, 1–86.

Jafari–Khouzani, K., Elisevich, K., Karvelis, K.C., & Soltanian–Zadeh, H. (2011). Quantitative multi-compartmental SPECT image analysis for lateralization of temporal lobe epilepsy. *Epilepsy Research*, *95*(1–2), 35–50.

Jea, A., Vachhrajani, S., Widjaja, E., Nilsson, D., Raybaud, C., Shroff, M., & Rutka, J.T. (2008). Corpus callosotomy in children and the disconnection syndromes: A review. *Child's Nervous System*, *24*(6), 685–92.

Johnston, M.V. (2009). Plasticity in the developing brain: Implications for rehabilitation. *Developmental Disabilities Research Review*, *15*(2), 94–101.

Kidwell, C.S., Chalela, J.A., Saver, J.L., Starkman, S., Hill, M.D., Demchuk, A.M., ... Warach, S. (2004). Comparison of MRI and CT for Detection of Acute Intracerebral Hemorrhage. *Journal of the American Medical Association*, *292*(15), 1823–1830.

Kim, S., Salamon, N., Jackson, H.A., Blüml, S., & Panigrahy, A. (2010). PET imaging in pediatric neuroradiology: Current and future applications. *Pediatric Radiology*, *40*(1), 82–96.

Kleinhans, N.M., Richards, T., Weaver, K., Johnson, L.C., Greenson, J., Dawson, G., & Aylward, E. (2010). Association between amygdala response to emotional faces and social anxiety in autism spectrum disorders. *Neuropsychologia*, *48*(12), 3665–70.

Koch, D., & Wagner, W. (2004). Endoscopic third ventriculostomy in infants of less than one year of age: Which factors influence the outcome? *Child's Nervous System*, *20*, 405–411.

Kou, Z., Wu, Z., Tong, K.A., Holshouser, B., Benson, R.R., Hu, J., & Haacke, E.M. (2010). The role of advanced MR imaging findings as biomarkers of traumatic brain injury. *Journal of Head Trauma Rehabilitation*, *25*(4), 267–82.

Kuhl, P., & Rivera-Gaxiola, M. (2008). Neural substrates of language acquisition. *Annual Review of Neuroscience*, *31*, 511–34.

Lewine, J.D., Davis, J.T., Bigler, E.D., Thoma, R., Hill, D., Funke, M., Sloan, J.H., ... Orrison, W.W. (2007). Objective documentation of traumatic brain injury subsequent to mild head trauma: Multimodal brain imaging with MEG, SPECT, and MRI. *Journal of Head Trauma Rehabilitation*, *22*(3), 141–55.

Liégeois, F., Cross, J.H., Polkey, C., Harkness, W., & Vargha–Khadem, F. (2008). Language after hemispherectomy in childhood: Contributions from memory and intelligence. *Neuropsychologia, 46*(13), 3101–7.

Liégeois, F., Morgan, A.T., Stewart, L.H., Helen Cross, J., Vogel, A.P., & Vargha–Khadem, F. (2010). Speech and oral motor profile after childhood hemispherectomy. *Brain Language, 114*(2), 126–34.

Limbrick, D.D., Narayan, P., Powers, A.K., Ojemann, J.G., Park, T.S., Bertrand, M., & Smyth, M.D. (2009). Hemispherotomy: Efficacy and analysis of seizure recurrence. *Journal of Neurosurgical Pediatrics, 4*(4), 323–32.

Lin, J.S., Lew, S.M., Marcuccilli, C.J., Mueller, W.M., Matthews, A.E., Koop, J.I., & Zupanc, M.L. (2011). Corpus callosotomy in multistage epilepsy surgery in the pediatric population. *Journal of Neurosurgical Pediatrics, 7*(2), 189–200.

Llinás, R.R., Ribary, U., Jeanmonod, D., Kronberg, E., & Mitra, P.P. (1999). Thalamocortical dysrhythmia: A neurological and neuropsychiatric syndrome characterized by magnetoencephalography. Proceedings of the *National Academy of Sciences USA, 96*(26), 15222–15227 .

Lodygensky, G.A., Vasung, L., Sizonenko, S.V., & Hüppi, P.S. (2010). Neuroimaging of cortical development and brain connectivity in human newborns and animal models. *Journal of Anatomy, 217*(4), 418–28. doi: 10.1111/j.1469–7580.2010.01280.x.

Lorson, C.L., Rindt, H., & Shababi, M. (2010). Spinal muscular atrophy: Mechanisms and therapeutic strategies. *Human Molecular Genetics, 15*(19, R1), R111–8.

Maria, B.L. (2008) *Current management in child neurology.* (4th ed.). Shelton, CT: PMPH-USA

Mbwana, J., Berl, M.M., Ritzl, E.K., Rosenberger, L., Mayo, J., Weinstein, S., … Gaillard, W.D. (2009). Limitations to plasticity of language network reorganization in localization related epilepsy. *Brain, 132*(Pt 2), 347–56.

McTague, A, & Appleton, R. (2011). Treatment of difficult epilepsy. *Archives of Diseases in Childhood, 96*(2), 200–4.

Mochida, G.H. (2009). Genetics and biology of microcephaly and lissencephaly. *Seminars in Pediatric Neurology, 16*(3), 120–6.

Ospina, L.H. (2009). Cortical visual impairment. *Pediatric Review, 30*(11), e81–90.

Paakki, J.J., Rahko, J., Long, X., Moilanen, I., Tervonen, O., Nikkinen, J., … Kiviniemi, V. (2010). Alterations in regional homogeneity of resting–state brain activity in autism spectrum disorders. *Brain Research 1321,* 169–179.

Panigrahy, A., Nelson, M.D. Jr, & Blüml. S, (2010). Magnetic resonance spectroscopy in pediatric neuroradiology: Clinical and research applications. *Pediatric Radiology, 40*(1), 3–30.

Pfeuffer, J., Tkac, I., Provencher, S.W., & Gruetter, R. (1999). Toward an in vivo neurochemical profile: quantification of 18 metabolites in short–echo–time (1) H NMR spectra of the rat brain. *Journal of Magnetic Resonance, 141,* 104–120.

Pitt, M. (2011). Paediatric electromyography in the modern world: A personal view. *Developmental Medicine and Child Neurology, 53*(2), 120–4. doi: 10.1111/j.1469–8749.2010.03831.x.

Rodriguez–Peña, A., Ibarrola, N., Iñiguez, M.A., Muñoz, A., & Bernal, J. (1993). Neonatal hypothyroidism affects the timely expression of myelin–associated glycoprotein in the rat brain. *Journal of Clinical Investigations, 91,* 812–818.

Rosenberger, L.R., Zeck, J., Berl, M.M., Moore, E.N., Ritzl, E.K., Shamim, S., … Gaillard, W.D. (2009). Interhemispheric and intrahemispheric language reorganization in complex partial epilepsy. *Neurology, 72*(21), 1830–6.

Ross, B.D., & Bluml, S. (1996). New aspects of brain physiology. *NMR in Biomedicine, 9,* 279–296.

Rubia, K., Halari, R., Cubillo, A., Smith, A.B., Mohammad, A.M., Brammer, M, & Taylor, E. (2011) Methylphenidate normalizes fronto–striatal underactivation during interference inhibition in medication–Naïve boys with attention–deficit/hyperactivity disorder. *Neuropsychopharmacology,* Mar 30.

Ruggiero, C., Cinalli, G., Spennato, P., Aliberti, F., Cianciulli, E., Trischitta, V., & Maggi, G. (2004). Endoscopic third ventriculostomy in the treatment of hydrocephalus in posterior fossa tumors in children. *Child's Nervous System, 20,* 828–833.

Saito, Y. (2009). Reflections on the brainstem dysfunction in neurologically disabled children. *Brain Development, 31*(7), 529–36.

Sandberg, D.I. (2008). Endoscopic management of hydrocephalus in pediatric patients: A review of indications, techniques, and outcomes. *Journal of Child Neurology, 23*(5), 550–60.

Schenone, A., Nobbio, L., Monti Bragadin, M., Ursino, G., & Grandis, M. (2011). Inherited neuropathies. *Current Treatment Options in Neurology, 13*(2), 160–79.

Shore, R.M. (2008). Positron emission tomography/computed tomography (PET/CT) in children. *Pediatric Annals, 37*(6), 404–12.

Siegal, M., & Varley, R. (2006). Aphasia, language, and theory of mind. *Society for Neuroscience, 1*(3–4), 167–74.

Spalice, A., Parisi, P., Nicita, F., Pizzardi, G., Del Balzo, F., & Iannetti, P. (2009). Neuronal migration disorders: clinical, neuroradiologic and genetics aspects. *Acta Paediatrica, 98*(3), 421–33.

Squire, L.R., Berg, D., Bloom, F., Du Lac, S., & Ghosh, A. (2006). *Fundamental neuroscience.* (3rd ed.). Salt Lake City, UT: Academic Press.

Sullivan, J.E., 3rd, Corcoran–Donnelly, M., & Dlugos, D.J. (2007). Challenges in pediatric video–EEG monitoring. *American Journal of Electroneurodiagnostic Technology, 47*(2), 127–39.

Sun, Y.F., Lee, J.S., & Kirby, R. (2010). Brain imaging findings in dyslexia. *Pediatrics & Neonatology 51*(2), 89–96. Review. Erratum in: *Pediatrics & Neonatology, 51*(3), 193.

Sunaga, S., Shimizu, H., & Sugano, H. (2009). Long–term follow–up of seizure outcomes after corpus callosotomy. *Seizure, 18*(2), 124–8.

Suskauer, S.J., & Huisman, T.A. (2009). Neuroimaging in pediatric traumatic brain injury: Current and future predictors of functional outcome. *Developmental Disabilities Research Review, 15*(2), 117–23.

Swaiman, K.F., Ashwal, S., & Ferriero, D.M. (2006) *Pediatric neurology: Principles and practice* (4th ed.). Maryland Heights, MO: Mosby.

Tanaka, T., & Gleeson, J.G. (2000). Genetics of brain development and malformation syndromes. *Current Opinion in Pediatrics, 12,* 523–528.

Tassëel Ponche, S., Ferrapie, A.L., Chenet, A., Menei, P., Gambart, G., Ménégalli Bogeli, D., … Richard, I. (2010). Intrathecal baclofen in cerebral palsy. A retrospective study of 25 wheelchair–assisted adults. *Annals of Physical Rehabilitation Medicine, 53*(8), 483–98.

Ten Donkelaar, H.J., & Lammens, M. (2009). Development of the human cerebellum and its disorders. *Clinical Perinatology, 36*(3), 513–30.

Tilton, A. (2009). Management of spasticity in children with cerebral palsy. *Seminars in Pediatric Neurology, 16*(2), 82–9.

Tripp, G., & Wickens, J.R. (2009). Neurobiology of ADHD. *Neuropharmacology, 57*(7–8), 579–89.

Vaidya, C.J., & Stollstorff, M. (2008). Cognitive neuroscience of attention-deficit/hyperactivity disorder: Current status and working hypotheses. *Developmental Disabilities Research Review, 14*(4), 261–7.

van der Knaap, M.S., Valk, J. (2005). Pattern recognition in white matter disorders. In M.S. Van der Knaap & J. Valk (Eds.), *Magnetic resonance of myelination and myelin disorders.* (3rd ed., pp. 881-904). Berlin, Germany: Springer.

van der Knaap, M.S., Valk, J., de Neeling, N., & Nauta, J.J. (1991). Pattern recognition in magnetic resonance imaging of white matter disorders in children and young adults. *Neuroradiology, 33,* 478–493.

van der Voorn, J.P., Pouwels, P.J., Hart, A.A., Serrarens, J., Willemsen,, M.A., Kremer, H.P., … van der Knaap, M.S. (2006). Childhood white matter disorders: Quantitative MR imaging and spectroscopy. *Radiology, 241*(2), 510–7.

van Schooneveld, M.M., Jennekens–Schinkel, A., van Rijen, P.C., Braun, K.P., & van Nieuwenhuizen, O. (2011). Hemispherectomy: A basis for mental development in children with epilepsy. *Epileptic Disorders, 13*(1), 47–55.

Varghese, G.I., Purcaro, M.J., Motelow, J.E., Enev, M., McNally, K.A., Levin, A.R., … Blumenfeld, H. (2009). Clinical use of ictal SPECT in secondarily generalized tonic–clonic seizures. *Brain, 132*(Pt 8), 2102–13.

Vazquez, E., & Mayolas, N. (2008). Developmental abnormalities of temporal lobe in children. *Seminars in Ultrasound CT MR, 29*(1), 15–39.

Verbruggen, K.T., Meiners, L.C., Sijens, P.E., Lunsing, R.J., van Spronsen, F.J., & Brouwer, O.F. (2009). Magnetic resonance imaging and proton magnetic resonance spectroscopy of the brain in the diagnostic evaluation of developmental delay. *European Journal of Paediatric Neurology, 13*(2), 181–190.

Verrotti, A., Spalice, A., Ursitti, F., Papetti, L., Mariani, R., Castronovo, A., … Iannetti, P. (2010). New trends in neuronal migration disorders. *European Journal of Paediatric Neurology, 14*(1), 1–12.

Vogel, A.C., Power, J.D., Petersen, S.E., & Schlaggar, B.L. (2010). Development of the brain's functional network architecture. *Neuropsychological Review, 20*(4), 362–75.

Volpe, J.J. (2008). *Neurology of the newborn* (54th ed.). Philadelphia, PA: W.B. Saunders.

Welsh, R.C., Chen, A.C., & Taylor, S.F. (2010). Low-frequency BOLD fluctuations demonstrate altered thalamocortical connectivity in schizophrenia. *Schizophrenia Bulletin, 36*(4), 713–722.

Waxman, S.G., & de Groot, J. (2009). *Correlative Neuroanatomy* (26th ed.). Norwalk, CT: Appleton and Lange. McGraw-Hill Medical.

Wee, C.D., Kong, L, & Sumner, C.J. (2010). The genetics of spinal muscular atrophies. *Current Opinions in Neurology, 23*(5), 450–458.

Xu, V., Chan, H., Lin, A.P., Sailasuta, N., Valencerina, S., Tran, T., … , Ross, B.D. (2008). MR spectroscopy in diagnosis and neurological decision–making. *Seminars in Neurology, 28,* 407–422.

Yim, S.Y., Lee, I.Y., Park, C.H., Sailasuta, N., Valencerina, S., Tran, T., … Ross, B.D. (2000). A qualitative analysis of brain SPECT for prognostication of the gross motor development in children with cerebral palsy. *Clinical Nuclear Medicine, 25*(4), 268–272.

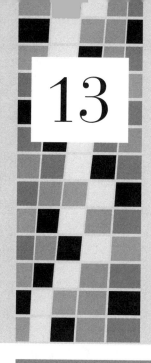

13

Muscles, Bones, and Nerves

Peter B. Kang

Upon completion of this chapter, the reader will

- Understand how the neuromuscular and musculoskeletal systems function and are integrated

- Recognize common signs and symptoms of neuromuscular and musculoskeletal disorders

- Be familiar with some of the most common neuromuscular and musculoskeletal diseases of childhood and their treatments

---

■ ■ ■ CASE REPORT

A 4-month-old female infant is brought in to be evaluated and treated for concerns of floppiness and poor weight gain. She was born full-term after an uncomplicated gestation, but her parents report that she feeds poorly and that milk sometimes pools in her mouth. During the examination, she has a weak cry and has trouble lifting her head from the exam table. Her muscle tone seems diminished when she is picked up, both in vertical and prone positions.

1. What should be the overall assessment of this case?

2. Does this infant appear to have a central nervous system or peripheral nervous system disease? What features of the clinical presentation help sort this out?

3. What categories of disease merit the greatest concern?

4. What types of therapies would be applicable to this case, regardless of the underlying diagnosis?

COMPONENTS OF THE NEUROMUSCULAR AND MUSCULOSKELETAL SYSTEMS

The neuromuscular system is the neurological network that connects the brain and spinal cord to the musculoskeletal system. It consists of 1) the **anterior horn cells** (lower motor neurons) in the spinal cord, 2) the peripheral nerves in the extremities, 3) the **neuromuscular junction** (which joins the nerves and muscles), and 4) the skeletal muscles (Figure 13.1). The musculoskeletal system consists of the skeletal muscles, tendons, bones, joints, and ligaments.

In order for a muscle to produce voluntary movement across a joint, an electrical signal originates in the cortex of the brain (within an

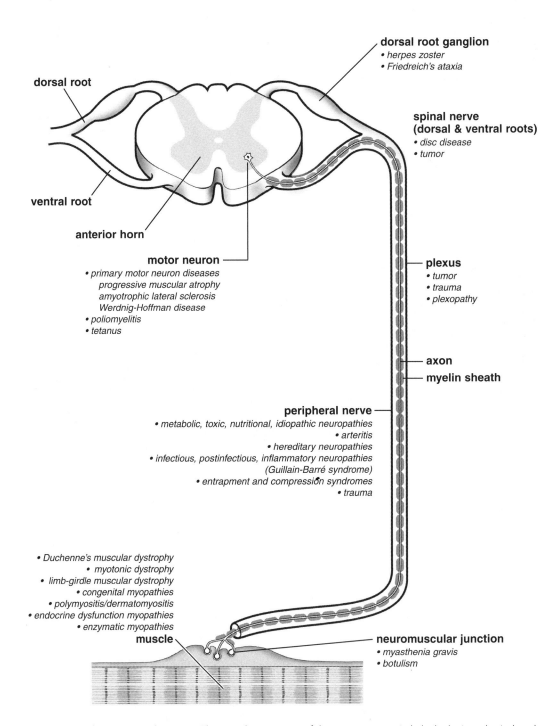

Figure 13.1. The neuromuscular system. The central components of the nervous system include the brain and spinal cord. Descending corticospinal pathways carry signals from the brain through the spinal cord to motor neurons in the anterior horns of the spinal cord. The motor neurons are generally regarded as being the first segment of the peripheral nervous system. Signals are transmitted from the motor neurons down the peripheral nerves, then across the neuromuscular junction to skeletal muscle. These signals initiate muscle contraction, leading to movement of the musculoskeletal system. Sensory signals are transmitted from the sensory nerves to the spinal cord, and then to the brain, which continuously integrates this information to monitor the state of the environment and the neuromuscular and musculoskeletal systems.

upper motor neuron), then passes through the spinal cord to an anterior horn cell whose axon extends down a peripheral nerve until the axon ends at a neuromuscular junction. The electrical impulse jumps across the gap (synapse) at this junction, using the neurotransmitter acetylcholine. The acetylcholine binds to receptors in the muscle fiber; these receptors generate a new electrical signal and stimulate the muscle to contract. The **sarcomere** is the basic contractile unit in the muscle fiber; it is composed of a number of proteins that bind to each other in a dynamic manner. As the musculoskeletal system moves (e.g., during walking), signals are sent to the brain through the sensory system, providing information about the body's position in space.

The main function of skeletal muscle is to contract by shortening, thereby causing the limbs to move across joints. **Agonist** muscles reinforce each others' movements, while antagonist muscles oppose one another. For example, when an individual flexes an arm at the elbow, the biceps contracts, as does the **brachialis**; the triceps, however, relaxes. If all these muscles contracted simultaneously, the arm would be held stiffly in an **isometric contraction** (i.e., muscular contraction against resistance in which the length of the muscle remains the same). Thus, when the brain tells the arm to move, it generates contraction of some muscles and relaxation of others.

The bones of the skeleton form the body's internal scaffolding. They range in size from the ½-inch-long **phalanges** (bones of the finger) to the **femur** (thigh bone), which is roughly 18 inches long in adults. As growth takes place and the bone is subject to different stresses, the bone responds by changing its shape, a process called remodeling. These changes usually increase the tensile strength and stability of the bone, making it less susceptible to fracture. On average, a given portion of a child's bone turns over around once annually. In an adult, the reshaping continues even though growth has stopped. The average bone segment of an adult turns over about every 7 years.

Together, the neuromuscular and musculoskeletal systems are responsible for our ability to sit, stand, and move; impairments of these systems are major causes of developmental disability in childhood. This chapter explores how to recognize the signs and symptoms of neuromuscular and musculoskeletal disorders, and how an integrated health care and school system can improve the lives of children affected by such disorders.

SYMPTOMS AND SIGNS OF NEUROMUSCULAR AND MUSCULOSKELETAL DISORDERS

Respiratory and Cardiac Issues

In most cases, respiratory and cardiac issues do not arise from neuromuscular or musculoskeletal disorders. But in rare instances, they may be early manifestations of such conditions. Examples include late-onset Pompe disease (a genetic lysosomal storage disorder), in which respiratory distress is an early symptom, and Becker muscular dystrophy, in which cardiomyopathy is sometimes the first sign of disease. Some neuromuscular disorders affect the respiratory muscles, resulting in an abnormal sleep pattern or sleep apnea (brief periods of respiratory arrest). These children may suffer from daytime somnolence and often appear fatigued or easily distractible.

Muscle Bulk, Tone, and Strength

Pseudohypertrophy (abnormal muscle enlargement), especially of the calves and in conjunction with weakness, may be a sign of Duchenne muscular dystrophy (DMD). Muscle atrophy is found in neuropathies such as Charcot-Marie-Tooth disease (CMT), but may also be seen in some myopathies and muscular dystrophies.

It is important to differentiate between tone abnormalities and strength abnormalities. Tone is the muscle's passive ability to respond to stretch, whereas strength represents the force that the muscle exerts actively. Children can have **hypertonia** (high tone and an overreactive response to a normal stimulus) or **hypotonia** (low tone, with a lesser response to a stimulus). Many neuromuscular or musculoskeletal disorders are linked to disturbances in tone. Hypertonia and spasticity are seen primarily in central nervous system (CNS) disorders, which affect the upper motor neuron or its axons in the brain and spine, whereas hypotonia can be seen not only in lesions of the CNS (upper motor neuron), but also in peripheral nervous system (lower motor neuron) involvement. In infants, preserved strength in the setting of hypotonia is usually associated with a central nervous system process, whereas weakness in conjunction with hypotonia is usually associated with a peripheral nervous system process.

Muscle weakness may be **proximal** (involving muscles or body segments closer to the center of the body) or **distal** (involving muscles or body segments farther from the center of the body). Proximal muscle weakness affects the shoulder and hip girdle muscles (often seen in **myopathies**, which are primary disorders of muscle); children with weak shoulder girdle muscles have difficulty reaching objects on a high shelf, climbing jungle gyms, or doing push-ups. Testing the ability of the child to grasp and manipulate objects demonstrates selective control, a skill necessary to operate hand controls; children with distal muscle weakness may thus have trouble holding a pen or pencil, finishing long writing activities on time, or using scissors. Proximal or distal lower extremity weakness often causes gait abnormalities (see following sections).

Sensation

Sensory symptoms such as numbness, **paresthesias** (skin sensations: e.g., burning, prickling, itching, tingling), and pain may result from disorders of the peripheral sensory nerves (e.g., peripheral neuropathies) or from CNS disorders. Sensory nerve fibers tell the brain where the body is in space, so these children may have an **ataxia**, clumsy gait, or even feel unsteady in the dark, requiring visual input for balance.

Scoliosis, Kyphosis, and Lordosis

Scoliosis is a lateral curvature of the spinal column; **kyphosis** is an excessive anterior (forward) curvature of the spine; and **lordosis** is an excessive posterior (backward) curvature. Isolated scoliosis in an otherwise healthy child or adolescent is usually not associated with a neuromuscular or musculoskeletal condition. **Idiopathic** scoliosis occurs frequently during the adolescent growth spurt, especially in females. However, scoliosis, kyphosis, lordosis, or a combination of these may be complications of numerous neuromuscular and musculoskeletal disorders. The appearance of these abnormalities in a younger child or of one of them in conjunction with other concerning findings should prompt careful evaluation.

Because spinal curves are best managed before they become severe, the spine of a child at greater risk (e.g., a child with meningomyelocele or muscular dystrophy) should be examined regularly. Early clues suggesting scoliosis are unequal heights of the shoulders or a slanting of the waist. Also, as the ribs attach to the thoracic (upper) spine, they may follow the curve of the vertebrae, causing a rib rise or "rib hump" when the child bends forward. School screening examinations for scoliosis are designed to look for these physical findings to detect scoliosis as early as possible.

Contractures and Gait Abnormalities

If a neuromuscular or musculoskeletal disorder prevents full range of motion around a joint for a prolonged period of time, a joint **contracture** (shortening of the soft tissue around a joint) can develop, resulting in a fixed loss of joint motion. In an ankle joint contracture, the Achilles tendon shortens and the child walks on his or her toes. Toe-walking, limping, walking with a wide-based gait, or other gait abnormalities should prompt medical evaluation.

In an ambulatory child, observing the gait pattern is a valuable part of the physical examination. During normal gait, the head and trunk should be level, with minimal sway from side to side. The child should be able to maintain balance while standing on one leg and swinging the opposite leg through. The leg that is swinging should clear the ground, and the foot should not drag.

Strong pelvic muscles are needed for the child to rise from a seated position and to climb stairs. Children with hip girdle weakness often need to pull on a handrail to walk up steps or to push off with their hands in order to rise from a chair. To get up from the floor, such children often use a Gowers maneuver: first they turn to face the floor, then use their hands on the floor to support part of their weight as they straighten their knees, and finally they push their hands on their thighs to achieve an erect posture.

Distal muscle weakness (often seen in neuropathies, which are primary disorders of peripheral nerves) affects the hands and feet (i.e., distal extremities). These children may trip and fall frequently because they cannot lift their feet or toes when walking. They also may not be able to walk on their heels and may "slap" their feet while walking (a condition called *foot drop*). Orthotic devices may stabilize distal leg weakness and lessen the frequency and severity of falls.

Joint Abnormalities

Range of motion is passive, so the patient should be relaxed while the examiner moves the extremities. The upper extremities should be examined for range of motion of the shoulders, elbows, and hands. The examiner should be able to lift the arms above the head. The elbows should straighten fully. All fingers should be able to be straightened and brought out of the palm.

The hip exam, like the spine exam, should be performed often, as early treatment of hip problems gives the best outcome. The examiner should be able to **abduct** (spread apart) the hips easily and symmetrically. Loss of hip abduction may indicate a hip dislocation or **subluxation**. Another means of assessing whether the hip is dislocated is to look at the knee heights with the hips and knees flexed and the ankles together.

The knee must be straight for standing but must flex to 90 degrees for comfortable sitting and flex even farther for easy stair climbing. Tightness of the hamstring muscles can limit knee movement and impair the ability to stand.

The ankle should be examined for **plantarflexion** (downward motion of the foot) and **dorsiflexion** (upward movement of the foot). The ability to dorsiflex beyond a neutral position is important for both walking and sitting and should be tested with the knee both extended and flexed. A child should be able to maintain the feet in a **plantargrade** (flat on the floor) position while walking, and maintain as much flexibility in the feet as possible.

LABORATORY TESTING AND RADIOGRAPHY

Serum Testing

Muscle enzymes are some of the most useful laboratory tests in the evaluation of potential neuromuscular disorders. The most well-known of these is the creatine phosphokinase (CPK), also known as the creatine kinase (CK) level. Aldolase is also useful as an adjunctive muscle enzyme marker. Three liver enzymes, alanine aminotransferase (ALT), aspartate aminotransferase (AST), and lactate dehydrogenase (LDH), are also found in small quantities in muscle and may show mild elevations in some muscle diseases, especially muscular dystrophy.

Genetic Testing

Genetic testing has been a boon to diagnosing inherited diseases, including neuromuscular and musculoskeletal disorders, and is sparing an increasing number of patients from invasive and painful diagnostic procedures such as electromyography and biopsies (see following sections). However, genetic testing can mislead, especially when the ordering physician is unsure how to interpret ambiguous genetic test results or does not interpret such results in the clinical context.

Electrophysiology

Nerve conduction studies and **electromyography** (EMG, a recording of electric currents associated with muscle contractions) are useful in diagnosing a variety of neuromuscular disorders, including anterior horn cell disease, neuropathies, neuromuscular junction disorders, and some myopathies. Advances in genetic testing and immunohistochemistry of biopsy specimens has resulted in changed distribution of pediatric patients who are referred for these studies (Darras et al., 2000). In particular, Duchenne and Becker muscular dystrophies are now primarily diagnosed with genetic testing and these patients are rarely referred to the EMG laboratory. Spinal muscular atrophy is usually diagnosed with genetic testing now, though in some instances where the diagnosis must be confirmed rapidly, EMG still plays a significant role in evaluating these patients. EMG, especially in children, is technically demanding, and should be performed only by an electromyographer experienced in performing these studies in children. This is important both for diagnostic accuracy and for the comfort of the child, as the procedure involves electrical stimulations during the nerve conduction studies, followed by needle examination of the muscle.

Biopsy

Muscle, nerve, and skin biopsies have traditionally been essential to the diagnosis of many neuromuscular and musculoskeletal disorders. Genetic testing, however, has changed the profile of patients who are referred for these tests; patients with Duchenne and Becker muscular dystrophies rarely need muscle biopsies anymore as they can usually be diagnosed by identification of mutations in blood. Advances in genetics and biochemistry also have enhanced the sophistication of biopsy interpretation, as immunohistochemistry of biopsy sections can detect protein deficiencies that may indicate a specific genetic defect.

Radiography

Abnormal musculoskeletal exam findings can be illuminated by plain x rays of the involved areas, which can help detect movement limitations caused by bony deformity. X rays are helpful in detecting the shapes of bones but are a poor gauge of the quality of bone because bone loss will not be apparent until at least one third of the bone has been lost. Bone density is best measured by a bone density scan.

Ultrasonography and magnetic resonance imaging (MRI) have only recently been applied to the evaluation of possible muscle disorders, but certain myopathies show distinct patterns of muscle involvement that may be detected by such methods (Jungbluth et al., 2004). These tests have the potential to spare some children from undergoing invasive diagnostic procedures such as muscle biopsy.

DISORDERS OF THE NEUROMUSCULAR SYSTEM

Anterior Horn Cells: Spinal Muscular Atrophy

The nerve cells (neurons) in the spinal column that control movement are called anterior horn cells. In the past, the most well-known disease associated with damage to the anterior horn cell was paralytic poliomyelitis. Fortunately, thanks to the polio vaccine, this viral illness is rare, though not extinct due to pockets of persistent infection in certain developing countries. A handful of children in the United States adopted from these countries have motor difficulties that are highly suspicious for prior poliomyelitis infection (McMillan et al., 2009).

Currently, the most common disorder affecting the anterior horn cell in children is **spinal muscular atrophy** (SMA; Darras et al., 2007). SMA is characterized by degeneration of α-motor neurons in the brainstem and spinal cord, leading to progressive weakness that is nearly always predominantly proximal (involving the muscles closest to the trunk) and symmetrical; intelligence is preserved (von Gontard et al., 2002). Most cases are associated with homozygous deletions in the *SMN1* gene, making this an autosomal recessive disorder (Lefebvre et al., 1995; Melki et al., 1994). Currently, SMA is the most common inherited cause of death in infancy, with an estimated incidence of 1 in 6,000 to 1 in 10,000 live births (Merlini et al., 1992; Pearn, 1978; Pearn, 1973).

SMA has traditionally been divided into three clinical variants, based primarily on the milestones attained. Patients with SMA I (previously known as Werdnig-Hoffman disease) have onset typically before 6 months of age and are never able to sit or walk. In SMA II, patients sit at some point during childhood but never walk, and the onset is usually between 6 and 18 months. Patients with SMA III are able to sit and walk, and usually have onset of motor difficulties after 18 months of age but before adulthood.

Infants with SMA I develop diffuse hypotonia and weakness with **areflexia** (lack of deep tendon reflexes). Swallowing and breathing difficulties are serious, life-threatening complications that may occur at any time. Without interventions, affected children rarely survive beyond 2 years of age and often die much earlier. More recently, the placement of gastrostomy feeding tubes and respiratory interventions, including both noninvasive and invasive options, have become more common in these children, extending their life expectancy, sometimes for years. If a gastrostomy tube is to be placed, it should be done as early as possible. Lung interventions may include pulmonary toilet, supplemental oxygen, noninvasive pressure support, and tracheostomy with full mechanical ventilation. Families and physicians should decide collaboratively on a treatment plan based on their ethical judgment about the quality of life they feel is best.

Infants and toddlers with SMA II typically present with hypotonia, areflexia, and delayed motor milestones. They are also susceptible to difficulties swallowing and breathing, but these complications tend to occur later and progress more slowly than in SMA I. Nutritional and respiratory therapies are similar to those used in SMA I. Scoliosis is a frequent and disabling complication in these children, for which spine surgery is often helpful. Depending on the severity of the individual case and the level of intervention, life expectancy ranges from late childhood through early adulthood.

Children with SMA III often present with gait difficulties, proximal weakness, and areflexia, sometimes severe enough to cause delayed motor milestones. The weakness is almost always symmetrical, though some exceptions have been described (Kang et al., 2006). Hypotonia, while present, is not as prominent a feature. Difficulties swallowing and breathing are rare, and life expectancy is usually not affected.

Disorders of the Peripheral Nerves: Charcot-Marie-Tooth Disease

The terms *neuropathy* and *peripheral neuropathy* are general terms that imply that some damage to the nerve has occurred. Neuropathies may be motor, sensory, or sensorimotor (a combination of the two). The term *mononeuropathy* implies that only a single nerve is damaged, whereas *polyneuropathy* refers to a generalized process that affects all or most nerves, albeit with varying degrees of severity. Because acute autoimmune neuropathy (Guillain-Barré syndrome) usually does not lead to prolonged disability, it will not be discussed in detail here.

Charcot-Marie-Tooth (CMT) disease is the most common inherited polyneuropathy, affecting 1 in 2,500 individuals in the United States. An alternative term for this disorder, *hereditary motor and sensory neuropathy* (HMSN), has been recently introduced. CMTs are classified based on their inheritance pattern (autosomal dominant or recessive) and physiology (demyelinating or axonal). **Demyelination** refers to a disease process in which the myelin insulation surrounding nerve axons is stripped off, whereas axonal loss refers to a process where the axons themselves degenerate. The major categories of polyneuropathies are CMT1 (dominant, demyelinating), CMT2 (dominant, axonal), CMT4 (recessive, demyelinating), and AR CMT2 (axonal, recessive). Déjerine-Sottas disease was previously known as CMT3, and is a rare, early-onset form of CMT. The most common form of CMT is CMT1A, which is caused by a duplication in the *PMP22* gene (Lupski et al., 1991). Hereditary neuropathy with liability to pressure palsies (HNPP) is a related disorder in which patients are susceptible to compression neuropathies after minor trauma. HNPP is typically caused by a deletion of the *PMP22* gene rather than a duplication.

Onset of CMT depends on the specific type and may occur at birth or not until adulthood, but many cases are diagnosed in the first two decades of life. Patients with CMT typically present with weakness and wasting of the foot and lower leg muscles, which may result in foot drop and a high-stepping gait with frequent tripping and falling. Foot deformities, such as **pes cavus** (high arches) and hammertoes (a condition in which the ends of the toes curl downward), result from weakness of the intrinsic foot muscles. Some children can present with **pes planus** (flat feet) and need arch supports. The degeneration of myelin, axons, or both, results in muscle weakness and atrophy in the extremities, and the degeneration of sensory nerves results in a reduced ability to feel heat, cold, and pain. Because of the muscle weakness, contractures develop with time, especially at the heel cords, and sometimes curvature of the spine may occur (Shy, 2004).

In general, CMT is slowly progressive, and people with most forms of CMT have a normal life expectancy. There is currently no cure, but physical therapy, occupational therapy, braces and other orthopedic devices, and orthopedic surgery can help individuals with CMT finish school, work, and live functional lives despite the disabling symptoms of the disease (Bertorini et al., 2004; McDonald, 2001; Shy, 2004).

Diseases of the Neuromuscular Junction: Myasthenia Gravis

The peripheral nerves end at the neuromuscular junction. For a nerve impulse to cross the synapse separating the nerve and muscle, the chemical neurotransmitter acetylcholine must be released from the nerve terminal, cross the space between the nerve and muscle, bind to its receptor on the muscle membrane (much like a key fitting into a keyhole), and generate the muscle membrane impulse that will transmit the signal to the contractile structures within the muscle cell. Impairment of any of these mechanisms prevents the impulse from generating muscle movement and results in disorders called myasthenic syndromes (from *myo* meaning muscle and *asthenia* meaning fatigability). In rare instances myasthenic syndromes are genetic in origin (congenital myasthenic syndrome), but they are most often acquired as autoimmune disorders. In children and adolescents, acquired autoimmune myasthenia is typically referred to as juvenile myasthenia gravis. The most common symptoms are **diplopia** (double vision), **ptosis** (drooping eyelid), **dysphagia** (difficulty swallowing), **dysarthria** (changes in voice) including nasal speech, and extremity weakness. These symptoms result from cranial nerve involvement which is almost invariably present. The symptoms tend to worsen with activity and towards the end of the day. In the most severe cases breathing may be impaired (Chiang et al., 2009).

Treatment of juvenile myasthenia gravis generally targets improving neuromuscular transmission and increasing muscle strength while suppressing the production of abnormal antibodies. Pyridostigmine is a drug that is a common first-line therapy. It is an acetylcholinesterase inhibitor, which means that it prevents acetylcholine from being metabolized at the neuromuscular junction, raising its effective levels. At high doses, pyridostigmine can cause cholinergic side effects (excessive secretions and sometimes worsening of myasthenia symptoms), but in general it is well-tolerated. Its main drawback is that it is a relatively weak therapy, and often patients will need immunomodulatory therapy as well.

There are three standard immunomodulatory therapies available for myasthenia gravis: plasmapheresis, intravenous immunoglobulin, and steroids. Plasmapheresis requires central venous access (a surgically placed central line) in younger children and others with small-caliber peripheral veins, but in older children and adolescents with large-caliber veins, the treatments may be performed through a peripheral vein (standard intravenous therapy). Intravenous immunoglobulin has also been used in some cases. Steroid therapy is perhaps the most traditional approach, but is associated with significant side effects when used on a long-term basis, especially in children and adolescents. Thymectomy is a surgical procedure that removes the **thymus**, a gland in the chest which plays a key role in regulating immune responses. This procedure appears to induce partial or complete remission in some cases of juvenile myasthenia gravis (Kogut et al., 2000).

Disorders of Muscle: Muscular Dystrophies and Myopathies

The two major categories of inherited muscle disease in childhood are the muscular dystrophies and the congenital myopathies. Muscular dystrophies are characterized by the progressive destruction of muscle tissue, whereas congenital myopathies typically involve either the abnormal accumulation of certain proteins or other developmental abnormalities in the muscle fibers. These findings can be observed on microscopic examination of skeletal muscle tissue obtained at biopsy. Muscular dystrophies tend to be progressive, whereas the clinical course in congenital myopathies varies. There is a vast array of muscular dystrophies, including limb-girdle muscular dystrophies, congenital muscular dystrophies, facioscapulohumeral muscular dystrophy, and Emery-Dreifuss muscular dystrophy. Genetic etiologies have been defined for each of these categories of disease.

Duchenne Muscular Dystrophy

Duchenne muscular dystrophy is the most common form of muscular dystrophy in childhood. It is a progressive skeletal muscle disorder caused by mutations in the X-linked *DMD* gene, resulting in the absence of dystrophin, a major muscle protein (Hoffman et al., 1987; Monaco et al., 1986). The incidence of Duchenne muscular dystrophy is approximately 1 in 3,300 male births (Jeppesen et al., 2003). This disorder is associated with a high spontaneous mutation rate (van Essen et al., 1992), so

a significant number of boys with Duchenne muscular dystrophy have no family history of the disease.

The disease manifests in early childhood, although abnormal muscle creatine phosphokinase (CPK) levels and microscopic signs of muscle damage may be observed at birth. Delayed walking and frequent falls are characteristic initial symptoms. Boys with Duchenne muscular dystrophy often walk on their tiptoes, and manifestations of proximal hip girdle muscle weakness become apparent by 3–5 years of age, when the child starts having difficulties climbing in the playground, getting up from the floor, climbing stairs, and running. Weakness in the quadriceps and gluteus maximus muscles makes it difficult to rise from the floor to a standing position, and affected boys use the Gowers maneuver to compensate. Weakness in the gluteus medius muscles leads to a Trendelenberg (waddling) gait. Pseudohypertrophy of various muscles occurs, most commonly at the calves (Figure 13.2). The term *pseudohypertrophy* is used because the enlargement is due primarily to fibrosis and fatty infiltration of muscle, rather than a true increase in muscle fiber diameter or numbers.

Accelerated deterioration in strength and balance often results from intercurrent disease

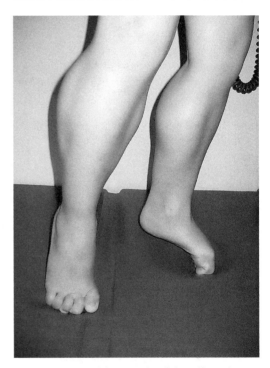

Figure 13.2. Pseudohypertrophy of the calf muscles in a 5-year-old boy with Duchenne muscular dystrophy, characterized by a deletion in *exon 45* in *DMD*, the dystrophin gene. (Courtesy of Peter B. Kang, M.D.)

or surgically induced immobilization. If tendon releases are performed, mobilization in a walking splint or cast is needed as soon as possible to prevent decrease in muscle strength from disuse. When ambulation is no longer possible, typically by the ages of 10–12 years, contractures in the lower extremities become more pronounced and may involve the shoulders. Daily physical therapy and occupational therapy services at school and daily stretching exercises at home are imperative.

Steroid treatment of Duchenne muscular dystrophy should start early, though the optimal age for initiation of this therapy remains controversial (Dubowitz et al., 2002; Kinali et al., 2002b). Oral prednisone (a steroid medication) stabilizes or improves strength and in many cases prolongs the ambulatory phase of the disease by 1–3 years (Griggs et al., 1993). The synthetic steroid Deflazacort, which is not currently approved by the U.S. Food and Drug Administration, is preferred by some clinicians and families as the side effects are milder than with prednisone in some cases. The one exception is asymptomatic cataract formation, which tends to be worse with Deflazacort (Biggar et al., 2001; Campbell et al., 2003; Moxley et al., 2005). Dietary supplements have generally been found not to improve outcome (Escolar et al., 2005).

Kyphoscoliosis may develop at any time but typically accelerates after ambulation is lost. This complication not only causes pain and postural problems, but also exacerbates pulmonary issues due to loss of effective lung volume. Baseline spine x ray images should be obtained for comparison with future studies to monitor the development of scoliosis. Using solid seat and back inserts in properly fitted wheelchairs helps slow the progression of scoliosis by keeping truncal posture erect. For some boys with Duchenne muscular dystrophy, long-leg braces can be fitted to allow braced upright standing to prevent curvature. Both manual and power wheelchairs are useful. When the kyphoscoliosis is severe enough, usually at 30–50 degrees of curvature, spinal fusion surgery with rod placement may be warranted to help preserve lung function and improve posture (Brook et al., 1996). The optimal time for surgical intervention is while lung and cardiac functioning is satisfactory (Finder et al., 2004). Failure to repair scoliosis at this point can result in increased hospitalization rates, worsening of pulmonary function, and poor quality of life (Finder et al., 2004).

Cardiac and respiratory complications are almost universal in the later stages of the disease, and one of these constitutes the immediate cause of death in most cases. Cardiac manifestations include cardiomyopathy and cardiac arrhythmias; the progression of cardiomyopathy may be slowed by the use of certain drugs. Progressive respiratory failure occurs from a combination of decreased lung capacity and function. Noninvasive ventilatory support is now commonly recommended to counteract this decline.

Lower-than-average IQ scores have been reported in individuals with Duchenne muscular dystrophy, although results have not been consistent and many children have typical cognition (Felisari et al., 2000). Certain cognitive areas such as verbal memory, digit span, and auditory comprehension are more affected than others (Hinton et al., 2000). Deletions localized in specific part of the dystrophin gene are preferentially associated with cognitive impairment (Giliberto et al., 2004). Similarly, the incidence of behavioral issues, ranging from attention-deficit/hyperactivity disorder (ADHD) to autism spectrum disorder (ASD), seems to be increased in boys with Duchenne muscular dystrophy (Hendriksen et al., 2008; Wu et al., 2005).

The life expectancy for patients with Duchenne muscular dystrophy without significant interventions was previously less than two decades. The supportive and medical therapies described above, including spinal fusion surgery, steroids, cardiac medications, and noninvasive ventilatory support, have together helped lengthen the life expectancy in many cases to the fourth decade, and in some cases to the fifth decade. Treatment by a multidisciplinary neuromuscular team is critical to implementing such a care plan.

Congenital Myopathies

Congenital myopathies usually present in infancy with marked hypotonia and weakness, feeding difficulties, and respiratory insufficiency. Within each type of congenital myopathy, there is a spectrum of severity (Dubowitz et al., 1995; Ryan et al., 2003). In contrast to muscular dystrophies, congenital myopathies are more likely to be associated with cranial nerve involvement (facial weakness, eye movement abnormalities, or both) and early respiratory complications.

The classic congenital myopathies include centronuclear myopathy (including X-linked myotubular myopathy), nemaline myopathy, central core disease, and congenital fiber type disproportion (Riggs et al., 2003). These diseases are listed in order of decreasing overall severity, although there is phenotypic overlap among these subtypes.

Causative mutations in various genes that encode structural muscle proteins, often localizing to the sarcomere, have been linked with each type of congenital myopathy. Mutations in *MTM1* gene cause myotubular myopathy (Laporte et al., 1996), and centronuclear myopathy has been associated with two genes to date: *DNM2* (Bitoun et al., 2005) and *BIN1* (Nicot et al., 2007). Nemaline myopathy has been associated with mutations in 6 different genes: *ACTA1* (Nowak et al., 1999), *CFL2* (Agrawal et al., 2007), *NEB* (Pelin et al., 1999), *TNNT1* (Johnston et al., 2000), *TPM2* (Donner et al., 2002), and *TPM3* (Laing et al., 1995). Central core disease and isolated malignant hyperthermia have been associated with mutations in the *RYR1* gene (Quane et al., 1993; Zhang et al., 1993). The phenotypic spectrum of *RYR1* has expanded recently, and mutations in this gene have been associated with other myopathies as well.

Caring for a child with a congenital myopathy will depend on specific complications. Respiratory interventions include invasive and noninvasive supports, depending on the individual case. A range of orthotic devices and orthopedic procedures may be helpful at various stages. Nutritional support may also be needed. No pharmacological treatment currently exists for any form of the disorders. These children generally have typical cognitive development, so education should be provided at the appropriate age and grade level. However, some children may have difficulty speaking due to facial and tongue weakness, and sometimes due to a tracheostomy, so an augmentative/alternative communication evaluation is essential. Rehabilitation focuses on improving daily living skills.

DISORDERS OF THE MUSCULOSKELETAL SYSTEM

Musculoskeletal disorders may involve abnormalities of just one limb or joint or the entire skeleton. This section discusses the different types of musculoskeletal disorders, providing an example of each.

Joint Disorders: Arthrogryposis

The term *arthrogryposis* refers to congenital joint contractures, and *arthrogryposis multiplex congenita* is a syndrome in which arthrogryposis is present in at least two major joints, with an incidence estimated to range from 1 in 3,000 to 1 in 12,000 live births (Darin et al., 2002). The final common pathway for this condition is significant prolonged fetal immobility (Gordon, 1998). Over 150 distinct causes of arthrogryposis multiplex congenita have been identified (Hall, 1997). The etiologies may be divided into *endogenous* and *exogenous* categories. Endogenous causes are often genetic in nature, and include multiorgan system genetic syndromes, connective tissue diseases, and central and peripheral nervous system disorders. Exogenous causes are typically maternal, and include structural uterine problems, placental insufficiency, maternal myasthenia gravis, and maternal multiple sclerosis (Livingstone et al., 1984). When a neuromuscular cause of arthrogryposis multiplex congenita is suspected, electrophysiological testing and muscle biopsy are complementary and should both be pursued when possible (Kang et al., 2003).

Although spinal deformity at birth is uncommon for infants with arthrogryposis, 30%–67% of children with arthrogryposis will develop scoliosis during childhood. Most curves are resistant to bracing. Physical therapy and occupational therapy, however, are helpful in maintaining joint motion and maximizing functional development. In cases of arthrogryposis associated with other congenital anomalies, the child may have additional medical problems that must be addressed.

Long-term orthopedic management is directed at maximizing function. Because arthrogryposis can be caused by many disorders, there is no single management plan. The common goals are independent ambulation or wheelchair mobility, self-care, and the ability to be employed and live independently. The initial treatment of any contracture involves gentle stretching and range-of-motion exercises. Once the joint is in a proper position, a lightweight splint may help prevent recurrence. If a joint's range of motion is not acceptable, casting or soft-tissue release followed by casting may improve it. The limitations of surgical interventions should be kept in mind in this patient population (Lahoti et al., 2005).

Skeletal Dysplasias: Achondroplasia

The skeletal dysplasias are a large, genetically diverse group of conditions characterized by abnormalities in the development, growth, and maintenance of the skeleton. Many of these disorders result in disproportionate short stature (Savarirayan et al., 2002). There are approximately

175 different skeletal dysplasias (OMIM, 2011; Orioli et al., 1986; Stoll et al., 1989).

Achondroplasia is the most common form of short stature associated with disproportionately shortened limbs. It occurs in 1 of every 15,000–25,000 live births, and has been found to result from a point mutation in the gene coding for fibroblast growth factor receptor 3 or *FGFR3* (Matsui et al., 1998). The condition is inherited as an autosomal dominant trait, and most individuals have the same genetic mutation, so the condition's physical manifestations tend to be similar across individuals (Bellus et al., 1995). It is important to monitor affected children for potentially serious complications such as hydrocephalus, craniocervical junction compression, upper airway obstruction, and kyphosis (Trotter et al., 2005).

Thoracolumbar kyphosis (curvature of the mid-lower spine in the front to back plane) is present to some degree in most infants with achondroplasia as a result of their enlarged heads, hypotonia, and **ligamentous laxity** (double jointedness). The kyphosis typically improves spontaneously once the child begins to walk, but 10%–15% of children require bracing or surgical correction of the curvature (Ain & Browne, 2004; Ain & Shirley, 2004). Careful monitoring is essential, and support for the back, particularly in the very young child, may be helpful.

The major impairments of the extremities are short limbs, limited elbow and hip extension, and knee and leg deformities that can impede locomotion. **Genu verum** (bowed legs) occurs in 40% of individuals with achondroplasia, but only 25% will experience a clinically significant deformity that requires surgical correction (Beals et al., 2005). Significant advances have been made in limb-lengthening procedures, but it still takes about 3 years to achieve the desired lengthening. Growth hormone therapy has achieved only limited success in people with achondoplasia (Hagenas et al., 2003).

Connective Tissue Disorders: Osteogenesis Imperfecta

Connective tissue disorders are caused by the mechanical failure of collagen, which results in joint hypermobility and, in the case of children with osteogenesis imperfecta (OI), brittle bones. Other examples of connective tissue disorders include Ehlers-Danlos syndrome and Marfan syndrome (see Appendix B).

Osteogenesis imperfecta (OI) is caused by a failure of formation of type I collagen, the scaffolding on which bone mineral is laid down. Blue **sclera** (the part of the eye that is normally white) and poor dentition, along with fractures and bone deformity, are OI's most common characteristics. The clinical diagnosis of OI is supported by a skin biopsy to test for the underlying genetic defect (Minch et al., 1998). OI has a prevalence of 1 in 20,000 births. Although hundreds of genetic variants have been identified, most result from a mutation in the *COL1A1* (on chromosome 17) and *COL1A2* (on chromosome 7) genes.

Orthopedic care has been the mainstay in managing OI and involves measures to prevent fractures, to treat acute fractures, and to correct bony deformities. People with OI are particularly susceptible to disuse **osteoporosis** (bone weakness); therefore, promoting mobility in both daily life and after an injury is essential. Placing rods inside the bones for support at the time of a fracture or in conjunction with **osteotomies** (surgical cuts through the bone to correct deformities) can improve the bone alignment, shorten rehabilitation time, and help prevent future fractures. Deformity of the spine occurs in 40%–80% of individuals with OI. Because thoracic curves can decrease lung capacity (Widmann et al., 1999), orthopedic consultation is recommended for monitoring curve progression, with spine fusion surgery performed if necessary (Engelbert et al., 1998).

The bone fragility seen in OI is due to disturbed organization of bone tissue, decreased bone mass, and altered bone geometry. While healthy-growing children form 7% more bone than they **resorb** (lose) during growth and remodeling, children with mild OI only form 3% more bone than they resorb. Children with moderate to severe OI form essentially the same amount of bone as they resorb. This imbalance informs the rationale for treating affected children with bisphosphonates (e.g., alendronate, typically used to treat osteoporosis in postmenopausal women), because this medication reduces osteoblast-mediated bone resorption (Shaw et al., 2005; Zeitlin et al., 2003). Recent data suggest that these agents are most effective in younger children with severe forms of the disorder. However, older children on bisphosphonate therapy do report a reduction in bone pain and improvement in confidence and general well-being (Pizones et al, 2005).

PRINCIPLES FOR THE MANAGEMENT OF NEUROMUSCULAR AND MUSCULOSKELETAL DISORDERS

Recommended standards of care have been published recently for Duchenne muscular dystrophy (Bushby et al., 2010a; Bushby et al., 2010b) and spinal muscular atrophy (Wang et al., 2007), and provide greater detail regarding the care of such disorders. These standards are by no means the last word on the subjects, but they summarize what is currently known about caring for children with these conditions and what gaps in knowledge persist.

Medical Care

The autoimmune neuromuscular disorders, including Guillain-Barré syndrome, chronic inflammatory demyelinating polyradiculo-neuropathy, and myasthenia gravis, typically respond to immunomodulatory therapies such as plasmapheresis, intravenous immunoglobulin, and steroids. One major exception is Guillain-Barré syndrome, which responds to the first two therapies but not to steroids.

Two important precautions apply to patients with primary muscle diseases. First, **rhabdomyolysis** (breakdown of muscle tissue) and **myoglobinuria** (the resulting spillage of myoglobin into the urine) may occur in isolation, or in the context of certain muscle diseases (Mathews et al., 2011), especially in the context of strenuous exercise, dehydration, or both. Whenever this reaction occurs, the individual should be taken to the nearest emergency department immediately, as the myoglobinuria aspect of the reaction has the potential to cause permanent kidney damage. Intravenous fluids will avert renal injury in most cases. Second, the risk of malignant hyperthermia with certain anesthetic agents may occur in association with *RYR1* mutations (MacLennan et al., 1990; McCarthy et al., 1990)or in the setting of muscle diseases, including muscular dystrophies and congenital myopathies such as *RYR1*-associated central core disease (Quane et al., 1993; Zhang et al., 1993).

Medical therapies for the inherited neuromuscular disorders are often limited, but there are some important medications for certain disorders. Albuterol (an asthma medication) appeared to increase patients' strength in two studies involving patients with SMA II (Kinali et al., 2002a; Pane et al., 2008) and some clinicians now prescribe this for certain SMA patients; however, its efficacy has not been proven in a randomized controlled trial. Steroids have been shown to improve the motor outcome in Duchenne muscular dystrophy, as discussed above. Also, specific subtypes of congenital myasthenic syndrome respond to various medications.

It is important for children with neuromuscular disease to have routine immunizations as recommended by the American Academy of Pediatrics (2010), especially when there is a high risk of pulmonary complications. They should also receive the pneumococcal and annual influenza (flu) vaccine. Certain immunizations may need to be deferred for some patients, such as those with active or recent episodes of Guillain-Barré syndrome and patients with active cases of chronic inflammatory demyelinating polyradiculoneuropathy. Parents of such patients should discuss the advisability of having certain vaccinations with the child's physicians.

Children with myopathies and muscular dystrophies are at increased risk for sleep apnea. Symptoms may be noticeable during daytime and often involve fatigue, falling asleep during class, or morning headaches. A **polysomnogram** (sleep study) with continuous carbon dioxide monitoring is the best way to assess the need for ventilatory support. Provision of noninvasive nocturnal ventilation can significantly increase quality of life and lengthen life expectancy (Baydur et al., 2000).

Rehabilitation Management

It is believed that physical therapy and rehabilitation play an important role in maximizing functional status and tone, and may even slow the progression of some diseases, though this effect is subtle and difficult to prove. Data are sparse regarding the effectiveness of physical therapy, stretching exercises, and braces in patients with neuromuscular disorders.

In muscular dystrophies there is a consensus that high-resistance exercises, especially those involving eccentric contractions (i.e., weight lifting, abdominal crunches), are damaging to the muscle cell membrane and should be avoided (Ansved, 2003). However, the impact of a sedentary life is equally negative (McDonald, 2002). Therefore, active, nonresistive exercises are encouraged; swimming is a good example (with the proper safeguards). An active lifestyle will also prevent excessive weight gain, especially if the child is receiving steroids. Daily walks help maintain strength and slow contracture formation.

Both the nature and quantity of activity should be modified so that fatigue does not remain after a night's sleep. Wheelchair games can be played when ambulation is lost. Children with neuromuscular disorders who are confined to bed because of the disease, injury, or surgery require physical therapy, including range-of-motion exercises, with prompt progression to more active exercise, including walking when possible. In the event of leg fractures, walking casts should be used as soon as possible (Siegel, 1977), and every effort should be made to limit the amount of time the child spends in a cast.

For those children who develop difficulty with activities of daily living, occupational therapy evaluation at school is essential to assess self-feeding, self-care, torso positioning within the classroom, and writing. A keyboard should be provided to complete school tasks, and an assistive technology evaluation should be completed. A voice recorder is useful for taking notes or a note-taker can be appointed. Some students may require a classroom aide in order to participate fully in the academic environment and safely navigate the school building.

Contractures

Stretching exercises, nighttime splinting, or both together should be recommended as soon as tightness of the heel cords is noticed (Hyde et al., 2000). A standing board tilted at an appropriate angle may be used for limited periods during the day to help stretch the Achilles tendon in children who do not ambulate. If stretching and orthoses (bracing) are not effective, surgical release of tight heel cords may be beneficial (Goertzen et al., 1995). Temporary bracing after tendon surgery is necessary for optimal results. Further details on orthoses may be found in Chapter 33.

Bone Health

In children with neuromuscular and musculoskeletal disorders, a fracture can occur with little or no trauma (e.g., from gentle range-of-motion exercises during physical therapy). Such fractures are called pathologic fractures and may result from bone fragility (especially osteogenesis imperfecta), as a secondary effect of a medication (e.g., steroids, antiepileptic drugs), or as weakness from disuse (Sambrook et al., 1995). Children with pathological fractures may have swelling and increased warmth of the fractured extremity. Weight-bearing activities are important for maintaining bone density, as bones have internal receptors that recognize weight-bearing activity and send signals to make bones stronger in response. Similarly, it is

essential that these children be given diets rich in calcium and vitamin D, with supplementation of vitamin D in some cases depending on the specific disease and the stage of illness.

Educational Services

Children with acute neuromuscular disorders such as myasthenia gravis or inflammatory myopathies may require prolonged admissions to the hospital, which can entail extended absences from school. Some require homebound instruction during convalescence. Once the child returns to school, supportive measures such as physical therapy and occupational therapy may be very helpful (Table 13.1). Children with fluctuating disorders such as myasthenia gravis may require rest periods or a shortened school day. Children with chronic disorders such as congenital and hereditary progressive myopathies, as well as chronic polyneuropathies, require specialized rehabilitation care.

Steroids are used in neuromuscular diseases such as Duchenne muscular dystrophy, chronic inflammatory demyelinating polyradiculoneuropathy, and myasthenia gravis. Two side effects, behavior problems and weight gain,

Table 13.1. School accommodations for children with neuromuscular and musculoskeletal disorders

Physical and occupational therapy
Stretching
Range-of-motion exercises
Muscle cramp massage
Safety training (on stairs and playground)
Hallway safety
Accommodating activities of daily living to changing physical needs (e.g., toileting, lunchtime/cafeteria safety)
Adapted or modified physical education and sports for individuals with disabilities
Consultation for body positioning, seating, and gross- and fine-motor function
Assistive technology

Specialized accommodations
Provision of an additional set of textbooks to avoid having to transport books from one classroom to another
Access to an elevator
Consideration of students' physical needs when designing class schedule
Preferential seating in the classroom
Consideration of students' physical needs when developing a school emergency evacuation plan
Consideration of students' needs when planning field trips and school events

may occur shortly after starting the medication and may persist. Changes in behavior related to the chronic treatment could impact school performance and personal relationships. Steroids can cause depression, hyperactivity, and behavioral changes, including in rare instances psychosis. Sometimes adjusting the dose can improve these symptoms, but in other cases the side effects are severe enough that the medication needs to be discontinued.

A child receiving steroids also tends to have increased appetite and weight gain, as well as slowing of linear growth. Unwanted weight gain can be especially detrimental in children with neuromuscular disease, especially those with muscular dystrophies. The increased body weight burdens the already weak muscles, and this can obscure the benefits of steroid treatment. This problem can sometimes be avoided or mitigated, however, if the child follows a healthy diet. Children on steroids should bring lunch to school whenever possible in order to follow their diet, and they should avoid snacks between meals.

SUMMARY

The neuromuscular and musculoskeletal systems support the physical structure of the body and help carry out essential movements. Diseases affecting these systems have a significant impact on a child's functional capacity and independence. Though cures have been elusive to date, treatments are available that may substantially alter the course of disease in many cases. The child's care team should include family members, primary care physicians, as well as medical specialists such as child neurologists, orthopaedic surgeons, therapists, and rehabilitative specialists. The goals are to gain or retain function, conserve energy, prolong life expectancy when possible, and improve quality of life. Attempts to reach these goals may involve a combination of medical and nonmedical therapies, including medications, bracing, physical therapy, occupational therapy, seating systems, adaptive equipment, and, when necessary, surgery. These disorders are under active investigation, with the goal of developing new treatment approaches, including the repair of genetic material, more effective medications, and improved surgical techniques.

REFERENCES

Agrawal, P.B., Greenleaf, R.S., Tomczak, K.K., Lehto-kari, V.L., Wallgren-Pettersson, C., Wallefeld, W.,

... Beggs, A.H. (2007). Nemaline myopathy with minicores caused by mutation of the CFL2 gene encoding the skeletal muscle actin–binding protein, cofilin–2. *American Journal of Human Genetics, 80,* 162–167.

Ain, M.C., & Browne, J.A. (2004). Spinal arthrodesis with instrumentation for thoracolumbar kyphosis in pediatric achondroplasia. *Spine, 29,* 2075–2080.

Ain, M.C., & Shirley, E.D. (2004). Spinal fusion for kyphosis in achondroplasia. *Journal of Pediatric Orthopedics,* 2004; *24,* 541–545.

American Academy of Pediatrics. (2010). Policy statement—Recommended childhood and adolescent immunization schedules—United States, 2010. *Pediatrics, 125,* 195–196.

Ansved, T. (2003). Muscular dystrophies, influence of physical conditioning on the disease evolution. *Current Opinion in Clinical Nutrition and Metabolic Care, 6,* 435–439.

Baydur, A., Layne, E., Aral, H., Krishnareddy, N., Topacio, R., Frederick, G., & Bodden, W. (2000). Long term non–invasive ventilation in the community for patients with musculoskeletal disorders, 46 year experience and review. *Thorax, 55,* 4–11.

Beals, R.K., & Stanley, G. (2005). Surgical correction of bowlegs in achondroplasia. *Journal of Pediatric Orthopedics, B14,* 245–249.

Bellus, G.A., Hefferon, T.W., Ortiz de Luna, R.I., Hecht, J.T., Horton, W.A., Machado, M., ... Francomano, C.A. (1995). Achondroplasia is defined by recurrent G380R mutations of FGFR3. *American Journal of Human Genetics, 56,* 368–373.

Bertorini, T., Narayanaswami, P., & Rashed, H. (2004). Charcot–Marie–Tooth disease (hereditary motor sensory neuropathies) and hereditary sensory and autonomic neuropathies. *Neurologist, 10,* 327–337.

Biggar, W.D., Gingras, M., Fehlings, D.L., Harris, V.A., & Steele, C.A. (2001). Deflazacort treatment of Duchenne muscular dystrophy. *Journal of Pediatrics, 138,* 45–50.

Bitoun, M., Maugenre, S., Jeannet, P.Y., Lacène, E., Ferrer, X., Laforêt, P., ... Guichenev, P. (2005). Mutations in dynamin 2 cause dominant centronuclear myopathy. *Nature Genetics, 37,* 1207–1209.

Brook, P.D., Kennedy, J.D., Stern, L.M., Sutherland A.D., Foster, B.K. (1996). Spinal fusion in Duchenne's muscular dystrophy. *Journal of Pediatric Orthopedics, 16,* 324–331.

Bushby, K., Finkel, R., Birnkrant, D.J., Case, L.E., Clemens, P.R, Cripe, L., ... DMD Care Considerations Working Group. (2010a). Diagnosis and management of Duchenne muscular dystrophy, part 1, diagnosis, and pharmacological and psychosocial management. *Lancet Neurology, 9,* 77–93.

Bushby, K., Finkel, R., Birnkrant, D.J., Case, L.E., Clemens, P.R, Cripe, L., ... DMD Care Considerations Working Group. (2010b). Diagnosis and management of Duchenne muscular dystrophy, part 2, implementation of multidisciplinary care. *Lancet Neurology, 9,* 177–189.

Campbell, C., & Jacob, P. (2003). Deflazacort for the treatment of Duchenne Dystrophy, a systematic review. *BMC Neurology, 3,* 7.

Chiang, L.M., Darras, B.T., & Kang, P.B. (2009). Juvenile myasthenia gravis. *Muscle & Nerve, 39,* 423–31.

Darin, N., Kimber, E., Kroksmark, A.K., & Tulinius, M. (2002). Multiple congenital contractures, birth prevalence, etiology, and outcome. *Journal of Pediatrics, 140,* 61–67.

Darras, B.T. & Jones, H.R. (2000). Diagnosis of pediatric neuromuscular disorders in the era of DNA analysis. *Pediatric Neurology, 23,* 289–300.

Darras, B.T., & Kang, P.B. (2007). Clinical trials in spinal muscular atrophy. *Current Opinions in Pediatrics, 19,* 675–679.

Donner, K., Ollikainen, M., Ridanpaa, M., Christen, H.J., Goebel, H.H., de Visser, M., ... Wallgren-Pettersson, C. (2002). Mutations in the beta–tropomyosin (TPM2) gene—A rare cause of nemaline myopathy. *Neuromuscular Disorders, 12,* 151–158.

Dubowitz, V., & Fardeau, M. (1995). Proceedings of the 27th ENMC sponsored workshop on congenital muscular dystrophy. 22–24 April 1994, The Netherlands. *Neuromuscular Disorders, 5,* 253–258.

Dubowitz, V., Kinali, M., Main, M., Mercuri, E., & Muntoni, F. (2002). Remission of clinical signs in early duchenne muscular dystrophy on intermittent low–dosage prednisolone therapy. *European Journal of Paediatric Neurology, 6,* 153–159.

Engelbert, R.H., Pruijs, H.E., Beemer, F.A., & Helders, P.J. (1998). Osteogenesis imperfecta in childhood, treatment strategies. *Archives of Physical Medicine and Rehabilitation, 79,* 1590–1594.

Escolar, D.M., Buyse, G., Henricson, E., Leshner, R., Florence, J., Mayhew, J., ... CINRG Group. (2005). CINRG randomized controlled trial of creatine and glutamine in Duchenne muscular dystrophy. *Annals of Neurology, 58,* 151–155.

Felisari, G., Martinelli Boneschi, F., Bardoni, A., Sironi, M., Comi, G.P., Robotti, M., ... Bresolin, N. (2000). Loss of Dp140 dystrophin isoform and intellectual impairment in Duchenne dystrophy. *Neurology, 55,* 559–564.

Finder, J.D., Birnkrant, D., Carl, J., Farber, H.J., Gozal, D., Iannoccone, S.T., ... American Thoracic Society. (2004). Respiratory care of the patient with Duchenne muscular dystrophy, ATS consensus statement. *American Journal of Respiratory and Critical Care Medicine, 170,* 456–465.

Giliberto, F., Ferreiro, V., Dalamon, V., & Szijan, I. (2004). Dystrophin deletions and cognitive impairment in Duchenne/Becker muscular dystrophy. *Neurological Research, 26,* 83–87.

Goertzen, M., Baltzer, A., & Voit, T. (1995). Clinical results of early orthopaedic management in Duchenne muscular dystrophy. *Neuropediatrics, 26,* 257–259.

Gordon, N. (1998). Arthrogryposis multiplex congenita. *Brain & Development, 20,* 507–511.

Griggs, R.C., Moxley, R.T., 3rd, Mendell, J.R., Fenichel, G.M., Brooke, M.H., Pestronk, A., ... Pandya, S. (1993). Duchenne dystrophy, randomized, controlled trial of prednisone (18 months) and azathioprine (12 months). *Neurology, 43,* 520–527.

Hagenas, L., & Hertel, T. (2003). Skeletal dysplasia, growth hormone treatment and body proportion, comparison with other syndromic and non–syndromic short children. *Hormone Research, 60*(3), 65–70.

Hall, J.G. (1997). Arthrogryposis multiplex congenita, etiology, genetics, classification, diagnostic approach, and general aspects. *Journal of Pediatric Orthopedics, 6,* 159–166.

Hendriksen, J.G., & Vles, J.S. (2008). Neuropsychiatric disorders in males with duchenne muscular dystrophy, frequency rate of attention–deficit/hyperactivity disorder (ADHD), autism spectrum disorder, and obsessive—compulsive disorder. *Journal of Child Neurology, 23,* 477–481.

Hinton, V.J., De Vivo, D.C., Nereo, N.E., Goldstein, E., & Stern, Y. (2000). Poor verbal working memory across intellectual level in boys with Duchenne dystrophy. *Neurology, 54,* 2127–2132.

Hoffman, E.P., Brown, R.H., Jr., & Kunkel, L.M. (1987). Dystrophin, the protein product of the Duchenne muscular dystrophy locus. *Cell, 51,* 919–928.

Hyde, S.A., Fłytrup, I., Glent, S., Kroksmark, A.K., Salling, B., Steffensen, B.F., ... Erlandsen, M. (2000). A randomized comparative study of two methods for controlling Tendo Achilles contracture in Duchenne muscular dystrophy. *Neuromuscular Disorders, 10,* 257–263.

Jeppesen, J., Green, A., Steffensen, B.F., & Rahbek, J. (2003). The Duchenne muscular dystrophy population in Denmark, 1977–2001, prevalence, incidence and survival in relation to the introduction of ventilator use. *Neuromuscular Disorders, 13,* 804–812.

Johnston, J.J., Kelley, R.I., Crawford, T.O., Morton, D.H., Agarwala, R., Koch, T., ... Biesecker, L.G. (2000). A novel nemaline myopathy in the Amish caused by a mutation in troponin T1. *American Journal of Human Genetics, 67,* 814–821.

Jungbluth, H., Davis, M.R., Muller, C., Counsell, S., Allsop, J., Chattopadhyay, A., ... Muntoni, F. (2004). Magnetic resonance imaging of muscle in congenital myopathies associated with RYR1 mutations. *Neuromuscular Disorders, 14,* 785–790.

Kang, P.B., Krishnamoorthy, K.S., Jones, R.M., Shapiro, F.D., & Darras, B.T. (2006). Atypical presentations of spinal muscular atrophy type III (Kugelberg–Welander disease). *Neuromuscular Disorders, 16,* 492–494.

Kang, P.B., Lidov, H.G., David, W.S., Torres, A., Anthony, D.C., Jones, H.R., & Darras, B.T. (2003). Diagnostic value of electromyography and muscle biopsy in arthrogryposis multiplex congenita. *Annals of Neurology, 54,* 790–795.

Kinali, M., Mercuri, E., Main, M., De Biasia, F., Karatza, A., Higgins, R., ... Muntoni, F. (2002a). Pilot trial of albuterol in spinal muscular atrophy. *Neurology, 59,* 609–610.

Kinali, M., Mercuri, E., Main, M., Muntoni, F., & Dubowitz, V. (2002b). An effective, low–dosage, intermittent schedule of prednisolone in the long–term treatment of early cases of Duchenne dystrophy. *Neuromuscular Disorders, 12*(1), S169–S174.

Kogut, K.A., Bufo, A.J., Rothenberg, S.S., & Lobe, T.E. (2000). Thoracoscopic thymectomy for myasthenia gravis in children. *Journal of Pediatric Surgery, 35,* 1576–1577.

Lahoti, O. & Bell, M.J. (2005). Transfer of pectoralis major in arthrogryposis to restore elbow flexion, deteriorating results in the long term. *Journal of Bone and Joint Surgery, British Volume 87,* 858–860.

Laing, N.G., Wilton, S.D., Akkari, P.A., Dorosz, S., Boundy, K., Blumbergs, P., ... Love, D.R. (1995). A mutation in the alpha tropomyosin gene TPM3 associated with autosomal dominant nemaline myopathy. *Nature Genetics, 9,* 75–79.

Laporte, J., Hu, L.J., Kretz, C., Mandel, J.L., Kioschis, P., Coy, J.F., ... Dahl, N. (1996). A gene mutated in X–linked myotubular myopathy defines a new putative tyrosine phosphatase family conserved in yeast. *Nature Genetics, 13,* 175–182.

Lefebvre, S., Burglen, L., Reboullet, S., Clermont, O., Burlet, P., Viollet, L., ... Zeviani, M. (1995). Identification and characterization of a spinal muscular atrophy–determining gene. *Cell, 180,* 155–165.

Livingstone, I.R., & Sack, G.H., Jr. (1984). Arthrogryposis multiplex congenita occurring with maternal multiple sclerosis. *Archives of Neurology, 41*, 1216–1217.

Lupski, J.R., de Oca–Luna, R.M., Slaugenhaupt, S., Pentao, L., Guzzetta, V., Trask, B.J., ... Patel, P.I. (1991). DNA duplication associated with Charcot–Marie–Tooth disease type 1A. *Cell, 66*, 219–232.

MacLennan, D.H., Duff, C., Zorzato, F., Fujii, J., Phillips, M., Korneluk, R.G., ... Worton, R.G. (1990). Ryanodine receptor gene is a candidate for predisposition to malignant hyperthermia. *Nature, 343*, 559–561.

Mathews, K.D., Stephan, C.M., Laubenthal, K., Winder, T.L., Michele, D.E., Moore, S.A., & Campbell, K.P. (2011). Myoglobinuria and muscle pain are common in patients with limb–girdle muscular dystrophy 2I. *Neurology, 76*, 194–195.

Matsui, Y., Yasui, N., Kimura, T., Tsumaki, N., Kawabata, H., & Ochi, T. (1998). Genotype phenotype correlation in achondroplasia and hypochondroplasia. *Journal of Bone and Joint Surgery, British Volume 80*, 1052–1056.

McCarthy, T.V., Healy, J.M., Heffron, J.J., Lehane, M., Deufel, T., Lehmann-Horn, F., ... Johnson, K. (1990). Localization of the malignant hyperthermia susceptibility locus to human chromosome 19q12–13.2. *Nature, 343*, 562–564.

McDonald, C.M. (2001). Peripheral neuropathies of childhood. *Physical Medicine and Rehabilitation Clinics of North America, 12*, 473–490.

McDonald, C.M. (2002). Physical activity, health impairments, and disability in neuromuscular disease. *American Journal of Physical Medicine and Rehabilitation, 81*, S108–S120.

McMillan, H.J., Darras, B.T., Kang, P.B., Saleh, F., & Jones, H.R. (2009). Pediatric monomelic amyotrophy, evidence for poliomyelitis in vulnerable populations. *Muscle & Nerve, 40*, 860–863.

Melki, J., Lefebvre, S., Burglen, L., Burlet, P., Clermont, O., Millasseau, P., ... Le Paslier, D. (1994). De novo and inherited deletions of the 5q13 region in spinal muscular atrophies. *Science, 264*, 1474–1477.

Merlini, L., Stagni, S.B., Marri, E., & Granata, C. (1992). Epidemiology of neuromuscular disorders in the under–20 population in Bologna Province, Italy. *Neuromuscular Disorders, 2*, 197–200.

Minch, C.M., & Kruse, R.W. (1998). Osteogenesis imperfecta, a review of basic science and diagnosis. *Orthopedics, 21*, 558–67; quiz 568–569.

Monaco, A.P., Neve, R.L., Colletti–Feener, C., Bertelsen, C.J., Kurnit, D.M., & Kunkel, L.M. (1986). Isolation of candidate cDNAs for portions of the Duchenne muscular dystrophy gene. *Nature, 323*, 646–650.

Moxley, R.T., 3rd, Ashwal, S., Pandya, S., Connolly, A., Florence, J., Mathews, K., ... Wade, C. (2005). Practice parameter, corticosteroid treatment of Duchenne dystrophy, report of the Quality Standards Subcommittee of the American Academy of Neurology and the Practice Committee of the Child Neurology Society. *Neurology, 64*, 13–20.

Nicot, A.S., Toussaint, A., Tosch, V., Kretz, C., Wallgren-Petterson, C., Iwarsson, E., ... Laporte, J. (2007). Mutations in amphiphysin 2 (BIN1) disrupt interaction with dynamin 2 and cause autosomal recessive centronuclear myopathy. *Nature Genetics, 39*, 1134–1139.

Nowak, K.J., Wattanasirichaigoon, D., Goebel, H.H., Wilce, M., Pelin, K., Donner, K., ... Laing, N.G.

(1999). Mutations in the skeletal muscle alpha–actin gene in patients with actin myopathy and nemaline myopathy. *Nature Genetics, 23*, 208–212.

OMIM (Online Mendelian Inheritance in Man). (2011). McKusick-Nathans Institute of Genetic Medicine, Johns Hopkins University, Baltimore, MD. Retrieved from http://omim.org/

Orioli, I.M., Castilla, E.E., & Barbosa–Neto, J.G. (1986). The birth prevalence rates for the skeletal dysplasias. *Journal of Medical Genetics, 23*, 328–332.

Pane, M., Staccioli, S., Messina, S., D'Amico, A., Pelliccioni, M., Mazzone, E.S., ... Mercuri, E. (2008). Daily salbutamol in young patients with SMA type II. *Neuromuscular Disorders, 18*, 536–540.

Pearn, J. (1978). Incidence, prevalence, and gene frequency studies of chronic childhood spinal muscular atrophy. *Journal of Medical Genetics, 15*, 409–413.

Pearn, J.H. (1973). The gene frequency of acute Werdnig–Hoffmann disease (SMA type 1). A total population survey in North–East England. *Journal of Medical Genetics, 10*, 260–265.

Pelin, K., Hilpela, P., Donner, K., Sewry, C., Akkari, P.A., Wilton, S.D., ... Wallgren-Pettersson, C. (1999). Mutations in the nebulin gene associated with autosomal recessive nemaline myopathy. *Proceedings of the National Academy of Sciences of the USA, 96*, 2305–10.

Pizones, J., Plotkin, H., Parra–Garcia, J.I., Alvarez, P., Gutierrez, P., Bueno, A., & Fernandez-Arroyo, A. (2005). Bone healing in children with osteogenesis imperfecta treated with bisphosphonates. *Journal of Pediatric Orthopedics, 25*, 332–335.

Quane, K.A., Healy, J.M., Keating, K.E., Manning, M.B., Couch, F.J., Palmucci, L.M., ... McCarthy, V. (1993). Mutations in the ryanodine receptor gene in central core disease and malignant hyperthermia. *Nature Genetics, 5*, 51–55.

Riggs, J.E., Bodensteiner, J.B., & Schochet, S.S., Jr. (2003). Congenital myopathies/dystrophies. *Neurological Clinics, 21*, 779–794; v–vi.

Ryan, M.M., Ilkovski, B., Strickland, C.D., Schnell, C., Sanoudou, D., Midgett, C., ... Beggs, A.H. (2003). Clinical course correlates poorly with muscle pathology in nemaline myopathy. *Neurology, 60*, 665–673.

Sambrook, P.N., & Jones, G. (1995). Corticosteroid osteoporosis. *British Journal of Rheumatology, 34*, 8–12.

Savarirayan, R., & Rimoin, D.L. (2002). The skeletal dysplasias. *Best Practice & Research of Clinical Endocrinology & Metabolism, 16*, 547–560.

Shaw, N.J., & Bishop, N.J. (2005). Bisphosphonate treatment of bone disease. *Archives of Diseases in Childhood, 90*, 494–499.

Shy, M.E. (2004). Charcot–Marie–Tooth disease, an update. *Current Opinion in Neurology, 17*, 579–85.

Siegel, I.M. (1977). Fractures of long bones in Duchenne muscular dystrophy. *Journal of Trauma, 17*, 219–222.

Stoll, C., Dott, B., Roth, M.P., & Alembik, Y. (1989). Birth prevalence rates of skeletal dysplasias. *Clinical Genetics, 35*, 88–92.

Trotter, T.L., & Hall, J.G. (2005). Health supervision for children with achondroplasia. *Pediatrics, 116*, 771–783.

van Essen, A.J., Busch, H.F., te Meerman, G.J., & ten Kate, L.P. (1992). Birth and population prevalence of Duchenne muscular dystrophy in The Netherlands. *Human Genetics, 88*, 258–266.

von Gontard, A., Zerres, K., Backes, M., Laufersweiler-Plass, C., Wendland, C., Melchers, P., ... Rudnik-Schöneborn, S. (2002). Intelligence and cognitive function in children and adolescents with spinal muscular atrophy. *Neuromuscular Disorders, 12*, 130–136.

Wang, C.H., Finkel, R. S., Bertini, E.S., Schroth, M., Simonds, A., Wong, B., ... Trela, A. (2007). Consensus statement for standard of care in spinal muscular atrophy. *Journal of Child Neurology, 22*, 1027–1049.

Widmann, R.F., Bitan, F.D., Laplaza, F.J., Burke, S.W., DiMaio, M.F., & Schneider, R. (1999). Spinal deformity, pulmonary compromise, and quality of life in osteogenesis imperfecta. *Spine, 24*, 1673–1678.

Wu, J.Y., Kuban, K.C., Allred, E., Shapiro, F., & Darras, B.T. (2005). Association of Duchenne muscular dystrophy with autism spectrum disorder. *Journal of Child Neurology, 20*, 790–795.

Zeitlin, L., Fassier, F., & Glorieux, F.H. (2003). Modern approach to children with osteogenesis imperfecta. *Journal of Pediatric Orthopaedics B, 12*, 77–87.

Zhang, Y., Chen, H.S., Khanna, V.K., De Leon, S., Phillips, M.S., Schappert, K., ... MacLennan, D.H. (1993). A mutation in the human ryanodine receptor gene associated with central core disease. *Nature Genetics, 5*, 46–50.

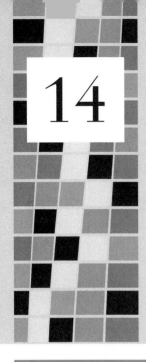

14

Patterns in Development and Disability

Louis Pellegrino

Upon completion of this chapter, the reader will

- Understand the clinical definitions of development and disability

- Comprehend individual and contextual contributions to development and disability

- Recognize how typical and atypical patterns of development are assessed

- Be able to explain how disturbances in expected patterns of development lead to the diagnosis of specific developmental disabilities

■ ■ ■ **BJ**

BJ is a 3-year-old boy who demonstrates skills significantly below his age level. He sat independently at 12 months of age (typical age, 6 months) and walked for the first time at 22 months of age (typical age, 12 months). He began using single words at 24 months of age (typical age, 12 months) and just recently started putting words together. BJ responds inconsistently to single-step commands and is beginning to point out body parts following verbal direction. He is mainly interested in exploratory play and is starting to show an interest in simple pretend play. He can remove his socks and shoes but is otherwise dependent on his parents for dressing and undressing. Although BJ is not yet toilet-trained, he is beginning to show interest in it, but is inconsistent in indicating when a diaper change is needed. His parents say that his skills are most like those of a 1½-year-old.

BJ and other children who have significant developmental delays raise concerns about the possibility that they may have a developmental disability. The terms *development* and *disability* are frequently used together to describe a range of problems that are usually recognized in childhood but that may have lifelong functional implications. Both terms have become so much a part of common usage that it is easy to lose sight of their precise meaning, when used either separately or together. This chapter describes how disability arises from disturbances in typical patterns of development.

DEFINING DISABILITY

The term *disability*, like the term *development*, is both widely used and widely misunderstood. At its most basic level, *disability* refers

231

to a decrement in the ability to perform some action, engage in some activity, or participate in some real-life situation or setting. Like development, disability can be thought of with respect to person-specific factors (e.g., the inability to walk as a result of a neuromuscular disorder) or to environment-contingent factors (barriers or obstacles that lead to functional limitations for individuals). Historically, the tendency has been to define disability mainly in terms of an individual's physical, cognitive, or psychological impairment. The trend more recently, however, has been to define disability in relation to the ecological and environmental context.

Behavioral and Functional Considerations

Clinically, disability is most often described and defined (diagnosed) with reference to an individual's functional and behavioral traits. As described in this chapter, specific disability diagnoses are defined based on the pattern of strengths and weaknesses observed within and among several functional domains, without explicit reference to the medical, genetic, or environmental factors that may relate to the formation and expression of that disability. The *Diagnostic and Statistical Manual of Mental Disorders, Fourth Edition, Text Revision (DSM-IV-TR;* APA, 2000) and the *International Classification of Mental and Behavioral Disorders* (WHO, 2007) provide standardized definitions of many disability diagnoses based on functional and behavioral characteristics, although these classification schemes are imperfect in their representation of diagnostic nuances, do not attempt to describe variations in function, and do not consider environmental aspects that influence function.

Etiologic Considerations in the Definition of Disability

An etiological diagnosis defines the exact cause of an illness or disorder (*etiology* refers to the cause of a medical condition). In contrast to a disability diagnosis (which is based on functional and behavioral characteristics), an etiological diagnosis often involves specialized medical testing (e.g., genetic tests, brain imaging studies; see Chapters 1, 12, and 17). For children with developmental issues, both developmental disability and etiological diagnoses must be considered. When a child is diagnosed with a developmental disability, such as cerebral palsy or an autism spectrum disorder (ASD), it is natural to wonder what caused the disability. It is important to recognize that although the processes involved

in diagnosing disability differ qualitatively from those involved in diagnosing etiology, they do occur in parallel, and the results of one diagnostic process tend to shed light on the other. For example, specific brain imaging findings are often associated with spastic cerebral palsy in preterm infants (see Chapter 24).

The relationship between etiological diagnoses and disability diagnoses is complex. For example, Down syndrome (see Chapter 18) is a specific etiological diagnosis known to be a cause of intellectual disability. Many other specific genetic, neurological, and medical conditions have also been associated with intellectual disability. Conversely, intellectual ability also varies in the general population, and individuals at the lower end of ability may meet the functional criteria for an intellectual disability. For these individuals, there is often no discrete, medically defined pathological cause for their disability. In these cases, learning and cognitive disabilities tend to "run in the family," that is, may be influenced more by environmental factors; the disabilities may not be associated with a definable neurological or genetic abnormality.

Cerebral palsy and some forms of learning disability provide an important counterpoint to this. Cerebral palsy can result from a number of causes, but in all cases, it is thought to be the consequence of a discrete pathological process that disrupts normal brain function (see Chapter 24). In other words, cerebral palsy would not be found as a variant of motor function in the general population. By contrast, some forms of learning disability represent variations in information processing that exist in the general population. Certain types of learning disability thus may not result from a discrete pathological process at all. For example, studies of children with reading disabilities suggest that reading decoding skills vary on a continuum and that reading disability or dyslexia represents a difference of degree (e.g., typically developing children with very weak reading skills) rather than a difference of kind (e.g., atypically developing children whose reading skills differ fundamentally from those of other children; Shaywitz, Morris & Shaywitz, 2008).

A specific etiological diagnosis may be made based on the medical and physical examination findings alone, but additional laboratory testing is required to identify or confirm a diagnosis in many instances. Genetic and neurological tests are most relevant to diagnosing etiology when evaluating developmental disabilities. In general, selecting tests must be determined on a case-by-case basis (see Chapter 17).

Societal, Cultural, and Therapeutic Considerations

Various classification schemes have emerged over several decades in attempts to better define disability and place it into a meaningful conceptual framework. Two frequently referenced models of disability are 1) the National Center for Medical Rehabilitation Research (NCMRR; National Institutes of Health, 1993) Model of Disability; and 2) the World Health Organization (WHO) International Classification of Functioning, Disability and Health (ICF; 2001). These models are summarized in Table 14.1.

The NCMRR model sees disability as including elements associated with the individual on the one hand, and the societal and cultural context on the other. *Pathophysiology*, *impairment*, and *function limitation* refer to the individual's characteristics that affect function, and *societal limitation* refers to environmental characteristics that do so. In this scheme, *disability* is the point of interaction between the individual and environmental components of function. For example, a person with cerebral palsy may have damaged or disrupted motor control pathways in the brain (pathophysiology) that result in difficulties with muscle tone and control (impairment) that in turn prevent the movements required for walking (functional limitation). Reduced mobility (disability) is a function both of the difficulties with walking and with environmental barriers. For example, lack of wheelchair access or financial support to purchase a wheelchair (societal limitations) contribute to loss of mobility. The NCMRR model is especially helpful in planning therapeutic

interventions, which are likely to be most effective if multiple levels in the disability hierarchy are addressed.

As the name implies, the International Classification of Functioning, Disability, and Health (*ICF*, for short) considers ability, disability, and health as being intimately related and subject to considerable variation based on multiple variables. Several broad categories (see Table 14.1) involving body functions and structures, activities and participation, and environmental factors are included in many subdivisions and qualifications, allowing function and disability to be characterized within a matrix of individual and environmental elements (an online version of the classification scheme is available at http://apps.who.int/classifications/icfbrowser/). The ICF is intended to complement traditional classification schemes that focus on disease and diagnosis rather than health and function. In 2007, a child-focused version of ICF, known as the International Classification of Functioning, Disability and Health for Children and Youth (ICF–CY), was introduced. This version accounts for the developmental aspects of function and disability that were not adequately addressed in the original ICF (Simeonsson et al., 2003; WHO: ICF-CY, 2007).

Legal Considerations

Legal definitions of disability are narrowly constructed based on the presence or absence of functional impairments as they relate to legal mandates to address these deficits. For example, under the Individuals with Disabilities Education Improvement Act (IDEA) of 2004 (PL 108-446), a disability exists only if "special

Table 14.1. Biopsychosocial models of disability

National Center for Medical Rehabilitation Research (NCMRR) Model of Disability (NIH; 1993)	World Health Organization International Classification of Functioning, Disability and Health (ICF; WHO, 2001)
Pathophysiology: Interruption or interference with normal physiology or development	*Body Functions & Structures*: Functional characteristics of various body systems and structures
Impairment: Losses or abnormalities of cognitive, emotional, physiological, or anatomical structure or function	*Activities*: Tasks and actions of an individual
Functional Limitation: Restriction or lack of ability to perform an action within expected parameters for a particular organ or organ system	*Participation*: Integration of activities and involvement in real-life settings
Disability: An inability or limitation in performing tasks, activities, and roles to levels expected within the physical and social context	*Environmental Factors*: Aspects of the physical, societal and cultural environment that influence function
Societal Limitation: Restrictions attributable to societal or physical barriers which prevent access to opportunities for full participation in society	

instruction" is required. Likewise, under the U.S. Social Security Act, disability is recognized if it affects an adult's capacity for employment; in a child it applies if the disability significantly limits activities (US-SSA, 2011).

What follows is a description, in general terms, of what constitutes typical and atypical development.

DEFINING DEVELOPMENT

Development in a generic sense can refer to anything that changes over time (e.g., a photographic negative *develops*), but it most often describes an organic process of change. For the purposes of this book, the term *development* is used with reference to changes in human thought, behavior, and function. Development is distinguished from *growth*, which refers more specifically to physical increases in height, weight, head size, and sexual maturation. Although the concepts *growth* and *development* are obviously connected, the techniques used to measure and describe them tend to be separate.

As applied to the individual human being, the term *development* can possess different meanings. On the one hand, a person changes in response to a specific set of life circumstances and experiences. In this sense every human being has a unique developmental history that can never be replicated. On the other hand, it is well-known that individuals experience changes in cognition, emotion, and in specific abilities that likely indicate a common "blueprint" that transcends individual life histories or cultures. For example, walking is begun and mastered at about the same age and seems to follow a fairly consistent sequence. Similarly, children universally and spontaneously learn to speak their native language and do so in a predictable sequence of steps without any explicit instruction in vocabulary or grammar. Additional general changes in behavior and social-emotional responses also occur on a predictable timeline and in predictable ways. Infants begin to exhibit "stranger anxiety" at about 8 or 9 months of age. Toddlers demonstrate limit-testing behavior as part of increased autonomy. School-age children become enamored of rules and enjoy a sense of industrious accomplishment. Preteens and teens experience a sense of independence and identity in the context of intensified peer relations.

Human development is wonderfully varied but reasonably predictable, and for the purposes of this discussion, may be defined as follows: *Development* refers to the characteristic,

predictable ways that behavior changes during the human life cycle. At its most basic level, *behavior* refers to any action that a person can perform and another can observe. Moving a leg, sneezing, saying a word, or composing a symphony are all forms of human behavior. Behavior can be characterized as simple (moving an arm) or complex (playing a concerto). Some forms of behavior are inherently more meaningful than others (e.g., talking versus coughing). With regard to the definition of development, behavior that is most directly relevant to real-life situations tends to be of greatest interest. Behavior is also used as a proxy for aspects of cognition and emotion that are critically important to development but that cannot be observed directly. Observing and interpreting behavior is, in fact, the main focus in developmental assessment.

Development and the Nervous System

Development is dependent on the brain, and the predictable behavioral changes that characterize development occur in parallel with the maturation of the central nervous system (CNS; Figure 14.1). Functional and structural changes in the human nervous system are most dramatically evident during fetal life and early childhood but continue into adulthood (see Chapters 2 and 12). Early brain development is dominated by a genetically predetermined series of events resulting in the formation of basic brain structures. By the end of the second trimester of pregnancy, the maximum number of neurons (brain cells) that an individual will possess in his or her lifetime have already formed in the fetal brain. Subsequent brain development is dominated by processes that increase the connectivity and functionality of existing neuronal elements.

Myelination is a process that involves elaboration of supportive structures that improve transmission of electrical impulses from one part of the nervous system to another. Myelination is most exuberant during early childhood (especially during the first 3 years) but continues into adulthood. Synaptogenesis is the elaboration of connections, or synapses, between individual neurons. This process peaks between 7 and 8 years of age; thereafter, there is a drop-off in the total number of synapses, related to a "pruning back" of underutilized connections (Volpe, 2008).

These processes promote and are intimately connected to developmental change.

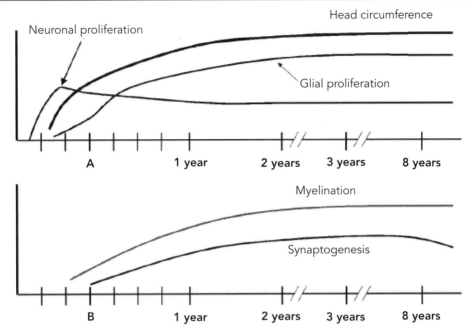

Figure 14.1. Patterns in brain maturation (*Source:* Volpe, 1995). A) During the first trimester of pregnancy, central nervous system development is dominated by formation of basic brain structures in association with proliferation of brain cells (neurons). The peak number of neurons is achieved at the end of this period. Proliferation of supporting elements (glial cells) begins by the end of the second trimester and continues through early childhood. B) Myelination (formation of the "insulation" of neuronal connections) proceeds in parallel with the development of glial cells and continues into adult life. Synaptogenesis (formation of the network of connections between neurons) is most exuberant during early childhood and begins to level off in late childhood.

For example, myelination of key **corticospinal pathways** (pathways from the cortex of the brain to the spinal cord that orchestrate movement) during the first year of life is one of the main determinants of early gross motor development (i.e., rolling over, sitting, and crawling; Volpe, 2008). Critical changes in the brain's functional organization occur toward the end of the second year of life that create an opportunity for explosive language development that typically occurs between 18 and 24 months of age (Redclay et al., 2008). Changing nervous system **plasticity** (the ability of the nervous system to change or adapt) over the course of the human life cycle also creates opportunities and constraints on development. One example of this is the well-known observation that young children much more easily attain fluency in a foreign language than adults or older children (beyond 8 or 9 years of age) do. Indeed, there appears to be a sensitive period for language acquisition during these early years; children who miss this opportunity will most likely never develop fluency in any language (Kuhl, 2010). The good news for adults is that although there is decreased brain plasticity with age, learning continues unabated through the entire life cycle. The brain works by creating a rich

network of functional connections within and across many cortical and subcortical domains, and these networks are continually enhanced and elaborated throughout the life span.

Development in Context

Developmental change is driven from both within and without. Neurological maturation is the internal driving force; the environment represents external influences. The "environment" is actually not a single entity; it consists of the physical environment and the social context. The physical environment is the Newtonian universe of light and heat, cause and effect, friction and gravity to which all organisms must adapt. The social context consists of the people, activities, and social settings that surround the developing individual and that are defined by history and culture. Various developmental theories have tended to emphasize these different influences to a greater or lesser extent.

Developmental Theories

Gesell (per Knobloch & Pasamanick, 1974) emphasized the maturational aspects of development; Piaget (1990) focused on the development of cognitive and problem solving abilities relative to the physical environment; and Vygotsky (1986) identified the importance of the sociocultural system in providing the basis for the development of higher cognitive processes. Bronfenbrenner (1979) took this a step further by describing the developmental settings within which the individual is immersed and that serve as the engine for developmental change.

Bronfenbrenner's model is appealing because it provides a way of thinking about developmental change as it occurs in real-life settings. For example, language development would be viewed emerging within the context of the home and the parent–child relationship, and not simply as something that "happens" to the child. Bronfenbrenner also recognized that the development process involves *everyone* embedded within a particular developmental setting (i.e., the child is not the only person who develops). Development is seen to be a property of the social landscape as much as a property of the individual, and Bronfenbrenner recognizes cultural differences that influence both the nature and interpretation of developmental change. The individual is a nexus of potential action that is only actuated when placed in this larger social and cultural context.

Newer developmental theories attempt to transcend older distinctions by conceptualizing the human organism as an amalgam of functional components or systems that cooperate in an ongoing process of adaptation to changing environmental circumstances. Dynamic systems theory, in particular, emphasizes that behavior is task-specific and focuses on process rather than product when describing the determinants of developmental change (Spencer, 2006). For example, motor development is usually seen as directly resulting from neurological maturation; in this sense, milestones such as rolling, sitting, and walking are considered to be genetically and neurologically "preprogrammed" events.

Dynamic systems theory places neurologic maturation on par with several other cooperating systems, including musculoskeletal components, sensory integrative mechanisms, and individual-specific characteristics such as body and head size. Developmental sequences, rather than being rigidly predetermined, are in a sense discovered through a dynamic process of adaptation. Skills are self-assembled as a child engages in a series of trial-and-error processes, drawing upon relevant functional systems and

organized around a specific task. In this connection, dynamic systems theory provides a more satisfying explanation for variations in development that are difficult to explain otherwise. For example, many infants who are otherwise typical in their motor development may show unexpected departures from the expected sequence of motor milestones. Healthy preterm infants are especially known for this; many exhibit transient differences in muscle tone in early infancy that result in relatively low muscle tone (looseness) in the trunk or torso and relatively high muscle tone (stiffness) in the legs. This pattern makes it relatively difficult for them to maintain a sitting posture but tends to affect other activities to a lesser degree. Infants who are unable to sit may be able to crawl or even pull themselves up to stand, in apparent defiance of the expected sequence of milestones. Maturational theories cannot easily explain this phenomenon. Dynamic systems theory would suggest that muscle tone differences make certain tasks more difficult (in this example, sitting) but have less of an effect on other tasks (e.g., crawling, pulling-to-stand).

Another example relates to the well-researched recommendation that infants should sleep on their backs to reduce the risk of sudden infant death syndrome (SIDS; American Academy of Pediatrics, 2005). Implementing the recommendation resulted in the desired effect of reducing SIDS, but it also resulted in changes in the expected pattern of motor development during the first year of life (Majnemer & Barr, 2006). Infants who sleep on their backs (supine position) tend to learn to roll, sit, crawl, and pull to stand later than infants who sleep on their bellies (prone position). Infants in both groups walk independently at about the same time. A purely maturationalist perspective cannot explain this difference. Dynamic systems theory would suggest that the prone position offers mechanical advantages over the supine position relative to the emergence of these motor activities. Infants who spend more time on their backs are therefore at a temporary disadvantage with regard to early motor development (the dramatic advantage of the supine position—reducing the rate of SIDS—clearly outweigh any short-term disadvantages, however).

Dynamic systems theory offers a conceptual framework for explaining both expected patterns of development and normal variations in these patterns. It allows for the possibility that similar functional outcomes can be arrived at by different pathways and that each individual pursues a unique developmental trajectory that can never be exactly replicated.

PATTERNS IN DEVELOPMENT

Developmental Strands, Streams, and Domains

In order to make reproducible observations of development, it is necessary to break it down into component parts. The component parts have been variously described as developmental strands, streams, and domains (Table 14.2). Most developmental screening and psychometric instruments rely on this fragmentation of development into domains; however, how these domains are defined can vary.

Development may be defined in terms of two schemes. One addresses development in terms of broad functional domains; this type of scheme tends to emphasize adaptation to real-life situations (e.g., whether a child can get dressed, walk to school, give a report, or play with friends at recess). The other scheme addresses the idea of specific skill sets. These skill sets tend to refer to specific abilities that are easily observed and tested in children, such as speech (putting words together to form a phrase), gross motor skills (jumping in place), symbolic play (engaging in pretend play with dolls), and academic skills (reading at grade level).

These two schemes are not mutually exclusive; in fact, skill sets make specific contributions to larger functional domains, and functional domains provide a frame of reference for specific skill sets. For example, the ability to manipulate small objects (a specific type of fine motor skill) contributes to the ability to work with buttons and zippers when getting dressed (a broad functional category). In practice, both types of schemes are deployed in different contexts to help characterize a particular child's developmental pattern.

Developmental Milestones

Reproducibility when observing developmental change also requires defining specific markers, or milestones, that can be generally agreed upon and reliably reproduced. Much of the early work in defining a variety of milestones was done by Arnold Gesell and his colleagues at Yale University in the early to mid-20th century (Knobloch & Pasamanick, 1974). Gesell amassed an enormous amount of information regarding a wide range of skills and abilities in various domains at different ages. He was able to gather from this a finite list of specific behaviors that were easily observed and that emerged during a relatively narrow range of ages. These items have become familiar components of many development screening and assessment instruments (Capute & Accardo, 2005; Squires & Bricker, 2005).

Milestones are useful, as referencing particular milestones allows a description of a child's pattern of skills, and also provide a means for tracking developmental progress. Milestones can become problematic, however, if they are misapplied or misinterpreted. Although many milestones reflect intrinsically important functional accomplishments, others are not critically important in and of themselves. For example, walking independently and speaking in sentences are intrinsically important milestones, whereas stacking blocks or placing a peg in a pegboard are useful proxies for other, more important skills (e.g., using utensils, writing with a pencil). Therapeutic interventions should not be directed toward achieving milestones per se, but rather toward achieving meaningful functional goals that are represented by milestones.

Table 14.2. Defining developmental domains

By functional domains	Communication/socialization
	Conversation skills
	Literacy (reading and writing)
	Social engagement
	Activities of daily living
	Dressing skills
	Toileting skills
	Feeding skills
	Electronic/computer literacy
	Mobility
	Ambulatory skills
By skill sets	Language
	Expressive language
	Receptive language
	Problem solving
	Visual-spatial skills
	Visual-motor skills
	Social and play
	Sensory
	Vision
	Hearing
	Motor
	Fine motor
	Gross motor
	Oral motor
	Attention and impulse control
	Academic

Another pitfall in interpreting milestones is the mistaken notion that a particular milestone is associated with an exact age. Stating that children walk at a year of age is actually providing only an estimate of that skill's age of onset. Based on a more precise, standardized assessment of this milestone, a more exact statement can be articulated (Figure 14.2). According to one assessment tool (Piper et al., 1994), a small minority of children take their first step between 8 and 9 months of age, 50% have taken their first step by 11 months of age, 75% by about 12½ months of age, and 90% by 13½ months of age. So a more precise statement would be "a majority of children start walking by 12 months of age" or "almost all typically developing children can walk by 14 months of age." Standardized measures of development tend to use 75% of children achieving a milestone as the typical age for that skill and use the 90% mark as the age beyond which a child is said to be late or delayed in achieving that skill.

Developmental Delay

Developmental delay is often described in terms of how many months or years a child is behind in the attainment of a particular milestone or set of skills. For example, a child who begins walking at 18 months of age is said to be "6 months delayed" for developing that skill. In this sense the developmental "gap" can be defined as the chronological age minus the developmental age (in this case, 18 months − 12 months = 6 months). It is often more useful, however, to conceptualize development as a percentage of expected attainment. In the previous example, the child would be said to be developing at about 67% of the expected rate for walking (12 months / 18 months × 100 = 67).

Defining development spotlights the rate of development. Focusing on rate gives a clearer picture of developmental change over time. A child who is 6 months delayed at 18 months (developing at 67% of the expected rate) has a more serious delay than a child who is 6 months delayed at 4 years of age (developing at 88% of the expected rate). Using rates of development allows us to track and compare degrees of delay across a range of ages. The rate of development at any given moment in time can be estimated by calculating the developmental quotient, which is defined as follows:

Developmental quotient =
Developmental age / Chronological age × 100

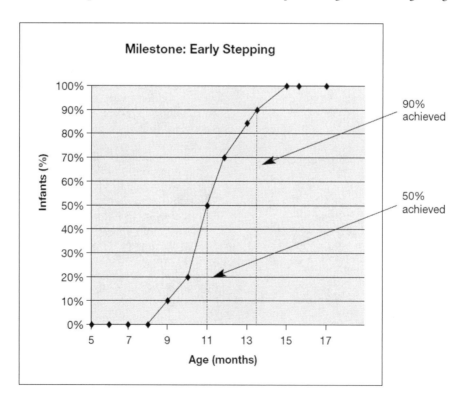

Figure 14.2. Milestone: Early stepping. 50% of children take their first independent steps by 11 months; 90% have achieved this milestone by 13.5 months. (From Piper, M.C., & Darrah, J. [1994]. *Motor assessment of the developing infant* [p. 165]. Philadelphia, PA: W.B. Saunders; Copyright © 1994 Elsevier; adapted by permission.)

In practice, the developmental age usually represents an average level of attainment across a variety of skills and domains, rather than an estimate of the level of attainment for a single skill, and chronological age may be adjusted for prematurity (e.g., the age of a child born at 28 weeks' gestation, or 3 months early, would be an adjusted chronological age of 15 months). Conceptualizing development as a rate phenomenon provides the basis for analyzing developmental trajectories and contributes to diagnostic and prognostic statements.

Developmental rates are used to assess differential patterns of function and behavior; this in turn yields data useful to the diagnostic process. For example, recognizing that a child's speech is developing at 50% of the expected rate, with age-appropriate development in all other areas, suggests that the child may have a specific language impairment. Rates also provide a key element in determining prognosis and outcome (Figure 14.3). If a child is developing at a slower rate, over time he or she will tend to fall further and further behind other children who are developing at a more typical rate. In order to "catch up," a child with developmental delays must show a significant acceleration in the attainment of new skills. In general, the slower a child's rate of development (especially if the developmental quotient falls well below 50), the more difficult, and thus less likely, it is for that child to catch up developmentally.

In order to get a true picture of a child's development, it is necessary to describe the evolution of skills over a sufficient interval of time. This can be done by directly assessing a child on multiple occasions or by eliciting historical information about a child's development from an involved and observant caregiver, teacher, or therapist. Making diagnostic or prognostic judgments based on a one-time direct observation of a child's skills is often problematic; in contrast, following a child over time leads to a clearer picture of the child's developmental trajectory. For example, if a child with delays gains 6 months of new skills at the 6-month reexamination, he or she is tracking at a typical rate and, although still delayed, may well catch up over time. If that child gains only 3 months, it would suggest that the delay may evolve into a disability.

DISTURBANCES IN DEVELOPMENT

From a clinical perspective, *developmental disabilities* are conditions that are first recognized as departures from expected patterns of development during early childhood. These departures can occur in three ways (Accardo, 2008).

First, a child may experience delays. *Delay* refers simply to a slower-than-expected rate in skills acquisition, usually defined with reference to widely accepted developmental milestones. A child with delays demonstrates skills that are typical of a younger child.

Second, a child may *deviate* from an expected developmental path. In this case, a child demonstrates functional or behavioral characteristics

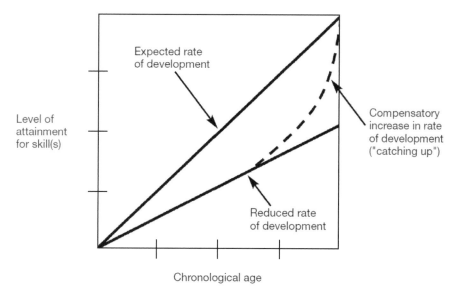

Figure 14.3. Developmental rates. If a child is developing at a slower than expected rate, compensatory acceleration in acquisition of skills is necessary for the child to "catch up."

that are not typical for any child at any age.

Third, a child may demonstrate an uneven pattern of skills, progress being fairly typical in some areas (developmental domains) but showing significant departure (delay or deviation) from the expected course in other areas. This unevenness phenomenon is referred to as *dissociation*.

The following examples illustrate delay, divergence, and dissociation in development.

BJ: The Child With Delayed Development

BJ, the 3-year-old described at the beginning of this chapter, provides an example of global development delay, or delay that involves multiple developmental domains. BJ exhibits a significantly delayed rate of development, and as his parents suggest, his current skills are most consistent with those usually observed in children between 18 and 20 months of age (this is consistent with an estimated developmental quotient of 53%). If he continues to develop at a persistently delayed rate, concern would be merited that his global delays represent an early manifestation of a long-term intellectual disability (i.e., mental retardation; see Chapter 17).

▇ ▇ ▇ JAKE: THE CHILD WITH DIVERGENT DEVELOPMENT

Jake is a 4-year-old with a history of difficulties with language, communication, and socialization skills. He was slightly late in beginning to speak but was using complete sentences by 3 years of age. Despite a large vocabulary and well-developed grammatical skills, Jake has trouble with social communication. He rarely uses speech to communicate wants and needs, and instead prefers to drag people by the hand to get their attention or to help him obtain a desired object. Jake's spontaneous speech consists mainly of repeated phrases from television shows. He seems oblivious to the feelings of others and tends to treat people as though they were objects. Jake is obsessively interested in letters and numbers and has poor imitative and pretend play skills. He can dress himself, was toilet-trained by 3 years of age, and recently taught himself to ride a bicycle without training wheels.

Although demonstrating age-appropriate skills in many areas, Jake displays a significant disturbance in communication, socialization, and play skills consistent with an ASD (see Chapter 21). Although some delays are evident, the most prominent features in Jake's profile of skills are those social and behavioral deviations from expected patterns that are not typical for any child at any age.

▇ ▇ ▇ SARAH: THE CHILD WITH DISSOCIATED DEVELOPMENT

Sarah is a 7-year-old who attends second grade in a public school. She had some mild difficulties with early speech development (mainly problems with pronouncing certain words), which have since resolved. She was on time or early in attaining and reaching all other skills and milestones. She was very successful in preschool, being consistently described by her teachers as exceptionally mature and intelligent. She began experiencing difficulties with reading decoding skills in first grade and was diagnosed with dyslexia by the beginning of second grade. She now receives resource room support for reading and is doing better. She continues to excel in other academic areas.

Sarah's problems with reading stand out against a background of well-developed social, cognitive, and academic skills. Other children may have specific weakness in other academic or functional domains (e.g., children with specific difficulties in learning math or in the area of attention and impulse control). The unevenness in Sarah's profile of skills is an example of developmental dissociation. More complex patterns of dissociation are frequently seen with children who have a variety of academic and functional difficulties; these are referred to collectively as *learning disabilities* (see Chapter 23).

These cases illustrate relatively pure examples of the three disturbances in development. Most children with developmental problems are more complex, frequently exhibiting elements of all three types of developmental disturbance. Given this complexity, it can be challenging to accurately analyze and describe the pattern of skills exhibited by a particular child, and more challenging still to encapsulate this in diagnosis form. In the process of assessing children with developmental difficulties, certain fairly consistent themes, constellations of behavioral characteristics, and patterns of skills emerge that make specific diagnoses possible. A particular developmental diagnosis, or developmental disability, is defined by these recognizable patterns (see Table 14.3).

As a clinical concept, *developmental disability* integrates what is known about typical and

Table 14.3. Patterns of development associated with specific developmental disabilities

Developmental diagnosis	Delays	Divergence	Dissociation
Intellectual disability	Significant early delays across developmental domains associated with long-term dysfunction	Atypical behavior patterns (e.g., self-injurious behavior), especially in severe or profound intellectual disability	Language skills tend to be more severely affected than other areas
Cerebral palsy	Significant delays in motor skills and mobility	Significantly pathological motor control, muscle tone, and involuntary motor responses in some	Motor and mobility dysfunction most prominent
Autism spectrum disorders	Delays in language, play and basic social skills common	Prominent disturbances in social communication and socialization skills; atypical play interests and behavioral patterns	Relatively few difficulties with problem-solving, self-care and motor skills, in many
Communication disorders	Delays in language skills most prominent	Atypical communication skills in some (pragmatic language dysfunction)	Relatively few difficulties with nonlanguage skills
Learning disability	Delays and dysfunction of specific aspects of learning (e.g., reading, math, writing)	Mildly atypical social and behavioral characteristics occasionally observed	Prominent discrepancy between areas of weakness and areas of strength
Attention-deficit/hyperactivity disorder (ADHD)	Delayed/weak attention, response inhibition, and executive function	Mildly atypical social and behavioral characteristics occasionally observed	Prominent discrepancy between areas of weakness and areas of strength
Hearing impairment	Delays in language and communication skills of variable degree, related to severity and timing of hearing loss and type of interventions	Prominent, pathological disturbance in the hearing apparatus	Relatively few difficulties with nonlanguage domains

atypical development into a cogent diagnostic framework and may be defined as follows: A *developmental disability* is a specific diagnostic entity characterized by a disturbance in or departure from expected patterns of development that results in predictable patterns of impairment, functional limitation, and disadvantage with regard to participation in real-life situations and settings. Section III of this book, Developmental Disabilities, describes specific forms of developmental disability in detail.

SUMMARY

Human development is a complex phenomenon that may be operationally defined with respect to the characteristic patterns of behavioral change and functional adaptation that occur during the course of the human life cycle. The precise determinants of these behavioral changes have

been the subject of intense scientific and philosophical debate. Developmental disabilities are clinically characterized as unexpected departures from typical patterns of development. Specific diagnoses are based on the recognition of 1) patterns of disturbance within and among specific developmental domains, and 2) the predictable functional consequences that arise from these disturbances. Developmental disabilities are further understood with reference to etiologic, social, cultural, therapeutic, and legal considerations. Although understanding of the complex nature of developmental disabilities continues to improve, it is still far from complete.

REFERENCES

Accardo, P.J. (Ed.). (2008). *Capute & Accardo's Neurodevelopmental disabilities in infancy and childhood* (3rd ed.). Baltimore, MD: Paul H. Brookes Publishing Co.

American Academy of Pediatrics Task Force on Sudden Infant Death Syndrome. (2005). The changing concept of sudden infant death syndrome: Diagnostic coding shifts, controversies regarding the sleeping environment, and new variables to consider in reducing risk. *Pediatrics, 166,* 1245–1255.

American Psychiatric Association. (2000). *Diagnostic and Statistical Manual of Mental Disorders, Fourth Edition, Text Revised (DSM-IV-TR).* Washington, DC: American Psychiatric Association.

Bronfenbrenner, U. (1979). *The ecology of human development.* Cambridge, MA: Harvard University Press.

Capute, A.J., & Accardo, P.J. (2005). *The Capute Scales: Cognitive adaptive test/clinical linguistic and auditory milestone scale (CAT/CLAMS).* Baltimore, MD: Paul H. Brookes Publishing Co.

Individuals with Disabilities Education Improvement Act (IDEA) of 2004, PL 108–446, 20 U.S. §§1400 et seq.

Knobloch, H., & Pasamanick, B. (Eds.). (1974). *Gesell and Amatruda's developmental diagnosis* (3rd ed.). New York, NY: Harper & Row.

Kuhl, P.K. (2010). Brain mechanisms in early language acquisition. *Neuron, 67*(5), 713–727.

Majnemer, A., & Barr, R.G. (2006). Association between sleep position and early motor development. *Journal of Pediatrics, 149*(5), 623–629.

National Institutes of Health. (1993). *Research plan for the National Center for Medical Rehabilitation Research.* (NIH Publication No. 93–3509). Bethesda, MD: Author.

Piaget, J. (1990). *The child's conception of the world.* New York, NY: Littlefield Adams Quality Paperbacks.

Piper, M.C., & Darrah, J. (1994). *Motor assessment of the developing infant.* Philadelphia, PA: W.B. Saunders.

Redcay, E., Haist, F., & Courchesne, E. (2008). Functional neuroimaging of speech perception during a pivotal period in language acquisition. *Developmental Science, 11*(2), 237–252.

Shaywitz, S.E., Morris, R., & Shaywitz, B.A. (2008). The education of dyslexic children from childhood to young adulthood. *Annual Review of Psychology, 59,* 451–475.

Simeonsson, R.J., Leonardi, M., Lollar, E., Bjorck-Akesson, E., Hollenweger, J., & Martinuzzi, A. (2003). Applying the International Classification of Functioning, Disability and Health (ICF) to measure childhood disability. *Disability and Rehabilitation, 25*(11–12), 602–610.

Spencer, J.P., Clearfield, M., Corbetta, D., Ulrich, B., Buchanan, P., & Schöner, G. (2006). Moving toward a grand theory of development: In memory of Esther Thelen. *Child Development, 77*(6), 1521–1538.

Squires, J., & Bricker, D. (2005). *Ages & Stages Questionnaires, Third Edition (ASQ-3).* Baltimore, MD: Paul H. Brookes Publishing Co.

United States Social Security Administration. (2011). *Social Security.* Retrieved April 11, 2011, Government Web site: http://www.ssa.gov/

Volpe, J. (Ed.). (1995). *Neurology of the newborn* (3rd ed.). Philadelphia, PA: W.B. Saunders.

Volpe, J. (Ed.). (2008). *Neurology of the newborn* (5th ed.). Philadelphia, PA: W.B. Saunders.

Vygotsky, L. (1986). *Thought and language* (A. Kozulin, Trans.). Cambridge, MA: The MIT Press.

World Health Organization. (2001). *ICF Browser.* Retrieved April 11, 2011, from Health Web site: http://apps.who.int/classifications/icfbrowser/

World Health Organization. (2001). *International Classification of Functioning, Disability and Health (ICF).* Retrieved April 11, 2011, from Health Web site: http://www.who.int/classifications/icf/en/

World Health Organization. (2007). *International Classification of Functioning, Disability and Health for Children and Youth (ICF–CY).* Retrieved April 11, 2011, from Health Web site: http://www.who.int/mediacentre/news/releases/2007/pr59/en/

World Health Organization. (2007). *International Statistical Classification of Diseases and Related Health Problems 10th Revision.* Retrieved April 11, 2011, from Health Web site: http://apps.who.int/classifications/apps/icd/icd10online/

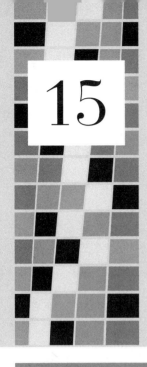

15

Diagnosing Developmental Disabilities

Scott M. Myers

Upon completion of this chapter, the reader will

- Recognize the major streams of development and their role in defining the spectrum and continuum of developmental disabilities

- Understand atypical patterns of development including delay, dissociation, deviance, and regression and their role in developmental diagnosis

- Be familiar with the components of the developmental diagnostic evaluation and how they contribute to the diagnostic formulation

Children typically present for developmental diagnostic evaluation because of concerns about not attaining cognitive, motor, or social/adaptive milestones, or about the presence of aberrant behaviors. These concerns may be raised spontaneously by parents or other caregivers, or may be elicited by health care providers through developmental surveillance and screening (American Academy of Pediatrics Council on Children with Disabilities et al., 2006). The diagnostic process enables the clinician to begin to answer the four fundamental questions that most parents have when they seek evaluation: 1) What is wrong with my child? (diagnosis), 2) What is going to happen to my child? (natural history/prognosis), 3) What can be done to improve my child's condition? (treatment), and 4) What caused my child's condition? (etiology).

In this chapter, general principles and processes involved in diagnosis of developmental disabilities are reviewed. Details about each of the specific disabilities and procedures such as developmental or psychological testing are available in other chapters in this volume and in other current textbooks in the field (e.g., Accardo, 2008; Carey, Crocker, Coleman, Elias, & Feldman, 2009; Voigt, Macias, & Myers, 2011; Wolraich, Drotar, Dworkin, & Perrin, 2008). The focus is on developmental disabilities caused by brain dysfunction, rather than those caused by sensory deficits such as blindness or deafness, orthopedic impairments, or disorders of the spinal cord, peripheral nervous system, or muscle.

■ ■ ■ NOAH

Before his second birthday, Noah's parents and pediatrician had concerns about delayed gross motor and speech milestones, which were initially attributed to his frequent ear and sinus infections. They were disappointed when his speech did not improve dramatically after placement of **tympanostomy** tubes at 23 months of age. Neurodevelopmental assessment at 28 months of age revealed significant global developmental delay, mild **hypotonia**, and neurobehavioral abnormalities including motor **stereotypy**, insomnia, and self-injurious behavior. He was short in stature and was noted to have minor **dysmorphic** features and a gruff voice. His family was guided to early intervention services, including habilitative therapies and behavioral intervention, which proved very helpful. Noah continued to make developmental progress at about 50% of the typical rate and the *global developmental delay* diagnosis was refined to *moderate intellectual disability* by the time he entered elementary school, where he thrived with special education supports and was known for his outgoing personality, sense of humor, and tendency to cross his arms and squeeze as if hugging himself when happy or excited.

At the time of his initial diagnostic evaluation, several genetic syndromes were in the differential diagnosis, and chromosomal microarray analysis revealed a 17p11.2 microdeletion, confirming that the etiology of Noah's developmental disability was Smith-Magenis syndrome (SMS; see Appendix B). His parents were relieved to learn that this was a *de novo* (new) **microdeletion** (see Chapter 1), so the chance that their subsequent children would have SMS was less than 1%. His family became very active in a support group and found it very helpful to meet other children and families affected by SMS. Because the cause of his intellectual disability was known, his pediatrician was able to assess and monitor him closely for associated medical problems, leading to the additional diagnosis of myopia and later **hypercholesterolemia** (elevated cholesterol levels in blood). In the preschool period, he developed insomnia characterized by markedly fragmented sleep, and challenging behaviors such as tantrums, self-injury, and aggression became more prominent. His sleep problems and daytime behavior improved substantially when he was treated with a beta-blocker in the morning and melatonin at night, based on the known abnormal pattern of melatonin secretion associated with SMS and the reported efficacy of this treatment in other affected individuals.

DEVELOPMENTAL PRINCIPLES

Development is an end product of neural function that unfolds over time as a result of 1) innate factors determined by the DNA sequence and

heritable epigenetic modifications that make up an individual's biological endowment, and 2) experiential influences that either affect neurodevelopment beneficially (e.g., environmental enrichment) or deleteriously (e.g., traumatic or **hypoxic-ischemic** brain insults or environmental deprivation) during sensitive periods of neuromaturation (Wang, 2011). The complex, dynamic processes that make up child development can be described clinically by quantifiable milestones and qualitative features and can be divided into three primary "streams" of development: motor, cognitive, and neurobehavioral. Each of the three primary streams can be broken down into narrower streams of development which can be assessed independently (Table 15.1). The motor stream includes gross and fine motor skills as well as oral motor function (chewing, swallowing, and motor aspects of speech). The cognitive or central processing stream includes receptive and expressive language abilities and nonlanguage cognition (problem-solving). The neurobehavioral stream includes fundamental aspects of social and emotional behavior, self-regulation, and mental status such as development of reciprocal social interaction, impulse control, attention, an appropriately varied repertoire of interests and activities, and adaptive regulation of mood and anxiety.

ATYPICAL PATTERNS OF DEVELOPMENT

Based on careful study of the development of thousands of infants and children, Gesell observed that typical development is methodical, orderly (sequential), timed, and therefore largely predictable (Gesell & Amatruda, 1947). This

Table 15.1. Streams of development

Motor
Gross motor
Fine motor
Oral motor

Cognitive (or central processing)
Language
Receptive
Expressive
Problem-solving/nonlanguage cognition

Neurobehavioral
Social behavior
Adaptive emotional behavior, self-regulation, and mental status

principle is the basis for using developmental milestones and tests as markers of neuromaturation. Independent assessment of skills within each stream of development facilitates recognition of patterns of atypical development. The terms *delay, dissociation,* and *deviance* describe variations in the attainment of developmental milestones as manifestations of underlying brain dysfunction, and analysis of these three types of variation is helpful in distinguishing among diagnostic possibilities (Accardo, Accardo, & Capute, 2008; see Chapter 14).

Developmental delay refers to a significant lag in the attainment of milestones in one or more areas of development; milestones are attained in the typical sequence, but at a slower rate. Traditionally, a delay of ≥ 25% in the rate of development, or performance that is 1.5 to 2 standard deviations or more below the norm, has been considered to be significant. The developmental quotient (DQ) is a useful means of quantifying development within a stream as a percentage of normal. The DQ is therefore a ratio; that is, the child's developmental age (DA) in a particular area of development divided by his or her chronological age (CA) and multiplied by 100 to yield a percentage (DQ = DA/CA × 100). For example, a 20-month-old child whose gross motor skills are at the level expected of a typically developing 12 month old has a DQ in the motor stream of 12/20 × 100 = 60. This child can thus be said to be exhibiting a 40% delay in gross motor development or to be progressing at 60% of the typical rate within the gross motor stream. The functional developmental age equivalent (developmental age) is determined based on normal milestones in a particular area of development, using tables of normal milestones that are available in textbooks (Accardo, 2008) and review articles (Gerber, Wilks, & Erdie-Lalena, 2010; Wilks, Gerber, & Erdie-Lalena, 2010) or assessment instruments that yield age equivalents in different streams of development, such as the Capute Scales (Cognitive Adaptive Test/Clinical Linguistic and Auditory Milestone Scale; CAT/CLAMS; Accardo & Capute, 2005), Parents Evaluation of Developmental Status: Developmental Milestones (PEDS:DM; Brothers et al., 2008), and Child Development Inventory (CDI; Ireton, 1992).

Developmental dissociation refers to a significant difference in developmental rates between two of the major areas of development: gross motor, fine motor, problem-solving, expressive language, receptive language, and social/adaptive. Typical sequences of development

are maintained, but there is asynchrony, resulting in one or more areas of development being significantly out of phase with other areas. By convention, a developmental quotient or rate discrepancy of greater than 15 percentage points between two major areas of development is typically considered to represent dissociation in infants or young children. In older children, a discrepancy of more than 1 or 1.5 standard deviations on standardized measures traditionally defines a significant discrepancy between academic achievement and intellectual ability (American Psychiatric Association, 2000; Shaywitz, Morris, & Shaywitz, 2008).

Developmental deviance refers to nonsequential unevenness in the achievement of milestones within one or more streams of development. This phenomenon is typically described qualitatively, rather than as a rate, quotient, or standard score. Typical developmental sequences are not maintained, and deviance is intrinsically abnormal. Whereas children exhibiting delay and dissociation attain milestones in a manner that would be expected for a younger typically developing child, deviance is not typical for any age.

The term *global developmental delay* (GDD), although not a diagnosis that appears in widely utilized classification systems (Wolraich & Drotar, 2008), has been defined in the literature as significant delays in two or more of the following domains: gross motor/fine motor, speech/language, cognition, social/personal, and activities of daily living (ADL; Riou, Ghosh, Francoeur & Shevell, 2009; Shevell et al., 2003). According to this definition, a child with cerebral palsy causing isolated motor delay and secondary difficulty with ADL and an infant exhibiting 25% delays in expressive language and gross motor skills (with average receptive language and problem-solving abilities) would both be considered to have GDD. The assumption that having delays in any two domains is equivalent to having general intellectual delay is inherently problematic, and Riou and colleagues (2009) demonstrated that 73% of a group of preschoolers had IQ greater than 70 despite concurrent GDD using this definition, and 20% had average intelligence.

In the alternate definition of *global developmental delay,* the term is restricted to children with significant delays in both language and cognition (problem solving) accompanied by deficits in adaptive behavior (activities of daily living). This definition more closely approximates applying the concept of intellectual disability to children who may be too young to obtain a valid and reliable IQ measurement. In these children, continued development at the same trajectory would predict functioning within the intellectual disability range. Of course, this does not mean that all children with GDD will ultimately have intellectual disability because developmental trajectories may change, but the greater the degree of global developmental delay, the higher the predictive validity of an early childhood diagnosis (VanderVeer & Schweid, 1974). There is general agreement that GDD should only be used as a diagnostic label until the child is old enough for evaluators to confidently make a more specific diagnosis, such as intellectual disability.

Once specific areas of delay have been identified, the concept of dissociation becomes particularly important in defining and distinguishing among the various developmental disability diagnoses (Table 15.2). Mixed receptive and expressive language disorders, for example, are defined by language development that is delayed and dissociated from other streams of development, especially problem solving/nonlanguage cognition. In the case of expressive language disorders, there is dissociation between the expressive and receptive components of the language stream; expressive language development is delayed but receptive language and nonlanguage cognition are intact. Specific learning disabilities are also determined by dissociation, or discrepancy; academic difficulty in a specific area (e.g., reading, mathematics, or written expression) is unexpected because the child appears to have all of the factors (i.e., intelligence, motivation, and exposure to reasonable instruction) present to achieve but continues to struggle (Shaywitz et al., 2008). In this case, the discrepancy is between academic achievement and intellectual ability or between actual and expected response to intervention (Fuchs & Fuchs, 2006; Shaywitz et al., 2008). Absolute developmental delay does not have to be present for dissociation to be significant since, for example, a child with an IQ of 125 whose standard scores on measures of various aspects of reading achievement are 85–90 could certainly have a specific reading disability.

Developmental deviance may present in young children as failure to accomplish simple tasks or skills in a given developmental sequence while passing more difficult items. For example, a 2-year-old child who can use single words to label more than 50 different objects or pictures and correctly identify colors and shapes yet does not use words to make requests, does not say "mama" or "dada," and still engages in immature jargoning is exhibiting significantly deviant language development. Strong rote memory skills accompanied by weak comprehension and pragmatic (social) language skills may contribute to this deviant profile, which may suggest the presence of an ASD (Myers & Challman, 2011). Most individually administered standardized psychometric tests include items that are arranged hierarchically, so in order to be able to administer only the appropriate portion of the test to a particular child, a "basal" and a "ceiling" must be established. This means that the child must answer a certain number of consecutive items correctly to establish a basal, and the test is stopped when the child answers a certain number of consecutive items incorrectly (ceiling). Developmental deviance, especially in older children with learning disorders, may be suggested by a much wider than average number of items between the basal and the ceiling on a particular test or subtest, or even the presence of "double basals" or "double ceilings" because of tending to pass more advanced items in the hierarchy while failing easier items (Accardo et al., 2008). **Dysarthria**, which is a motor speech disorder that is the result of paralysis, muscle weakness, or poor coordination, is intrinsically qualitatively abnormal and may also be considered to be an example of developmental deviance.

Another phenomenon that may be detected by history-taking or serial assessments is *developmental regression*, which is the loss of previously attained milestones. A child who has truly regressed developmentally is no longer capable of performing previously mastered skills. Loss of language and/or social skills occurs in a substantial minority of young children with ASDs (16%–41%), typically between 15 and 24 months of age, and may occur following typical development but is more commonly superimposed on preexisting atypical development (Baird et al., 2008; Meilleur & Fombonne, 2009). This type of regression is not unique to children with ASDs, although it appears to be most frequent in this population (Baird et al., 2008). Rare conditions such as acquired epileptic aphasia (Landau-Kleffner syndrome) and childhood disintegrative disorder are characterized by loss of language skills, which can also occur occasionally in children with intellectual disabilities, language disorders, congenital blindness, or acquired or progressive hearing loss (Rogers, 2004). Global regression involving language, motor, and cognitive skills may

Table 15.2. Key defining areas of relative impairment in selected developmental disabilities

	Intellectual disability	Specific learning disabilities	Cerebral palsy	Dysarthria	Mixed receptive and expressive language disorder	Expressive language disorder	Autistic disorder	Asperger disorder	ADHD
Motor									
Gross			X						
Fine			X						
Oral				X					
Language									
Expressive	X				X	X	X		
Receptive	X				X		X		
Pragmatic							X	X	
Problem-solving/non-language cognition	X								
Academic achievement		X							
Adaptive behavior (self-care)	X								
Social reciprocity							X	X	
Attention, impulse control, regulation of activity level (relative to developmental level)									X

Key: X signifies relative delay or impairment present by definition; ADHD, attention-deficit/hyperactivity disorder.

indicate the presence of certain inborn errors of metabolism, neurogenetic disorders, brain tumor, or subclinical seizures. Global regression always warrants investigation.

Specific types of isolated regression in motor skills, such as deterioration in gait in someone with a known disability, may be explained by the history and physical exam and warrant further evaluation and/or treatment. For example, deterioration in gait in a child or adolescent with spastic **diplegia** (a form of cerebral palsy) may be due to the mechanics of linear growth and weight gain in the setting of abnormal tone and the development of contractures requiring medical or surgical intervention. Similar deterioration in gait accompanied by increasing spasticity in the legs, change in bowel and bladder function, and progressive scoliosis in a patient with spina bifida would prompt evaluation for tethering or **syrinx** of the spinal cord (see Chapter 25).

Spectrum and Continuum of Developmental Disabilities

The various developmental disorders that result from neurologically based abnormalities in cognitive, motor, and neurobehavioral function have been referred to as the *spectrum* of developmental disabilities (Accardo et al., 2008).

Within each group of disorders, there also exists a spectrum of severity and prevalence. These conditions range from high prevalence, low-severity conditions such as dyslexia/specific reading disability, developmental coordination disorder (DCD), and attention-deficit/hyperactivity disorder (ADHD), to low-prevalence, high-severity conditions such as intellectual disability and cerebral palsy (Accardo et al., 2008; Voigt, 2011). Severity is determined by the degree of developmental delay, dissociation, and/or deviancy and, as with most other pathology, the milder forms are more common than the most severe forms.

In contrast to focal neurologic deficits that occur in the mature nervous system as a result of insults such as cerebrovascular accidents, developmental brain dysfunction tends to be diffuse, resulting in observable manifestations in cognitive, motor, and neurobehavioral functioning (Figure 15.1). Clinical neurodevelopmental disability syndromes may be primarily cognitive (e.g., intellectual disability, language disorder, learning disability), motor (e.g., cerebral palsy, DCD), or neurobehavioral (e.g., ASD, ADHD) conditions, but careful examination typically reveals additional impairments in the other streams of development. In fact, the presence of additional impairments or coexisting (comorbid) disorders is the rule rather than

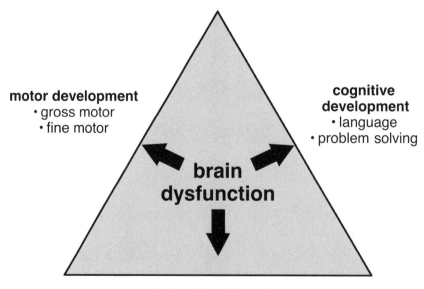

Figure 15.1. Adaptation of Capute's triangle: Developmental brain dysfunction impacts all three major streams of development. (*Source:* Capute, 1991.)

the exception. This concept is referred to as the *continuum* of developmental disabilities.

The epidemiology of developmental disabilities supports the concept of a continuum across streams of development, as essentially all developmental disorders co-occur with other developmental disorders much more frequently than expected by chance. For example, data from population-based epidemiologic studies suggest that 31%–65% of children with cerebral palsy (CP) also have an IQ less than 70 (Pakula, Van Naarden Braun, & Yeargin-Alsopp, 2009). Even among those individuals with CP but without intellectual disability, the prevalence of below-average IQ, learning disabilities, speech and language disorders, and ADHD is high (Odding, Roebroeck, & Stam, 2006). Data from the Metropolitan Atlanta Developmental Disability Surveillance Program (2006) indicate that 9% of 8-year-old children with CP also had an ASD diagnosis (Pakula et al., 2009). Insults causing brain dysfunction severe enough to result in CP also increase the risk of other neurological and sensory dysfunction; also increased in this population are rates of epilepsy (20%–46%), visual impairment (2%–19%), and hearing impairment (2%–6%) (Pakula et al., 2009). In addition, the neuromotor impairment associated with CP often leads to secondary associated conditions, such as orthopedic deformities, chronic constipation, gastroesophageal reflux, malnutrition, poor growth, **osteopenia**, and skin breakdown (see Chapter 24).

The developmental profile can be conceptualized as an iceberg, with one or more visible tips representing the defining features of the primary diagnoses, and the submerged portion representing the larger continuum of manifestations of underlying brain dysfunction (Accardo et al., 2008). For example, a child with ADHD by definition exhibits symptoms of inattention and/or hyperactivity/impulsivity that are inappropriate for age and developmental level, and interfere significantly with functioning. However, the ADHD symptoms (tip of the iceberg) are usually accompanied by other signs and symptoms below the surface, such as motor coordination deficits, tics, neurologic "subtle" or "soft" signs on exam, learning deficits, pragmatic language impairment, social skills deficits, sleep problems, obsessive and/or compulsive behaviors, anxiety, depressed or irritable mood, and disruptive behaviors. These are manifestations of the underlying mild brain dysfunction and its interaction with environmental influences/experiences. Often, some of these symptoms of neurological dysfunction are prominent enough to meet diagnostic criteria for one or more other disorders such as specific learning disability, developmental coordination disorder, Tourette syndrome, obsessive-compulsive disorder, or oppositional-defiant disorder (additional visible tips of the iceberg). Other symptoms may remain subthreshold in terms of additional diagnoses but may still be important to address when planning treatment. Comorbidity among developmental disorders is primarily due to the diffuse nature of the underlying brain dysfunction, which is often genetic in origin, although environment and experience may be important modifiers of this effect. For example, studies of twins have shown that reading disorder (RD), math disorder (MD), and ADHD are familial and heritable and that the etiology of the co-morbidity between RD and MD (28%–64%), RD and ADHD (10%–40%), and MD and ADHD (12%–36%) is primarily explained by common genetic influences (Willcutt et al., 2010). A genetic abnormality may result in different phenotypes due to incomplete penetrance, variable expressivity, or interactions between genes and the environment. A gene/environment (G × E) interaction is said to occur if environmental circumstances modify the expression of an individual's genetic background, either strengthening or weakening the phenotype. Significant G × E interactions have been described in psychiatric conditions such as conduct disorder and depression and are being explored in developmental disabilities such as ADHD and ASD (Willcutt et al., 2010).

DIAGNOSTIC CLASSIFICATION

Diagnostic labels, whether *disease* names that imply a known etiology or pathophysiology or *disorder* names that are defined by clusters of attributes or symptoms less closely related to a single cause, are the usual means by which clinicians access the relevant medical literature to guide management decisions and communicate about conditions with patients, families, and colleagues. Diagnostic classification is important not only for treatment planning, prognostication, and other aspects of clinical care for an individual patient, but also for etiologic and outcomes research and societal allocation of resources (Table 15.3).

In most branches of medicine, systematic classification systems based on etiology and pathophysiology predominate; conditions are differentiated first by cause (e.g., infectious, genetic, neoplastic, autoimmune, traumatic) and second by how these processes disturb

Table 15.3. Importance of diagnostic classification

Clinical care
Parent/caregiver education
Treatment planning
Etiologic investigation
Identification of associated deficits
Genetic counseling
Prognostication
Reimbursement

Research
Epidemiology
Etiology
Natural history
Treatment efficacy/outcomes

Societal resource allocation
Planning, funding, and distribution of services and supports
Identification and correction of gaps in knowledge and service delivery
Training of health care and other professionals
Education and prevention efforts
Research funding

organ structure and function (e.g., pneumonia, skeletal dysplasia, leukemia, hepatitis, brain injury). In developmental medicine and psychiatry, however, conditions are described primarily phenomenologically as disorders or symptom-cluster syndromes rather than as diseases with known causes. While a definitive etiologic diagnosis can be made in a subset of individuals with any developmental disorder, there is not a 1:1 correspondence between developmental disorder diagnosis and etiologic diagnosis. Most developmental disorders can have many different causes, and most etiologic diagnoses can result in a variety of different clinical disorders.

Autistic disorder, for example, is defined clinically by early childhood onset of a cluster of symptoms that include qualitative impairment in reciprocal social interaction, deficits in communication, and a restricted, repetitive repertoire of interests and behaviors (Myers & Challman, 2011; see Chapter 21). In 15%–20% of individuals, a specific etiology (usually genetic) can be identified; the remaining 80%–85% of cases are currently considered to be idiopathic (Abrahams & Geschwind, 2008). Many different defined genetic syndromes, mutations, and *de novo* or inherited copy number variants (see Chapter 1) have been shown to cause autistic disorder, but no individual genetic disorder accounts for more than 1%–2% of

cases. Copy number variants (microdeletions or microduplications) at 16p11.2, for example, have been identified in 1% of individuals with ASDs, but also in 1.5% of individuals with unexplained intellectual disability (Weiss et al., 2008; McCarthy et al., 2009). In addition, the 16p11.2 microduplication has been associated with schizophrenia. In fact, at least 7 recurrent, pathogenic copy number variants are now known to be associated with autism or intellectual disability and also with schizophrenia (Moreno-De-Luca et al., 2010).

Levels of Diagnosis

Disorders of development and behavior can be described at three different levels, each of which has clinical significance (Figure 15.2; Table 15.4). This conceptualization is shown in Figure 15.2 as an inverted triangle, with the broad first level (specific impairments) at the top, narrower second level (categorical diagnoses) in the middle, and very narrow third level (etiologic diagnosis) at the bottom. An individual patient may have many specific impairments or symptoms which identify a smaller number of categorical disorders or symptom-cluster syndromes that are due to one underlying etiology or a very small number of distinct etiologies.

Specific Impairments

The first level of diagnosis, which is descriptive and may not be traditionally thought of as representing a diagnosis at all, is the level of identifying and labeling pertinent signs and symptoms as specific impairments or deficits. In addition to being a prerequisite for formulating categorical diagnoses (disorders or symptom-cluster syndromes), delineation of functionally impairing symptoms is essential for treatment planning, since educational, behavioral, and psychopharmacologic interventions most often address these specific impairments rather than the categorical diagnostic classification or etiologic diagnosis (Myers, Johnson, & the Council on Children with Disabilities, 2007). Even psychopharmacologic treatments are sometimes determined more by the specific impairments or target symptoms than by categorical or etiologic diagnoses. The traditional psychiatric model of psychopharmacologic decision making involves first making the diagnosis of a specific disorder, such as ADHD or depression, and then choosing a medication based on that diagnosis. However, because symptoms exist on a continuum and occur across different disorders, and modifications of diagnostic criteria

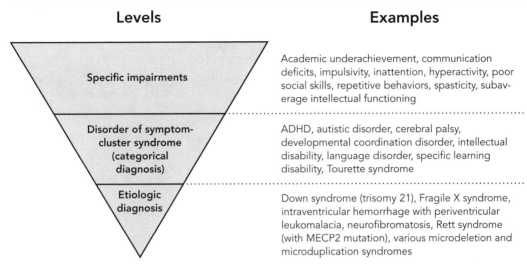

Levels	Examples
Specific impairments	Academic underachievement, communication deficits, impulsivity, inattention, hyperactivity, poor social skills, repetitive behaviors, spasticity, subaverage intellectual functioning
Disorder of symptom-cluster syndrome (categorical diagnosis)	ADHD, autistic disorder, cerebral palsy, developmental coordination disorder, intellectual disability, language disorder, specific learning disability, Tourette syndrome
Etiologic diagnosis	Down syndrome (trisomy 21), Fragile X syndrome, intraventricular hemorrhage with periventricular leukomalacia, neurofibromatosis, Rett syndrome (with MECP2 mutation), various microdeletion and microduplication syndromes

Figure 15.2. Levels of diagnosis. *(Key: ADHD, attention-deficit/hyperactivity disorder.)*

are necessary in order to apply many psychiatric diagnoses to individuals with more severe disabilities, the value of categorical distinctions in selecting pharmacologic treatment is often unclear. Therefore, a target-symptom approach is often the most appropriate treatment strategy (Bostic & Rho, 2006; Myers, 2007).

In addition to considering impairments that are intrinsic to the individual, it is important to also consider the child's abilities and the practical impact of environmental, early experiential, and societal factors. The International Classification of Functioning, Disability, and Health for Children and Youth (ICF-CY) classification system focuses on impairment and enablement in body structures and functions, activities, and participation/involvement as well as the influences of environmental and personal factors, which would be described at this level of diagnosis (Msall & Msall, 2008; Wolraich and Drotar, 2008).

Categorical Diagnoses: Disorders, Symptom-Cluster Syndromes

The second level of diagnosis involves recognizing patterns of specific impairments as disorders or clusters of symptoms that represent clinical syndromes (e.g., ADHD, autism, intellectual disability, mixed receptive-expressive language disorder), and categorizing them as such. This is the primary way that developmental disability diagnoses are classified using the World Health Organization ICD-10 (1992) and American Psychiatric Association DSM-IV-TR (2000)

diagnostic classification systems. Identification of the categorical diagnoses is important for guiding treatment, identifying associated problems, providing a prognosis, and communicating information to patients, families, and treatment providers including educators, habilitative therapists, psychologists, and healthcare providers. Epidemiologic information is also most often collected at this level of diagnosis, and this information can be used to guide resource allocation.

Etiologic Diagnosis

The third level of diagnosis, the etiologic diagnosis, involves identifying the specific underlying cause of the developmental disorder, which may be genetic, metabolic, teratogenic, infectious, hypoxic-ischemic, traumatic, a combination of more than one of these, or unknown/idiopathic. This etiologic level of diagnosis currently can be determined in only a minority of individuals with brain-based developmental disabilities but much more commonly in those with disorders of the spinal cord, peripheral nervous system, or sensory deficits (such as blindness or deafness). In general, the more severe the brain-based developmental disability, the more likely a specific etiologic diagnosis can be identified. For example, among individuals with intellectual disability, a specific etiology is much more likely to be determined if the cognitive impairment is severe (defined as IQ under 50) than if it is mild (e.g., 43% versus 13% in a metropolitan Atlanta cohort), but the vast majority

Table 15.4. Significance of each level of diagnosis

Level of diagnosis	Importance					
	Treatment		Genetic counseling	Identification of associated medical problems	Prognosti-cation	Resource allocation
	Behavioral, Educational	Psychophar-macologic				
Specific impairments	++	++	−	−/+	+/++	+
Disorder of symptom-cluster syndrome (categorical diagnoses)	+	+	+	+	++	++
Etiologic diagnosis	−	−/+*	++	++	+	−/+

Key: − minimal or no importance, + important, ++ very important
* emerging importance (may become very important with future advances)

of people with intellectual disability have an IQ above 50 (Yeargin-Allsopp et al., 1997).

The etiologic diagnosis is important, especially in the case of genetic disorders for which accurate counseling regarding recurrence risk can be provided and, in some cases, associated medical problems can be identified as a result of their known association with the genetic abnormality. For example, a patient who is found to have a 22q11.2 deletion (velocardiofacial syndrome; see Appendix B) as the cause of his intellectual disability or ASD is at increased risk for cardiac, palatal, immune, and renal anomalies as well as psychiatric disorders, and there is a 6%–10% chance that one of his parents has the deletion (McDonald-McGinn & Sullivan, 2011). If a parent is affected, he or she has a 50% chance of passing the deletion to each of his or her children.

The value of determining an etiologic diagnosis is not limited to genetic disorders that directly affect neurological function, and genetic tests are not the only valuable studies. For example, brain imaging may reveal an infarct as the cause of a young child's hemiplegia. This would prompt further evaluation that might identify a genetic coagulopathy (clotting disorder such as Factor V Leiden thrombophilia) for which additional treatment, stroke recurrence risk counseling, and family genetic counseling are available. An infant with congenital cytomegalovirus (CMV) infection requires serial assessments for hearing loss, which may be delayed in onset and/or progressive. In the case of certain inborn errors of metabolism, neuroprotective or even curative treatment can

be provided if the diagnosis is made early (see Chapter 19).

All of these important aspects of medical management are more closely linked to etiologic diagnosis than to categorical (level 2) diagnoses or specific impairments (Table 15.4). Discoveries about the neurobiology of genetic neurodevelopmental disorders have led to pharmacological interventions to improve cognitive function in animal models of various disorders, and with recent clinical drug trials in humans with fragile X syndrome, we have entered the era of neuroscience-driven pharmacotherapy that depends on the etiologic diagnosis rather than the disorder- or symptom-level diagnosis (Levenga, de Vrij, Oostra, & Willemsen, 2010; Wetmore & Garner, 2010).

THE DIAGNOSTIC PROCESS

Similar to other areas of medicine, the diagnostic process in developmental medicine consists of taking a history, examining the patient, generating a differential diagnosis, planning tests and investigations, formulating a provisional or definitive diagnosis, and developing a management plan. However, in developmental medicine the examination of the patient includes developmental and/or psychoeducational testing as an extension of the neurologic exam. In addition, there are essentially two levels of differential diagnosis: one addressing the categorical diagnosis (e.g., intellectual disability or autistic disorder) and the other addressing the etiologic diagnosis (e.g., a chromosomal microdeletion or fragile X syndrome). Laboratory tests and other investigations such as neuroimaging and neurophysiologic studies primarily address the etiologic differential diagnosis or medical conditions that may be associated with the categorical diagnosis.

The diagnostic evaluation format will vary depending on the availability of local resources and clinician preferences. One approach involves employing an interdisciplinary or multidisciplinary team specializing in developmental disabilities. This includes individuals from a variety of disciplines including psychology, speech-language pathology, occupational therapy, physical therapy, special education, social work, audiology, and various medical subspecialties. Alternatively, the diagnostic evaluation may be conducted by an individual clinician-specialist who is capable of interpreting and integrating information from various disciplines and comfortable with making developmental diagnoses even if there is not an interdisciplinary team that meets in-person. Most often, this is a neurodevelopmental pediatrician, developmental-behavioral pediatrician, pediatric psychologist, child and adolescent psychiatrist, or pediatric neurologist. The diagnostic evaluation should incorporate the following elements (Myers & Challman, 2011, p. 268):

1. Caregiver interview, with thorough medical history and review of systems, developmental and behavioral history, social history, and family history.

2. Review of pertinent medical and educational records, including any available standardized testing done by early intervention evaluators, psychologists, speech-language pathologists, occupational therapists, physical therapists, and special educators.

3. Direct clinical assessment, including physical examination (with an emphasis on the neurologic examination and dysmorphologic evaluation), developmental and/or psychological testing (appropriate for age and level of ability), and neurobehavioral examination. In the case of team evaluations, the developmental or psychoeducational testing is often completed by someone other than the physician. In some cases, even a physician diagnostician who is working independently will review and interpret the results of current standardized testing performed by professionals in other disciplines in lieu of directly administering tests her- or himself.

4. Determination of categorical diagnoses, most often using current criteria from *Diagnostic and Statistical Manual of Mental Disorders* (DSM-IV-TR; American Psychiatric Association, 2000) or International Classification of Diseases (ICD-10; World Health Organization, 1992), although the diagnostician is not limited to these classification systems.

5. Consideration of etiologic possibilities and determination of appropriate investigations to evaluate these etiologic possibilities and/or associated medical conditions.

Many clinicians choose to gather some historical information in advance by having parents complete medical, developmental, and family history questionnaires, which allows consultation time to be used for more focused questioning. This process may also increase the accuracy of historical information because it gives families the opportunity to reflect on the questions without pressure or time constraints, review milestones in baby books or journals, and ask relatives about family history. In some practice models, the diagnostic process involves more than one office visit.

Chief Complaint and Age of Presentation

In all branches of medicine, the physician starts the diagnostic process by asking about the presenting symptoms and concerns, or "chief complaint." In the field of developmental disabilities, the age of presentation/referral to the developmental specialist is closely tied to the nature of the chief complaint and developmental diagnosis (Lock, Shapiro, Ross, & Capute, 1986; Shapiro & Gwynn, 2008). Although caregivers may detect severe hearing or vision impairment in infants at 3–6 months of age based on a lack of appropriate response to sounds or visual tracking, concerns arising in the first 6 months of life are usually based not on developmental delays but on medical risk factors. These include major congenital anomalies, obvious dysmorphic features, failed newborn hearing screening, or known central nervous system insults such as severe intraventricular hemorrhage or hypoxic-ischemic encephalopathy. Physiologic instability resulting from frequent seizures, feeding dysfunction, or poor weight gain may also trigger concerns about development in early infancy.

Concerns presenting at 6–18 months of age are most often related to delayed attainment of gross motor milestones, and common diagnoses include cerebral palsy and other types of neuromotor dysfunction, including central hypotonia and neuromuscular disorders (Crawford, 1996; Lock et al., 1986).

Patients with delayed language development tend to present at 18–36 months of age, and common diagnoses among this group include language disorders, global developmental delay/intellectual disability, and ASD. Toddlers with both delayed language and problem-solving skills (global developmental delay) tend to present for diagnostic evaluation slightly earlier than those with primary language disorders (median ages 27 months and 32 months, respectively; Lock et al., 1986). Among 17–36 month old children with ASDs receiving early intervention services in Louisiana, the most common first concern reported by parents was delayed communication (74%), followed by challenging behaviors (24%) and social skills deficits (12%; Kozlowski, Matson, Horovitz, Worley, & Neal, 2011). However, communication impairment was also the most frequent initial concern reported by parents of toddlers with other developmental disorders (81%), and no single area of concern distinguished ASDs from other developmental disorders.

Disruptive behaviors including tantrums, oppositional and defiant behaviors, impulsivity, hyperactivity, and aggressive or destructive behavior tend to present over a wide range of ages, from 24 months to school-age and beyond. These behaviors are associated with a variety of developmental and behavioral diagnoses. Whereas the hyperactivity and impulsivity of ADHD of the combined type (ADHD-C) may prompt referral in the preschool period, children with predominantly inattentive type ADHD (ADHD-I) typically do not present until inattention, distractibility, and poor organizational skills interfere with academic functioning in elementary school or later. Individuals with ADHD-I tend to manifest impairment later (after age 7 in 43%), have primarily academic problems, and exhibit fewer social and behavioral problems than those with ADHD-C (Applegate et al., 1997). Concerns about academic achievement or school performance may present as early as age 3–5 years in these children, but these issues more commonly arise as problems in the elementary school years or later. As a result,

learning disorders or disabilities are primarily diagnosed in school-age children or adolescents with ADHD.

Information Gathering

The Medical History

A careful prenatal and perinatal history may identify risk factors such as toxic or teratogenic exposure, premature birth, or maternal complications (e.g., infection, gestational diabetes mellitus, pregnancy-induced hypertension, hypothyroidism, or other significant illness; Whitaker & Palmer, 2008). In addition to eliciting any potential history of perinatal hypoxic-ischemic insult, the clinician may identify markers of fetal abnormality such as hypoactive or hyperactive fetal movements, evidence of distress noted on fetal monitoring, breech presentation, or abnormal brain/somatic growth (i.e., microcephaly, macrocephaly, and small for gestational age status). The neonatal history is focused on identifying pertinent complications and treatments, especially in infants who were born prematurely and/or had medical or surgical problems requiring intensive care, and eliciting evidence of nonspecific neurobehavioral or neuromotor abnormalities that may provide insight into the integrity of the central nervous system (CNS). Examples of the latter include excessive quietness, irritability, persistent colic, altered sleep-wake cycle, feeding problems, jitteriness, floppiness, and stiffness. Complications such as intraventricular or **parenchymal** CNS hemorrhage, periventricular leukomalacia, neonatal seizures, severe hyperbilirubinemia, chronic lung disease associated with prematurity (especially with early postnatal steroid treatment), and retinopathy of prematurity should be noted (see Chapters 6 and 7).

The medical history beyond the neonatal period is also helpful in establishing risk and providing clues to the etiology of developmental problems (Whitaker & Palmer, 2008). Pertinent findings include past acute medical conditions (e.g., meningitis, encephalitis, traumatic brain injury), chronic illnesses that have the potential to impact development and behavior (e.g., malnutrition, recurrent infections, cancer, sickle-cell anemia, chronic renal disease), and environmental exposures (e.g., lead). Clues suggesting the possibility of a metabolic disorder (e.g., episodic neurological dysfunction, unusual prostration with illness, or intolerance of fasting) or genetic syndrome (e.g., congenital anomalies such as congenital heart defects, cleft palate, or hypospadias) may also be elicited. Specific prompts are often required to elicit all of the pertinent issues from parents; important medical problems may be omitted by parents unless there is a specific review of systems and inquiry about hospitalizations or other medical consultants who have participated in the child's care. Sometimes anomalies that were surgically corrected are not mentioned by parents until the clinician inquires specifically about previous surgical procedures.

Developmental and Behavioral History

A thorough and accurate developmental and behavioral history requires substantial skill, experience, and time to complete but is usually the most informative aspect of the neurodevelopmental diagnostic assessment (Leppert, 2011; Montgomery, 2008; Whitaker & Palmer, 2008). The components of the developmental and behavioral history are outlined in Table 15.5. Developmental milestones are the cornerstones of the developmental and behavioral history. They provide the information necessary to identify developmental delays and atypical patterns of development including dissociation, deviance, and regression, as described previously.

Useful milestones must have precise definitions, occur within a narrow normative timeframe, be clinically observable and useful to the child, and have predictive validity (Accardo et al., 2008; Shapiro & Gwynn, 2008). Questions about current abilities should seek more detail than those on past milestones, which should focus on more notable milestones that are easier to recall by parents. When eliciting a current history of babbling in an infant, for example, the clinician must first define for the parent that babbling is consonant-vowel combinations. Then they can explore where the child is in the hierarchy of babbling which normally progresses from single syllables ("da") to reduplicative strings ("dadada") of varying length. This is followed by an increased repertoire of reduplicative strings ("dadada," "bababa," "gagaga") and then nonreduplicative strings ("badabagaba"). If the patient were a 3 year old who is speaking in phrases, the clinician would not go into this level of detail about babbling while eliciting the expressive language history because this is not something that parents would be likely to recall. The clinician would instead focus on milestones such as when the first meaningful words were spoken and when

the child began to use novel two-word combinations. More detailed questions are reserved for current abilities (e.g., vocabulary, length and content of phrases and sentences, use of pronouns, use of plurals, intelligibility).

The experienced diagnostician not only has a thorough knowledge of the average age of attainment of milestone in all areas of development, but is able to improve parent recall of developmental achievements by linking them to important family events. This might include asking about function during past holidays, birthdays, or summer vacations (e.g., How was your child moving around on her first birthday? Was she crawling, pulling up to a standing position, cruising along furniture, or walking independently?). Each area of development is reviewed chronologically to ascertain the age at which specific important milestones were attained as well as the current level of functioning (Leppert, 2011; Whitaker & Palmer, 2008). This approach allows retrospective analysis of developmental rate in each stream and recognition of changes in trajectory over time, such as improving trajectory ("catch-up"), plateau, or regression. This is analogous to obtaining past growth measurements and plotting them on appropriate growth curves to facilitate recognition of important patterns, such as crossing percentiles due to a plateau in linear or head circumference growth or loss of weight.

It is also important to thoroughly explore whether there are challenging or maladaptive behaviors and, if so, to obtain specific descriptions of the problem behaviors (Table 15.5). Standardized checklists or rating scales may be helpful in eliciting and quantifying various aspects of behavior from different sources, including parents and teachers, but they are not independently diagnostic and should not replace the clinician interview (American Academy of Pediatrics, Task Force on Mental Health, 2010). If the child exhibits problematic disruptive behaviors such as tantrums or aggressive outbursts, for example, it is important to specifically describe 1) the specific behaviors (e.g., screaming, crying, throwing things, hitting, kicking, dropping to the floor and flailing arms and legs); 2) their frequency, intensity, and duration; 3) exacerbating factors/triggers (e.g., time, setting/location, demand situations, denials, transitions); 4) ameliorating factors and response to behavioral interventions; 5) time trends (increasing, decreasing, stable); and 6) degree of interference with functioning.

Table 15.5.   Developmental and behavioral history

Age of developmental milestone attainment and current functioning

Gross motor skills
Fine motor skills
Communication/language skills (receptive, expressive, pragmatic)
Problem-solving skills/nonlanguage cognition
Academic achievement (strengths, weaknesses)
Social skills
Adaptive skills (self-care; activities of daily living)
Play/leisure skills and interests

Identification of abnormal developmental patterns

Delay, dissociation, deviance
Regression

Adaptive and maladaptive emotional behavior, self-regulation, and mental status

Temperament
Problem behaviors
  Inattention
  Disorganization
  Hyperactivity
  Impulsivity
  Noncompliance, oppositional and defiant behavior
  Tantrums, emotional outbursts
  Aggression
  Self-injurious behavior
  Repetitive behaviors
    Stereotypy
    Obsessions
    Compulsions
    Perseveration
    Rituals, nonfunctional routines
    Tics
  Sensory modulation issues
    Over responsivity
    Under responsivity
    Sensation-seeking, unusual sensory exploration
  Food- or meal-related problems, pica
  Sleep problems
    Difficulty falling asleep, bedtime resistance
    Nightwakings
    Early morning awakening
    Snoring, gasping, apnea
    Excessive sleep
  Anxiety
  Mood problems
    Depression, mania, irritability, lability
  Conduct problems
    Lying, stealing, truancy, vandalism, cruelty to animals, fire setting
  Enuresis, encopresis

In this way, it is often possible to determine the function of the behaviors and what aspects of the environment are maintaining these behaviors through inadvertent operant conditioning (see Chapter 32). Ultimately, after the child's developmental functioning in all major streams has been assessed, it is possible to judge whether the behaviors that concern the parent are inappropriate for the child's developmental level or whether they are actually typical behaviors once understood in the context of the child's developmental level of functioning or "developmental age." For example, parents who express concern and frustration about their 6-year-old child's inattention, impulsivity, tantrums in response to denials, and nocturnal enuresis may begin to understand the behaviors and approach them more appropriately when they are put in the context of the child's developmental age of 3 years.

Family History

The primary goal of the family history, which should include at least three generations, is to identify genetic risk and clues to specific genetic etiology, including pattern of inheritance. Parental ages at conception, history of prior fetal losses, educational levels, early educational difficulties, and major medical problems should be queried. Family history should include developmental and neurological disorders such as intellectual disability, ASD, cerebral palsy (CP), muscular dystrophies, ADHD, learning disorders, language disorders, developmental delays, epilepsy, hearing loss, and blindness. It is also often helpful to ask about whether any family members were slow learners, required special education services or any extra help in school, needed a wheelchair for mobility, or weren't able to live independently as adults. Psychiatric conditions such as schizophrenia, depression, bipolar disorder, anxiety disorders, obsessive-compulsive disorder, and substance abuse should also be explored.

The pattern of individuals with intellectual disability in a family, for example, may suggest autosomal dominant, autosomal recessive, X-linked, or mitochondrial inheritance (see Chapter 1). Even in the absence of any other family members with major developmental disabilities, the presence of other conditions may point to a specific genetic etiology. For example, a history of anxiety and difficulty with math in the mother and an undiagnosed tremor and ataxia syndrome in the maternal grandfather of a boy with global developmental delay, hyperactivity, and gaze avoidance raises the possibility of fragile X syndrome. Factors such as ethnicity, consanguinity, and history of multiple fetal losses, infant deaths, progressive or neurodegenerative disorders, or conditions associated with abnormal energy metabolism (e.g., myopathy, myoclonic epilepsy, cardiomyopthy, retinitis pigmentosa, ophthalmoplegia, sensorineural deafness, peripheral neuropathy) may suggest an increased risk of metabolic disease (Kelley, 2008).

Social History

Potential protective and deleterious psychosocial and socioeconomic factors should be explored. Parental education, cultural beliefs, family support systems, and previous experience with people with disabilities may impact the ability and willingness of parents or grandparents and extended family members to accept the diagnosis and treatment recommendations (see Chapter 37). A history of abuse or neglect of the child may be particularly relevant to the interpretation of the child's behavior, attachment, and social functioning; and previous involvement with child protective service agencies or foster care should be queried. Psychosocial stressors such as recent crises or transitions, financial or marital difficulties, and mental health or substance abuse issues may impact the child's development and behavior and the ability of the family to access resources and comply with treatment recommendations. If there are behavioral concerns about the child, it is important to determine the parents' expectations and behavior management strategies.

The child's educational/habilitative intervention history is also important. This includes utilization of early intervention services, preschool programs (including Head Start), and special education services. Any history of grade retention should be noted. Details of the current educational program should always be explored because a significant mismatch between educational expectations or demands and the child's current abilities is likely to result in poor progress and often behavioral or emotional problems, especially in school-age children. The timing and types of concerns voiced by the teachers and other school staff should be noted, along with previous disciplinary actions such as frequent loss of recess or other privileges, after-school detention, or suspension from school.

Physical Examination

The diagnostic evaluation should include a complete general physical and neurological examination. Particularly important aspects of the general physical examination include assessment for abnormal growth, dysmorphic features, evidence of **visceral** storage such as **hepatomegaly** (enlarged liver) and **spleno-megaly** (enlarged spleen), and skin manifestations of neurocutaneous disorders or other genetic syndromes.

Aberrations in growth such as short stature, tall stature, obesity, microcephaly, and macrocephaly may provide important clues to the etiology of the developmental disability. For some underlying causes, such as hypothyroidism, effective treatment is available. Important alterations in the trajectory or velocity of growth may be exposed by plotting serial measurements on normal population growth curves, revealing crossing of multiple percentile lines. For example, an infant with a rapidly increasing head circumference may have hydrocephalus and require surgical intervention. A plateau in head growth after 6 months of age resulting in acquired microcephaly in a female infant in the second year of life may be a manifestation of Rett syndrome. The visible change over time on the growth curve is much more informative than just a single measurement at the time of evaluation.

The child also should be examined for congenital anomalies, which can be classified as major or minor. Major anomalies usually require medical or surgical intervention, whereas minor anomalies generally do not require intervention but may be of cosmetic concern and diagnostic significance (Toriello, 2008). Major and minor anomalies occur much more commonly in children with developmental disabilities than in typically developing children. In individuals with three or more minor anomalies the chance of having a major anomaly, a dysmorphic syndrome, or both, increases greatly (Kirby, 2002; Toriello, 2008). Measurements should be recorded and compared to normative values in order to confirm or refute clinical impressions of abnormal size, proportions, or spacing of body parts (Hall et al., 2007). A clinical impression of hypotelorism (eyes close together), for example, should be confirmed by measurements because it is a strong indicator of abnormal brain development. Findings such as a **submucosal** cleft palate are important not only because of the treatable impact on speech, feeding, and conductive hearing loss, but also as a clue to an underlying genetic syndrome such as 22q11.2 deletion syndrome. Documentation of detailed descriptions of anomalies is useful for later searching the literature and online databases for potential diagnoses, which can in turn lead to a reasonable approach to laboratory testing (Toriello, 2008).

Coarse facial features, large tongue, corneal clouding, hepatomegaly, and splenomegaly may be due to **lysosomal storage diseases** (e.g., mucopolysaccharidoses, Gaucher disease; Kelley, 2008; see Appendix B). In all children the skin should be carefully examined, along with the other accessible ectodermal derivatives (hair, teeth, and nails). Hyperpigmented or hypopigmented lesions, vascular anomalies, and other lesions such as various types of **fibromas** and **hamartomas** are prominent aspects of neurocutaneous (i.e., skin and nervous system) syndromes such as neurofibromatosis, tuberous sclerosis, Sturge-Weber syndrome, ataxia-telangiectasia, and incontinentia pigmenti (Thiele & Korf, 2006; see Appendix B). Linear streaks or whorls of hypopigmentation, sometimes referred to as hypomelanosis of Ito, are often associated with **mosaicism** for a variety of chromosomal abnormalities (Kuster & Honig, 1999; see Chapter 1).

The neurologic examination of children with developmental disabilities includes standard evaluation of cranial nerve function, posture/station, muscle strength, muscle tone, deep tendon reflexes, cerebellar function, gait, coordination, and sensation. Abnormalities such as unusual movements, pathological reflexes, and significant asymmetry of function, strength, tone, or deep tendon reflexes are recorded. In infants and young children, markers of neuromotor maturation such as primitive reflexes and postural reactions should be examined (Blasco, 1992). Older children are assessed for markers of neuromaturation and neurodysfunction, such as upper extremity posturing during stressed gait maneuvers and finger-tapping tasks (Montgomery, 2008). Neurologic "subtle" or "soft" signs such as dysrhythmia and overflow movements, which are unintentional and unnecessary movements that accompany voluntary activity, are often detected. Mirror overflow, for example, includes movements that occur on the opposite side of the body during tasks such as sequential finger-tapping (Cole, Mostofsky, Gidley Larson, Denckla, & Mahone, 2008; Mostofsky, Newschaffer, & Denckla, 2003). Although most basic motor skills are mastered by age 6 or 7, some subtle signs may persist in typically developing children until about age 10

(Larson et al., 2007). However, prominent persistence into late childhood or adolescence may indicate atypical neurological development. These subtle signs are more common in children and adolescents with developmental disabilities, including ADHD, learning disorders, and high-functioning autism, and are related to inhibitory control (Cole et al., 2008; Mostofsky et al., 2003).

Developmental Testing and Neurobehavioral Status Exam

In addition to assessing each stream of development by history, the diagnostician evaluates each child by direct observation and elicitation (Leppert, 2011; Montgomery, 2008; Stein & Lukasik, 2009). Formal testing is either completed by the clinician or the results of current testing done by professionals in other disciplines are reviewed, or both. Language and nonlanguage/problem-solving aspects of cognition are measured directly. Age-appropriate quantifiable visual-motor measures, such as those that assess figure copying, drawing, and written output, and those that do not require pencil and paper (e.g., block design tasks) are included, and the qualitative aspects of the child's performance (e.g., pencil grasp, tremor or overflow movements, and qualitative features of the final product) are carefully observed and recorded. In older preschoolers and school-age children, academic achievement is also typically measured using standardized instruments.

A review of the many specific developmental and psychoeducational tests available is contained in Chapter 16, and more thorough reviews are available elsewhere (Aylward, 2011; Feldman & Messick, 2008; Montgomery, 2008; Stein & Lukasik, 2009). In general, physicians who perform independent evaluations tend to use tests that are relatively brief to administer such as the Capute Scales (CAT/CLAMS; Accardo & Capute, 2005), Battelle Developmental Inventory (BDI-2; Newborg, 2005), Mullen Scales of Early Learning (MSEL; Mullen, 1995), Stanford-Binet Intelligence Scales for Early Childhood (Early SB5; Roid, 2005), Young Children's Achievement Test (YCAT; Hresko, Peak, Herron, & Bridges, 2000), Peabody Picture Vocabulary Test (PPVT-4; Dunn & Dunn, 2007), Kauffman Brief Intelligence Test (KBIT-2; Kaufman & Kaufman, 2004), and Wide Range Achievement Test (WRAT-4; Wilkinson & Robertson, 2006). They also use portions or subtests of various measures such as the Gesell Developmental Schedules (Gesell & Amatruda, 1947; Gesell, Halvorsen, & Amatruda, 1940) and others to assess different domains of development.

Adaptive functioning is usually quantified using standardized interviews such as the Vineland Adaptive Behavior Scales, Second Edition (VABS-2; Sparrow, Balla, & Cichetti, 2005), or caregiver-completed rating scales such as the Adaptive Behavior Assessment System-II (ABAS-II; Harrison & Oakland, 2003), but may be supplemented by direct observation and elicitation. Criterion-referenced functional measures such as the broad-based Functional Independence Measure for Children (WeeFIM; Msall et al., 1994) and the motor domain-specific Gross Motor Function Classification System (Palisano et al., 2007) are useful for determining an individual's current ability to perform the tasks of daily living and to fulfill expected social roles. These evaluations can often be used as meaningful outcome measures and to suggest supports necessary for successful progress (Msall & Msall, 2008).

Social behavior is often quantified as part of a broad adaptive measure such as the VABS-2 or the ABAS-II, but must be directly assessed as well. Appropriate toys should be available to the child so that spontaneous independent play can be observed (often while the clinician is conducting the parent interview) and interactive play can be elicited by the examiner or spontaneously initiated by the child. Eye contact, including referential gaze shifts, response to joint attention bids, and initiation of social communicative interactions such as bringing/showing toys to the parents to share interest and positive affect, and commenting should be assessed. Direct assessment measures specific to certain disorders are often utilized when needed to further evaluate clinical suspicion or narrow the differential diagnosis. For example, the appropriate module of the Autism Diagnostic Observation Schedule (ADOS; Lord, Rutter, DiLavore, & Risi, 1999) or the standard or high-functioning versions of the Childhood Autism Rating Scale, Second Edition (CARS2-ST or CARS2-HF; Schopler, Van Bourgondien, Wellman, & Love, 2010) may be administered.

Maladaptive behavior is also typically quantified using standardized rating scales completed by parents or teachers to supplement the history obtained by interview and review of records. The American Academy of Pediatrics Task Force on Mental Health (2010) has published a comprehensive review of available informal tools and standardized instruments, including broad measures (some of which include adaptive behaviors as well) and narrow measures targeting specific disorders or types of symptoms (e.g., ADHD, depression, conduct problems). Important information can also be gained from qualitative assessment of anxiety, attention, distractibility, impulse control, activity level, compliance, and atypical repetitive behaviors or resistance to change during the interview, testing, and physical examination. Deviations from the norm may be readily apparent upon observation of the child's behavior during the various aspects of the evaluation. It is common, however, not to witness problem behaviors such as tantrums, self-injury, aggression, and irritability during the evaluation, and even a child with significant ADHD may exhibit few overt symptoms. This does not negate the history provided by the parents, especially when verified by documentation from teachers, therapists, or other family members such as grandparents, since many children are able to temporarily modify their behavior for a few hours, especially in a one-on-one or very small group setting. In contrast, the history is suspect if the child clearly exhibits skills such as appropriate imaginative play and reciprocal social interaction during the evaluation despite parental report that the child never exhibits these behaviors at home or in other settings.

Diagnostic Formulation

Ultimately, the diagnostic process is an exercise in the reduction of uncertainty through information gathering, serial hypothesis generation and testing, and deductive reasoning. The developmental evaluation should culminate in a diagnostic formulation, which in turn guides etiologic investigation and management recommendations. All of the information-gathering in the form of the history-taking, record review, and direct clinical assessment provides the input which the clinician then has to compare to existing scientific knowledge of normal and abnormal development and behavior to identify the pertinent problems and develop hypotheses to explain these problems in a list called a differential diagnosis.

For over a century, the Oslerian paradigm of formulating a differential diagnosis has been pivotal to best-practice medicine (Pearn, 2011). The differential diagnosis is defined as a list of conditions consistent with the patient's history and observed signs arranged in ranked order of decreasing likelihood. It is constantly modified throughout the evaluation process as additional information becomes available, with potential diagnoses being added, eliminated, and moved up or down on the list. The quality of differential diagnosis depends on clinician history-taking and examination skills, ability to assign relative weights of importance to specific symptoms and signs, and knowledge of disorders of development and behavior and their causes (Pearn, 2011).

The clinician has actually formulated and modified the differential diagnosis throughout the history-taking process. This is further refined by considering the direct clinical assessment, and it may be helpful to tabulate the data obtained from the developmental testing, physical examination, and neurobehavioral status examination (Figure 15.3) to facilitate identifying the pertinent problems and narrowing the differential diagnosis through pattern recognition (such as discrepancies suggesting developmental dissociation).

Because developmental disabilities result from diffuse brain dysfunction, the set of problems identified through the thorough evaluation process is likely to include cognitive, motor, and neurobehavioral manifestations (refer to Figure 15.1) and sometimes CNS morphologic anomalies (e.g., microcephaly, structural malformation on brain imaging) or neurophysiologic abnormalities (e.g., seizures, abnormal EEG). This may lead to the tendency to arrive at a long list of diagnoses that is essentially the same list of concerns that the parents had expressed, except that it has been translated into medical terminology. Such an approach is not very helpful or very satisfying to parents. Over 40 years ago, McKusick (1969) used the terms *lumping* and *splitting* to describe two positions on the origin of genetic diseases, and emphasized that both had an important place: lumping in connection with pleiotropism ("many from one"—multiple phenotypic features arising from one etiologic factor) and splitting in connection with heterogeneity ("one from many"—the same or almost the same phenotype arising from several different etiologic factors). In developmental disabilities, although splitting is emphasized in the information-gathering process, etiologic diagnosis, and identification of specific impairments to be addressed in treatment, lumping is the key to parsimonious diagnostic classification at the disorder or syndrome level. The diagnostician must emphasize the importance of the forest over the trees.

For example, a particular child may exhibit deficits in language and nonlanguage cognition, self-help skills/activities of daily living, phonology, semantic and pragmatic aspects of language, socialization with peers, reading comprehension, math computation, written output, and motor coordination. The child may

Domain	Test(s)	Age level	SS or DQ	Grade level	Pertinent qualitative information
Language, verbal IQ				—	
Problem-solving, nonverbal IQ				—	
Working memory, processing speed, other					
Visual-motor, fine motor				—	
Gross motor				—	
Reading					
- Decoding					
- Comprehension					
- Fluency					
Mathematics					
Spelling					
Writing					
Other academic or pre-academic achievement					
Adaptive behavior				—	
Social-emotional behavior				—	
Maladaptive behavior (rating scales)				—	
General physical exam	—	—	—	—	
Neurologic exam	—	—	—	—	
Neurobehavioral status exam	—			—	

Figure 15.3.   Sample format for tabulating neurodevelopmental assessment data. (Key: DQ developmental quotient, SS standard score.)

also have problem behaviors including inattention, impulsivity, hyperactivity, tantrums, noncompliance, preference for structure and routine, and perseveration on certain topics or questions. All of these findings can be explained by the single diagnosis of moderate intellectual disability rather than a list of diagnoses including moderate intellectual disability, ASD, ADHD, global learning disabilities, phonological disorder, developmental coordination disorder, and oppositional defiant disorder. Alternatively, she may be appropriately and meaningfully diagnosed with several categorical disorders (e.g., moderate intellectual disability, ASD, and disruptive behavior disorder not otherwise specified), yet there is likely a single underlying etiology, which may or may not be identified through laboratory investigations. Even when a relatively long list of diagnoses is appropriate, it is important to emphasize that the child has one problem, brain dysfunction, and that these diagnoses represent the most parsimonious description of the manifestations of that brain dysfunction.

Once the diagnostic evaluation has been completed, the diagnoses and recommendations for treatment and further evaluation are presented to the family. Often, referrals are made to specialists in other disciplines, such as special education, speech-language therapy, occupational therapy, or physical therapy (usually within the early intervention or education systems) in order to develop and implement specific treatment plans. In some cases, further evaluation is required to delineate the diagnoses, and referral to a neuropsychologist, clinical psychologist, or speech-language pathologist for additional testing may be necessary.

When explaining the developmental profile and diagnostic formulation to parents, one can start with writing *brain dysfunction* in the center of a blank piece of paper, followed by listing beneath it the child's pertinent problems (impairments), divided into the three categories: *cognitive, neuromotor, neurobehavioral,* and sometimes a fourth category, *anatomic/physiologic* (used when there are CNS-related anomalies, such as microcephaly or macrocephaly, or known

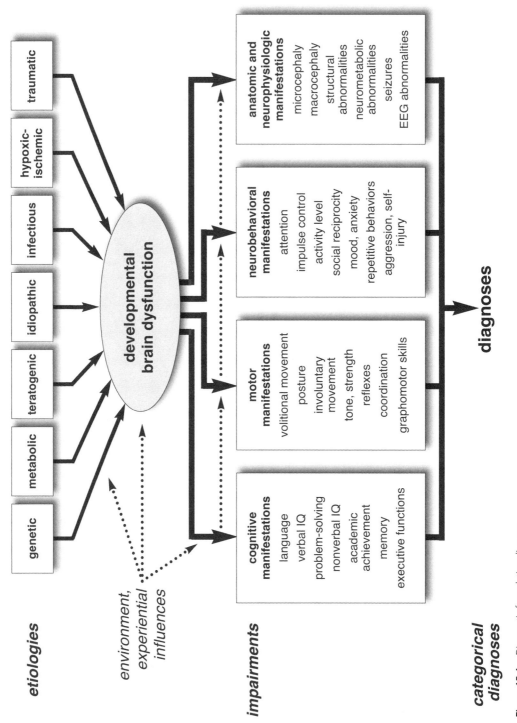

Figure 15.4. Diagnostic formulation diagram.

neurophysiologic abnormalities, such as seizures or abnormal EEG). Below the three or four parallel columns of impairments, the categorical diagnoses are listed while explaining the meaning of each. Next, one can go back to the top of the paper and diagram the various causes of brain dysfunction, followed by crossing out those that do not pertain to the child and arriving at those that should be further investigated. This leads to a discussion of recommendations for laboratory tests, imaging studies, and/or other additional evaluations (or brief discussion of why further investigation is not necessary). The potential influence of environmental and experiential influences fits well into the discussion at this point. All of this leads to a piece of paper looking like something similar to Figure 15.4, but specific to the individual patient. The diagnosis list and profile of impairments can also be referred to during discussion of treatment recommendations.

The specific recommendations regarding etiologic investigations depend on the specific diagnoses (especially presence or absence of global developmental delay or intellectual disability), physical examination findings, neurobehavioral profile, and family history. Less severe disabilities such as language disorders, learning disabilities, and ADHD usually do not require etiologic investigation unless the history and/or physical examination suggest the possibility of a specific etiology that requires further evaluation (such as vision or hearing impairment, obstructive sleep apnea, thyroid dysfunction, lead toxicity or physical stigmata of a genetic syndrome). Clinical practice guidelines for the etiologic evaluation of global developmental delay/intellectual disability (Moeschler, Shevell, & the Committee on Genetics, 2006; Shevell et al., 2003), autism spectrum disorders (Johnson, Myers, & the Council on Children with Disabilities), and cerebral palsy (Ashwal et al., 2004) have been published. Unfortunately, the specific test recommendations tend to become rapidly outdated due to the development of new technology, and the publication of new guidelines may lag several years behind state-of-the-art care (Manning & Hudgins, 2010; Miller et al., 2010; Myers & Challman, 2011). It is important to note, for example, that the current standard of care for genetic testing of individuals with apparently nonsyndromic global developmental delay/intellectual disability, autism spectrum disorders, or multiple anomalies that are not specific to a well-delineated syndrome is chromosomal microarray analysis for copy number variants (Manning & Hudgins, 2010;

Miller et al., 2010; see Chapter 1). Some families decline etiologic investigation for various reasons including concerns about cost or insurance coverage, potential assignment of responsibility or "guilt" to one parent, issues of future insurability of the child, lack of curative treatment based on etiology, and not wanting to put the child through any discomfort or risk associated with tests.

SUMMARY

Developmental brain dysfunction, whether genetic or due to other pathology, varies in severity and is manifested as a spectrum/continuum of disorders ranging from high-prevalence, low-severity conditions such as ADHD, learning disabilities, and developmental coordination disorder to low-prevalence, high-severity conditions such as intellectual disability and cerebral palsy. Developmental diagnosis includes delineation of the specific developmental disorder(s), quantification of severity, identification of associated deficits, and a search for an underlying etiology. The developmental profile compiled during diagnostic evaluation is vital for determining prognosis and guiding treatment planning.

REFERENCES

Abrahams, B.S., & Geschwind, D.H. (2008). Advances in autism genetics: On the threshold of a new neurobiology. *Nature Reviews Genetics, 9*, 341–355.

Accardo, P.J. (2008). *Capute & Accardo's neurodevelopmental disabilities in infancy and childhood. Vol. I: Neurodevelopmental diagnosis and treatment*, (3rd ed). Baltimore, MD: Paul H. Brookes Publishing Co.

Accardo, P.J., & Capute, A.J. (2005). *The Capute Scales: Cognitive adaptive test/clinical linguistic & auditory milestone scale (CAT/CLAMS)*. Baltimore, MD: Paul H. Brookes Publishing Co.

Accardo, P.J., Accardo, J.A., & Capute, A.J. (2008). A neurodevelopmental perspective on the continuum of developmental disabilities. In P.J. Accardo (Ed.), *Capute & Accardo's neurodevelopmental disabilities in infancy and childhood: Vol. I: Neurodevelopmental diagnosis and treatment* (3rd ed, pp. 3–25). Baltimore, MD: Paul H. Brookes Publishing Co.

American Academy of Pediatrics, Council on Children With Disabilities, Section on Developmental Behavioral Pediatrics, Bright Futures Steering Committee, & Medical Home Initiatives for Children With Special Needs Project Advisory Committee. (2006). Identifying infants and young children with developmental disorders in the medical home: An algorithm for developmental surveillance and screening. *Pediatrics, 118*, 405–420.

American Academy of Pediatrics, Task Force on Mental Health. (2010). Supplemental appendix S12: Mental health screening and assessment tools for primary care. *Pediatrics, 125*, S173–S192.

American Psychiatric Association. (2000). *Diagnostic and statistical manual of mental disorders* (4th ed., text rev.). Washington, DC: American Psychiatric Association.

Applegate, B., Lahey, B.B., Hart, E.L., Biederman, J., Hynd, G.W., Barkley, R.A., ... Shaffer, D. (1997). Validity of the age-of-onset criterion for ADHD. A report from the DSM-IV field trials. *Journal of the American Academy of Child & Adolescent Psychiatry, 36,* 1211–1221.

Ashwal, S., Russman, B.S., Blasco, P.A., Miller, G., Sandler, A., Shevell, M., & Stevenson, R. (2004). Practice parameter: Diagnostic assessment of the child with cerebral palsy: Report of the Quality Standards Subcommittee of the American Academy of Neurology and the Practice Committee of the Child Neurology Society. *Neurology, 62,* 851–863.

Aylward, G.P., & Psychoeducational testing. (2011). In R.G. Voigt, M.M. Macias, S.M. Myers (Eds.), *AAP Developmental and Behavioral Pediatrics* (pp. 293–311). Elk Grove Village, IL: American Academy of Pediatrics.

Baird, G., Charman, T., Pickles, A., Chandler, S., Loucas, T., Meldrum, D., ... Simonoff, E. (2008). Regression, developmental trajectory, and associated problems in disorders in the autism spectrum: The SNAP study. *Journal of Autism and Developmental Disorders, 38,* 1827–1836.

Blasco, P.A. (1992). Normal and abnormal motor development. *Pediatric Rounds, 1,* 1–6.

Bostic, J.Q., & Rho, Y. (2006). Target-symptom psychopharmacology: Between the forest and the trees. *Child and Adolescent Psychiatric Clinics of North America, 15,* 289–302.

Brothers, K.B., Glascoe, F.P., & Robertshaw, N.S. (2008). PEDS: Developmental milestones—an accurate brief tool for surveillance and screening. *Clinical Pediatrics, 47,* 271–279.

Capute, A. (1991). The expanded Strauss syndrome: MBD revisited. In P.J. Accardo, Blondis, T.A., & Whitman, B.Y (Eds.), *Attention deficit disorders and hyperactivity.* New York, NY: Marcel Dekker.

Carey, W.B., Crocker, A.C., Coleman, W.L., Elias, E.R., & Feldman, H.M. (2009). *Developmental-behavioral pediatrics* (4th ed.). Philadelphia, PA: Saunders.

Cole, W.R., Mostofsky, S.H., Gidley Larson, J.C., Denckla, M.B., & Mahone, E.M. (2008). Age-related changes in motor subtle signs among girls and boys with ADHD. *Neurology, 71,* 1514–1520.

Crawford, T.O. (1996). Neuromuscular Disorders. In A.J. Capute & P.A. Accardo (Eds.), *Developmental disabilities in infancy and childhood:* (2nd ed. Vol. II: *The Spectrum of developmental disabilities* pp.151–162). Baltimore, MD: Paul H. Brookes Publishing Co.

Dunn, L.M., & Dunn, D.M. (2007). *Peabody picture vocabulary test, fourth edition manual.* Minneapolis, MN: NCS Pearson.

Feldman, H.M., & Messick, C. (2008). Assessment of speech and language. In M.L. Wolraich, D.D. Drotar, P.H. Dworkin, & E.C. Perrin (Eds), *Developmental-behavioral pediatrics: evidence and practice* (pp. 177–190). Philadelphia, PA: Mosby.

Fuchs, D. & Fuchs, L. (2006). Introduction to response to intervention: What, why, and how valid is it? *Reading Research Quarterly, 41,* 93–99.

Gerber, R.J., Wilks, T., & Erdie-Lalena, C. (2010). Developmental milestones: Motor development. *Pediatrics in Review, 31,* 267–276.

Gesell, A., & Amatruda, C.S. (1947). *Developmental diagnosis: Normal and abnormal child development.* New York, NY: Paul B. Hoeber.

Gesell, A.L., Halverson, H,M., & Amatruda, C.S. (1940). *The first five years of life: A guide to the study of the preschool child, from the Yale clinic of child development.* New York, NY: Harper.

Hall, J.G., Allanson, J.E., Gripp, K.W., & Slavotinek, A.M. (2007). *Handbook of physical measurements* (2nd ed.). New York, NY: Oxford.

Harrison, P., & Oakland, T. (2003). *Adaptive behavior assessment system-II.* San Antonio, TX: Harcourt Assessment.

Hresko, W.P., Peak, P.K., Herron, S.R., & Bridges, D.L. (2000). *Young children's achievement test.* Austin, TX: PRO-ED.

Individuals with Disabilities Education Improvement Act (IDEA) of 2004, PL 108–446, 20 U.S. §1400 et seq.

Ireton, H. (1992). *Child development inventory manual.* Minneapolis, MN: Behavior Science Systems.

Johnson, C.P., Myers, S.M., & the Council on Children with Disabilities. (2007). Identification and evaluation of children with autism spectrum disorders. *Pediatrics, 120,* 1183–1215.

Kaufman, A.S., & Kaufman, N.L. (2004). *Kaufman brief intelligence test: Second edition manual.* Minneapolis, MN: NCS Pearson.

Kelley, R.I. (2008). Metabolic diseases and developmental disabilities. In P.J. Accardo (Ed.), *Capute & Accardo's Neurodevelopmental disabilities in infancy and childhood: (3rd ed., Volume I: Neurodevelopmental diagnosis and treatment* pp. 115–145). Baltimore, MD: Paul H. Brookes Publishing Co.

Kirby, R.S. (2002). Co-occurrence of developmental disabilities with birth defects. (2002). *Mental Retardation and Developmental Disabilities Research Reviews, 8,* 182–187.

Kozlowski, A.M., Matson, J.L., Horovitz, M., Worley, J.A., & Neal, D. (2011). Parents' first concerns of their child's development in toddlers with autism spectrum disorders. *Developmental Neurorehabilitation, 14,* 72–78.

Kuster, W., & Konig, A. (1999). Hypomelanosis of Ito: No entity, but a cutaneous sign of mosaicism. *American Journal of Medical Genetics, 85,* 346–350.

Larson, J., Mostofsky, S.H., Goldberg, M.C., Cutting, L.E., Denckla, M.B., & Mahone, E.M. (2007). Effects of gender and age on motor exam in developing children. *Developmental Neuropsychology, 32,* 543–562.

Leppert, M.L. (2011). Neurodevelopmental assessment and medical evaluation. In R.G. Voigt, M.M. Macias, S.M. Myers (Eds.), *AAP Developmental and behavioral pediatrics* (pp. 93–119). Elk Grove Village, IL: American Academy of Pediatrics.

Levenga, J., de Vrij, F.M.S., Oostra, B.A., & Willemsen, R. (2010). Potential therapeutic interventions for fragile X syndrome. *Trends in Molecular Medicine, 16,* 516–527.

Lock, T.M., Shapiro, B.K., Ross, A., & Capute, A.J. (1986). Age of presentation in developmental disability. *Journal of Developmental and Behavioral Pediatrics, 7,* 340–345.

Lord, C., Rutter, M., DiLavore, P., & Risi, S. (1999). *Autism diagnostic observation schedule-WPS edition.* Los Angeles, CA: Western Psychological Services.

Manning, M., & Hudgins, L., for the Professional Practice and Guidelines Committee. (2010). Array-based technology and recommendations for utilization in medical genetics practice for detection of chromosomal abnormalities. *Genetics in Medicine, 12*, 742–745.

McCarthy, S.E., Makarov, V., Kirov, G., Addington, A.M., McClellan, J, Yoon, S., ... Sebat, J. (2009). Microduplications of 16p11.2 are associated with schizophrenia. *Nature Genetics, 41*, 1223–1227.

McDonald-McGinn, D.M., & Sullivan, K.E. (2011). Chromosome 22q11.2 deletion syndrome (DiGeorge syndrome/velocardiofacial syndrome). *Medicine, 90*, 1–18.

McKusick, V.A. (1969). On lumpers and splitters, or the nosology of genetic disease. *Perspectives in Biology and Medicine, 12*, 298–312.

Mefford, H.C., Batshaw, A.L., & Hoffman, E.P. (2012). Genomics, intellectual disability, and autism. *New England Journal of Medicine, 366*, 733–743.

Meilleur, A.-A.S., & Fombonne, E. (2009). Regression of language and non-language skills in pervasive developmental disorders. *Journal of Intellectual Disability Research, 53*, 115–124.

Miller, D.T., Adam, M.A., Aradhya, S., Biesecker, L.G., Brothman, A.R., Carter, N.P., ... Ledbetter, D.H. (2010). Consensus statement: Chromosomal microarray is a first-tier clinical diagnostic test for individuals with developmental disabilities or congenital anomalies. *American Journal of Human Genetics, 86*, 749–764.

Moeschler, J.B., Shevell, M., & the Committee on Genetics. (2006). Clinical genetic evaluation of the child with mental retardation or developmental delays. *Pediatrics, 117*, 2304–2316.

Montgomery, T. (2008). Neurodevelopmental assessment of school-age children. In P.J. Accardo (Ed.), *Caputo & Accardo's neurodevelopmental disabilities in infancy and childhood: (3rd ed., Vol. I: Neurodevelopmental diagnosis and treatment* pp. 405–417). Baltimore, MD: Paul H. Brookes Publishing Co.

Moreno–De–Luca, D, SGENE Consortium, Mulle, J.G., Simons Simplex Collection Genetics Consortium, Kaminsky, E.B., Sanders, S.J., ... Ledbetter, D.H. (2010). Deletion 17q12 is a recurrent copy number variant that confers high risk of autism and schizophrenia. *American Journal of Human Genetics, 87*, 618–630.

Mostofsky, S.H., Newschaffer, C.J., & Denckla, M.B. (2003). Overflow movements predict impaired response inhibition in children with ADHD. *Perceptual & Motor Skills, 97*, 1315–1331.

Msall, M.E., DiGuadio, K., Rogers, B.T., LaForest, S., Lyon, N., Campbell, J., ... Duffy, L.C. (1994). The Functional Independence Measure for Children (WeeFIM): Conceptual basis and pilot use in children with developmental disabilities. *Clinical Pediatrics, 33*, 421–430.

Msall, M.E., & Msall, E.R. (2008). Functional assessment in neurodevelopmental disorders. In P.J. Accardo (Ed.), *Caputo & Accardo's neurodevelopmental disabilities in infancy and childhood: (3rd ed., Vol. I: Neurodevelopmental diagnosis and treatment* pp. 419–444). Baltimore, MD: Paul H. Brookes Publishing Co.

Mullen, E.M. (1995). *Mullen Scales of Early Learning Manual.* Circle Pines, MN: American Guidance Service.

Myers, S.M. (2007). The status of pharmacotherapy for autism spectrum disorders. *Expert Opinion on Pharmacotherapy, 8*, 1579–1603.

Myers, S.M., & Challman, T.D. (2011). Autism Spectrum Disorders. In R.G. Voigt, M.M. Macias, S.M. Myers (Eds.), *AAP Developmental and behavioral pediatrics* (pp. 249–291). Elk Grove Village, IL: American Academy of Pediatrics.

Myers, S.M., Johnson, C.P., & the Council on Children with Disabilities. (2007). Management of children with autism spectrum disorders. *Pediatrics, 120*, 1162–1182.

Newborg, J. (2005). *Battelle Developmental Inventory* (Second ed.). Itasca, IL: Riverside Publishing.

Odding, E., Roebroeck, M.E., & Stam, H.J. (2006). The epidemiology of cerebral palsy: Incidence, impairments and risk factors. *Disability & Rehabilitation, 28*, 183–191.

Pakula, A.T., Van Naarden Braun, K., & Yeargin-Alsopp, M. (2009). Cerebral palsy: Classification and epidemiology. *Physical Medicine & Rehabilitation Clinics of North America, 20*, 425–452.

Palisano, R., Rosenbaum, P., Bartlett, D.J., & Livingston M. (2007). *Gross Motor Function Classification System: Expanded and Revised* (GMFCS-E&R). Available at http://motorgrowth.canchild.ca/en/GMFCS/resources/GMFCS–ER.pdf. Accessed May 3, 2011.

Pearn, J. (2011). Differentiating diseases: The centrum of differential diagnosis in the evolution of Oslerian medicine. *Fetal and Pediatric Pathology, 30*, 1–15.

Rogers, S.J. (2004). Developmental regression in autism spectrum disorders. *Mental Retardation and Developmental Disabilities Research Reviews, 10*, 139–143.

Roid, G. (2005). *Stanford-Binet Intelligence Scales for Early Childhood.* Itasca, IL: Riverside Publishing.

Riou, E.M., Ghosh, S., Francoeur, E., & Shevell, M.I. (2009). Global developmental delay and its relationship to cognitive skills. *Developmental Medicine & Child Neurology, 51*, 600–606.

Schopler, E., Van Bourgondien, M.E., Wellman, G.J., & Love, S.R. (2010). *Childhood Autism Rating Scale, Second edition manual.* Los Angeles, CA: Western Psychological Services.

Shapiro, B.K., & Gwynn, H. (2008). Neurodevelopmental assessment of infants and young children. In P.J. Accardo (Ed.), *Caputo & Accardo's neurodevelopmental disabilities in infancy and childhood: (3rd ed., Vol. I: Neurodevelopmental diagnosis and treatment* pp. 367–382). Baltimore, MD: Paul H. Brookes Publishing Co.

Shaywitz, S.E., Morris, R., & Shaywitz, B.A. (2008). The education of dyslexic children from childhood to young adulthood. *Annual Review of Psychology, 59*, 451–475.

Shevell, M., Ashwal, S., Donley, D., Flint, J., Gingold, M., Hirtz, D., ... Practice Committee of the Child Neurological Society. (2003). Practice parameter: evaluation of the child with global developmental delay: Report of the Quality Standards Subcommittee of the American Academy of Neurology and the Practice Committee of the Child Neurology Society. *Neurology, 60*, 367–380.

Sparrow, S.S., Balla, D.A., & Cichetti, D.V. (2005). *Vineland Adaptive Behavior Scales-2 manual.* Circle Pines, MN: American Guidance Service.

Stein, M.T., & Lukasik, M.K. (2009). Developmental screening and assessment: Infants, toddlers, and preschoolers. In W. B. Carey, A.C. Crocker, W.L. Coleman, E.R. Elias, & H.M. Feldman (Eds.), *Developmental-behavioral pediatrics* (4th ed., pp. 785–796). Philadelphia, PA: Saunders.

Thiele, E.A., & Korf, B.R.. (2006). Phakomatoses and allied conditions. In K.F. Swaiman, S. Ashwal, & D.M. Ferriero (Eds.), *Pediatric neurology: Principles & practice, Fourth edition, Volume I* (pp. 771–796). Philadelphia, PA: Mosby.

Toriello, H.V. (2008). Role of the dysmophologic evaluation in the child with developmental delay. *Pediatric Clinics of North America, 55,* 1085–1098.

VanderVeer, B., & Schweid E. (1974). Infant assessment: Stability of mental functioning in young retarded children. *American Journal of Mental Deficiency, 79,* 1–4.

Voigt, R.G. (2011). Developmental and behavioral diagnoses: The spectrum and continuum of developmental–behavioral disorders. In R.G. Voigt, M.M. Macias, S.M. Myers (Eds.), *AAP Developmental and behavioral pediatrics* (pp. 121–145). Elk Grove Village, IL: American Academy of Pediatrics.

Voigt, R.G., Macias, M.M., & Myers, S.M. (2011). *AAP Developmental and behavioral pediatrics.* Elk Grove Village, IL: American Academy of Pediatrics.

Wang, P.P. (2011). Nature, nurture, and their interactions in child development and behavior. In R.G. Voigt, M.M. Macias, S.M. Myers (Eds.), *AAP Developmental and behavioral pediatrics* (pp. 5–21). Elk Grove Village, IL: American Academy of Pediatrics.

Weiss, L.A., Shen, Y., Korn, J.M., Arking, D.E., Miller, D.T., Fossdal, R., ... Autism Consortium. (2008). Association between microdeletion and microduplication at 16p11.2 and autism. *New England Journal of Medicine, 358,* 667–675.

Wetmore, D.Z., & Garner, G.C. (2010). Emerging pharmacotherapies for neurodevelopmental disorders. *Journal of Developmental and Behavioral Pediatrics, 31,* 564–581.

Whitaker, T.M., & Palmer, F.B. (2008). The developmental history. In P.J. Accardo (Ed.), *Capute & Accardo's neurodevelopmental disabilities in infancy and childhood: (3rd ed. Vol. I: Neurodevelopmental diagnosis and treatment* pp. 297–310). Baltimore, MD: Paul H. Brookes Publishing Co.

Wilkinson, G.S., & Robertson, G.J. (2006). *Wide range assessment test, Fourth edition manual.* Lutz, FL: Psychological Assessment Resources.

Willcutt, E.G., Pennington, B.F., Duncan, L., Smith, S.D., Keenan, J.M., Wadsworth, S., ... Olson, R.K. (2010). Understanding the complex etiologies of developmental disorders: Behavioral and molecular genetic approaches. *Journal of Developmental and Behavioral Pediatrics, 31,* 533–544.

Wilks, T., Gerber, R.J., & Erdie–Lalena, C. (2010). Developmental milestones: Cognitive development. *Pediatrics in Review, 31,* 364–367.

Wolraich, M.L. & Drotar, D.D. (2008). Diagnostic classification systems. In M.L. Wolraich, D.D. Drotar, P.H. Dworkin, & E.C. Perrin (Eds.), *Developmental-behavioral pediatrics: Evidence and practice* (pp 109–122). Philadelphia, PA: Mosby.

Wolraich, M.L., Drotar, D.D., Dworkin, P.H., & Perrin, E.C. (2008). *Developmental-Behavioral Pediatrics: Evidence and Practice.* Philadelphia, PA: Mosby.

World Health Organization. (1992). *The ICD-10 classification of mental and behavioral disorders.* Geneva: World Health Organization.

Yeargin–Allsopp, M., Murphy, C.C., Cordero, J.F., Decoufle, P., & Hollowell, J.G. (1997). Reported biomedical causes and associated medical conditions for mental retardation among 10-year-old children, metropolitan Atlanta, 1985 to 1987. *Developmental Medicine & Child Neurology, 39,* 142–149.

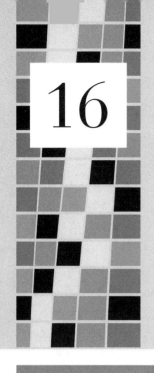

16

Understanding and Using Neurocognitive Assessments

Lauren Kenworthy and Laura Gutermuth Anthony

Upon completion of this chapter, the reader will

- Understand the purpose of neuropsychological assessment

- Be able to describe a model of neuropsychological assessment that incorporates development, brain, and context

- Be familiar with the domains of functioning that neuropsychological assessments address

- Understand how to formulate referral questions and interpret testing results in order to inform treatment

- Know how to maximize the impact of an assessment through effective dissemination of findings and recommendations

- Be able to apply these concepts to a specific case

This chapter focuses on general principles and practical aspects of neuropsychological/cognitive assessment. In order to ensure that the application of this topic is clear, we will refer to a specific case (see John, Parts 1–10) throughout to illustrate key points.

■ ■ ■ JOHN, PART 1

John is an 8-year-old boy in the second grade who was referred for a neuropsychological evaluation following difficulties with socialization and schoolwork. He had previously been diagnosed with a sensory integration disorder, motor delay, and anxiety but received an Asperger Disorder diagnosis as a result of his neuropsychological evaluation. John is a boy with many strengths,

including precocious math and science abilities. His parents also report that he has a good sense of humor, likes to learn, and is devoted to a few important people in his life. But he is socially isolated, rude to his teacher, inflexible, and produces poor written work.

THE PURPOSE OF NEUROPSYCHOLOGICAL ASSESSMENT

There are currently no medical treatments for the core symptoms of many neurodevelopmental disabilities. For example, primary interventions for intellectual and learning disabilities (ID/LD) and autism spectrum disorders (ASDs) are linguistic, behavioral, and cognitive. In the case of attention-deficit/hyperactivity disorder (ADHD) there are potent medications that target core symptoms, but they are most effective when used in combination with behavioral and cognitive interventions (Jensen et al., 2001). Because children with neurodevelopmental disabilities are frequently educated in mainstream environments, interventions are best applied in school settings. As such, adjunctive therapies and the development of an appropriate school and therapeutic program is typically a fundamental step to a comprehensive treatment plan (Klin & Volkmar, 2000; Wolraich & DuPaul, 2010). In addition, there is a great deal of variability within the cognitive profiles of children with neurodevelopmental disabilities. For these two reasons, a neuropsychological evaluation that delineates cognitive strengths and weaknesses and makes specific recommendations regarding classroom placement, accommodations, and special education and therapy needs can serve as the cornerstone of an effective treatment plan for a child with a neurodevelopmental disability.

Over the last several decades, neuropsychology has evolved to better meet the needs of children with neurodevelopmental disabilities. The advent of brain imaging and other sophisticated diagnostic techniques has shifted neuropsychology's role from diagnosis and lesion location to the determination of functional capacities and needs in real world settings, such as home and school (Burgess et al., 2006; Chaytor & Schmitter-Edgecombe, 2003; Kenworthy, Yerys, Anthony, & Wallace, 2008; Manchester et al., 2004). Matarazzo documented this shift in his seminal paper distinguishing *psychological testing*, which is focused on producing test scores, from *psychological assessment*, which incorporates test scores into a broadly based assessment of a child's abilities and environment. Bernstein (2000) elaborated on this, saying "The primary goal of a comprehensive clinical assessment [of a child] is ... to produce a comfortable, competent 25 year old" (p. 408), which requires an assessment designed to promote optimum fit between an individual child's cognitive, social, and behavioral profile and the environments in which that child learns and develops (Baron, 2004). This is typically what parents most want from an assessment; however, when evaluations are geared toward the presentation of "test results" or performance on specific criterion-based testing, as within school settings, it is easy for this goal to become lost.

A MODEL FOR DEVELOPMENTAL NEUROPSYCHOLOGICAL ASSESSMENT

The developmental neuropsychological assessment model described by Bernstein (2000) is ideally suited to the needs of children with neurodevelopmental disabilities because it emphasizes identification of diagnostic behavioral clusters or domains, which pose specific risks to the developing child in specific contexts (e.g., elementary school). Bernstein's model of assessment has three key interacting variables: 1) development, 2) brain, and 3) context.

Development is the first key variable. An understanding of development in typical children and in the specific child being assessed is a hallmark of a good assessment. This means not only knowing that reversing letters when writing is typical in 5 year olds and not expected in 8 year olds, for example, but also understanding an individual child's developmental trajectory and how a neurodevelopmental disorder may alter brain functions that in turn change the way a child learns and develops other abilities. Piaget (1952) first provided this understanding of children as constructing knowledge through experience. A child's development occurs in the context of his or her own specific brain and environment interacting together. Joint attention is a good example of a neurocognitive ability that influences how a child benefits from his or her environment. Joint attention, or the ability to share attention between another person and an object, plays an early developing "self-organizing role" in helping children learn from their social environment (Mundy & Newell, 2007). Impairments in joint attention, as occur in autism, have downstream effects on language, intelligence, and social abilities (Mundy & Neal, 2001; Pennington, 2002). Assessment of a developing brain also requires an appreciation of plasticity and consideration of possible brain reorganization following injury. An understanding of the typical course of development, the timing of the insult or injury and its potential effects on brain structure, and the ability to benefit from context are all important (Baron, 2004; see John, Part 2).

■ ■ ■ JOHN, PART 2

Developmental variables are key to understanding John's neuropsychological profile. The development of his preacademic skills was precocious, he could recite the alphabet at 18 months of age, demonstrating a facility for memorizing discrete units of information. At 5 years of age he demonstrated very strong expressive and receptive language skills, and he achieved a superior verbal IQ score, but at 8 years of age John is expected to formulate multiple sentences on a topic of his teacher's choosing and his precocious vocabulary and verbal memorization do not support him on this higher order academic language task. It does, however, allow him to tell his teacher in very sophisticated language what is wrong with her assignments.

The brain is Bernstein's second key variable for assessment. Assessment of a child with a neurodevelopmental disability occurs in the context of an understanding of the neural substrate, or brain structure/function, expected in the specific disorder and observed in the individual child being assessed. It can be very powerful for parents and the treatment team to understand which components of the child's behavior are related to brain-based differences in processing, understanding, and producing information/behavior, as opposed to behaviors which may be learned, or even willful on the child's part. Distinguishing between these two sources of behavior is what helps a family distinguish when a child "can't"—as opposed to "won't"—do what they expect. In the case of "can't," parents and treatment teams can clearly understand that changes in the demand or context will be needed (see John, Part 3). For example, most children with ADHD and ASDs struggle with executive dysfunction and disorganization. Many of them cannot sit down on their own initiative at home to begin homework, but if the context is altered to be more supportive, through the provision of a written schedule, checklist, breaks, and rewards, they are successful.

■ ■ ■ JOHN, PART 3

In John's case, discussion of his brain-based deficits in executive function, organization, and flexibility abilities was essential for helping his teacher understand that this bright boy with an oversized vocabulary really *couldn't* organize words into written responses on specific topics of her choosing, unless he was taught a highly structured writing rubric. Like most of us, until instructed otherwise, she assumed that a boy with John's core language abilities and

considerable intelligence must be *choosing* not to write.

This leads directly to the final key variable in assessment, which is the context in which the child, with his or her specific brain, is developing (see Figure 16.1). Context is important for many reasons. It is essential to understand how a child's context to date affects his or her performance during an assessment. For example, impaired vocabulary in a 7-year-old child who comes from a home in which books were read to him daily throughout his development, raises concerns regarding abnormalities in left frontal-temporal brain networks and the need for specialized therapy; the same vocabulary in a child whose family speaks a different language than that in which the assessment was administered may simply indicate the need for increased exposure to English words (family and culture). The context of the assessment itself is vital as well. The 7-year-old child with impaired vocabulary may be reacting poorly to the assessment setting. Perhaps the examiner was unable to develop adequate rapport with the child, who became very anxious and provided only minimal responses. Many children behave differently in school, home, and clinical settings, and thus information must be gathered about performance in each setting to create a complete picture. Finally, an understanding of future contexts is important for an assessment to effectively predict risk and make recommendations. For example, a 4-year-old child with impaired phonological awareness and segmentation abilities may be thriving in a nonacademic preschool, but is at great risk of failure to

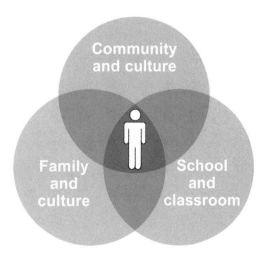

Figure 16.1. Viewing the child in context.

succeed in a kindergarten setting where reading skills are emphasized. Likewise, a very bright but disorganized fifth grader is at great risk for increased difficulties when he or she makes the transition to middle school with its demands for managing multiple subjects, teachers, and longer assignments (school and classroom). Delineation of risks is what drives practical recommendations for intervention (Baron, 2000). Development and successful recommendations for enhancing development do not exist in a vacuum. They occur within specific contexts that can affect the course and prognosis of the child's difficulties, the way they are expressed, and the success of treatment. For this reason, tests should not be used nor interpreted in isolation (see John, Part 4).

■ ■ ■ JOHN, PART 4

In John's case, consideration of context was important for many reasons. For example, although his parents were concerned about his lack of social skills, John had a close friend his age who did not have any neurodevelopmental disabilities. He saw this person frequently and at first review his ability to sustain this friendship raised questions about whether he had greater social interaction abilities than his parents gave him credit for. Review of the context revealed, however, that this friend was a member of a family that socialized with John's whole family on a regular basis, and so John was not sustaining the friendship independently, but rather benefiting from a highly supported social context.

Assessment requires the integration of 1) test performance, behavioral observations, and contextual information provided by parents, teachers, and treatment team; 2) principles of development; and 3) knowledge of brain function. This information is integrated across the span of the child's development and across the settings the child inhabits. Baron (2004) terms this process *convergence profile analysis*, highlighting the fact that one test score or reported behavior is insufficient to generate an accurate cognitive profile. For example, take an assessment designed to answer whether or not a child has an attention deficit. All of the following questions must be answered before a determination can be made:

1. Is there a history of problems paying attention or is it a new problem?

2. Is the child inattentive to all types of stimuli (people, words, and pictures) or just some types?

3. Is the child inattentive at home, at school, and in the clinician's office, or just in some settings?

4. What are the demands being placed on the child to pay attention and what attention demands will he or she confront in the future?

5. What other cognitive, emotional, or contextual factors are affecting the child's ability to pay attention?

6. Have medical sources of attention problems, such as sleep disturbance and thyroid abnormalities, been ruled out?

A comprehensive neuropsychological assessment should provide a thorough investigation of each of the domains of functioning that are described in the next section of this chapter to identify: a pattern of cognitive and behavioral strengths and weaknesses; the risks posed by the child's profile in the contexts he or she inhabits; and recommendations to ameliorate those risks through accommodations or special teaching/therapies (see John, Part 5).

■ ■ ■ JOHN, PART 5

Convergence profile analyses were essential for interpreting John's attention data. He was reported by parents to have considerable difficulty maintaining focused attention at home, but he performed well on a computerized "attention" task during the assessment. His attention to the examiner's spoken directions was somewhat less consistent, but he usually knew exactly what to do before she had finished giving directions anyway. He was least attentive in the assessment when the examiner tried to chat with him about her own interests and experiences. Teacher report of attention indicated problems with attention to her instructions, class discussion, and tasks he found to be boring, although the report also indicated excellent ability to focus, once engaged in independent work, on a task that interested him. John also experienced problems with anxiety and sleep. Integration of this data across contexts and tasks indicates several things: John does not experience pervasive attention problems but has increasing difficulty attending as the context becomes less structured and predictable and the executive function demands increase (home versus school) and as the social content of the material increases (good attention to a computerized task or in independent work, but poor attention when people are talking to him). This points to executive and social deficits as the primary problem, not attention. John's strength in terms of his remarkable intelligence is another key factor affecting attention as he typically understands information very quickly and thus is more easily bored. Finally, both sleep problems and anxiety may contribute to John's attention problems, a finding that has important implications for treatment strategies.

DOMAINS OF FUNCTIONING ASSESSED IN NEUROPSYCHOLOGICAL EVALUATIONS

A comprehensive neuropsychological assessment includes a description of strengths and weaknesses. For each neuropsychological domain, the assessment should provide a clear summary statement describing the child's abilities and an integration of data from multiple sources. A full assessment includes multiple methods, such as parent and child clinical interviews, norm-referenced rating scales from the parent, teacher, and child (self-report), behavioral observations, standardized, norm-referenced tests in relevant domains, and projective techniques (subjective measures). Although the specific neuropsychological domains and their labels can vary somewhat depending on the examiner, the most commonly referenced domains of functioning are defined below. Table 16.1 also lists these domains, indicates neurodevelopmental disabilities that may be associated with deficits in each domain, and gives examples of relevant data sources regarding each domain. There is also a table listing many common tests associated with each of these domains in the appendix at the end of this chapter.

General Intelligence

General intelligence is commonly discussed in neuropsychological assessments and is often considered the benchmark against which other cognitive abilities are measured. For example, a child with an overall IQ score that is in the intellectually deficient range would not be identified as having a specific visual processing deficit

unless difficulties in that domain were greater than what would be expected, based on his or her IQ. That having been said, it is important to recognize that general intelligence scores have narrower implications for a child's ability to become a successful and happy 25-year-old than is often assumed by parents. Intelligence testing originated in early 20th century France as a method to predict which children would succeed in school. Its development in 20th century America included the delineation of separate factors in intelligence with a strong emphasis on verbal knowledge and spatial performance as key factors in determining overall intellectual abilities. Crystallized (use of knowledge and experience) versus fluid (solving novel problems) intelligence is another common dichotomy. Processing speed has played an increasing role in our understanding of performance on IQ tests, particularly in children with congenital or acquired brain abnormalities (see Baron, 2004). In any case, Gardner's (1983) seminal book on multiple intelligences serves as an important reminder that IQ scores capture only a fraction of the many abilities that govern a person's performance in the real world. Other caveats regarding measures of general intelligence are that 1) crystallized and verbal knowledge measures are affected by the home and school environment, 2) IQ scores are unstable in young children and are not necessarily predictive of later performance on intelligence tests, and 3) the causes of poor performance have been oversimplified. For example, Wechsler Processing Speed Index scores are heavily reliant on fast processing but also fast motor output, a demand that is not recognized by their name. The Wechsler Arithmetic subtest requires listening to a word problem and then performing arithmetic operations, without paper, to produce an answer. As a result, the task includes auditory processing (listening to the question), verbal processing (identifying the quantities and operations required), working memory (maintaining the key elements in working memory and performing operations on them), and exposure to arithmetic (Sattler, 2001).

Attention

Attention is closely associated with, and sometimes even subsumed under, executive functioning. Common subdomains within the concept of attention include orienting, focusing, shifting, and sustaining attention. Attention relies on complex distributed networks in the brain

Table 16.1. Common neurocognitive domains and associated neurodevelopmental disorders

Domain	Examples of associated neurodevelopmental disorders	Examples of key data sources
General intelligence	Intellectual disability	Standardized IQ tests
Attention	Attention deficit disorder Emotional disorders (anxiety, depression, trauma) Traumatic brain injury Epilepsy	Parent and teacher rating scales and qualitative report Observations during assessment Standardized tests
Executive function	Attention deficit disorder Autism Reading disability Prematurity Nonverbal learning disability Traumatic brain injury	Parent and teacher rating scales and qualitative report Observations during assessment Standardized tests
Language	Language-based learning disabilities (reading, writing) Developmental language disorders Autism Hearing impairment	Observations during assessment Standardized tests School work Qualitative parent and teacher report
Visual perceptual	Nonverbal learning disability Prematurity Visual impairment	Standardized tests Observations during assessment
Learning/memory	Autism Attention deficit disorder Learning disabilities Developmental language disorders Nonverbal learning disability Traumatic brain injury Intellectual disability Epilepsy	Standardized tests Observations during assessment Qualitative parent and teacher report
Social cognition	Autism Nonverbal learning disability	Parent and teacher rating scales and qualitative report Structured interview observations Standardized tasks
Motor/sensory	Cerebral palsy Attention-deficit/hyperactivity disorder Autism Nonverbal learning disability	Standardized tests Observations during assessment Work samples
Emotional adjustment	Depression Anxiety disorder Trauma Adjustment problems Bipolar disorder Attention deficit disorder Medical disorders	Parent and teacher rating scales and qualitative report Observations and self-report during assessment Projective measures
Adaptive/academic	All	Parent teacher qualitative report and report on standardized adaptive behavior interviews Standardized academic tests/tasks Work samples

(Mesulam, 2000) with indications of specific right hemisphere involvement (Stefanatos & Wasserstein, 2001). Attention is affected by a diverse array of factors including anxiety, arousal (most sleepy people are inattentive), difficulty of the task (e.g., dyslexic children are inattentive specifically on reading-related tasks), motivation (e.g., interest level in the material), and the novelty, as well as the type, of the situation. A finding of impaired attention should be based on data showing difficulty paying attention in several different contexts (home and school), on a variety of tasks, and in the absence of other interfering mental states.

Executive Function

Executive function is an umbrella term that captures a set of cognitive abilities that govern behavior regulation and goal-oriented activity (Welsh & Pennington, 1988). These cognitive processes include working memory, inhibition, flexibility, monitoring, planning, and generativity (Rogers & Bennetto, 2000). Executive functions rely on complex interconnected brain networks emphasizing frontal and subcortical nodes (D'Esposito, 2007; Miller & Cohen, 2001; Stuss & Benson, 1984). Executive functions are notoriously difficult to capture in the standard test-based assessment, as the assessments are usually conducted in a quiet room with one highly supportive adult examiner prompting performance. In this structured arrangement, the examiner provides the plan, organizes the activities, gives explicit instructions and cues regarding performance, probes for elaboration, presents tasks one at a time, and generally supports executive control (Bernstein & Waber, 1990; Gioia & Isquith, 2004). Such support makes it difficult to reveal deficits in this area. Therefore, intact performance on an executive function (EF) test should not be considered adequate evidence of intact EF. Often some subdomains of EF are intact while others are impaired in a child with a neurodevelopmental disability. By school age, delineation of performance in specific subdomains (e.g., inhibition/impulse control versus planning or self monitoring) is informative for targeting specific interventions (e.g., interventions to support and improve weak working memory are quite different than those targeting impulse control or flexibility; see John, Part 6).

■ ■ ■ JOHN, PART 6

John, like many children with high-functioning autism spectrum disorders, had specific EF deficits affecting his ability to organize, integrate, and plan with complex information or multistep tasks, which affected his ability to write essays at school. He required interventions targeted at helping him to learn to use a specific writing rubric that provided familiarity and structure to this otherwise open-ended, overwhelming task. John also struggled with cognitive inflexibility and needed to learn routines and scripts to help him be more flexible. On the other hand, John's ability to manipulate numbers in working memory was remarkable, and he generally had adequate impulse control.

Language

This domain addresses the ability to understand language, use language to express needs and wants, establish social relationships, and make the sounds of speech (see Chapter 20). Often subsumed under the language domain are a full range of communicative abilities, including motor speech capacities and pragmatic nonverbal communications such as gestures. At its core, the language domain involves the phonological, semantic, syntactic, and formulation abilities that enable us to distinguish and combine sounds, build a vocabulary, and combine words into sentences and longer utterances. Language abilities rely heavily on frontotemporal brain networks, typically in the left hemisphere. Language skills are often divided between receptive or comprehension abilities and expressive abilities, which can be divergent. Although most neurocognitive evaluations screen basic language abilities and can be helpful in differentiating the unique contributions of attention, executive function, social cognition, and language difficulties to a problem in the child's functioning, a significant concern regarding language abilities typically also merits a full speech and language assessment (see John, Part 7).

■ ■ ■ JOHN, PART 7

In John's case, basic language abilities related to phonology, semantics, and syntax were very strong and supported fluent reading, decoding, excellent vocabulary, and a sophisticated use and understanding of words and sentence syntax. His communication deteriorated, however, as executive demands to organize and integrate information into paragraphs or as pragmatic language demands to use gestures and eye contact increased. Finally, inflexibility drove him to be overly precise in his use of language and interfered with his ability to maintain a conversation about topics that were not intrinsically interesting to him.

Visual Processing

The brain supports a variety of visual processing abilities, including perception and spatial location. Right hemisphere posterior brain structures are frequently involved, although the neural underpinnings of visual processing are complex (see Baron, 2004, for review). Visual processing is closely associated with visual construction skills, which also require motor output; perception of visual gestalts; and visual pattern recognition, often associated with visual reasoning. All of these skills rely on intact or corrected vision. Isolated deficits in this domain are not common in neurodevelopmental disabilities, and it is important to recognize that a significantly lower Wechsler Performance IQ score than Verbal IQ score cannot be interpreted in isolation to indicate a perceptual deficit (see John, Part 8). Such a discrepancy can result from many different conditions, including executive dysfunction and highly enriched verbal teaching at home and at school. A true deficit in this domain should be confirmed with performance data other than IQ scores, such as scores on tests of visual learning and memory.

■ ■ ■ JOHN, PART 8

John's IQ scores showed a significant discrepancy between very superior Verbal IQ and average Performance IQ. Yet, he was a gifted math student and had strong visual learning abilities. Observation of John's approach to the tasks that constitute the Performance IQ revealed that his inflexibility and tendency to focus on details slowed his performance and reduced his score, implicating executive dysfunction, not a perceptual deficit.

Learning and Memory

While true memory impairments are relatively rare in children with neurodevelopmental disabilities, learning deficits are common (Baron, 2004). Learning can be impaired for visual or verbal information in the context of core deficits in language or visual processing. Executive dysfunction also typically interferes with effective information retrieval in response to open-ended queries (e.g., "How was your day?") and learning larger amounts of information, but not information retrieval in structured conditions

(e.g., multiple choice) and learning simpler data. A neuropsychological evaluation should provide specific insight into how a child learns best and in which learning conditions the child will require extra support (for example, only during lectures, written responses, or independent reading). Optimizing learning is a key intervention for all children, since their major academic task is to learn new information (see John, Part 9).

■ ■ ■ JOHN, PART 9

In John's case it was useful to delineate the difference between his prodigious learning and memory abilities for small chunks of information, such as words, facts, and mathematic operations, but much greater difficulty learning and retrieving from memory large chunks of information. In the assessment he struggled with learning and remembering a large, complex abstract figure, and in his daily life he struggled to learn from his experiences.

Social Cognition

Current research reveals that social perception and cognition rely on fronto-temporal brain networks and that the brain makes specific contributions to a person's ability to perceive social stimuli, such as faces, facial expressions, voice intonation, and body language. The brain also reasons with social information, such as understanding human relationships and having a theory of mind; this social reasoning ability is commonly referred to as social cognition (for reviews see Frith & Frith, 2007, 2010; Pelphrey & Carter, 2008). However, our ability to measure social cognition with standardized tools is still quite limited. With the exception of basic social perception tasks that measure learning, memory for faces, and recognition of facial expression, measuring social cognition largely relies on parent and teacher report, observation, and responses in structured interviews. For planning successful interventions, it is essential to have an understanding of whether a child with a neurodevelopmental disability can accurately perceive and express social cues, have a theory of mind, and reason with social information.

Motor/Sensory

The motor sensory domain encompasses a broad range of gross and fine motor abilities as well as sensory perception. Standardized motor tasks eliciting speed, strength, and dexterity, such as quickly placing pegs in a board, tracing a curvy line, or imitating a gait or hand movement, all can provide information about the subtle motor impairments often seen in neurodevelopmental disabilities. These impairments can profoundly affect a child's ability to produce written work at school, carry out key activities of daily living, or simply stay sitting upright in his or her chair. A complex or pervasive motor difficulty often merits a physical and/or occupational therapy evaluation. Sensory information regarding visual, auditory, and tactile perception can also be collected with standardized assessments and can be particularly important for children with focal brain damage. Over- and undersensitivity to sensory stimuli is a prominent finding in autism and is best assessed by observation and parent or teacher report.

Emotional Adjustment

Emotional adjustment should be evaluated in any comprehensive assessment because it has a major impact on the child's overall functioning level, the intervention plan, and specific neurocognitive functions. Mood, anxiety, and any other emotional difficulties interfering with the child's functioning and ability to regulate mood and behavior should all be assessed. These data may inform diagnosis of comorbid psychiatric disorders. They may also indicate alternative explanations for cognitive impairments. For example, working memory can be impaired by anxiety; depression slows down motor response and generally impairs performance on tasks requiring cognitive effort; and even hallucinations occur in a small number of children, which certainly interfere with attention (Eysenck, Derakshan, Ferreri, & Lapp, 2011; Porter, Bourke, & Gallagher, 2007; Santos & Calvo, 2007). Parent, teacher, and child report on standardized measures, as well as a qualitative report of symptoms and concerns, are useful. In addition to an interview with the child, which can be play-based with a younger child, the child's response to projective measures is also often used. Projective measures present incomplete or ambiguous stimuli (such as drawings, sentence beginnings, or inkblots) and are designed to elicit information about the child's internal state.

Adaptive/Academic

Adaptive and academic functioning are best thought of as outcomes of the pattern of strengths and weaknesses in a child's core cognitive domains, combined with the full range of contextual factors described above. They reflect how successfully the child is coping with the demands of daily living (e.g., showing age-appropriate toileting, dressing, grooming, communication and social skills) and accumulating academic knowledge and skills.

ENSURING THAT ASSESSMENT INFORMS MANAGEMENT

Useful Assessments Are Driven by Appropriate Referral Questions

Neuropsychological assessment can answer or provide input on a wide range of questions, but there are at least as many questions that it cannot, or should not, answer. A comprehensive neuropsychological assessment can often provide input in the following areas: 1) diagnostic clarification, 2) the child's level of developmental or cognitive functioning, 3) patterns of strengths and weaknesses, 4) school placement or program eligibility determinations, 5) progress or deterioration over time, 6) forensic issues, and 7) suggestions for treatment. Assessment can rarely definitively answer questions such as "What caused this to happen?"

A good referral request asks a clear, answerable question. Some examples of appropriate questions would be whether the child has autism, whether the child's difficulties are due to language or attention problems, or whether the child is receiving appropriate services and making the expected level of progress. Providing the evaluator with information about the strengths and weaknesses of the child, the family system, and the current educational plan will increase the utility of the assessment. Specifying which exact tests should be given is not useful. There may be very good reasons for not giving a certain test, such as any of the threats to validity described below.

An Understanding of the Purpose and Limits of Psychometric Data Informs Effective Use of Assessment Results

When selected, administered and scored appropriately, standardized test instruments provide important normative benchmarks against which to compare performance. They complement nonstandardized data and provide key information about how a child's abilities compare with same-age typically developing children. One study (Meyer et al., 2001) compared psychological tests with medical tests like magnetic resonance imaging, Pap smears, and electrocardiograms and found that psychological tests generally predict outcomes just as well as medical tests do.

The term *psychometrics* refers to the branch of psychology addressing the design, administration, and interpretation of quantitative (numerical) tests for the measurement of psychological factors such as intelligence, aptitude, and personality traits (Upton & Cook, 2008). Psychometric approaches have proven to be extraordinarily useful over time but have been criticized for being overly reductionistic. The inherent limitations in the psychometric approach are part of why standards typically are set for training and experience for professionals to meet in order to be able to purchase psychological tests and be licensed to administer and interpret those tests (American Educational Research Association, American Psychological Association, & National Council of Measurements in Education, 1999). This sets a very high standard for the appropriate interpretation of any test score and should caution unqualified people against attempting to interpret scores.

Psychometric measures should be interpreted with caution for many reasons. Psychometrics do not model the neural substrate (e.g., a test score does not map neatly onto brain regions or functions) or place behavior in context. Further, psychological tests are rarely pure (e.g., they do not measure only the domain they are supposed to measure), are not completely objective (e.g., variability in examiners or cultural factors can have a significant impact on scores), and are not always reliable and even less often valid. The results of any psychometric measure are only as good as the measure itself. The largest factors that contribute to score accuracy include 1) the use of standardized procedures; 2) the reliability of the test; 3) the validity of the test; and 4) the quality, size, recency, and diversity of the normative sample (Anastasi & Urbina, 1997; Pedhazur & Schmelkin, 1991; Streiner & Norman, 1995). Described below are some of the most important psychometric factors a neuropsychologist considers.

What Does It Mean for a Test to be Standardized?

A test is standardized if 1) it has exact procedures for administration, including the qualifications of the administrator; 2) it has instructions and questions that must be repeated in exactly the same way every time (i.e., the administrator must "stick to the script"), 3) the exact same materials are used every time; and 4) rules for scoring are specifically defined and are not subjective (Sattler, 2001).

What Does It Mean for a Test to be Reliable?

Reliability is a measure of how consistent a score is over time (test-retest reliability), between examiners (inter-rater reliability), across different forms of the test (alternate forms reliability), and within the items of the test (internal consistency). Reliability can be affected by the length of the test, variability in the normative sample, the difficulty range of the items (it is important that items are neither too difficult nor too easy), and how well the administration and scoring procedures are described.

Most children with neurodevelopmental disabilities receive neurocognitive testing repeatedly to monitor their development and the efficacy of the interventions they receive. The evaluator should always review the child's previous testing and compare the results to the current scores. Yet, even a cognitive test with good test-retest reliability may produce different scores over time. More score consistency should be expected as the child gets older. The 2-year stability of scores on a cognitive skill is likely to be greater for a school-age child than for a toddler, for example (Youngstrom et al., 2010). Changes in standard scores can occur for a variety of reasons, including 1) administration of newer versions of tests with more up-to-date normative data; 2) increased demands within tests for specific skills such as executive functions as children get older; 3) cumulative effects of lost learning opportunities due to an undertreated learning disability; 4) natural variability in a child's performance on tests, which is particularly common in children with developmental disabilities like ADHD and autism; and 5) in very rare cases, a progressive neurological process. In the last situation, other signs of decline typically are present, such as parent and teacher report of reduced performance at home and at school and declines in adaptive behavior. Any concern about drops in scores should be carefully reviewed with the conductor of the assessment in order to evaluate possible causes.

What Does It Mean for a Test to be Valid?

A test is valid if it accurately measures what it is supposed to measure. A well-standardized test has undergone many different types of checks for validity under controlled situations.

However, most tests are used outside of these controlled situations, and therefore the evaluator should tell the reader of the report how valid he or she believes the child's assessment to be, and how predictive the assessment is likely to be of the child's functioning. For instance, most individually administered tests (such as IQ tests) are not valid if repeated within 6–12 months because practicing the tasks improves performance on those tasks. Child-specific factors can also reduce the validity of a test result. Was the child hungry, tired, ill, or distracted? Was the child taking any medication that could affect results? Cultural factors should always be considered as a potential threat to validity; a test's questions may contain content and assume knowledge that are foreign to the child's environment. For example, a child from Taiwan may not be able to correctly categorize the fruits we typically eat in the United States. Poor performance relates to the child's culture, not to her categorization or abstract thinking ability. Sometimes a certain child will need accommodations during testing, or will need to be given special tests, and the report should acknowledge these factors, and how they affect validity. A child with cerebral palsy (CP) or other physical disabilities may need to be given motor-free tests, and even verbal tests should not be timed. When a child with a language disorder is assessed in other domains, nonverbal tests should be given (such as the Leiter or the Comprehensive Test of Non-Verbal Intelligence). A child who speaks a different language should either receive nonverbal tests or a test that has been translated and standardized in the child's native language. Some testing accommodations are less dramatic, such as allowing the child to stand or move around the room, instituting reward systems, and breaking the testing up into several sessions. But these accommodations should be noted in the report, as the validity of the findings may be tied to them. Practically speaking it is also helpful to alert teachers and parents to specific accommodations that are likely to improve performance at home and at school.

Why Is It Important for a Test to be Norm-Referenced?

A test is norm-referenced if it has been given to a large number of people (the sample) who are representative of the population of interest. An individual child's performance is measured against the performance of all others the child's age in the normative sample in order to generate a standard score. The larger and more diverse the normative sample is, the more useful this standard score is. Cultural, linguistic, and physical factors that the child does not share with the normative sample will reduce its utility. The normative sample also must be recent, as children's scores in the population change over time. For example, cognitive intelligence scores have been shown to increase by about three standard score points per decade (Flynn, 1999).

What Is a Standardized Score (How to Interpret a Score)?

Standardized scores are statistically derived from the normative sample during test development. All standardized scores assume that the scores range according to a normal distribution (see Figure 16.2). There are several types of standardized scores. Test scores can be expressed as follows:

1. *Age or grade equivalents.* Performance is typical of a specific age group or grade level in the normative sample. Age and grade equivalents should not be used for making diagnostic or placement decisions because of their low reliability and validity (Bracken, 1988; Reynolds, 1981). Unfortunately, these flawed scores are the most intuitive of the standardized scores and are the most easily understood by parents and teachers.

2. *Percentiles.* Rank of the child's relative position in the normative sample. For example, a child's score at the 80th percentile means that the child performed better than 80% of children in the sample.

3. *Deviation scores.* The child's performance in relation to the distance from the mean in terms of standard deviations *(SD)*. The standard deviation of a score is a measure of how much variability there is in scores in terms of distance from the mean (average). Standard Scores, Scale Scores, T Scores, and Z scores are all deviation scores. Standard Scores typically have a mean of 100 and a *SD* of 15. Scale Scores typically have a mean of 10 and a *SD* of 3. T Scores have a mean of 50 and a *SD* of 10, and Z Scores have a mean of 0 and a *SD* of 1.

Most children (about 68%) obtain scores within 1 *SD* of the mean. These scores are considered "average." The further a score is away from the mean, the fewer children obtain that score. Figure 16.2 represents what is commonly referred to as the "Bell curve" or the normal

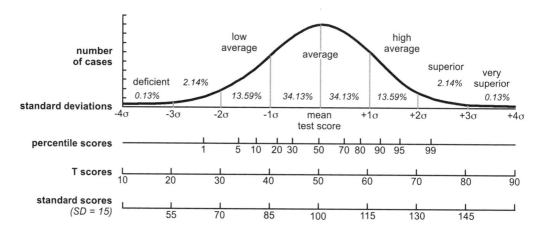

Figure 16.2. The normal curve.

distribution of scores in a group of individuals. The area under the curve represents the number of children obtaining that score. If Figure 16.2 represents a total of 1,000 children, then 680 children would obtain scores in the area of the curve representing the "average range." However, only one child would obtain a score in the small area under the curve in the "very superior range," which is the area of the curve 4 *SD*s above the mean. The general labels used to describe scores are depicted on Figure 16.2, but each test may also use their own descriptive labels, depending on what the test is measuring. For example, a child who scores very low on an anxiety measure, such as a T Score of 20, is not said to be "deficient" of anxiety symptoms. Instead, a T Score of 70 on the anxiety measure may be described as "clinically significant," meaning that the score indicates noteworthy anxiety symptoms.

Effective Feedback and Dissemination of Findings

A recent meta-analysis (Poston & Hanson, 2010) shows that when psychological assessment and the sharing of assessment results is done in a collaborative fashion with the patient/family, and the feedback is offered in a sensitive, clinically meaningful manner, the assessment process itself functions as a therapeutic intervention. Effective communication of assessment results is essential for optimizing the power of an assessment as an intervention tool. When a child is referred for a medical specialist's consult, the professional making the referral wants the specialist's interpretation and integration of information to answer the referral question and to suggest avenues of treatment, if needed. The

same is true in referrals for neuropsychological assessments. Presentation of cognitive strengths and weaknesses, appropriate diagnoses, primary risks, and recommendations should all be communicated in a collaborative conversation and in language that both the referring professional and the parents can understand.

An assessment's utility is determined by its usefulness and intelligibility to family and treatment team of the child being assessed.

Often the largest intervention resulting from an assessment is simply to see the child's behavior in a new light. For example, a child who was described by the teacher as unmotivated can now be seen as a child with short-term memory problems, an attention disorder, or depression. This reframing of the problem can then lead to teachers, parents, and other adults changing their intervention strategies and interactions with and expectations of the child. In turn, this can then lead to a difference in how the child sees him- or herself. The first step in this reframing process is to confirm that the parents understand the assessment results. Follow-up questions regarding what was communicated during the assessment feedback session are important because misunderstandings are common. Provision of resources that will help the family move towards a greater understanding of their child's strengths, weaknesses, risks, needed interventions and accommodations, and prognosis may enable parents to be their child's best advocate.

Implementation of Recommendations

The next step is to make sure that a plan is in place so that all necessary recommendations can be implemented. This can be an over-whelming process for parents, particularly if their child needs multiple types of interventions and accommodations. It is important to help parents recognize that many assessments provide recommendations meant to be implemented over a period of several years. Prioritizing among recommendations and identifying key initial targets for intervention can be helpful. Very often, recommendations will call for changes in both school-based and home/outpatient-based services (see John, Part 10).

▨ ▨ ▨ JOHN, PART 10

John's assessment report led to several significant changes. Perhaps most importantly, his parents and teachers became better able to distinguish his "can'ts" from his "won'ts." He was provided with some social coaching to help him read social cues and understand how his behavior can seem rude to others. He got an IEP in school, which allowed him to use extra supports for writing assignments and provided specialized speech and language therapy targeting language pragmatic and formulation skills and special education services targeting executive functions and writing. In addition, he got help from a peer buddy on the playground to ensure inclusion in games and activities. John's school services were supplemented by outpatient services in social skills training and anxiety reduction techniques by a skilled therapist. His parents also received some coaching in how to organize John's day and to set up a comprehensive reward system.

School-Based Recommendations

School-based services in private schools are up to the discretion of the school. Some private schools offer specialized services to students, but they are not required to do so and may charge an additional fee. There are three options for services in public schools: 1) informal supports and accommodations negotiated with the child's teacher and/or the student support team, 2) a 504 plan to provide formalized accommodations that will allow a student with a disability to access the general curriculum, or 3) an individualized educational plan (IEP) to formulate specific and measurable goals. In order to make progress towards meeting those goals, formalized services must usually be provided to the student (e.g., special education or

speech-language therapy), and those services may be provided in a mainstream classroom, resource room, special classroom, or special school, depending on the student's needs. Every student has a right to an appropriate education in the least restrictive environment possible (See Chapter 31). School-based services are generally well-coordinated across disciplines. The quality of school-based services varies widely, however, from county to county and sometimes even from one school to another. Having an outside professional review the services a child is receiving and monitor the progress the child is making is helpful for many families. If the family needs extra help navigating the school-based meetings, they may want to hire an educational specialist/advocate, a professional who knows the laws and the local schools, or a special education attorney if the family is heading towards mediation or due process. The free-access web site http://www.wrightslaw.com has more information on advocating for special education services.

Home/Outpatient-Based Services

Getting services through a disconnected service system, as most out-of-school systems are, requires active advocacy skills from parents. Parents often find themselves filling multiple roles, including case manager and treatment coordinator, as well as having to obtain insurance authorizations, schedule and transport their child, and act as a treatment provider at home. Many parents need help in this process regarding the identification and coordination of treatment team members. Every treatment provider and key school personnel should see the assessment report. Contact is vital among the team through e-mail or other means to coordinate response to the assessment and the care plan. If the child's needs are complicated, a short conference call is useful to make sure that everyone has the same information and there is consistency across settings. Over time, it is useful to review recommendations and discuss suggestions that have not yet been tried, or next steps in treatment. Risk factors identified in the report should also be monitored. Too often, an evaluation is reviewed once and then ignored, when in fact it should contain data relevant to the treatment plan for a school child for several years after the assessment. The final step of effective implementation of an assessment is following up at the appropriate time for recommended reevaluations.

SUMMARY

The primary purpose of neuropsychological assessment is to educate the child, his or her family, and the treatment and educational team about the child's profile of cognitive strengths and weaknesses, and emotional and behavioral functioning. This profile is used to identify where the child is at risk of difficulty and to develop a plan for making environmental accommodations or for teaching the child missing skills so that those risks can be mitigated. A successful model of neuropsychological assessment requires the integration of understanding brain structure and function, development, and context. Understanding the neural substrate available to a child at his or her stage of development, and the demands placed by the contexts the child inhabits, informs the description of the child's neuropsychological profile and treatment plan. The neuropsychological profile typically addresses multiple domains of functioning, including general intelligence, attention, executive, language, visual, learning and memory, social cognition, sensory, motor, emotional, adaptive, and academic performance. Appropriate referral questions, followed by thorough assessment and effective dissemination of findings and recommendations to families and treatment teams, maximizes the impact of neuropsychological assessment on children's lives.

REFERENCES

American Educational Research Association, American Psychological Association, & National Council of Measurements in Education (1999). *Standards for educational and psychological testing.* Washington, DC: Author.

Anastasi, A., & Urbina, S. (1997). *Psychological testing* (7th ed.). New York, NY: Macmillan Publishers.

Baron, I. (2000). Clinical implications and practical applications of child neuropsychological evaluations. *Pediatric neuropsychology: Research, theory, and practice* (pp. 439–456). New York, NY: Guilford Press.

Baron, I. (2004). *Neuropsychological evaluation of the child.* New York, NY: Oxford University Press.

Bernstein, J. (2000). Developmental neuropsychological assessment. *Pediatric neuropsychology: Research, theory, and practice* (pp. 405–438). New York, NY: Guilford Press.

Bernstein, J.H., & Waber, D.P. (1990). Developmental neuropsychological assessment: The systemic approach. In A.A. Boulton, G.B. Baker, M. Hiscock (Eds.), *Neuropsychology: Neuromethods* (311–371). Clifton, NJ: Humana Press.

Bracken, B. (1988). Ten psychometric reasons why similar tests produce dissimilar results. *Journal of School Psychology, 26*(2), 155–166. doi:10.1016/0022-4405(88)90017-9

Burgess, P., Alderman, N., Forbes, C., Costello, A., Coates, L., Dawson, D., ... Channon, S. (2006). The case for the development and use of 'ecologically valid' measures of executive function in experimental and clinical neuropsychology. *Journal of the International Neuropsychological Society, 12*(2), 194–209. doi:10.1017/S1355617706060310

Castaneda, A., Tuulio-Henriksson, A., Marttunen, M., Suvisaari, J., & Lönnqvist, J. (2008). A review on cognitive impairments in depressive and anxiety disorders with a focus on young adults. *Journal of Affective Disorders, 106*(1–2), 1–27. doi:10.1016/j.jad.2007.06.006

Chaytor, N., & Schmitter-Edgecombe, M. (2003). The ecological validity of neuropsychological tests: A review of the literature on everyday cognitive skills. *Neuropsychology Review, 13*(4), 181–197. doi:10.1023/B:NERV.0000009483.91468.fb

D'Esposito, M. (2007). From cognitive to neural models of working memory. *Philosophical Transactions of the Royal Society B: Biological Sciences, 362*(1481), 761–772. doi: 10.1098/rstb.2007.2086

Eysenck, M., Derakshan, N., Santos, R., & Calvo, M. (2007). Anxiety and cognitive performance: Attentional control theory. *Emotion, 7*(2), 336–353. doi:10.1037/1528-3542.7.2.336

Ferreri, F., & Lapp, L.K. (2011). Current research on cognitive aspects of anxiety disorders. *Current Opinion in Psychiatry, 24*(1), 49–54.

Flynn, J.R. (1994). Searching for justice: The discovery of IQ gains over time. *American Psychologist, 54*, 5–20.

Frith, C.D., & Frith, U. (2007). Social cognition in humans. *Current Biology, 17*(16), R724–32.

Frith, U., & Frith, C.D. (2010). The social brain: Allowing humans to boldly go where no other species has been. *Philosophical Transactions of the Royal Society B: Biological Sciences, 365*(1537), 165–176.

Gioia, G.A., & Isquith, P.K. (2004). Ecological assessment of executive function in traumatic brain injury. *Developmental Neuropsychology, 25*(1), 135–158. doi: 10.1207/s15326942dn2501&2_8

Gardner, H. (1983). *Frames of mind: The theory of multiple intelligences.* New York, NY: Basic Books.

Jensen, P., Hinshaw, S., Kraemer, H., Lenora, N., Newcorn, J., Abikoff, H., ... Vitiello, B. (2001). ADHD comorbidity findings from the MTA study: Comparing comorbid subgroups. *Journal of the American Academy of Child & Adolescent Psychiatry, 40*(2), 147–158. doi:10.1097/00004583-200102000-00009

Kenworthy, L., Yerys, B., Anthony, L., & Wallace, G. (2008). Understanding executive control in autism spectrum disorders in the lab and in the real world. *Neuropsychology Review, 18*(4), 320–338. doi:10.1007/s11065-008-9077-7

Klin, A., & Volkmar, F. (2000). Treatment and intervention guidelines for individuals with Asperger syndrome. *Asperger syndrome* (pp. 340–366). New York, NY: Guilford Press.

Manchester, D., Priestley, N., & Jackson, H. (2004). The assessment of executive functions: Coming out of the office. *Brain Injury, 18*(11), 1067–1081. doi:10.1080/02699050410001672387

Matarazzo, J. (1990). Psychological assessment versus psychological testing: Validation from Binet to the school, clinic, and courtroom. *American Psychologist, 45*(9), 999–1017. doi:10.1037/0003-066X.45.9.999

Mesulam, M.M. (2000). *Principles of behavioral and cognitive neurology.* New York, NY: Oxford University Press.

Meyer, G., Finn, S., Eyde, L., Kay, G., Moreland, K., Dies, R., ... Reed, G.M. (2001). Psychological testing and psychological assessment: A review of evidence and issues. *American Psychologist, 56*(2), 128–165. doi:10.1037/0003-066X.56.2.128.

Miller, E.K., & Cohen J.D. (2001). An integrative theory of prefrontal cortex function. *Annual Review of Neuroscience, 24*(1), 167–202. doi: 10.1146/annurev. neuro.24.1.167

Mundy, P., & Neal, A. (2001). Neural plasticity, joint attention, and a transactional social-orienting model of autism. *International review of research in mental retardation: Autism* (Vol. 23, pp. 139–168). San Diego, CA: Academic Press.

Mundy, P., & Newell, L. (2007). Attention, joint attention, and social cognition. Current Directions in *Psychological Science, 16*(5), 269–274. doi:10.1111/j.1467–8721.2007.00518.x

Pedhazur, E., & Schmelkin, L. (1991). *Measurement, design, and analysis: An integrated approach* (Student ed.). Hillsdale, NJ: Lawrence Erlbaum Associates, Inc.

Pelphrey, K., & Carter, E. (2008). Brain mechanisms for social perception: Lessons from autism and typical development. *Learning, skill acquisition, reading, and dyslexia* (pp. 283–299), NY: Wiley-Blackwell.

Pennington, B. (2002). *The development of psychopathology: Nature and nurture.* New York, NY: Guilford Press.

Piaget, J. (1952) *The origins of intelligence in children.* New York, NY: International Universities Press.

Porter, R., Bourke, C., & Gallagher, P. (2007). Neuropsychological impairment in major depression: Its nature, origin, and clinical significance. *Australian and New Zealand Journal of Psychiatry, 41*(2), 115–128. doi:10.1080/00048670601109881

Poston, J.M., & Hanson, W.E. (2010). Meta-analysis of psychological assessment as a therapeutic intervention. *Psychological Assessment, 22*(2), 203–212. doi: 10.1037/a0018679

Reynolds, C.R. (1981). The fallacy of 'two years below grade level for age' as a diagnostic criterion for reading disorders. *Journal of School Psychology, 19*(4), 350–358. doi: 10.1016/0022-4405(81)90029-7

Rogers, S.J., & Bennetto, L. (2000). Intersubjectivity in autism: The roles of imitation and executive function. In A. P. Wetherby & B. Prizant (Eds.), *Autism spectrum disorders: A transactional developmental perspective* (pp. 79–107). Baltimore, MD: Paul H. Brookes Publishing Co.

Sattler, J.M. (2001). *Assessment of children: Cognitive applications* (4th ed.). La Mesa, CA: Jerome M. Sattler Publisher.

Stefanatos, G.A., & Wasserstein, J. (2001). Attention deficit/hyperactivity disorder as a right hemisphere syndrome: Selective literature review and detailed neuropsychological case studies. *Annals of the New York Academy of Sciences, 931*(1), 172–195. doi: 10.1111/j.1749-6632.2001.tb05779.x

Streiner, D.L., & Norman, G.R. (1995). *Health measurement scales: A practical guide to their development and use,* (2nd ed.). New York, NY: Oxford University Press.

Stuss, D.T., & Benson, D.F. (1984). Neuropsychological studies of the frontal lobes. *Psychological Bulletin, 95*(1), 3–28. doi: 10.1037/0033-2909.95.1.3

Upton, G., & Cook, I. (2008). *A dictionary of statistics,* (2nd ed. rev.) New York, NY: Oxford University Press.

Welsh, M., & Pennington, B. (1988). Assessing frontal lobe functioning in children: Views from developmental psychology. *Developmental Neuropsychology, 4*(3), 199–230. doi:10.1080/87565648809540405.

Wolraich, M.L., & DuPaul, G.J. (2010). *ADHD diagnosis and management: A practical guide for the clinic and the classroom.* Baltimore, MD: Paul H. Brookes Publishing Co.

Youngstrom, E., LaKind, J.S., Kenworthy, L., Lipkin, P.H., Goodman, M., Squibb, K., … Anthony, L.G. (2010). Advancing the selection of neurodevelopmental measures in epidemiological studies of environmental chemical exposure and health effects. *International Journal of Environmental Research and Public Health, 7,* 229–268

Chapter 16 Appendix Examples of widely used neurodevelopmental measures organized by functional domain [1].

Measure	Scale name	Age range (yrs unless otherwise indicated)	Admin. time	Advantages	Disadvantages	References
General intelligence						
Bayley Scales of Infant Development, Third Edition (Bayley-III)	Adaptive Behavior, Cognitive, Language Composite, Motor Composite	1–42 months	50–90 min	One of the only instruments available in the age range, recently restandardized, extended floors and ceilings, improved evidence of reliability and validity	Difficult to administer and confounded by significant language demands	[2]
Mullen Scales of Early Learning (AGS Edition)	Early Learning Composite Gross Motor; Visual Reception; Fine Motor; Receptive Language; Expressive Language	Birth to 68 months	~15 min (for 1-year-olds) to 60 min (for 5-year-olds)	Limited language demands	Old normative data	[3]
Wechsler Intelligence Scales for Children—Fourth Edition (WISC-IV)	Full Scale, Verbal Comprehension, Perceptual Reasoning, Working Memory, Processing Speed	6–16	60–90 min	Most widely used test of cognitive ability in children and adolescents; excellent norms; familiar; stronger measurement of working memory than previous	Not tied to strong theory of intelligence; relatively weak assessment of processing speed	[4]
Wechsler Adult Intelligence Scales (WAIS-III)	Full Scale Verbal, Performance, Verbal Comprehension, Perceptual Organization, Working Memory, Processing Speed	16–89	60–90 min	Reliable, good norms, commonly administered	Not tied to strong theory of intelligence; relatively weak assessment of processing speed and working memory	[5]
Wechsler Abbreviated Scale of Intelligence (WASI)	Full Scale, Verbal, Performance	6–89	30 min	Validated as a brief measure of verbal, nonverbal, and general cognitive ability; very precise scores; Matrix Reasoning can be administered nonverbally	No coverage of processing speed, working memory, or other aspects of cognitive ability	[6]

Instrument	Age range	Time	Strengths	Limitations	
Comprehensive Test of Nonverbal Intelligence (CTONI-2)	6–89 years 11 months	40–60 min	Pictorial Analogies, Geometric Analogies, Pictorial Categories, Geometric Categories, Pictorial Sequences, Geometric Sequences	Minimizes cultural bias, good for children with language disorders	Less predictive of some aspects of functioning than verbally loaded scales	[7]
Leiter International Performance Scale–Revised	2–21	40–90 min	Visualization & Reasoning (VR); Attention & Memory (AM)	Covers wide age range; minimal bias across cultures; strong theoretical model guiding revision	Special training may be needed for good standardization; AM subtests not very stable over time	[8]
Differential Abilities Scale–II (DAS-II)	2.5–17 years 11 months	60 min	General Cognitive Ability, Verbal Ability, Nonverbal Ability, Spatial Ability	Good norms, conceptual model, strong psychometrics, nonverbal subtests can be administered without language	No working memory or processing speed	[9]

Attention

Instrument	Age range	Time	Strengths	Limitations	
Conners' Continuous Performance Test (3rd ed)	6–18	5–20 min	Total Score (also a short form, a DSM form, and a global form)	Parent, teacher, and youth forms; includes DSM-IV content; extensive research base; includes validity scales	Cumbersome to score without computer software; short forms validated in embedded version (not separate administration)	[10]
Continuous Performance Test–II (CPT)	3+	15–20 min	Sustained attention, Omissions, d Prime, Commissions, Variability, Standard Error	Standardized task that measures multiple performance facets of attention	Relatively small number of minorities included in the norm sample; overall mild correlations between CPT and ADHD rating scales	[11]

Executive functioning

Instrument	Age range	Time	Strengths	Limitations	
Behavior Rating Inventory of Executive Functioning (BRIEF)	2 to adult	10–15 min	Global Executive Composite	Parent and teacher forms; inexpensive; collateral source of information about executive functioning. Comprehensive coverage of subdomains of executive functioning; ecologically valid measure; used extensively in research with good sensitivity; easy to administer and complete	Parent ratings are susceptible to bias; report of everyday executive function does not necessarily accurately parse subdomains of executive function. Normative sample not nationally representative; variable correlations between scores and underlying processes	[12]

(continued)

Measure	Scale name	Age range (yrs unless otherwise indicated)	Admin. time	Advantages	Disadvantages	References
			Executive functioning (continued)			
Rey Complex Figure Test	Copy Strategy	6–89	45 min, including 30 min delayed interval	New manual (1996) improves scoring criteria and guidelines, as well as norms. Developmental scoring norms capture problem-solving strategy (as opposed to outcome score), which is a key correlate of executive functions that is often not addressed	Wide developmental variation and limited normative sample compromise sensitivity. Scoring system is complex and prone to error; requires specific training for adequate accuracy	[13]
Wisconsin Card Sorting Test (WCST)	Perseverative Errors	6.5–89 years 11 months	20–30 min	Relevant construct for neuro-toxicity	Difficult to reliably score if not using computer administration; not representative norms; complex relationship between scales and executive function	[14]
			Language			
Goldman–Fristoe Test of Articulation, 2nd Edition	Sounds in Words; Sounds in Sentences; Stimulability	2–21	15–30 min	Strong standardization sample; good norm-referenced scores	Technical information based on administrations by speech pathologists; unclear how results would vary with less trained raters; use with caution with speakers of nonstandard English	[15]
Preschool Language Scale, 4th Edition (PLS)	Auditory Comprehension; Expressive Communication	Birth to 6 years 11 months	20–45 min	New norms; Spanish version available (though less technical data available)	Standardized only in English; no information about how bilingual status influences performance (though ~7% of sample was bilingual); potential for marked variability in administration and scoring means that a high degree of training is needed for consistency	[16]

Test	Subtests/Domains	Age range	Time	Advantages	Disadvantages	Ref
Clinical Evaluation of Language Fundamentals (4th edition) (CELF)	Expressive Language, Receptive Language	5–21 (preschool version also available)	30–45 min	Easy to learn; computer-assisted scoring; focuses on specific skills and areas of functioning (versus achievement)	18 subtests if do full battery; low reliability for a few subtests	[17]
California Verbal Learning Test (CVLT)	Verbal learning, memory	5 to adult	30–50 min	Widely used test of verbal learning and memory, short, measures recognition and recall		[18]
Test of Problem Solving Child and Adolescent (TOPS 3 Elementary)	Pragmatic Language	6–12 years 11 months	35 min	Assesses language-based critical thinking skills	Lengthy to administer	[19]
Visual perceptual						
Beery Visual Motor Integration (5th edition)	Total Score, Visual, Motor	2–18 for full form	10–15 min	Culture free, easy to administer, used in many countries	Scoring somewhat difficult	[20]
Performance subtests from IQ measures (e.g., WISC, DAS)	Block Design, Digit Cancellation, Copy, etc.	Various	Various	Well-normed; clear scoring; readily available	Not validated as stand-alone tests; scores on single scale driven by multiple factors	[4, 9]
Learning/Memory						
Wide Range Assessment of Memory and Learning (WRAML-2)	Visual Memory Index, Verbal Memory Index, Attention/Concentration, General Memory Index, Screening Memory Index	5–84 years 11 months	60 min for all core subtests	Wide age range; new norms; stronger factor structure than earlier version	Lengthy administration time; often only specific subtests are used	[21]
Social cognition						
Social Responsiveness Scale (SRS) Parent and teacher forms	Total, Social Cognition, Social Communication, Social Awareness, Autistic Mannerisms	4–18	15 min	Exceptional evidence of construct validity; inexpensive to administer	Norms not fully nationally representative	[22]
Autism Diagnostic Observation Schedule (ADOS)	Communication, Social, Repetitive interests/behaviors	Toddler to adult	45 min	Language-based modules, good validity, play- and interview-based assessment	Difficult to administer and score reliably, extensive training needed	[23]
Autism Diagnostic Interview, Revised (ADI)	Communication, Social, Repetitive interests/behaviors	4 to adult	1½ to 2½ hours	Comfortable for parents, thorough	Retrospective parent report, difficult to administer and score reliably, extensive training needed, lengthy	[24]

(continued)

Measure	Scale name	Age range (yrs unless otherwise indicated)	Admin. time	Advantages	Disadvantages	References
Motor/Sensory						
Peabody Developmental Motor Scales	Fine Motor Quotient, Gross Motor Quotient, plus 9 subtest scores	Birth to 72 months	2–3 hours (20–30 min per subtest)	Minimal training needed because of clear instructions and objective scoring; easy to administer	Limited data on children with special needs; kit does not include all materials needed for administration; small objects are a choke hazard and need cleaning if mouthed	[25]
Digital Finger-tapping	Digital Finger Tapping	Various norms; college student for digital version	10 min with scoring	Easy to administer; electronic counter enhances accuracy	Poor norms; limited psychometric data; primarily suited to research use with comparison groups	[26]
Finger Tapping (Halstead-Reitan)	Finger Tapping	15–64	10 min with scoring	Easy to administer; widely recognized test	Small and dated norms	[27]
Finger Tapping (Findeis and Weight Meta-Norms)	Finger Tapping	5–14	10 min with scoring	Easy to administer	Pools data from 20 different studies to create "norms"	[28]
Emotional adjustment						
Achenbach Child Behavior Checklist	Total Problems, Externalizing, Internalizing, Attention Problems	1.5 to young adult	10–15 min	Multiple versions, multiple informants, forms and norms for multiple age ranges, large research and clinical literature with wide variety of medical conditions	Omits some content likely to be relevant, including theory of mind, mania scale; scales do not map directly onto psychiatric diagnoses	[29]
Aberrant Behavior Checklist (ABC)	Irritability, Lethargy, Stereotypy, Hyperactivity, Inappropriate Speech	5–51+	~5 min for a rater familiar with subject's behavior	Good content coverage; sensitive to treatment effects	Manual provides incomplete psychometric information; although often used as parent or teacher rating, less validation of these formats	[30]

Measure	Content/Subtests	Age range	Time	Features	Notes	Ref
Infant-Toddler Social and Emotional Assessment (ITSEA)	Problem Total; Competence Total; also Externalizing, Internalizing, Dysregulation, Competence, and Maladaptive Item Clusters	12–35 months	20–30 min	Parent form, parent interview form, and child care provider form; Spanish translation available; brief screening version (BITSEA)	Little technical information about child care provider or Spanish forms	[31]

Measure	Content/Subtests	Age range	Time	Features	Notes	Ref
Adaptive Behavior Assessment System–II (ABAS)	Parent Form Global Assessment of Competence	Birth to adult	15–20 min	Multiple versions for different ages and parents and day care providers; extensive construct validity	Like any parent checklist, ABAS is susceptible to misinterpretation and bias	[32]
Vineland Adaptive Behavior Scale–II (VABS)	Parent Interview Edition Parent Form Teacher Form	0–18 2–21	20–60 minutes 15–20 min	Well validated in multiple clinical groups Self-report version; multiple versions for different ages and parents and day care providers; extensive construct validity	Time and expertise intensive measure for the interview version; can take more than 1 hour to complete. Administration of interview version requires expertise gained through graduate level training programs in psychology or social work	[33]
Wide Range Achievement Test 4 (WRAT-4)	Word Reading, Sentence Comprehension, Reading Composite, Spelling, Math Computation	5–94 years 11 months	15–25 min for ages 5 to 7 for whole test; 30–45 min for over age 7 for whole test	Short, alternative forms allows retesting, part can be administered in group format	Captures basic learning difficulties with reading decoding, and math computation, but is not sensitive to learning disabilities associated with executive function, processing speed, motor output, reading comprehension, or written expression	[34]
Woodcock-Johnson–III	Academic Fluency Subtests	2–90+	Variable, ~5 min per test	Relatively easy to administer; sensitive to the effects of processing speed and motor output deficits on academics	Moderately old norms	[35]

Source: Adapted from Youngstrom, E., LaKind, J.S., Kenworthy, L., Lipkin, P.H., Goodman, M., Squibb, K.,... Anthony, L.G. (2010). Advancing the selection of neurodevelopmental measures in epidemiological studies of associations between environmental chemical exposure and adverse health Effects. *International Journal of Environmental Research and Public Health, 7*, 229–268. doi:10.3390/ijerph7010229. © 2010 by the authors; licensee Molecular Diversity Preservation International, Basel, Switzerland. This article is an open-access article distributed under the terms and conditions of the Creative Commons Attribution license (http://creativecommons.org/licenses/by/3.0/).

REFERENCES FOR APPENDIX

1. Youngstrom, E., LaKind, J.S., Kenworthy, L., Lipkin, P.H., Goodman, M., Squibb, K., ... Anthony, L.G. (2010). Advancing the selection of neurodevelopmental measures in epidemiological studies of associations between environmental chemical exposure and adverse health effects. *International Journal of Environmental Research and Public Health, 7,* 229–268; doi:10.3390/ijerph7010229
2. Bayley, N. (2006). *Bayley Scales of Infant and Toddler Development: Technical manual.* San Antonio, TX: Harcourt Brace and Company.
3. Mullen, E.M. (1995). *Mullen Scales of Early Learning.* Circle Pines, MN: American Guidance Service.
4. Wechsler, D. (2003). *Wechsler Intelligence Scale for Children—Fourth Edition: Technical and interpretive manual.* San Antonio, TX: The Psychological Corporation.
5. Wechsler, D. (1997). *Wechsler Adult Intelligence Scale–Third Edition, Wechsler Memory Scale-Third Edition technical manual.* San Antonio, TX: The Psychological Corporation.
6. The Psychological Corporation. (1999). *Wechsler Abbreviated Scale of Intelligence Manual.* San Antonio, TX: Harcourt Brace and Company.
7. Hammill, D.D., Pearson, N.A., & Wiederholt, J.L. (2009). *Comprehensive Test of Nonverbal Intelligence-Second Edition.* Austin, TX: PRO-ED
8. Roid, G.H., & Miller, L.J. (1998). *Leiter International Performance Scale-Revised.* Wood Dale, IL: Stoelting Co.
9. Elliott, C.D. (2007). *Differential Ability Scales-Second Edition, administration & scoring manual.* San Antonio, TX: Psychological Corporation.
10. Conners, C.K. (2008). *Conners' Continuous Performance Test* (3rd ed). North Tonawanda, NY: Multi-Health Systems.
11. Conners, C.K., & MHS Staff. (2004). *Conners' Continuous Performance Test (CPT II).* North Tonawanda, NY: Multi-Health Systems.
12. Gioia, G.A., Isquith, P.K., Guy, S.C., & Kenworthy, L. (2000). Behavior Rating Inventory of Executive function. *Child Neuropsychology, 6,* 235–238.
13. Meyers, J.E., & Meyers, K.R. (1996). *Rey Complex Figure Test and recognition trial.* Odessa, FL: Psychological Assessment Resources.
14. Heaton, R.K., Chelune, G.J., Talley, J.L., Kay, J.H., & Curtiss, G. (1993). *Wisconsin Card Sorting Test manual.* Odessa, FL: Psychological Assessment Resources.
15. Goldman, R., & Fristoe, M. (2000). *Goldman Fristoe Test of Articulation* (2nd ed.) Circle Pines, MN: American Guidance Service.
16. Zimmerman, I.L., Steiner, V.G., & Pond, R.E. (2002). *Preschool Language Scale* (4th ed.) San Antonio, TX: Harcourt Brace Jovanovich.
17. Semel, E., Wiig, E., Secord, W.A. (2003). *Clinical Evaluation of Language Fundamentals, Fourth Edition.* San Antonio, TX: The Psychological Corporation.
18. Delis, D.C., Kramer, J.H., Kaplan, E., & Ober, B.A. (1994). *California Verbal Learning Test—Children's Version.* San Antonio, TX: Harcourt Brace and Company
19. Bowers, L., Huisingh, R., & LoGiudice, C. (2005). *Test of Problem Solving 3: Elementary.* East Moline, IL: LinguiSystems.
20. Beery, K.E., & Beery, N.A. (2004). *The Beery-Buktenica Developmental Test of Visual-Motor Integration.* 5th edition. Minneapolis, MN: NCS Pearson.
21. Sheslow, D., & Adams, W. (2003). *Wide Range Assessment of Memory and Learning, Second Edition.* Lutz, Fl: PAR.
22. Constantino, J.N., & Gruber, C.P. (2005). *Social Responsiveness Scale (SRS).* Los Angeles, CA: Western Psychological Services
23. Lord, C., Rutter, M., DiLavore, P.C., Risi, S. (2001). *The Autism Diagnostic Observation Schedule.* Los Angeles, CA: Western Psychological Services
24. Rutter, M., Le Couteur, A. Lord, C. (2003). *Autism Diagnostic Interview—Revised.* Los Angeles, CA: Western Psychological Services
25. Folio, M.R., & Fewell, R.R. (2000). *Peabody Developmental Motor Scales-Second Edition.* Austin, TX: PRO-ED.
26. Brandon, A.D., & Bennett, T.L. (1989). *Digital Finger Tapping Test.* Los Angeles, CA: Western Psychological Services
27. Reitan, R.M. (1979). *Halstead-Reitan Neuropsychological Test Battery.* Tucson, AZ: Reitan Neuropsychology Laboratory/Press.
28. Baron, I.S. (2004). *Neuropsychological Evaluation of the Child.* New York, NY: Oxford University Press
29. Achenbach, T.M., & Rescorla, L.A. (2001). *Manual for the ASEBA school-age forms & profiles.* Burlington, VT: University of Vermont.
30. Aman, M.G., & Singh, N.N. (1986). *Aberrant Behavior Checklist.* East Aurora, NY: Slosson Educational Publications.
31. Briggs Gowan, M.J., & Carter, A.S. (2006). *ITSEA/BITSEA: Infant-Toddler and Brief Infant-Toddler Social and Emotional Assessment.* San Antonio, TX: The Psychological Corporation.
32. Harrison, P.L., & Oakland, T. (2003). *Adaptive Behavior Assessment System (ABAS.* 2nd ed.). San Antonio, TX: The Psychological Corporation.
33. Sparrow, S., Balla, D.A., & Cicchetti, D. (2005). *Vineland Adaptive Behavior Scales, 2nd Edition: Survey forms manual.* San Antonio, TX: Pearson.
34. Wilkinson, G.S., & Robertson, G.J. (2006). *Wide Range Achievement Test 4 (WRAT4).* Lutz, FL: PAR.
35. Woodcock, R.W., McGrew, K.S., & Mather, N. (2005). *Woodcock-Johnson Psychoeducational Battery—III NU complete.* Rolling Meadows, IL: Riverside Publishing Company.

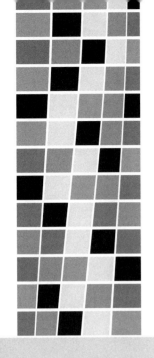

III

Developmental Disabilities

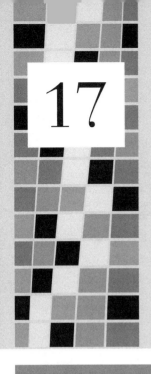

17

Developmental Delay and Intellectual Disability

Bruce K. Shapiro and Mark L. Batshaw

Upon completion of this chapter, the reader will

■ Understand the definition of *developmental delay* and implications of the terms *mental retardation* and *intellectual disability*

■ Be aware of the various causes of intellectual disability

■ Recognize the various interventions in intellectual disability

■ Be aware of the different levels of functioning and independence that individuals with intellectual disability can achieve

The term **global developmental delay** is most commonly used as a temporary diagnosis in young children at risk for developmental disabilities, especially intellectual disabilities. In this context, it indicates a failure to achieve age-appropriate neurodevelopmental milestones in the areas of language, motor, and social-adaptive development (Beirne-Smith, Patton, & Kim, 2005). It is often but not always predictive of a future diagnosis of intellectual disability (Riou, Ghosh, Francoeur, & Shevell, 2009).

■■■ DANIEL

Daniel's mother, Marina, noticed many signs in his early development that indicated atypical development. (In the following paragraphs, the typical ages for these developmental milestones are indicated in parentheses after the age at which Daniel achieved them.)

As an infant, Daniel showed little interest in his environment and was not very alert. Although Marina tried to breastfeed him, his suck was weak, and he frequently regurgitated his formula. He was floppy and had poor head control. His cry was high pitched, and he was difficult to comfort. He would sit in an infant seat for hours without complaint.

In social and motor development, Daniel lagged behind the norm. In language skills, he did not start babbling until 13 months (6 months). He smiled at 5 months (2 months) and was not very responsive to his parents' attention. In terms of gross motor development, Daniel could hold his head up at 4 months (1 month), roll over at 8 months (5 months), and sit up at 14 months (6 months). He transferred objects from one hand to the other at 14 months (5 months).

When evaluated with the Bayley Scales of Infant Development—Third Edition (BSID-III; Bayley, 2006) at 16 months of age, Daniel's mental age was found to be 7 months, and he received a mental developmental index (MDI; similar to an IQ score) of less than 50.

291

He progressed from an early intervention program to a special preschool program. Prior to school entry at age 6, Daniel was retested on the Stanford-Binet Intelligence Scales, Fifth Edition (SB5; Roid, 2003). His score indicated a mental age of 2 years 8 months, and an IQ score of 40. Concomitant impairments in adaptive behavior were demonstrated by the Vineland Adaptive Behavior Scales, Second Edition (Vineland-II; Sparrow, Bella, & Chrichetti, 2005), which revealed communicative, self-care, and social skill challenges.

EARLY IDENTIFICATION OF DEVELOPMENTAL DELAY

Global developmental delay is recognized by the failure to meet age-appropriate expectations based on the typical sequence of development. In the first months of life, delayed development can be manifested by a lack of visual or auditory response, an inadequate suck, and/or floppy or spastic muscle tone. Later in the first year, lack of language and motor delays in sitting and walking may suggest developmental delay. When a child continues to show significant delays in all developmental areas, intellectual disability is the most likely diagnosis. Unfortunately some medical practitioners continue to use the term global developmental delay long after a more specific diagnosis of intellectual disability can be made. Although developmental delay is the most common presenting concern in children who turn out to have an intellectual disability, sensory impairment, an autism spectrum disorder (ASD), or cerebral palsy, it does not always indicate a developmental disability. Isolated mild delays in expressive language (particularly in boys) or in gross-motor abilities usually resolve over time. These mild early delays, however, often signal an increased risk of the child developing academic or behavioral difficulties by school age.

Early identification of atypical development is more likely to occur with more severe impairments. In order to facilitate early identification, all children should receive developmental surveillance as part of their routine pediatric care (King et al., 2010; Rydz, Shevell, Majnemer, & Oskoui, 2005). This includes obtaining a history of developmental concerns from the parents, recording developmental milestones, and performing a screening test (e.g., the Ages & Stages Questionnaires® [ASQ; Bricker, Squires, & Mounts, 1999], or

the Parent Evaluations of Developmental Status [PEDS; Glascoe, 1997; see also http://www.pedstest.com]). In 2006, The American Academy of Pediatrics et al. developed a system of developmental surveillance and screening to be employed in primary care settings. Unfortunately, many children come from underserved populations and do not have a "medical home" with systematic screening, assessment, and family supports (Balogh, Ouellette-Kuntz, Bourne, Lunsky, & Colantonio, 2008). Furthermore, the available developmental screening tests themselves are not sufficiently sensitive to detect many developmental disabilities.

It is important to emphasize that screening tests are not designed to supplant a formal neurodevelopmental and psychological assessment (Shapiro & Batshaw, 2011). They are designed for use in the general population in order to identify individuals at risk. The usefulness of a screening instrument is determined by its ability to appropriately classify children who do or do not have significant developmental delays—that is, its sensitivity and specificity, respectively. Sensitivity is the ability to detect affected children (measured by the true-positive rate). Specificity is the ability to classify typical children as typical (measured by the true-negative rate). The ideal screening instrument would detect all of the children who require further assessment (no false negatives) and none of those who do not (no false positives). Unfortunately, many screening instruments misclassify too many children to be clinically useful, which speaks to the importance of clinical judgment.

Given these difficulties, the best approach to early identification is multifaceted (Beirne-Smith et al., 2005). Infants at high risk should be closely monitored and entered into early intervention programs if appropriate (Shapiro & Batshaw, 2011; see Chapter 30). High-risk conditions include the following:

1. Prematurity (see Chapter 7)

2. Low birth weight (Anderson & Doyle, 2008)

3. Perinatal complications

4. Chronic physical health conditions

5. Exposure to environmental hazardous substances (Frederick & Stanwood, 2009)

6. Maternal functioning compromised by depression (Tronick & Reck, 2009), substance abuse (Bandstra, Morrow, Mansoor, & Accornero, 2010), lack of education (Chapman, Scott, & Stanton-Chapman, 2008), child neglect/abuse (Ayoub et al.,

2006; Hibbard, Desch, American Academy of Pediatrics Committee on Child Abuse and Neglect, & American Academy of Pediatrics Council on Children with Disabilities, 2007), or domestic violence (Koenen, Moffitt, & Caspi, 2003)

7. Low socioeconomic family background (Huston & Bentley, 2010)

In addition, all parents should be educated to look for and report delays in developmental achievement. Clinic staff and primary providers should routinely note achievement of developmental milestones, much like they note height and weight. In addition, children should receive neonatal hearing screening and evaluation of development, behavior, hearing, and vision in conjunction with each well-child visit (American Academy of Pediatrics et al., 2006; Gifford, Holmes, & Bernstein, 2009; Shapiro, 2011).

Parents usually seek an evaluation for developmental delay once their child fails to meet specific developmental milestones (Table 17.1). In early infancy, these include a lack of responsiveness, unusual muscle tone or posture, and feeding difficulties (Bear, 2004). Between 6 and 15 months of age, motor delay is the most common complaint. Language and behavior problems are the most common concerns after 18 months. If there is evidence of a significant developmental lag over time, the child should be sent for a comprehensive evaluation. Ideally, this evaluation should include an examination by at least a physician (pediatrician, neurodevelopmental pediatrician, developmental-behavioral pediatrician, child psychiatrist, geneticist, or pediatric neurologist) experienced in early childhood development and/or developmental disabilities, preferably in tandem with a clinical/educational psychologist and a social worker.

Depending on the child's age and impairments, he or she also may need to be seen for early intervention assessment by an early childhood educator, advanced practice nurse, speech-language pathologist, and/or an audiologist. If the child displays motor impairments, physical therapists, occupational therapists, and possibly a physiatrist should also be involved. Following the assessment, an individual family service plan (IFSP) is developed in the context of an early intervention program (see Chapter 30).

DEFINING INTELLECTUAL DISABILITY

The term **intellectual disability** has been gradually replacing the classic term **mental retardation**. This change was codified in federal legislation in 2010, when Rosa's Law was enacted. Rosa's Law changed the term used in federal legislation from mental retardation to intellectual disability. The definition of the term itself, however, did not change and comes from the Individuals with Disabilities Education Act (IDEA) of 2004 (PL 108–446). It defines intellectual disability as "significantly subaverage general intellectual functioning, existing concurrently with deficits in adaptive behavior and manifested during the developmental period, that adversely affects a child's educational performance."

Intellectual Functioning

There is general agreement the definition of intellectual disability requires that a person must have significantly subaverage intellectual functioning and impairments in adaptive abilities with onset during the developmental period; however, disagreements over the details of this

Table 17.1. Presentations of intellectual disability by age

Age	Area of concern
Newborn	Dysmorphisms (structural abnormalities)
	Major physiologic dysfunction (e.g., eating, breathing)
2–4 months	Failure to interact with the environment (e.g., parent suspects child is deaf or has a visual impairment)
6–18 months	Gross motor delay (e.g., sitting, crawling, walking)
18 months to 3 years	Language
3–5 years	Language
	Behavior (including play)
	Fine motor (e.g., cutting, coloring)
5+ years	Academic achievement
	Behavior (e.g., attention, anxiety, mood, conduct)

Source: Shapiro and Batshaw (2002).

definition have arisen for both biological and philosophical reasons. The first controversial issue in that the definition involves the assessment of intellectual functioning. The average level of intellectual functioning in a population corresponds to the apex of a bell-shaped curve. Two standard deviations on either side of the mean encompass 95% of a population sample and approximately defines the range of typical intellectual functioning (Figure 17.1). By definition, the average intelligence quotient (IQ score) is 100, and the standard deviation (a statistical measure of dispersion from the mean) of most IQ tests is 15 points. Historically, a person scoring more than 2 standard deviations below the mean, or below an IQ of 70, has been considered to have an intellectual disability.

Statisticians, however, point out that there is a measurement variance of approximately 5 points in assessing IQ by most psychometric tests. In other words, repeated testing of the same individual will produce scores that vary by as much as 5 points (American Academy of Pediatrics, 2000). Using this schema, intellectual disability would be diagnosed in an individual with an IQ score between 70 and 75, who exhibits significant impairments in adaptive

behavior, whereas it would not be diagnosed in an individual with an IQ of 65–70 who demonstrates adaptive skills in the typical range.

Beyond any measurement variability, a more fundamental concern of some theorists is the underlying value of an IQ score. Gardner (1983) challenged the dichotomous (verbal versus performance) structure of intelligence assessed by many IQ tests. He proposed that intelligence comprises a wider range of abilities, not only the traditional linguistic and logical-mathematical skills, but also musical, spatial, bodily–kinesthetic, and interpersonal characteristics as well. This approach has not gained wide acceptance, as it does not have a clear neuropsychological or neuroanatomical basis. Although it is acknowledged that a single IQ score averages a person's cognitive abilities and may not capture all forms of intelligence, there is evidence that a significantly subnormal IQ score is a meaningful predictor of future cognitive functioning.

However, it must be emphasized that cognitive functioning is not always uniform across all neurodevelopmental domains. An example is found in the study by Wang and Bellugi (1993) comparing neuropsychological testing results in children with Down syndrome and Williams syndrome. Although the Full-Scale IQ scores in both groups were similar, the pattern of cognitive strengths and weaknesses was very different. The individuals with Williams syndrome had much stronger skills in language but much poorer visual-perceptual abilities than did the children with Down syndrome. When volumetric analysis of magnetic resonance imaging (MRI) scans was performed, the cortical areas involved in language acquisition were much more developed in individuals with Williams syndrome; conversely the basal ganglia area that is involved in visual-perception was more developed in individuals with Down syndrome.

Finally, there are the concerns over predictive validity and cultural bias. Infant psychological tests are notoriously poor predictors of adult IQ scores, although they clearly differentiate severe impairments from typical functioning. In addition, cultural bias has been suggested as one explanation for differences in IQ scores found among individuals from various racial, ethnic, and socioeconomic groups.

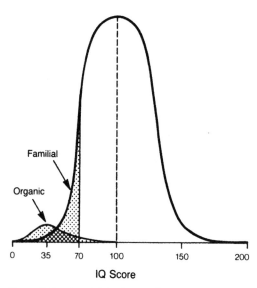

Figure 17.1. Bimodal distribution of intelligence. The mean IQ score is 100. An IQ score of less than 70, or 2 standard deviations below the mean, can indicate intellectual disability. The second, smaller curve takes into account individuals who have intellectual disability because of birth trauma, infection, inborn errors, or other organic causes. This explains why more individuals have severe to profound intellectual disability than are predicted by the familial curve alone. (From Zigler, E. [1967]. Familial retardation: A continuing dilemma. *Science, 155,* 292–298. http://www.aaas.org Reprinted with permission from AAAS.)

Adaptive Impairments

Individuals fulfilling the diagnosis of intellectual disability not only must have limitations in their intellectual abilities, but these deficits must also impair their ability to adapt or function in daily life, when compared with peers of similar age or culture. Indeed, it is the deficits in adaptive function that bring children to our attention. These impairments limit or restrict participation and performance in one or more aspects of daily life activities, such as communication, social participation, function at school or work, or personal independence at home or in community settings. The limitations result in the need for ongoing support at school, work, or independent life. Typically, adaptive behavior is measured using individualized, standardized, culturally appropriate, and psychometrically sound tests (American Psychiatric Association, 2011).

The American Association on Intellectual and Developmental Disability (AAIDD; Schalock, Borthwick-Duffy, Buntinx, Coulter, & Ellis, 2009) divided adaptive function into three domains: conceptual, practical, and socialization. Conceptual skills include such things as language and literacy; money, time, and number concepts; and self-direction. Practical skills include the activities of daily living, occupational skills, health care, travel/transportation, schedules/routines, safety, use of money, and use of the telephone. Social skills encompass interpersonal skills, social responsibility, self-esteem, gullibility, naïveté, social problem solving, the ability to follow rules/obey laws, and to avoid being victimized. The AAIDD definition of intellectual disability requires deficits to exist in one of the three domains of adaptive behavior.

CLASSIFICATION OF INTELLECTUAL DISABILITY

Intellectual disability is a heterogeneous group of conditions that arise from many different causes and that have many different expressions. Although the diagnosis of intellectual disability is important, the classification of intellectual disability is as important. Etiologic evaluation, neurobiological mechanisms, management, planning, and prognosis are all predicated on the ability to classify the disorder. There are many methods for classification, but this chapter focuses on four: degree of intellectual impairment, required supports, domains of disability, and etiology.

Degree of Intellectual Impairment

There is controversy about classifying the levels of intellectual disability. Per the APA (2000), an individual is classified as having mild intellectual disability if his or her IQ level is 50 to approximately 70; moderate intellectual disability if his or her IQ level is 35 to approximately 50; severe intellectual disability if his or her IQ level is 20 to approximately 35; and profound intellectual disability if his or her IQ level is below 20–25. This classification has met with widespread acceptance in the medical community, but it should be noted that classification solely on the basis of IQ is incomplete and does not describe all of an individual's abilities.

It has also been suggested that intellectual disability should be simply dichotomized into mild (IQ score of 50 to approximately 70) and severe (IQ score below 50). This suggestion is based on the discrete biological division between mild intellectual disability and the more severe forms, with different etiologies and outcomes. This dichotomy has not been widely accepted for clinical purposes because the medical, educational, and habilitative needs are quite different between individuals with moderate impairments and those with profound impairments.

Required Supports

The AAIDD takes a different approach in defining the degree of severity of intellectual disability, relying not on IQ scores but rather on the patterns and intensity of needed support (i.e., requiring intermittent, limited, extensive, or pervasive support). This definition marks a philosophical shift from an emphasis on degree of impairment to a focus on the abilities of individuals to function in an inclusive environment. This shift is controversial because it assumes that adaptive behaviors can be independent of cognition and does not provide clear guidelines for establishing diagnostic eligibility of children with IQ scores in the upper limits of the range connoting intellectual disability. This chapter (and other chapters throughout this book) uses the APA's categories in discussing medical issues and the AAIDD's categories in discussing educational and other interventions, emphasizing the capabilities rather than the impairments of individuals with intellectual disability.

Domains of Disability

Another way to classify intellectual disability is to use the terminology developed by the National Center for Medical Rehabilitation Research (Msall, 2005). This model defines five domains: pathophysiology, impairment, functional limitation, disability, and societal limitation (Table 17.2). Pathophysiology focuses on the cellular, structural, or functional events resulting from injury, disease, or genetic abnormality that underlie the developmental disability. Impairment refers to the losses that result from the pathophysiological event. Functional limitation describes the restriction or lack of ability to perform a normal function. Disability is the inability to perform activities or limitation in the performance of activities. Societal limitations focus on barriers to full participation in society. Table 17.2 illustrates how this system can be applied to children with Prader-Willi syndrome, fetal alcohol spectrum disorder, and Down syndrome. The advantage of this approach is that it leads directly from diagnosis to treatment and focuses on how to overcome limitations. It also acknowledges the change in emphasis in the diagnosis of intellectual disability from impairment and functional limitations to disability and societal limitations. This is consistent with the move from focusing on the intensity of the disability (e.g., severe) to the support needed to function in society (e.g.,

requiring extensive support). This approach is also in keeping with the process for developing an individualized education program (IEP) for a school-age child (see Chapter 31).

PREVALENCE OF INTELLECTUAL DISABILITY

Based on the previous discussion, the prevalence of intellectual disability depends on the definition used, the method of ascertainment, and the population studied. The prevalence of intellectual disability ranges between 6.7 (Boyle et al., 2011) and 10.37 (Maulik, Mascarenhas, Mathers, Dua, & Saxena, 2010) per 1,000. According to statistics, 2.5% of the population could be predicted to have intellectual disability, and another 2.5% could be predicted to have superior intelligence (Figure 17.1). Of individuals with intellectual disability, the IQ scores of 85% should fall 2–3 standard deviations below

Table 17.2. Relationship between disabilities domains and treatment in Prader-Willi syndrome, fetal alcohol spectrum disorder, and Down syndrome

Pathophysiology	Impairment	Functional limitation	Disability	Societal limitation	Treatment
Deletion in chromosome 15	Prader-Willi syndrome	Intellectual disability Feeding disorder	Learning and adaptive skills below age level Obesity	Noninclusive school settings Stereotyping because of obesity and intellectual disability Underestimating abilities	Education Activities to promote weight loss
In utero alcohol exposure	Fetal alcohol spectrum disorder	Intellectual disability Behavioral disturbances	Learning and adaptive skills below age level but variable Severe hyperactivity common	Noninclusive school settings Stigma because of etiology Overestimating abilities because of variable cognitive profile	Education Mental health Interventions as required
Trisomy 21	Down syndrome	Intellectual disability	Learning and adaptive skills below age level	Noninclusive school settings Stereotyping because of intellectual disability Underestimating abilities	Education Programs to raise societal awareness

Source: Msall, Avery, Tremont, Lima, Rogers, and Hogan (2003).

Note: Even though each child may have similar degrees of intellectual disability, the pattern of disability and type of treatments may vary widely.

the mean, in the range of mild intellectual disability. If individuals who score low on IQ tests because of cultural or societal disadvantage are excluded from the count of those with mild intellectual disability; however, the prevalence is only about half these predictions, somewhere between 0.8% and 1.2% (Heikura et al., 2003; McLaren & Bryson, 1987). Whatever the prevalence, intellectual disability appears to peak at 10–14 years of age, acknowledging that children with mild impairments are identified significantly later than those with more severe impairments. Overall, the recurrence risk in families with one child who has severe intellectual disability of unknown origin is 3%–9% (De Souza, Halliday, Chan, Bower, & Morris, 2009; Van Naarden Braun, Autry, & Boyle, 2005). Recurrence risk for intellectual disability of known origin, however, varies according to the cause. A family whose child has intellectual disability following neonatal meningitis does not have a significantly increased risk of having future affected children, whereas a woman who has had one child with a fetal alcohol spectrum disorders has a 30%–50% risk of having other affected children if she continues to abuse alcohol during pregnancy. The risk of recurrent Down syndrome ranges from less than 1% for trisomy 21 to more than 10% for a balanced translocation (see Chapter 1; De Souza et al., 2009). If the cause of intellectual disability is a Mendelian disorder (see Chapter 1), such as neurofibromatosis (an autosomal dominant trait), Hurler syndrome (an autosomal recessive trait), or fragile X syndrome (an X-linked trait), the recurrence risk ranges from 0%–50%, depending on the inheritance pattern of the specific disorder.

Etiology

The epidemiology of intellectual disability suggests that there are two overlapping populations: Mild intellectual disability is more likely to be associated with racial, social, and familial factors (Heikura et al., 2005; Leonard & Wen, 2002; Noble, Tottenham, & Casey, 2005), whereas severe intellectual disability is more typically linked to a biological/genetic origin (Ropers, 2008; Strømme & Hagberg, 2000; Yeargin-Allsopp, Murphy, Cordero, Decouflé, & Hollowell, 1997). There is often, however, an interaction between nature and nurture. Postnatal environmental influences mediate biological processes through mechanisms that may be indirect (e.g., epigenetics; see Chapter 1) and not fully understood at present. In addition, postnatal environmental factors may affect the expression of the

neurodevelopmental dysfunction. For example, a child may have an initial biological insult (e.g., intrauterine growth restriction [IUGR]) that can be compounded by postnatal environmental variables (e.g., poor nutrition, parental neglect). Mothers who never finished high school are four times more likely to have children with mild intellectual disability than are women who completed high school (Mendola, Selevan, Gutter & Rice, 2002). The explanation for this is unclear but may involve a genetic component (i.e., inheritance of a cognitive impairment) and socioeconomic factors (e.g., poverty, poor nutrition). Application of early intervention services to high-risk infants who are also at socioeconomic risk has resulted in improved cognitive outcomes (see Chapter 30).

The specific origins of mild intellectual disability are identifiable in less than half of affected individuals (Moeschler, Shevell, & the Committee on Genetics, 2006). The most common biological causes are certain genetic/chromosomal syndromes—for example, velocardiofacial syndrome (VCFS), Klinefelter syndrome, fetal deprivation (e.g., IUGR), perinatal complications (e.g., encephalopathy, infection), and intrauterine exposure to drugs of abuse, especially alcohol (Kodituwakku, 2009). Although definite genetic causes are less common (5% versus 47% in severe intellectual disability), familial clustering of mild intellectual disability is common (Heikura et al., 2005).

In children with severe intellectual disability, a biological origin can be identified in about three quarters of cases. The most common identifiable causes are Down syndrome, fragile X syndrome, and fetal alcohol spectrum disorders, which together account for almost one third of all currently detectable cases of severe intellectual disability (Kodituwakku, 2009; Moser, 1995).

One way of dividing the biological origins of intellectual disability is by their timing in the developmental sequence; in general, the earlier the problem, the more severe its consequences. This is consistent with finding a prenatal cause in about three quarters of individuals with an identifiable cause of severe intellectual disability (Acosta, Gallo, & Batshaw, 2002; Gropman & Batshaw, 2010; Squier & Jansen, 2010; Weindling, 2010). Chromosomal disorders (e.g., Down syndrome, Prader-Willi syndrome, 22q11 syndrome), certain single gene defects (e.g., Rubinstein-Taybi syndrome, Hurler syndrome), and abnormalities of brain development (e.g., holoprosencephaly) that affect early embryogenesis are the most common and severe examples of biologic origin. Together, these groups of genetically based causes of severe intellectual disability account for more than two thirds of identifiable causes and encompass more than 500 disorders (see http://www.ncbi.nlm.nih.gov/omim for more information). Insults occurring in the first and second trimesters as a result of substance abuse (e.g., fetal alcohol spectrum disorders), infections (e.g., cytomegalovirus), and other pregnancy problems (e.g., IUGR) occur in 10% of cases. Fetal deprivation in the third trimester due to placental damage, preeclampsia, or hemorrhage (see Chapter 2) and problems in the perinatal period (see Chapter 6) now account for less than 10% of identifiable causes of severe intellectual disability. Five percent are the result of postnatal brain damage, most commonly meningitis/encephalitis and traumatic brain injury (see Chapter 26).

ASSOCIATED IMPAIRMENTS

An intellectual disability is often accompanied by other impairments called comorbid conditions. Although a mild intellectual disability is frequently an isolated disorder, it may be paired with motor or communication impairments that affect the child's developmental outcome. The prevalence of these associated impairments correlates with the severity of the disability (Allen, 2008; Cooper & van der Speck, 2009; Fletcher, Loschen, Stavrakaki, & First, 2007; Jansen, Krol, Groothoff, & Post, 2004; Kerr, Turky, & Huber, 2009; Oliver & Richards, 2010). These comorbid conditions include cerebral palsy, seizure disorders, communication disorders, sensory impairments (hearing and/or visual deficits), and psychological/behavioral disorders (e.g., mood disorders, autism spectrum disorders, attention-deficit/hyperactivity disorder [ADHD], self-injury, aggression, conduct

Table 17.3. Percentage of children with Intellectual Disability (ID) who have associated chronic health conditions

Epilepsy	22.0
Cerebral palsy	19.8
Hearing problems	4.5
Vision problems	2.2–26.8
Down syndrome	11.0
Fragile X	1.9
Autistic disorder	10.1
PDD	7.1
ADHD/hyperkinetic disorder	9.5
Conduct disorder	5.1
Oppositional defiant disorder	12.4
Anxiety disorder	17.1

Source: Osesburg, Dijkstra, Groothoff, Reijneveld, and Jansen (2011).

Key: PDD, Pervasive developmental disorder; ADHD, attention-deficit/hyperactivity disorder

disorders; Table 17.3). Communication deficits (speech-language impairments), beyond those related to the cognitive impairment, also are frequent. Approximately 20% of children with severe intellectual disability have cerebral palsy, which may also be associated with feeding problems and failure to thrive. Seizure disorders also occur in about 20% of children with intellectual disability. Finally, psychological and behavior disorders occur in up to half of children with intellectual disability (Cooper & van der Speck, 2009). In considering intervention strategies, identifying these comorbid conditions and working toward their treatment is essential in order to obtain an optimal outcome.

Associated impairments may make it difficult to distinguish intellectual disability from other developmental disabilities. Certain distinguishing features, however, usually exist

Table 17.4. Developmental delays in various developmental disabilities during preschool years

Disorder	Developmental area			
	Motor	Language	Problem solving (nonverbal reasoning)	Social-adaptive
Intellectual disability	Variable	2	2	2
Autism spectrum disorder	N/A	3	Variable	3
Cerebral palsy	3	Variable	Variable	2
Language disorder/ deafness	N/A	2	N/A	Variable
Blindness	1	N/A	Variable	1

Key: 3, severe impairment; 2, moderate impairment; 1, mild impairment; N/A, not affected.

(Table 17.4). In isolated intellectual disability, language and nonverbal reasoning skills are significantly delayed, whereas gross motor skills tend to be less affected. Conversely, in cerebral palsy, motor impairments are more prominent than cognitive impairments. In communication disorders, expressive and/or receptive language skills are more delayed than nonverbal reasoning skills. In autism spectrum disorders, social skills impairments and atypical behaviors are superimposed on cognitive (especially communication) impairments. In some instances, repeated assessments may be necessary to determine the primary developmental disability.

MEDICAL DIAGNOSTIC TESTING

No single method exists for detecting all causes of intellectual disability (American Academy of Pediatrics et al., 2006; Moeschler et al., 2006; see Chapter 15). As a result, diagnostic testing should be based on the medical history and a physical examination. For example, a child with an unusual facial appearance, a history of other affected family members, or multiple congenital anomalies should be referred to a geneticist. With the increased ability to identify genetic disorders, even minor anomalies may be worth pursuing with chromosomal microarray analysis (Miller et al., 2010; Qiao et al., 2010; see Chapter 1). A male with unusual physical features and/or a family history of intellectual disability and/or autism spectrum disorder should probably have molecular studies for fragile X syndrome. A child with a progressive neurological disorder will need extensive metabolic investigation, and a child with seizurelike episodes should have an electroencephalogram. Finally, children with abnormal head growth or asymmetrical neurological findings may warrant an MRI scan. These tests, however, should not be seen as screening tools to be used in all children with intellectual disability because their yield of useful results is low unless there is a specific reason for performing the study. Table 17.5 lists tests that may be used to investigate intellectual disability and how commonly they are likely to reveal a cause.

Although these are the most common reasons for performing diagnostic tests, it now seems clear that some children with subtle physical or neurological findings also may have determinable biological origins of their intellectual disability. It has been shown that a significant percentage of unexplained intellectual disability can be accounted for by microdeletions (very minute chromosomal abnormalities)

that can be evaluated by chromosomal microarray analysis. Here abnormalities have been found in 15%–20% of samples from individuals with intellectual disability who were tested (Miller et al., 2010). In addition, MRI scans have been found to document a significant number of subtle markers of cerebral malformations in about 10% of children with intellectual disability (Barkovich & Raybaud, 2004).

How intensively one should investigate the cause of a child's intellectual disability is based on a number of factors. First, what is the degree of intellectual disability? One is less likely to find a biological cause in a child with mild intellectual disability than in a child with a severe disability. Second, is there a specific diagnostic path to follow? If there is a medical history, a family history, or physical findings pointing to a specific cause, a diagnosis is more likely to be made. Conversely, in the absence of these indicators, it is difficult to choose specific tests to perform. Third, are the parents planning to have additional children? If so, clinicians are more likely to intensively seek disorders for which prenatal diagnosis or a specific early treatment option is available (e.g., for many inborn errors of metabolism). Finally, and most important, what are the parents' wishes? Different parents have different levels of investment in searching for the cause of the intellectual disability. Some focus exclusively on treatment while others are so directed on obtaining a diagnosis that they have difficulty accepting intervention until a specific cause has been determined. Both extremes and every perspective in between must be respected, and supportive anticipatory guidance should be provided in the context of parent education for the "here and now" as well as for the future.

PSYCHOLOGICAL TESTING

The routine evaluation for intellectual disability should include an individual intelligence test (see Chapter 16). The most commonly used test in children are the Bayley Scales of Infant Development—Third Edition (BSID-III; Bayley, 2006), the Stanford Binet Intelligence Scales—Fifth Edition (Roid, 2003) and the Wechsler scales: the Wechsler Preschool and Primary Scale of Intelligence—Third Edition (WPPSI-III; Wechsler, 2002) and the Wechsler Intelligence Scale for Children—Fourth Edition (WISC-IV; Wechsler, 2003).

As noted in the APA definition of intellectual disability, in addition to testing intelligence, adaptive skills (including social functioning)

Table 17.5.   Suggested evaluation of the child with intellectual disability

Test	Yield	Comment
In-depth history		Prenatal, perinatal, and postnatal events (including seizures)
		Developmental attainments
		Three-generation pedigree in family history
Physical examination		Particular attention to minor/subtle abnormalites
		Neurological examination for focality and skull abnormalities
		Behavioral phenotype
Vision/hearing evaluation		Physiologic measures may be required if behavioral responses cannot be reliably assessed.
Chromosomal microarray analysis	15%–20%	May not detect some balanced rearrangements or low-level mosaicism
		Technology and interpretation of results is evolving
Karyotype	3.7%	Now replaced in most cases by microarray analysis, which has a higher yield
Fragile X screen	2.6%	Preselection on clinical grounds may increase yield to 7.6%
Neuroimaging (magnetic resonance imaging preferred)	40%–55%	Positives increased by abnormalities of skull contour or size, or focal neurological examination
		Identification of specific etiologies is rare
		Most conditions that are found do not alter treatment plan
		Need to weigh risk of sedation against possible yield
Thyroid/thyroid stimulating hormone	~4%	Near 0% in settings with universal newborn screening program
Serum lead	?	Performed in the presence of identifiable risk factors for excessive environmental lead exposure
Metabolic testing	~1%	Urine organic acids
		Plasma
		Amino acids
		Ammonia
		Lactate
		Capillary blood gas
		Focused testing based on clinical findings warranted
MECP2 for Rett syndrome	?	Females with severe ID
Electroencephalogram	~1%	May be deferred in absence of history of seizures

Sources: Curry et al. (1997); Miller et al. (2010); Shevell et al. (2003).

also should be measured. The most commonly used test of adaptive behavior is the Vineland-II (Sparrow et al., 2005). Other tests of adaptive behavior that are used commonly include the Scales of Independent Behavior—Revised (Bruininks, Woodcock, Weatherman, & Hill, 1996) and the Adaptive Behavior Assessment System—Second Edition (ABAS-II; Harrison & Oakland, 2003).

Interpretation of Test Results

In infants and young children with typical development, there is substantial variability in IQ scores on repeated cognitive testing and consequently poor predictive validity until around 10 years of age. Accuracy is enhanced if repeated testing confirms a stable rate of cognitive development. The predictive value of infant tests is further limited because such tests are primarily dependent on nonlanguage items, whereas language skills remain the best predictors of future IQ scores. These tests do permit the differentiation of infants with severe intellectual disability from typically developing infants but are less helpful in distinguishing between a typically developing child and one with a mild intellectual disability. In general, however, there is less variability seen with cognitive growth in children with intellectual disability, so predictive validity is enhanced compared with children with typical development.

Although children with intellectual disability usually score below average on all subscale scores, they may score in the typical range in one or more performance areas in the Wechsler Scales (Wechsler, 2002, 2003). Overall, these scales are quite accurate in predicting adult IQ scores when administered to school-age children. The evaluator, however, must ensure that situations that may lead to falsely low IQ scores do not confound the test performance. Conditions such as motor impairments, communication disorders, sensory impairments, speaking a language other than English, extremely low birth weight, or insufficient schooling may invalidate certain intelligence tests and require modification of others, and the presence of such conditions always requires caution with regard to interpretation.

There is usually, but not always, a good correlation between scores on the intelligence and adaptive scales (Bloom & Zelko, 1994). Adaptive abilities, however, are more responsive to intervention efforts than is the IQ score. They are also more variable, which may relate to the underlying condition and to environmental expectations. For example, although individuals with Prader-Willi syndrome have stability of adaptive skills through adulthood, individuals with fragile X syndrome may have increasing impairments over time (Jacquemont et al., 2004).

TREATMENT APPROACHES

The most useful treatment approach for children with intellectual disability consists of multimodal efforts directed at many aspects of the child's life—education, social, and recreational activities; behavior problems; and associated impairments (Harris, 2010; Shapiro & Batshaw, 2011). Support for parents, siblings, and other caregivers (both family members and unrelated caregivers) is also important (see Chapter 37).

Educational Services

Education is the single most important discipline involved in intervention for children with intellectual disability and their families (see Chapters 30 and 31). The achievement of good outcomes in an educational program is dependent on the interaction between the student and teacher. Educational programs must be relevant to the child's needs and address the child's individual strengths and challenges. The child's developmental level and his or her requirements for support and goals for independence provide a basis for establishing an individualized family service plan (IFSP) or an individualized education program (IEP).

It also needs to be remembered that children's learning begins in a family context that later is shared with the educational system. Education for infants and toddlers (early intervention, birth to 3 years) usually takes place in the home. Although home is also the primary

educational setting for 3–4 year olds, some of these children attend out-of-home center-based or preschool environments. At age 5, most children enter kindergarten for half- or full-day sessions and are introduced to a more formal learning environment. Formal special education services are provided in the school setting thereafter.

Leisure and Recreational Needs

In addition to education, the child's physical, social, and recreational needs should be addressed (Patel & Greydanus, 2010; van Naarden Braun, Yeargin-Allsopp, & Lollar, 2009; Verdonschot, de Witte, Reichrath, Buntinx & Curfs, 2009). Children's peer socialization in play and recreational activities constitutes an important part of their social-emotional development and builds resilience. As such, children's socialization competenci and experiences (e.g., dealing with social co flict, managing anger, making needs kno expressing affection or unhappiness) can ex significant influence upon their developm outcomes and school readiness and part tion, and it eventually also can influence dren's future success in adult life. In the world, children with intellectual disability w d participate as equals in all recreation and leisure activities. Although young children with intellectual disability are not usually excluded from play activities, parents still may have a difficult time finding age- and skill-appropriate adaptive play equipment (cost can be a significant factor) or socially oriented play groups (transportation costs and availability of inclusive programs are additional compromising factors). Furthermore, adolescents with an intellectual disability are often not included by their typically developing peers in extracurricular sports and social activities (Patel & Greydanus, 2010). Yet, participation in sports or related exercise regimens should be encouraged with all children (as functionally appropriate) because it offers many immediate and long-term benefits, including weight management, development of physical coordination, maintenance of cardiovascular fitness, and improvement of self-image (see Chapter 34). For some individuals, these needs can be met through the Special Olympics.

Social activities are equally important to the social and emotional development of youth with intellectual disabilities. Such activities should include those with adolescents of the opposite gender and with typically developing youth. These activities, however, need to be based on the youth's functionally adaptive age-appropriate behaviors. Examples of normalizing activities include participation in summer camps; school dances; school or family trips; dating or socialization in youth groups or school clubs; visits to movies, restaurants, and other socializing establishments; and other typical recreational events. These activities should also include opportunities for increasing social-emotional independence away from direct parental oversight. They should also involve exposure to novel experiences in which the individual has the opportunity to test, grapple with, and practice his or her overall adaptive competencies (see Chapter 40). While parental oversight may diminish during this period, sufficient supports are needed to ensure that the adolescent with intellectual disability is not targeted or bullied in these settings.

Behavior Therapy

Although most children with intellectual disability do not have behavior disorders, these problems do occur with a greater frequency in this population than among children with typical development (Allen, 2008). To facilitate the child's socialization and not limit academic opportunities, significant behavior problems must be addressed (Chapter 32). Behavior problems may result from organic problems (e.g., ADHD), primary or associated secondary psychiatric disorders (e.g., mood disorders), unrealistic parental expectations, and/or other family difficulties and school-related adjustment difficulties (Deutsch, Dube, & McIlvane, 2008). Often, behavior problems represent attempts by the child to communicate, gain attention, or avoid frustration. In assessing the problematic behavior, one must first consider whether the behavior is appropriate for the child's "cognitive" age rather than for his or her chronological age. The child's chronological age, however, needs to be considered in order to address the manifested behavior in the environmental context of the child's functioning. When intervention is needed, an environmental change, such as a more appropriate classroom environment, may improve behavior problems for some children. For other children, behavior management techniques (see Chapter 32) and/or the use of psychotropic medication may be appropriate.

Use of Medication

Medication is not useful in treating the core symptoms of intellectual disability; no drug has been found to improve cognitive function in these individuals. Medication may be helpful, however, in treating comorbid behavioral and emotional disorders (Risen, Accardo, & Shapiro, 2010). These drugs are generally directed at specific symptom complexes, including ADHD (e.g., stimulants, alpha-2-adrenergic agonists), self-injurious behavior or aggression (e.g., mood stabilizers, neuroleptics), and mood and/or obsessive-compulsive disorders (e.g., selective serotonin reuptake inhibitors). The properties of these psychopharmaceutical drugs are outlined in Appendix C. Before long-term therapy with any drug is initiated, a short trial should be conducted. Even if a medication proves successful, its use should be reevaluated at least yearly to assess the need for continued treatment.

Treating Comorbid Conditions

Comorbid conditions—for example, cerebral palsy; sensory impairments; seizure disorders; speech disorders; ADHD; autism spectrum disorders; and other disorders of language, behavior, or perception—must be treated to achieve an optimal outcome for the child with intellectual disability. This may require ongoing physical therapy, occupational therapy, speech-language therapy, behavioral therapy, adaptive equipment, eyeglasses, hearing aids, medication, and so forth. Failure to adequately identify and treat these problems may negatively influence functional outcomes and result in difficulties in the home, school, or neighborhood environment.

Family Counseling

All families benefit from anticipatory guidance regarding their child's health and development, but this is especially true for those families who have children with intellectual disability (Coren, Hutchfield, Tomae, & Gustafsson, 2010). Many families adapt well to having a child with intellectual disability, but some have significant problems. Among the factors that have been associated with family coping skills are the severity of the child's disability, number of siblings, stability of the parents' relationship, parental age, mental and physical health of the family, financial stability, expectations and acceptance of the child's diagnosis, supportiveness of the extended family, and availability of community resources and respite care services. In families in which the emotional demands of having a child with intellectual disability are great, family counseling should be an integral part of the treatment plan (see Chapter 37).

Periodic Reevaluation

The needs of children and their families change over time. As a result, children's health, learning, adaptive, and behavioral goals must be reassessed and developmentally based; furthermore, school-related programming needs to be adjusted. A periodic review should include information about the child's health status as well as his or her functioning at home, at school, and in other social contexts. Other information, such as formal **psychoeducational** testing, may be needed. Reevaluation should be undertaken at routine intervals, at any time the child is not meeting expectations, and when he or she is moving from one service provision system to another. Reevaluations are needed during early childhood and preschool years to ensure that the program remains appropriate as the child matures. Transition programs are especially necessary during adolescence to prepare for the move to adulthood (Neece, Kraemer, & Blacher, 2009; see Chapter 40).

OUTCOME

Save in individuals with severe–profound intellectual disability, IQ scores alone are not good predictors of outcome. Outcome for an individual with intellectual disability depends on the interplay of many factors including the underlying cause; the degree of functional disability; the presence of comorbid conditions and behavior problems; the capabilities of the family; and the supports, community services, and training provided to the child and family (Patel, Greydanus, Calles, & Pratt, 2010; Turnbull, Summers, Lee, & Kyzar, 2007). As adults, many people with mild intellectual disability are able to gain functional literacy and some economic and social independence and only require intermittent supports (Seltzer et al., 2009). Such adults may, however, need periodic assistance, especially when under social or economic stress. Some marry and live successfully in the community, either independently or in supervised settings (Aylward, 2002; Felce et al., 2008). Life expectancy usually is not adversely affected.

For individuals with moderate intellectual disability, the goals of education are to enhance adaptive abilities, functional academics, and vocational skills so that these individuals are better able to live in the adult world (Cummins, 2001; Totsika, Felce, Kerr, & Hastings, 2010). Contemporary gains including supported employment have benefited these individuals

the most. Supported employment challenges the view that prerequisite skills must be taught before there can be successful vocational adaptation. Instead, individuals are trained by a coach to do a specific job in the setting in which the person is to work. This approach bypasses the need for extended time mastering "prerequisite skills" and has resulted in successful work adaptation in the community for many people with intellectual disability. Outcome studies have documented the benefits and effectiveness of this approach (Stephens, Collins, & Dodder, 2005). People with intellectual disability requiring limited support (e.g., individuals with Down syndrome) generally live at home or in a supervised setting in the community.

As adults, people with intellectual disability requiring extensive to pervasive support (severe–profound intellectual disability) may perform simple tasks in supervised settings. These individuals, however, may have comorbid conditions such as cerebral palsy and sensory impairments that further limit their adaptive functioning. Yet most people with this level of intellectual disability are able to live in the community with supportive adaptations in their environment and with supervisory oversight (see Chapter 40). Family-based, community-supported care is preferable to institutional care for these individuals, but it is often difficult to achieve for a variety of reasons (e.g., parents' advanced ages, lack of financial support, familial or community resistance, comorbid conditions). As a result, some of these individuals with severe medical problems, behavioral disturbances, or disrupted families require out-of-home living in such settings as foster homes, alternative living units, group homes, nursing homes, or residential schools. People who require extensive or pervasive supports have increased utilization of medical and behavioral health care and often have a shortened life span (Katz, 2003; Kilgour, Starr, & Whalley, 2010).

SUMMARY

Development is an ordered process that is linked to the maturation of the central nervous system. With intellectual disability, development is altered so that intellectual and adaptive skills are impaired. In most cases of mild intellectual disability, the underlying cause is unclear and may be tied to environmental effects. In three quarters of individuals with severe intellectual disability, however, there is a definable biologic cause. Most people with intellectual disability have a mild degree, require only intermittent support, and are often able to achieve some economic and social independence. The early identification of a global developmental delay is important to ensure appropriate treatment and to enable the child to develop and use all of his or her capabilities. Treatment should be multi-modal, supporting the education, mental and physical health, adaptive behavior, and communication skills of individuals with intellectual disability.

REFERENCES

Acosta, M., Gallo, V., & Batshaw, M.L. (2002). Brain development and the ontogeny of developmental disabilities. *Advances in Pediatrics, 49*, 1–57.

Allen, D. (2008). The relationship between challenging behaviour and mental ill-health in people with intellectual disabilities: A review of current theories and evidence. *Journal of Intellectual Disabilities, 12*(4), 267–294.

American Academy of Pediatrics, Council on Children with Disabilities, Section on Developmental Behavioral Pediatrics; Bright Futures Steering Committee; and Medical Home Initiatives for Children with Special Needs Project Advisory Committee. (2006). Identifying infants and young children with developmental disorders in the medical home: An algorithm for developmental surveillance and screening. *Pediatrics 118*(1), 405–420. Erratum in *Pediatrics 118*(4), 1808–1809.

American Psychiatric Association. (2000). *Diagnostic and statistical manual of mental disorders* (4th ed., text rev.). Washington, DC: Author.

Anderson, P.J., & Doyle, L.W. (2008). Cognitive and educational deficits in children born extremely preterm. *Seminars in Perinatology, 32*(1), 51–58.

Aylward, G.P. (2002). Cognitive and neuropsychological outcomes: More than IQ scores. *Mental Retardation and Developmental Disability Research Reviews, 8*(4), 234–340.

Ayoub, C.C., O'Connor, E., Rappolt-Schlichtmann, G., Fischer, K.W., Rogosch, F.A., Toth, S.L., & Cicchetti, D. (2006). Cognitive and emotional differences in young maltreated children: A translational application of dynamic skill theory. *Developmental Psychopathology, 18*(3), 679–706.

Balogh, R., Ouellette-Kuntz, H., Bourne, L., Lunsky, Y., & Colantonio, A. (2008). Organising health care services for persons with an intellectual disability. *Cochrane Database of Systematic Reviews, 8*(4), CD007492.

Bandstra, E.S., Morrow, C.E., Mansoor, E., & Accornero, V.H. (2010). Prenatal drug exposure: Infant and toddler outcomes. *Journal of Addictive Disease, 29*(2), 245–258.

Barkovich, A.J., & Raybaud, C.A. (2004). Malformations of cortical development. *Neuroimaging Clinics of North America, 14*(3), 401–423.

Batshaw, M.L., Shapiro, B.K., & Farber, M.L.Z. (2007). Developmental delay and intellectual disability. In M.L. Batshaw, L. Pelligrino, N.J. Roizen (Eds.), *Children with Disabilities* (6th edition). Baltimore, MD: Paul H. Brookes Publishing Co.

Bayley, N. (2006). *Bayley Scales of Infant Development: Third edition manual*. San Antonio, TX: Harcourt Assessment.

Bear, L.M. (2004). Early identification of infants at risk for developmental disabilities. *Pediatric Clinics of North America, 51*(3), 685–701.

Beirne-Smith, M., Patton, J.M., & Kim, S.H. (2005). *Mental retardation: An introduction to intellectual disability* (7th ed). Upper Saddle River, NJ: Prentice Hall.

Bloom, A.S., & Zelko, F.A. (1994). Variability in adaptive behavior in children with developmental delay. *Journal of Clinical Psychology, 50*, 261–265.

Boyle, C.A., Boulet, S., Schieve, L.A., Cohen, R.A., Blumberg, S.J., Yeargin-Allsopp, M., ... Kogan, M.D. (2011). Trends in the prevalence of developmental disabilities in US children, 1997–2008. *Pediatrics, 127*(6), 1034–42.

Bricker, D., Squires, J., & Mounts, L., (1999). *Ages & Stages Questionnaires (ASQ): A Parent-Completed, Child-Monitoring System* (2nd ed.). Baltimore, MD: Paul H. Brookes Publishing Co.

Bruininks, R.H., Woodcock, R.W., Weatherman, R.F., & Hill, B.K. (1996). *Scales of Independent Behavior–Revised (SIB-R)*. Chicago, IL: Riverside Publishing.

Centers for Disease Control and Prevention. (1996). State-specific rates of mental retardation—United States, 1993. *Morbidity and Mortality Weekly Report, 45*(3), 61–65.

Chapman, D.A., Scott, K.G., & Stanton-Chapman, T.L. (2008). Public health approach to the study of mental retardation. *American Journal of Mental Retardation, 113*(2),102–16.

Cooper, S.A., & van der Speck, R. (2009). Epidemiology of mental ill health in adults with intellectual disabilities. *Current Opinion in Psychiatry, 22*(5), 431–436.

Coren, E., Hutchfield, J., Thomae, M., & Gustafsson, C. (2010). Parent training support for intellectually disabled parents. *Cochrane Database of Systematic Reviews, 16*(6), CD007987.

Cummins, R.A. (2001). Living with support in the community: Predictors of satisfaction with life. *Mental Retardation and Developmental Disabilities Research Reviews, 7*(2), 99–104.

Curry, C.J., Stevenson, R.E., Aughton, D., Byrne, J., Carey, J.C., Cassidy, S., ... Opitz, J. (1997). Evaluation of mental retardation: Recommendations of a consensus conference. American College of Medical Genetics. *American Journal of Medical Genetics, 72*, 468–477.

De Souza, E., Halliday, J., Chan, A., Bower, C., & Morris, J.K. (2009). Recurrence risks for trisomies 13, 18, and 21. *American Journal of Medical Genetics Part A, 149A*(12), 2716–2722.

Deutsch, C.K., Dube, W.V., & McIlvane, W.J. (2008). Attention deficits, attention-deficit/hyperactivity disorder, and intellectual disabilities. *Developmental Disabilities Research Reviews, 14*(4), 285–292.

Felce, D., Perry, J., Romeo, R., Robertson, J., Meek, A., Emerson, E., & Knapp, M. (2008). Outcomes and costs of community living: Semi-independent living and fully staffed group homes. *American Journal of Mental Retardation, 113*(2), 87–101.

Fletcher, R., Loschen, E., Stavrakaki, C., & First, M. (2007). *Diagnostic Manual-Intellectual disability (DM-ID): A clinical guide for diagnosis of mental disorders in persons with intellectual disability*. Kingston, NY: NADD Press.

Frederick, A.L., & Stanwood, G.D. (2009). Drugs, biogenic amine targets, and the developing brain. *Developmental Neuroscience, 31*(1–2), 7–22.

Gardner, H. (1983). *Frames of mind: The theory of multiple intelligences*. New York, NY: Basic Books.

Gifford, K.A., Holmes, M.G., & Bernstein, H.H. (2009). Hearing loss in children. *Pediatrics in Review*, *30*(6), 207–15.

Glascoe, F. (1997). Parents' concerns about children's development: Prescreening technique or screening test. *Pediatrics*, *99*, 522–528.

Gropman, A.L., & Batshaw, M.L. (2010). Epigenetics, copy number variation, and other molecular mechanisms underlying neurodevelopmental disabilities: New insights and diagnostic approaches. *Journal of Developmental and Behavioral Pediatrics*, *31*(7), 582–591.

Harris, J.C. (2010). *Intellectual disability: A guide for families and professionals*. Oxford, UK: Oxford University Press.

Harrison, P.L., & Oakland, T. (2003). *Adaptive Behavior Assessment System-II*. San Antonio, TX: Pearson.

Heikura, U., Linna, S.L., Olsén, P., Hartikainen, A.L., Taanila, A., & Järvelin, M.R. (2005). Etiological survey on intellectual disability in the northern Finland birth cohort 1986. *American Journal of Mental Retardation*, *110*(3), 171–180.

Heikura, U., Taanila, A., Olsen, P., Hartikainen, A.L., von Wendt, L., & Järvelin, M.R. (2003). Temporal changes in incidence and prevalence of intellectual disability between two birth cohorts in Northern Finland. *American Journal of Mental Retardation*, *108*(1), 19–31.

Hibbard, R.A., Desch, L.W., American Academy of Pediatrics Committee on Child Abuse and Neglect, & American Academy of Pediatrics Council on Children With Disabilities. (2007). Maltreatment of children with disabilities. *Pediatrics*, *119*(5), 1018–1025.

Huston, A.C., & Bentley, A.C. (2010). Human development in societal context. *Annual Review of Psychology*, *61*, 411–37. C1.

Individuals with Disabilities Education Improvement Act (IDEA) of 2004, PL 108–446, 20 U.S.C. §§ 1400 *et seq.*

Jacquemont, S., Farzin, F., Hall, D., Leehey, M., Tassone, F., Gane., & ...Hagerman, R.J. (2004). Aging in individuals with the FMR1 mutation. *American Journal on Mental Retardation*, *109*(2), 154–164.

Jansen, D.E., Krol, B., Groothoff, J.W., & Post, D. (2004). People with intellectual disability and their health problems: A review of comparative studies. *Journal of Intellectual Disability Research*, *48*(2), 93–102.

Katz, R.T. (2003). Life expectancy for children with cerebral palsy and mental retardation: Implications for life care planning. *NeuroRehabilitation*, *18*(3), 261–270.

Kerr, M.P., Turky, A., & Huber, B. (2009). The psychosocial impact of epilepsy in adults with an intellectual disability. *Epilepsy & Behavior*, *15*(Suppl. 1), S26–S30.

Kilgour, A.H., Starr, J.M., & Whalley, L.J. (2010). Associations between childhood intelligence (IQ), adult morbidity and mortality. *Maturitas*, *65*(2), 98–105.

King, T.M., Tandon, S.D., Macias, M.M., Healy, J.A., Duncan, P.M., Swigonski, N.L., ... Lipkin, P.H. (2010). Implementing developmental screening and referrals: Lessons learned from a national project. *Pediatrics*, *125*(2), 350–360.

Kodituwakku, P.W. (2009). Neurocognitive profile in children with fetal alcohol spectrum disorders. *Developmental Disabilities Research Reviews*, *15*(3), 218–224.

Koenen, K.C., Moffitt, T.E., Caspi, A., Taylor, A., & Purcell, S. (2003). Domestic violence is associated with environmental suppression of IQ in young children. *Development and Psychopathology*, *15*(2), 297–311.

Leonard, H., & Wen, X. (2002). The epidemiology of mental retardation: Challenges and opportunities in the new millennium. *Mental Retardation and Developmental Disabilities Research Reviews*, *8*(3), 117–134.

Maulik, P.K., Mascarenhas, M.N., Mathers, C.D., Dua, T., & Saxena, S. (2011). Prevalence of intellectual disability: A meta-analysis of population-based studies. *Research in Developmental Disabilities*, *32*(2), 419–436.

McLaren, J., & Bryson, S.E. (1987). Review of recent epidemiological studies of mental retardation: Prevalence, associated disorders, and etiology. *American Journal of Mental Retardation*, *92*(3), 243–354.

Mendola, P., Selevan, S.G., Gutter, S., & Rice, D. (2002). Environmental factors associated with a spectrum of neurodevelopmental deficits. *Mental Retardation and Developmental Disabilities Research Reviews*, *8*(3), 188–197.

Miller, D.T., Adam, M.P., Aradhya, S., Biesecker, L.G., Brothman, A.R., Carter, N.P., ... Ledbetter, D.H. (2010). Consensus statement: Chromosomal microarray is a first-tier clinical diagnostic test for individuals with developmental disabilities or congenital anomalies. *American Journal of Medical Genetics*, *85*(5), 749–764.

Michelson, D.J., Shevell, M.I., Sherr, E.H., Moeschler, J.B., Gropman, A.L., & Ashwal, S. (2011). Evidence report: Genetic and metabolic testing on children with global developmental delay: Report of the Quality Standards Subcommittee of the American Academy of Neurology and the Practice Committee of the Child Neurology Society. *Neurology*, *77*, 1629–1635.

Moeschler, J.B., Shevell, M., & the Committee on Genetics. (2006). Clinical genetic evaluation of the child with mental retardation or developmental delays. *Pediatrics*, *117*, 2304–2316.

Moser, H.W. (1995). A role for gene therapy in mental retardation. *Mental Retardation and Developmental Disabilities Research Reviews*, *1*, 4–6.

Msall, M.E. (2005). Measuring functional skills in preschool children at risk for neurodevelopmental disabilities. *Mental Retardation and Developmental Disability Research Reviews*, *11*(3), 263–273.

Neece, C.L., Kraemer, B.R., & Blacher, J. (2009). Transition satisfaction and family well being among parents of young adults with severe intellectual disability. *Intellectual and Developmental Disabilities*, *47*(1), 31–43.

Noble, K.G., Tottenham, N., & Casey, B.J. (2005). Neuroscience perspectives on disparities in school readiness and cognitive achievement. In C. Rouse, J. Books-Gunn, & S. McLanahan (Eds.), *The future of the children: School readiness*, *15*(1), 71–89.

Oeseburg, B., Dijkstra, G.J., Groothoff, J.W., Reijneveld, S.A., & Jansen, D.E. (2011). Prevalence of chronic health conditions in children with intellectual disability: A systematic literature review. *Intellectual and Developmental Disabilities*, *49*(2), 59–85.

Oliver, C., & Richards, C. (2010). Self-injurious behaviour in people with intellectual disability. *Current Opinion in Psychiatry*, *23*(5), 412–416.

Patel, D.R., & Greydanus, D.E. (2010). Sport participation by physically and cognitively challenged young athletes. *Pediatric Clinics of North America*, *57*(3), 795–817.

Patel, D.R., Greydanus, D.E., Calles, J.L. Jr., & Pratt, H.D. (2010). Developmental disabilities across the lifespan. *Disease-a-Month*, *56*(6), 304–397.

Qiao, Y., Harvard, C., Tyson, C., Liu, X., Fawcett, C., Pavlidis, P., ... Rajcan-Separovic, E. (2010). Outcome of array CGH analysis for 255 subjects with intellectual disability and search for candidate genes using bioinformatics. *Human Genetics, 128*(2), 179–194.

Riou, E.M., Ghosh, S., Francoeur, E., & Shevell, M.I. (2009). Global developmental delay and its relationship to cognitive skills. *Developmental Medicine and Child Neurology, 5*(8), 600–606.

Risen, S., Accardo, P.J., & Shapiro, B.K., (2010). A clinical approach to the pharmacological management of behavioral disturbance in intellectual disability. In B.K. Shapiro & P.J. Accardo (Eds.), *Neurogenetic syndromes: Behavioral issues and their treatment.* Baltimore: Paul H. Brookes Publishing Co.

Roid, G. (2003). *Stanford-Binet Intelligence Scales, Fifth Edition (SB5).* Chicago, IL: Riverside Publishing.

Ropers, H.H. (2008). Genetics of intellectual disability. *Current Opinion in Genetics and Development, 18*(3), 241–50.

Rydz, D., Shevell, M.I., Majnemer, A., & Oskoui, M. (2005). Developmental screening. *Journal of Child Neurology, 20*(1), 4–21.

Schalock, R., Borthwick-Duffy, S.A., Buntinx, W.H.E., Coulter, D.L., & Ellis, M.C. (2009). *Intellectual disability: Definition, classification, and systems of support (11th Edition).* Washington, DC: American Association on Intellectual and Developmental Disabilities.

Seltzer, M.M., Floyd, F.J., Greenberg, J.S., Hong, J., Taylor, J.L., & Doescher, H. (2009). Factors predictive of midlife occupational attainment and psychological functioning in adults with mild intellectual deficits. *American Journal of Intellectual and Developmental Disability, 114*(2), 128–143.

Shapiro, B.K. (2011). Reflections on early identification. In Eidelman, S. (Vol. Ed.). Contemporary policy and practices landscape. In C. J. Groark (Series Ed.), *Early childhood intervention: Shaping the future for children with special needs and their families, three volumes: Vol. 1.* Santa Barbara, CA: ABC-CLIO, Praeger.

Shapiro, B.K., & Batshaw, M.L. (2011). Intellectual disability. In R.M. Kliegman, B.M.D. Stanton, J.W. St. Geme, N.F. Schor, R.E. Behrman (Eds.), *Nelson's textbook of pediatrics* (19th ed., pp. 122–129). Philadelphia, PA: Saunders Elsevier.

Shevell. M., Ashwal, S., Donley, D., Flint, J., Gingold, M., Hirtz, D., ... Quality Standards Subcommittee of the American Academy of Neurology, & Practice Committee of the Child Neurology Society. (2003). Practice parameter: Evaluation of the child with global developmental delay: Report of the quality standards subcommittee of the american academy of neurology and the practice committee of the child neurology society. *Neurology, 60,* 367–380.

Sparrow, S.S., Bella, D.A., & Crichetti, D.V. (2005). *Vineland Adaptive Behavior Scales, Second Edition (Vineland-II).* Circle Pines, MN: AGS.

Squier, W., & Jansen, A. (2010). Abnormal development of the human cerebral cortex. *Journal of Anatomy, 217*(4), 312–323. doi: 10.1111/j.1469-7580 .2010.01288.x

Stephens, D.L., Collins, M.D., & Dodder, R.A. (2005). A longitudinal study of employment and skill acquisition among individuals with developmental disabilities. *Research in Developmental Disabilities, 26*(5), 469–486.

Strømme, P., & Hagberg, G. (2000). Aetiology in severe and mild mental retardation: A population-based study of Norwegian children. *Developmental Medicine and Child Neurology, 42,* 76–86.

Totsika, V., Felce, D., Kerr, M., & Hastings, R.P. (2010). Behavior problems, psychiatric symptoms, and quality of life for older adults with intellectual disability with and without autism. *Journal of Autism and Developmental Disorders, 40*(10), 1171–1178.

Tronick, E., & Reck, C. (2009). Infants of depressed mothers. *Harvard Review of Psychiatry, 17*(2), 147–156.

Turnbull, A.P., Summers, J.A., Lee, S.H., & Kyzar, K. (2007). Conceptualization and measurement of family outcomes associated with families of individuals with intellectual disabilities. *Mental Retardation and Developmental Disability Research Reviews, 13*(4), 346–356.

Van Naarden Braun, K., Autry, A., & Boyle, C. (2005). A population-based study of the recurrence of developmental disabilities—Metropolitan Atlanta Developmental Disabilities Surveillance Program, 1991–1994. *Paediatric and Perinatal Epidemiology, 19*(1), 69–79.

Van Naarden Braun, K., Yeargin-Allsopp, M., & Lollar, D. (2009). Activity limitations among young adults with developmental disabilities: A population-based follow-up study. *Research in Developmental Disabilities, 30*(1), 179–191.

Verdonschot, M.M., de Witte, L.P., Reichrath, E., Buntinx, W.H., & Curfs, L.M. (2009). Community participation of people with an intellectual disability: A review of empirical findings. *Journal of Intellectual Disability Research, 53*(4), 303–318.

Wang, P.P., & Bellugi, U. (1993). Williams syndrome, Down syndrome, and cognitive neuroscience. *American Journal of Diseases of Childhood, 147,* 1246–1251.

Wechsler, D. (2002). *Wechsler Preschool and Primary Scale of Intelligence–Third Edition (WPPSI-III).* San Antonio, TX: Harcourt Assessment.

Wechsler, D. (2003). *Wechsler Intelligence Scale for Children–Fourth Edition (WISC-IV).* San Antonio, TX: Harcourt Assessment.

Weindling, M. (2010). Insights into early brain development from modern brain imaging and outcome studies. *Acta Paediatrica, 99*(7), 961–966.

Yeargin-Allsopp, M., Murphy, C.C., Cordero, J.F., Decouflé, P., & Hollowell, J.G. (1997). Reported biomedical causes and associated medical conditions for mental retardation among 10-year-old children, metropolitan Atlanta, 1985 to 1987. *Developmental Medicine & Child Neurology, 39,* 142–149.

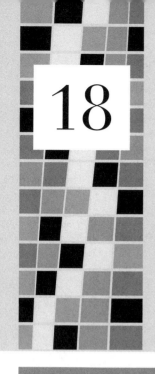

18

Down Syndrome (Trisomy 21)

Nancy J. Roizen

Upon completion of this chapter, the reader will

■ Recognize the physical characteristics of Down syndrome

■ Understand the medical complications of this disorder

■ Know the typical cognitive, developmental, and behavioral characteristics of a child with Down syndrome

■ Have knowledge regarding educational and other types of interventions

Down syndrome was one of the first symptom complexes associated with intellectual disability to be identified as a syndrome. In fact, evidence of this syndrome dates back to ancient times. Archaeological excavations have revealed a skull from the 7th century A.D. that displays the physical features of an individual with Down syndrome. Portrait paintings from the 1500s depict children with a Down syndrome–like facial appearance. In 1866, Dr. John Langdon Down, for whom the syndrome is named, published the first complete physical description of Down syndrome, including the similarity of facial features among affected individuals. In 1959, researchers identified the underlying chromosomal abnormality (an additional chromosome 21) that causes Down syndrome (Lejeune, Gautier, & Turpin, 1959).

■ ■ ■ JASON AND CHRIS

In many ways, Jason is like the typically developing 8-year-olds in the neighborhood. He plays soccer, skates, swims, participates in Boy Scouts, and is in the second grade. Jason has a great sense of humor and is a bit mischievous. His mother makes every effort to provide him with a balance of social and academic opportunities. But in some ways, Jason's experience is unique. He has Down syndrome, a unilateral hearing loss, moderate intellectual disability, and attention-deficit/hyperactivity disorder (ADHD). His reading skills are at a kindergarten level. At the local Down syndrome family support group, Jason's mother is inspired by Chris, who also has Down syndrome and has done well. Chris, who is 30 years old, graduated from high school with an equivalency certificate, lives at home, and takes public transportation to the office where he has worked for the last 9 years.

PREVALENCE

From 1979 to 2003, the prevalence of Down syndrome births increased from 9.0 to 11.8 per 10,000 births in the United States (Shin et al.,

2009). Increasing maternal age has been consistently linked to an increased chance of having a child with Down syndrome. At 20 years of age, women have about a 1 in 1,600 chance of having a child with trisomy 21; at 45 years of age, the likelihood increases to 1 in 50 (Wald & Leck, 2000). There is no increased risk of translocation Down syndrome (defined in the following section) with increased maternal age. However, one third of individuals with translocation Down syndrome inherit the translocation from a typically unaffected parent who is a carrier but has only one copy of the genetic material of chromosome 21 (Bull & the American Academy of Pediatrics Committee on Genetics, 2011; Jones, 2006). Chromosome analysis can identify parents who are at risk of having children with translocation Down syndrome.

CHROMOSOMAL FINDINGS

Three types of chromosomal abnormalities result in extra copies of the Down syndrome area of chromosome 21 and can lead to Down syndrome: trisomy 21 (which accounts for about 95% of individuals with the disorder), translocation (4%–5%), and mosaicism (1%–2%; Bull & the American Academy of Pediatrics Committee on Genetics, 2011; Jones, 2006). Trisomy 21 results from nondisjunction, most commonly during meiosis I of the egg (see Chapter 1, Figure 1.3). Translocation Down syndrome involves the attachment of the long arm of an extra chromosome 21 to chromosome 14, 21, or 22 (see Chapter 1, Figure 1.5). Mosaic trisomy implies that some, but not all cells, have the defect. This results from nondisjunction during mitosis of the fertilized egg.

Studies indicate that children with translocation Down syndrome do not differ cognitively or medically from those with trisomy 21. Children with mosaic Down syndrome, perhaps because their trisomic cells are interspersed with normal cells, typically score higher on IQ tests than those with trisomy 21 or translocation Down syndrome (Fishler & Koch, 1991; see Chapter 1). Medical complications tend to be similar among the three groups (McClain et al., 1996).

EFFECTS OF TRISOMY 21

Down syndrome results from an extra copy of the long arm of human chromosome 21 (HSA21q), which results in increased expression of the genes on HSA21q, due to having 3 copies of those genes instead of 2 copies. The complete genomic sequence of HSA21q was completed in 2000 (Hattori et al., 2000) and a recent review identified more than 500 genes on HSA21q which belong to a wide variety of functional classes (Gardiner, 2009). Magnetic resonance imaging (MRI) studies of individuals with an extra copy of HSA21q reveal reduced overall brain volume with smaller frontal and temporal areas, cerebellum, and notably the hippocampus, which is critical for long-term storage of memory. Alterations of these different regions of the brain likely have a convergent impact on learning (Lott & Dierssen, 2010). On the cellular level, neuropathologic abnormalities include fewer neurons, decreased neuronal density, and abnormal neuronal distribution. After 6 months of age, dendritic branching decreases steadily, becoming significantly subnormal after 2 years of age. This may result in a reduced connected neuronal network that limits information processing and decreases synaptic plasticity (Lott & Dierssen, 2010). The impairment of connectivity of the fronto-cerebellar structures, which are involved in articulation and verbal working memory, may be related to the lower performance of individuals with Down syndrome in both linguistic and visual-spatial tasks. The hippocampal dysfunction may be a cause of reduced long-term memory skills (Lott &Dierssen, 2010).

EARLY IDENTIFICATION

The American College of Obstetricians and Gynecologists recommend that, regardless of age, all pregnant women should be offered screening and diagnostic testing for Down syndrome. First trimester screening incorporates maternal age, nuchal (neck) translucency, ultrasonography, and maternal blood tests and has a detection rate of 82%–87%. Second trimester screening, which is often called the "quad screen" and includes measurement of four elements in the maternal serum, has a detection rate of 80%. Integrated screening that includes a combination of first and second trimester screening has a detection rate of 95% (Bull & the American Academy of Pediatrics Committee on Genetics, 2011; see Chapter 5). If Down syndrome is identified and the pregnancy is continued, the parents can be provided with counseling regarding the disorder and planning for appropriate medical evaluation of the newborn infant.

Because of the distinctive pattern of physical features, infants with Down syndrome can be identified fairly easily. Common characteristics at birth include the distinctive facial appearance, Brushfield spots (colored speckles in the iris of the eye), short ear length, increased neck skinfold, congenital heart disease, and widely spaced first toes (Rex & Preus, 1982). Individuals with other syndromes, however, may bear a physical resemblance to individuals with Down syndrome in the newborn period (Jones, 2006). Therefore, all children suspected of having Down syndrome should have a chromosomal analysis performed to ensure correct diagnosis and to allow for the provision of accurate genetic counseling about future pregnancies.

MEDICAL COMPLICATIONS IN DOWN SYNDROME

Children with Down syndrome have an increased risk of abnormalities in almost every organ system (Roizen & Patterson, 2003; van Trotsenburg, Heyman, Tijssen, de Vijlder, & Vulsma, 2006). Knowledge of these possible medical complications enables the health care provider to evaluate the child for the more common conditions and to monitor, prevent, and be vigilant for other medical problems.

Congenital Heart Defects

In a population-based study of infants with Down syndrome, 44% had congenital heart defects, the most common being **ventricular septal defect** (a connection between the two lower chambers; 43%), followed by **atrial septal defect** (a connection between the two upper chambers; 42%), and **endocardial cushion defect** (resulting in connection between the atria and ventricles; 39%; Freeman et al., 2008). A major complication of congenital heart disease is **pulmonary vascular obstructive disease**. This leads to increased back pressure in the arteries that connect the heart to the lungs and results in congestive heart failure. Progression of this potentially fatal complication is more rapid in children with Down syndrome than in children with the same heart defects and normal chromosomes (Suzuki et al., 2000).

Sensory Impairments

Vision and hearing problems occur with an increased frequency in children with Down syndrome. Deficits in visual acuity occur in 30%–62% of Down syndrome cases, with **amblyopia** ("lazy eye") occurring in 3%–20% of Down syndrome cases. Disorders of eye movement such as **strabismus** (crossed eyes; 20%–60%) and **nystagmus** (jiggling of the eyes; 10%–20%), as well as **blepharitis** (inflammation of the eyelids), tear duct obstruction, **cataracts**, and **ptosis** (droopy eyelids) are also found more commonly among people with Down syndrome than in the general population (Creavin & Brown, 2009). In children with no ophthalmic abnormalities observed during pediatric checkups, 35% are subsequently found to have an identifiable disorder when examined by an ophthalmologist (Roizen, Mets, & Blondis, 1994; see Chapter 11).

Hearing loss occurs in as many as two thirds of children with Down syndrome. It can be **conductive** (middle ear conduction of sound), **sensorineural** (involving the cochlea or auditory nerve), or combined; in addition, it can be unilateral or bilateral (see Chapter 10). Conductive hearing problems develop as a result of recurrent **otitis media** (middle ear infections) related to narrowed ear and throat passages and immune variation (Shott, 2006). Chapman, Seung, Schwartz, and Bird (1998) estimated that 10% of the language impairment in children with Down syndrome is attributable to hearing losses.

Endocrine Abnormalities

Congenital **hypothyroidism** resulting from impaired development of the thyroid gland is found in 0.8%–1.8% of newborns with Down syndrome, a rate 28–54 times that seen in the general population (Fort et al., 1984; Tuysuz & Beker, 2001). In addition, beyond the neonatal period, 25%–40% of children with Down syndrome manifest compensated hypothyroidism, in which there is an elevated level of thyroid stimulating hormone (TSH) but normal thyroid hormone levels (Rubello et al., 1995). In one study of 1257 children on Medicaid with Down syndrome, 11% of children between 1 and 18 years of age were treated with thyroid hormone replacement (thryoxine), most commonly before 3 years of age and between 12 and 18 years of age (Carroll et al., 2008). In addition, type 1 (juvenile) diabetes occurs at a rate that is 4.2 times that found in the general population of children (Bergholdt, Eising, Nerup, & Pociot, 2006).

Growth and Obesity Problems

Children with Down syndrome are at great risk for becoming overweight. A major factor in the development of obesity among children with Down syndrome is the presence of a lower resting metabolic rate, which results in requiring fewer calories to gain weight (Bauer et al.,

2003). In general, newborns with Down syndrome have proportional weight for height; in the first year of life, they tend to become light for their height. During the next few years, however, the children gain relatively more weight than height, and by early childhood, half are overweight. In addition to being overweight, individuals with Down syndrome have short stature. The average adult height is 5 feet in males and 4½ feet in females with the syndrome (Toledo et al., 1999).

Orthopedic Problems

Children with Down syndrome have an increased prevalence of orthopedic problems that are probably related to abnormally loose ligaments. These problems include **atlantoaxial subluxation** (partial dislocation of the upper spine; Figure 18.1); **patellar** (knee cap) instability; and pes planus (flat feet). These children also can develop juvenile **idiopathic arthritis**, which is associated with joint subluxation in half of the cases and is usually diagnosed about 2 years after symptoms develop (Juj & Emery, 2009).

Atlantoaxial subluxation is the most controversial and perplexing of these problems, occurring in approximately 15% of children with Down syndrome (Cohen, 2006). This condition involves the partial displacement of the upper vertebra as measured by x ray, and potentially can lead to spinal nerve entrapment. An easy, accurate, and cost-effective way to screen for subluxation has not been identified. Fortunately, only 2% of children with atlantoaxial subluxation develop symptoms of spinal cord compression, and it rarely leads to paralysis (Cohen, 2006). Symptoms of subluxation can include the following: easy fatigability, difficulties in walking, abnormal gait, neck pain, limited neck mobility, **torticollis** (painful head tilt), a change in hand function, the new onset of urinary retention or incontinence, incoordination and clumsiness, sensory impairments, and spasticity (Cohen, 2006).

Dental Problems

The most serious dental problem common among children with Down syndrome is early-onset **periodontal disease** (disease of tissue

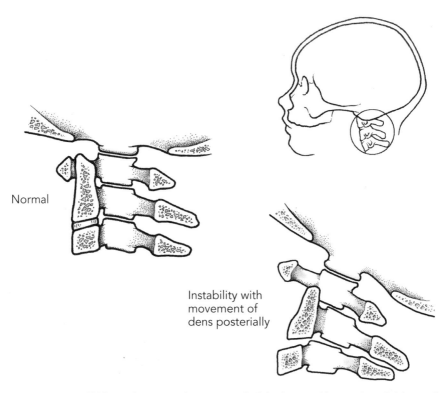

Figure 18.1.   Children with Down syndrome are at risk of developing subluxation (partial dislocation) of the atlantoaxial or atlanto-occipital joint, as shown in this illustration (right side). A typical neck region is shown for comparison (left side). This subluxation predisposes these children to spinal injury with trauma. This abnormality can be detected by x ray or magnetic resonance imaging scan of the neck.

surrounding the teeth) that can rapidly progress (Hennequin, Faulks, Veyrune, & Bourdiol, 1999). This involves both gingivitis (gum inflammation) and regression of the bone that anchors the teeth (see Chapter 35). Periodontal disease is common, probably as part of a manifestation of the immune variations in children with Down syndrome. In addition to having periodontal disease, almost all children with Down syndrome have **malocclusions** (abnormal contact of opposing teeth), and many have dental anomalies (e.g., fused teeth, microdontia [small teeth], missing teeth). In addition, **primary** and permanent teeth erupt later than usual. Interestingly, dental cavities occur less often in children with Down syndrome than in the general population; the reason for this is unclear but is probably related to differences in immunity and tooth shape.

Gastrointestinal, Renal, and Urinary Tract Anomalies and Problems

Gastrointestinal malformations are found in approximately 6.7% of children with Down syndrome. Most of these abnormalities present with symptoms in the newborn period such as poor feeding, vomiting, or aspiration pneumonia. The malformations include **stenosis** (narrowing) or **atresia** (blockage) of the duodenum (the first section of the small intestine; 3.9%), **imperforate** (closed) anus (1.0%), **Hirschsprung disease** (congenitally enlarged colon; 0.8%), tracheoesophageal fistula (an abnormal connection between the trachea and esophagus) or **esophageal atresia** (0.4%), and pyloric stenosis (narrowing of the stomach outlet; 0.3%; Freeman et al., 2009). **Gastroesophageal reflux disease** (GERD; acid reflux) also is known to be common among children with Down syndrome. **Celiac disease** (sensitivity to wheat and other grains) has been found in 1%–7% of children with Down syndrome (Bull & the American Academy of Pediatrics Committee on Genetics, 2011; Cohen, 2006). Children with Down syndrome are also at an increased risk for renal and urinary tract anomalies (3.2%) compared with the general population (0.7%; Kupferman, Druschel, & Kupchik, 2009).

Epilepsy

Epilepsy occurs in 6% of individuals with Down syndrome (Johannsen, Christensen, Goldstein, Nielsen, & Mai, 1996). This is more common than in the general population but about average for children with moderate intellectual disability. Seizure types include generalized tonic-clonic (55% of all seizures in children with Down syndrome), infantile spasms (13%), myoclonic (6%), atonic plus tonic-clonic (6%), and simple partial (6%; see Chapter 27). Seizures are diagnosed most commonly in individuals younger than 3 years and older than 13 years of age. 62% of the seizures have an identifiable cause, the most common being infections and hypoxia (resulting from congenital heart disease). Children with Down syndrome who have infantile spasms have a better outcome than children with infantile spasms who do not have Down syndrome (Goldberg-Stern et al., 2001; Stafstrom & Konkol, 1994).

Hematologic Disorders

Leukemias are the most common malignancy in individuals with Down syndrome and account for 97% of the malignancies in children with Down syndrome under 15 years of age. Individuals with Down syndrome have a 10- to 20-fold higher relative risk than the general population, with a cumulative risk of 2% by 5 years of age and 2.7% by 30 years of age (Rabin & Whitlock, 2009). Children with Down syndrome experience three types of leukemia, and, as in the typically developing population of children, the most common type is acute lymphoblastic leukemia (ALL). Newborns with Down syndrome have a 3%–10% chance of having elevated numbers of white blood cells (transient myeloproliferative disease [TMD]; Pine et al., 2007; Rabin & Whitlock, 2009). Of children with TMD, 10%–20% will subsequently develop acute megakaryocytic leukemia (AMKL; Ahmed et al., 2004). AMKL is associated with a mutation in the gene that encodes for GATA-1, which is required for the development of young platelets (Ahmed et al., 2004; Malinge, Izraeli, & Crispino, 2009).

Children with Down syndrome have low dietary intake of iron (Luke, Sutton, Schoeller, & Roizen, 1996), and iron deficiency or iron deficiency anemia are found in 10% of this population (Dixon et al., 2010).

Skin Conditions

Several skin conditions, mostly of immune origin, are observed more frequently in individuals with Down syndrome than in the general population. Some of these conditions noticeably affect the appearance and therefore the quality of life of children with Down syndrome, therefore requiring treatment. By puberty, half or more of these individuals will experience

eczema (atopic dermatitis), **cheilitis** (inflammation of the lips), **ichthyosis** (dry and scaly skin), **onychomycosis** (fungal infection of the nails), **seborrheic dermatitis** (dandruff), **vitiligo** (patches of depigmentation), and/or **xerosis** (dryness of eyes; Ercis, Balci, & Atakan, 1996). Less common skin diseases found among children with Down syndrome are **syringomas** (sweat gland cysts) and **alopecia** (hair loss).

NEURODEVELOPMENT AND BEHAVIOR

Infants with Down syndrome typically have central hypotonia (floppiness without weakness) and delayed, though typically sequenced, gross-motor development (Lott & Dierssen, 2010). Most children with Down syndrome do not sit up until 11 months of age or walk until 19 months of age (Winders, 1997). Boys with Down syndrome generally reach developmental milestones slightly later than girls with the syndrome. By school age, children with Down syndrome learn to run, ride bicycles, and participate in sports.

Children with Down syndrome often do not speak their first word until 18 months of age. By 2 years of age, significant language delays have become evident (Kumin, 2001). Their receptive language is generally better than their expressive language. One frequently used method of bridging the gap between receptive and expressive language is to teach children with Down syndrome sign language. Even after children with Down syndrome learn to speak in sentences, problems with intelligibility interfere with effective communication; in fact, speech therapy that addresses the development of expressive speech and intelligibility is often needed for many years (Chapman, Schwartz, & Kay-Raining Bird, 1991; Chapman et al., 1998; Kumin, 2001; Miller, Leddy, & Leavitt, 1999). Intellectual testing reveals standard scores of 80 at 6 months of age; however this score steadily decreases and is 45 at 4 years of age (Carr, 1988). These children generally have relative weakness in expressive language, syntactics, and verbal working memory (Silverman, 2007). This cognitive pattern is consistent with the macro and micro brain morphology described earlier.

Children with Down syndrome are stereotyped as being amiable and happy. Temperament studies, however, have shown them to have profiles comparable to typically developing children (Chapman & Husketh, 2000). Compared with the general population, individuals with Down syndrome are at increased risk for experiencing behavioral, emotional, and psychiatric problems (18%–23%) but compared with other children with intellectual disabilities, children with Down syndrome are at decreased risk (30%–40%). Children and youth with Down syndrome have been found to have low levels of extreme aggression (e.g., 6% fighting) but high rates of provocative behaviors and low-level aggressive behaviors (e.g., 73% disobedient, 65% argumentative, 50% demanding attention). In addition, 6%–8% of children with Down syndrome are diagnosed with ADHD, like Jason in our case study. About 10% of children with Down syndrome fall on the autism spectrum (Dykens, 2007). About half of the children with Down syndrome who have an autism spectrum disorder (ASD) experience a late regression, with loss of language around 5 years of age (Castillo et al., 2008). Studies have also reported a delay in the diagnosis of ASDs among children who have Down syndrome compared with the general population of children (Rasmussen, Borjesson, Wentz, & Gillberg, 2001).

Some individuals with Down syndrome may experience a deterioration of cognitive or psychological functioning in adolescence, often manifested as worsening of behavior or academic performance. Many times, this deterioration can be attributed to unrecognized hypothyroidism or depression. If such diagnoses are confirmed, medical and psychiatric treatment can reverse these problems. When an etiology and related intervention are not found, this phenomenon is sometimes referred to as childhood disintegrative disorder (Prasher, 2002). It appears, however, that virtually all individuals with Down syndrome have the characteristic neuropathology of Alzheimer's disease by 45 years of age. They have an increased concentration of brain amyloid, which is associated with neurofibrillary tangles. A number of genes on chromosome 21 have been implicated in Alzheimer's disease. Despite the Alzheimer neuropathology, clinical signs of dementia do not occur in all adults with Down syndrome. It should be noted, however, that 75% of individuals with Down syndrome who live beyond 65 years of age meet the criteria for dementia (Lott & Dierssen, 2010).

EVALUATION AND TREATMENT

Several of the medical conditions discussed above occur with sufficient frequency that an organized approach to medical management is indicated. Some conditions require routine monitoring: congenital heart disease, hearing loss, vision deficits, thyroid disorders, and celiac disease. Gum disease and obesity are to be prevented. And vigilance must be maintained for disorders that occur more frequently in children with Down syndrome than in the general population, such as diabetes, seizures, arthritis, and leukemia. The American Academy of Pediatrics (Bull & the American Academy of Pediatrics Committee on Genetics, 2011) has developed guidelines for medical management of individuals with Down syndrome (Figure 18.2). Several other reports have focused on providing medical care to children with Down syndrome in specific age groups, including infants and young children (Saenz, 1999), adolescents (Roizen, 2002), and adults (Smith, 2001).

Congenital heart disease in children with Down syndrome may be difficult to identify based on physical findings alone because it is not always accompanied by a cardiac murmur, nor does it commonly produce a "blue baby." However, because children with Down syndrome tend to develop pulmonary vascular disease sooner than other children with the same defect, early identification and treatment are essential. Although children with Down syndrome were once considered poor risks for cardiac surgery, data now indicate that they have a similar mortality as other children with the same heart defect (Fudge et al., 2010), but they have more postoperative complications. An echocardiogram is recommended for the newborn with Down syndrome, even if there has been a prior fetal echocardiogram (Bull & the American Academy of Pediatrics Committee on Genetics, 2011).

Within the first 6 months of life, a pediatric ophthalmologist should evaluate newborns with Down syndrome for cataracts, strabismus, and nystagmus (see Chapter 11). Subsequently, these children should be evaluated yearly from 1–5 years of age; every 2 years from 5–13 years of age; and every 3 years from 13–21 years of age (Bull & the American Academy of Pediatrics Committee on Genetics, 2011) to detect refractive errors and other ophthalmic disorders that may develop after the first decade of life (Creavin & Brown, 2009).

Infants with Down syndrome who have an abnormal newborn hearing screen will need a hearing evaluation by 3 months of age. If they have a hearing loss, by 6 months of age they will need hearing aids and additional early intervention services that address the hearing loss. Not all losses are present at birth; children with Down syndrome are at increased risk for recurrent middle-ear infections leading to conductive hearing losses and possibly even sensorineural hearing losses (Shott, 2006). Therefore, the child with Down syndrome should have an ear cleaning, a check for middle ear fluid, and a hearing evaluation every 6 months from birth to 5 years of age and then annually from 5–21 years of age (Cohen, 1999; Shott, 2006).

At least 57% of 3-year-olds with Down syndrome have evidence of obstructive sleep apnea when evaluated by **polysomnograms** (sleep study). Of the 69% of parents who report no sleep problems in their child with Down syndrome, 54% of their children were found to have abnormal sleep studies (Shott et al., 2006). Because of this data, it is recommended that all children with Down syndrome have polysomnograms by 4 years of age. If the diagnosis is confirmed and found to be associated with enlarged adenoids, antibiotic treatment is used and the adenoids are subsequently removed surgically. If the adenoidectomy does not correct the mechanical obstruction, other surgical procedures can be considered in order to enlarge the airway (Wootten & Shott, 2010). Sleeping with continuous positive airway pressure (CPAP) or, infrequently, a **tracheostomy** may be necessary to keep the airway open (Shott, 2006).

As with all newborns, children with Down syndrome are routinely screened for congenital hypothyroidism. In addition, they should have a TSH (thyroid stimulating hormone) test performed at 6 months of age, at 1 year, and then annually (Bull & the American Academy of Pediatrics Committee on Genetics, 2011). More frequent thyroid function tests are indicated if the child displays accelerated weight gains, behavior problems, plateauing of height, or an unexpected lack of cognitive progress. If there is clinical and laboratory evidence of hypothyroidism, treatment with thyroxine is indicated.

The AAP Committee on Genetics (2011) recommends that children with Down syndrome who have symptoms of celiac disease be screened using tissue transglutaminase IgA and quantitative IgA. At this time, growth should be monitored using growth charts for typical children (Centers for Disease Control, n.d.) using weight-for-height (dividing their actual weight by the weight at the 50th percentile of their height age) and BMI (body mass index; see Chapter 8).

Figure 18.2. Recommendations for preventive health care for children and adolescents with Down syndrome. (*Source:* Bull and American Academy of Pediatrics Committee on Genetics, 2011.)

	Birth to 1 month	Infancy months						Early childhood years					Late childhood years									
		2	4	6	8	10	12	1	2	3	4	5	5	7	9	11	13	13	15	17	19	21
Karyotype	•																					
Echocardiogram	•																					
Hearing screen and follow-up	•																					
Audiological[1]				•			Every 6 months															
Ear specific audiogram[1]												Annually										
Eye exam for cataracts[2]	•																					
Ophthalmology referral		Once in 1st 6 mo						Annually						Every 2 years					Every 3 years			
TSH (Thyroid Stimulating Hormone)	•			•			•								Annually							
CBC[3] (complete blood count) and differential	•						•															
Hb[4] (hemoglobin)												Annually										
Hb only																Annually						
Radiographic swallowing assessment[5]		If symptomatic																				
Lateral neck x ray in neutral position[6]								If symptomatic														
Tissue transglutaminase IgA and quantitative IgA[7]														If symptomatic								
Echocardiogram[8]														If symptomatic								

1. If normal hearing established, do behavioral audiogram and tympanometry until bilateral ear specific testing possible. Refer child with abnormal hearing to otolaryngologist.
2. Referral to ophthalmologist who has experience with Down syndrome to assess for strabismus, cataracts, and nystagmus.
3. To rule out transient myeloproliferative disorder; polycythemia.
4. Hb annually; CRP (c-reactive protein) and ferritin or CHr (reticulocyte hemoglobin content) if possible risk of iron deficiency or Hb < 11 g.
5. If marked hypotonia, slow feeding, choking with feeds, recurrent or persistent respiratory symptoms, failure to thrive.
6. If myelopathic symptoms: obtain neutral position spine films and, if normal, obtain flexion and extension films and refer to pediatric neurosurgeon or orthopedic surgeon with expertise in evaluation and treating atlanto-axial instability.
7. If symptoms of celiac disease are present.
8. If symptoms of acquired mitral or aortic valve disease such as increased fatigue, shortness of breath, or exertional dyspnea or abnormal physical examination findings such as a new murmur or gallop.

Because of the high prevalence of periodontal disease, daily cleaning of teeth should begin as soon as they erupt. As with all children, regular dental visits should also begin at this time. Orthodontic intervention is needed by most children with Down syndrome and becomes possible when the child is able to cooperate with and tolerate the therapy.

The radiographic evaluation of children for atlantoaxial subluxation is reserved for those who are symptomatic. Signs and symptoms of spinal cord compression include the onset of weakness in gait, torticollis (wry neck), neck pain, or bowel and bladder incontinence. The AAP recommends a cautious sequence of evaluation, beginning with plain cervical spine films in the neutral position (Bull & the American Academy of Pediatrics Committee on Genetics, 2011). If there are no radiological abnormalities, flexion and extension films should be done, followed by referral to a pediatric neurosurgeon or orthopedic surgeon with expertise in the evaluation and treatment of atlantoaxial subluxation. Children with radiologic findings indicating neck instability of an unacceptable degree and children with symptomatic subluxation are treated surgically with a neck fusion. The Special Olympics (see Chapter 34) have specific requirements for radiological assessment for participation of children with Down syndrome. These requirements focus on sports, such as diving, that may put stress on the neck (Special Olympics, Inc., 2004).

Several other medical problems, such as diabetes and leukemia, occur more frequently in children with Down syndrome than in the general population. Although screening for these disorders is not routinely performed, it is appropriate to lower the threshold for evaluation for individuals with Down syndrome. The clinician also should be alert to symptoms of behavioral and psychiatric disorders (e.g., autism, depression, psychosis, ADHD) and refer the individual for appropriate evaluation and treatment when indicated (see Chapter 29 and Chapter 22).

INTERVENTION

The parents of a newborn with Down syndrome should be provided with a balanced view of the condition. They should be given up-to-date print materials on infants with Down syndrome, the telephone number of the point-of-entry to the early intervention system, local and national parent support/advocacy programs such as the National Down Syndrome Society and the National Down Syndrome Congress (see Appendix D), respite care options, and Supplemental Security Income (SSI; see Chapter 41; Skotko, Capone, & Kishnani, 2009). Children with Down syndrome have a long history of involvement in early intervention programs (see Chapter 30). Studies of early intervention in Down syndrome indicate improved development especially in fine-motor, social, and self-help skills (Guralnick, 1997).

The educational program of the child with Down syndrome needs to provide the optimal environment for learning. A balance of inclusion in learning environments with typical children and therapeutic interventions needs to be planned for each child (Chapter 31). The individualized education program (IEP) needs to consider the child's opportunities for socialization in the home and community and his or her developmental and educational strengths and needs. Most frequently, children with Down syndrome have strengths in visual motor skills and weakness in verbal short-term memory (Wang, 1996). A visual approach that uses aids such as written instructions, visual organizers, and schedules employs this strength. Such plans need to be reviewed and altered at regular intervals.

In their role as advocates for their child with Down syndrome, most parents consider using alternative and complementary therapies for improvement of cognitive function and appearance (Prussing, Sobo, Walker, & Kurtin, 2005; see Chapter 38). Eighty-seven percent of these parents do at some time treat their child with an alternative therapy, most commonly combination nutritional therapy (e.g., Nutrivene; Prussing, Sobo, Walker, Dennis, & Kurtin, 2004). Although there are many studies of alternative therapies in individuals with Down syndrome, few meet even the minimal methodology criteria of scientific studies (Roizen, 2005). Alternative therapies often include mixtures and individual vitamins (e.g., vitamins A, C, E), minerals (e.g., selenium, zinc), and hormones (e.g., growth, thyroid); cell therapy or injections of fetal lamb brains; facial plastic surgery; and drugs (e.g., piracetam). None of these has been shown to be effective (Ellis et al., 2008; Roizen, 2005). Some studies in children and adults with Down syndrome treated with donepezil (a drug that increases the level of acetylcholine, which is thought to be decreased in Alzheimer's disease) show improvement in language and other function (Kishnani, 2009; Spiridigliozzi et al., 2007).

OUTCOME

Since the 1970s, the prognosis for a productive and positive life experience for individuals with Down syndrome has increased significantly, largely due to the efforts of parent advocacy groups. Children with Down syndrome were among the first children with disabilities to be "mainstreamed" in public schools, and they have been the pioneers in the trend toward inclusion. In a 25-year follow-up study, however, parents reported that inclusive educational placements and services became less common as their children neared and attained adulthood at age 21. The most difficult challenges included medical complications, bullying or ostracism, disappointments in their child's ability to achieve certain adult milestones (e.g., obtaining a driver's license), and a lack of adequate services and supports in adulthood (Hanson, 2003).

Due to improved medical care over the past 45 years, the life expectancy of individuals with Down syndrome is estimated to have increased from 12 to 60 years (Bittles, Bower, & Hussain, 2006). Improved treatment of congenital heart defects, hypothyroidism, and leukemia, which were causes of death out of proportion to the general population accounts for much of this increased lifespan (Yang, Rasmussen, & Friedman, 2002).

With the introduction in the 1980s of supported employment (in which individuals with disabilities have a job coach), adults with Down syndrome often hold jobs with improved pay, improved benefits, and better working conditions. To succeed in supported employment, a person needs a healthy sense of self-esteem that is nurtured from early childhood, the ability to complete tasks without assistance, a willingness to separate emotionally from his or her parents and family members, and access to personal recreational activities (see Chapter 40). All of these should be goals of educational and transition programs for individuals with Down syndrome.

SUMMARY

Down syndrome is characterized by a recognizable pattern of physical features, an increased risk for specific medical problems, and intellectual disability requiring intermittent to significant support. Because children with Down syndrome are usually identified at birth, they are frequently the youngest enrollees in the early intervention system. Although much remains to be learned and accomplished, the educational and medical systems are probably more knowledgeable and comfortable with the special needs of children with Down syndrome than with any other single diagnostic disability group.

The American Academy of Pediatrics Committee on Genetics (Bull & the American Academy of Pediatrics Committee on Genetics, 2011) recommended standards of medical care that include evaluation, periodic monitoring, and vigilance for signs and symptoms of the medical conditions that occur frequently in children with Down syndrome. With optimal audiologic, cardiac, endocrinologic, ophthalmologic, and orthopedic functioning, children with Down syndrome have the opportunity for good health and developmental functioning.

REFERENCES

Ahmed, M., Sternberg, A., Hall, G., Thomas, A., Smith, O., O'Marcaigh, A., ... Vyas, P. (2004). Natural history of GATA1 mutations in Down syndrome. *Blood, 103*, 2480–2489.

Bauer, J., Teufel, U., Doege, C., Hans-Juergen, G., Beedgen, B., & Linderkamp, O. (2003). Energy expenditure in neonates with Down syndrome. *Journal of Pediatrics, 143*, 264–266.

Bergholdt, R., Eising, S., Nerup, J., & Pociot, F. (2006). Increased prevalence of Down's syndrome in individuals with type 1 diabetes in Denmark: A nationwide population-based study. *Diabetologia, 49*, 1179–1182.

Bittles, A.H., Bower, C., & Hussain, R. (2006). The four ages of Down syndrome. *European Journal of Public Health, 17*, 221–225.

Bull, M.J., & the American Academy of Pediatrics Committee on Genetics. (2011). Clinic report: Health supervision for children with Down syndrome. *Pediatrics, 128*, 393–404.

Carr, J. (1988). Six weeks to twenty-one years old: A longitudinal study of children with Down syndrome and their families. *Journal of Child Psychology and Psychiatry, 29*, 407–431.

Carroll, K.N., Arbogast, P.F., Dudley, J.A., & Cooper, W.O. (2008). Increase in incidence of medically treated thyroid disease in children with Down syndrome after rerelease of American Academy of Pediatrics Health Supervision Guidelines. *Pediatrics, 122*, e493–e498.

Castillo, H., Patterson, B., Hickey, F., Kinsman, A., Howard, J.M., Mitchell, T., & Molloy, C.A. (2009). Difference in age at regression in children with autism with and without Down syndrome. *Journal of Developmental & Behavioral Pediatrics, 29*, 89–93.

Centers for Disease Control and Prevention. (n.d.). National Center for Health Statistics Growth Charts. Retrieved from www.cdc.gov/growthcharts.

Chapman, R.E., Schwartz, S.E., & Kay-Raining Bird, E. (1991). Language skills of children and adolescents with Down syndrome, I: Comprehension. *Journal of Speech, Language, and Hearing Research, 34*, 1106–1120.

Chapman, R.E., Seung, H.-K., Schwartz, S.E., & Kay-Raining Bird, E. (1998). Language skills of children and adolescents with Down syndrome, II: Production deficits. *Journal of Speech, Language, and Hearing Research, 41*, 861–873.

Chapman, R.S., & Hesketh, L.J. (2000). Behavioral phenotype of individuals with Down syndrome. *Mental Retardation and Developmental Disabilities Research Reviews, 6*, 84–95.

Cohen, W.I. (2006). Current dilemmas in Down syndrome clinical care: Celiac disease, thyroid disorders, and atlanto-axial instability. *American Journal of Medical Genetics Part C (Seminars in Medical Genetics) 142C*, 141–148.

Cohen, W.I., for the Down Syndrome Medical Interest Group. (1999). Health care guidelines for individuals with Down syndrome: 1999 revision (Down syndrome preventive medical checklist). *Down Syndrome Quarterly, 4*, 1–15.

Creavin, A.L., & Brown, R.D. (2009). Ophthalmic abnormalities in children with Down syndrome. *Journal of Pediatric Ophthalmology and Strabismus, 46*, 76–82.

Dixon, N.E., Crissman, B.G., Smith, P.B., Zimmerman, S.A., Worley, G., & Kishnani, P.S. (2010). Prevalence of iron deficiency in children with Down syndrome. *Journal of Pediatrics, 157*, 967–971.

Down, J.L.H. (1866). Observations on an ethnic classification of idiots. *Clinical Lecture Reports, London Hospital, 3*, 559.

Dykens, E.M. (2007). Psychiatric and behavioral disorders in persons with Down syndrome. *Mental Retardation and Developmental Disabilities Research Reviews, 13*, 272–278.

Ellis, J.M., Tan, H.K., Gilbert, R.E., Muller, D.P.R., Henley, W., Moy, R., ... Logan, S. (2008). Supplementation with antioxidants and folinic acid for children with Down's syndrome: Randomized controlled trial. *British Medical Journal, 336*(7644), 594–597.

Ercis, M., Balci, S., & Atakan, N. (1996). Dermatological manifestations of 71 Down syndrome children admitted to a clinical genetics unit. *Clinical Genetics, 50*, 317–320.

Fishler, K., & Koch, R. (1991). Mental development in Down syndrome mosaicism. *American Journal on Mental Retardation, 96*, 345–351.

Fort, P., Lifshitz, F., Bellisario, R., Davis, J., Lanes, R., Pugliese, M., ... David, R. (1984). Abnormalities of thyroid functioning in infants with Down syndrome. *Journal of Pediatrics, 104*, 545–549.

Freeman, S.B., Bean, L.H., Allen, E.G., Tinker, S.W., Locke, A.E., Druschel, C., ... Sherman, S.L. (2008). Ethnicity, sex, and the incidence of congenital heart defects: A report for the National Down Syndrome Project. *Genetics in Medicine, 10*, 173–180.

Freeman, S.B., Torfs, C.P., Romitti, P.A., Royle, M.H., Druschel, C., Hobbs, C.A., & Sherman, S.L. (2009). Congenital gastrointestinal defects in Down syndrome: A report from the Atlanta and National Down Syndrome Projects. *Clinical Genetics, 75*, 180–186.

Fudge, J.C. Jr., Li, S., Jaggers, J., O'Brien, S.M., Peterson, E.D., Jacobs, J.P., ... Pasquali, S.K. (2010). Congenital heart surgery outcomes in Down syndrome: Analysis of a national clinical database. *Pediatrics, 126*, 314–322.

Gardiner, K.J. (2009). Molecular basis of pharmacotherapies for cognition in Down syndrome. *Trends in Pharmacological Sciences, 31*, 66–73.

Goldberg-Stern, H., Strawsburg, R.H., Patterson, B., Hickey, F., Bare, M., Gadoth, N., & Degrauw, T.J. (2001). Seizure frequency and characteristics in children with Down syndrome. *Brain Development, 23*, 375–378.

Guralnick, M.J. (Ed.). (1997). *The effectiveness of early intervention.* Baltimore, MD: Paul H. Brookes Publishing Co.

Hanson, M. (2003). Twenty-five years after early intervention: A follow-up of children with Down syndrome and their families. *Infants and Young Children, 16*, 354–365.

Hattori, M., Fujiyama, A., Taylor, T.D., Watanabe, H., Yada, T., Park, H.-S., ... Yaspo, M.-L. (2000). The DNA sequence of human chromosome 21. *Nature, 405*, 311–319.

Hennequin, M., Faulks, D., Veyrune, J.-L., & Bourdiol, P. (1999). Significance of oral health in persons with Down syndrome: A literature review. *Developmental Medicine and Child Neurology, 41*, 275–283.

Johannsen, P., Christensen, J.E., Goldstein, H., Nielsen, V.K., & Mai, J. (1996). Epilepsy in Down syndrome: Prevalence in three age groups. *Seizure, 5*, 121–125.

Jones, K.L. (2006). *Smith's recognizable patterns of human malformation* (6th ed.). Philadelphia, PA: Elsevier Saunders.

Juj, H., Emery, H. (2009). The arthropathy of Down syndrome: An underdiagnosed and under-recognized condition. *The Journal of Pediatrics, 154*, 234–238.

Kishnani, P.S., Sommer, B.R., Handen, B.L. Seltzer, B., Capone, G.T., Spiridigliozzi, G.A., ... McRae, T. (2009). The efficacy, safety, and tolerability of donepezil for the treatment of young adults with Down syndrome. *American Journal of Medical Genetics. Part A, 149A*, 1641–1654.

Kumin, L. (2001). Speech intelligibility in individuals with Down syndrome: A framework for targeting specific factors for assessment and treatment. *Down Syndrome Quarterly, 6*, 1–8.

Kupferman, J.C., Druschel, C.M., & Kupchik, G.S. (2009). Increased prevalence of renal and urinary tract anomalies in children with Down syndrome. *Pediatrics, 124*, e615–e621.

Lejeune, J., Gautier, M., & Turpin, R. (1959). Etude des chromosomes somatiques de neufenfants mongoliens. [Study of somatic chromosomes of new children with mongolism] *CompteRendud'Academy Science, 248*, 1721–1722.

Lott, I.T., & Dierssen, M. (2010). Cognitive deficits and associated neurological complications in individuals with Down syndrome. *The Lancet Neurology, 9*, 623–633.

Luke, A., Sutton, M., Schoeller, D., & Roizen, N. (1996). Nutrient intake and obesity in prepubescent children with Down syndrome. *Journal of the American Dietetic Association, 96*, 1262–1267.

Malinge, S., Izraeli, S., & Crispino, J.D. (2009). Insights into the manifestations, outcomes, and mechanisms of leukemogenesis in Down syndrome. *Blood, 113*, 2619–2628.

McClain, A., Bodertha, J., Meyer, J., et al. (Eds.). (1996). *Mosaic Down syndrome.* Richmond, VA: Richmond Medical College of Virginia/Virginia Commonwealth University.

Miller, J.F., Leddy, M., & Leavitt, L.A. (Eds.). (1999). *Improving the communication of people with Down syndrome.* Baltimore, MD: Paul H. Brookes Publishing Co.

Pine, S.R., Guo, Q., Yin, C., Jayabose, S., Druschel, C.M., & Sandoval, C. (2007). Incidence and clinical implications of GATA1 mutations in newborns with Down syndrome. *Blood, 110,* 2128–2131.

Prasher, V.P. (2002). Disintegrative syndrome in young adults with Down syndrome. *Irish Journal of Psychological Medicine, 19,* 101–102.

Prussing, E., Sobo, E.J., Walker, E., Dennis, K., & Kurtin, P.S. (2004). Communication with pediatricians about complementary/alternative medicine: Perspectives from parents of children with Down syndrome. *Ambulatory Pediatrics, 4,* 488–494.

Prussing, E., Sobo, E.J., Walker, E., & Kurtin, P.S. (2005). Between "desperation" and disability rights: A narrative analysis of complementary/alternative medicine use by parents for children with Down syndrome. *Society of Scientific Medicine, 60,* 587–598.

Rabin, K.R., & Whitlock, J.A. (2009). Malignancy in children with trisomy 21. *The Oncologist, 14,* 164–173.

Rasmussen, P., Borjesson, O., Wentz, E., & Gillberg, C. (2001). Autistic disorders in Down syndrome: Background factors and clinical correlates. *Developmental Medicine and Child Neurology, 43,* 750–754.

Rex, A.P., & Preus, M. (1982). A diagnostic index for Down syndrome. *The Journal of Pediatrics, 100,* 903–906.

Roizen, N.J. (2002). Medical care and monitoring for the adolescent with Down syndrome. *Adolescent Medicine: State of the Art Reviews, 13,* 345–357.

Roizen, N.J. (2005). Complimentary and alternative medicine in Down syndrome. *Mental Retardation and Developmental Disabilities Research Reviews, 11,* 149–155.

Roizen, N.J., Mets, M.B., & Blondis, T.A. (1994). Ophthalmic disorders in children with Down syndrome. *Developmental Medicine and Child Neurology, 36,* 594–600.

Roizen, N.J., & Patterson, D. (2003). Down's Syndrome. *The Lancet, 361,* 1281–1289.

Rubello, D., Pozzan, G.B., Casara, D., Girelli, M.E., Boccato, S., Rigon, F., ... Busnardo, B. (1995). Natural course of subclinical hypothyroidism in Down's syndrome: Prospective study results and therapeutic considerations. *Journal of Endocrinologic Investigation, 17,* 35–40.

Saenz, R.B. (1999). Primary care of infants and young children with Down syndrome. *American Family Physician, 59,* 381–390, 392, 395–396.

Shin, M., Besser, L.M., Kucik, J.E., Lu, C., Siffel, C., Correa, A., & the Congenital Anomaly Multistate Prevalence and Survival (CAMPS) Collaborative. (2009). Prevalence of Down syndrome among children and adolescents in 10 regions of the United States. *Pediatrics, 124,* 1565–1571.

Shott, S.R. (2006). Down syndrome: Common otolaryngologic manifestations. *American Journal of Medical Genetics Part C (Seminars in Medical Genetics) 142C,* 131–140.

Shott, S.R., Amin, R., Chini, B., Heubi, C., Hotze, S., & Akers, R. (2006). Obstructive sleep apnea: Should all children with Down syndrome be tested? *Archives of Otolaryngology, Head, and Neck Surgery, 132,* 432–436.

Silverman, W. (2007). Down syndrome: Cognitive phenotype. *Mental Retardation and Developmental Disabilities Research Reviews, 13,* 228–236.

Skotko, B., Capone, G.T., & Kishnani, P.S. for the Down Syndrome Diagnosis Study Group. (2009). Postnatal diagnosis of Down syndrome: Synthesis of the evidence on how best to deliver the news. *Pediatrics, 124,* e751–e758.

Smith, D.S. (2001). Health care management of adults with Down syndrome. *American Family Physician, 64,* 1031–1038.

Special Olympics. (2004). Participation by individuals with down syndrome who have atlanto-axial instability. *Special Olympics Official General Rules, Section 6.02 (g).* Washington, DC: Special Olympics.

Spiridigliozzi, G.A., Heller, J.H., Crissman, B.G., Sullivan-Saarela, J.A., Eells,R., Dawson, D., ... Kishnani, P.S. (2007). Preliminary study of the safety and efficacy of donepezil hydrochloride in children with Down syndrome: A clinical report series. *American Journal of Medical Genetics. Part A, 143A,* 1408–1413.

Stafstrom, C.E., & Konkol, R.J. (1994). Infantile spasms in children with Down syndrome. *Developmental Medicine and Child Neurology, 36,* 576–585.

Suzuki, K., Yamaki, S., Mimori, S., Murakami, Y., Katsuhiko, M., Takahashi, Y., & Kikuchi, T. (2000). Pulmonary vascular disease in Down's syndrome with complete atrioventricularseptal defect. *American Journal of Cardiology, 86,* 434–437.

Toledo, C., Alembik, Y., Aguirre Jaime, A., & Stoll, C. (1999). Growth curves of children with Down syndrome. *Annals of Genetics, 42,* 81–90.

Tuysuz, B., & Beker, D.B. (2001). Thyroid dysfunction in children with Down's syndrome. *ActaPaediatrics, 90,* 1389–1393.

van Trotsenburg, A.S., Heymans, H.S., Tijssen, J.G., de Vijlder, J.J.M., Vulsma, T. (2006). Comorbidity, hospitalization, and medication use and their influence on mental and motor development of young infants with Down syndrome. *Pediatrics, 118,* 1633–1639.

Wald, N.J., & Leck, I. (Eds.). (2000). *Antenatal and Neonatal Screening* (2nd ed.). Oxford, UK: Oxford University Press.

Wang, P. (1996). A neuropsychological profile of Down syndrome: Cognitive skills and brain morphology. *Mental Retardation and Developmental Disabilities Research Reviews, 2,* 102–108.

Winders, P.C. (Ed.). (1997). *Gross motor skills in children with Down syndrome: A guide for parents and professional.* Bethesda, MD: Woodbine House.

Wooten, C.T., & Shott, S.R. (2010). Evolving therapies to treat retroglossal and base-of-tongue obstruction in pediatric obstructive sleep apnea. *Archives of Otolaryngology, Head, & Neck Surgery, 136,* 983–987.

Yang, Q., Rasmussen, S.A., & Friedman, J.M. (2002). Mortality associated with Down's syndrome in the USA from 1983 to 1997: A population-based study. *The Lancet, 359,* 1019–1025.

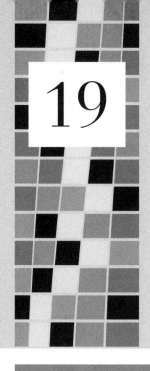

19

Inborn Errors of Metabolism

Mark L. Batshaw and Brendan Lanpher

Upon completion of this chapter, the reader will

- Understand the term *inborn error of metabolism*

- Know the differences among a number of these inborn errors, including amino acid disorders, organic acidemias, fatty acid oxidation defects, mitochondrial disorders, peroxisomal disorders, and lysosomal storage diseases

- Identify the characteristic clinical symptoms and diagnostic tests for these disorders

- Know which of these disorders have newborn screening tests available

- Recognize different approaches to treatment

- Understand the outcome and range of developmental disabilities associated with inborn errors of metabolism

The food we eat contains fats, proteins, and carbohydrates that must be broken down into smaller components and then metabolized by hundreds of enzymes that maintain body functions. Approximately 1 in 2,500 children are born with a deficiency in one of the enzymes that normally **catalyzes** an important biochemical reaction in the cells (Online Mendelian Inheritance in Man, 2010). These children are said to have an inborn error of metabolism. Such an enzyme deficiency can result in the accumulation of a toxic chemical compound behind the enzyme block or lead to a deficiency of a product normally produced by the deficient enzyme (Figure 19.1). The result may be organ damage/dysfunction (often the brain), various degrees of disability, or even death. For

example, children with phenylketonuria (PKU) have a deficiency in the enzyme that normally converts one amino acid (phenylalanine) to another (tyrosine). An inherited deficiency of this enzyme (phenylalanine hydroxylase) leads to the accumulation of phenylalanine, which at high levels is toxic to the brain (Antshel, 2010; van Spronsen, 2010). If PKU is not recognized and treated soon after birth, severe intellectual disability ensues (Figure 19.1). In contrast, in children with congenital adrenal hypoplasia, an inherited enzyme deficiency leads to decreased production of certain steroid hormones (e.g., cortisol) that are essential for normal body function. Females with this deficiency may be born with ambiguous genitalia because they produce abnormal amounts of male steroid sex hormone (testosterone) *in utero* (Antal & Zhou, 2009; Nimkarn & New, 2010). Fortunately, for these disorders and others, newborn screening tests and early treatment have permitted children who are affected to grow up with typical intelligence and normal physiological functioning. Not all inborn errors of metabolism can be as effectively treated, however, because of delays in diagnosis or lack of an effective intervention. This chapter provides examples from a range of inborn errors of metabolism to explain diagnostic and therapeutic advances that are improving the outcome of patients with these disorders.

▓ ▓ ▓ LISA

Lisa was discharged from the hospital at 3 days of age. Her parents were surprised and upset when they were called back a week later, after doctors reported that she had abnormal results for her screening test for PKU. Amino acid studies confirmed the diagnosis of PKU, and Lisa was placed on a formula that was low in phenylalanine. As Lisa grew, her parents could hardly believe there was a problem because Lisa looked and acted like a typically developing child and achieved her developmental milestones on time. The visits to the metabolism clinic were difficult reminders of her "silent disorder." Once Lisa entered elementary school, she began resisting her dietary restrictions, and her parents had difficulty maintaining good metabolic control. Lisa was born in 1970, when the importance

of strict metabolic control for life in PKU was not widely appreciated. Her parents stopped her low-phenylalanine diet at age 7. Psychometric testing at 10 years of age showed that Lisa had an IQ score of 85. Despite some learning and behavioral difficulties, she graduated from high school and began working. When she became pregnant, however, she refused to go back on a phenylalanine-restricted diet, despite her parents' and health care providers' explanation of the serious risks to her baby. Her child was born with a small head, and at age 5 had an intellectual disability.

▓ ▓ ▓ DARNEL

Darnel babbled at 6 months and sat without support shortly thereafter. His parents became concerned, however, when at 1 year of age he had made no further progress. If anything, he seemed less steady in sitting and was uninvolved with his surroundings. His pediatrician worried that Darnel might have an autism spectrum disorder. By 18 months, there were graver concerns. Darnel was no longer able to roll over; he was very floppy and did not appear to respond to light or sound. His pediatrician referred Darnel to a genetics clinic, where an extensive workup eventually diagnosed him as having Tay-Sachs disease, a genetic disorder affecting lipid metabolism in the brain. Over the next 3 years, Darnel slipped into an

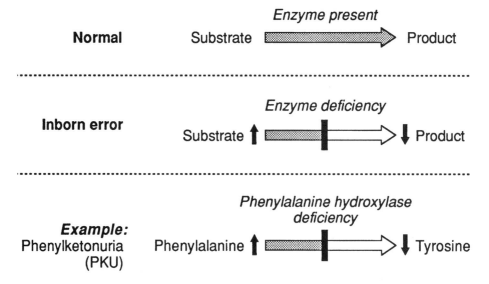

Figure 19.1. Inborn errors of metabolism are genetic disorders involving an enzyme deficiency. This enzyme block leads to the accumulation of a toxic substrate and/or the deficient synthesis of a product needed for normal body function. In phenylketonuria (PKU) there is a toxic accumulation of phenylalanine behind the deficient enzyme, phenylalanine hydroxylase.

unresponsive condition and required tube feeding. He finally succumbed to aspiration pneumonia. As a result of the diagnosis, his parents decided to undergo prenatal diagnosis in subsequent pregnancies. They now have two healthy children, and his mother underwent one termination of a fetus that was affected.

TYPES OF INBORN ERRORS OF METABOLISM

Inborn errors of metabolism are a rather recently discovered group of diseases. PKU, one of the first disorders of this type to be identified, was described by Fölling in 1934. About 300 additional disorders have been identified since the 1950s, and a number of new ones are described each year (Online Mendelian Inheritance in Man, 2010). The majority of these enzyme deficiencies are inherited as autosomal recessive traits, in which both parents carry a genetic change on one of their two copies of the gene. These carriers are healthy and develop typically, due to the normal second copy of the gene. Patients who are affected typically inherit two abnormal genes and have no normal version. A few metabolic disorders are transmitted as X-linked disorders or through mitochondrial inheritance (see Chapter 1). Prenatal diagnosis is available for most of these disorders (see Chapter 4).

Although there are many different ways of categorizing these disorders, inborn errors of metabolism are often divided into 1) those that are clinically "silent" for a relatively long period before being recognized, 2) those that produce acute metabolic crises, and 3) those that cause progressive organ damage or dysfunction (Table 19.1).

Among the silent disorders are certain abnormalities involving amino acids (e.g., PKU) or hormones (e.g., congenital hypothyroidism). Disorders producing acute toxicity include certain inborn errors in the metabolism of small molecules, including ammonia, amino acids, organic acids, fatty acids, lactic acid, and carbohydrates (Levy, 2009a, 2009b). Inborn errors of metabolism causing progressive disorders include most **glycogen** storage and peroxisomal and lysosomal storage disorders. The specific names of the disorders are often derived from their deficient enzyme (e.g., **ornithine transcarbamylase [OTC] deficiency**, a disorder of nitrogen metabolism).

Silent disorders such as PKU do not manifest life-threatening crises, but if untreated,

Table 19.1. Examples of inborn errors of metabolism

Type I: Silent disorders
   Phenylketonuria (PKU)
   Congenital hypothyroidism

Type II: Disorders presenting in acute metabolic crisis
   Urea cycle disorders (ornithine transcarbamylase [OTC] deficiency)
   Organic acidemias (multiple carboxylase deficiency)

Type III: Disorders with progressive neurological deterioration
   Tay-Sachs disease
   Gaucher disease
   Metachromatic leukodystrophy

lead to brain damage and developmental disabilities. These disorders contrast with inborn errors that cause episodic symptoms, such as OTC deficiency, that may be acutely life threatening with each decompensation, typically starting in early infancy. In both cases, an infant who is affected is generally protected in the womb because the maternal circulation can remove the toxic chemical or provide the missing product. After birth, however, the infant must rely on his or her own metabolic pathways, and if they are abnormal, toxicity occurs rapidly or over time, depending on the severity of the defect. In progressive disorders, there is the gradual accumulation of large molecules. These molecules are stored in the cells of various body organs, including the brain, where they ultimately cause damage, leading to physical and/or neurological deterioration. Many of the small molecular disorders, both those that are silent and those with acute symptoms, are treatable with fairly good outcome. The large molecular disorders, with a few notable exceptions, have been far more difficult to treat, and their outcome generally remains poor.

Clinical Manifestations

The clinical manifestations of the various inborn errors of metabolism fall along a spectrum, from lack of overt symptoms to life-threatening episodes.

The silent disorders (e.g., PKU) do not manifest symptoms such as lethargy, coma, or regression of skills. Instead, children who are untreated develop very slowly and are typically not identified as having intellectual disability until later in childhood.

Life-threatening crises characterize the second group of inborn errors of metabolism. Infants with these disorders appear to be unaffected at birth, but by a few days of age they develop vomiting, respiratory distress, and lethargy before slipping into coma. These symptoms, however, mimic those observed in other severe newborn illnesses such as sepsis (bloodborne infection), brain hemorrhage, heart and lung malformations, and gastrointestinal obstruction, making the correct diagnosis difficult to identify. If specific metabolic testing of the blood and urine is not performed, the disease will go undetected. Undiagnosed and untreated, virtually all children who are affected will die quickly. One study reported that 60% of children with newborn onset inborn errors of the **urea** cycle (causing elevated ammonia level) had at least one sibling who died before the disorder was correctly diagnosed in a subsequent child (Batshaw et al., 1982). Even with "heroic" treatment, which may include **dialysis** to "wash out" the toxin (ammonia), many infants do not survive, and severe developmental disabilities may occur in those who do (Krivitzky et al., 2009).

In children with neonatal-onset disease, DNA analysis typically shows mutations that cause the absence of the enzyme or the formation of a completely nonfunctional enzyme. Enzyme activity levels are generally undetectable (see Chapter 1). Some children with the same inborn error of metabolism, however, have less severe mutations that result in reduced (rather than absent) amount of enzymes or that result in enzymes that are only partially dysfunctional. These children typically have later onset of clinical signs and more variable or subtle symptoms. Here, symptoms of behavioral changes and cyclical vomiting and lethargy are often provoked by excessive protein intake or intercurrent infections (Seminara et al., 2010). Although these children generally have a better outcome than those with neonatal-onset disease, they remain at risk for life-threatening metabolic crises throughout life. In addition, although their developmental disabilities may be less severe than those in children with neonatal-onset disease, children with later onset disease rarely escape without some residual cognitive impairment, ranging from attention-deficit/hyperactivity disorder (ADHD) and learning disabilities to intellectual disability.

The third clinical presentation of inborn errors of metabolism is in the form of a large molecule, slowly progressive disorder. Examples include the following:

- Lysosomal storage disorders, such as Gaucher and Tay-Sachs disease (Jardim, Villanueva,

de Souza, & Netto, 2010; Martins, Valadares, et al, 2009; Pastores et al., 2000)

- Ceroid lipofuscinosis such as Batten disease (Jalanko & Braulke, 2009; Rakheja, Narayan, & Bennett, 2007)

- Mucopolysaccharide disorders (Martins, Dualibi, et al., 2009; Muenzer, Wraith, & Clarke., 2009)

- Metachromatic leukodystrophy (Biffi, Lucchini, Rovell, & Sessa, 2008; Gieselmann & Krägeloh-Mann, 2010)

- Peroxisomal disorders, including adreno-leukodystrophy (Fidaleo, 2009) and Zellweger syndrome (Steinberg et al., 2006)

In the more severe of these disorders, there is a gradual and progressive loss of motor and/or cognitive skills beginning in infancy or early childhood that, if left untreated, commonly leads to death in childhood. In the case of Tay-Sachs disease (Darnel's disorder in the previous case study), the child who is affected appears to develop typically until 3–6 months of age, at which point skill development halts. For the next 1–2 years, the child gradually loses all skills; begins having seizures; and exhibits decreased muscle tone, vision, hearing, and cognition. Death usually results from malnutrition or aspiration pneumonia. Unfortunately, no effective treatment currently exists for this disorder.

Enzyme replacement therapy, however, has been recently found to be successful in treating several lysosomal disorders (Gaucher disease, Fabry disease, and Hunter syndrome) in which target organs other than the brain are accessible to the recombinant enzyme (El Dib & Pastores, 2010; Grubb, Vogler, & Sly, 2010; Hollak, de Fost, van Dussen, Vom Dahl, & Aerts, 2009; Lim-Melia & Kronn, 2009; Wraith, 2009). However, the synthetic enzyme does not cross the blood–brain barrier, (the network of blood vessels and cells around the brain that act as a filter for blood flowing to the central nervous system) so it does not halt or reverse the cognitive effects of these disorders. Stem-cell and bone-marrow transplantation have been somewhat helpful in certain mucopolysaccharidoses and leukodystrophies and curative in nonneuronopathic Gaucher (though the enzyme replacement therapy for Gaucher has been successful enough to obviate the need for bone marrow transplantation in most patients; Orchard & Tolar, 2010; Prasad & Kurtzberg, 2010; Shihabuddin & Aubert, 2010).

MECHANISM OF BRAIN DAMAGE

The causes of brain damage in the various inborn errors of metabolism are not completely understood. Research is starting to provide some clues that may eventually lead to improved treatment. For example, thyroid hormone has been found to be necessary for the normal growth of neurons, their processes, and surrounding myelin in the brain. Untreated, a congenital thyroid hormone deficiency is thought to lead to poor postnatal brain growth and result in microcephaly (Chen & Hetzel, 2010). Fortunately there is neonatal screening available for this disorder, and early treatment is protective of brain development (Lafranchi, 2010).

Neurotoxins appear to play a role in certain other metabolic disorders. For example, in nonketotic hyperglycinemia, an inborn error of amino acid metabolism, there is an accumulation of **glycine**, leading to uncontrolled seizures (Hamosh, Scharer, & Van Hove, 2009). Glycine appears to produce excitotoxicity at a neurotransmitter receptor, leading to the influx of calcium ions and water into the neuron. This causes swelling and, eventually, cell death. Experimental drugs are being tested to block this receptor from being overstimulated (Suzuki, Kure, Oota, Hino, & Fukuda, 2010). In Lesch-Nyhan syndrome, which is caused by a defect in **purine** metabolism, deficits in the **dopamine** neurotransmitter system are associated with self-injurious behavior (Nyhan, O'Neill, Jinnah, & Harris, 2010).

In some disorders, more than one neurotoxin may be involved. Scientists believe that in inborn errors of the urea cycle, the accumulating toxins, ammonia and/or glutamine, directly cause nerve cells to swell and indirectly cause excitotoxic damage to the brain (Braissant, 2010; Lichter-Konecki, Mangin, Gordish-Dressman, Hoffman, & Gallo, 2008). If children are rescued from the ammonia-induced coma within a day or two, the neurotoxic effect can subside and outcome can be fairly good (Krivitzky et al., 2009). If the coma is prolonged, however, irreversible brain damage occurs.

ASSOCIATED DISABILITIES

The toxic accumulation of metabolic compounds or the deficient synthesis of essential products results in a range of developmental disabilities in children with inborn errors of metabolism. The most common are intellectual disability and cerebral palsy. However, in certain inborn errors, there are also rather specific impairments. These are sometimes associated with distinctive pathological features in the brain, which may eventually permit a better understanding of brain development and function. For example, boys with the X-linked Lesch-Nyhan syndrome exhibit choreoathetosis (a movement disorder), dyskinetic cerebral palsy (see Chapter 24) and compulsive, self-injurious behavior (Nyhan et al., 2010). Children with glutaric acidemia type I, other organic academia, and/or mitochondrial disorders can have dyskinetic cerebral palsy associated with calcifications of the basal ganglia (Falk, 2010; Gitiaux et al., 2008; Gouider-Khouja, Kraoua, Benrhouma, Fraj, & Rouissi, 2010). In Zellweger syndrome, a disorder of the **peroxisome** formation, children exhibit multiple malformations that are more commonly associated with chromosomal abnormalities, including an abnormal facial appearance, kidney cysts, and congenital heart defects (Fidaleo, 2009). This indicates a prenatal origin of the abnormalities, unlike the other disorders described above where abnormalities occur as a result of an accumulation of a toxin or lack of a needed product after birth.

DIAGNOSTIC TESTING

All children with significant developmental disabilities of unknown origin should be referred for a genetic evaluation. As a part of that evaluation, particular attention will be paid to potential metabolic disorders if a child displays any of the following signs or symptoms: cyclical behavioral changes, vomiting and lethargy, enlargement of the liver or spleen, evidence of neurological deterioration, and/or a family history suggestive of an inherited disorder (Kamboj, 2008). An increasing number of clinically available biochemical and molecular tests can lead to a specific diagnosis. In some disorders, early diagnosis leads to therapy with an improved outcome. Even in currently untreatable disorders, a specific diagnosis may permit effective genetic counseling. A metabolic evaluation is not required, however, for all children with intellectual disability. It is expensive, and the diagnostic yield is quite low.

Diagnosis of an inborn error of amino acid or organic acid metabolism relies primarily on blood and urine tests to detect toxins and/or biochemical markers. The most common blood tests are for blood ammonia, lactic acid, acylcarnitines, and amino acids; urine is principally tested for organic acids. The metabolic evaluations are individualized based on the specific biochemical pathway that is suspected to be involved. OTC deficiency, the most common inborn error of the urea cycle, illustrates one such defective pathway (Figure 19.2). When proteins are broken down into their amino acids components, the amino acids that are not reused for making new proteins are degraded to produce energy. During this process, nitrogen waste is normally released as ammonia, which is then converted into the nontoxic product urea through six enzymatic steps, the urea cycle (OTC is the second enzyme in the cycle). Urea is then excreted in the urine, safely eliminating waste nitrogen. If any one of the six enzymes is deficient, ammonia will accumulate and can cause devastating neurological symptoms (Gropman, Summar, & Leonard, 2007). In those individuals with some residual enzyme activity, the disorder may only manifest under certain environmental stresses (e.g., severe infections, a large dietary protein load), and the disorders may only be correctly diagnosed during those acute episodes. To diagnose this disorder, levels of ammonia and amino acids are measured in blood, and orotic acid is measured in the urine. Many other inborn errors of amino acid and organic acid metabolism can be identified using similar blood and urine tests.

Brain degenerative conditions such as lysosomal storage disorders are typically diagnosed by measuring the suspected deficient enzyme activity in the blood or cultured skin cells (Martins et al., 2009b). Direct mutation analysis in suspected genes may lead to the diagnosis more rapidly in some disorders. Imaging studies (e.g., magnetic resonance imaging [MRI], magnetic resonance spectroscopy [MRS], computed tomography [CT] scan, electroencephalogram [EEG]), and other neurological measures (e.g., nerve conduction velocity, electromyography) may also prove helpful in diagnosing these disorders.

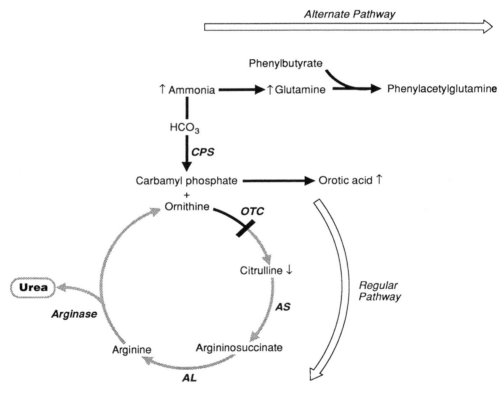

Figure 19.2. The urea cycle and alternate pathway therapy. There are five enzymes in this cycle that convert toxic ammonia, a breakdown product of protein, to nontoxic urea, which is excreted in the urine. The enzymes, shown in boldface italic type, are CPS (carbamyl phosphate synthetase), OTC (ornithine transcarbamylase), AS (argininosuccinate synthetase), AL (argininosuccinate lyase), and arginase. Inborn errors at each step of the urea cycle have been described, with the most common being OTC deficiency. In OTC deficiency, behind the block there is accumulation of ammonia, glutamine, and orotic acid and deficient production of citrulline. Treatment has been directed at providing an alternate pathway for waste nitrogen excretion by giving the drug sodium phenylbutyrate, which combines with glutamine to form phenylacetylglutamine, a nontoxic product that can be excreted in the urine. This results in a decrease in the accumulation of ammonia.

NEWBORN SCREENING

Because individual inborn errors of metabolism are rare (typically occurring in fewer than 1 in 10,000 births) and the diagnosis is easily missed, efforts have been directed at developing newborn mass screening methods for the detection of the more common and treatable disorders (Fernhoff, 2009; Pitt, 2010). As explained previously, rapid diagnosis and treatment are essential in achieving a favorable outcome. As a result, screening efforts have focused on newborn infants. The first newborn screening test was developed for PKU in 1959, and it was successful in detecting more than 90% of infants who are affected. Subsequently, methods have been established for screening other disorders, including congenital hypothyroidism, galactosemia, homocystinuria, biotinidase deficiency, maple syrup urine disease, and fatty acid oxidation defects, as well as certain other genetic disorders that are not associated with developmental disabilities, including cystic fibrosis, adrenal insufficiency, sickle-cell disease, and alpha$_1$-antitrypsin deficiency (a disorder affecting the liver and lungs). This expanded testing, now employing tandem mass spectrometry in state-run screening laboratories, can measure more than 30 inborn errors of metabolism and is offered to families in the newborn nurseries (Sahai & Marsden, 2009). The specific inborn errors of metabolism tested for vary among states based on local legislation. State-specific

information is provided on the National Newborn Screening and Genetics Resource Center web site (http://genes-r-us.uthscsa.edu).

To perform the newborn screening test, a few drops of blood are drawn from the infant's heel and placed on a filter paper. The dried blood sample is mailed to the screening laboratory, where results are obtained within a few days. Although these tests have proved to be remarkably effective, parents should be reminded that a positive test only indicates a higher than normal likelihood of a genetic disorder that needs to be confirmed or ruled out by additional confirmatory testing in the specialized clinic. In addition, the tests detect only a fraction of disorders that cause developmental disabilities, whereas parents might incorrectly assume that these tests are diagnostic for all disorders (see Newborn Screening in Chapter 5).

THERAPEUTIC APPROACHES

Figure 19.3 illustrates the varying approaches to treating inborn errors of metabolism. These methods include 1) **substrate** deprivation (dietary restriction of a potentially toxic material normally metabolized by the defective enzyme), 2) externally supplying the deficient product (e.g. thyroid hormone), 3) stimulating an alternative pathway around the enzyme block, 4) providing a vitamin cofactor to stimulate the deficient enzyme, 5) replacing the enzyme with the infusion of a synthesized enzyme,

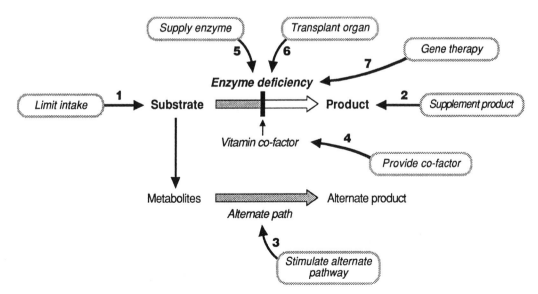

Figure 19.3. Approaches to treatment of inborn errors of metabolism. Treatment can be directed at 1) limiting the intake of a potentially toxic compound, 2) supplementing the deficient product, 3) stimulating an alternate metabolic pathway, 4) providing a vitamin co-factor to activate residual enzyme activity, 5) supplying the enzyme itself, 6) transplanting a body organ containing the deficient enzyme, and 7) gene therapy.

6) transplanting an organ that has normal enzyme activity, and 7) using gene therapy to substitute for the abnormal gene that is causing the disease. With the exception of gene therapy, which is not yet a clinical option, each of these approaches is illustrated by specific disorders in Table 19.2.

Substrate Deprivation (Dietary Restriction)

A relatively straightforward method of treating an inborn error of metabolism is to establish dietary restrictions that limit the child's intake of a potentially toxic amino acid. For example, children with PKU are placed on a phenylalanine-restricted diet in order to prevent the phenylalanine accumulation that is associated with brain damage (Poustie & Wildgoose, 2010). This involves a diet consisting of a special phenylalanine-restricted formula combined with low-protein foods. It is important to note that the diet for patients with PKU cannot be completely free of phenylalanine. Phenylalanine is an essential amino acid, and a small amount is necessary for normal growth and development. Close monitoring of essential amino acids is an important component of the management of patients on controlled diets for metabolic disorders.

Fortunately, phenylalanine-restricted diets are quite effective for patients with PKU. A classic study showed that the IQ scores of children who began this treatment within the first month of life were around 100, whereas the scores of those initially treated later in childhood were 20–50 points lower (Hanley, Linsao, & Netley, 1971).

Scientists initially thought that only those children with PKU who were younger than 6 years needed to follow a phenylalanine-restricted diet, as was done with Lisa. For older children, it was thought that phenylalanine would be much less toxic. In addition, the high cost and rejection of this rather unpleasant and restrictive diet made continuation difficult. Initial studies to determine whether children with PKU experienced a loss in intellectual functioning following dietary treatment discontinuation suggested that IQ scores did not decline over time (Waisbren, Mahon, Schnell, & Levy, 1987). In a subsequent study, however, researchers found that children with PKU who maintained the diet through age 10 actually experienced a modest gain in IQ scores compared with children who stopped the diet at age 6. The differences in IQ scores between the two groups were statistically significant (Michals, Azen, Acosta, Koch, & Matalon, 1988). Thus, metabolic specialists now suggest that the

Table 19.2.   Examples of treatment approaches for inborn errors of metabolism

Approaches	Disorder	Specific treatment
Substrate deprivation	Phenylketonuria (PKU)	Phenylalanine restriction
	Maple syrup urine disease	Branch chain amino acid restriction
	Galactosemia	Galactose restriction
Externally supplementing the deficient product	Congenital hypothyroidism	Thyroid hormone (Synthroid)
	Glycogen storage disease	Cornstarch
	Urea cycle disorders (except argininemia)	Arginine
Stimulating an alternative pathway	Urea cycle disorders	Phenylbutyrate (Buphenyl)
	Organic acidemias	Carnitine
	Isovaleric acidemia	Glycine
	Tyrosinemia	NTBC
Providing a vitamin co-factor	Multiple carboxylase deficiency	Biotin
	Homocystinuria	Pyridoxine
	Methylmalonic acidemia	Vitamin B12
Replacing an enzyme	Fabry disease	Agalsidase beta (Fabrazyme)
	Gaucher disease	Alglucerase (Ceredase)
	Hurler disease	Alpha-L-iduronidase (laronidase [Aldurazyme])
Transplanting an organ	Metachromatic leukodystrophy	Bone marrow transplant
	Ornithine transcarbamylase (OTC) deficiency	Liver transplant

phenylalanine-restricted diet be continued indefinitely.

An elevated maternal phenylalanine level poses a serious threat for the fetus of a woman with PKU who is without dietary control, as described with Lisa (Lee, Ridout, & Walter, 2005). Before newborn screening and effective treatment were available, men and women with PKU had severe intellectual disability and did not often bear children. Since effective treatment became available, most women with PKU became mothers. These women, however, had typically stopped following the phenylalanine-restricted diet during childhood. Unexpectedly, almost all of the children born to these women were found to have microcephaly, intellectual disability, and other congenital abnormalities, including congenital heart disease, cleft lip and palate, and gastrointestinal and urinary abnormalities. These children, however, do not have PKU; they are only carriers. Instead, the intellectual disability and other abnormalities are caused by the **teratogenic** (interfering with normal embryonic development) effect of the mother's high phenylalanine levels on the developing fetus. Studies have shown that lowering the phenylalanine levels in the pregnant mother with PKU significantly improves the chances for typical development of offspring. As a result, it is now advised that women with PKU resume a phenylalanine-restricted diet prior to conception (American College of Obstetricians and Gynecologists Committee on Genetics, 2009).

Another example of substrate deprivation therapy has shown promise in animal models of PKU. Here, the use of a recombinant enzyme to degrade phenylalanine in the intestine before its absorption could reduce the phenylalanine load and allow less severe dietary restriction (Sarkissian et al., 2008). In certain lysosomal storage disorders, inhibition of glycosphingolipid synthesis would have the analogous effect of reducing lysosomal products that are toxic to the brain (Jakobkiewicz-Banecka et al., 2007; McEachern et al., 2007).

Externally Supplementing the Deficient Product

Some children with inborn errors of metabolism are given replacements for the enzyme product they are missing. For example, children with congenital hypothyroidism receive a thyroid supplement to compensate for the thyroid hormone they lack. Similarly, children with congenital adrenal hyperplasia receive steroid hormone replacement. Children with hypothyroidism who are treated in the first months of life develop typical intelligence; however, as with children who have PKU, these children have some residual impairment in attention and learning (van der Sluijs Veer, Kempers, Last, Vulsma, & Grootenhuis, 2008). The medical formulas for PKU are enhanced in tyrosine, the product of the deficient enzyme. Tyrosine is an important precursor for a number of neurotransmitters. The goals of PKU management include both controlling phenylalanine elevations and ensuring adequate tyrosine.

Stimulating an Alternative Pathway

Physicians are now able to treat some metabolic disorders by stimulating an alternative pathway that detours around the enzymatic block. For example, children with inborn errors of the urea cycle cannot convert toxic ammonia to nontoxic urea. Treatment by dietary protein restriction alone has proven unsuccessful because the degree of restriction required to prevent an accumulation of ammonia does not allow a sufficient diet to permit sustained growth or prolonged survival (Shih, 1976). A different approach is to use the drug sodium phenylbutyrate to stimulate an alternate pathway for ammonia excretion. By providing a detour around the enzymatic block and converting the ammonia to an alternate nontoxic product, phenylacetylglutamine, instead of urea (Figure 19.2), this drug allows the majority of children with urea cycle disorders to survive, although many have developmental disabilities (Enns et al., 2010).

Another example of using a detour is the inhibition of a pathway upstream to prevent the formation of toxic products behind the enzymatic block. In hereditary tyrosinemia type I, the drug NTBC, an herbicide derivative, was found to inhibit tyrosine degradation in children who were affected, preventing the formation of a toxic compound that is suspected to cause liver and kidney disease and liver cancer in these children (Masurel-Paulet et al., 2008; Sniderman King, Trahms, & Scott, 2008). Similarly, miglustat, used for the treatment of Gaucher disease, inhibits the formation of glucosylcermide, reducing the accumulated substrate load and improving clinical outcome (Pastores, Giraldo, Chérin, & Mehta, 2009). It is being tested for other lysosomal storage disorders as well (Niemann-Pick Type C, Late

Onset Tay-Sachs, and Type 3 Gaucher disease; Pineda et al, 2010; Shapiro, Pastores, Gianutsos, Luzy, & Kolodny, 2009).

Providing a Vitamin Cofactor

For certain patients with metabolic diseases, providing a large dose of a vitamin cofactor results in amplification of residual enzyme activity or enhanced enzyme stability and clinical improvement. This approach has been used most effectively in treating children with an organic acidemia called biotinidase deficiency (Wolf, 2010). These children, who develop symptoms of acidosis and coma because of a defect in the enzyme biotinidase, show remarkable improvement if the vitamin biotin is provided at a very high (but nontoxic) dosage. The primary defect in biotinidase deficiency is the inability of the body to recycle the vitamin biotin. Biotin is an essential cofactor for a number of critical enzymes in multiple metabolic pathways. By supplying patients with large doses of biotin, these enzymes are normalized. In other disorders, the mutation may affect the binding site for enzyme cofactors. In some of these cases, providing large quantities of a vitamin cofactor may stabilize and even normalize enzyme activity. This type of vitamin therapy can help children with certain forms of another organic acidemia called methylmalonic aciduria (using vitamin B_{12}; Froese, Zhang, Healy, & Gravel, 2009) and an amino acid disorder called homocystinuria (using vitamin B_6; Clayton, 2006; Picker et al., 2006). Certain patients with PKU respond well to an analogue of tetrahydrobiop-terin (Blau et al., 2009). Vitamin therapy has unfortunately spawned a "quick-fix" approach to treating everything from cancer to Down syndrome and schizophrenia, although there is no evidence that megavitamin therapy is effective in treating these disorders (Braganza, 2005; Nutrition Committee of the Canadian Paediatric Society, 1990).

Replacing an Enzyme

The previously discussed methods of therapy use indirect approaches to improve the child's condition. Supplying the missing enzyme is a more direct approach to actually correct the inborn error. Injections of a synthetic enzyme first proved successful in treating the lysosomal storage disorder Gaucher disease, which is associated with the accumulation of glucocerebroside in cells of the liver, spleen, and bone marrow. With severe infantile Gaucher disease,

the glucocerebroside accumulates in the brain as well. Individuals who receive biweekly injections of the deficient enzyme showed marked improvements, including significant shrinkage of the liver and spleen (Charrow, 2009; Hollak et al., 2009). This enzyme, however, cannot cross the blood–brain barrier, making replacement therapy ineffective for those children with severe infantile Gaucher disease. As of 2010, specific enzyme replacement therapy has been approved for Fabry disease, mucopolysaccharidosis type I (Hurler disease), mucopolysaccharidosis type II (Hunter disease), mucopolysaccharidosis type VI (Maroteaux-Lamy syndrome), and glycogen storage disease II (Pompe disease), and this therapy is being tested for other lysosomal storage diseases (Lim-Melia & Kronn, 2009).

Although replacement therapy seems ideal, it is not without shortcomings. These synthetic enzymes are some of the most expensive drugs in the world. In addition, the enzyme must be injected at frequent intervals throughout the individual's life, and antibodies can develop against the foreign protein, just as antibodies against insulin develop in some individuals with diabetes. Many patients experience hypersensitivity reactions to their infusions, ranging from mild flushing and nausea to severe, life-threatening anaphylactic reactions.

Transplanting an Organ

Some deficient enzymes can be replaced by transplanting a body organ that contains the enzyme. For example, bone marrow, cord blood, and stem cell transplantation have been done in individuals with certain lysosomal and peroxisomal storage disorders, including juvenile metachromatic leukodystrophy, adrenoleukodystrophy, and Hurler syndrome. These disorders, marked by neurological and physical deterioration and early death, are caused by the deficiency of enzymes found in many body organs, including bone marrow cells. In a number of studies, transplantation has resulted in the arrest of or improvement in symptoms, although it is questionable whether it has an effect on brain function (Biffi et al., 2008; Cartier & Aubourg, 2008; Orchard & Tolar, 2010; Prasad & Kurtzberg, 2010; Semmler, Köhler, Jung, Weller, & Linnebank, 2008).

In addition to bone-marrow, stem-cell, and cord-blood transplants, liver transplantation has been used to treat certain inborn errors of amino acid metabolism, most notably newborn-onset OTC deficiency and hereditary tyrosinemia type I. It has been associated with biochemical correction and improvement in symptoms (Campeau et al., 2010; Moini, Mistry, & Schilsky, 2010; Sniderman King, Trahms, & Scott, 2008). In some cases of methylmalonic acidemia, liver transplant in conjunction with kidney transplant has been effective. Organ transplantation does carry a certain risk of mortality and morbidity, and transplant recipients require immunosuppression therapy for life.

Using Gene Therapy

In theory, an ideal treatment for an inborn error of metabolism would involve the insertion of a normal gene to compensate for a defective one. This insertion would allow for the production of a normal enzyme, thereby permanently correcting or curing the disorder. In clinical research studies, however, gene therapy trials have not yet been successful or have been associated with severe adverse events (Cavazzana-Calvo, Lagresle, Hacein-Bey-Abina, & Fischer, 2005; Raper et al., 2003). In addition, for brain-based disorders, there is the problem of getting across the blood–brain barrier. There is the potential for therapeutic application of hematopoietic stem cell gene therapy with intracerebral gene transfer (brain gene therapy) in patients with metachromatic leukodystrophy and adrenoleukodystrophy (Sevin, Cartier-Lacave, & Aubourge, 2009).

OUTCOME

The range of outcomes in inborn errors of metabolism varies enormously. In most disorders that can be detected by newborn screening, such as PKU, children who are affected have generally done well. Their intellectual functioning generally falls within the typical range, if somewhat lower than that of their parents. They are, however, at increased risk for having learning disabilities and ADHD (Antshel, 2010; Gentile, Ten Hoedt, & Bosch, 2010). Less favorable outcomes occur in other inborn errors of amino acid and organic acid metabolism. Although these children are surviving longer now, many manifest developmental disabilities. Among children with metabolic disorders associated with progressive neurological disorders, such as certain lysosomal storage diseases, there has been only limited improvement in mortality and morbidity (Jardim et al., 2010; Orchard & Tolar, 2010).

SUMMARY

Although inborn errors of metabolism are rare, their consequences are often devastating. Fortunately, therapy is effective for a number of these disorders. Children who are affected, however, often must continue treatment for the rest of their lives, which may prove difficult. For therapy to succeed, it must be started early. Researchers continue to look for new therapeutic strategies for these diseases. It is hoped that these new therapeutic approaches will continue to improve the outcome for children with inborn errors of metabolism. The expansion in the number of disorders that are tested by newborn screening also bodes well for early identification and treatment with the possibility of improved outcome.

REFERENCES

American College of Obstetricians and Gynecologists Committee on Genetics. (2009). ACOG committee opinion no. 449: Maternal phenylketonuria. *Obstetrics and Gynecology, 114*(6), 1432–1433.

Antal, Z., & Zhou, P. (2009). Congenital adrenal hyperplasia: Diagnosis, evaluation, and management. *Pediatrics in Review, 30*(7), e49–e57.

Antshel, K.M. (2010). ADHD, learning, and academic performance in phenylketonuria. *Molecular Genetics and Metabolism, 99*(Suppl. 1), S52–S58.

Batshaw, M.L., Brusilow, S., Waber, L., Blom, W., Brubakk, A.M., Burton, B.K., ... Schafer, I.A. (1982). Treatment of inborn errors of urea synthesis: Activation of alternative pathways of waste nitrogen synthesis and excretion. *The New England Journal of Medicine, 306*(23), 1387–1392.

Blau, N., Bélanger-Quintana, A., Demirkol, M., Feillet, F., Giovannini, M., MacDonald, A., ... van Spronsen, F.J. (2009). Optimizing the use of sapropterin [BH(4)] in the management of phenylketonuria. *Molecular Genetics and Metabolism, 96*, 158–163.

Biffi, A., Lucchini, G., Rovelli, A., & Sessa, M. (2008). Metachromatic leukodystrophy: An overview of current and prospective treatments. *Bone Marrow Transplant, 42*(Suppl. 2), S2–S6.

Braganza, S.F., & Ozuah, P.O. (2005). Fad therapies. *Pediatrics in Review, 26*(10), 371–376.

Braissant, O. (2010). Current concepts in the pathogenesis of urea cycle disorders. *Molecular Genetics and Metabolism, 100*(Suppl. 1), S3–S12.

Campeau, P.M., Pivalizza, P.J., Miller, G., McBride, K., Karpen, S., Goss, J., & Lee, B.H. (2010). Early orthotopic liver transplantation in urea cycle defects: Follow up of a developmental outcome study. *Molecular Genetics and Metabolism, 100*(Suppl. 1), S84–S87.

Cartier, N., & Aubourg, P. (2008). Hematopoietic stem cell gene therapy in Hurler syndrome, globoid cell leukodystrophy, metachromatic leukodystrophy and X-adrenoleukodystrophy. *Current Opinion in Molecular Therapeutics, 10*(5), 471–478.

Cavazzana-Calvo, M., Lagresle, C., Hacein-Bey-Abina, S., & Fischer, A. (2005). Gene therapy for severe combined immunodeficiency. *Annual Review of Medicine, 56*, 585–602.

Charrow, J. (2009). Enzyme replacement therapy for Gaucher disease. *Expert Opinion on Biological Therapy*, 9(1), 121–131.

Chen, Z.P., & Hetzel, B.S. (2010). Cretinism revisited. *Best Practice and Research: Clinical Endocrinology and Metabolism*, 24(1), 39–50.

Clayton, P.T. (2006). B_6-responsive disorders: A model of vitamin dependency. *Journal of Inherited Metabolic Disease*, 29(2–3), 317–326.

El Dib, R.P., & Pastores, G.M. (2010). Enzyme replacement therapy for Anderson-Fabry disease. *Cochrane Database System Review*, 12(5),CD006663.

Enns, G.M. (2010). Nitrogen sparing therapy revisited: 2009. *Molecular Genetics and Metabolism*, 100(Suppl. 1), S65–S71.

Falk, M.J. (2010). Neurodevelopmental manifestations of mitochondrial disease. *Journal of Developmental and Behavioral Pediatric*, 31(7), 610–621.

Fernhoff, P.M. (2009). Newborn screening for genetic disorders. *Pediatric Clinics of North America*, 56(3), 505–513.

Fidaleo, M. (2009). Peroxisomes and peroxisomal disorders: The main facts. *Experimental and Toxicological Pathology*, 62(6), 615–625.

Folling, A. (1934). Excretion of phenylalanine in urine: An inborn error of metabolism associated with intellectual disability. *Hoppe-Seyler's Zeitschrift fur physiologische Chemie*, 227, 169–176.

Froese, D.S., Zhang, J., Healy, S., & Gravel, R.A. (2009). Mechanism of vitamin B_{12}-responsiveness in cblC methylmalonic aciduria with homocystinuria. *Molecular Genetics and Metabolism*, 98(4), 338–343.

Gentile, J.K., Ten Hoedt, A.E., & Bosch, A.M. (2010). Psychosocial aspects of PKU: Hidden disabilities—A review. *Molecular Genetics and Metabolism*, 99(Suppl. 1), S64–S67.

Gieselmann, V., & Krägeloh-Mann, I. (2010). Metachromatic leukodystrophy: An update. *Neuropediatrics*, 41(1), 1–6.

Gitiaux, C., Roze, E., Kinugawa, K., Flamand-Rouvière, C., Boddaert, N., Apartis, E., … Bahi-Buisson, N. (2008). Spectrum of movement disorders associated with glutaric aciduria type 1: A study of 16 patients. *Movement Disorders*, 23(16), 2392–2397.

Gouider-Khouja, N., Kraoua, I., Benrhouma, H., Fraj, N., & Rouissi, A. (2010). Movement disorders in neuro-metabolic diseases. *European Journal of Paediatric Neurology*, 14(4), 304–307.

Gropman, A.L., Summar. M., & Leonard, J.V. (2007). Neurological implications of urea cycle disorders. *Journal of Inherited Metabolic Disease*, 30(6), 865–879.

Grubb, J.H., Vogler, C, & Sly, W.S. (2010). New strategies for enzyme replacement therapy for lysosomal storage diseases. *Rejuvenation Research*, 13(2–3), 229–236.

Hamosh, A., Scharer, G., & Van Hove, J. (2009). Glycine Encephalopathy. In R.A. Pagon, T.C. Bird, C.R. Dolan, & K. Stephens (Eds.), *GeneReviews 1993*. Seattle, WA: University of Washington. Retrieved from http://www.ncbi.nlm.nih.gov/bookshelf/br.fcgi?book=gene&part=nkh.

Hanley, W.B., Linsao, L.S., & Netley, C. (1971). The efficacy of dietary therapy for phenylketonuria. *Canadian Medical Association Journal*, 104(12), 1089–1091.

Hollak, C.E., de Fost, M., van Dussen, L., Vom Dahl, S., & Aerts, J.M. (2009). Enzyme therapy for the treatment of type 1 Gaucher disease: Clinical outcomes and dose-response relationships. *Expert Opinion on Pharmacotherapy*, 10(16), 2641–2652.

Jakóbkiewicz-Banecka, J., Wegrzyn, A., & Wegrzyn, G. (2007). Substrate deprivation therapy: A new hope for patients suffering from neuronopathic forms of inherited lysosomal storage diseases. *Journal of Applied Genetics*, 48(4), 383–388.

Jalanko, A., & Braulke, T. (2009). Neuronal ceroid lipofuscinoses. *Biochim Biophys Acta*, 1793(4), 697–709.

Jardim, L.B., Villanueva, M.M., de Souza, C.F., & Netto, C.B. (2010). Clinical aspects of neuropathic lysosomal storage disorders. *Journal of Inherited Metabolic Disease*, 33(4), 315–329.

Kamboj, M. (2008). Clinical approach to the diagnoses of inborn errors of metabolism. *Pediatric Clinics of North America*, 55(5), 1113–1127, viii.

Krivitzky, L., Babikian, T., Lee, H.S., Thomas, N.H., Burk-Paull, K.L., & Batshaw, M.L. (2009). Intellectual, adaptive, and behavioral functioning in children with urea cycle disorders. *Pediatric Research*, 66(1), 96–101.

Lafranchi, S.H. (2010). Newborn screening strategies for congenital hypothyroidism: An update. *Journal of Inherited Metabolic Disease*, 33(2), S225–233.

Lee, P.J., Ridout, D., & Walter, J.H. (2005). Cockburn, F. Maternal phenylketonuria: Report from the United Kingdom Registry 1978–97. *Archives of Disease in Childhood*, 90(2), 143–146.

Levy, P.A. (2009a). Inborn errors of metabolism: Part 1: Overview. *Pediatrics in Review*, 30(4), 131–137.

Levy, P.A. (2009b). Inborn errors of metabolism: Part 2: Specific disorders. *Pediatrics in Review*, 30(4), e22–e28.

Lichter-Konecki, U., Mangin, J.M., Gordish-Dressman, H., Hoffman, E.P., & Gallo, V. (2008). Gene expression profiling of astrocytes from hyperammonemic mice reveals altered pathways for water and potassium homeostasis in vivo. *Glia*, 56(4), 365–377.

Lim-Melia, E.R., & Kronn, D.F. (2009). Current enzyme replacement therapy for the treatment of lysosomal storage diseases. *Pediatric Annals*, 38(8), 448–455.

Martins, A.M., Dualibi, A.P., Norato, D., Takata, E.T., Santos, E.S., Valadares, E.R., …Guedes, Z.C. (2009). Guidelines for the management of mucopolysaccharidosis type I. *The Journal of Pediatrics*, 155(4 Suppl), S32–S46.

Martins, A.M., Valadares, E.R., Porta, G., Coelho, J., Semionato Filho, J., Pianovski, M.A., … Brazilian Study Group on Gaucher Disease and other Lysosomal Storage Diseases. (2009). Recommendations on diagnosis, treatment, and monitoring for Gaucher disease. *The Journal of Pediatrics*, 155(4 Suppl), S10–S18.

Masurel-Paulet, A., Poggi-Bach, J., Rolland, M.O., Bernard, O., Guffon, N., Dobbelaere, D., …Touati, G. (2008). NTBC treatment in tyrosinaemia type I: Long-term outcome in French patients. *Journal of Inherited Metabolic Disease*, 31(1), 81–87.

McEachern, K.A., Fung, J., Komarnitsky, S., Siegel, C.S., Chuang, W.L., Hutto, E., … Marshall, J. (2007). A specific and potent inhibitor of glucosylceramide synthase for substrate inhibition therapy of Gaucher disease. *Molecular Genetics and Metabolism*, 91(3), 259–267.

Michals, K., Azen, C., Acosta, P., Koch, R., & Matalon, R. (1988). Blood phenylalanine levels and intelligence of 10-year-old children with PKU in the National Collaborative Study. *Journal of the American Diabetic Association, 88*(10), 1226–1229.

Moini, M., Mistry, P., & Schilsky, M.L. (2010). Liver transplantation for inherited metabolic disorders of the liver. *Current Opinion in Organ Transplant, 15*(3), 269–276.

Muenzer, J., Wraith, J.E., Clarke, L.A., & International Consensus Panel on Management and Treatment of Mucopolysaccharidosis I. (2009). Mucopolysaccharidosis I: management and treatment guidelines. *Pediatrics, 123*(1), 19–29.

Nimkarn, S., & New, M.I. (2010). Congenital adrenal hyperplasia due to 21-hydroxylase deficiency: A paradigm for prenatal diagnosis and treatment. *Annuals of the New York Academy of Sciences, 1192*(1), 5–11.

Nutrition Committee of the Canadian Paediatric Society. (1990). Megavitamin and megamineral therapy in childhood. *Canadian Medical Association Journal, 143*, 1009–1013.

Nyhan, W.L., O'Neill, J.P., Jinnah, H.A., & Harris, J.C. (2010). *Lesch-Nyhan syndrome.* 2000 Sep 25 [updated 2010 Jun 10]. In R.A. Pagon, T.C. Bird, C.R. Dolan, & K. Stephens (Eds.), GeneReviews 1993. Seattle, WA: University of Washington. Retrieved from http://www.ncbi.nlm.nih.gov/bookshelf/br.fcgi?book=gene&part=lns

Online Mendelian Inheritance in Man. (2010). McKusick-Nathans Institute of Genetic Medicine, Johns Hopkins University and National Center for Biotechnology Information, National Library of Medicine. Retrieved from: http://www.ncbi.nlm.nih.gov/Online Mendelian Inheritance in Man/

Orchard, P.J., & Tolar, J. (2010). Transplant outcomes in leukodystrophies. *Seminars in Hematology, 47*(1), 70–80.

Pastores, G.M., Giraldo, P., Chérin, P., & Mehta, A. (2009). Goal-oriented therapy with miglustat in Gaucher disease. *Current Medical Research Opinion, 25*(1), 23–37.

Pastores, G.M., & Hughes, D.A. (2000, July). Gaucher Disease. [updated 2008 Mar 13] In R.A. Pagon, T.C. Bird, C.R. Dolan, & K. Stephens. (Eds.), GeneReviews 1993-. Seattle, WA: University of Washington. Retrieved from http://www.ncbi.nlm.nih.gov/bookshelf/br.fcgi?book=gene&part=gaucher.

Picker, J.D., & Levy, H.L. (2006, March). Homocystinuria Caused by Cystathionine Beta-Synthase Deficiency. Jan 15 [updated 2006 Mar 29]. Seattle, WA: University of Washington. In R.A. Pagon, T.C. Bird, C.R. Dolan, & K. Stephens (Eds.), GeneReviews 1993-. Seattle, WA: University of Washington. Retrieved from http://www.ncbi.nlm.nih.gov/bookshelf/br.fcgi?book=gene&part=homocystinuria

Pineda, M., Perez-Poyato, M.S., O'Callaghan, M., Vilaseca, M.A., Pocovi, M., Domingo, R., ... Coll, M.J. (2010). Clinical experience with miglustat therapy in pediatric patients with Niemann-Pick disease type C: A case series. *Molecular Genetics and Metabolism, 99*(4), 358–366.

Pitt, J.J. (2010). Newborn screening. *Clinical Biochemistry Review, 31*(2), 57–68.

Poustie. V.J., & Wildgoose, J. (2010). Dietary interventions for phenylketonuria. *Cochrane Database of Systematic Reviews, 20*(1), CD001304.

Prasad, V.K., & Kurtzberg, J. (2010). Transplant outcomes in mucopolysaccharidoses. *Seminars in Hematology, 47*(1), 59–69.

Rakheja, D., Narayan, S.B., & Bennett, M.J. (2007). Juvenile neuronal ceroid-lipofuscinosis (Batten disease): A brief review and update. *Current Molecular Medicine, 7*(6), 603–608.

Raper, S.E., Chirmule, N., Lee, F.S., Wivel, N.A., Bagg, A., Guang-ping, G., ... Batshaw, M.L. (2003). Fatal systemic inflammatory response syndrome in an ornithine transcarbamylase deficient patient following adenoviral gene transfer. *Molecular Genetics and Metabolism, 80*(1–2), 148–158.

Sahai, I., & Marsden, D. (2009). Newborn screening. *Critical Review of Clinical Labratory Science, 46*(2), 55–82.

Sarkissian, C.N., Gámez, A., Wang, L., Charbonneau, M., Fitzpatrick, P., Lemontt, J.F., ... Scriver, C.R. (2008). Preclinical evaluation of multiple species of PEGylated recombinant phenylalanine ammonia lyase for the treatment of phenylketonuria. *Proceedings of the National Academy of Sciences of the United States of America, 105*(52), 20894–20899.

Seminara, J., Tuchman, M., Krivitzky, L., Krischer, J., Lee, H.S., Lemons, C., ...Batshaw, M.L. (2010). Establishing a consortium for the study of rare diseases: The Urea Cycle Disorders Consortium. *Molecular Genetics and Metabolism, 100*(Suppl. 1), S97–S105.

Semmler, A., Köhler, W., Jung, H.H., Weller, M., & Linnebank, M. (2008). Therapy of X-linked adrenoleukodystrophy. *Expert Review of Neurotherapeutics, 8*(9), 1367–1379.

Sevin, C., Cartier-Lacave, N., & Aubourg, P. (2009). Gene therapy in metachromatic leukodystrophy. *International Journal of Clinical Pharmacology and Therapeutics, 47*(Suppl. 1), S128–131.

Shapiro, B.E., Pastores, G.M., Gianutsos, J., Luzy, C., & Kolodny, E.H. (2009). Miglustat in late-onset Tay-Sachs disease: A 12-month, randomized, controlled clinical study with 24 months of extended treatment. *Genetics in Medicine, 11*(6), 425–433.

Shih, V.E. (1976). Hereditary ura-cycle disorders. In S. Grisolia, R. Baguena & E. Mayor (Eds.), *The urea cycle* (pp. 367–414). Hoboken, NY: John Wiley & Sons.

Shihabuddin, L.S., & Aubert, I. (2010). Stem cell transplantation for neurometabolic and neurodegenerative diseases. *Neuropharmacology, 58*(6), 845–854.

Sniderman King, L., Trahms, C., & Scott, C.R. (2006). *Tyrosinemia type 1.* 2006 Jul 24 [updated 2008 Oct 21]. In R.A. Pagon, T.C. Bird, C.R. Dolan, & K. Stephens (Eds.), GeneReviews 1993-. Seattle, WA: University of Washington. Retrieved from http://www.ncbi.nlm.nih.gov/books/NBK1116/

Steinberg, S.J., Dodt, G., Raymond, G.V., Braverman, N.E., Moser, A.B., & Moser, H.W. (2006). Peroxisome biogenesis disorders. *Biochimica et Biophysica Acta, 1763*(12),1733–1748.

Suzuki, Y., Kure, S., Oota, M., Hino, H., & Fukuda, M. (2010). Nonketotic hyperglycinemia: Proposal of a diagnostic and treatment strategy. *Pediatric Neurology, 43*(3), 221–224.

van der Sluijs Veer, L., Kempers, M.J., Last, B.F., Vulsma, T., & Grootenhuis, M.A. (2008). Quality of life, developmental milestones, and self-esteem of young adults with congenital hypothyroidism diagnosed by neonatal screening. *Journal of Clinical Endocrinology and Metabolism, 93*(7), 2654–2661.

van Spronsen, F.J. (2010). Phenylketonuria: A 21st century perspective. *Nature Reviews Endocrinology, 6*(9), 509–514.

Waisbren, S.E., Mahon, B.E., Schnell, R.R., & Levy, H.L. (1987). Predictors of intelligence quotient and intelligence quotient change in persons treated for phenylketonuria early in life. *Pediatrics, 79*(3), 351–355.

Wolf, B. (2010). Clinical issues and frequent questions about biotinidase deficiency. *Molecular Genetics and Metabolism, 100*(1), 6–13.

Wraith, J.E. (2009). Enzyme replacement therapy for the management of the mucopolysaccharidoses. *International Journal of Clinical Pharmacology and Therapeutics, 47*(Suppl. 1), S63–S65.

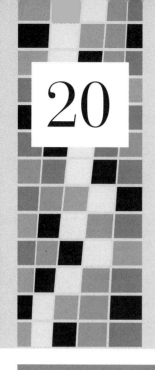

20

Speech and Language Disorders

Sheela Stuart

Upon completion of this chapter, the reader will

- Be able to describe the different elements of speech and of language
- Be familiar with the biological processes that underlie speech and language
- Understand the typical course of language development
- Understand considerations in bilingual language acquisition
- Know the major types of speech and language disorders and their causes
- Be aware of the methods of speech and language assessment
- Recognize the treatment approaches for these communication disorders

As humans, one of the major means of participating in our lives is through communication. We complain, calm, greet, request, inform, question, praise, compliment, argue, demand, order, correct, beg, invite, cajole (and so the list continues). Although there are many different elaborate, sophisticated, versatile, and creative ways of communicating (e.g., body language, signing), the means most frequently used is talking. Therefore, families herald a child's first words with joy, and when there is a problem in the development of the child's ability to talk, anxiety occurs. The following letter is an example of this situation.

▪ ▪ ▪ LETTER FROM A WORRIED GRANDMOTHER

Dear Pediatric Speech Pathologist: My grandson, David, is 2½ years old. Although as an infant he cooed and babbled and began walking at 12 months, he has never talked. He often grunts and points to things he wants, and he has begun to consistently make a few sounds for "mama," "daddy," "up," "bow wow," and "cup." He has never been seriously ill, and an audiological evaluation revealed normal hearing.

He was evaluated by a speech-language pathologist (SLP). During this evaluation, the therapist played with David. She tried to get him to say words and imitate animal sounds that she made, and they spent some time looking in the mirror while she tried to get him to imitate facial expressions. She also asked him to look at pictures in a book and do things she requested (point to the picture of the baby, put the block in the box, behind the bear, and so forth). In addition, she used a long interview sheet. She asked David's mother about how he plays, what he does to interact with her and with other children, whether he follows directions, and so forth. Her report concluded that David's receptive language was at approximately the 18- to 20-month level, and his expressive language was at approximately the 9- to 12-month level at 30 months chronological age. We still have many questions. What causes this type of problem? Will David eventually talk? If his parents decide to have another child, is this type of problem likely to reoccur?

This chapter approaches Grandmother's questions by describing the physiological aspects of talking (i.e., speech and language), what can go wrong, and how to evaluate and treat impairments. We have included the typical developmental pathway/timeline used as a guideline in determining delays and/or disorders (see Table 20.1). Acknowledging that there is no single way children learn to communicate, we have also included information about bilingualism and cultural influences in language acquisition. We discuss the underlying causes of speech and language disorders, including findings of genetic links to specific communication disorders. Finally, we address the various types of therapy and compensatory approaches used to overcome communication disorders.

COMPONENTS OF COMMUNICATION

Communication has been studied by many different professionals including linguists, psychologists, anthropologists, literature scholars, SLPs, neuropsychologists, and even engineers and biologists. Because each profession's interest in communication comes from a different perspective, the resulting information includes a variety of terminology and at times contrasting viewpoints.

Regardless of the perspective, it is recognized that the human brain is the underlying mechanism that supports and coordinates the separate processes of communication. The brain is a dynamic organ, the function of which varies depending upon the age, personal experiences, and even gender of the individual. The brain includes interconnecting pathways among areas that regulate, integrate, and formulate communicative messages. Many of the specific functions related to hearing, speech, and language are found in the cerebrum (cerebral cortex). The frontal lobe of the cerebrum contains the primary motor and Broca's speech production areas. The temporal lobe contains

Table 20.1. Indications for speech-language evaluation

Age for referral	Indications for referral
Birth to 6 months	Does not respond to environmental sounds or voices
3–4 months	Does not gesture or make sounds to indicate he or she wants you to do something
	Has no interactive eye gaze
1 year	Does not follow simple commands or understand simple questions (e.g., "Roll the ball," "Kiss the doll," "Where's your shoe?")
	Does not say 8–10 words spontaneously
	Does not identify three body parts on self or doll
2 years	Does not use some one- or two-word questions (e.g., "Where kitty?" "Go bye-bye?" "What's that?")
	Does not use at least 50 understandable, different words
	Does not refer to self by name or pronoun (e.g., "me," "mine")
3 years	Does not understand differences in meaning (e.g., go/stop, in/on, big/little, up/down)
	Does not respond to wh-questions (e.g., who, what, where)
	Does not tell you about something in two- or three-word "sentences"
4 years	Has difficulty learning new concepts and words
	Still echoes speech
	Has unclear speech
	Does not explain events

the primary auditory and Wernicke's speech comprehension areas. The occipital lobe is concerned with vision, and the parietal lobe controls somatesthetic (bodily) sensations. It is important to state that this description may give an impression that is deceptively simple. In an article by Ross (2010), an argument is made to suggest that functional localization of behavior related to specific areas of the brain (such as language) is a much more robust, dynamic, and four-dimensional process. Ross further states that localization of such functions as language are a learned phenomenon driven over time by large-scale, spatially distributed, neural networks that process, store and manipulate information for cognitive and behavioral operations.

It is useful to understand some general information about the complex activities of understanding (receptive) and producing (expressive) language. An example of receptive language functioning occurs when a person hears the word "cup." The sound signal is transmitted along the auditory pathway, which then sends it to Wernicke's area, in which neurons that correspond to that particular combination of sounds are activated. Other neurons are then activated to store a visual picture of a cup, and additional ones store concepts about how cups are used. If a person wishes to name the object "cup," he or she would first activate the internal visual picture of a cup (e.g., shape, uses, materials used for cups). These ideas would be channeled through the speech area of the brain (Broca's area). Here, these thoughts are converted into patterns of motor movement, then transmitted to the motor strip located in the frontal lobe of the cerebrum, in which impulses for the muscle movement needed to produce the sound /cup/ are transmitted.

To answer David's grandmother's questions, it will be important to discuss aspects of specific areas involved in the process of listening and talking. We provide a brief summary of the general components of the communication process and remind the reader that this is a complex process in which components work interactively (Figure 20.1).

Hearing

To develop typical speech, children must perceive speech sounds. Normal hearing (see Chapter 10) is essential to this process so that children have an active model based on what they hear and can monitor and modify what they say. Infants actually begin listening to speech and language *in utero* (Sohmer, Perez, Sichel, Priner, & Freeman,

2001). As related to speech and language, hearing includes being able to perceive the sounds (auditory perception) and being able to decode the different sounds for meaning (auditory processing). At birth, infants are able to listen to and discriminate among different speech sounds. The newborn immediately begins to listen to the stream of speech sounds within his or her environment and begins attaching meaning to these sounds. The infant also becomes both sensitive to speech sound contrasts that make up the native language and insensitive to unimportant phonetic contrasts

Speech

Speech involves the production of sounds and syllables according to language rules. Voice is the sound source for producing words. Breath from the lungs is channeled through the larynx and provides the power source to set the vocal folds vibrating, producing sound. The sound is shaped into specific patterns by a series of rapid movements of various structures in the mouth, including the tongue and lips, a process called articulation.

Prosody

Prosody involves the use of pitch, loudness, tempo, and rhythm in speech to convey information about the structure and meaning of an utterance. Achieving the goal of communication through talking requires that a child produce words in a particular easy fluid manner. This process involves the joining of sounds, syllables, words, and phrases within oral language without hesitations or repetitions. It involves rate, rhythm, stress, and the use of suprasegmentals. This area of speech production is commonly called *fluency*.

Language

Language includes three major components (form, content, and use), each containing basic rule systems. Form includes the processes syntax, morphology, and phonology that connect sounds and symbols (words) in order. Content includes meaning or semantics, and use includes the area called pragmatics.

When we talk, the following occurs according to the rules for each component: We have an idea and encode it (semantics) into a symbol (e.g., sound/word). To produce this word we select appropriate sound units (phonology), appropriate word beginnings and endings to further define meaning (morphology), and appropriate word order (syntax).

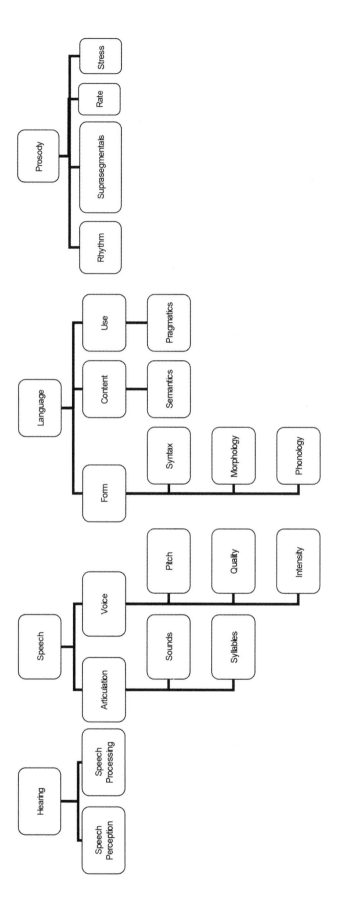

Figure 20.1. Components of human communication.

Finally, the purpose of talking is to accomplish a functional goal as we participate in life. Pragmatics provides the rules for using language contextually to achieve functions. For example, to request, comment, repair/clarify, reject/protest, and question we must adhere to the rules of form and content, and pragmatics (Beukelman & Mirenda, 2005).

TYPICAL DEVELOPMENT OF SPEECH AND LANGUAGE

At birth babies cry, coo, and then begin to babble, but these are reflexive, nonreflexive, and vegetative sounds. A very young infant cries out of distress or discomfort. The infant is not crying with the desire of conveying a message. Therefore, the productions at this time are termed preintentional communications (Sachs, 2005.)

However, Harding (1983) noted that the mother assigns a meaning/message to the preintentional communications and responds to the infant's needs. The response (including the mother talking to the child in an engaging, encouraging manner) creates the possibility for the child to begin using different cries to communicate different messages. During the first year, the infant progresses to become an intentional communicator, and by the second year the communicative intent becomes encoded into words and language.

An infant's first words are produced around 12 months and are related to the world of objects and events. Research has revealed that the process of acquiring words and expanding language is highly correlated to joint attention, social cognition, and cultural influences (Strauss & Ziv, 2001; Tomasello, 2000). The joint attention/social cognition behaviors have been incorporated into a concept called "Theory of Mind" that addresses the development of a child's ability to understand the mental states and behaviors of others. Miller (2006) states that although Theory of Mind requires several years to develop, it begins with the infant's joint attention or joint reference.

In typical development, a child's own preferences and tendencies, as well as the caregivers' use of language and the course of communication/interactions throughout each day contribute to the language acquisition process. Maternal behaviors often involve repetitive routines and sequences/games (Owens, 2008a). The mother might say, "How big are you?" "SOOOO Big!" "That big?" Repetitions such as this maintain joint attention while offering opportunities for turn-taking and unique child expression.

Although speech and language learning continues throughout life, language learners generally go through two waves of language acquisition: 1) developing form-function or "rule" knowledge, and 2) refining skills involving increased speed of verbal communication and processing. Cummins (1991) discussed the need for English language learners to develop conversational competence that he called basic interpersonal communication skills (BICS) and competence in communicating within the classroom called cognitive academic language proficiency (CALP). Knowledge about each of the developmental stages provides the basis for the formal testing used in assessing language skills, with a caveat that "typical development" includes wide individual variability.

BILINGUALISM

In 2010, the U.S. Census Bureau reported that 16.8% of children between 5 and 17 years of age (or about 9 million) were bilingual, speaking English "very well" alongside another language spoken at home (U.S. Census Bureau, 2010). Children learning two languages follow the general acquisition patterns previously described, but there are additional factors to be considered. The child is not only learning two languages but also two cultures, a process called *language socialization*. This socialization involves ways in which language learning reflects and is used to further develop personhood, status, and authority (Genesee, Paradis, & Crago, 2004; Paugh, 2005). The second language may be learned simultaneously or successively. In simultaneous acquisition both languages develop prior to age 3. This is characterized by initial language mixing, followed by a slow division of vocabulary and form-function rules. In successive acquisition a child learns one language (L1) at home followed by a second language (L2) at school after the age of 3 years (Owens, 2008b).

It is a common assumption that bilingual children are at a disadvantage or delayed in their language development. Although there can be these effects, the reality is much more complex. Kohnert (2004) studied typically developing bilingual children and found that the two languages may develop at similar rates and in a similar direction, or they may diverge so that the skill in one language increases at the same time that the skill in the other language reaches a plateau or decreases. Variability in the timeframes and patterns of language acquisition, as well as variability in the child's resulting competence in each language, has become the norm of developing bilingualism (Kohnert & Goldstein, 2005). True balanced bilingualism (skill level comparable in both languages) is rare.

COMMUNICATION DISORDERS

By first grade, 5% of children in the United States are identified as having some type of a communication disorder (National Institute on Deafness and other Communication Disorders [NIDCD], 2010). In some instances this is an associated impairment, secondary to underlying hearing loss, trauma, autism, cognitive disability, or genetic syndrome. For the majority of children, however, the cause is unknown. Genetic associations with various communication disorders are being identified (Kang et al., 2010; Shriberg et al., 2005, 2006) and may form the basis for interventions focused on remediating the underlying impairment.

ASSESSMENT

The process of the speech-language assessment includes a primary caregiver interview, an examination of the child's oral motor mechanism and functioning, testing of receptive and expressive language, and evaluation of speech sound production, voice, and fluency. It is important to include an audiological examination to determine the status of the child's hearing, preferably prior to a speech-language assessment.

The assessment includes the SLPs' clinical observations of the child's interactions during the session with people, toys, and books. In addition, the SLP will assess the child's abilities through the use of standardized tests and gather additional information with informal checklists. Standardized tests are designed to assist the examiner in determining if the child lags behind children of his or her age in the use of particular speech or language skills.

Table 20.2 is a listing of some frequently used formal measures of speech and language skills. There obviously are many more and different standardized instruments. The tests sample various aspects of speech and/or language performance. The SLP will make the choice of testing instruments based upon the testing focus.

TYPES OF COMMUNCATION DISORDERS

Speech Disorders

Speech disorders are caused by problems in making sounds correctly. These are most frequently due to 1) articulation difficulties—not making the sound in the proper area of the oral mechanism and/or proper movements of the oral mechanism (tongue, lips, teeth, jaw) to produce the sound properly; 2) phonological processing disorders—not learning the rules about which sounds go together in specific positions within words when sounds are voiced or voiceless; and 3) resonance disorders—atypical amounts of nasality, often caused by structural malformations such as enlarged adenoids and tonsils, or structural anomalies such as a deviated septum.

There is a developmental progression in the ability to accurately articulate phonemes. In English, the sounds /p/ and /b/ may be correctly produced by 12–24 months, but sounds such as /r/ and /l/ may take a child up to age 6 to correctly produce (Goldman & Fristoe, 2000). Sound patterns, such as vowel–consonant and consonant–vowel–consonant, require practice to produce correctly, especially when they are in different positions within words. The child's abilities depend on the interaction of their hearing/attending (listening to others produce the sounds and self-monitoring their productions) and the control and coordination of the movement and placement of tongue, lips, and jaw.

Language Disorders

Children with developmental disabilities struggle with language development. As in the previous discussion, there are many causes, hearing being one of the first considerations (see Chapter 10). The degree of hearing impairment (mild versus severe-profound) has a variable impact on acquiring speech and oral language. Without appropriate opportunities to learn language, however, children with hearing loss will fall behind their hearing peers in communication, cognition, reading, and social-emotional development (Joint Committee on Infant Hearing, 2007). It should be noted that the long-held belief that conductive hearing loss associated with middle ear infection (otitis media) can have long-term consequences for typically developing children has been disproved (Zumach, Gerrits, Chenault, & Anteunis, 2010).

Table 20.2. Frequently used measures of speech and language skills

Test	Ages	Description
Bankson-Bernthal Test of Phonology (BBTOP; Bankson & Bernthal, 1990)	2–16 years	Identifies error patterns according to distinctive features and phonological processes
Peabody Picture Vocabulary Test—4th Edition (PPVT-4, Dunn & Dunn, 2007).	2½–adult	Tests receptive vocabulary
MacArthur-Bates Communicative Development Inventories (CDIs), Second Edition (Fenson et al., 2007)	8–37 months	Develops a profile of communicative behaviors in words and gestures (CDI: Words and Gestures, 8–18 months); Spanish version available Develops a profile of communicative behaviors in words and sentences (CDI: Words and Sentences, 16–30 months); Spanish version available Measures expressive vocabulary and grammar (CDI-III, 30–37 months)
Expressive One-Word Picture Vocabulary Test–2000 Edition (EOWPVT-2000; Brownell, 2000)	2–15 years	Tests expressive vocabulary
Goldman-Fristoe Test of Articula-tion–2 (GFTA-2; Goldman & Fristoe, 2000)	2–16 years	Assesses articulation of consonant sounds
The Rossetti Infant-Toddler Language Scale (Rossetti, 2006).	Birth to 36 months	Develops a profile of communicative behaviors in six areas: interaction-attachment, pragmatics, gesture, play, language comprehension, and language expression
Clinical Evaluation of Language Fun-damentals, 4th Edition. (CELF-4, Semel, Wiig, & Secord, 2003).	6–21 years	Has multiple subtests of expressive and receptive language, tapping grammar semantics, phonology, sentence recall, and paragraph comprehension; Spanish version available
Clinical Evaluation of Language Fundamentals—Preschool-2 (CELF-Preschool 2; Wiig, Secord, & Semel, 2004).	3–6 years	Contains multiple subtests of receptive language, tapping semantics, morphology, syntax, and expressive language and assesses phonology, sentence recall, and auditory memory
Preschool language Scales, 5th Edi-tion. (PLS-5; Zimmerman, Steiner, & Pond, 2011)	Birth to 6 years	Has subscales on auditory comprehension and expressive communication; Spanish version avail-able

Regardless of the etiology of a language disorder, the manner and extent to which language development is affected varies from child to child. Ultimately, there is an effect on how the child is able to listen to talking within the environment, analyze it, associate it with a multitude of experiences, and use his or her communication system to respond and/or imitate. As examples, the child may 1) be slow to remember the specific names of objects, 2) not understand or use functional words (e.g., *the, am, to*), 3) not understand the implication of word endings (e.g., *-ing, -ed, -s*), and 4) be delayed in being able to produce multiword sentences. Children with autism spectrum disorder may be able to produce words that are imitated (echolalia) but may have difficulty spontaneously generating words to meet their communicative needs. Children with Asperger's Disorder may have accurately developed linguistic elements of language but make errors in pragmatics, such as turn-taking and topic-sharing during conversation. Some children experience problems in more than one area of language development.

Fluency Disorders

As children develop speech and language, they also develop the skill to produce the words in a smooth, flowing, and effortless manner. They are able to produce a series of words without hesitation, repetition, or sound prolongation. They pause at the conceptually appropriate time and continue talking without any evidence of a struggle to resume producing words. These children have achieved fluency.

Some children (usually between ages 2–4 years) experience a type of developmental disfluency. This is characterized by hesitations, repetitions of a sound (*b-b-but*), or repetitions of syllables or words (*but but but*) and/or fillers (*um, well, uh*). This speech behavior often appears during a period of rapid progress in language acquisition and is not considered to be a real communication disorder.

A small percentage of children demonstrate greater degrees of disfluency (both in frequency of occurrence and types of disfluencies). For example, they produce more part word repetitions than expected in typical child speech, and more than 10 repeated words, syllables, or sounds per hundred words (Bloodstein & Bernstein Ratner, 2007). Very importantly, as the child continues to experience disfluencies, he or she becomes increasingly aware of them and expresses frustration. These are the symptoms of stuttering.

Genetic studies have found that a susceptibility to stuttering may be inherited and that it is most likely to occur in boys (Kang et al., 2010; Yairi & Ambrose, 2005). Congenital brain damage is also suspected to be a predisposing factor in some cases. For the most part, however, children who stutter have neither a family history of the disorder nor clear evidence of brain damage. Brain imaging studies in adults who stutter show deactivation of the left-hemisphere sensorimotor centers and overactivation of the identical right-hemisphere structures during both stuttered and nonstuttered speech. The essential defect is hypothesized to be a lack of sensorimotor integration necessary to regulate the rapid movements of fluent speech (Ingham, 2003).

By age 7 more than half of all children who stutter as preschoolers are reported to have recovered (Bloodstein & Bernstein Ratner, 2007). Therapy (fluency shaping and stuttering modification) can be helpful for those children who continue to have difficulties producing fluent speech.

TREATMENT APPROACHES

A treatment plan and its supporting intervention techniques should be 1) based on findings during the assessment, 2) related to the most appropriate research (evidence-based practice), and 3) designed to meet the individual's needs (American Speech-Language-Hearing Association [ASHA], 2007). It requires discussions with the family, observation of interactive and play skills, and an ongoing collection of speech-language samples. Best practice also requires the SLP to spend considerable time discussing with the primary caregiver and, when possible, other team members, the general impressions from the assessment. During these discussions, the SLP will delineate the factors correlated with outcome from a communication disorder, including early identification and specific causes and severity of the communication impairment (Bashir & Scavuzzo, 1992).

In addition, it is understood that the "who, how, and where" of intervention is very important in achieving a good outcome. Building an intervention program that is carried out collaboratively with individuals who regularly interact with the child (parents, extended family, preschool staff), and consideration of places and activities in which the child is regularly involved is essential to success. Therapy in natural settings involving collaboration with caregivers achieves at least three major benefits for the child: 1) enhanced relationships among family members, therapists, educational staff, and parents; 2) modeling and support to facilitate caregivers in their work in addressing the child's problems; and 3) improved ability to assess a child's functioning and set appropriate, meaningful outcome goals (Bowen & Cupples, 2004; Hanft & Pikington, 2000). Therefore, the ideal approach for designing therapy involves creating a team approach that incorporates all the specialized knowledge about the child, the child's culture, and input from the key members of the child's environment.

Observing and recognizing opportunities for the child to use communication to participate in the activities and routines that occur within his or her environments will be critical to the intervention plan. The therapist's challenge will be to find creative ways to translate expertise and knowledge into meaningful interventions to support the child in learning while participating. This will mean that the speech-language intervention includes targeting words for modeling and imitation within joint attention activities and reinforcing all types of vocalization and word approximations as well as compensatory therapy approaches.

In a compensatory approach, strategies and supports are designed for children to bypass their communicative limitations. Because the goal for every child is functional communication that supports him or her in participating in all the activities of life, the compensatory approach may include signing, low-tech symbols, and speech-generating devices of various levels of complexity.

Parents often fear that the introduction of a compensatory approach will foster dependence on an artificial means of communication and further delay verbal development. The opposite has been found to be the case (Light & Drager, 2007). Even when it seems likely that oral speech may eventually develop, augmentative and alternative communication (AAC) is often used to prevent delayed communication development and to support communicative participation in daily activities.

AAC includes sign language, picture communication boards, object symbols, adapted books, and low-tech or high-tech speech-generating devices (see Chapter 36). Parents, preschool teachers, siblings, and friends all need to learn ways to use the specific customized AAC items when interacting with the child whose verbal speech is not adequate to his or her communicative needs. Each of these AAC approaches should be used within the naturally occurring routines of a child's daily activities. The specific signs, pictures on a board, object symbols and messages in a speech-generating device are chosen on the basis of what the child's needs are within activities.

Sign language (e.g., American Sign Language [ASL]), which is used with deaf individuals, can also provide a visual and tactile representation of spoken words that serves as a "ready" vocabulary for the child with limited verbal output due to a language disorder. The signs often include the names for favorite toys, activities, people, as well as phrases to control actions. For example, "want," "more," "please," and "thank you" have many applications over the course of a day. Most parents and teachers are encouraged to choose 20 or 30 signs that are relevant to their child and social situations. If the child is unable to make the signs perfectly, approximations are accepted. The goal is for the child to have an easy, consistent means of transferring information.

Picture boards and object symbols can be used to highlight simple vocabulary choices for home routines (e.g., cereal or milk) or to tell complex stories (e.g., a visit to the zoo). They can be organized to offer special tactile cues (for children with visual impairments) or to request individual interests (e.g., string enjoyed by a child with autism).

Speech-generating devices contain prerecorded messages in a single form or in combination. They can be simple or complex, depending on the child's abilities and needs. By touching a button or pressing a switch, the device will speak a message supporting the child in participating in academic games such as circle time, asking a question, or introducing him- or herself.

It is important that the AAC system be designed through collaboration with all the individuals who will interact with the child (caregivers, educators, professionals, and friends). However, the AAC system designer should take the lead in customizing the device to make certain it supports many communication functions, such as questions, jokes, commentary, and requests (Romski, Sevcik, Cheslock, & Barton, 2006).

It should be noted that there are no prerequisites (cognitive milestones, receptive language strengths, demonstrable communicative intent, or *yes/no* consistency) that must be met before the individual becomes a "candidate" for an AAC system. Also, children are never too young or have too severe disabilities or motor impairments to utilize AAC (National Joint Committee for the Communication Needs of Persons with Severe Disabilities [NJC], 2003).

SUMMARY

The ability to communicate provides a primary means of participating in our lives and the lives of others. Therefore, disorders of communication have a profound impact on the very essence of our being. Children who are not talking as early or in a manner expected by their caregivers should receive a speech-language and hearing assessment as soon as possible. The results of this evaluation will enable the SLP to design an intervention that is evidence based. This treatment program will incorporate an understanding of the child as an individual and include his or her caregivers and other important people from his or her environment as team members in the process.

REFERENCES

American Speech-Language-Hearing Association (ASHA; 2007). Scope of practice in speech-language pathology: Ad hoc committee on the scope of practice in speech-language pathology. Retrieved from http://www.asha.org/docs/html/SP2007-00283.html

Bashir, A.S., & Scavuzzo, A. (1992). Children with language disorders: Natural history and academic success. *Journal of Learning Disabilities, 25,* 53–65. doi:10.1177/002221949202500109

Bernthal, J.E., & Bankson, N.W. (1990). *Bankson-Bernthal Test of Phonology.* Austin, TX: Pro-Ed, Inc.

Beukelman, D., & Mirenda, P. (2005). Language learning and development. In D.R. Beukelman & P. Mirenda (Eds.), *Augmentative alternative communication supporting children & adults with complex communication needs* (3rd ed., pp. 327–350). Baltimore, MD: Paul H. Brookes Publishing Co.

Bloodstein, O., & Bernstein Ratner, N. (2007). *A handbook on stuttering* (6th ed.). Clifton Park, NY: Cengage.

Bowen, C., & Cupples, L. (2004). The role of families in optimizing phonological therapy outcomes. *Child Language Teaching and Therapy 20*(3), 245–260. doi:10.1191/0265659004ct274oa

Brownell, R. (2011). *Expressive One-Word Picture Vocabulary Test—2011 Edition.* Novato, CA: Academic Therapy Publications.

Cummins, J. (1991). Language development and academic learning. In L. Malaveand & G. Duquette (Eds.), *Language, culture and cognition.* Clevedon, England: Multilingual Matters.

Dunn, L.M., & Dunn, L.M. (2007). *Peabody Picture Vocabulary Test—4th Edition* (PPVT-IV). Circle Pines, MN: American Guidance Service (AGS).

Fenson L., Marchman, V.A., Thal, D.J., Dale, P.S., Reznick, J.S., & Bates, E. (2007). *MacArthur-Bates communicative development inventories: Users guide and technical manual* (2nd ed.). Baltimore, MD: Paul H. Brookes Publishing Co.

Genesee, F., Paradis, J., & Crago, M. (2004). *Dual language development and disorders.* Baltimore, MD: Paul H. Brookes Publishing Co.

Goldman, R., & Fristoe, M. (2000). *Goldman-Fristoe test of articulation 2.* Circle Pines, MN: American Guidance Service (AGS).

Hanft, B., & Pilkington, K. (2000). Therapy in natural environments: The means or end goal for early intervention. *Infants and Young Children, 12*(4), 1–13.

Harding, C.G. (1983). Setting the stage for language acquisition: Communication development in the first year. In R.M. Golinkoff (Ed.), *The transition from prelinguistic to linguistic communication* (pp. 93–115). Hillsdale, NJ: Erlbaum.

Ingham, R.J. (2003). Brain imaging & stuttering: Some reflections on current and future developments. *Journal of Fluency Disorders, 28*(4), 411–420. doi:10.1016/j.jfludis.2003.08.003

Joint Committee on Infant Hearing. (2007). Year 2007 position statement: Principles and guidelines for early hearing detection and intervention programs. *Pediatrics, 120*(4), 898–921. doi:10.1542/peds.2007-2333

Kang, C., Riazuddin, S., Mundorff, J., Krasnewich, D, Friedman, P., Mullikin, J., & Drayna, D. (2010). Mutations in the lysosomal enzyme-targeting pathway and persistent stuttering. *The New England Journal of Medicine, 362*(8), 677–685. doi:10.1056/NEJMoa0902630

Kohnert, K. (2004). Processing skills in early sequential bilinguals. In B. Goldstein (Ed.), *Bilingual language development and disorders in Spanish-English speakers* (pp. 53–76). Baltimore, MD: Paul H. Brookes Publishing Co.

Kohnert, K., & Goldstein, B. (2005). Speech, language, and hearing in developing bilingual children: From practice to research. *Language, Speech, and Hearing Services in Schools, 36,* 169–171. doi:10.1044/0161-1461(2005/018)

Light, J., & Drager, K. (2007). AAC technologies for young children with complex communication needs: State of the science and future research directions. *Augmentative and Alternative Communication, 23*(3), 204–216. doi:10.1080/07434610701553635

Miller, C.A. (2006). Developmental relationships between language and theory of mind. *American Journal of Speech-Language Pathology, 15,* 142–154. doi:10.1044/1058-0360(2006/014)

National Institute on Deafness and Other Communication Disorders (NIDCD). (2010). U.S. National Library of Medicine. *Medline Plus JCD, 5*(41), 444–457.

National Joint Committee for the Communication Needs of Persons with Severe Disabilities (NJC; 2003). *ASHA Supplement, 23,* 19–20.

Owens, R.E. (2008a). The social and communicative bases of early language and speech. In R.E. Owens (Ed.), *Language development* (7th ed.; pp. 141–144). Boston, MA: Pearson.

Owens, R.E. (2008b). Language differences: Bidialectism and bilingualism. In R.E. Owens (Ed.), *Language development* (7th ed.; pp. 409–413). Boston, MA: Pearson.

Paugh, A.L. (2005). Language socialization. In J. Cohen, K. McCalister, K. Rolstad, & J. MacSwan (Eds.), *Proceedings of the 4th international symposium on bilingualism* (pp. 1807–1820). Somerville, MA: Cascadilla Press.

Romski, M., Sevcik, R., Cheslock, M., & Barton, A. (2006). The system for augmenting language. In R.J. McCauley & M.E. Fey (Eds.), *Treatment of language disorders in children* (pp. 123–147). Baltimore, MD: Paul H. Brookes Publishing Co.

Ross, E.D. (2010). Cerebral localization of functions and the neurology of language: Fact versus fiction or is it something else? *The Neuroscientist, 16*(3), 222–243. doi:10.1177/1073858409349899

Rossetti, L. (2006). *The Rossetti Infant-Toddler Language Scale.* East Moline, IL: LinguiSystems.

Sachs, J. (2005). Communication development in infancy. In J. Berko Gleason (Ed.), *The development of language* (6th ed.; pp. 39–61). Boston, MA: Pearson, Allyn & Bacon.

Semel, E.M., Wiig, E.H., & Secord, W.A. (2004) *Clinical Evaluation of Language Fundamentals, 4th Edition.* San Antonio, TX: Psychological Corporation.

Shriberg, L., Ballard, K., Tomblin, J.B., Duffy, J., Odell, K., & Williams, C. (2006). Speech, prosody, and voice characteristics of a mother and daughter with a 7;13 translocation affecting FOXP2. *Journal of Speech, Language, and Hearing Research, 49,* 500–525. doi:10.1044/1092-4388(2006/038)

Shriberg, L., Lewis, B., Tomblin, J.B., McSweeny, J., Karlsson, H., & Scheer, A. (2005). Toward diagnostic and phenotype markers for genetically transmitted speech delay. *Journal of Speech, Language, and Hearing Research, 48,* 834–852. doi:10.1044/1092-4388(2005/058)

Sohmer, H., Perez, R., Sichel, J.Y., Priner, R., & Freeman, S. (2001). The pathway enabling external sounds to reach and excite the fetal inner ear. *Audiology and Neuro-Otology, 6*(3). 109–116. doi:10.1159/000046817

Strauss, S., & Ziv, M. (2001). Children request teaching when asking for names of objects. *Behavioral and Brain Sciences, 24*(6), 1118–1119. doi:10.1017/S0140525X01380135

Tomasello, M. (2000). First steps toward a usage-based theory of language acquisition. *Cognitive Linguistic, 11*(1–2), 61–82. doi:10.1515/cogl.2001.012

U.S. Census Bureau (2010). Age by Language Spoken at Home by Ability to Speak English for the Population 5 Years and over (Table C16004). 2010 American Community Survey 1–Year Estimates. Retrieved November 21, 2011, from http://factfinder2.census.gov/faces/tableservices/jsf/pages/productview.xhtml?pid=ACS 10 1YR C16004&prodType=table

Wiig, E.H., Secord, W.A. & Semel, E.M. (2004). *Clinical Evaluation of Language Fundamentals—Preschool-2.* San Antonio, TX: Psychological Corporation.

Yairi, E., & Ambrose, N. (2005). Early childhood stuttering. *Journal of Speech, Language, and Hearing Research, 42*, 1125–1135.

Zimmerman, I.L., Steiner, V.G., & Pond, R.E. (2011). *Preschool Language Scale 5 (PLS-5)*. San Antonio, TX: The Psychological Corporation.

Zumach, A., Gerrits, E., Chenault, M., & Anteunis, L. (2010). Long term effects of early life otitis media on language development. *Journal Speech Language & Hearing Research, 53*, 34–43. doi:10.1044/1092-4388(2009/08-0250)

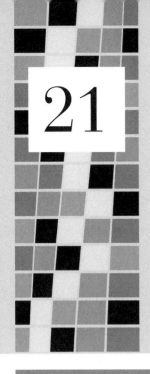

21

Autism Spectrum Disorders

Susan L. Hyman and Susan E. Levy

Upon completion of this chapter, the reader will

- Be familiar with the core features of autism spectrum disorders
- Know about the different studies seeking an etiology for autism spectrum disorders
- Be able to identify the conditions associated with autism spectrum disorders
- Be familiar with interventions and outcomes

Autism spectrum disorders (ASDs) are a class of neurodevelopmental disorders characterized by impairments in social reciprocity, atypical communication, and repetitive behaviors. The term *autism spectrum* indicates that the disorders in this category occur along a continuum. As of January 2012, the classification system for ASDs is in flux. The *Diagnostic and Statistical Manual of Mental Disorders, Fourth Edition, Text Revision* (*DSM-IV-TR*; American Psychiatric Association, 2000) uses the term *Pervasive Developmental Disorders* (PDDs) rather than ASDs because symptoms pervade all areas of development. Included in the *DSM-IV-TR* classification of PDDs are five specific diagnoses: Autistic Disorder, Asperger's Disorder, Rett's Disorder, childhood disintegrative disorder (CDD), and pervasive developmental disorder not otherwise specified (PDD-NOS). In contrast, the new edition of the *Diagnostic and Statistical Manual, DSM-5*, to be published in 2013, will label this group of disorders as autism spectrum disorders

rather than PDDs. Furthermore, *DSM-5* will no longer use the previously mentioned five diagnostic subcategories (Happé, 2011); it will instead include a description of severity level of the ASD. This change has been proposed because distinctions among the subtypes of ASDs in the past have been inconsistent (Lord et al., 2011). In this chapter, the term *ASD* will be used, except when research studies cited have included solely individuals with the more severe category. In these cases the term *Autistic Disorder* will be specifically used because the findings might be different for people with different severities of ASDs.

Although the classification system may be changing, there is general agreement that the symptoms of ASDs are neurologically based, that the disorder has a genetic predisposition, and that gene–environment interaction plays a role (Levy, Mandell, & Schultz, 2009; Muhle, Trentacoste, & Rapin, 2004). It is also recognized that ASDs can occur in conjunction with

1) other functionally defined diagnoses such as intellectual disability and learning disabilities; 2) genetic syndromes such as Rett, Prader Willi, and Williams syndrome; 3) biologically based behaviors, such as tics; and 4) medical conditions including epilepsy (Levy et al., 2010). As noted, *DSM-5* will address these dimensions by characterizing the heterogeneity of the autism spectrum disorders rather then continuing to divide them into subgroups of Autistic Disorder, Asperger's Disorder, and PDD-NOS.

■ ■ ■ JAMES

James is a 10-year-old boy with behavior difficulties that interfere with his progress. His mother reports that he is passive and avoidant at school and becomes agitated, aggressive, and noncompliant at home with her. James is in an autistic support class in third grade. His teacher reports that he has a variety of avoidant and/or self-stimulatory behaviors that are interfering with his progress in school. His avoidant behaviors are characterized by withdrawal (e.g., he shuts his eyes and does not respond to directions; he becomes difficult to engage or "flat"). His self-stimulatory behaviors include self-talk or jargoning and rubbing his eyes; he also seems to be sensitive to loud sounds. At home he has outbursts/meltdowns several times a day, and his mother is often the target. He will obsess/perseverate on parts of toys and will need to (obsessively) hold on to the toy everywhere. His neurodevelopmental pediatrician saw him in follow-up and reports that he is in good health and has a normal general examination. No specific etiology has been determined for his autism. His doctor recommended that he continue autistic support class placement, full time. She recommended that behavioral intervention strategies continue to be included into his curriculum to work on enhancing compliance and increasing engagement. She also proposed that he continue to receive speech-language therapy, occupational therapy, and physical therapy weekly in school. In addition, his physician suggested that he have a functional behavior analysis performed in order to develop and implement an appropriate behavioral treatment protocol focused on enhancing his engagement and compliance. Finally, his doctor discussed options for a trial of an atypical antipsychotic (e.g., risperidone) to assist in managing his disruptive and aggressive behaviors, thereby enabling him to benefit most from the behavioral treatment.

DIAGNOSTIC CATEGORIES WITHIN THE AUTISM SPECTRUM

ASDs are defined by the presence or absence of behaviors in three areas: social reciprocity, communication, and repetitive behaviors (American Psychiatric Association, 2000). The number and distribution of symptoms, the pattern of early language development, cognitive abilities, and the presence of regression all are used to make a specific diagnosis within this category of disorders. The terms *Autistic Disorder*, *PDD-NOS* and *Asperger's Disorder* are proposed to disappear in *DSM-5* within the new ASD classification system. The other two disorders that are listed as PDDs in *DSM-IV-TR*, Rett's Disorder and Childhood Disintegrative Disorder, will no longer be part of the ASD classification system. Rett syndrome is now known to be one of a number of genetic syndromes that have a high risk for manifesting symptoms of ASD (see text that follows). Regarding childhood disintegrative disorder, it is not clear if this is a discrete entity or rather a term that has been used as a placeholder for individuals with a neurodegenerative disorder with autistic features for which a specific genetic diagnosis has not yet been made. In the following paragraphs we will describe Autistic Disorder (ASD), PDD-NOS, and Asperger's Disorder.

Autistic Disorder

Autism (or Autistic Disorder, per the *DSM-IV-TR*) is defined by a pattern of at least six symptoms distributed across three domains (Table 21.1). At least two symptoms must be in the area of social reciprocity. Dr. Leo Kanner first described the syndrome of autism (derived from the Greek word for self-absorption; Kanner, 1943). He observed a series of individuals in his practice of child psychiatry that had social aloofness and a desire for "preservation of sameness." Although Kanner believed autism was an organic condition, throughout the 1950s most psychiatrists considered autism to be caused by poor parenting. Some thought it was a form of childhood schizophrenia. With improved behavior characterization, it became clear that the ASDs were discrete from schizophrenia and

Table 21.1. Diagnostic criteria for Autistic Disorder

A. A total of six (or more) items from the following groups:

Group 1[a]	Group 2[b]	Group 3[c]
1. Marked impairment in the use of multiple nonverbal behaviors such as eye-to-eye gaze, facial expression, body postures, and gestures to regulate social interaction	1. Delay in, or total lack of, the development of spoken language (not accompanied by an attempt to compensate through alternative modes of communication such as gesture or mime)	1. Encompassing preoccupation with one or more stereotyped and restricted patterns of interest that is abnormal either in intensity or focus
2. Failure to develop peer relationships appropriate to developmental level	2. In individuals with adequate speech, marked impairment in the ability to initiate or sustain a conversation with others	2. Apparently inflexible adherence to specific, nonfunctional routines or rituals
3. A lack of spontaneous seeking to share enjoyment, interests, or achievements with other people (e.g., by a lack of showing, bringing, or pointing out objects of interest)	3. Stereotyped and repetitive use of language or idiosyncratic language	3. Stereotyped and repetitive motor mannerisms (e.g., hand or finger flapping or twisting, complex whole-body movements)
4. Lack of social or emotional reciprocity	4. Lack of varied, spontaneous make-believe play or social imitative play appropriate to developmental level	4. Persistent preoccupation with parts of objects

B. Delays or abnormal functioning in at least one of the following areas with onset prior to age 3 years:

1. Social interaction
2. Language as used in social communication
3. Symbolic or imaginative play

C. The disturbance is not better accounted for by Rett's Disorder or Childhood Disintegrative Disorder.

Reprinted with permission from the *Diagnostic and Statistical Manual of Mental Disorders, Fourth Edition, Text Revision* (Copyright ©2000). American Psychiatric Association.

[a]Qualitative impairments in social interaction, as manifested by at least two criteria from Group 1.

[b]Qualitative impairments in communication, as manifested by at least one criterion from Group 2.

[c]Restricted, repetitive, and stereotyped patterns of behavior, interests, and activities, as manifested by at least one criterion from Group 3.

occurred along a gradient. Progressive modification of the *DSM* (American Psychiatric Association, 2000) has altered diagnostic criteria so that younger children and children with the full range of cognitive abilities (typical or impaired) can be identified as having an ASD.

Pervasive Developmental Disorder Not Otherwise Specified

The diagnosis of PDD-NOS is used to describe children who do not have the prerequisite number or distribution of symptoms for another diagnosis within the ASDs or have atypical presentation with functional impairments in the relevant areas. There is no minimum number of symptoms necessary to diagnose PDD-NOS, but there must be social impairment. This results in significant heterogeneity among individuals given this clinical diagnosis. The comorbidity of cognitive, language, and behavioral symptoms with PDD-NOS may result in significant functional impairment, even though fewer symptoms of autism may be present.

Asperger's Disorder

Dr. Hans Asperger was a contemporary of Dr. Kanner (Asperger, 1991). Asperger observed children with apparently typical language who had difficulties with socialization, could not conform to social demands, and had repetitive behaviors. The *DSM-IV-TR* indicates that Asperger's Disorder can be diagnosed if three symptoms—two related to social reciprocity and one to habitual behaviors—are present. Early language development must be grossly within typical limits, but pragmatic language impairments are common. Adaptive behaviors may be delayed. There is considerable overlap between the diagnosis of high-functioning autism (Autistic Disorder in someone with typical intelligence) and Asperger's Disorder (Szatmari et al., 2000). This is one of the factors leading to the change in the classification system of ASD in *DSM-5*. Children with Asperger's Disorder are often not diagnosed until school age, when the social demands of the classroom make the symptoms functionally apparent.

DIAGNOSTIC FEATURES OF AUTISM SPECTRUM DISORDERS

There is significant heterogeneity among individuals with ASDs, but they all share three core domains of symptoms that are discussed next: qualitative impairments in social reciprocity, atypical communication development, and atypical behavior.

Qualitative Impairments in Social Reciprocity

Impairments in social reciprocity, critical to the diagnosis of an ASD, reflect an intrinsic inability to read and comprehend the feelings, experiences, and motives of others. Typical social reciprocity skills allow the interpretation of verbal and nonverbal messages of others, including nuanced facial expression, vocal inflection, gestures, social intention, and emotional tone. Because of impaired social reciprocity skills, children with ASDs often have difficulties interacting with peers (Travis, Sigman, & Ruskin, 2001). The prototypical example of social reciprocity is eye contact; infants with typical development learn that eye contact with an adult leads to attention. In addition, the ability to share a common point of reference, called joint attention, starts to develop around 6 months of age and facilitates social interaction and sharing (Mundy & Newell, 2007).

In addition to maintaining a connection through eye contact and vocalization, social reciprocity involves understanding that other people have a different point of view, referred to as Theory of Mind. Individuals with ASD do not possess Theory of Mind. This basic impairment interferes with their capacity to understand social language and the intent of others (Rogers, 1998).

People without ASDs generally look at the eyes of a person to whom they are speaking, whereas most people with ASDs look at the person's mouth (Klin, Jones, Schultz, Volkmar, & Cohen, 2002). When people with ASD have eye gaze, it tends to be intense and without the social awareness of when to look away. Symptoms related to atypical social reciprocity are also closely tied to quality and atypicality of language function. In addition, people with ASDs may have difficulty in integrating verbal and nonverbal components of communication.

Although individuals with ASDs have varying degrees of difficulty in initiating, responding to, and maintaining social interactions, they may be highly responsive to specific individuals or situations (e.g., family members or favored television programs/movies). Patterns of relating to other people, however, tend to be atypical. They may have diminished eye contact, decreased use of facial expression, and exaggerated or absent gestures.

In terms of the underlying neurological impairments in ASD, there is evidence that mirror neurons in the brain, which permit imitation of what an individual sees, may be functionally atypical. This may affect facial imitation and use of expression as well as other motor imitation (Oberman & Ramachandran, 2007).

Atypical Communication Development

Difficulty with communication is present to varying degrees in most individuals with ASDs (Rapin & Dunn, 2003). Atypical language development may relate to comorbid intellectual disability or exist in isolation. Language delay is usually the first area of concern identified by most families whose children are later diagnosed with ASDs. Typical early language is often reported, including the emergence of single words. When early milestones are scrutinized, however, it becomes apparent that many children with ASDs have had atypical development in receptive and expressive language from infancy (Mars, Mauk, & Dowrick, 1998; Mitchell et al., 2006). Although language delay from infancy is the most common presentation, in about 25%–30% of children with ASD early language development is typical but is subsequently lost between 18 and 24 months (Parr et al., 2011; Rogers, 2004).

Early language of children with ASDs is often characterized by 1) imperative labeling (using words for naming instead of communicating), 2) echolalia (echoing speech), 3) atypical prosody (inflection), and 4) improper use of pronouns (referring to self in the third person). It should be noted that echoing adult words is common in typical development, as toddlers gain vocabulary and learn to process what is said to them. Echolalia, however, is usually gone before 2 years of age, whereas in children with ASDs it may persist in a **perseverative** (uncontrollable repetitious) fashion into childhood and beyond. It is speculated that the child with ASD may use perseverative language to provide structure and a known outcome in a social situation that the child does not understand. Once functional language is established, **prosody** (the use of pitch, loudness, tempo, and rhythm in speech) may be singsong, robotic, or imitative of the inflection used by the original speaker (e.g., imitating an announcer on TV). Young children with ASDs also may have difficulty using pronouns (i.e., saying "I want this" versus "Julie wants this") because they may not see how words need to be rearranged to have meaning to another person (Rapin & Dunn, 2003).

In addition to speech, communication requires a synthesis of many behaviors that are nonverbal. Children with ASDs may have a basic impairment in many of these nonverbal behaviors such as the ability to both perceive and imitate facial expression (Dawson, Webb, & McPartland, 2005). Studies have shown that the brains of people with Autistic Disorder process faces as if they were objects. As a result, every time the facial expression of the communication partner is changed, the person with an ASD must reidentify the face (Schultz, 2005). People with ASD may also have a decreased ability to simultaneously process speech and gesture that influences both social processing and pragmatic language (Silverman, Bennetto, Campana, & Tanenhaus, 2010) .

Receptive language problems may also affect communication. Learning may be more efficient with visual, rather than auditory cues. Unusual eye contact, body posture, gestures, and other nonverbal aspects of communication may have an impact on communication. Without specific intervention, nonverbal communication impairments may be problematic even with the development of conversational language.

Atypical Behavior

Although the differences in social "give and take" may be central to the diagnosis of ASDs, repetitive, perseverative, and stereotyped behaviors are often the most visible symptoms. Strict adherence to routines is common among people with ASDs. This can extend to food selectivity, rituals related to daily routines, and/or obsessions. Young children with ASDs may have attachments to unusual items, such as string, rather than to soft or cuddly toys. Children with ASDs may not use toys in their intended manner but may focus instead on a part of a toy—for example, the wheels on a toy truck, which they may spin repetitively. They may line things up, stare out of the corners of their eyes, or minutely inspect aspects of objects. In addition, pretend play may not develop spontaneously, and once taught, it may take on a rote quality.

Interruption of a ritual or preoccupation may upset a child with an ASD and lead to distress or a temper tantrum. Stereotyped movements such as pacing, spinning, running in circles, drumming, flipping light switches, rocking, hand waving, arm flapping, and toe walking are common. Self-injurious behavior, including biting and head banging, may also occur. Unusual responses to sensory input are commonly reported. These include insensitivity to pain or heat and overreaction to environmental noises, touch, or odors. For example, although the child may appear "deaf" to the language of others, he or she may be alert to or respond to sounds, or alternatively may cover his or her ears and scream because of hyperacusis (unusual sensitivity to certain sounds, such as a vacuum cleaner).

The core symptoms of ASD vary with age and ability. For example, some people with autism may have a total absence of language and communicative intent, whereas those with Asperger's Disorder may engage in "professorial" speech with little conversational regard for the interest of the listener. Challenges include development of more precise ways to elicit and quantify the core symptoms of ASD for early and accurate diagnosis. It is anticipated that additional guidance will be provided for the evaluator using *DSM-5* criteria.

CAUSES OF AUTISM SPECTRUM DISORDERS

ASDs have multiple etiologies. The weight of evidence now points to a genetic predisposition with environmental interactions.

The Genetics of Autism

The evidence for a genetic etiology for ASDs comes from both family and twin studies. The recurrence risk for an ASD in subsequent siblings of a child with ASD has been quoted to be 2%–8% (O'Roak & State, 2008). Data published in 2011, however, suggests it may be as high as 18% (Ozonoff et al., 2011) . This is tenfold higher than what would be expected in the general population. Recent analysis of 192 twin pairs with ASD in California reported concordance (i.e., both twins have ASD) of 77% for identical male twins and 31% for fraternal male twins. This data supports a genetic predisposition to autism but also points to a greater influence of the intrauterine environment on the development of autism than had been previously appreciated (Hallmayer et al., 2011). Genetic research has followed three strategies: family studies, candidate gene studies, and association with genetic disorders of known etiology.

Family Studies

In family studies, also called linkage analysis, patterns of genes or specific DNA markers in family members with and without Autistic Disorder or another ASD are investigated. This strategy has identified genes that may be related to ASDs on multiple chromosomes, including 2, 7, and 15 (O'Roak & State, 2008).

Candidate Genes Studies

Identification of a trait of interest allows specific investigation of associated genes in families with individuals with ASDs. A number of genes of interest relate to early brain development (Muhle et al., 2004). The interaction of genes and environmental events in early pregnancy is an area of active study. Candidate genes related to neurotransmitter generation and receptor function are of great interest because they may be a target for drug development (Scott & Deneris, 2005). In addition, genes responsible for early brain development have research implications for examining the "connectivity" of areas of the brain that underlies both processing and etiology in people with ASD (Jones et al., 2010; Minshew & Williams, 2007).

Association with Genetic Disorders of Known Etiology

ASDs tend to be associated with other genetic disorders that have known etiologies. It is understood that brain functioning in certain genetic disorders including Rett syndrome, Angelman syndrome, Prader-Willi syndrome, tuberous sclerosis, and fragile X syndrome places individuals at a greater risk for having ASDs (see Chapter 1 and Appendix B). It is intriguing that most of these disorders involve **epigenetics** (changes in gene expression caused by mechanisms other than changes in the underlying DNA sequence; see Chapter 1). This knowledge allows for investigation of the relationship among known biologic impairments and behaviors symptomatic of ASD.

Brain Structure and Function in Autism Spectrum Disorders

Neuroimaging techniques are used to study brain development and function (see Chapter 12). Although head circumference is normal at birth, about 60% of boys with ASDs have **macrocephaly** (large heads), with accelerated head circumference growth noted beginning between 4 and 12 months of age (Elder, Dawson, Toth, Fein, & Munson, 2008) followed by normal growth rates by school age. The reason for this is not yet known. Magnetic resonance imaging (MRI) studies of children with ASDs note a greater volume of white matter in cortex and cerebellum in early childhood. Genetic regulation of synaptic development and connections may be associated with this observation. The various MRI studies of brain anatomy do not consistently identify the same structural asymmetries or size differences. Improvements in imaging, such as diffusion tensor imaging (which images specific white matter tracts) should advance our understanding of brain structure and function.

Specialized neuroimaging studies such as functional MRI and spectroscopy can indirectly examine neurotransmitter activity and energy utilization in selected areas of the brain. Most studies published as of 2011 have involved adolescents and adults with Asperger's Disorder. One finding is that there is an impairment in Theory of Mind tasks requiring the networking of the medial prefrontal cortex, temporoparietal junction, and temporal poles with other brain regions (Vollm et al., 2006). Adolescents with Asperger's Disorder and high-functioning autism demonstrate impairments in processing faces in the fusiform gyrus (Schultz, 2005) and in processing the eye gaze of others in the superior temporal sulcus (Pelphrey, Morris, McCarthy, 2005). In addition, imitation may be impaired because mirror neurons do not communicate properly (Williams, Waiter, et al., 2005). A related technology, magnetoencephalography (MEG), has demonstrated delays in processing auditory information in people with ASD (Roberts et al., 2010).

Histological (anatomical study of the cellular structure of the brain) findings to date suggest that prenatal events alter cell number and density in the cerebellum and limbic system in ASD, but few studies have been published to confirm this. Atypical development of the brain stem nuclei and the inferior olive, as well as heterotopias (abnormally placed neurons) have been reported in isolated cases (Bailey et al., 1998). Modern techniques have identified additional pathological changes in some individuals' brains, including atypical inflammation and disordered cellular organization in the cortex (Casanova, 2006; Vargas, Nascimbene, Krishan, Zimmerman, & Pardo, 2005).

Obstetric Complications

Epidemiologic studies have not strongly associated any specific prenatal or birth complication with the development of ASDs. Obstetric optimality scores that reflect the overall health of the pregnancy, delivery, and newborn period, however, are lower in children with ASDs (Zwaigenbaum et al., 2002). The prenatal events that predispose a child to develop an ASD may compromise fetal well-being in subtle and inconsistent ways. An increased risk for ASD has been reported among premature infants (Limperopoulos, 2009; Schendel & Bhasin, 2008). An increased risk has also been reported to be present in women who become pregnant within 12 months of having a first child (Cheslack-Postava et al., 2011).

Environmental Exposures

It may be that environmental factors interact with genes to cause the symptoms of ASDs. To date, however, the only established environmental risk factors for ASDs are a few medications (discussed in the next section) that a mother might have been prescribed early in pregnancy (Landrigan, 2010). We describe below evidence for associations of teratogens, vaccines, and infections with ASDs.

Teratogens

Substances that result in an increased risk of birth defects in the developing fetus are termed *teratogens*. These include maternal medications, drugs of abuse, chemicals, and radiation. As one example, thalidomide, a drug that was used to treat nausea in pregnant women in the early 1960s, was associated with limb deformities in exposed fetuses. Many years later, ophthalmologists studying the impairments of eye movement in adults who were exposed to thalidomide *in utero* found that these individuals had a very high prevalence of ASDs (Stromland, Nordin, Miller, et al., 1994). In addition, increased rates of ASDs have been reported in children who were exposed during early pregnancy to valproic acid (an antiepileptic drug) and mesoprostol (used to induce early termination of pregnancy; Landrigan, 2010).

No known environmental or chemical exposure has been associated with an increased risk for ASDs to date (see Chapter 3). For example, an epidemiologic study that compared the rates of ASD in Brick Township, New Jersey (a site of the Superfund cleanup of toxic waste) to other communities in New Jersey did not identify an increased risk in that locale (Bertrand et al., 2001). Recent reports of increased airborne mercury in locations with higher rates of children with ASDs require further study

with more rigorous methodology that includes actual air sampling (Palmer, Blanchard, Stein, Mandell, & Miller, 2006). Additional environmental agents studied include PCBs, television exposure, and floor tiles (Landrigan, 2010). Although existing data do not implicate specific chemical agents, it is possible that substances to which mothers and newborns are exposed may affect brain development in a way that leads to ASDs in susceptible individuals. This needs to be further explored.

Vaccinations

Since the initial allegation of an association of the measles, mumps, and rubella (MMR) vaccine with developmental regression and ASDs, a large body of evidence has been published that has refuted the connection. The journal that published the article retracted the publication because of improper scientific practices (Retraction, 2010). Population-based studies, in fact, do not demonstrate an increase in the rate of diagnosis of ASDs with the introduction of MMR (Demicheli, Jefferson, Rivetti, & Price, 2005). Madsen et al. (2002) compared the rate of ASDs in more than 400,000 children in Denmark who received the MMR vaccine with about 100,000 children who did not get the vaccine. There was no difference in the rate of ASDs. Despite this evidence against a connection between vaccination and ASD, there continues to be a decreased rate of immunization by parents concerned about a possible association (Leask, Booy, & McIntyre, 2010). Families should be reassured that the immunization schedule advocated by the American Academy of Pediatrics is not associated with the development of autism.

A second hypothesis relates the ethylmercury-based preservative thimerosal (used as a preservative in pediatric vaccines prior to 2001) to symptoms of ASD in genetically susceptible children (Bernard, Enayati, Redwood, Roger, & Binstock, 2001). Yet, the rate of diagnosis of ASDs actually increased after removal of thimerosal from vaccines in Denmark (Madsen, Lauritsen, Pedersen, et al., 2003), although this could be attributed to the broadened diagnostic criteria and increased awareness of ASDs in families and providers. The neurologic symptoms that are known to be associated with specific types of mercury toxicity depend on the type of mercury and age at and length of exposure. Both the neurologic symptoms of ASDs and acute, chronic, and prenatal mercury toxicity affect sensory functions, motor abilities, and learning, but the specific symptoms of mercury toxicity are not the same as autism (Nelson & Bauman, 2003). In addition, methylmercury, the type of mercury ingested in fish and marine mammals, has not been found to be associated with autism in populations with high prenatal and postnatal exposure (Myers et al., 2003; Ng, Chan, Soo, & Lee, 2007).

In sum, no study provides scientific evidence of a causal relationship of thimerosal containing vaccines or methylmercury and ASDs. In addition, vaccines administered to children in the United States, other than some influenza vaccines, are typically thimerosal free. Despite these factors, chelation therapy to bind and excrete heavy metals including mercury is pursued as a clinical intervention by some families of children with ASDs. There is no evidence that chelation therapy is of value, and the safety of this practice is unclear (Levy & Hyman, 2005).

Infections

Prenatal infection with rubella increases the risk for cerebral palsy, intellectual disability, visual impairments, and ASDs, depending on the timing of the infection (Chess, 1971). Fortunately MMR vaccination-based immunity in women has all but eliminated this cause of ASDs in the United States. Other viruses and bacteria that commonly infect pregnant women are not routinely associated with ASDs in the offspring, although rare cases of ASD have been reported in children with congenital cytomegalovirus (CMV). A mother's own immunologic response to infections such as influenza, however, might cause subtle differences in brain development that hypothetically could predispose a susceptible fetus to an ASD (Croen, Grether, Yoshida, Odouli, & Van de Water, 2005; Zimmerman et al., 2007).

Another issue that has been raised is the possibility of infections in early childhood being associated with ASDs. In fact, children who have severe neurologic injury after meningitis or encephalitis may develop symptoms of ASDs. There is no evidence, however, to indicate that hypothetical overgrowth of intestinal yeasts or bacteria (Buie, Fuchs, et al., 2010) can cause ASDs.

Gender and Autism Spectrum Disorders

Autism affects more boys than girls, with gender ratios generally ranging from 2:1 to 5:1 (Centers for Disease Control and Prevention, 2009; Fombonne, 2003). The observed male-to-female ratio increases as IQ scores increase, ranging from close to 1:1 for children with IQ scores lower than 50 (Fombonne, 1999; Yeargin-Allsopp et al., 2003) to about 6:1 for children with high-functioning autism (Fombonne, 2003). Fetal testosterone exposure has been raised as one possible explanation for the increased number of affected boys with ASD (Auyeung et al., 2009). There is no scientific evidence to date to support that medically altering the onset of puberty (thereby delaying the increased production of testosterone) provides cognitive or behavior benefit to boys with ASD (Geier & Geier, 2006).

EPIDEMIOLOGY OF AUTISM SPECTRUM DISORDERS

There continues to be debate about the prevalence of ASDs and the reasons for the recently reported marked increase. Since 2009, studies have reported the prevalence of ASDs as approximately 1 in 110 children (Centers for Disease Control and Prevention, 2009; Kogan et al., 2009). Prevalence rates have varied in the past, but the reported rate in 2011 is tenfold what was reported a generation ago. This may be due to differences in methodology of surveillance, change in *DSM* criteria for ASDs, and changes in awareness and identification of children with the disorder (Maenner & Durkin, 2010; Parner et al., 2011; Pinborough-Zimmerman, Bilder, Satterfield, Hossain, & McMahon, 2010; Posserud, Lundervold, Lie, & Gillberg, 2010). However, evidence is accumulating that some of this change in prevalence represents a real increase in the number of children with ASD.

Prevalence in racial/ethnic minorities also varies, with some studies reporting decreased rates in African American children (Dyches, Wilder, Sudweeks, Obiakor, & Algozzine, 2004; Sanua 1984), whereas other studies have not found a significant difference in rates among races (Yeargin-Allsopp et al., 2003). It is possible that the variations actually reflect health care disparities (Mandell et al., 2009). On average, African American children are diagnosed 2 years later than Caucasian children (Mandell, Listerud, Levy, & Pinto-Martin, 2002; Mandell, Novak, & Zubritsky, 2005). Finally, advanced maternal and paternal ages have been associated with increased risk for an ASD diagnosis (Croen, Najar, Fireman, et al., 2007).

EARLY IDENTIFICATION OF AUTISM SPECTRUM DISORDERS

By the *DSM-IV-TR* definition, the symptoms of an ASD must be present by 3 years of age. Yet, even when parents are concerned about their child's early development, the diagnosis of an ASD may not be established for a few years (Howlin & Asgharian, 1999; Mandell et al., 2005). The age of diagnosis has decreased with increased awareness by pediatricians, parents, and preschool teachers. Children with Asperger's Disorder and high-functioning autism, however, tend to be diagnosed at school age.

Delayed language development, repetitive behaviors, and atypical social responsiveness are common early parental concerns. Systematic review of videotapes from the first year of life demonstrates differences in infants with ASDs. A child with ASD may not respond to his or her name and may be less interested in faces and voices than other infants. Infants later diagnosed with ASDs may have had poor eye contact, absence of a social smile, irritability, and a dislike of being held. As toddlers, they may have had sleep difficulties, limited diets, tantrums, and inattention to language. Because of limited response to the language of others, initial concerns may have been around hearing impairment.

Early diagnosis is based on recognition of core features of ASDs in early childhood. Atypical development of pretend play, pointing to share interest, use of eye gaze to engage another person in communication, and social interest can distinguish toddlers at high risk for ASD as young as 18 months of age. These observations are the basis for the Checklist for Autism in Toddlers (CHAT; Baron-Cohen et al., 2000) and the Modified Checklist for Autism in Toddlers (M-CHAT; Pandey et al., 2008; Robins, Fein, Barton, & Green, 2001). The M-CHAT is a brief parent questionnaire suitable for screening toddlers in a pediatrician's office. Although sensitive to symptoms of ASD, it is not specific unless the items endorsed by the family are examined further by interview. The M-CHAT authors have subsequently developed an interview used to confirm the screening questionnaire (Pandey et al., 2008).

Other tests that can be used to screen for ASDs in toddlers include the screening tool for autism (STAT; Stone, Coonrod, Ousley, 2000; Stone, McMahon, & Henderson, 2008;) and the Pervasive Developmental Disorder Screening Test–II (PDDST–II; Dumont-Mathieu & Fein, 2005). The routine use of general developmental and behavior screening tests and ongoing developmental surveillance by primary care providers, however, is likely to be the best screening mechanism to identify children with ASD. This approach identifies general delays and results in earlier referral for diagnostic and treatment services. Because of the importance of early diagnosis in leading to early intervention, there has been much interest in the accurate screening and diagnosis at younger and younger ages. Table 21.2 contains more information about screening tools.

Evaluation of the Child with an Autism Spectrum Disorder

Assessment for ASDs requires time, collaboration among health care and educational professionals, and knowledge about development. The evaluation follows directly from the diagnostic criteria that focus on impairments in social reciprocity, language, and restricted patterns of behavior (Filipek et al., 2000).

Multidisciplinary Assessment

Most children are initially referred to school-based assessment teams or early intervention services by their primary care providers or by their parents because of language delays (see Chapter 30). Initial multidisciplinary evaluation of developmental concerns should involve formal assessments of 1) receptive and expressive language, 2) cognitive function, 3) hearing, 4) fine and gross motor function, 5) social and emotional skills, and 6) adaptive skills.

If an ASD is suspected, referral should be made to a professional who is experienced in making the diagnosis, such as a neurodevelopmental pediatrician, developmental-behavioral pediatrician, child neurologist, child psychiatrist, child psychologist, or speech-language pathologist. The assessment should include a detailed medical history, with particular attention paid to 1) social development; 2) developmental milestones, especially in language; 3) other medical conditions; 4) family history, including behavioral, medical, neurologic, developmental, and psychiatric illnesses; and 5) current family functioning and circumstances. As noted previously, one quarter to one third of children with Autistic Disorder have a reported loss of language and/or social milestones in the second year of life. An underlying medical condition needs to be ruled out in these cases, as 10% of children with ASDs are reported to have medical conditions that might be etiologic (Chakrabarti & Fombonne, 2001).

Table 21.2. Screening and diagnostic tests for autism spectrum disorders (ASDs)

Screening tests for ASDs in toddlers

Modified Checklist for Autism in Toddlers (M-CHAT; Dumont-Mathew & Fein, 2005): ages 18–36 months

Screening Tool for Autism in Two-Year-Olds (STAT; Stone, Coonrod, Turner, & Pozdol, 2004.)

Pervasive Developmental Disorder Screening Test (PDDST II; Siegerl, 2004.)

Screening tests for older children

Social Communication Questionnaire (SCQ; Rutter, Bailey, & Lord, 2003): older than 3 years of age

Social Responsiveness Scale (Constantino, 2005): school age

Standardized tests that support a clinical diagnosis of autism

Childhood Autism Rating Scale (CARS2; Schopler, Van Bourgondien, Wellman, & Love, 2010): older than 2 years of age

Gilliam Autism Rating Scale, Second Edition (GARS 2; Gilliam, 2006): older than age 3

"Gold standard" companion measures designed to elicit symptoms of ASDs for diagnostic purposes

Autism Diagnostic Interview (ADI-R; Rutter, LeCouteur, & Lord-Revised, 2003): semistructured interview with the care giver that allows for scoring whether autism is present

Autism Diagnostic Observation Schedule (ADOS; Lord, Rutter, DiLavore, Risi, Gotham, & Bishop, 2012): structured interactions for children of different language abilities to allow for observation of symptoms of ASDs per the *Diagnostic and Statistical Manual of Mental Disorders, Fourth Edition, Text Revision* (*DSM-IV-TR*; American Psychiatric Association, 2000) criteria for both Autistic Disorder and Pervasive Developmental Disorder

The above two measures are often used together to characterize cases for research related to autism.

Note: Clinical application of the diagnostic criteria from *DSM-IV-TR* by an experienced clinician is the mainstay of diagnosis.

The identification of these conditions is independent of a history of regression (e.g., fragile X syndrome).

A general physical and neurological examination should occur to identify intercurrent medical conditions that might exacerbate behavior or underlying causes of the ASD. The physical examination should include an examination of the skin, as children with neurocutaneous syndromes (e.g., tuberous sclerosis) are at higher risk for ASDs. Head circumference should be monitored, with conventional neurologic assessment of macro and microcephaly.

Diagnostic Measures

As there are currently no specific biomarkers for ASDs, the diagnosis relies on the history and clinical observation. This requires input from parents, therapists, and teachers who are familiar with the child in multiple settings. A structured history through the Autism Diagnostic Inventory (ADI-R; Lord et al., 1994) and observation of symptoms through the Autism Diagnostic Observation Schedule (ADOS; Lord et al., 2000) are used to standardize clinical and research application of diagnostic criteria. The ADI-R is a lengthy standardized parental interview that is primarily used in research settings. The ADOS is a semistructured examiner directed evaluation of social interaction, communication, and imaginative play (Lord et al., 2000). The ADOS may be used in some clinical or educational settings to support the clinical diagnosis of an ASD but requires extensive training for reliability if used in research settings. Other questionnaires such as the Social Communication Questionnaire (SCQ) or Social Responsiveness Scale (SRS) are briefer parent report measures used to confirm the history of symptoms of ASD (Chandler et al., 2007; Constantino et al., 2003) and may be useful to support the clinical diagnosis of an ASD in the outpatient clinical setting.

Laboratory Testing and Neuroimaging

There is no standard medical workup for children with ASDs. Etiologic workup is determined by the history and physical examination (Johnson, Myers, the Council on Children with Disabilities, 2007). DNA analysis for fragile X syndrome is often recommended in children with cognitive limitations and symptoms of ASDs. Microarray has largely replaced high-resolution karyotype as the initial recommended test for evaluation for genetic etiologies for ASD (see Chapter 1). Atypical results are present in up to 10% of children with ASD. As the genes for ASD are identified, it is likely that testing for specific gene alterations will be routinely recommended.

Although impairments may be seen on MRI in children with ASDs, the yield for diagnostic or treatable conditions identified by routine neuroimaging studies is low. Similarly, in the absence of a history of seizures, routine screening with electroencephalography (EEG) is not indicated (Filipek et al., 2000). General metabolic screening rarely has positive results if the history and physical examination is negative. Although additional medical and biological evaluations are often pursued, there is no scientific evidence to support measurement of heavy metal levels in hair, blood, or urine; immunologic parameters in blood; stool flora; urine peptides; or yeast metabolites in urine in children with ASDs (Levy & Hyman, 2005).

ASSOCIATED CONDITIONS

ASDs are commonly associated with comorbid symptoms or conditions (Levy et al., 2010). These are discussed next.

Intellectual Disability

Older studies report that up to three quarters of individuals with Autistic Disorder also have an intellectual disability. Yeargin-Allsopp and colleagues (Yeargin-Allsopp et al., 2003) reported that 68% of the children between 3 and 10 years of age who were identified with ASDs in the Atlanta area had comorbid intellectual disability. In contrast, only 40% of preschool children diagnosed with ASDs were found to have intellectual disability at the time of their first evaluation (Chakrabarti & Fombonne, 2001). With more expanded diagnostic criteria for ASD, it is likely that both increasing numbers of individuals with typical cognitive abilities and with significant intellectual disability will be identified as having ASDs.

It is assumed that the reason that intellectual disability is so commonly associated with ASDs is that the brain insults responsible for causing ASDs disrupt other neurologic functions as well. Overlap of symptoms between intellectual disability and ASDs also complicates the diagnostic process. Careful clinical assessment is necessary to determine if social development is atypical for the child's mental age. Symptoms of ASD, such as a lack of interest in peer play, lack of pretend play, and repetitive behaviors may also be seen in people with severe intellectual disability without an underlying ASD (de Bildt et al., 2004).

Learning Disabilities

Learning disabilities are common among individuals who have an ASD and average intellectual function. Specific impairments in **executive function**—the cognitive tasks related to taking in, organizing, processing and acting on information—also may be present in people with ASDs, manifesting as learning differences and/or attention-deficit/hyperactivity disorder (ADHD) (Chan et al., 2009; Schmitz et al., 2006).

Epilepsy

Overall, epilepsy is reported in about 25% of individuals with ASDs and most commonly presents in infancy and adolescence (Trevathan, 2004; Tuchman & Rapin, 2002). There is also an increased likelihood of having an abnormal EEG without seizures in people with ASDs. The implications of this finding are unclear, and the role of antiepileptic drug treatment in the absence of seizures requires further study (Tuchman, 2004).

Tic Disorders

Up to 9% of children with ASDs have motor tics (brief involuntary movements), or Tourette syndrome. Tourette syndrome is diagnosed when both vocal and motor tics are present and last 12 months or more. Tourette syndrome, in addition, may be associated with inattention and hyperactivity, obsessions, and learning disabilities. Individuals who have Tourette syndrome but not an ASD will manifest appropriate social reciprocity (Ringman & Jankovic, 2000).

Sleep Disorders

Sleep disturbances are reported in 50%–70% of children with ASDs (Malow et al., 2006). Although often considered most problematic in the preschool years, symptoms persist into later childhood in many children. Night waking, delayed sleep onset, and early morning waking are all reported (Souders et al., 2009). Poor sleep may be associated with daytime inattention, irritability, and other difficulties (Malow, McGrew, Harvey, Henderson, & Stone, 2006). The underlying biologic causes may relate to abnormal melatonin synthesis and release or disordered sleep cycles. Until the etiology is better understood, the mainstay of treatment is behavioral intervention. Medical treatment with melatonin to augment behavioral treatment has increasing research support (Johnson & Malow, 2008).

Gastrointestinal Symptoms

Although high rates of gastrointestinal symptoms are reported among children with ASDs who attend subspecialty clinics, no increased rate of complaint was identified in studies examining primary care records in the United Kingdom. The subspecialty related problems included abdominal pain, gastroesophageal reflux, diarrhea, constipation, and bloating (Erickson et al., 2005). Abdominal discomfort may be responsible for acute behavior changes. In addition to abdominal discomfort, children with ASDs often have specific food aversions and rituals and are at risk for nutritional compromise. In sum, symptoms of gastrointestinal disease need to be assessed and treated in children with ASDs as with any other children (Buie, Campbell, et al., 2010; Buie, Fuchs, et al., 2010).

Psychiatric Conditions

Children with ASDs are at greater risk for depression, mood disorders, ADHD, and anxiety (Levy et al., 2010). Comorbid diagnosis may be most evident in adolescents with adequate language and insight to allow standard application of diagnostic criteria.

Genetic Disorders Associated with Autism Spectrum Disorders

ASDs occur with greater frequency among children with certain genetic disorders, and these children should be closely monitored for signs and symptoms of autism. Additional information about these syndromes may be found in Appendix B.

Tuberous Sclerosis

Tuberous sclerosis is an autosomal dominant disorder caused by a defect in the *TSC2* gene that codes for the protein tuberin. This neurocutaneous condition results in characteristic skin lesions (depigmented oblong patches called ash leaf spots), acne-like adenoma sebaceum, and benign growths (tubers) in the brain (Smalley, 1998). Intellectual disability and seizures are common features. Although only 1%–4% of people with ASDs are likely to have tuberous sclerosis, a substantial number of children with tuberous sclerosis have symptoms of autism. All children being evaluated for an ASD should be examined to rule out neurocutaneous conditions.

Fragile X Syndrome

At one time fragile X syndrome, the most prevalent cause of inherited intellectual disability, was believed to be a common genetic cause of ASDs. With careful clinical diagnosis, it has become clear that a large number of individuals with fragile X syndrome have many symptoms of ASDs but may not meet strict criteria for the diagnosis (Clifford et al., 2007; Hall, Lightbody, Hirt, Rezvani, & Reiss, 2010). Conversely, up to 2% of boys with an ASD have been found to have fragile X (Moss & Howlin, 2009).

Chromosome 15 Deletion

Prader-Willi syndrome and Angelman syndrome share a common region for chromosomal deletion on chromosome 15 (15q11-q13) (Kwasnicka-Crawford, Roberts, Scherer, 2007). People with Prader-Willi syndrome have profound obesity, short stature, skin picking behaviors, and mild cognitive limitations. Angelman syndrome is characterized by intellectual disability, happy affect, ataxic movements, hand clapping, and a characteristic facial appearance. A subgroup of children within ASD with a variable phenotype has been identified who also have a deletion or duplication in this region on chromosome 15 (Muhle et al., 2004; Peters, Beaudet, Madduri, & Bacino, 2004).

Other Syndromes Associated with Autism Spectrum Disorders

An increased rate of ASDs has been reported in Moebius syndrome (facial diplegia) and Joubert syndrome (cerebellar hypoplasia). Both of these syndromes involve disruption of early embryologic brain development. Other genetic syndromes that have been associated with ASDs include Down syndrome, *PTEN* mutation, CHARGE syndrome (coloboma and cranial nerve abnormalities, defects of the eyeball, heart defects, atresia of the choanae, retardation of growth and development, genital and urinary abnormalities, and ear abnormalities and hearing loss), and Smith-Lemli-Opitz syndrome. The co-occurrence, of these syndromes and the behaviors of autism may help researchers learn more about the neurobiology of ASDs (Kumar & Christian, 2009; O'Roak & State, 2008). Clinicians caring for children with syndromes that place them at increased risk for ASD should screen them for symptoms of autism through early childhood.

TREATMENT APPROACHES

It is important to diagnose children with ASDs early and accurately, as it is believed that treatment is most effective if started early. Early educational programs focus on teaching social language and enhancing appropriate behaviors. The National Research Council (2001) recommended intervention that is intensive, multidisciplinary, and continuous. Goals of autism treatment include 1) fostering development, 2) promoting learning, 3) reducing rigidity and stereotypy, 4) eliminating maladaptive behaviors, and 5) alleviating family distress (National Research Council, 2001; Rutter, 1985).

A comprehensive approach usually requires a combination of an individualized educational program (IEP), behavioral intervention and supports, social and pragmatic language skills development, and family support. Research on efficacy of treatments has focused on social communication and behavioral impairments, and the use of highly structured approaches that are integrated into the home, educational, and community environments (Warren et al., 2011). Most effective programs include a combination of developmental and behavioral approaches to address core impairments and ameliorate behavior difficulties.

Educational Approaches

A critical component of treatment is education (National Research Council, 2001). There are many different approaches to preschool education for children with ASDs. Successful programs share the characteristics of early entry, active participation in an intensive program offered daily throughout the year, planned teaching opportunities organized with the attention span of the child in mind, and sufficient adult staffing to meet the needs of the individual child and his or her program. An increase in tested IQ scores has been documented in young children with autism who participate in disorder-specific interventions (Harris, Handleman, Gordon, Kristoff, & Fuentes, 1991). This finding may be in part the result of maturation, and increased motivation to participate in testing. A recent randomized controlled trial of the Early Start Denver Model (ESDM), a comprehensive developmental behavioral intervention, reported improvement in IQ, adaptive behavior and autism diagnosis after 2 years of treatment that was initiated before 30 months of age (Dawson et al., 2010). Further study is needed to determine if the children sustain their gains and how these treatment strategies may be implemented more widely.

Although there are philosophical differences among some of the teaching strategies, most preschool programs utilize the following: 1) structured teaching periods, 2) reinforcement of spontaneous communication, 3) instruction of specific skills using principles of reinforcement, and 4) incidental learning (i.e., use of spontaneously occurring "teachable moments").

For children 3–21 years of age, Autistic Disorder is included as a special category of educational disability under the Individuals with Disabilities Education Improvement Act of 2004 (IDEA; PL 108–446). This law mandates that specific academic goals should relate to the child's cognitive and functional level, and the program should be provided in the least restrictive environment (see Chapter 31). The Handicapping Condition under federal law is Autism.

Children with ASDs should have their individualized needs addressed whether they are educated in small structured classrooms or in inclusive environments. Inclusive education allows for the child to model appropriate behaviors and learn how to participate in the community. Modifying educational materials may require consultant teacher support or team-taught classrooms. Some children with ASDs may benefit from a more structured environment with fewer sensory distractions. A specialized class setting could potentially be less restrictive for some children with ASDs because the predictability may result in less personal distress. Many educational strategies are used to enhance the success of children with ASDs in the classroom (Harrower & Dunlap, 2001; Jordan, 2005). Future studies need to determine which programs are most effective and for which students (White, Scahill, Klin, Koenig, & Volkmar, 2007).

TEACCH (Treatment and Education of Autistic and related Communication Handicapped Children) was one of the initial disorder-specific educational programs that recognized the need for an intensive and coordinated approach toward skill building and developing communication abilities (Mesibov & Shea, 2010; Panerai, Ferrante, & Zingale, 2002). It was designed to address the needs of the child and family across the school experience and includes classroom teaching, parent training, and other support services. The approach is eclectic and involves the use of behavioral strategies to enhance communication and social interaction, as well as visual organization and cuing. In addition, it emphasizes the parents' roles as cotherapists.

Behavioral Approaches

Applied Behavior Analysis

Most behavioral treatment programs are based on principals and procedures of applied behavior analysis (ABA). This involves combining principles of learning and motivation with an understanding that consequences of behavior (whether positive or negative) reinforce or extinguish subsequent behavior (Granpeesheh & Tarbox, 2009). Many types of ABA-based programs exist, with varying degrees of evidence for efficacy (Rogers & Vismara, 2008; Vismara & Rogers, 2010).

The behavioral principles of operant learning (see Chapter 32) were initially used in a program for preschool children with ASDs developed by Dr. Ivar Lovaas (1987). His studies demonstrated that intensive early intervention that specifically teaches the component skills necessary for development was associated with subsequent typical classroom performance in almost half of the 20 children with autism studied (McEachin, Smith, & Lovaas, 1993). This model initially tested a 40-hour per-week program that was based on individual therapy using discrete trial teaching, prompting, and reinforcement. Goals of the first year of treatment were to develop language skills, increase social use of language, increase social approach, promote play skills, and decrease behaviors that competed with the desired goals of therapy. In the second year of treatment, the goal was to extend intervention to a preschool environment in order to encourage interaction with peers and generalize the acquired skills. Later studies reported qualitative improvement even in children who do not have the dramatic response to behavioral treatment as a result of comorbid intellectual disability (Smith, Eikeseth, Klevstran, & Lovaas, 1997). Modifications in the delivery of ABA services have addressed teaching language skills and using a variety of behaviorally based strategies for skill development (Koegel, Koegel, & McNerney, 2001). Generalization of skills to the home and classroom are an important component of the treatment plan (Foxx, 2008). ABA has been particularly useful in children with ASD and intellectual disability.

Developmental-Individual Difference-Relationship Based Model

The Developmental-Individual Difference-Relationship Based model (DIR model) is a treatment strategy (Wieder & Greenspan, 2003) that builds on social communication learned in relationships with consistent and responsive adults. "Opening and closing circles of communication" in the context of child directed play is one focus of this intervention. It depends on participation by the family and educational team. This type of therapy has been demonstrated to contribute to developmental gains when used as part of an early intervention program (Mahoney & Perales, 2005). It seeks to build shared attention, leading to engagement.

Communication and problem solving are also practiced, and the adults shape the development of appropriate play and interaction.

Relationship Development Intervention

Relationship Development Intervention (RD; Gutstein, Burgess, & Montfort, 2007) is another approach that addresses social learning as an apprenticeship model. Adults lead the child through learning how to interact and respond in naturalistic settings. Parents are educated to understand the core impairments of ASDs so they can respond and shape their child's responses to language and social situations. There is little data currently available about the efficacy of this treatment.

Other Models

A combination of approaches has been studied in young children that address skill development using behavioral approaches. The Early Start Denver Model (ESDS) as previously described is a good example of this (Dawson et al., 2010).

Management of Maladaptive Behaviors

Behavioral support can be helpful in establishing daily routines, in extinguishing destructive behaviors, and in responding to tantrums. All behaviors carry meaning and should not be presumed to be random acts. For example, painful medical conditions and comorbid psychiatric conditions should be considered in cases of acute behavior deterioration. If the origin of the behavior is identified, it may be possible to teach more effective ways to achieve a similar result (e.g., comfort, communication) and to expand behaviors that increase social adaptability. A functional behavior analysis at school is indicated if behaviors interfere with classroom functioning (Dalton, 2002). This formal assessment determines why the behaviors are occurring. A functional behavior plan can then be developed to alter the environmental factors that precipitate the challenging behaviors or teach the child and staff other means of responding (see Chapter 30).

Pragmatic Language and Social Skills Training

Communication attempts by children with ASDs should be rewarded socially or in other ways to foster language development. It has been shown (Bondy & Frost, 1998) that organizing visual cues helps children with ASDs associate the spoken word with events. This helps them learn the role of communication in obtaining tangible items and can be built into a Picture Exchange Communication System (PECS; Bondy & Frost, 2001; Charlop-Christy, Carpente, Le, LeBlanc, & Kellet, 2002). Therapy may include a visual language system (picture or sign) that, in some cases, scaffolds the development of spoken communication. The use of augmentative and alternative communication (AAC) is different from facilitated communication (see Chapter 20). In AAC, children who do not have efficient oral speech (e.g., verbal apraxia) are taught to independently gain access to written, graphic, or computer-assisted technologies for independent communication. Facilitated communication is a technique whereby a facilitator guides the individual with an ASD to type responses. Subconscious guidance by the facilitator has been demonstrated under experimental conditions, and facilitated communication is not endorsed for clinical use (Mostert, 2001).

For children who have spoken language, an important objective is the promotion of language skills used in conversation. *Pragmatic language* refers to the integration of gesture, expression, proximity, and inflection of language to enhance interpersonal understanding of communication; and it is a core impairment in many individuals with ASD (Russell & Grizzle, 2008; Tesink et al., 2009). Pragmatics involves both production and understanding of these functions in the conversational partner. These skills can make the difference in permitting independent living, employment, and higher education. Encouraging social and pragmatic language development can be accomplished through a variety of approaches, including modeling by peers in inclusive settings, Social Stories (Chan & O'Reilly, 2008; Kokina and Kern, 2010), formal social skills curricula (Bellini & Peters, 2008), supervised social skills group experiences, and tutoring by typically developing peers (Rogers, 2000).

Children with ASDs may not generalize rehearsal that occurs in a group to other settings unless specifically taught to do so. Moreover, these techniques may not bridge the gap between social interactions and social relationships (Bauminger, Solomon, & Rogers, 2010). Therefore, educational objectives should address mastery of social skills in different settings and with different people.

Medication

There is no medication that corrects the underlying impairments in ASDs. However, medication may play a role in a comprehensive therapeutic program that also includes educational, developmental, and behaviorally based therapy. Treatment with medication should be directed at specific target behaviors or comorbid psychiatric or medical conditions.

Stimulant Medications

Hyperactivity and inattention are common symptoms in children with ASDs. If appropriate language and educational interventions are in place and inattention persists, treatment with conventional stimulant medications such as methylphenidate or mixed dextroamphetamine salts can have beneficial effects (Handen, Johnson, Lubetsky, 2000; see Appendix C). Side effects may include insomnia, decreased appetite, increased moodiness, and repetitive behaviors. Alpha-adrenergic agonists, guanfacine and clonidine, have been used for treatment of motor hyperactivity with some success (Handen, Sahl, & Hardan, 2008). General side effects of these two medications include hypotension and sedation. Because side effects of stimulant medications might include an increase in repetitive behaviors, moodiness, or appetite suppression with the use of stimulants, an alternative is the use of atomoxetine, which has similar benefits to stimulants. All of these drugs act on the neurotransmitters dopamine and norepinephrine, which have been shown to improve ADHD symptoms.

Selective Serotonin Reuptake Inhibitors

Because of some similarities between perseverative interests and obsessions, selective serotonin reuptake inhibitors (SSRIs) have been used to treat repetitive behaviors, irritability, and self-injury in people with ASDs (Moore, Eichner, & Jones, 2004). Decreasing anxiety may have additional benefits in enhancing language and social interactions. Side effects may include paradoxical hyperactivity or mood instability. Suicidal behaviors have very rarely been reported with drugs in this class when used to treat adolescent depression. Monitoring of mood and behavioral response is suggested. No benefit was noted in reduction of repetitive or agitated behaviors in a double blind trial of citalopram (King et al., 2009). Additional studies are necessary to determine if there is significant improvement in behaviors in children with ASD treated with SSRIs (Williams, Wheeler, Silove, & Hazell, 2010).

Atypical Neuroleptics

Well-designed trials have demonstrated that the atypical neuroleptics risperdone and aripiprazole significantly improve irritability, aggression, and self-stimulatory/self-injurious behaviors in children with ASDs and intellectual disability (Findling, Steiner, & Weller, 2005; McCracken et al., 2002; McDougle et al., 2005). The major side effect seen is weight gain, which can be considerable. Less common side effects from this class of medications include metabolic syndrome (a prediabetic state with hypertension and elevated blood lipids), tardive dyskinesia (a movement disorder), sedation, and hormonal imbalances. Routine monitoring for side effects is important.

Mood Stabilizers

Antiepileptic drugs used to treat bipolar disorder, such valproic acid and carbamazepine, have also been employed in the management of explosive behaviors in people with ASDs (Hollander, Dolgoff-Kaspar, Cartwright, Rawitt, & Novotny, 2001). Both medications need to be monitored with blood levels. By extension, newer antiepileptic drugs such as lamitrigane, topiramate, and oxycabemazepine are sometimes used.

Other Medications

Other types of medications are being investigated for treatment of symptoms of ASDs. Recent animal and human studies support further study of medications that act as agonists for GABA and excitatory amino acids. Advances in technology are likely to bring to market other medications designed to affect specific neural systems.

Complementary and Alternative Therapies

Almost two thirds of Americans receive treatments that fall into the category of complementary or alternative medicine (CAM; see Chapter 38). In ASDs the most common CAM therapies have involved dietary manipulation, vitamin supplements, and non–FDA-approved use of prescription medication (Levy & Hyman, 2003). Dietary treatment is particularly popular. Elimination of gluten and casein (wheat and milk proteins) has been hypothesized to result in decreased symptoms of autism and in decreased intestinal distress in some children with ASDs. Although there are many anecdotal reports of improvement, there is no scientific data to support the use of this intervention (Millward, Ferriter, & Connell-Jones, 2008). Despite this, the gluten- and casein-restricted diet remains popular. Families who decide to pursue it need to carefully monitor their child's nutritional needs; for example, when milk is removed from the diet, alternative sources of calcium, vitamin D, and protein need to be provided.

Vitamins are often used in doses far greater than the recommended daily intake in an attempt to effect behavior change. Vitamin B_6 taken with magnesium is one such treatment that has been used to enhance attention and language. Although several uncontrolled studies suggested benefit, two double-blind placebo-controlled studies did not demonstrate efficacy (Nye & Brice, 2005). Other nutritional treatments that enjoy popularity include supplementation with essential fatty acids, B_{12}, dimethylglycine, and carnosine (Levy & Hyman, 2008). Other types of CAM have been used to treat hypothesized infectious or immune imbalances such as yeast overgrowth in the colon and intestinal dysbiosis (Finegold et al., 2002); current scientific literature does not support these treatments. When using a CAM therapy children should have target behaviors identified and a monitoring system in place to determine if the treatment has a positive effect. Knowledge of potential side effects is also crucial.

Sometimes the non–FDA-approved use of a prescription medication becomes a CAM therapy. Secretin is one example. Secretin is a hormone that increases pancreatic secretion into the intestine and is usually employed to evaluate pancreatic function during endoscopy. The anecdotal observation of behavior improvement in three children who received secretin during an endoscopic procedure resulted in its subsequent widespread use. It should be noted, however, that more than 700 children with ASDs have been studied in double-blind placebo-controlled trials of secretin without confirmation of the original improvement (Williams, Wray, & Wheeler, 2005). As a result, secretin is not recommended for treatment of ASD.

Not all CAM therapies are biologic. Facilitated communication, auditory integration training, and optometric training are non-biologic examples of CAM that have been used in ASDs. The conventional medical literature does not support the use of these interventions. Sensory integration techniques are often used by occupational therapists to stimulate or calm children who demonstrate altered sensory and motor reactivity (Baranek, 2002). Although popular, there is little data to support general implementation of these strategies. With greater understanding of the neurobiology of sensory processing, effective sensory interventions may be developed and studied. Music therapy may be one such promising approach (Gold, Wigram, & Elefant, 2006). Until appropriately designed scientific studies are completed, each child must be evaluated by the family and therapy team for both positive and negative responses to CAM therapies that families choose to employ.

Family Supports

Families should be connected with appropriate parent support organizations at the time of diagnosis (Chapter 37). The stressors of receiving the diagnosis, making decisions, and addressing the child's needs may require referral for additional counseling services for other family members. The needs of siblings must also be addressed. It is encouraging to note that most studies indicate that siblings of children with disabilities are resilient (Kaminsky & Dewey, 2002).

OUTCOME

IQ scores that fall in the average range and the presence of language that can be used for conversation remain the best predictors of outcome for children with ASDs (Billstedt, Gillberg, & Gillberg, 2005). More than half of children diagnosed with autism acquire language that can be used for communication (Howlin, 2003). With the expansion of diagnostic criteria to include a large number of individuals with typical cognitive abilities among those with ASDs, the outcome for successful completion of education and community employment may be more optimistic.

It is as yet unknown how function is altered by intervention. Although diagnosis of an ASD at age 2 using standard measures is accurate (Lord et al., 2006), a recent parent-reported national survey found that up to one third of children who were given a diagnosis of autism earlier in childhood are no longer considered by parents to have the disorder by school age (Kogan et al., 2009). This may reflect resolution of symptoms, maturation of children diagnosed at young ages, diagnostic substitution, or improvement to the point that the child can be served in a general education setting. It is impossible to predict at the time of diagnosis which children will respond positively to intervention and which children will later be diagnosed with intellectual disability. Therefore, the need to provide an intensive, disorder-specific intervention program to all children with ASDs is imperative.

SUMMARY

ASDs are neurodevelopmental disorders with a genetic basis, the presentation of which might be modified by environmental factors. These disorders are characterized by impairments in communication, social interaction, and repetitive interests and behaviors. Children with ASDs may have associated intellectual disability and severe communication impairments. Individuals with typical cognitive abilities have symptoms related to social reciprocity and repetitive behaviors. Advances in early recognition and intervention have had a positive impact on outcome and quality of life for people with ASDs and their families. Individualized, multidimensional treatment is the standard of care and may be associated with notable improvements in symptoms.

REFERENCES

American Psychiatric Association. (2000). *Diagnostic and statistical manual of mental disorders (Fourth Edition, Text Revision)*. Washington, DC: American Psychiatric Association.

Asperger, H. (1991). Autisic psychopathy in childhood. In U. Frith (Ed.), *Autism and Asperger syndrome* (pp. 37–92). New York, NY: Cambridge University Press.

Auyeung, B.S., Baron-Cohen, S., Ashwin, E., Knickmeyer, R., Taylor, K., & Hackett, G. (2009). Fetal testosterone and autistic traits. *British Journal of Psychology, 100*(1), 1–22. doi:10.1348/000712608X311731

Bailey, A.P., Luthert, P., Dean, A., Harding, B., Janota, I., Montgomery, M., … Lantos, P. (1998). A clinicopathological study of autism. *Brain, 121*(5), 889–905. doi:10.1093/brain/121.5.889

Baranek, G. (2002). Efficacy of sensory and motor interventions for children with autism. *Journal of Autism and Developmental Disorders, 32*(5), 397–422.

Baron-Cohen, S., Wheelwright, S., Cox, A., Baird, G., Charman, T., Swettenham, J., … Doehring, P. (2000). Early identification of autism by Checklist for Autism in Toddlers (CHAT). *Journal of Royal Society of Medicine, 93*(10), 521–525.

Bauminger, N.M., Solomon, M., & Rogers, S.J. (2010). Predicting friendship quality in autism spectrum disorders and typical development. *Journal of Autism and Developmental Disorders, 40*(6), 751–761. doi:10.1007/s10803-009-0928-8

Bellini, S., & Peters, J.K. (2008). Social skills training for youth with autism spectrum disorders. *Child*

Adolescent Psychiatric Clinics of North America, 17(4), 857–873.

Bernard, S.A., Enayati, A., Redwood, L., Roger, H., & Binstock, T. (2001). Autism: A novel form of mercury poisoning. *Medical Hypotheses, 56*(4), 462–471. doi:10.1054/mehy.2000.1281

Bertrand, J.A., Mars, A., Boyle, C., Bove, F., Yeargin-Allsopp, M., & Decoufle, P. (2001). Prevalence of autism in a United States population: The Brick Township, New Jersey, investigation. *Pediatrics, 108*(5), 1155–1161. doi:10.1542/peds.108.5.1155

Billstedt, E.I., Gillberg, C., & Gillberg, C. (2005). Autism after adolescence: Population-based 13- to 22-year follow-up study of 120 individuals with autism diagnosed in childhood. *Journal of Autism and Developmental Disorders, 35*(3), 351–360. doi:10.1007/s10803-005-3302-5

Bondy, A.S., & Frost, L.A. (1998). The picture exchange communication system. *Seminars in Speech and Language, 19*(4), 373–388. doi:10.1055/s-2008-1064055

Bondy, A.S., & Frost, L.A. (2001). The picture exchange communication system. *Behavior Modification, 25*(5), 725–744. doi:10.1177/0145445501255004

Buie, T., Campbell, D.B., Fuchs III., G.J., Furuta, G.T., Levy, J., VandeWater, J., ... Winter, H. (2010). Evaluation, diagnosis, and treatment of gastrointestinal disorders in individuals with ASDs: A consensus report. *Pediatrics, 125*(Supplement 1), S1–S18. doi:10.1542/peds.2009-1878C

Buie, T., Fuchs III., G.J., Furuta, G.T., Koorosh, K., Levy, J., Lewis, J.D., ... Winter, H. (2010). Recommendations for evaluation and treatment of common gastrointestinal problems in children with ASDs. *Pediatrics, 125*(Supplement 1), S19–S29. doi:10.1542/peds.2009-1878D

Casanova, M.F. (2006). Neuropathological and genetic findings in autism: The significance of a putative minicolumnopathy. *The Neuroscientist, 12*(5), 435–441. doi:10.1177/1073858406290375

Centers for Disease Control and Prevention. (2009). Surveillance summaries: Prevalence of autism spectrum disorders—Autism and developmental disabilities monitoring network, United States 2006. *Morbidity and Mortality Weekly Report, 58*(No. SS-#), 1–24.

Chakrabarti, S., & Fombonne, E. (2001). Pervasive developmental disorders in preschool children. *The Journal of the American Medical Association, 285*(24), 3093–3099. doi:10.1001/jama.285.24.3093

Chan, A.S., Cheung, M.C., Han, Y.M.Y., Size, S.L., Leung, W.W., Man, H.S., & To, C.Y. (2009). Executive function deficits and neural discordance in children with autism spectrum disorders. *Clinical Neurophysiology, 120*(6), 1107–1115. doi:10.1016/j.clinph.2009.04.002

Chan, J.M., & O'Reilly, M.F. (2008). A social stories intervention package for students with autism in inclusive classroom settings. *Journal of Applied Behavior Analysis, 41*(3), 405–9.

Chandler, S., Charman, T., Baird, G., Simonoff, E., Loucas, T., Meldrum, D., ... Pickles, A. (2007). Validation of the social communication questionnaire in a population cohort of children with autism spectrum disorders. *Journal of the American Academy of Child & Adolescent Psychiatry, 46*(10), 1324–1332. doi:10.1097/chi.0b013e31812f7d8d

Charlop-Christy, M.H., Carpenter, M., Le, L., LeBlanc, L.A., & Kellet, K. (2002). Using the Picture Exchange Communication System (PECS) with children with autism: Assessment of PECS acquisition, speech, social-communicative behavior, and problem behavior. *Journal of Applied Behavior Analysis, 35*(3), 213–231. doi:10.1901/jaba.2002.35-213

Cheslack-Postava K., Liu, K., & Bearman, P.S. (2011). Closely spaced pregnancies are associated with increased incidence of autism in California sibling births. *Pediatrics, 127*(2), 246–53.

Chess, S. (1971). Autism in children with congenital rubella. *Journal of Autism and Child Schizophrenia, 1*(1), 33–47

Clifford, S., Dissanayake, C., Bui, Q.M., Huggins, R., Taylor, A.K., & Loesch, D.Z. (2007). Autism spectrum phenotype in males and females with fragile X full mutation and premutation. *Journal of Autism and Developmental Disorders, 37*(4), 738–747. doi:10.1007/s10803-006-0205-z

Constantino, J. (2005). *Social Responsiveness Scale*. Torrance, CA: Western Psychological Services.

Constantino, J. N., Davis, S.A., Todd, R.D., Schindler, M.K., Gross, M.M., Brophy, S.L., ... Reich, W. (2003). Validation of a brief quantitative measure of autistic traits: Comparison of the social responsiveness scale with the autism diagnostic interview—Revised. *Journal of Autism and Developmental Disorders, 33*(4), 427–433.

Croen, L.A., Grether, J.K., Yoshida, C.K., Odouli, R., & Van de Water, J. (2005). Maternal autoimmune diseases, asthma and allergies, and childhood autism spectrum disorders: A case-control study. *Archives of Pediatrics and Adolescent Medicine, 159*(2), 151–157. doi:10.1001/archpedi.159.2.151

Croen, L.A., Najjar, D.V., Fireman, B., & Grether, JK. (2007). Maternal and paternal age and risk of autism spectrum disorders. *Archives of Pediatric Adolescent Medicine, 161*(4), 334-40.

Dalton, M. (2002). Education rights and the special needs child. *Child & Adolescent Psychiatric, Clinics of North America, 11*(4), 859–868. doi:10.1016/S1056-4993(02)00021-4

Dawson, G., Rogers, S., Munson, J., Smith, M., Winter, J., Greenson, J., ...Varley, J. (2010). Randomized, controlled trial of an intervention for toddlers with autism: The Early Start Denver model. *Pediatrics, 125*(1), e17–e23. doi:10.1542/peds.2009-0958

Dawson, G., Webb, S.J., & McPartland, J. (2005). Understanding the nature of face processing impairment in autism: Insights from behavioral and electrophysiological studies. *Developmental Neuropsychology, 27*(3), 403–424. doi:10.1207/s15326942dn2703_6

de Bildt, A., Sytema, S., Ketelaars, C., Kraijer, D., Mulder, E., Volkmar, F., & Minderaa, R. (2004). Interrelationship between Autism Diagnostic Observation Schedule-Generic (ADOS-G), Autism Diagnostic Interview-Revised (ADI-R), and the *Diagnostic and Statistical Manual of Mental Disorders (DSM-IV-TR)* classification in children and adolescents with mental retardation. *Journal of Autism and Developmental Disorders, 34*(2), 129–137.

Demicheli, V., Jefferson, T., Rivetti, A., & Price, D. (2005). Vaccines for measles, mumps and rubella in children. *Cochrane Database of Systematic Reviews*. doi:10.1002/14651858.CD004407.pub2

Dumont-Mathieu, T., & Fein, D. (2005). Screening for autism in young children: The Modified Checklist for Autism in Toddlers (M-CHAT) and other measures. *Mental Retardation and Developmental Disabilities Research Reviews, 11*(3), 253–262. doi:10.1002/mrdd.20072

Dyches, T.T., Wilder, L.K., Sudweeks, R.R., Obiakor, F.E., & Algozzine, B. (2004). Multicultural issues in autism. *Journal of Autism and Developmental Disorders, 34*(2), 211–222. doi:10.1023/B:JADD.0000022611.80478.73

Elder, L.M., Dawson, G., Toth, K., Fein, D., & Munson, J. (2008). Head circumference as an early predictor of autism symptoms in younger siblings of children with autism spectrum disorder. *Journal of Autism and Developmental Disorders, 38*(6), 1104–1111. doi:10.1007/s10803-007-0495-9

Erickson, C.A., Stigler, K.A., Corkins, M.R., Posey, D.J., Fitzgerald, J.F., & McDougle, C.J. (2005). Gastrointestinal factors in autistic disorder: A critical review. *Journal of Autism and Developmental Disorders, 35*(6), 713–727. doi:10.1007/s10803-005-0019-4

Filipek, P., Accardo, P., Ashwal, S., Baranek, G.T., Cook, Jr., E.H., Dawson, G., ... Volkmar, F.R. (2000). Practice parameter: Screening and diagnosis of autism. *Neurology, 55*, 468–479.

Findling, R.L., Steiner, H., & Weller, E.B. (2005). Use of antipsychotics in children and adolescents. *Journal of Clinical Psychiatry, 66*(Supplement 7), 29–40.

Finegold, S.M., Molitoris, D., Song, Y., Liu, C., Vaisanen, M.-L., Bolte, E., ... Kaul, A. (2002). Gastrointestinal microflora studies in late-onset autism. *Clinical Infectious Diseases, 35*(Supplement 1), S6–S16. doi:10.1086/341914

Fombonne, E. (1999). The epidemiology of autism: A review. *Psychological Medicine, 29*(4), 769–786. doi:10.1017/S0033291799008508

Fombonne, E. (2003). Epidemiological surveys of autism and other pervasive developmental disorders: An update. *Journal of Autism and Developmental Disorders, 33*(4), 365–382.

Foxx, R.M. (2008). Applied behavior analysis treatment of autism: The state of the art. *Child and Adolescent Psychiatric Clinics of North America, 17*(4), 821–834. doi:10.1016/j.chc.2008.06.007

Geier, D.A., & Geier, M.R. (2006). A clinical trial of combined anti-androgen and anti-heavy metal therapy in autistic disorders. *Neuroendocrinology Letters, 27*(6), 833–838.

Gilliam, J.E. (2006). *Gilliam Autism Rating Scale 2*. Torrance, CA: Western Psychological Services.

Gold, C., Wigram, T., & Elefant, C. (2006). Music therapy for autistic spectrum disorder. *Cochrane Database of Systematic Reviews*. doi:10.1002/14651858.CD004381.pub2

Granpeesheh, D., & Tarbox, J. (2009). Applied behavior analytic interventions for children with autism: A description and review of treatment research. *Annals of Clinical Psychiatry, 21*(3), 162–173.

Gutstein, S.E., Burgess, A.F., & Montfort, K. (2007). Evaluation of the relationship development intervention program. *Autism, 11*(5), 397–411. doi:10.1177/1362361307079603

Hall, S.S., Lightbody, A.A., Hirt, M., Rezvani, A., & Reiss, A.L. (2010). Autism in fragile X syndrome: A category mistake? *Journal of the American Academy of Child and Adolescent Psychiatry, 49*(9), 921–933. doi:10.1016/j.jaac.2010.07.001

Hallmayer, J., Cleveland, S., Torres, A., Phillips, J., Cohen, B., Torigoe, T., ... Risch, N. (2011). Genetic heritability and shared environmental factors among twin pairs with autism. *Archives of General Psychiatry, 68*(11), 1095–1102. doi:10.1001/archgenpsychiatry.2011.76

Handen, B.L., Johnson, C.R., & Lubetsky, M. (2000). Efficacy of methylphenidate among children with autism and symptoms of attention-deficit/hyperactivity disorder. *Journal of Autism and Developmental Disorders, 30*(3), 245–255.

Handen, B.L., Sahl, R., & Hardan, A.Y. (2008). Guanfacine in children with autism and/or intellectual disabilities. *Journal of Developmental and Behavioral Pediatrics, 29*(4), 303–308. doi:10.1097/DBP.0b013e3181739b9d

Happé, F. (2011). Criteria, categories, and continua: Autism and related disorders in DSM-5. *Journal of the American Academy of Child and Adolescent Psychiatry, 50*(6), 540–542. doi:10.1016/j.jaac.2011.03.015

Harris, S.L., Handleman, J.S., Gordon, R., Kristoff, B., & Fuentes, F. (1991). Changes in cognitive and language functioning of preschool children with autism. *Journal of Autism and Developmental Disorders, 21*(3), 281–290. doi:10.1007/BF02207325

Harrower, J.K., & Dunlap, G. (2001). Including children with autism in general education classrooms. A review of effective strategies. *Behavior Modification, 25*(5), 762–784.

Hendry, C.N. (2000). Childhood disintegrative disorder: Should it be considered a distinct diagnosis? *Clinical Psychology Review, 20*(1), 77–90.

Hollander, E., Dolgoff-Kaspar, R., Cartwright, C., Rawitt, R., & Novotny, S. (2001). An open trial of divalproex sodium in autism spectrum disorders. *The Journal of Clinical Psychiatry, 62*(7), 530–534. doi:10.4088/JCP.v62n07a05

Howlin, P. (2003). Outcome in high-functioning adults with autism with and without early language delays: Implications for the differentiation between autism and Asperger syndrome. *Journal of Autism and Developmental Disorders, 33*(1), 3–13.

Howlin, P., & Asgharian, A. (1999). The diagnosis of autism and Asperger syndrome: Findings from a survey of 770 families. *Developmental Medicine and Child Neurology, 41*(12), 834–839. doi:10.1017/S0012162299001656

Johnson, C.P., Myers, S.M., & the Council on Children with Disabilities. (2007). Identification and evaluation of children with autism spectrum disorders. *Pediatrics, 120*(5), 1183–1215. doi:10.1542/peds.2007-2361

Johnson, K.P., & Malow, B.A. (2008). Assessment and pharmacologic treatment of sleep disturbance in autism. *Child and Adolescent Psychiatric Clinics of North America, 17*(4), 773–785. doi:10.1016/j.chc.2008.06.006

Jones, T.B., Bandettini, P.A., Kenworthy, L., Case, L.K., Milleville, S.C., Martin, A., & Birn, R.M. (2010). Sources of group differences in functional connectivity: An investigation applied to autism spectrum disorder. *NeuroImage, 49*(1), 401–414. doi:10.1016/j.neuroimage.2009.07.051

Jordan, R. (2005). Managing autism and Asperger's syndrome in current educational provision. *Developmental Neurorehabilitation, 8*(2), 104–112. doi:10.1080/13638490500054891

Kaminsky, L., & Dewey, D. (2002). Psychosocial adjustment in siblings of children with autism. *Journal of Child Psychology and Psychiatry, 43*(2), 225–232. doi:10.1111/1469-7610.00015

Kanner, L. (1943). Autistic disturbances of affective contact. *Nervous Child, 2*, 217–250.

King, B.H., Hollander, E., Sikich, L., McCracken, J.T., Scahill, L., Bregman, J.D., ... Ritz, L. (2009). Lack of efficacy of citalopram in children with autism spectrum disorders and high levels of repetitive behavior: Citalopram ineffective in children with autism. *Archives of General Psychiatry, 66*(6), 583–590. doi:10.1001/archgenpsychiatry.2009.30

Klin, A., Jones, W., Schultz, R., Volkmar, F., & Cohen, D. (2002). Visual fixation patterns during viewing of naturalistic social situations as predictors of social competence in individuals with autism. *Archives of General Psychiatry, 59*(9), 809–816. doi:10.1001/archpsyc.59.9.809

Koegel, R., Koegel, L., & McNerney, E.K. (2001). Pivotal areas in intervention for autism. *Journal of Clinical Child Psychology, 30*(1), 19–32. doi:10.1207/S15374424JCCP3001_4

Kogan, M.D., Blumberg, S.J., Schieve, L.A., Boyle, C.A., Perrin, J.M., Ghandour, R.M., ... van Dyck, P.C. (2009). Prevalence of parent-reported diagnosis of autism spectrum disorder among children in the US, 2007. *Pediatrics, 124*(5), 1395–1403. doi:10.1542/peds.2009- 1522

Kokina, A., & Kern, L. (2010). Social story interventions for students with autism spectrum disorders: A meta analysis. *Journal of Autism and Developmental Disorders, 40*(7), 812–26.

Kumar, R., & Christian, S. (2009). Genetics of autism spectrum disorders. *Current Neurology and Neuroscience Reports, 9*(3), 188–197. doi:10.1007/s11910-009-0029-2

Kwasnicka-Crawford, D.A., Roberts, W., & Scherer, S.W. (2007). Characterization of an autism-associated segmental maternal heterodisomy of the chromosome 15q11-13 region. *Journal of Autism and Developmental Disorders, 37*(4), 694–702. doi:10.1007/s10803-006-0225-8

Landrigan, P.J. (2010). What causes autism? Exploring the environmental contribution. *Current Opinion in Pediatrics, 22*(2), 219–225. doi:10.1097/MOP.0b013e328336eb9a

Leask, J., Booy, R., & McIntyre, P.B. (2010). MMR, Wakefield and The Lancet: What can we learn? *The Medical Journal of Australia, 193*(1), 5–7.

Levy, S.E., Giarelli, E., Lee, L.-C., Schieve, L.A., Kirby, R.S., Cunniff, C., ... Rice, C.E. (2010). Autism spectrum disorder and co-occurring developmental, psychiatric, and medical conditions among children in multiple populations of the United States. *Journal of Developmental and Behavioral Pediatrics, 31*(4), 267–275. doi:10.1097/DBP.0b013e3181d5d03b

Levy, S.E., & Hyman, S.L. (2003). Use of complementary and alternative treatments for children with autistic spectrum disorders is increasing. *Pediatric Annals, 32*(10), 685–691.

Levy, S.E., & Hyman, S.L. (2005). Novel treatments for autistic spectrum disorders. *Mental Retardation and Developmental Disabilities Research Reviews, 11*(2), 131–142. doi:10.1002/mrdd.20062

Levy, S.E., & Hyman, S.L. (2008). Complementary and alternative medicine treatments for children with autism spectrum disorders. *Child and Adolescent Psychiatric Clinics of North America, 17*(4), 803–820. doi:10.1016/j.chc.2008.06.004

Levy, S.E., Mandell, D.S., & Schultz, R.T. (2009). Autism. *Lancet, 374*(9701), 1627–1638.

Limperopoulos, C. (2009). Autism spectrum disorders in survivors of extreme prematurity. *Clinics in Perinatology, 36*(4), 791–805 doi:10.1016/j.clp.2009.07.010.

Lord, C., Petkova, E., Hus, V., Gan, W., Lu, F., Martin, D.M., ...Risi, S. (2011). A multisite study of the clinical diagnosis of autism spectrum disorders. *Archives of General Psychiatry.* 2011 Nov 7. [Epub ahead of print]

Lord, C., Risi, S., DiLavore, P.S., Shulman, C., Thurm, A., & Pickles, A. (2006). Autism from 2 to 9 years

of age. *Archives of General Psychiatry, 63*(6), 694–701. doi:10.1001/archpsyc.63.6.694

Lord, C., Risi, S., Lambrecht, L., Cook, E.H., Jr., Leventhal, B.L., Pickles, A., & Rutter, M. (2000). The ADOS-G (Autism Diagnostic Observation Schedule-Generic): A standard measure of social-communication deficits associated with autism spectrum disorders. *Journal of Autism and Developmental Disorders, 30*(3), 205–223.

Lord, C., Rutter, M., & LeCouteur, A. (1994). Autism Diagnostic Interview-Revised: A revised version of a diagnostic interview for caregivers of individuals with possible pervasive developmental disorders. *Journal of Autism and Developmental Disorders, 24*(5), 659–685. doi:10.1007/BF02172145

Lovaas, O. (1987). Behavioral treatment and normal educational and intellectual functioning in young autistic children. *Journal of Consulting and Clinical Psychology, 55*(1), 3–9. doi:10.1037//0022-006X.55.1.3

Madsen, K.M., Hviid, A., Vestergaard, M., Schendel, D., Wohlfahrt, J., Thorsen, P., ... Melbye, M. (2002). A population-based study of measles, mumps, and rubella vaccination and autism. *New England Journal of Medicine, 347*(19), 1477–1482

Madsen, K.M., Lauritsen, M.B., Pedersen, C.B., Thorsen, P., Plesner, A.M., Andersen, P.H, & Mortensen, P.B. (2003). Thimerosal and the occurrence of autism: Negative ecological evidence from Danish population-based data. *Pediatrics, 112*(3, Pt 1), 604–606.

Maenner, M.J., & Durkin, M.S. (2010). Trends in the prevalence of autism on the basis of special education data. *Pediatrics, 126*(5), e1018–e1025. doi:10.1542/peds.2010-1023

Mahoney, G., & Perales, F. (2005). Relationship-focused early intervention with children with pervasive developmental disorders and other disabilities: A comparative study. *Journal of Developmental and Behavioral Pediatrics, 26*(2), 77–85.

Malow, B.A., Marzec, M.L., McGrew, S.G., Wang, L., Henderson, L.M., & Stone, W.L. (2006). Characterizing sleep in children with autism spectrum disorders: A multidimensional approach. *Sleep, 29*(12), 1563–1571.

Malow, B.A., McGrew, S.G., Harvey, M., Henderson, L.M., & Stone, W.L. (2006). Impact of treating sleep apnea in a child with autism spectrum disorder. *Pediatric Neurology, 34*(4), 325–328. doi:10.1016/j.pediatrneurol.2005.08.021

Mandell, D.S., Listerud, J., Levy, S.E., & Pinto-Martin, J.A. (2002). Race differences in the age at diagnosis among Medicaid-eligible children with autism. *Journal of the American Academy of Child and Adolescent Psychiatry, 41*(12), 1447–1453. doi:10.1097/00004583-200212000-00016

Mandell, D.S., Novak, M.M., & Zubritsky, C.D. (2005). Factors associated with age of diagnosis among children with autism spectrum disorders. *Pediatrics, 116*(6), 1480–1486. doi:10.1542/peds.2005-0185

Mandell, D.S., Wiggins, L.D., Carpenter, L.A., Daniels, J., DiGuiseppi, C., Durkin, M.S., ... Kirby, R.S. (2009). Racial/ethnic disparities in the identification of children with autism spectrum disorders. *American Journal of Public Health, 99*(3), 493–498. doi:10.2105/AJPH.2007.131243

Mars, A.E., Mauk, J.E., & Dowrick, P.W. (1998). Symptoms of pervasive developmental disorders as observed in prediagnostic home videos of infants and toddlers. *The Journal of Pediatrics, 132*(3), 500–504. doi:10.1016/S0022-3476(98)70027-7

McCracken, J.T., McGough, J., Shah, B., Cronin, P., Hong, D., Aman, M.G., ... McMahon, D. (2002). Risperidone in children with autism and serious behavioral problems. *New England Journal of Medicine, 347*(5), 314–321. doi:10.1056/NEJMoa013171

McDougle, C.J., Scahill, L., Aman, M.G., McCracken, J.T., Tierney, E., Davies, M., ... Vitiello, B. (2005). Risperidone for the core symptom domains of autism: Results from the study by the autism network of the research units on pediatric psychopharmacology. *American Journal of Psychiatry, 162*(6), 1142–1148. doi:10.1176/appi.ajp.162.6.1142

McEachin, J.J., Smith, T., & Lovaas, O.I. (1993). Long-term outcome for children with autism who received early intensive behavioral treatment. *American Journal on Mental Retardation, 97*(4), 359–372.

Mesibov, G.B., & Shea, V. (2010). The TEACCH program in the era of evidence-based practice. *Journal of Autism and Developmental Disorders, 40*(5), 570–579. doi:10.1007/s10803-009-0901-6

Millward, C., Ferriter, M., & Connell-Jones, G. (2008). Gluten- and casein-free diets for autistic spectrum disorder. *Cochrane Database of Systematic Reviews.* doi:10.1002/14651858.CD003498.pub2

Minshew, N.J., & Williams, D.L. (2007). The new neurobiology of autism: Cortex, connectivity, and neuronal organization. *Archives of Neurology 64*(7), 945–950. doi:10.1001/archneur.64.7.945

Mitchell, S., Brian, J., Zwaigenbaum, L., Roberts, W., Szatmari, P., Smith, I., & Bryson, S. (2006). Early language and communication development of infants later diagnosed with autism spectrum disorder. *Journal of Developmental and Behavioral Pediatrics, 27*(Supp. 2), S69–S78. doi:10.1097/00004703-200604002-00004

Moore, M.L., Eichner, S.F., & Jones, J.R. (2004). Treating functional impairment of autism with selective serotonin-reuptake inhibitors. *Annals of Pharmacotherapy, 38*(9), 1515–1519. doi:10.1345/aph.1D543

Moss, J., & Howlin, P. (2009). Autism spectrum disorders in genetic syndromes: Implications for diagnosis, intervention and understanding the wider autism spectrum disorder population. *Journal of Intellectual Disability Research, 53*(10), 852–873. doi:10.1111/j.1365-2788.2009.01197.x

Mostert, M.P. (2001). Facilitated communication since 1995: A review of published studies. *Journal of Autism and Developmental Disorders, 31*(3), 287–313.

Muhle, R., Trentacoste, S.V., & Rapin, I. (2004). The genetics of autism. *Pediatrics, 113*(5), e472–e486. doi:10.1542/peds.113.5.e472

Mundy, P., & Newell, L. (2007). Attention, joint attention and social cognition. *Current Directions in Psychological Science, 16*(5), 269–274. doi:10.1111/j.1467-8721.2007.00518.x

Myers, G.J., Davidson, P.W., Cox, C., Shamlaye, C.F., Palumbo, D., Cernichiari, E., ... Clarkson, T.W. (2003). Prenatal methylmercury exposure from ocean fish consumption in the Seychelles child development study. *Lancet, 361*(9370), 1686–1692. doi:10.1016/S0140-6736(03)13371-5

National Research Council. (2001). *Educating children with autism.* Washington, DC: National Academy Press.

Nelson, K.B., & Bauman, M.L. (2003). Thimerosal and autism? *Pediatrics, 111*(3), 674–679. doi:10.1542/peds.111.3.674

Ng, D.K., Chan, C.-H., Soo, M.-T., & Lee, R.S.-Y. (2007). Low-level chronic mercury exposure in children and adolescents: Meta-analysis. *Pediatrics International, 49*(1), 80–87. doi:10.1111/j.1442-200X.2007.02303.x

Nye, C., Brice, A. (2005) Combined vitamin B6-magnesium treatment in autism spectrum disorders. *Cochrane Database of Systematic Reviews Oct 19*(4), CD003497.

O'Roak, B.J., & State, M.W. (2008). Autism genetics: Strategies, challenges, and opportunities. *Autism Research, 1*(1), 4–17. doi:10.1002/aur.3

Oberman, L.M., & Ramachandran, V.S. (2007). The simulating social mind: The role of the mirror neuron system and simulation in the social and communicative deficits of autism spectrum disorders. *Psychological Bulletin, 133*(2), 310–327. doi:10.1037/0033-2909.133.2.310

Ozonoff, S., Young, G.S., Carter, A., Messinger, D., Yirmiya, N., Zwaigenbaum, L., ... Stone, W.L. (2011). Recurrence risk for autism spectrum disorders: A baby siblings research consortium study. *Pediatrics, 128*(3), 2010–2825. doi: 10.1542/peds.2010-2825)

Palmer, R.F., Blanchard, S., Stein, Z., Mandell, D., & Miller, C. (2006). Environmental mercury release, special education rates, and autism disorder: An ecological study of Texas. *Health Place, 12*(2), 203–209. doi:10.1016/j.healthplace.2004.11.005

Pandey, J., Verbalis, A., Robins, D.L., Boorstein, H., Klin, A., Babitz, T., ... Fein, D. (2008). Screening for autism in older and younger toddlers with the Modified Checklist for Autism in Toddlers. *Autism, 12*(5), 513–535. doi:10.1177/1362361308094503

Panerai, S., Ferrante, L., & Zingale, M. (2002). Benefits of the treatment and education of autistic and communication handicapped children (TEACCH) programme as compared with a non-specific approach. *Journal of Intellectual Disability Research, 46*(4), 318–327. doi:10.1046/j.1365-2788.2002.00388.x

Parner, E.T., Thorsen, P., Dixon, G., de Klerk, N., Leonard, H., Nassar, N., ... Glasson, E.J. (2011). A comparison of autism prevalence trends in Denmark and Western Australia. *Journal of Autism and Developmental Disorders, 41*(12), 1601–1608. doi:10.1007/s10803-011-1186-0

Parr, J., Le Couteur, A., Baird, G., Rutter, M., Pickles, A., Fombonne, E., & Bailey, A.J. (2011). Early developmental regression in autism spectrum disorder: Evidence from an international multiplex sample. *Journal of Autism and Developmental Disorders, 41*(3), 332–340.

Pelphrey, K.A., Morris, J.P., & McCarthy, G. (2005). Neural basis of eye gaze processing deficits in autism. *Brain, 128*(5), 1038–1048. doi:10.1093/brain/awh404

Peters, S.U., Beaudet, A.L., Madduri, N., & Bacino, C.A. (2004). Autism in Angelman syndrome: Implications for autism research. *Clinical Genetics, 66*(6), 530–536. doi:10.1111/j.1399-0004.2004.00362.x

Pinborough-Zimmerman, J., Bilder, D., Satterfield, R., Hossain, S., & McMahon, W. (2010). The impact of surveillance method and record source on autism prevalence: Collaboration with Utah maternal and child health programs. *Maternal and Child Health Journal, 14*(3), 392–400. doi:10.1007/s10995-009-0472-3

Posserud, M., Lundervold, A.J., Lie, S.A., & Gillberg, C. (2010). The prevalence of autism spectrum disorders: Impact of diagnostic instrument and non-response bias. *Social Psychiatry and Psychiatric Epidemiology, 45*(3), 319–327. doi:10.1007/s00127-009-0087-4

Rapin, I., & Dunn, M. (2003). Update on the language disorders of individuals on the autistic spectrum. *Brain and Development, 25*(3), 166–172. doi:10.1016/S0387-7604(02)00191-2

Retraction—Ileal-lymphoid-nodular hyperplasia, non-specific colitis, and pervasive developmental disorder in children. (2010). *The Lancet, 375*(9713), 445. doi:10.1016/S0140-6736(10)60175-4

Ringman, J.M., & Jankovic, J. (2000). Occurrence of tics in Asperger's syndrome and autistic disorder. *Journal of Child Neurology, 15*(6), 394–400. doi:10.1177/088307380001500608

Roberts, T.P., Khan, S.Y., Rey, M., Monroe, J.F., Cannon, K., Blaskey, L. ... Edgar, J.C. (2010). MEG detection of delayed auditory evoked responses in autism spectrum disorders: Towards an imaging biomarker for autism. *Autism Research, 3*(1), 8–18.

Robins, D.L., Fein, D., Barton, M.L., & Green, J.A. (2001). The Modified Checklist for Autism in Toddlers: An initial study investigating the early detection of autism and pervasive developmental disorders. *Journal of Autism and Developmental Disorders, 31*(2), 131–144.

Rogers, S. (1998). Neuropsychology of autism in young children and its implications for early intervention. *Mental Retardation and Developmental Disabilities Research Reviews, 4*, 104–112. doi:10.1002/(SICI)1098-2779(1998)4:2<104::AID-MRDD7>3.0.CO;2-P

Rogers, S.J. (2000). Interventions that facilitate socialization in children with autism. *Journal of Autism and Developmental Disorders, 30*(5), 399–409.

Rogers, S.J. (2004). Developmental regression in autism spectrum disorders. *Mental Retardation and Developmental Disabilities Research Reviews, 10*(2), 139–143. doi:10.1002/mrdd.20027

Rogers, S.J., & Vismara, L.A. (2008). Evidence-based comprehensive treatments for early autism. *Journal of Clinical Child & Adolescent Psychology, 37*(1), 8–38. doi:10.1080/15374410701817808

Russell, R.L., & Grizzle, K.L. (2008). Assessing child and adolescent pragmatic language competencies: Toward evidence-based assessments. *Clinical Child and Family Psychology Review, 11*(1–2), 59–73. doi:10.1007/s10567-008-0032-1

Rutter, M. (1985). The treatment of autistic children. *Journal of Child Psychology and Psychiatry, 26*(2), 193–214. doi:10.1111/j.1469-7610.1985.tb02260.x

Rutter, M., Bailey, A., & Lord, C. (2003). *Social Communication Questionnaire.* Torrance, CA: Western Psychological Services.

Rutter, M., LeCouteur, A., Lord, C. (2003). *Autism Diagnostic Interview–Revised.* Torrance, CA: Western Psychological Services

Sanua, V.D. (1984). Is infantile autism a universal phenomenon? An open question. *International Journal of Social Psychiatry, 30*(3), 163–177. doi:10.1177/002076408403000301

Schendel, D., & Bhasin, T.K. (2008). Birth weight and gestational age characteristics of children with autism, including a comparison with other developmental disabilities. *Pediatrics, 121*(6), 1155–1164. doi:10.1542/peds.2007-1049

Schmitz, N., Rubia, K., Daly, E., Smith, A., Williams, S., & Murphy, D.G.M. (2006). Neural correlates of executive function in autistic spectrum disorders. *Biological Psychiatry, 59*(1), 7–16. doi:10.1016/j.biopsych.2005.06.007

Schopler, E., Van Bourgonden, M.E., Wellman, G.J., & Love, S.R. (2010). *Childhood Autism Rating Scale 2.* Torrance, CA: Western Psychological Services.

Schultz, R.T. (2005). Developmental deficits in social perception in autism: The role of the amygdala and fusiform face area. *International Journal of Developmental Neuroscience, 23*(2–3), 125–141. doi:10.1016/j.ijdevneu.2004.12.012

Scott, M.M., & Deneris, E.S. (2005). Making and breaking serotonin neurons and autism. *International Journal of Developmental Neuroscience, 23*(2–3), 277–285. doi:10.1016/j.ijdevneu.2004.05.012

Seigel, B. (2004). *Pervasive Developmental Disorder Screening Test II.* San Antonio, TX: Pearson, Psych Corp.

Silverman, L.B., Bennetto, L., Campana, E., & Tanenhaus, M.K. (2010). Speech-and-gesture integration in high functioning autism. *Cognition, 115*(3), 380–393. doi:10.1016/j.cognition.2010.01.002

Smalley, S.L. (1998). Autism and tuberous sclerosis. *Journal of Autism and Developmental Disorders, 28*(5), 407–414.

Smith, T., Eikeseth, S., Klevstran, M., & Lovaas, O.I. (1997). Intensive behavioral treatment for preschoolers with severe mental retardation and pervasive developmental disorder. *American Journal on Mental Retardation, 102*(3), 238–249. doi:10.1352/0895-8017(1997)102<0238:IBTFPW>2.0.CO;2

Souders, M.C., Mason, T.B., Valladares, O., Bucan, M., Levy, S.E., Mandell, D.S., ... Pinto-Martin, J. (2009). Sleep behaviors and sleep quality in children with autism spectrum disorders. *Sleep, 32*(12), 1566–1578.

Stone, W.L., Coonrod, E.E., & Ousley, O.Y. (2000). Brief report: Screening Tool for Autism in Two-year-olds (STAT): Development and preliminary data. *Journal of Autism and Developmental Disorders, 30*(6), 607.

Stone, W.L., McMahon, C.R., & Henderson, L.M. (2008). Use of the Screening Tool for Autism in Two-year-olds (STAT) for children under 24 months: An exploratory study. *Autism, 12*(5), 557–573. doi:10.1177/1362361308096403

Strömland, K., Nordin, V., Miller, M., Akerström, B., & Gillberg, C. (1994). Autism in thalidomide embryopathy: A population study. *Developmental Medicine and Child Neurology, 36*(4), 351-6.

Szatmari, P., MacLean, J.E., Jones, M.B., Bryson, S.E., Zwaigenbaum, L., Bartolucci, G., ... Tuff, L. (2000). The familial aggregation of the lesser variant in biological and nonbiological relatives of PDD probands: A family history study. *Journal of Child Psychology and Psychiatry, 41*(5), 579–586. doi:10.1111/1469-7610.00644

Tesink, C.M., Buitelaar, J.K., Petersson, K.M., van der Gaag, R.J., Kan, C.C., Tendolkar, I., & Hagoort, P. (2009). Neural correlates of pragmatic language comprehension in autism spectrum disorders. *Brain, 132*(7), 1941–1952. doi:10.1093/brain/awp103

Travis, L., Sigman, M., & Ruskin, E. (2001). Links between social understanding and social behavior in verbally able children with autism. *Journal of Autism and Developmental Disorders, 31*(2), 119–130.

Trevathan, E. (2004). Seizures and epilepsy among children with language regression and autistic spectrum disorders. *Journal of Child Neurology, 19*(Supp. 1), S49–S57. doi:10.1177/08830738040190010601

Tuchman, R. (2004). AEDs and psychotropic drugs in children with autism and epilepsy. *Mental Retardation and Developmental Disabilities Research Reviews, 10*(2), 135–138. doi:10.1002/mrdd.20026

Tuchman, R., & Rapin, I. (2002). Epilepsy in autism. *Lancet Neurology, 1*(6), 352–358. doi:10.1016/S1474-4422(02)00160-6

Vargas, D.L., Nascimbene, C., Krishnan, C., Zimmerman, A.W., & Pardo, C.A. (2005). Neuroglial activation and neuroinflammation in the brain of patients with autism. *Annals of Neurology, 57*(1), 67–81. doi:10.1002/ana.20315

Vismara, L.A., & Rogers, S.J. (2010). Behavioral treatments in autism spectrum disorder: What do we know? *Annual Review of Clinical Psychology, 6*(1), 447–468. doi:10.1146/annurev.clinpsy.121208.131151

Vollm, B.A., Taylor, A.N., Richardson, P., Corcoran, R., Stirling, J., McKie, S., ... Elliot, R. (2006). Neuronal correlates of theory of mind and empathy: A functional magnetic resonance imaging study in a nonverbal task. *NeuroImage, 29*(1), 90–98. doi:10.1016/j.neuroimage.2005.07.022

Warren, Z., McPheeters, M.L., Sathe, N., Foss-Feig, J.H., Glasser, A., & Veenstra-VanderWeele, J. (2011). A systematic review of early intensive intervention for autism spectrum disorders. *Pediatrics, 127*(5), e1303–e1311. doi:10.1542/peds.2011-0426

White, S.W., Scahill, L., Klin, A., Koenig, K., & Volkmar, F.R. (2007). Educational placements and service use patterns of individuals with autism spectrum disorders. *Journal of Autism and Developmental Disorders, 37*(8), 1403–1412. doi:10.1007/s10803-006-0281-0

Wieder, S., & Greenspan, S.I. (2003). Climbing the symbolic ladder in the DIR model through floor time/interactive play. *Autism, 7*(4), 425–435. doi:10.1177/1362361303007004008

Williams, J.H., Waiter, G.D., Gilchrist, A., Perrett, D.I., Murray, A.D., & Whiten, A. (2006). Neural mechanisms of imitation and 'mirror neuron' functioning in autistic spectrum disorder. *Neuropsychologia, 44*(4), 610-21.

Williams, K., Wheeler, D.M., Silove, N., & Hazell, P. (2010). Selective serotonin reuptake inhibitors (SSRIs) for autism spectrum disorders (ASD). *Cochrane Database of Systematic Reviews, 8*, CD004677.

Williams, K.W., Wray, J.J., & Wheeler, D.M. (2005). Intravenous secretin for autism spectrum disorder. *Cochrane Database of Systematic Reviews, 3*, CD003495. doi:10.1002/14651858.CD003495

Yeargin-Allsopp, M., Rice, C., Karapurkar, T., Doernberg, N., Boyle, C., & Murphy, C. (2003). Prevalence of autism in a US metropolitan area. *Journal of American Medical Association, 289*(1), 49–55. doi:10.1001/jama.289.1.49

Zimmerman, A.W., Connors, S.L., Matteson, K.J., Lee, L.-C., Singer, H.S., Castaneda, J.A., & Pearce, D.A. (2007). Maternal antibrain antibodies in autism. *Brain, Behavior, and Immunity, 21*(3), 351–357. doi:10.1016/j.bbi.2006.08.005

Zwaigenbaum, L., Szatmari, P., Jones, M.B., Bryson, S.E., Maclean, J.E., Mahoney, W.J., ... Tuff, L. (2002). Pregnancy and birth complications in autism and liability to the broader autism phenotype. *Journal of the American Academy of Child and Adolescent Psychiatry, 41*(5), 572–579. doi:10.1097/00004583-200205000-00015

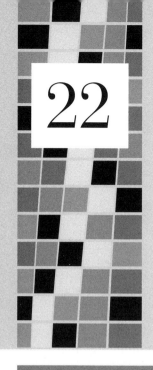

22

Attention Deficits and Hyperactivity

Marianne Glanzman and Neelam Sell

Upon completion of this chapter, the reader will

■ Be familiar with the characteristics of attention-deficit/hyperactivity disorder

■ Be aware of some of the causes of inattention and hyperactivity

■ Understand the components of the diagnostic process

■ Know the different approaches to management

■ Be aware of the natural history and outcomes for this disorder

Attention-deficit/hyperactivity disorder (ADHD) is one of the most prevalent neurodevelopmental/ mental health conditions in childhood. It is characterized by developmentally inappropriate levels of inattention and distractibility and/or hyperactivity and impulsivity that cause impairment in adaptive functioning at home, school, and in social situations. Treatment improves short-term academic, social, and adaptive functioning (Multimodal Treatment Study of ADHD [MTA] Cooperative Group, 2004a). Comprehensive management leads to some documented long-term benefits for children with ADHD, though much work remains to be done to improve their outcomes. We now understand that the condition and its impact tend to persist into adolescence and adulthood in a substantial percentage of individuals (Spencer, Biederman, & Mick, 2007).

▪ ▪ ▪ RICKY

Ricky, age 7, is in second grade. His teacher reports that he is having great difficulty learning to read. He also is quite disruptive in class, frequently not listening to directions, getting out of his seat, making silly comments, and talking out of turn. His first-grade teacher reported similar problems, but these difficulties were attributed to him having to adjust to the new school, as he attended a Montessori kindergarten previously. His parents and soccer coach have also noticed problems with his ability to follow directions and pay attention. Ricky was adopted shortly after birth, so there is no family history available. He has, however, always had a "difficult" temperament. He was a colicky infant with poor sleep patterns. As a preschooler, he was demanding and would exhaust all those around him. His parents and teachers feel that he is still quite immature and demanding, as he requires much more attention than other children his age.

A comprehensive evaluation revealed that Ricky has ADHD combined type and a learning disability in reading, though he is intellectually gifted. Ricky is at significant risk for both academic and behavior difficulties, so a multimodal treatment plan was put into place. Stimulant medication has been dramatically helpful at school and is used on weekends and school vacations as well for improved functioning in social situations and activities of daily living. His counseling focuses on the development of a consistent behavior management plan at home and school and social skill instruction. At school, he receives resource room assistance for reading and language arts, enrichment programming in math, and weekly meetings with the school counselor for a social skills group.

DIAGNOSIS AND ATTENTION-DEFICIT/HYPERACTIVITY DISORDER SUBTYPES

ADHD is a neurobehavioral syndrome; as of 2011, there are no available medical or psychological tests to definitively make the diagnosis. Instead, the diagnosis depends on "ruling in" symptoms of ADHD and "ruling out" other causes of the symptoms. Through the use of interviews and rating scales to systematically collect information from parents, teachers, and (older) children, the clinician must determine whether 1) significant ADHD symptoms are present in more than one setting; 2) they result in functional impairment; and 3) they are the result of another psychiatric, medical, or social condition rather than ADHD (American Academy of Pediatrics, 2011; Pelham, Fabiano, & Massetti, 2005). The current diagnostic criteria consist of two major clusters of symptoms: inattention and hyperactivity/impulsivity. These criteria, outlined in the *Diagnostic and Statistical Manual-IV* (*DSM-IV-TR*) of the American Psychiatric Association (APA), are shown in Table 22.1 (American Psychiatric Association [APA], 2000).

Children who display a significant number (>6) of symptoms from both clusters have ADHD combined type (ADHD-C), provided: 1) the symptoms were evident before age 7; 2) they have persisted for at least 6 months; and 3) they occur across multiple settings (i.e., both school and home), cause impairment, and cannot be better accounted for by another disorder. The selection of 7 years as the age at which symptoms must have been present is controversial because some children who meet all other criteria for ADHD do not demonstrate functionally impairing symptoms before later elementary or middle school (Barkley, 2010; Stefanatos & Baron, 2007).

ADHD-C is the most commonly diagnosed and studied form of ADHD. It is associated with social impairment, increased prevalence of coexisting internalizing (anxiety and mood) disorders, and externalizing (oppositional defiant and conduct) disorders, as well as academic underachievement (Baeyens, Roeyers, & Walle, 2006; Spencer, Biederman, et al., 2007).

The second most common subtype, ADHD predominately inattentive type (ADHD-I), refers to individuals who do not display significant levels of hyperactivity but have significant problems in maintaining attention. There is some evidence to suggest that the specific nature of inattention in this subtype may differ from the inattention shown by those with the combined subtype. A "slow" cognitive tempo is characteristic in ADHD-I. The ratio of girls to boys with this subtype is slightly higher than for the other subtypes, and it is usually identified at a later age. The pattern of psychiatric comorbidity also differs from that of ADHD-C type with fewer oppositional or conduct disorders, but with more anxiety and mood disorders. Educational impairments are the most prominent difficulty experienced by this group (Baeyens et al., 2006; Barkley, 1998; Stefanatos & Baron, 2007).

The third subtype, ADHD predominantly hyperactive/impulsive type (ADHD-HI), was first identified in *DSM-IV* and refers to children who do not display significant levels of attention problems in the presence of hyperactivity and impulsivity. This subtype is most often diagnosed in preschool age boys and may change over time to the combined subtype as young children may have not yet reached an age at which attention problems are impairing (Greenhill, Posner, Vaughan, & Kratochvil, 2008). The developmental course of this subtype and its response to treatment continue to be explored.

Finally, ADHD not otherwise specified (ADHD-NOS) can be used for individuals who have significant functional impairment from the symptoms of ADHD but may not meet strict criteria for the diagnosis based on number of symptoms present or age of onset criteria. Any of the subtypes can be used with the phrase "in partial remission" when symptoms are present but have improved such that the individual no longer meets strict criteria.

Table 22.1. Current *Diagnostic and Statistical Manual of Mental Disorders, Fourth Edition, Text Revision* criteria for attention-deficit/hyperactivity disorder (ADHD)

A. Inattention/distractibility

1. Often fails to give close attention to details or makes careless mistakes in schoolwork, work, or other activities
2. Often has difficulty sustaining attention in tasks or play activities
3. Often does not seem to listen when spoken to directly
4. Often does not follow through on instructions and fails to finish schoolwork, chores, or duties in the workplace (not due to oppositional behavior or failure to understand instructions)
5. Often has difficulty organizing tasks and activities
6. Often avoids, dislikes or is reluctant to engage in tasks that require sustained mental effort (e.g., schoolwork, homework)
7. Often loses things necessary for tasks or activities (e.g., toys, school assignments, pencils, books, tools)
8. Is often easily distracted by extraneous stimuli
9. Is often forgetful in daily activities

B. Hyperactivity

1. Often fidgets with hands or feet or squirms in seat
2. Often leaves seat in classroom or in other situations in which remaining seated is expected
3. Often runs about or climbs excessively in situations in which it is inappropriate (in adolescents or adults, may be limited to subjective feelings of restlessness)
4. Often has difficulty playing or engaging in leisure activities quietly
5. Is often "on the go" or acts as if "driven by a motor"
6. Often talks excessively

Impulsivity

1. Often blurts out answers before the questions have been completed
2. Often has difficulty awaiting turn
3. Often interrupts or intrudes on others (e.g., butts into conversations or games)

To make a diagnosis

A. At least 6 symptoms from just Category A (ADHD, Inattentive subtype) or just Category B (ADHD, Hyperactive-impulsive subtype), or at least 6 symptoms from both categories (ADHD, Combined subtype)

B. Symptoms are chronic (some symptoms were functionally-impairing from before the age of 7), are clearly significantly impairing (in social, academic, or occupational functioning), are present across settings

C. Symptoms do not occur exclusively during the course of a pervasive developmental disorder, schizophrenia or other psychotic disorder, and are not better-accounted for by another mental disorder (e.g., mood, anxiety, dissociative, or personality disorder).

Reprinted with permission from the *Diagnostic and Statistical Manual of Mental Disorders, Fourth Edition, Text Revision* (Copyright ©2000). American Psychiatric Association.

There is ongoing research regarding the two major symptom domains and subtypes of ADHD. Some research suggests that the inattentive subtype and hyperactive subtype have different genetic influences, although both are highly heritable (Nikolas & Burt, 2010). Proposed revisions to the *DSM-5* further clarify hyperactive and impulsive symptoms separately and delineate more clearly the diagnosis of the three subtypes.

PREVALENCE AND EPIDEMIOLOGY

Although diagnostic practices, service utilization, and prevalence rates differ widely across and within cultures, when similar diagnostic procedures are utilized, ADHD has been detected in 7%–10% of children in the United States (Froelich et al., 2007; Pelham et al., 2005; Visser, Lesesne, & Perou, 2007) and has a pooled prevalence of 5% worldwide (Polanzyck, de Lima, Horta, Beiderman, & Rohde, 2007). The diagnosis is estimated to persist into adulthood in 2%–5% of the population in the United States (Barkley, 2010; Fayyad et al., 2007; Simon, Czobor, Balint, Meszaros, & Bitter, 2009). In clinic-referred samples, the ratio of boys:girls diagnosed with ADHD ranges from 6:1 to 12:1, though in community samples that ratio is closer to 3:1 (Biederman et al., 2005). It is thought that boys may be referred more often due to a higher rate of co-occurring aggressive behavior, oppositional and conduct disorders. Girls may be more likely to be referred because of the inattentive subtype and associated learning and internalizing disorders (mood and anxiety disorders) as well as disordered eating (Quinn, 2008; Rucklidge, 2010).

CLINICAL PRESENTATION

The presenting symptoms of ADHD differ with age. During the preschool years, excessive activity level and impulsivity are typically the most prominent symptoms. This is often accompanied by "intense" temperament and cognitive inflexibility. In combination, these symptoms may lead to impulsive aggression toward peers. Given the high activity level and short attention span of the typical preschooler, only children severely affected with ADHD will differ sufficiently from the developmental norm to fully meet the criteria for the disorder. Children in this age group who meet diagnostic criteria for ADHD have a greater rate of developmental delay, coordination disorders, language disorders and comorbid internalizing and externalizing disorders (Chacko, Wakschlag, Hill, Danis, & Espy, 2009; Greenhill et al., 2008). In order to make an accurate diagnosis, children who present in the preschool period should be carefully assessed for language, cognitive, sensory, and autistic spectrum disorders, all of which have some similarities in presentation to ADHD (Daley, Jones, Hutchings, & Thompson, 2008). Future research into the treatment of preschool children with ADHD will likely include the impact of early intervention before the social and academic problems commonly seen at school age occur (Sonuga-Barke & Halperin, 2010).

Upon entering elementary school, problems with listening and compliance, task completion, work accuracy, and socializing are common concerns of parents and teachers. In adolescence, observable hyperactivity may decline significantly (Faraone, Biederman, & Mick, 2006). Concerns then often focus around work completion, organization, and following rules. Approximately 65% of children with ADHD diagnosed early in childhood continue to meet the criteria for the disorder in adolescence, while an additional group will meet criteria for ADHD, not otherwise specified because of a reduced number of symptoms. Occasionally, individuals are not diagnosed with ADHD until adolescence, though they must have had symptoms by history that were impairing in childhood in order to meet current diagnostic criteria. Children who were able to cope during the early grades, typically

because of low levels of hyperactivity/impulsivity, strong intellectual skills, social, athletic, or other strengths, and supportive families and school personnel, may present in adolescence. Their attentional/executive systems may finally be overwhelmed by the demands for processing increased volumes of reading and writing, as well as the complex social, time management, organizational, and higher-order thinking and language processing skills required of them in high school.

COMMON COEXISTING CONDITIONS

There are several conditions that commonly coexist with ADHD, typically referred to as "comorbid" or "coexisting" conditions. Less frequently, another condition mimics ADHD and is the primary cause of inattentive or hyperactive symptoms rather than coexisting with ADHD (see The Evaluation Process in a following section). Coexisting conditions are important to identify during an evaluation because 1) they will often require additional or different treatment, and 2) unless treated, they may prevent adequate treatment of ADHD.

Up to two thirds of children and adolescents with ADHD presenting to a specialty clinic will have a coexisting disorder, including internalizing disorders (mood and anxiety disorders), externalizing disorders, learning disorders, and/or tic disorders (Pliszka, 2000; Singer, 2005). More than half of children with ADHD have an externalizing behavior disorder, such as oppositional defiant disorder (~60%; characterized by noncompliance and defiance of authority) or conduct disorder (~20%; characterized by more serious antisocial behaviors) (Conner, Steeber, & McBurnett, 2010). There is an association between hyperactive/impulsive symptoms and oppositionality (Wood, Rijsdijk, Asherson, & Kuntsi, 2009). Estimates of mood disorders (depression, anxiety, or bipolar disorder) in ADHD vary considerably from study to study, ranging from 14%–83%. Childhood bipolar disorder has been examined in several cross-sectional studies at tertiary care centers, with rates ranging from 11%–23%. Children with bipolar disorder are likely to have episodic irritability or atypical mood, intermittent explosiveness, psychomotor agitation characterized by talkativeness or motor restlessness, and signs of disordered thinking (Galanter & Leibenluft, 2008). Anxiety disorders occur in approximately 15%–35% of children with ADHD and may include separation anxiety, generalized anxiety, phobic, or obsessive-compulsive disorders (OCD; Schatz & Rostain, 2006). Comorbid anxiety and ADHD may lead to increased school problems and functional impairment as compared with either disorder alone (Hammerness et al., 2009).

The prevalence of learning disorders in children with ADHD ranges from 10%–40%, depending on which test and criteria for learning disabilities are utilized (Kronenberger & Dunn, 2003). Although the prevalence of specific reading disability (the most common type of learning disability) among students with ADHD is unclear because of variability in how each diagnosis is made, it is estimated to be about 30% (Fletcher, Shaywitz, & Shaywitz, 1999).

Tic disorders, including transient, chronic, or Tourette syndrome are seen in at least 6% of children in a community sample over the course of a year, with transient tics being the most common (approximately 5%) and Tourette syndrome being the least common (< 1%; Khalifa & von Knorring, 2005). Group data show no increase in rates of tic disorders in children with ADHD on psychostimulant medications, but tics may occur on an individual basis (Erenberg, 2006). Persistent tics are often associated with ADHD, as well as other neuropsychiatric conditions, most notably OCD (Pollak et al., 2009). Tics can occur on a spectrum from mild (which may not even be reported by parents) to the more severe (in which tics have important physical, emotional, and social impact). In children with ADHD and Tourette syndrome, ADHD typically causes greater functional impairment than does the tic disorder itself (Denkla, 2006; Singer, 2005). Nonetheless, the clinician must look for tic disorders by history and exam in the child presenting for an evaluation for ADHD, and in family members, as it may have implications for treatment.

Proposed revisions to *DSM-5* also allow the diagnosis of ADHD in the presence of autism spectrum disorders (ASDs), which was previously an exclusion criterion (APA, 2010). Children with ASDs frequently have attentional issues and high percentages meet *DSM-IV* criteria for ADHD as well as an ASD (Lee & Ousley, 2006).

ASSOCIATED IMPAIRMENTS

Individuals with ADHD often have associated impairments that are neither directly described by the core features of ADHD, nor indicative of one of the common coexisting diagnoses above.

Nonetheless, they can be significantly impairing and may require additional interventions. These include impairments in executive, language, social, academic, and adaptive functions, as well as altered sleep patterns and motor coordination.

Although ADHD is defined and diagnosed based on the presence of observed behavior, neuropsychological investigations suggest that impairments in executive functioning based in the frontal/prefrontal cortex may in part underlie the characteristic observed behaviors in many children with ADHD (Weyandt, 2005; Willcutt, Doyle, Nigg, Faraone, & Pennington, 2005). Executive functions include sustaining and shifting attention, being able to hold and manipulate information in order to complete a task (working memory), organizing and prioritizing incoming information, planning ahead, self-monitoring, and inhibiting responses (Martinussen, Hayden, Hogg-Johnson & Tannock, 2005). It should be noted that executive function impairments are also found in other developmental disabilities, including autism and learning disabilities. Impairments in auditory processing can also occur with symptoms of ADHD and contribute to academic underachievement (Dawes & Bishop, 2009).

Executive function impairments contribute independently from ADHD symptoms to academic difficulties. According to one meta-analysis, 21% of children with ADHD have no executive function impairments, depending on the measures used (Castellanos, Sonuga-Barke, Milham, & Tannock, 2006; Willcutt, Doyle, et al., 2005). Other neuropsychological impairments, such as motivation and altered responses to reinforcement, are also thought to contribute to the underlying symptoms of ADHD (Nigg, 2005; Tripp & Wickens, 2009). However, individuals with ADHD do not have a single, uniform neuropsychological profile (Doyle, 2006).

Academic underachievement is a concern of many parents of school-age children with ADHD, even in the absence of criteria for a learning disability. Difficulty with verbal memory, listening comprehension, and organization of verbal and written output occur in children with ADHD, even in the absence of specific language impairments (McInnes, Humphries, Hogg-Johnson, & Tannock, 2003). Difficulty reading (most often in the form of problems with fluency, comprehension, or engagement and retention of written material) often occurs in students with ADHD, even in the absence of a diagnosed reading disability (Ghelani, Sidhu, Jain, & Tannock, 2004; Willicut, Pennington, Olson, Chabildas, & Hulslander, 2005).

Many children with ADHD have social difficulties and face peer rejection, an important risk factor for later negative outcomes. These difficulties persist even after reduction in symptoms of ADHD with stimulants or behavioral intervention (Hoza, 2007; McQuade & Hoza, 2008; Nijmeijer et al, 2007). They have difficulty "reading" the nuances of social behavior or inhibiting impulsive responses. They may react excessively or overly negatively to the behavior of others, leading some peers to enjoy "pushing their buttons" to get a reaction. Some children with ADHD have difficulty initiating or sustaining the verbal turn-taking or other reciprocal aspects of peer relations and may find themselves passively or actively ignored and without the deeper friendships that older school children begin to develop. They may be inflexible or perfectionistic, leading to "bossiness" with peers. Children with ADHD tend to overestimate their social competency and don't recognize and adjust maladaptive behavior (Owens, Goldfine, Evangelista, Hoza, & Kaiser, 2007). Although not well studied, there also appears to be a high rate of pragmatic language difficulties in children with ADHD (Armstrong & Nettleton, 2004). Pragmatic language refers to the use of language for socially appropriate communication.

Research has supported a link between ADHD and sleep disturbances (Owens, 2005). Children with ADHD have inconsistent sleep patterns compared with controls, with greater variability in sleep initiation combined with shorter duration and less sleep overall (Grueber, 2009). They also have difficulty with awakening and maintaining daytime alertness. Although stimulant medication treatment can contribute to insomnia, sleep disturbance occurs in nonmedicated children with ADHD as well. Increased latency to sleep time (time it takes to fall asleep), increased nighttime activity, decreased rapid eye movement sleep, and significant daytime somnolence, have all been identified as problematic sleep issues (Tsai & Huang, 2010). The underlying pathophysiologic mechanism that leads to the association between ADHD and disturbed sleep is presently unknown although behavioral, circadian, and genetic models have been suggested (Grueber, 2009; Konofal, Lecendreux, & Cortes, 2010). Furthermore, sleep disorders can also contribute to ADHD symptoms. There is an increased rate of periodic limb movements and restless legs syndrome in individuals with ADHD. While there does not appear to be an increased incidence of obstructive sleep apnea in individuals with ADHD, when present its treatment can improve daytime somnolence, concentration, and behavioral regulation (Grueber, 2009; Konofal et al., 2010; Tsai & Huang, 2010).

Children with ADHD also have an increased incidence of problems with motor coordination, which may impair written work in school and social participation in athletic activities (Martin, Piek, & Hay, 2006). Half of children with ADHD will also meet criteria for developmental coordination disorder, characterized by poor motor performance to a degree that causes functional impairment (Cairney, Veldhuizen, & Szatmari, 2010). Impairments in visual-spatial organization and cerebellar function are thought to be common underlying mechanisms for these two disorders (Piek & Dyck, 2004).

CAUSES OF ATTENTION-DEFICIT/HYPERACTIVITY DISORDER

Genetics

The most common etiological factor in the development of ADHD is heredity. Siblings of children with ADHD are between 5–7 times more likely to be diagnosed with ADHD than children from unaffected families. Each child of a parent with ADHD has a 25% chance of having ADHD (Faraone et al., 2005; Sharp, McQuillen, & Gurling, 2009). Between 55%–92% of identical twins will be concordant for ADHD, and heritability is estimated at 76% (Faraone et al., 2005).

Multiple candidate genes have been found to relate to susceptibility to ADHD including genes related to the dopamine, norepinephrine, serotonin, acetylcholine, GABA, and glutamate neurotransmitter systems, as well as genes associated with neurotransmitter release and neuroimmunology (see Chapter 12).

Dopamine-related genes are candidate genes for investigating the basis for ADHD, because a variety of types of evidence indicates that dopamine is involved in the modulation of attention and behavioral regulation in the frontal cortex and its connections, particularly the striatum. Norepinephrine is another neurotransmitter that plays an important role in orienting attention and regulating alertness in the frontal cortex and in other areas of the cortex and lower brain. Medications that are effective in ameliorating ADHD symptoms have consistently been shown to affect one or both of these neurotransmitters (Banaschewski, Becker,

Scherag, Franke, & Coghill, 2010; Kieling, Goncalves, Tannock, & Castellanos, 2008).

We all have all of these genes. There are a few, slightly different forms of each of these genes, called alleles (see Chapter 1). In molecular genetic studies of families (linkage analysis), a specific allele of each of these genes has been found to occur at a higher frequency in the individuals in the family who have ADHD than can be explained by chance alone. Different alleles tend to be present in those individuals within the family who do not have ADHD. This suggests that specific alleles of these genes may confer susceptibility to ADHD and can be used to identify candidate genes that we suspect in ADHD.

Those genes that have been found to be associated with ADHD in more than one study sample include the dopamine transporter, the dopamine type 4 and 5 receptors, dopamine beta hydroxylase (an enzyme which is involved in the conversion of dopamine to norepinephrine), the serotonin transporter, the serotonin 1B receptor subtype, tryptophan hydroxylase (a precursor to serotonin), and SNAP-25 (synaptosomal-associated protein), a membrane protein involved in synaptic release of neurotransmitters (Banaschewski et al., 2010; Franke, Neale & Faraone, 2009; Sharp et al., 2009).

The genes thus far identified do not account for the majority of the variation in ADHD symptoms, however, suggesting that other as yet unidentified genes are important. Genome wide association studies (GWAS) using advances in genetic technology developed over the last 5 years assess variants throughout the entire genome that are associated with ADHD. More recent GWAS also implicate genes involved in neuronal migration and plasticity, cell adhesion, and division (Banaschewski et al., 2010).

Specific genotypes that are associated with ADHD are being explored to assess their relationship to associated diagnoses and impairments, persistence of symptoms, treatment response, and outcome (Froehlich, McGough, & Stein, 2010). Epigenetic phenomena (gene–environment interactions) may also play a role in the clinical phenotype of ADHD (Franke et al., 2009; Kieling et al., 2008; see Chapter 1).

Other Etiologic Factors

Although the most common etiology of ADHD is genetic, other conditions known to affect brain development may result in ADHD symptoms or increase the risk of those genetically

at risk for the disorder. These include prenatal exposures to cigarette smoking, lead at even low levels (Ha et al., 2009; Nicolescu et al., 2010), alcohol, cocaine, antidepressants (Figueroa, 2010), prematurity, intrauterine growth retardation, brain infections, and inborn errors of metabolism (Banerjee, Middleton, & Faraone, 2007). Sex chromosome abnormalities (including Klinefelter syndrome, Turner syndrome, and fragile X syndrome) and other syndromes that may be inherited or genetic (e.g., neurofibromatosis type 1, Williams syndrome, 22q11 deletion syndrome; see Appendix B) are associated with attention problems or overactivity/impulsivity (reviewed by Lo-Castro, D'Agati, & Curatolo, 2010). In children who do not have a family history of ADHD, there is an increased incidence of complications during labor, delivery, and infancy (Sprich-Buckminster, Biederman, Milberger, Faraone, & Lehman, 1993). Premature infants with evidence for low cerebral blood flow were found at 12–14 years of age to have an increased risk for ADHD and motor reaction time impairments that were associated with alterations in dopamine type 2/3 receptor binding. This suggests that cerebral ischemia may contribute to long-term changes in dopamine neurotransmission that are related to ADHD motor and behavioral symptoms (Lou et al., 2004). Children who undergo surgery for congenital heart disease also may have decreased cerebral blood flow and have a higher risk for subsequent attention problems (Shillingford et al., 2009). Other large studies of premature children confirm the increased risk for ADHD with low birth weight and prematurity (Delobel-Ayoub et al., 2009; Indredavik et al., 2005). Acquired traumatic brain injury can also result in ADHD symptoms and exacerbate predisposing behavioral traits (Chapman et al., 2010; Yeates et al., 2005).

Structural and Functional Differences in the Brain

Multiple lines of evidence suggest that structural and functional differences exist in the brains of individuals with ADHD (Kelly, Margulies, & Castellanos, 2007; Makris, Biederman, Monuteaux, & Siedman, 2009). Magnetic resonance imaging (MRI) scans have shown important differences when the shape, thickness, and volume of specific areas are compared. Five regions have shown consistent differences—frontal lobes, including the dorsolateral prefrontal cortex and dorsal anterior cingulate cortex, inferior parietal cortex, basal ganglia, including the caudate nucleus and globus pallidus, corpus callosum (particularly anteriorly), and the posterior inferior cerebellar vermis. Networks in the frontal cortex serve as the "executive center," processing incoming stimuli, connecting to other structures and coordinating appropriate cognitive, emotional, and motor responses (Arnsten, 2009). The cerebellum and basal ganglia are thought to be involved because these areas are critical to motor planning, behavioral inhibition, and motivation. Compared with controls, these regions are 3%–4% smaller in subjects with ADHD, involve both gray and white matter, and are present early in childhood (Makris et al., 2009; Shaw & Rabin, 2009). Studies of the amygdala and hippocampus, part of the limbic system, have also shown anomalies in shape and volume in children with ADHD (Shaw & Rabin, 2009).

Functional magnetic resonance imaging (fMRI) is a noninvasive technique that is used to evaluate variations in regional oxygen uptake in the brain, which correlates with cellular activity. fMRI studies indicate that subjects with ADHD have hypoactivation of the prefrontal cortex, parietal cortex, cerebellum, and caudate nucleus, and that stimulant medication can increase activation in these areas (Casey, Nigg, & Durston, 2007). In particular, the dorsal anterior cingulate cortex and striatum are repeatedly shown to have hypofunction/hypoperfusion in children and adults with ADHD. This is consistent with structural and neuropsychological findings. Differences in the activation of the temporal and parietal cortex as well as the thalamus are more recent areas of investigation (Kelly et al., 2007).

Positron emission tomography (PET) and single photon emission tomography (SPECT) scans provide information about brain neurotransmitters but are more invasive, involving injection of a radioactive tracer molecule and so have limited use in children. PET/SPECT scans provide information about regional perfusion, oxygen and glucose metabolism, or about a particular neurotransmitter system. This provides neurochemically specific regional information. Early studies indicated globally decreased glucose metabolism in children with ADHD. Multiple studies in children and adults document underperfusion of frontal-striatal regions, though the specific findings within these areas differ among studies (Glanzman, 2006; Glanzman & Elia, 2006). Several studies document abnormalities in the fronto-striatal dopamine system, including alterations in dopamine uptake in the prefrontal cortex in adults and right

midbrain and striatum in children. In both adults and children, studies report increased dopamine receptor availability and increased binding to the dopamine transporter (Zimmer, 2009).

Structural and functional imaging scans are presently important research tools, but they have not been shown to be sufficiently sensitive or specific to be used diagnostically (American Academy of Pediatrics, 2011; Bush 2008; Glanzman & Elia, 2006).

THE EVALUATION PROCESS

Evaluating a child for ADHD requires assessment of four areas: 1) symptoms of ADHD; 2) different conditions that might cause the same symptoms; 3) coexisting conditions; and 4) any associated medical, psychosocial, or learning issues that may not reach the threshold for a specific diagnosis but may nonetheless influence the treatment plan. In order to cover these four areas, a comprehensive history, physical/neurological examination, and academic assessment must be completed. Findings in these examinations may prompt additional investigations, including consultation from specialists.

The history, generally taken from the parents, with the child's participation depending on age, includes current status and concerns, previous treatments and their effects, prenatal and perinatal events, medical history, developmental, psychiatric and behavioral history, educational course, social and family circumstances, and biological family history for ADHD symptoms and associated disorders. The main pediatric and child psychiatric professional organizations—the American Academy of Pediatrics (AAP) and the American Academy of Child and Adolescent Psychiatry (AACAP)—provide guidelines for the assessment of ADHD, and both emphasize the importance of adhering to the *DSM-IV-TR* diagnostic criteria. Information from teachers, typically in the form of standardized rating scales, should be included to document impairment in the school setting (AACAP, 2007; AAP, 2011).

The medical examination should focus on growth parameters and physical signs of sensory, genetic, chronic medical, and neurologic disorders, as well as mental status, informal communicative ability and insight, and motor skills.

Educational testing (including intellectual, achievement, and processing measures) will be necessary for many children and should focus on the careful assessment for learning disabilities, memory and processing, and areas of academic weakness that may not meet criteria for a learning disability. Additional support may allow the child to make better academic progress rather than falling further behind. This should include assessments of reading mechanics and comprehension, spelling, mathematical concepts and computation, and writing. Tests of verbal and visual memory and processing efficiency can be useful in identifying reasons for intellectual achievement discrepancies and can inform choices about educational remediation strategies.

Obtaining information about symptoms of ADHD and related conditions, comparing the level of symptoms to age- and gender-matched peers, and assessing the level of functional impairment is frequently facilitated by the use of standardized interview formats and rating scales for parents and teachers. In addition, rating scales designed for teachers allow the required collection of information from more than one setting. Commonly used rating scales to specifically assess ADHD symptoms include the ADHD-IV Rating Scale, the Conners Rating Scales, the SNAP, and the Vanderbilt Rating Scale (AACAP, 2007; AAP, 2000; Pelham et al., 2005).

Structured diagnostic interviews are quite time-consuming and require training for standardized administration; therefore, they are most often used in psychiatric and research settings. Commonly used structured diagnostic interviews include the Diagnostic Interview for Children and Adolescents, Revised (DICA-R), the Diagnostic Interview Schedule for Children (DISC), and the Kiddie Schedule for Affective Disorders and Schizophrenia (K-SADS; Pelham et al., 2005).

Because comprehensive information is required, several professionals are typically involved (e.g., physician, psychologist, teacher). The primary person responsible for formulating the diagnosis and communicating the findings and recommendations to the family must be experienced with the range of coexisting conditions. This person is typically a physician (pediatrician, neurodevelopmental or developmental-behavioral pediatrician, neurologist and/or psychiatrist) or psychologist. Additional professionals, such as speech-language pathologist and occupational therapists, may be asked to provide input. While such a complex evaluation can be coordinated through a primary care setting, there are also a number of barriers related to knowledge, time, resources, and medical/mental health insurance coverage that limit access to a thorough evaluation for many children (Rushton, Fant, & Clark, 2004).

TREATMENT OF ATTENTION-DEFICIT/HYPERACTIVITY DISORDER

Most treatment plans for ADHD will include education about the disorder and one or more of the following interventions: behavioral and family counseling, special education services, and medication. Often a combination of treatments is used because of the chronicity and multiple types of impairment caused by ADHD (AAP, 2001).

Education About Attention-Deficit/Hyperactivity Disorder and Emotional Support for Families

Parents and older children need to learn as much as possible about ADHD so that they can be effective decision makers and advocates. The clinician can provide some information directly but should also guide the family toward resources such as national support and advocacy organizations, books and online resources, and parent support groups (see Appendix D). Growing up with and parenting a child with ADHD are significant challenges. Although providing emotional support alone is not likely to result in significant improvements, without emotional support parents and children may not be able to perform the difficult work needed to address the consequences of ADHD.

Behavioral Counseling and Social Skill Intervention

Behavior therapy is the type of counseling intervention with the best documented efficacy in preschoolers (Greenhill et al., 2008; Murray, 2010) and school-age children (Young & Amarasinghe, 2010) with ADHD, especially if there are additional disruptive behaviors (Eyberg, Nelson, & Boggs, 2008). Studies also suggest efficacy of behavior therapy in adolescents with ADHD, though additional psychosocial interventions are more often necessary in this age group (Robin, 2008; Young & Amarasinghe, 2010). Behavior therapy changes behavior by altering the antecedents to, or consequences of, the behavior in such a way that it increases the chances that the child will successfully engage in the desired behaviors and reduces the chances that the child will engage in unwanted behaviors (see Chapter 32).

Behavior therapy can be done in individual or group sessions and forms the basis for most parent training and classroom management programs for children with ADHD. Studies have consistently found that these interventions result in at least short-term improvements in the behavior (Pelham & Fabiano, 2008; Young & Amarasinghe, 2010) and homework problems (Langberg et al., 2010) of children with ADHD. A study of a very intensive behavioral intervention that also included social skill-building and emotional support found some persistent benefit from this intervention 15 months after the intervention ended (MTA Cooperative Group, 2004a); however, this level of treatment intensity in unlikely to be widely available (Young & Amarasinghe, 2010). Factors that may interfere with successful parent training in behavior management include parental depression or ADHD, high levels of marital discord (Chronis, Chacko, Fabiano, Wymbs, & Pelham, 2004), low maternal parental self-efficacy, and multiple coexisting conditions in the child (van den Hoofdakker et al., 2010).

There is insufficient evidence to recommend family therapy as a specific treatment for core ADHD symptoms (Bjornstad & Montogomery, 2005); however, disruptive behavior can lead to increasingly negative and coercive patterns of parent–child interaction (Deault, 2010). Family therapy can help to mitigate the effects of parenting a child with ADHD on the marital relationship and sibling interactions. Family therapy may be necessary when parents cannot agree on an intervention plan or other family stressors interfere with implementation of a treatment plan.

Cognitive-behavior therapy changes behavior by helping individuals to change self-defeating thought and behavior patterns. It is a well-documented treatment for depression and anxiety and has recently been shown to be effective in the treatment of adult ADHD (Safren et al., 2010; Solanto et al., 2010; Young & Amarasinghe, 2010). Children and teens with ADHD frequently hold negative or inaccurate attributions that can interfere with the use of productive strategies to face challenges. Whether or not cognitive-behavior therapy will be effective in teens and older children with inaccurate attributions or other unproductive thought and behavior patterns is just beginning to be studied. Individual psychotherapy or play therapy may be helpful for children with coexisting mood, anxiety, or self-esteem problems but is not effective in treating the core symptoms of ADHD (Barkley, 2004).

Coaching is an emerging approach to improve the daily functioning of teens and adults with ADHD. It involves regular meetings between the individual with ADHD and his or her coach to identify executive function impairments leading to problems in daily functioning and to develop systems and strategies to address them. Coaching is most likely to be successful when the individual recognizes the problems and wishes to address them but cannot seem to do it without help. It does not address core symptoms of ADHD, coexisting conditions, or motivational or emotional problems. Coaches are typically psychologists, educators, social workers, or successful adults with ADHD. A recent positive step in the field has been the development of professional standards and certification procedures (Murphy, Ratey, Maynard, Sussman, & Wright, 2010).

Interpersonal difficulties such as peer victimization (bullying) and/or social isolation are common in individuals with ADHD (Hoza, 2007; Nijmeijer et al., 2007); thus social-skill interventions may be recommended as part of a comprehensive treatment plan. Social skill groups are often conducted in school or other group settings and teach by modeling, practicing, and reinforcing prosocial behaviors. When social skills interventions for children with ADHD are evaluated as a single intervention, however, the results have generally been disappointing (Abikoff et al., 2004; Barkley, 2004). It seems that children "know" or can be taught appropriate skills but do not apply them when needed. The social skills interventions that seem to be the most effective are conducted in naturalistic settings (i.e., at a camp or school rather than in a clinic) and are combined with behavioral parent training (Pelham & Fabiano, 2008).

Educational Treatment

Appropriate school programs are extremely important for children with ADHD, many of whom have coexisting learning disabilities. Even those children without a specific learning disability may require substantial repetition or alternate methods of instruction. Unfortunately, their difficulty in sustaining mental effort and their weak working memory often result in resistance to the repeated practice they require. A well-trained teacher who is able to provide special help and an educational program suited to the needs of the child is invaluable to the student with ADHD. The teacher may need to use environmental modifications and behavior management techniques to maintain the child's attention to tasks and decrease unwanted behavior. The child may need the teacher's assistance to develop organizational skills and support comprehension. Classwork or assignments may need to be modified to emphasize the child's strengths, help manage the child's learning weaknesses or disabilities, and compensate for problems with initiation or slow work production. Tutoring outside of school will be helpful in some cases, especially to ensure that basic concepts that serve as building blocks for more advanced work have been learned thoroughly and that effective approaches are used for comprehension, memorization, studying for tests, and organizing written work and materials.

When children with ADHD are in need of more assistance than is typically provided in the classroom, they may qualify for modification within their general education classes or in special education settings under either Section 504 of the Rehabilitation Act of 1973 (PL 93-112 Section 504) or the Individuals with Disabilities Education Act [IDEA](Education for All Handicapped Children Act of 1975, PL-94-142 see Chapter 31).

A child with ADHD who needs modification of curricular materials, demands, or teaching methods should have an individualized education program (IEP; http://www.idea.ed.gov). Although ADHD is not one of the disabilities specifically included under IDEA, some children with ADHD will have an IEP under a coexisting condition such as specific learning disability, speech-language impairment, or emotional disturbance. Others will be provided an IEP under the IDEA category of "Other Health Impaired." A child with ADHD who is less educationally impaired by his or her symptoms may still be eligible for accommodations through a "Section 504 Plan" (http://www2.ed.gov/about/offices/list/ocr/504faq.html). Accommodations allow the child with ADHD to successfully "access" the regular education environment and may include (but are not limited to) regular home–school communication; a behavior program to support desired behaviors; a plan to insure that the student understands and is following through on instructions; modifications of testing time, format, or environment; an extra set of materials at home; and technological assistance such as the use of recording devices and word processors.

Pharmacological Treatment

Stimulant medications are the most effective and most commonly prescribed medications for ADHD. Atomoxetine and sustained-release guanfacine and clonidine are the only nonstimulant medications approved by the Food and Drug Administration (FDA) for the treatment of ADHD. Non–FDA-approved medications that have been used to treat ADHD include antidepressants (bupropion and tricyclics) and immediate-release or short-acting guanfacine and clonidine. Combinations of medications are also used, though research lags behind practice in this area. See Appendix C for information on medication dosages and side effects.

Stimulant Medication

Stimulant medications, including methylphenidate and amphetamine (see Table 22.2) have been used for the treatment of children with disruptive behaviors for over 60 years and have been more frequently used and more thoroughly studied than any other psychopharmacologic treatment in children. In the United States, approximately 1 in 25 children and adolescents take medication for ADHD (Scheffler, Hinshaw, Modrek, & Levine, 2007). Stimulants are statistically more effective than nonstimulant options (Biederman, Wigal, Spencer, McGough, & Mays, 2006) and appear to work equally well in the inattentive and combined subtypes (Solanto et al., 2009), in boys and girls, and from early school-age through adulthood (Cornforth, Sonuga-Barke, & Coghill, 2010). Preschoolers appear to have a somewhat less beneficial effect/side effect ratio than older children (see Stimulants in Preschoolers).

Beneficial Effects

Stimulant medications significantly reduce symptoms in 70%–90% of children and adolescents correctly diagnosed with ADHD (Wigal, 2009). They result in a rapid and often dramatic improvement in attention and distractibility and a decrease in impulsivity and hyperactivity. In addition, they improve academic productivity and accuracy, improve parent–child interactions, and decrease aggression. Stimulants also improve driving performance in adolescents and young adults with ADHD (Barkley & Cox, 2007). The effect of stimulants on academic achievement and executive function is modest compared with their effects on behavior, indicating that additional interventions are needed in these areas (Jitendra, DuPaul, Someki, & Tresco, 2008; MTA Cooperative Group, 2004a, b; Raggi & Chronis, 2006). The positive effects of stimulants on executive function appear to be limited to those measures most related to attention and verbal learning; whereas measures of interference control, processing speed, and organization/planning remain impaired (Abikoff et al., 2009; Biederman, Monuteaux, et al., 2008). Stimulants have "normalizing" effects on biological parameters that differentiate individuals with ADHD from controls, including activation patterns in corical-striatal-cerebellar attentional networks, basal ganglia surface morphology, and event-related brain (electrical) potentials (Bush et al., 2008; Ozdag, Yorbik, Ulas, Hamamcioglu, & Vural, 2004; Rubia et al., 2009; Sobel et al., 2010).

Although beneficial effects on behavior are very clearly demonstrated in short to intermediate term studies, the long-term efficacy of stimulants is not nearly as well studied (May & Kratochvil, 2010; See Outcome). It should also be noted that response to stimulant treatment is not diagnostic of ADHD, since individuals with other psychiatric or developmental disorders, as well as controls, display similar effects when given stimulant medication (Rapaport et al., 1978).

Formulations

Methylphenidate and amphetamine come in a variety of formulations as shown in Table 22.2. The beneficial effects and side effects of these two types of stimulants are nearly identical, although 30%–40% of children may respond better to one medication than the other (May & Kratochvil, 2010). A recent meta-analysis indicates that amphetamine may improve symptoms to a slightly greater degree than methylphenidate, but tolerability was not taken into account (Faraone & Buitelaar,

Table 22.2. Stimulant medications commonly used to treat attention-deficit/hyperactivity disorder

Brand name	Generic name of active medicine	Usual duration of action (hours)	Dosages available (mg)	Other
Ritalin	D,L-methylphenidate	3–4	Tablets–5, 10, 20	
Focalin	D-methylphenidate	3–4	Tablets–2.5, 5, 10	Contains only the active isomer of methylphenidate; typical dose is ½ that of D,L-methylphenidate
Focalin XR	D-methylphenidate	8–12 (12 for 20 mg dose)	Capsules–5, 10, 20, 30	Capsule can be opened and sprinkled
Methylin	D,L-methylphenidate	3–4	Tablets–2.5, 5, 10 Suspension–5 mg/5ml and 10mg/5ml	Tablets are grape flavored and chewable
Metadate CD	D,L-methylphenidate	6–8	Capsules–10, 20, 30, 40, 50, 60	Capsule can be opened and sprinkled 30% of dose immediately released
Ritalin LA	D,L-methylphenidate	6–8	Capsules–10, 20, 30, 40, 50, 60	Capsule can be opened and sprinkled 50% of dose immediately released
Concerta	D,L-methylphenidate	10–12	Capsule–18, 27, 36, 54	Must be swallowed whole 22% of dose immediately released
Daytrana	D,L-methylphenidate	Up to 12	Patch–10, 15, 20, 30	Duration depends on timing of removal
Dexedrine	Dextroamphetamine	3–6	Tablet–5	
Dexedrine Spansules	Dextroamphetamine	6–8	Capsule–5, 10, 15	
Adderall	Mixed salts of amphetamine	3–6	Tablets–5, 7.5, 10, 12.5, 15, 20, 30	
Adderall XR	Mixed salts of amphetamine	8–10	Capsule–5, 10, 15, 20, 25, 30	Capsule can be opened and sprinkled 50% of dose immediately released
Vyvanse	Lisdexamfetamine	12	Capsule–20, 30, 40, 50, 60, 70	Inactive until lysine cleaved from amphetamine in the gastrointestinal tract

2010). Amphetamine-based stimulants are typically given at half to two thirds the dose of the methylphenidate-based stimulants to account for differences in the potency of the two medications. Likewise, dex-methylphenidate, the isolated, more effective d-isomer, has approximately twice the potency of d,l-methylphenidate and is given at approximately half the dose. Lisdexamfetamine is the only prodrug formulation, requiring cleavage of the attached lysine by gastrointestinal enzymes for activation.

The onset of action of immediate-release forms of methylphenidate and amphetamine is usually within 30 minutes of taking the dose. Based on the technology used to extend the duration of release, different formulations vary in how much of the medication is released immediately and time to onset, how the remainder is released (in a later bolus versus continuously), and duration of effect. Although Table 22.2 gives the typical duration of effect for the various formulations, there is significant variation among individuals. The methylphenidate patch is the only formulation that gives individuals the capacity to vary the duration of action on a daily basis (up to 12 hours) based on the timing of patch removal (Shire Pharmaceuticals).

Side Effects

The most common adverse effects of stimulants are decreased appetite, headaches, stomachaches, and sleep problems (May & Kratochvil, 2010; Wigal, 2009). As headaches, stomachaches, and sleep problems are common in untreated children with ADHD, it is important to determine the nature and frequency of these symptoms prior to starting the medication. Preexisting sleep problems predict sleep problems on long-acting methylphenidate; however, they may not be substantially different than in children receiving placebo (Faraone et al., 2009). Decreased appetite is reported in 50%–60% of children, but it is typically limited to lunchtime hours, with compensation at breakfast and dinner. A much smaller percentage of children have more extensive appetite suppression and weight loss. These children may benefit from caloric and nutrient supplementation to prevent weight loss and maintain adequate nutrition, or they may be able to eat in between doses of shorter-acting formulations. Appetite suppression and dyspepsia will prevent some children from tolerating stimulants or atomoxetine. It may be that this minority has an underlying gastrointestinal condition that renders them prone to related side effects, such as gastroesophageal reflux, gastritis, or other inflammatory condition. Treatment of the underlying condition may then allow such children to tolerate pharmacologic treatment for ADHD. Less common but potentially more problematic side effects include "rebound" effects, tics, and social withdrawal. *Rebound* refers to a temporary worsening of symptoms, including irritability, increased activity, and/or mood swings, when the medication wears off. Although it is estimated that 30% of school-age children experience some rebound effects, they are significant enough to require altering the medication regimen in only about 10% of cases (Carlson & Kelly, 2003). Preliminary results suggest that some young adults may have increased driving errors during rebound (Cox et al., 2008). Some children do become withdrawn on stimulant medication. This may improve with dose adjustment or switching to another medication. The best ways to mitigate medication side effects is an area that has not been systematically researched and is typically based on common clinical experience rather than scientific evidence.

Tics have been reported to occur in approximately 10% of children treated with stimulants (Lipkin, Goldstein, & Adesman, 1994), but they have also been reported in a similar percentage of community control samples (22% of preschoolers, 8% of elementary school children, and 3.4% of adolescents; Gadow & Sverd, 2006). Early reports suggested that stimulants induced or exacerbated tics, but more recent research indicates that this is less common than originally thought (Gadow & Sverd, 2006; Palumbo, Spencer, Lynch, CoChien, & Faraone, 2004). In addition, tics that appear to be stimulant-induced or exacerbated usually subside with time, after the dose is reduced, or when treatment is discontinued. In rare cases, tics that appear to have been induced by stimulants do not resolve, or may even worsen over time. Given that tics and ADHD commonly co-occur (Denkla, 2006; Gadow & Sverd, 2006), it is possible that those individuals whose tics appear to be induced by stimulants have a biological predisposition to develop tics.

Growth velocity slows by approximately 1.2 cm/yr on average in prepubertal children during at least the first 2 years of continuous treatment with stimulants (MTA Cooperative Group, 2004b). In preschoolers, growth was 20% less and weight gain 55% less than expected over the first year of treatment (Swanson et al., 2006). When school-age children are followed for up to 3 years, however, slowed growth rates tend to stabilize, though growth rebound does not occur (Swanson et al., 2007). Short- to intermediate-term treatment does not seem to have a significant effect on adult height (Faraone, Biederman, Morley, & Spencer, 2008); however, continuous treatment into adulthood has not been studied.

Other side effects include elevations of pulse or blood pressure, and rarely, activation of mania or psychosis. Methylphenidate, amphetamine, and atomoxetine all cause statistically, but rarely clinically significant increases in pulse, blood pressure and corrected QT interval on the EKG (prolonged QTc interval is a risk factor for serious arrhythmia; Elia & Vetter, 2010; Hamerness, Wilens, et al., 2009; Silva, Skimming, & Muniz, 2010). Significant elevations are so rare that they should prompt an investigation for underlying medical causes that may be exacerbated by the medication. Recent reports of sudden death in children on stimulants raised concerns that stimulants might be causative, but careful review showed that approximately two thirds of the cases had previously undetected cardiac abnormalities. The Food and Drug Administration (FDA) and Health Canada have recommended that stimulants not be used in individuals with known heart disease such as structural heart problems, rhythm abnormalities, and hypertension. Relevant professional organizations in pediatrics, psychiatry, and cardiology are in agreement about the importance of a careful personal and family history for risk factors for sudden death. These include palpitations, syncope or near-syncope, the presence of congenital structural abnormalities, hypertrophic cardiomyopathy, Marfan syndrome, long QT syndrome, and Wolff-Parkinson-White syndrome. During treatment, there should be regular monitoring of interim cardiovascular history, including concomitantly used medications with cardiovascular effects, and pulse and blood pressure checks (Vetter et al., 2008; Warren et al., 2009). In the absence of risk factors, the value of additional cardiac assessment or monitoring is unclear and controversial at this time. Though it appears that stimulants can increase the vulnerability to serious cardiac events in those already vulnerable as a result of underlying cardiac disease, the relative risk to those without underlying cardiac disease appears so low that treatment of ADHD should not be withheld in the absence of risk factors (Elia & Vetter, 2010; Newcorn & Donnelly, 2009).

Potential for Substance Abuse

Stimulants are classified as controlled substances by the Drug Enforcement Agency (DEA). When injected or taken intranasally they can produce a "high." However, oral stimulants for ADHD do not induce euphoria or dependence due to their relatively slow uptake into the brain (Volkow & Swanson, 2003). The use of slow release forms, in which the medication is mixed with other substances and released slowly, makes abuse even less likely to occur (Faraone & Upadhyaya, 2007).

While prescribed stimulants are relatively ineffective for producing euphoria, diversion of stimulants for the purpose of staying awake for prolonged periods of study or other activities is much more common. Approximately 7% of college students report using stimulants that were not prescribed to them for ADHD in this manner (DuPaul, Weyandt, O'Dell, & Varejao, 2009; Setlik, Bond, & Ho, 2009). Coaching adolescents about managing their medication before they go to college, and providing anticipatory guidance about how they will manage requests from peers to share their medication, are important aspects of clinical practice for prescribing physicians.

ADHD has been shown to be a risk factor for later substance use disorders, most clearly in the presence of conduct disorder (Biederman, Monuteaux, Spencer, Wilens, & Faraone, 2009; Merkel & Kuchibhatla, 2009). However, multiple studies indicate that the use of stimulant medication does not increase this risk (Biederman et al., 2009; Mannuzza et al., 2008), and may, in some cases, be protective (Katusic et al., 2005).

Given the high rate of comorbidity of ADHD and substance abuse, physicians will need to consider how to best treat such individuals. Current recommendations include psychosocial treatments for both ADHD and substance abuse, careful monitoring, and pharmacological treatment of ADHD with a nonstimulant. However, the use of a long-acting stimulant when the nonstimulants are ineffective can be considered (Schubiner, 2005; Upadhyaya, 2007; Wilson, 2007).

Initiating and Monitoring Therapy

Medication should be but one part of a comprehensive treatment plan (AACAP, 2007). Considerations regarding medication include duration of coverage needed, specific targets for improvement, and any previous treatment experience. In most circumstances, a stimulant will be used as a first-line agent (AAP, 2001). School day (8–9 hours) or 12-hour coverage options exist in both stimulant categories. Immediate-release products lasting 3–5 hours may be used after school on certain days: 1) if 12-hour coverage is not required on a daily basis; 2) if shorter weekend coverage is desired; or 3) in the morning with a long-acting formulation, if it reaches an effective level too slowly to be effective for the first class. Optimal dose is determined by the effectiveness and side effects profile and is best determined by a dose titration protocol so that a variety of dosage levels can be evaluated. During a dose titration protocol, it is important for parents, students, and teachers to have sufficient opportunity to observe for effects and side effects and to provide feedback. Typically, a new medication or dose will be started on the weekend, so parents have the opportunity to monitor their child before sending him or her to school, and each dose will be monitored for a week. Standardized rating scales should be obtained before starting and at the end of the week on each dose. Most standardized rating scales focus on the core symptoms or *DSM-IV-TR* criteria. It is also helpful to obtain feedback about functional changes in the areas of completion of activities of daily living, quality of social interaction, and academic accuracy and productivity. When parent and teacher rating scale results do not agree, it is important to consider reasons for this. It may signal additional diagnoses or symptoms and the need for additional interventions such as parent training or specialized instruction. If a child does not respond or has significant side effects on one stimulant, it is reasonable to try a stimulant from the other class (methylphenidate versus amphetamine; AACAP, 2007). Sometimes, a child will show a better response to one formulation or release pattern over another, even within the same stimulant category; and some children who do not tolerate or respond to either stimulant category may respond to atomoxetine. Certain side effects, such as prominent tics, significant anxiety, and persistent irritability may lead to consideration of a nonstimulant trial, or medication combination. Lack of response to a series of rationally considered trials should prompt a reevaluation of the diagnosis, evaluation for coexisting conditions, and an assessment of compliance and other medical or psychosocial factors that may interfere with effective treatment (AACAP, 2007; AAP, 2001).

School achievement, behavior, relationships, mood, vital signs, and growth velocity should be monitored at baseline, after medication or dose adjustments, and at regular intervals (typically every 3–6 months) to assure continued beneficial responses and the absence of significant adverse effects. No specific laboratory tests are indicated as part of the monitoring. Clinical history and exam may lead a clinician to order tests to rule out abnormalities that may coexist, exacerbate symptoms, limit effectiveness of medication treatment, or relate to observed side effects. These include ferritin (iron binding protein) and thyroid hormone levels, celiac panel, sleep study, electroencephalography (EEG), and bone age x ray. During childhood it is important to periodically assess whether medication is still providing a benefit. Since most children will continue to benefit throughout their school years, it is important to consider with parents and teachers how to best do such an assessment without substantially compromising the student's functioning, if the medication is still helpful.

As children become adolescents and young adults, additional targets for medication management become important that make a longer duration of coverage relevant. These include more hours spent doing homework and extracurricular activities, after-school jobs, the requirement for social decision making with increasingly serious implications, and the need for consistent concentration while driving. Driving performance (but not knowledge) has been shown to be impaired in individuals with ADHD, and effective medication treatment has been shown to improve performance (Barkley & Cox, 2007).

Stimulants in Preschoolers

Stimulants have been used increasingly in children 3–5 years of age. The range of effective doses in mg/kg is similar to that found in school-age children, but the percentage of preschool children having a beneficial response may be slightly lower than in elementary school-age children, and side effects, particularly adverse emotional reactivity and growth rate reductions, may be more common (Kratochvil, Greenhill, March, Burke, & Vaughn, 2004; Swanson et al., 2006; Wigal et al., 2006). Effectiveness was maintained over 10 months of follow up, but with an almost 50% dose increase required (Vitiello et al., 2007). Although methylphenidate has been studied more frequently than dextroamphetamine or mixed salts of amphetamine in preschool children with ADHD, methylphenidate is not FDA approved for children under 6 years of age, while the amphetamine products are approved for children over 3 years of age. Typically, immediate-release methylphenidate up to three times daily has been the treatment regimen used in most studies; thus there is little information about the use of long-acting formulations in preschoolers. Preliminary open-label studies suggest effectiveness for a longer-acting beaded methylphenidate formulation (Maayan et al., 2009). Behavior management training is recommended as a first-line treatment for preschoolers, although only about 13% of families enrolled in a recently completed, large multisite study of ADHD treatment in preschoolers felt that it was sufficient (Greenhill et al., 2006).

Nonstimulant Medications for Attention-Deficit/Hyperactivity Disorder

Between 10%–30% of children with ADHD will not benefit from stimulants or will have adverse side effects that preclude their use. Nonstimulant medications may be helpful in this group. These medications fall into three categories: norepinephrine reuptake inhibitors, antidepressants, and alpha-2-adrenergic agonists.

Norepinephrine Reuptake Inhibitors

Atomoxetine is the only norepinephrine reuptake inhibitor that is FDA approved for the treatment of ADHD (in individuals 6 years of age and over). It is, however, less often effective than extended-release methylphenidate or amphetamine (Garnock-Jones & Keating, 2009). At least 11 double-blind, placebo-controlled trials in children, teens, and adults have demonstrated that atomoxetine improves parent and teacher rating of attention and decreases their ratings of hyperactivity and impulsivity at doses of 1.2–1.4 mg/kg/day. Benefits persist in the absence of serious adverse effects for 2–4 years (the longest duration thus far reported) without development of tolerance, or progressive ineffectiveness over time (Donnelly et al., 2009; Garnock-Jones & Keating, 2009; Kratochvil et al., 2006). It is effective for ADHD in children and adolescents with a variety of coexisting conditions and does not worsen (or may improve) coexisting symptoms, including tics and anxiety (Garnock-Jones & Keating, 2009). A preliminary study suggests effectiveness in preschoolers (Ghuman, Aman, Ghuman et al., 2009). Nonetheless, it does not appear to be more effective in children with internalizing disorders than those without internalizing disorders (Scott, Ripperger-Suhler, Rajab, & Kjar, 2010). Preliminary evidence suggests that the

benefits of atomoxetine may exceed effects on core symptoms to include improvements in reading and executive function skills (Maziade et al., 2009).

Atomoxetine may take a few days before one begins to see effects and several weeks to reach the maximum effect. Similarly, beneficial effects may dissipate gradually when it is discontinued, and some children remain improved over baseline (Buitelaar et al., 2007); there is no adverse effect of abrupt discontinuation (Wernicke et al., 2004). It is generally given once daily in the morning but can be given twice daily to extend coverage into the evening. Fatigue and gastrointestinal upset are relatively common side effects, but atomoxetine is unlikely to cause sleep disturbance. Gastrointestinal upset is typically prevented by giving the medication with food; foods containing protein or fat are particularly effective for this purpose. Some children experience weight loss during the first few months of treatment, but the average reduction in height and weight percentiles was maximal after 18 months of continued use, was about 2% at 2 years, and resolved by 5 years in all except the largest children (Spencer, Kratochvil, et al., 2007). Other side effects include dizziness, irritability, somnolence, and allergic reactions. Increases in pulse and blood pressure do occur, but these are typically not clinically significant. Other, more significant cardiovascular events have not been reported. Prescribing information includes a black box warning about the increased risk of suicidal ideation, thus monitoring for depression, mood instability, and behavioral activation is critical. Atomoxetine is metabolized by cytochrome P450 (CYP2D6), and levels may be affected in individuals who are rapid or slow metabolizers, and by other medications that inhibit CYP2D6. Although genotyping for these variants is not currently a routine practice, dose reduction should be considered in those with prominent early side effects (ter Laak et al., 2010).

Antidepressants

Several types of antidepressants have been found to be effective in children with ADHD, though they are not FDA-approved for this purpose. More than 20 placebo-controlled studies of tricyclic antidepressants (TCAs; including desipramine, imipramine, and nortriptyline) have demonstrated that they improve ADHD symptoms in children, although they are not as effective as stimulants for the majority of children (AACAP, 2007; Banaschewski, Roessner, Dittman, Santosh, & Rothenberger, 2004).

About two thirds of children with ADHD who do not respond to a stimulant will improve with a tricyclic antidepressant (Biederman, Baldessarini, Wright, Knee, & Harmatz, 1989).

Compared with stimulants, tricyclic antidepressants have advantages that are similar to those of atomoxetine. They have a longer duration of action, low abuse potential, and tend not to exacerbate tics. However, they have many more potentially problematic cardiovascular, neurologic (tingling, incoordination, tremors) and anticholinergic (blurred vision, dry mouth) side effects that limit their use. Drug levels should be checked, as there can be large interindividual differences in metabolism of these medications (Banaschewski et al., 2004). Electrocardiograms (EKGs) must be obtained at baseline and monitored for cardiovascular changes. Overdoses can be lethal and a few cases of sudden death, presumably from cardiac arrhythmias, have occurred in children taking appropriate doses of desipramine, although causality could not be clearly established (Popper, 2000).

Bupropion is a chemically distinct antidepressant whose precise mechanism of action in ADHD treatment remains unknown. It is a weak dopamine reuptake inhibitor; this may explain its benefit. It has been shown to improve ADHD symptoms in both children and adults with ADHD. Beneficial effects may be detected as early as 3 days after initiation of treatment, but maximum effects may not be seen until 4 weeks of treatment (Conners et al., 1996). On average the magnitude of the effects is similar to or slightly less than those of stimulants (Conners et al., 1996; Verbeeck, Tuinier, & Bekkering, 2009). Gastrointestinal complaints, drowsiness, and rashes are the most common side effects; insomnia can also occur. Bupropion treatment is associated with a slightly increased risk of drug-induced seizures (about 4 per 1,000 individuals). Use of high doses, a previous history of seizures, and the presence of an eating disorder seem to increase the risk for seizures. Bupropion also may exacerbate tic disorders. An extended release formulation (XL) has been shown to provide extended symptom control throughout the day in adults (Wilens et al., 2005); it has not been studied in children.

Alpha-2-Adrenergic Agonists

Despite relatively limited studies, the alpha-2-adrenergic agents, clonidine and guanfacine, have been used for the treatment of ADHD since the 1980s. Clonidine, in particular, has also been used for aggression and insomnia

(Banaschewski et al., 2004). As with other medications that affect primarily the noradrenergic system, clonidine and guanfacine do not tend to exacerbate tics and may reduce them (Bloch, Panza, Landeros-Weisenberger, & Leckman, 2009). Disadvantages of the immediate-release forms of these medications include 1) sedation and dry mouth, 2) rapid peaking of levels, and 3) decreased compliance as a result of the need for frequent dosing (reviewed in Sallee, 2010). In 2009, the FDA approved a long-acting form of guanfacine (Intuniv) for the treatment of ADHD in children and adolescents. Two placebo-controlled trials (Biederman, et al., 2008; Sallee, McGough, et al., 2009) documented the efficacy of extended release guanfacine on both inattentive and hyperactive/impulsive symptoms in 6–17 year olds. The most common side effects were somnolence-related, and tended to subside over time (studies above and Faraone & Glatt, 2010). Cardiovascular changes were mild and not clinically significant. Open-label continuation demonstrated safety and effectiveness for up to 2 years (Biederman, et al., 2008; Sallee, Lyne, et al., 2009). Although there is a theoretical concern about rebound hypertension with abrupt discontinuation, this was not found in a study of abrupt discontinuation in healthy young adults (Kisicki, Fiske, & Lyne, 2007). A clonidine patch changed weekly has been available since 1984, though it is not yet FDA approved for the treatment of ADHD. In 2010, a twice-daily, extended release clonidine tablet (Kapvay, Shionogi, Inc.) was approved for use alone or with stimulant medication for children and adolescents aged 6–17.

TREATMENT WITH COEXISTING CONDITIONS

Treatment of Children with Attention-Deficit/Hyperactivity Disorder and Intellectual Disabilities

ADHD can be diagnosed in the presence of intellectual disability when inattention or hyperactivity and impulsivity exceed expectations for the child's delayed developmental level and cause additional functional impairment. Studies suggest that methylphenidate can be effective for ADHD symptoms and cognitive task performance in preschoolers and school-age children with intellectual disability; however, they have a lower response rate (around 50%) and an increased risk for side effects, such as stereotypic behavior and emotional lability (Deutsch, Dube, & McIlvane, 2008; Ghuman, et al., 2009; Handen & Gilchrist, 2006). The likelihood of a positive response appears to vary directly with IQ; that is, the higher the IQ, the better the response (Aman, Buican, & Arnold, 2003). An initial double-blind, placebo-controlled study of guanfacine in a small number of children with intellectual disability, autism, or both who previously failed methylphenidate treatment showed improvements in hyperactivity and aberrant behavior but not in attention (Handen, Sahl, & Hardan, 2008). Atypical antipsychotics, particularly risperidone (Risperdal) may also be helpful for hyperactivity and disruptive behaviors in children with intellectual disability (Filho et al., 2005; Handen & Gilchrist, 2006; Olfson, Crystal, Huang, & Gerhard, 2010); however, there are few studies using double-blind, placebo-controlled methods (Thompson, Maltezos, Paliokosta, & Xenitidis, 2009). An open-label study in children and adolescents showed continued effectiveness for up to 2 years (Reyes, Croonenberghs, Augustyns, & Eerdekends, 2006). The development of metabolic syndrome (the combination of obesity, hypertension, high cholesterol, and high blood sugar levels) is a significant risk with the use of atypical antipsychotics (Weiss et al., 2009).

Treatment of Attention-Deficit/Hyperactivity Disorder and Autism Spectrum Disorders

Older studies of children with autism suggested that the benefit to side effects ratio of stimulants (primarily methylphenidate) was not sufficient to warrant their use in this population; however, newer studies show positive effects (Abanilla, Hannahs, Wechsler, & Silva, 2005). Since a higher IQ is associated with better response, more recent inclusion of individuals with milder autism spectrum symptoms and higher IQ may have shifted the results.

Methylphenidate has been shown to improve hyperactivity in about 50% of children with autism spectrum disorders (ASDs), with less robust effects on attention, and significant variability in dose response (Posey et al., 2007). Positive effects have also been reported on attention to social interaction and self-regulation (Jahromi et al., 2009). Methylphenidate does not appear to help rigidity or stereotypic behavior, and an increased susceptibility to side effects is seen compared with the rates seen in children with ADHD in the absence of ASD or intellectual disability (Handen, Johnson, & Lubetsky, 2000).

Preliminary studies suggest that atomoxetine may be safe and effective for hyperactivity in 5–15 year olds with ASD, with similar effectiveness to methylphenidate, and fewer intolerable side effects (Arnold et al., 2006). There are a limited number of studies of clonidine and guanfacine in this population, with a small number of participants and variable results (Handen et al., 2008). If using these medications, clinicians must be vigilant for both positive and negative changes in behavior, and physical side effects.

Risperidone has been shown to improve irritability, aggression, and stereotyped behavior in children with autism (Arnold et al., 2010; McDougle et al., 2005). It may improve hyperactivity (Posey, Stigler, Erickson, & McDougle, 2008) but the presence of hyperactivity is one of several predictors of less positive response in core autism symptoms (Arnold et al., 2010). There is less evidence for effectiveness of antidepressants, anxiolytics, and mood stabilizers (Aman, Farmer, Hollway, & Arnold, 2008).

Treatment of Attention-Deficit/Hyperactivity Disorder and Externalizing Disorders (Oppositional Defiant Disorder and Conduct Disorder)

Individuals with ADHD and conduct disorder are at much higher risk of developing substance abuse or antisocial personality disorder and of being involved in criminal activity than individuals with ADHD alone (Turgay, 2009). Oppositional defiant disorder (ODD) and conduct disorder (CD) are difficult to treat, but typically respond best to comprehensive approaches involving counseling, educational interventions, and medication (Connor et al., 2010). About 60% of individuals with ODD will develop CD (Turgay, 2009).

Pharmacologic studies may evaluate individuals with ODD and CD separately or as one experimental group. Furthermore, some studies identify the characteristic of aggression rather than a specific diagnosis as the independent variable. The term *externalizing disorders* will be used hereafter to refer to all of these conditions collectively.

Individuals with ADHD and externalizing disorders respond well to stimulants for their ADHD symptoms. In addition, the externalizing symptoms are likely to improve, so stimulants should be considered the first-line pharmacologic treatment for externalizing disorders with ADHD (List & Barzman, 2010; Pliszka et al., 2006; Turgay, 2009). When children with aggression appear to be stimulant nonresponders, a systematic, carefully monitored titration protocol to identify optimal dose, in combination with behavior therapy, may show sufficient improvement in up to 50% to remain on stimulant monotherapy (Blader, Pliszka, Jensen, Schooler, & Kafantaris, 2010). Atomoxetine has been shown to be equally efficacious for ADHD symptoms with or without additional externalizing disorders (Dell'Agnello et al., 2009), but its effect on oppositional symptoms remains controversial (Biederman et al., 2007; Connor et al., 2010). Both stimulants and atomoxetine have a small but finite risk of exacerbating depression, mood lability, and/or aggression, so these symptoms should be monitored with regular follow-up visits. Additional medications that demonstrate effectiveness for some individuals with externalizing disorders include mood stabilizers (such as lithium or divalproex sodium), alpha-adrenergic agonists (guanfacine and clonidine), SSRIs, and atypical antipsychotics (Connor et al., 2010; Nevels, Dehon, Alexander, & Gontkovsky, 2010; Pliszka et al., 2006). Medication combinations may eventually prove to be most useful for this group of children, but require further study before they can be FDA-approved (McBurnett & Pfiffner, 2009; Spencer, 2009).

Treatment of Attention-Deficit/Hyperactivity Disorder and Internalizing Disorders

The treatment of children with ADHD and anxiety can be challenging because the ADHD core symptoms may not respond as well to methylphenidate (Ter-Stepanian, Grizenko, Zappitelli, & Joober, 2010) or because anxiety may be exacerbated by stimulants. Although anxiety may inhibit impulsivity, it also may make working memory impairments worse (Schatz & Rostain, 2006). Psychosocial intervention has been shown to be particularly efficacious in children with coexisting anxiety disorders and may be a critical component of treatment in this group of children (MTA Cooperative Group, 1999b). One algorithm derived by expert consensus (The Texas Children's Medication Algorithm) recommends initiating treatment with a stimulant and then adding an SSRI if anxiety does not improve sufficiently when the ADHD symptoms are treated effectively (Pliszka et al., 2006). Atomoxetine may be helpful for both ADHD and anxiety (Geller et al., 2007; Kratochvil et al., 2005) and may allow some children to be treated with one rather than two medications. When symptoms of depression are present, the more severe disorder should be treated first, with an SSRI being used for depression and a stimulant for ADHD (Pliska et al., 2006). Other antidepressants that also treat ADHD symptoms (tricyclic antidepressants and bupropion) are options if a stimulant is not tolerated or is not effective. The finding that SSRIs and other antidepressants can increase suicidal ideation in individuals with depression underscores the need for close monitoring (March et al., 2004).

Treatment of Attention-Deficit/Hyperactivity Disorder with Tic Disorders

Although the presence of tics or a personal or family history of Tourette syndrome are listed as contraindications to stimulant use by the pharmaceutical companies that manufacture these medications, this stance appears to be unnecessarily restrictive (see Side Effects). ADHD symptoms may cause much more functional impairment than the tics and thus be the priority for treatment (AACAP, 2007; Denkla, 2006). Most children do not have significant tic exacerbations in response to therapeutic stimulant doses (Gadow & Sverd, 2006; Palumbo et al., 2004). Nonstimulant medications (atomoxetine, guanfacine, clonidine) can be tried first and may improve existent tics (Bloch et al., 2009). Tricyclic antidepressants may also treat ADHD without inducing or exacerbating tics, but their safety profile is a limitation. If stimulants are the only effective medication and do exacerbate tics, the addition of guanfacine or clonidine is recommended (AACAP, 2007). If these are not effective, risperidone or pimozide may be used for tic suppression (Pliszka et al., 2006). The antiepileptic medication topiramate may also be an effective tic suppressant, though further study is needed (Jankovic, Jiminez-Shahed, & Brown, 2010).

Treatment of Attention-Deficit/Hyperactivity Disorder with Medication Combinations

As described previously, it is common for individuals with ADHD to have one or more coexisting conditions. Medications approved for the treatment of ADHD do not typically address the coexisting symptoms, with some exceptions—atomoxetine may have positive effects on anxiety (Kratochvil et al., 2005; Spencer, 2009) and ODD (Bangs et al., 2008; Newcorn, Spencer, Biederman, Milton, & Michelson, 2005) and alpha-adrenergic agonists may improve aggression (Connor et al., 2010; Sallee, 2010) and tics (Bloch et al., 2009; Pliszka et al., 2006).

Combinations of methylphenidate with alpha-adrenergic agonists (Spencer, Greenbaum, Ginsberg, & Murphy, 2009), SSRIs, (Spencer, 2009), atomoxetine (Kratochvil et al., 2005; Wilens et al., 2008), and atypical antipsychotics have all shown some benefit for individuals with ADHD and coexisting conditions (Sallee, 2010; Spencer, 2009). Preliminary investigation indicates that atomoxetine with fluoxetine is a safe and effective combination for ADHD with coexisiting anxiety or depressive symptoms. The safety information is important given that both medications are substrates for P450–CY2D6 liver metabolism (Kratochvil et al., 2005). Partial responders to atomoxetine show improvements when methylphenidate is added (Wilens et al., 2008) but adverse effects are also increased (Hammerness et al., 2009). In spite of increasing evidence for effectiveness, and widespread need for optimal management of ADHD with coexisting conditions, there are only two recent FDA-approved medication combinations for ADHD or ADHD with coexisting conditions, sustained-release clonidine (Kapvay, Shionogi, Inc.) or sustained release guanfacine (Intuniv, Shire, Inc.) with a stimulant.

ALTERNATIVE THERAPIES

Elimination diets, nutrient supplementation, and brain training techniques are the most-often studied alternative treatments for ADHD. Dietary treatments include two different approaches, either the elimination of certain foods or additives or nutrient supplementation. Presently, there is more evidence in favor of the former. The two most commonly identified additive-free diets are the Feingold Program (elimination of artificial colors and flavors, the preservatives BHA, BHT, and TBHQ, and naturally occurring salicylates found in some fruits and vegetables), and a British version (elimination of artificial colors and the preservative sodium benzoate). There are, in fact, no accurately designed studies of the Feingold diet. Studies in the early 1970s, which purported to test this hypothesis, contained methodological flaws that would have minimized

positive results. Nonetheless, 10%–20% of children were noted to respond, and preschoolers were noted to have a much higher response rate (Bateman et al., 2004; Kaplan, McNichol, Conte, & Moghadam, 1989). Studies focusing on the role of artificial colors and sodium benzoate in the general population of children (not selecting for those identified as having ADHD-related symptoms) have revealed small, but significant detrimental effects of these substances on the behavior of 3 and 8–9 year old children (Bateman et al., 2004; McCann et al., 2007). The adverse effect of additives in this group was moderated by polymorphisms in histamine degradation genes, suggesting that histamine response may play a role in the effects of additives on behavior (Stevenson et al., 2010). A meta-analysis of double-blind placebo-controlled elimination diet trials found positive effects, though with overall small effect sizes (Schab & Trinh, 2004). With the addition of more recent studies, additive-free elimination diets are considered to have similar levels of evidence for treatment effects in preschoolers, as does behavior management (Ghuman, Arnold, & Anthony, 2008).

The elimination of specific foods may also improve ADHD-related symptoms. Commonly allergenic foods are typically most often implicated, and children who reacted to foods also reacted to artificial colors (Carter et al., 1993; Egger, Carter, Graham, Gumley, & Soothill, 1985; Schmidt et al., 1997). A recent controlled, though not blinded, study of this approach in young children with ADHD resulted in an approximately 50% improvement on parent and teacher ADHD rating scales (Pelsser et al., 2008). The mechanism for this observation is unknown, but case reports document improvement in ADHD symptoms when IgG-mediated food reactions are eliminated (Ritz & Lord, 2005), though there are no well-controlled studies at this time. The elimination of sugar has not been found to be an effective intervention (Wolraich, Wilson, & White, 1995).

Children with ADHD may be relatively deficient in iron, zinc, and magnesium (Arnold et al., 2005; Glanzman, 2009). Small, open label studies of supplementation with these minerals have demonstrated partial improvement in ADHD symptoms (Rucklidge, Johnstone, & Kaplan, 2009). Recently a large, double-blind placebo-controlled study of zinc found improvements in hyperactive and impulsive behaviors but not inattention. Approximately 29% of the zinc-treated group versus 20% of the placebo group was judged to be responders, and those with lower zinc levels at baseline were more likely to respond (Bilici et al., 2004). Zinc status was also shown to correlate with parent and teacher ratings of inattention, but not hyperactivity in middle-class Americans (Arnold et al., 2005). Multinutrient supplementation has not been studied in ADHD specifically, or in well-controlled trials, but should be since multiple nutrients are involved in neurochemical reactions, and individuals deficient in one nutrient may be more likely to be deficient in others. There is some open-trial evidence that multinutrient formulas can improve ADHD symptoms (Harding, Judah, & Gant, 2003) and mood/conduct in children or adults with mental health diagnoses (Frazier, Fristad, & Arnold, 2009; Rucklidge, Gately, & Kaplan, 2010), including adults with ADHD (Rucklidge, Taylor, & Whitehead, 2010). "Megadoses" of vitamins or minerals can have toxic effects and are not indicated.

Essential fatty acids (EFAs) are lower in children with ADHD than controls, and supplementation has shown positive effects in a number of mental health disorders, but treatment effects in ADHD have been weak (reviewed in Chalon, 2009; Raz & Gabis, 2009). Earlier studies tended to be negative and to use one type of EFA (omega-3 or omega-6). More recent studies have shown positive results (Johnson, Östlund, Fransson, Kadesjö, & Gillberg, 2009; Richardson & Montgomery, 2005; Sinn & Bryan, 2007) using eicosapentaenoic (EPA, omega-3), docosahexaenoic (DHA, omega-3) and linoleic acid (LA, omega-6) or gama-linoleic acid (GLA, omega 6) together, suggesting that a combination of omega-3 and omega-6 may be necessary. Since children with ADHD appear to be deficient due to altered metabolism of EFAs rather than decreased intake (Colter, Cutler, & Meckling, 2008), initial measurement followed by individualized treatment may be a more appropriate way to assess the effects of supplementation. For example, a recent study in which EPA treatment alone did show positive effects also found higher levels of arachidonic acid (an omega-6 EFA) among responders (Gustafsson et al., 2010).

Several techniques that "train" brain activity with the goal of improving attention and working memory are under investigation. EEG biofeedback is the treatment that has been studied most extensively, though there are only a few well-controlled trials. Quantitative EEG studies indicate that subjects with ADHD tend to have a lower level of those waves (alpha and beta) associated with alert, thinking states, and a higher level of those waves associated with drowsiness (theta). EEG biofeedback uses computer technology to train the individual to produce more of the brain wave patterns associated with concentration and to suppress those associated with overarousal or underarousal (Monastra, 2008). There is some evidence for its effectiveness (Friel, 2007; Holtman & Stadler, 2006), though more methodologically sound studies are needed. A recent randomized, controlled trial found positive effects that persisted at a 6 month follow-up (Gevensleben et al., 2010), but another double-blind study that included a sham neurofeedback control condition did not show effects on ADHD ratings or continuous performance and stop signal tasks (Logemann, Lansbergen, Van Os, Böcker, & Kenemans, 2010).

Other types of computerized training programs that purport to improve attention and/or working memory show promising initial results (Beck, Hanson, Puffenberger, Benninger, & Benninger, 2010; Holmes, Dunning, & Gathercole, 2009; Klingberg et al., 2005; Rabiner, Murray, Skinner, & Malone, 2010; Shalev, Tsal, & Mevorach, 2007). A multicenter, randomized, controlled, double-blind study of 53 children with ADHD who were not on stimulant medication showed improvements in working memory, response inhibition, reasoning, and parent-rated inattention (Klingberg et al., 2005). A functional magnetic resonance study showed task-dependent enhancement of brain activation in expected regions after training, but not in children who received control training (Hoekzema et al., 2010).

OUTCOME

Symptoms of ADHD decline over time; yet about 15% of young adults continue to meet full criteria and about 65% meet criteria for ADHD in partial remission (Faraone et al., 2006). Overall, up to 78% have some evidence of persistence (Biederman, Petty, Evans, Small, & Faraone, 2010). Unfortunately, even with a reduction in symptom burden, longitudinal follow-up studies indicate that functional impairments persist 10 years later in the majority of individuals diagnosed at 6–17 years of age (Biederman, Monuteaux, et al., 2006).

Young adults with ADHD have lower educational and employment performance and attainment, fewer friendships and more social problems, poorer driving records, and a higher chance of sexually transmitted disease and unplanned pregnancy (Barkley, Fischer,

Smallish, & Fletcher, 2006; Biederman, Monu-teaux, et al., 2006; Fischer, Barkley, Smallish, & Fletcher, 2007; Wehmeier, Schacht, & Bar-kley, 2010). Youth with ADHD are at higher risk for emerging coexisting conditions in their young adult years, including antisocial, addic-tive, mood, and anxiety disorders (Biederman, Monuteaux, et al., 2006). Girls with ADHD are also at higher risk for eating disorders (Bieder-man et al., 2010). The presence of a conduct disorder predicts some of the most severe out-come risks, including failure to graduate high school, early sexual activity and parenthood, antisocial behavior, and substance use (Barkley et al., 2006).

Understanding the effects of current treatment options in ameliorating the subop-timal outcomes faced by youth with ADHD is hampered by the difficulty in performing well-controlled, prospective, long-term studies, but some consistent information is emerging based on a combination of different types of studies. The MTA study is the largest clinical trial of ADHD treatments to date (MTA Coopera-tive Group, 1999a). This prospective multisite treatment study of 576 children with ADHD-C between the ages of 7 and 9 years random-ized children to one of four treatment groups: medication management, intensive behavioral treatment, medication and intensive behavioral treatment, and standard community care. The medication management group received pri-marily methylphenidate titrated to the best of three doses. The behavioral treatment involved 35 group and individual sessions for parents, a summer program for children, teacher con-sultation, and 60 days of a part-time behavior-ally trained paraprofessional working with the child in school. The combined treatment group received both of these interventions, while the standard community care group were evalu-ated and referred back to providers in their own community for treatment. (About 67% of this group received some type of medication treat-ment). The main disadvantage of this study for outcome assessment is that treatment was lim-ited to 14 months, and subsequent treatment during the follow-up phase was not systemati-cally evaluated.

After 14 months of treatment, medication alone was found to be nearly as effective as the combined treatment for improving core ADHD symptoms, although those receiving the com-bined treatment achieved these outcomes on lower doses of medication. Both the combined and medication-only treatments were more effective in improving core ADHD symptoms than behavioral treatment or community care. For academic achievement, anxiety/depressive symptoms, oppositional/aggressive symptoms, social skills, and parent–child relationships, there were benefits of combined treatment compared with medication alone (Jensen et al., 2001). Children with anxiety disorders responded as well to the psychosocial treatment as they did to medication alone.

At 24 months (10 months after the end of treatment), about half of the advantage provided by medication at 14 months had dissipated. This was most likely due to failure to main-tain effective treatment and some "shifting" of groups; for example some in the combination and medication treatment groups discontinued medication, and some in the behavioral treat-ment group initiated medication treatment (Murray et al., 2008; Swanson et al., 2008). Behavioral treatment, either alone or in combi-nation with medication management, provided a sustained advantage in ameliorating parent-reported homework problems (Langberg et al., 2010).

At 36 months (22 months after the end of treatment), there were no longer any differ-ences in the variety of outcome measures used among any of the treatment groups. All groups were doing better across all measures compared with baseline, but all were worse off than com-munity controls. Outcome was related to the initial pattern of treatment response rather than to the specific treatment itself. There were three patterns of initial response: 1) about 34% of subjects showed an initial mild improve-ment that gradually increased over time, 2) 52% showed an initial substantial improve-ment that was maintained over time, 3) about 14% had an initial substantial improvement and then deteriorated over time. The second group had the most favorable outcome. They were less impaired at baseline, had less psycho-social adversity, and were more frequently in the medication or combined treatment groups. The third group had the poorest outcome. They had increased severity at baseline, lower IQs, decreased social skills, more coexisting conditions, and more psychosocial risk factors. The first group showed an intermediate out-come, and in this group, those who continued to take medication did better (Murray et al., 2008; Swanson et al., 2008). One might inter-pret these findings to mean that medication treatment does not provide long-term benefit; however, it is also more likely that those with the most severe symptoms were most likely to remain on medication.

At the 6–8 year follow-up, the importance of the initial pattern of response continued. Outcome measures were collected from parents, teachers, and subjects, and additional variables that were appropriate for adolescents, such as grades earned, arrests, and psychiatric hospitalizations, were included. Although a majority of the group had initial treatment gains that were maintained, MTA participants remained disadvantaged compared with community controls on 91% of the variables measured (Molina et al., 2009). The MTA data were further examined to evaluate the role of moderators and mediators of treatment outcome. Moderators are uncontrolled variables present at baseline that influence response to intervention, whereas mediators are variables that are present during treatment that may explain how treatments work or do not work. MTA-identified moderators include coexisting anxiety disorder, public assistance, severity of ADHD symptoms, IQ, and parental depressive symptoms. Negative or ineffective parent discipline was a key mediator (Hinshaw, 2007).

Other outcome studies of medication effects indicate slight benefits in social skills and self-esteem (Hechtman & Greenfield, 2003), and decreased risk for depression and other psychiatric disorders (Biederman et al., 2009; Daviss, Birmaher, Diler, & Mintz, 2008). Academic benefits can be identified in adolescence, even when medication treatment was only provided in childhood, on variables such as grade retention, high school grade point average (GPA), and WIAT II subtest scores (Powers, Marks, Miller, Newcorn, & Halperin, 2008). There is no clear evidence for an effect of childhood medication treatment on later substance use risk (Biederman et al., 2008), but there is evidence that a significant percentage of older adolescents and young adults with ADHD are using substances to "self-medicate" (Wilens et al., 2007), suggesting that optimal medication treatment for ADHD may ameliorate this risk.

In summary, the MTA study indicates that optimally managed medication treatment is effective, that the addition of behavioral treatment may be particularly important in subgroups with coexisting symptoms and psychosocial adversity, and that children with coexisting anxiety disorders are a particularly treatment-responsive subgroup of children with ADHD, at least during the initial treatment phase. However, clinical presentation in childhood (including symptom severity, conduct symptoms, intellect, and social advantage), and the degree of response to any treatment are better predictors of adolescent functioning than the type of 14-month treatment received during childhood. Other studies suggest that carefully managed medication treatment can improve specific functional outcomes, even when not provided continuously into later adolescence and young adulthood. The role of continued medication and optimal prescribing practices remains to be determined. There is a critical need for studies to determine the best ways to mitigate adverse moderators and mediators and to improve, rather than simply accommodate, the executive function impairments that are known to contribute to academic and adult functional impairment.

SUMMARY

ADHD is a prevalent neurodevelopmental condition that has a significant impact on the lives of affected children, their families, and the educational and medical/mental health systems. The core features of difficulty sustaining mental effort, hyperactivity, and impulsivity lead to impairment in academic, occupational, social, and adaptive functions without effective intervention. Coping with ADHD is made more complicated by commonly coexisting conditions, including learning disorders, oppositional defiant disorder, and anxiety disorders. ADHD is highly genetic, but adverse conditions in the prenatal and perinatal period can contribute to symptoms. Multiple lines of evidence suggest a biological basis involving frontal cortical-basal ganglia-cerebellar pathways and biogenic amine neurotransmitters, particularly dopamine and norepinephrine. Treatments include counseling, particularly that focusing on behavior management; accommodations in the classroom; addressing coexisting conditions; and medication. Fortunately, the knowledge and resources presently available, and the increases in these areas that are sure to occur over the next generation, offer children growing up with ADHD the opportunity to experience success.

REFERENCES

Abanilla, P.K., Hannahs, G.A., Wechsler, R., & Silva, R.R. (2005). The use of psychostimulants in pervasive developmental disorders. *Psychiatric Quarterly*, 76, 271–281. doi:10.1007/s11126-005-2980-7

Abikoff, H., Hechtman, L., Klein, R.G., Gallagher, R., Fleiss, K., Etcovitch, J., & Pollack, S. (2004). Social functioning in children with ADHD treated with long-term methylphenidate and multimodal psychosocial treatment. *Journal of the American Academy of Child & Adolescent Psychiatry, 43,* 820–829. doi:10.1097/01.chi.0000128797.91601.1a

Abikoff, H., Nissley-Tsiopinis, J., Gallagher, R., Zambenedetti, M., Seyffert, M., Boorady, R., & McCarthy, J. (2009). Effects of MPH-OROS and the organizational, time management, and planning behaviors of children with ADHD. *Journal of the American Academy of Child and Adolescent Psychiatry, 48,* 166–175. doi:10.1097/CHI.0b013e3181930626

Aman, M.G., Buican, B., & Arnold, L.E. (2003). Methylphenidate treatment in children with borderline IQ and mental retardation: Analysis of three aggregated studies. *Journal of Child & Adolescent Psychopharmacology, 13,* 29–40. doi:10.1089/104454603321666171

Aman, M.G., Farmer, C.A., Hollway, J., & Arnold, L.E. (2008). Treatment of inattention, overactivity, and impulsiveness in autism spectrum disorders. *Child & Adolescent Psychiatric Clinics of North America, 17,* 713–738. doi:10.1016/j.chc.2008.06.009

American Academy of Pediatrics. (2011). Clinical practice guideline: ADHD: Clinical practice guideline for the diagnosis, evaluation, and treatment of attention-deficit/hyperactivity disorder in children and adolescents. *Pediatrics, 128,* 1–16.

American Academy of Child and Adolescent Psychiatry. (2007). Practice parameter for the use of stimulant medications in the treatment of children, adolescents, and adults. *Journal of the American Academy of Child and Adolescent Psychiatry, 46,* 894–921.

American Psychiatric Association. (2000). *Diagnostic and statistical manual of mental disorders* (4th ed., text rev.).

American Psychiatric Association. (2010). *DSM-5: The future of psychiatric diagnosis.* Retrieved from http://www.DSM5.org

Armstrong, M.B., & Nettleton, S.K. (2004). Attention deficit hyperactivity disorder and preschool children. *Seminars in Speech and Language, 25,* 225–232. doi:10.1055/s-2004-833670

Arnold, L.E., Aman, M.G., Cook, A.M., Witwer, A.N., Hall, K.L., Thompson, S., & Ramadan, Y. (2006). Atomoxetine for hyperactivity in autism spectrum disorders: Placebo-controlled crossover pilot study. *Journal of the American Academy of Child & Adolescent Psychiatry, 45,* 1196–1205.

Arnold, L.E., Bozzolo, H., Holloway, J., Cook, A., DiSilvestro, R.A., Bozzolo, D.R., ... Williams, C. (2005). Serum zinc correlates with parent- and teacher-rated inattention in children with attention-deficit/hyperactivity disorder. *Journal of Child & Adolescent Psychopharmacology, 15,* 628–636. doi:10.1089/cap.2005.15.628

Arnold, L.E., Farmer, C., Kraemer, H.C., Davies, M., Witwer, A., Chuang, S., ... Swiezy, N.B. (2010). Moderators, mediators, and other predictors of risperidone response in children with autistic disorder and irritability. *Journal of Child & Adolescent Psychopharmacology, 20,* 83–93. doi:10.1089/cap.2009.0022

Arnsten, A.F.T. (2009). Toward a new understanding of attention-deficit hyperactivity disorder pathophysiology: An important role for prefrontal cortex dysfunction. *CNS Drugs, 23*(Supp. 1), 33–41.

Baeyens, D., Roeyers, H., & Walle, J.V. (2006). Subtypes of attention-deficit/hyperactivity disorder (ADHD): Distinct or related disorders across measurement levels? *Child Psychiatry & Human Development, 36,* 403–417. doi:10.1007/s10578-006-0011-z

Banaschewski, T., Becker, K., Scherag, S., Franke, B., & Coghill, D. (2010). Molecular genetics of attention-deficit/hyperactivity disorder: An overview. *European Child & Adolescent Psychiatry, 19,* 237–257. doi:10.1007/s00787-010-0090-z

Banaschewski, T., Roessner, V., Dittman, R.W., Santosh, P.J., & Rothenberger, A. (2004). Non-stimulant medications in the treatment of ADHD. *European Child & Adolescent Psychiatry, 13*(Supp. 1), 102–116. doi:10.1007/s00787-004-1010-x

Banerjee, T.D., Middleton, F., & Faraone, S.V. (2007). Environmental risk factors for attention-deficit hyperactivity disorder. *Acta Paediatrica, 96,* 1269–1274. doi:10.1111/j.1651-2227.2007.00430.x

Bangs, M.E., Hazell. P., Danckaerts, M., Hoare, P., Coghill, D.R., Wehmeier, P.M., ... Levine, L. (2008). Atomoxetine for the treatment of attention-deficit/hyperactivity disorder and oppositional defiant disorder. *Pediatrics, 121,* e314–e320. doi:10.1542/peds.2006-1880

Barkley, R.A. (1998). Attention-deficit hyperactivity disorder. *Scientific American, 279,* 66–71. doi:10.1038/scientificamerican0998-66

Barkley, R.A. (2004). Adolescents with attention-deficit/hyperactivity disorder: An overview of empirically-based treatments. *Journal of Psychiatric Practice, 10,* 39–56. doi:10.1097/00131746-200401000-00005

Barkley, R.A. (2010). Against the status quo: Revising the diagnostic criteria for ADHD. *Journal of the American Academy of Child & Adolescent Psychiatry, 49,* 205–207. doi:10.1016/j.jaac.2009.12.005

Barkley, R.A., & Cox, D. (2007). A review of driving risks and impairment associated with attention-deficit/hyperactivity disorder and effects of stimulant medication on driving performance. *Journal of Safety Research, 38,* 113–128. doi:10.1016/j.jsr.2006.09.004

Barkley, R.A., Fischer, M., Smallish, L., & Fletcher, K. (2006). Young adult outcome of hyperactive children: Adaptive functioning in major life activities. *Journal of the American Academy of Child & Adolescent Psychiatry, 45,* 192–202. doi:10.1097/01.chi.0000189134.97436.e2

Bateman, B., Warner, J.O., Hutchinson, E., Dean, T., Rowlandson, P., Gant, C., ... Stevenson, J. (2004). The effects of a double-blind, placebo controlled, artificial food colorings and benzoate preservative challenge on hyperactivity in a general population sample of preschool children. *Archives of Diseases in Children, 89,* 506–511. doi:10.1136/adc.2003.031435

Beck, S.J., Hanson, C.A., Puffenberger, S.S., Benninger, K.L., & Benninger, W.B. (2010). A controlled trial of working memory training for children and adolescents with ADHD. *Journal of Clinical Child & Adolescent Psychology, 39,* 825–836. doi:10.1080/15374416.2010.517162

Biederman, J., Baldessarini, R.J., Wright, V., Knee, D., & Harmatz, J.S. (1989). A double-blind placebo controlled study of desipramine in the treatment of ADD: I. Efficacy. *Journal of the American Academy of Child and Adolescent Psychiatry, 28,* 777–784. doi:10.1097/00004583-198909000-00022

Biederman, J., Kwon, A., Aleardi, M., Chouinard, V.A., Marino, T., Cole, H., ... Faraone, S.V. (2005).

Absence of gender effects on attention deficit hyperactivity disorder: Findings in non-referred subjects. *American Journal of Psychiatry, 162*, 1083–1089.

Biederman, J., Melmed, R.D., Patel, A., McBurnett, K., Donahue, J., & Lyne, A. (2008). Long-term, open-label extension study of guanfacine extended release in children and adolescents with ADHD. *CNS Spectrums, 13*, 1047–1055.

Biederman, J., Melmed, R.D., Patel, A., McBurnett, K., Konow, J., Lyne, A., & Scherer, N. (2008). A randomized, double-blind, placebo-controlled study of guanfacine extended release in children and adolescents with attention-deficit hyperactivity disorder. *Pediatrics, 121*, e73–e84. doi:10.1542/peds.2006-3695

Biederman, J., Monuteaux, M.C., Mick, E., Spencer, T., Wilens, T.E., Silva, J., ... Faraone, S.V. (2006). Young adult outcome of attention deficit hypeactivity disorder: A controlled 10-year follow-up study. *Psychological Medicine, 36*, 167–179. doi:10.1017/S0033291705006410

Biederman, J., Monuteaux, M.C., Spencer, T., Wilens, T.E., & Faraone, S.V. (2009). Do stimulants protect against psychiatric disorders in youth with ADHD? A 10-year follow-up study. *Pediatrics, 124*, 71–78. doi:10.1542/peds.2008-3347

Biederman, J., Monuteaux, M.C., Spencer, T., Wilens, T.E., Macpherson, H.A., & Faraone, S.V. (2008). Stimulant therapy and risk for subsequent substance use disorders in male adults with ADHD: A naturalistic controlled 10-year follow-up study. *American Journal of Psychiatry, 165*, 597–603.

Biederman, J., Petty, C.R., Evans, M., Small, J., & Faraone, S.V. (2010). How persistent is ADHD? A controlled 10-year follow-up study of boys with ADHD. *Psychiatry Research, 177*, 299–304. doi:10.1016/j.psychres.2009.12.010

Biederman, J., Petty, C.R., Monuteaux, M.C., Fried, R., Byrne, D., Mirto, T., ... Faraone, S.V. (2010). Adult psychiatric outcomes of girls with attention deficit hyperactivity disorder: 11-year follow-up in a longitudinal case-control study. *American Journal of Psychiatry, 167*, 409–417. doi:10.1176/appi.ajp.2009.09050736

Biederman, J., Seidman, L.J., Petty, C.R., Fried, R., Dolye, A.E., Cohen, D.R., ... Faraone, S.V. (2008). Effects of stimulant medication on neuropsychological functioning in young adults with attention-deficit/hyperactivity disorder. *Journal of Clinical Psychiatry, 69*, 1150–1156. doi:10.4088/JCP.v69n0715

Biederman, J., Spencer, T.J., Newcorn, J.H., Gao, H., Milton, D.R., Feldman, P.D., & Witte, M.M. (2007). Effect of comorbid symptoms of oppositional defiant disorder on responses to atomoxetine in children with ADHD: A meta-analysis of controlled clinical trial data. *Psychopharmacology, 190*, 31–41. doi:10.1007/s00213-006-0565-2

Biederman, J., Wigal, S.B., Spencer, T.J., McGough, J.J., & Mays, D.A. (2006). A post hoc subgroup analysis of an 18-day randomized controlled trial comparing the tolerability and efficacy of mixed amphetamine salts extended release and atomoxetine in school-age girls with attention-deficit/hyperactivity disorder. *Clinical Therapeutics, 28*, 280–293. doi:10.1016/j.clinthera.2006.02.008

Bilici, M., Yildirim F, Kandil, S., Bekaroglu, M., Yildirmis S., Deger, O., ... Aksu, H. (2004). Double-blind, placebo-controlled study of zinc sulfate in the treatment of attention deficit hyperactivity disorder.

Progress in Neuro-Psychopharmacology & Biological Psychiatry, 28, 181–190. doi:10.1016/j.pnpbp.2003.09.034

Bjornstad, G., & Montogomery, P. (2005). Family therapy for attention-deficit disorder or attention-deficit/hyperactivity disorder in children and adolescents. *Cochrane Database of Systematic Reviews.* doi:10.1002/14651858.CD005042.pub2

Blader, J.C., Pliszka, S.R., Jensen, P.S., Schooler, N.R., & Kafantaris, V. (2010). Stimulant-responsive and stimulant-refractory aggressive behavior among children with ADHD. *Pediatrics, 126*, e796–e806. doi:10.1542/peds.2010-0086

Bloch, M.H., Panza, K.E., Landeros-Weisenberger, A., & Leckman, J.F. (2009). Meta-analysis: Treatment of attention-deficit/hyperactivity disorder in children with comorbid tic disorders. *Journal of the American Academy of Child & Adolescent Psychiatry, 48*, 884–893. doi:10.1097/CHI.0b013e3181b26e9f

Buitelaar, J.K., Michelson, D., Danckaerts, M., Gillberg, C., Spencer, T.J., Zuddas, A., ... Biederman, J. (2007). A randomized, double-blind study of continuation treatment for attention-deficit/hyperactivity disorder after 1 year. *Biological Psychiatry, 61*, 694–699. doi:10.1016/j.biopsych.2006.03.066

Bush, G. (2008). Neuroimaging of attention deficit hyperactivity disorder: Can new imaging findings be integrated into clinical practice? *Child & Adolescent Psychiatric Clinics of North America, 17*, 385–404.

Bush, G., Spencer, T., Holmes, J., Shin, L.M., Valera, E.M., Seidman, L.J., ... Biederman, J. (2008). Functional magnetic resonance imaging of methylphenidate and placebo in attention-deficit/hyperactivity disorder during the multi-source interference task. *Archives of General Psychiatry, 65*, 102–114. doi:10.1001/archgenpsychiatry.2007.16

Cairney, J., Veldhuizen, S., & Szatmari, P. (2010). Motor coordination and emotional-behavioral problems in children. *Current Opinion in Psychiatry, 23*, 324–329. doi:10.1097/YCO.0b013e32833aa0aa

Carlson, G.A., & Kelly, K.L. (2003). Stimulant rebound: How common is it and what does it mean? *Journal of Child and Adolescent Psychopharmacology, 13*, 137–142. doi:10.1089/104454603322163853

Carter, C.M., Urbanowicz, M., Hemsley, R., Mantilla, L., Storbel, S., Graham, P.J., & Taylor, E. (1993). Effects of a few foods diet in attention deficit disorder. *Archives of Diseases in Childhood, 69*, 564–568. doi:10.1136/adc.69.5.564

Casey, B.J., Nigg, J.T., & Durston, S. (2007). New potential leads in the biology and treatment of attention deficit-hyperactivity disorder. *Current Opinions in Neurology, 20*, 119–124. doi:10.1097/WCO.0b013e3280a02f78

Castellanos, F.X., Sonuga-Barke, E.J.S., Milham, M.P., & Tannock, R. (2006). Characterizing cognition in ADHD: Beyond executive dysfunction. *Trends in Cognitive Science, 10*, 117–123. doi:10.1016/j.tics.2006.01.011

Chacko, A., Wakschlag, L., Hill, C., Danis, B., & Espy, K.A. (2009). Viewing preschool disruptive behavior disorders and attention-deficit/hyperactivity disorder through a developmental lens: What we know and what we need to know. *Child & Adolescent Psychiatric Clinics of North America, 18*, 627–643. doi:10.1016/j.chc.2009.02.003

Chalon, S. (2009). The role of fatty acids in the treatment of ADHD. *Neuropharmacology, 57*, 636–639. doi:10.1016/j.neuropharm.2009.08.012

Chapman, L.A., Wade, S.L., Walz, N.C., Taylor, H.G., Stancin, T., & Yeates, K.O. (2010). Clinically significant behavior problems during the 18 months following early childhood traumatic brain injury. *Rehabilitation Psychology*, 55, 48–57. doi:10.1037/a0018418

Chronis, A.M., Chacko, A., Fabiano, G.A., Wymbs, B.T., & Pelham, W.E. Jr. (2004). Enhancements to the behavioral parent training paradigm for families of children with ADHD: Review and future directions. *Clinical Child & Family Psychology Review*, 7, 1–27. doi:10.1023/B:CCFP.0000020190.60808.a4

Colter, A.L., Cutler, C., & Meckling, K.A. (2008). Fatty acid status and behavioral symptoms of attention deficit hyperactivity disorder in adolescents: A case-control study. *Nutrition Journal*, 7, 8. doi:10.1186/1475-2891-7-8

Conners, C.K., Casat, C.D., Gualtieri, C.T., Weller, E., Reader, M., Reiss, A., ... Ascher, J. (1996). Bupropion hydrochloride in attention deficit disorder with hyperactivity. *Journal of the American Academy of Child and Adolescent Psychiatry*, 35, 1314–1321. doi:10.1097/00004583-199610000-00018

Connor, D.F., Steeber, J., & McBurnett, K. (2010). A review of attention-deficit/hyperactivity disorder complicated by symptoms of oppositional defiant disorder or conduct disorder. *Journal of Developmental & Behavioral Pediatrics*, 31, 427–440. doi:10.1097/DBP.0b013e3181e121bd

Cornforth, C., Sonuga-Barke, E., & Coghill, D. (2010). Stimulant drug effects on attention deficit/hyperactivity disorder: A review of the effects of age and sex of patients. *Current Pharmaceutical Design*, 16, 2424–2433. doi:10.2174/138161210791959827

Cox, D.J., Moore, M., Burket, R., Merkel, L.R., Mikami, A.L., & Kovatchev, B. (2008). Rebound effects with long-acting amphetamine or methylphenidate stimulant medication preparations among adolescent male drivers with attention-deficit/hyperactivity disorder. *Journal of Child & Adolescent Psychopharmacology*, 18, 1–10. doi:10.1089/cap.2006.0141

Daley, D., Jones, K., Hutchings, J., & Thompson, M. (2008). Attention deficit hyperactivity disorder in pre-school children: Current findings, recommended interventions and future directions. *Child: Care, Health and Development*, 35, 754–766. doi:10.1111/j.1365-2214.2009.00938.x

Daviss, W.B., Birmaher, B., Diler, R.S., & Mintz, J. (2008). Does pharmacotherapy for attention-deficit/hyperactivity disorder predict risk of later major depression? *Journal of Child & Adolescent Psychopharmacology*, 18, 257–264. doi:10.1089/cap.2007.0100

Dawes, P., & Bishop, D. (2009). Auditory processing disorder in relation to developmental disorders of language, communication and attention: A review and critique. *International Journal of Language & Communication Disorders*, 44, 440–465. doi:10.1080/13682820902929073

Deault, L.C. (2010). A systematic review of parenting in relation to the development of comorbidities and functional impairments in children with attention-deficit/hyperactivity disorder (ADHD). *Child Psychiatry and Human Development*, 41, 168–192. doi:10.1007/s10578-009-0159-4

Dell'Agnello, G., Zuddas, A., Masi, G., Curatolo, P., Besana, D., & Rossi, A. (2009). Use of atomoxetine in patients with attention-deficit hyperactivity disorder and co-morbid conditions. *CNS Drugs*, 23, 739–753. doi:10.2165/11314350-000000000-00000

Delobel-Ayoub, M., Arnaud, C., White-Koning, M., Casper, C., Pierrat, V., Garel. M., ... Larroque, B. (2009). Behavioral problems and cognitive performance at 5 years of age after very preterm birth: The EPIPAGE study. *Pediatrics*, 123, 1485–1492. doi:10.1542/peds.2008-1216

Denkla, M.B. (2006). Attention deficit hyperactivity disorder: The childhood comorbidity that most influences the burden of disability. In J.T. Walkup, J.W. Mink, & P.J. Hollenbeck (Eds.), *Advances in Neurology: Volume 99: Tourette Syndrome* (pp. 17–21). Philadelphia, PA: Lippincott Williams & Wilkins.

Deutsch, C.K., Dube, W.V., & McIlvane, W.J. (2008). Attention deficits, attention-deficit hyperactivity disorder, and intellectual disabilities. *Developmental Disabilities Research Reviews*, 14, 285–292. doi:10.1002/ddrr.42

Donnelly, C., Bangs, M., Trzepacz, P., Jin, L., Zhang, S., Witte, M.M., ... Spencer, T.J. (2009). Safety and tolerability of atomoxetine over 3 to 4 years in children and adolescents with ADHD. *Journal of the American Academy of Child & Adolescent Psychiatry*, 48, 176–185. doi:10.1097/CHI.0b013e318193060e

Doyle, A.E. (2006). Executive functions in attention-deficit/hyperactivity disorder. *Journal of Clinical Psychiatry*, 67(Supp. 8), 21–26.

DuPaul, G.J., Weyandt, L.L., O'Dell, S.M., & Varejao, M. (2009). College students with ADHD. *Journal of Attention Disorders*, 13, 234–250. doi:10.1177/1087054709340650

Education for All Handicapped Children Act of 1975, PL 94-142, 20 U.S.C. §§1400 *et seq.*

Egger, J., Carter, C.M., Graham, P.J., Gumley, D., & Soothill, J.F. (1985). Controlled trial of oligoantigenic treatment in the hyperkinetic syndrome. *The Lancet*, 325(8428), 540–546. doi:10.1016/S0140-6736(85)91206-1

Elia, J., & Vetter, V.L. (2010). Cardiovascular effects of medications for the treatment of attention-deficit hyperactivity disorder: What is known and how should it influence prescribing in children? *Pediatric Drugs*, 12, 165–175.

Erenberg, G. (2006). The relationship between Tourette syndrome, attention-deficit hyperactivity disorder, and stimulant medication: A critical review. *Seminars in Pediatric Neurology*, 12, 217–221. doi:10.1016/j.spen.2005.12.003

Eyberg, S.M., Nelson, M.M., & Boggs, S.R. (2008). Evidence-based psychosocial treatments for children and adolescents with disruptive behavior. *Journal of Clinical Child & Adolescent Psychology*, 37, 215–237. doi:10.1080/15374410701820117

Faraone, S.V., Biederman, J., & Mick, E. (2005). The age-dependent decline of attention deficit hyperactivity disorder: A meta-analysis of follow-up studies. *Psychological Medicine*, 36, 159–165. doi:10.1017/S003329170500471X

Faraone, S.V., Biederman, J., Morley, C.P., & Spencer, T.J. (2008). Effect of stimulants on height and weight: A review of the literature. *Journal of the American Academy of Child & Adolescent Psychiatry*, 47, 994–1009. doi:10.1097/CHI.ObO13e31817eOea7

Faraone, S.V., & Buitelaar, J. (2010). Comparing the efficacy of stimulants for ADHD in children and adolescents using meta-analysis. *European Child & Adolescent Psychiatry*, 19, 353–364. doi:10.1007/s00787-009-0054-3

Faraone, S.V., & Glatt, S.J. (2010). Effects of extended-release guanfacine on ADHD symptoms and sedation-related adverse events in children with ADHD. *Journal of Attention Disorders, 13,* 532–538. doi:10.1177/1087054709332472

Faraone, S.V., Glatt, S.J., Bukstein, O.G., Lopez, F.A., Arnold, L.E., & Findling, R.L. (2008). Effects of once-daily oral and transdermal methylphenidate on sleep behavior of children with ADHD. *Journal of Attention Disorders, 12,* 308–315. doi:10.1177/1087054708314844

Faraone S.V., Perlis R.H., Doyle A.E., Smoller J.W., Goralinick J.J., Holmgren M.A., & Sklar, P. (2005). Molecular genetics of attention-deficit/hyperactivity disorder. *Biological Psychiatry, 57,* 1313–1323. doi:10.1016/j.biopsych.2004.11.024

Faraone, S.V., & Upadhyaya, H.P. (2007). The effect of stimulant treatment for ADHD on later substance abuse and the potential for medication misuse, abuse, and diversion. *Journal of Clinical Psychiatry, 68,* e28. doi:10.4088/JCP.1107e28

Fayyad, J., De Graaf, R., Kessler, R., Alonso, J., Angermeyer, M., Demyttenaere, K., ... Jin, R. (2007). Cross-national prevalence and correlates of adult attention-deficit hyperactivity disorder. *British Journal of Psychiatry, 190,* 402–409. doi:10.1192/bjp.bp.106.034389

Figueroa, R. (2010). Use of antidepressants during pregnancy and risk of attention-deficit/hyperactivity disorder in the offspring. *Journal of Developmental Behavioral Pediatrics, 31,* 1–8.

Filho, A.G.C., Bodanese, R., Silva, T.L., Alvares, J.P., Aman, M., & Rohde, L.A. (2005). Comparison of risperidone and methylphenidate for reducing ADHD symptoms in children and adolescents with moderate mental retardation. *Journal of the American Academy of Child & Adolescent Psychiatry, 44,* 748–755.

Fischer, M., Barkley, R.A., Smallish, L., & Fletcher, K. (2007). Hyperactive children as young adults: Driving abilities, safe driving behavior, and adverse driving outcomes. *Accident Analysis & Prevention, 39,* 94–105. doi:10.1016/j.aap.2006.06.008

Fletcher, J.M., Shaywitz, S.E., & Shaywitz, B.A. (1999). Comorbidity of learning and attention disorders: Separate but equal. *Pediatric Clinics of North America, 46,* 885–897.

Franke, B., Neale, B.N., & Faraone, S.V. (2009). Genome-wide association studies in ADHD. *Human Genetics, 126,* 13–50. doi:10.1007/s00439-009-0663-4

Frazier, E.A., Fristad, M.A., & Arnold, L.E. (2009). Multinutrient supplement as treatment: Literature review and case report of a 12-year-old boy with bipolar disorder. *Journal of Child & Adolescent Psychopharmacology, 19,* 453–460. doi:10.1089/cap.2008.0157

Friel, P.N. (2007). EEG biofeedback in the treatment of attention deficit hyperactivity disorder. *Alternative Medicine Reviews, 12,* 146–151.

Froelich, T.E., Lanphear, B.P., Epstein, J.N., Barbaresi, W.J., Katusic, S.K., & Kahn, R.S. (2007). Prevalence, recognition and treatment of attention-deficit/hyperactivity disorder in a national sample of US children. *Archives of Pediatric and Adolescent Medicine, 161,* 857–864. doi:10.1001/archpedi.161.9.857

Froehlich, T.E, McGough, J.J., & Stein, M.A. (2010). Progress and promise of attention-deficit hyperactivity disorder pharmacogenetics. *CNS Drugs, 24,* 99–117. doi:10.2165/11530290-000000000-00000

Gadow, K.D., & Sverd, J. (2006). Attention-deficit/hyperactivity disorder, chronic tic disorder, and methylphenidate. In J.T. Walkup, J.W. Mink, & P.J. Hollenbeck (Eds.), *Advances in neurology: Vol. 99: Tourette syndrome* (pp. 197–207). Philadelphia, PA: Lippincott Williams & Wilkins.

Galanter, C.A., & Leibenluft, E. (2008). Frontiers between attention deficit hyperactivity disorder and bipolar disorder. *Child & Adolescent Psychiatric Clinics of North America, 17,* 325–346. doi:10.1016/j.chc.2007.11.001

Garnock-Jones, K.P., & Keating, G.M. (2009). Atomoxetine: A review of its use in attention-deficit hyperactivity disorder in children and adolescents. *Pediatric Drugs, 11,* 203–226.

Geller, D., Donnelly, C., Lopez, F., Rubin, R., Newcorn, J., Sutton, V., ... Sumner, C. (2007). Atomoxetine treatment for pediatric patients with attention-deficit/hyperactivity disorder with comorbid anxiety disorder. *Journal of the American Academy of Child & Adolescent Psychiatry, 46,* 1119–1127. doi:10.1097/chi.0b013e3180ca8385

Gevensleben, H., Holl, B., Albrecht, B., Schlamp, D., Kratz, O., Studer, P., & Heinrich, H. (2010). Neurofeedback training in children with ADHD: 6-month follow-up of a randomized controlled trial. *European Journal of Child & Adolescent Psychiatry, 19,* 715–724. doi:10.1007/s00787-010-0109-5

Ghelani, K., Sidhu, R., Jain, U., & Tannock, R. (2004). Reading comprehension and reading related abilities in adolescents with reading disabilities and attention-deficit/hyperactivity disorder. *Dyslexia: The Journal of the British Dyslexia Association, 10,* 364–384. doi:10.1002/dys.285

Ghuman, J.K., Aman, M.G., Ghuman, H.S., Reichenbacher, T., Gelenberg, A., Wright, R., ... Fort, C. (2009). Prospective, naturalistic, pilot study of open-label atomoxetine treatment in preschool children with attention-deficit/hyperactivity disorder. *Journal of Child & Adolescent Psychopharmacology, 19,* 155–166. doi:10.1089/cap.2008.054

Ghuman, J.K., Aman, M.G., Lecavalier, L., Riddle, M.A., Gelenberg, A., Wright, R., & Fort, C. (2009). Randomized, placebo-controlled, crossover study of methylphenidate for attention-deficit/hyperactivity disorder symptoms in preschoolers with developmental disorders. *Journal of Child & Adolescent Psychopharmacology, 19,* 329–339. doi:10.1089/cap.2008.0137

Ghuman, J.K., Arnold, L.E., & Anthony, B.J. (2008). Psychopharmacological and other treatments in pres-school children with attention-deficit/hyperactivity disorder: Current evidence and practice. *Journal of Child & Adolescent Psychopharmacology, 18,* 413–447.

Glanzman, M. (2006). Genetics, imaging, and neurochemistry in attention deficit hyperactivity disorder (ADHD). In P. Accardo, B. Whitman, T. Blondis, & M. Stein (Eds.), *Attention deficits and hyperactivity in children and adults.* Baltimore, MD: Paul H. Brookes Publishing Co.

Glanzman, M. (2009). ADHD and nutritional supplements. *Current Attention Disorders Reports, 1,* 75–81. doi:10.1007/s12618-009-0011-6

Glanzman, M., & Elia, J. (2006). Neurodevelopmental and neuropsychiatric disorders. In M. Charron (Ed.), *Practical Pediatric PET Imaging.* New York, NY: Springer.

Greenhill, L.L., Kollins, S., Abikoff, H., McCracken, J., Riddle, M., Swanson, J., ... Cooper, T. (2006). Efficacy and safety of immediate-release methylphenidate treatment for preschoolers with ADHD.

Journal of the American Academy of Child & Adolescent Psychiatry, 45, 1284–1293. doi:10.1097/01.chi.0000235077.32661.61

Greenhill, L.L., Posner, K., Vaughan, B.S., & Kratochvil, C.J. (2008). Attention-deficit/hyperactivity disorder in preschool children. *Child and Adolescent Psychiatric Clinics of North America, 17*, 347–366. doi:10.1016/j.chc.2007.11.004

Gruber, R. (2009). Sleep characteristics of children and adolescents with attention-deficit hyperactivity disorder. *Child & Adolescent Psychiatric Clinics of North America, 18*, 863–876. doi:10.1016/j.chc.2009.04.011

Gustafsson, P.A., Birberg-Thornberg, U., Duchen, K., Landgren,M., Malmberg, K., Pelling, H., & Karlsson, T. (2010). EPA supplementation improves teacher-rated behavior and oppositional symptoms in children with ADHD. *Acta Paediatrica, 99*, 1540–1549. doi:10.1111/j.1651-2227.2010.01871.x

Ha, M., Kwon, H.J., Lim, M.H., Jee, Y.K., Hong, Y.C., Leem, J.H., ... Jo, S.-J. (2009). Low blood levels of lead and mercury and symptoms of attention deficit hyperactivity in children: A report of the children's health and environment research (CHEER). *Neurotoxicology, 30*, 31–36. doi:10.1016/j.neuro.2008.11.011

Hammerness, P., Geller, D., Petty, C., Lamb, A., Bristol, E., & Biederman, J. (2009). Does ADHD moderate the manifestation of anxiety disorders in children? *European Child & Adolescent Psychiatry, 19*, 107–112. doi:10.1007/s00787-009-0041-8

Hammerness, P., Georgiopoulos, A., Doyle, R.L., Utzinger, L., Schillinger, M., Martelon, M., ... Wilens, T.E. (2009). An open study of adjunt OROS-methylpheniate in children who are atomoxetine partial responders: II. Tolerability and pharmacokinetics. *Journal of Child & Adolescent Psychopharmacology, 19*, 493–499. doi:10.1089/cap.2008.0126

Hammerness, P., Wilens, T., Mick, E., Spencer, T., Doyle, R., McCreary, M., ... Biederman, J. (2009). Cardiovascular effects of longer-term, high-dose OROS methylphenidate in adolescents with attention deficit hyperactivity disorder. *Journal of Pediatrics, 155*, 84–89. doi:10.1016/j.jpeds.2009.02.008

Handen, B.L., & Gilchrist, R. (2006). Practitioner review: Psychopharmacology in children and adolescents with mental retardation. *Journal of Child Psychology & Psychiatry, 47*, 871–882. doi:10.1111/j.1469-7610.2006.01588.x

Handen, B.L., Johnson, C.R., & Lubetsky, M. (2000). Efficacy of methylphenidate among children with autism and symptoms of attention-deficit hyperactivity disorder. *Journal of Autism & Developmental Disorders, 30*, 245–255.

Handen, B.L., Sahl, R., & Hardan, A.Y. (2008). Guanfacine in children with autism and/or intellectual disabilities. *Journal of Developmental & Behavioral Pediatrics, 29*, 303–308. doi:10.1097/DBP.0b013e3181739b9d

Harding, K.L., Judah, R.D., & Gant, C.E. (2003). Outcome-based comparison of Ritalin versus food-supplement treated children with AD/HD. *Alternative Medicine Review, 8*, 319–330.

Hechtman, L., & Greenfield, B. (2003). Long-term use of stimulants in children with attention deficit hyperactivity disorder: Safety, efficacy, and long-term outcome. *Pediatric Drugs, 5*, 787–794.

Hinshaw, S.P. (2007). Moderators and mediators for treatment outcome for youth with ADHD: Understanding for whom and how interventions

work. *Journal of Pediatric Psychology, 32*, 664–675. doi:10.1093/jpepsy/jsl055

Hoekzema, E., Carmona, S., Tremols, V., Gispert, J.D., Guitart, M., Fauquet, J., ... Villarroya, O. (2010). Enhanced neural activity in frontal and cerebellar circuits after cognitive training in children with attention-deficit/hyperactivity disorder. *Human Brain Mapping, 31*(12), 1942–1950. doi:10.1002/hbm.20988

Holmes,J., Dunning, D., & Gathercole, S. (2009). Adaptive training leads to sustained enhancement of poor working memory in children. *Developmental Science, 12*, F9–F15. doi:10.1111/j.1467-7687.2009.00848.x

Holtmann, M., & Stadler, C. (2006). Electroencephalographic biofeedback for the treatment of attention-deficit hyperactivity disorder in childhood and adolescence. *Expert Review of Neurotherapeutics, 6*, 533–540. doi:10.1586/14737175.6.4.533

Hoza, B. (2007). Peer functioning in children with ADHD. *Journal of Pediatric Psychology, 32*, 655–663. doi:10.1093/jpepsy/jsm024

Indredavik, M.S., Skranes, J.S., Vik, T., Heyerdahl, S., Romundstad, P., Myhr, G.E., & Brubakk, A.-M. (2005). Low-birth-weight adolescents: Psychiatric symptoms and cerebral MRI abnormalities. *Pediatric Neurology, 33*, 259–266. doi:10.1016/j.pediatrneurol.2005.05.002

Jahromi, L.B., Kasari, C.L., McCracken, J.T., Lee, L.S., Aman, M.G., McDougle, C.J., ... Posey, D.J. (2009). Positive effects of methylphenidate on social communication and self-regulation in children with pervasive developmental disorders and hyperactivity. *Journal of Autism & Developmental Disorders, 39*, 395–404. doi:10.1007/s10803-008-0636-9

Jankovic, J., Jiminez-Shahed, J., & Brown, L.W. (2010). A randomised, double-blind, placebo-controlled study of topiramate in the treatment of Tourette syndrome. *Journal of Neurology, Neurosurgery, & Psychiatry, 81*, 70–73. doi:10.1136/jnnp.2009.185348

Jensen, P.S., Hinshaw, S.P., Swanson, J.M., Greenhill, L.L., Conners, C.K., Arnold, L.E., ... Wigal, T. (2001). Findings from the NIMH Multimodal Treatment Study of ADHD (MTA): Implications and applications for primary care providers. *Journal of Developmental & Behavioral Pediatrics, 22*, 60–73. doi:10.1097/00004703-200102000-00008

Jitendra, A.K., DuPaul, G.J., Someki, F., & Tresco, K.E. (2008). Enhancing academic achievement for children with attention-deficit hyperactivity disorder: Evidence from school-based intervention research. *Developmental Disabilities Research Reviews, 14*, 325–330. doi:10.1002/ddrr.39

Johnson, M., Östlund, S., Fransson, G., Kadesjö, B., & Gillberg, C. (2009). Omega-3/omega-6 fatty acids for attention deficit hyperactivity disorder: A randomized placebo-controlled trial in children and adolescents. *Journal of Attention Disorders, 12*, 394–401. doi:10.1177/1087054708316261

Kahbazi, M., Ghoreishi, A., Rahiminejad, F., Mohammadi, M.R., Kamalipour, A., & Akhondzadeh, S. (2009). A randomized, double-blind and placebo-controlled trial of modafinil in children and adolescents with attention deficit and hyperactivity disorder. *Psychiatry Research, 168*, 234–237. doi:10.1016/j.psychres.2008.06.024

Kaplan, B.J., McNicol, J., Conte, R.A., & Moghadam, H.K. (1989). Dietary replacement in preschool-aged hyperactive boys. *Pediatrics, 83*, 7–17.

Katusic, S.K., Barbaresi, W.J., Colligan, R.C., Weaver, A.L., Leibson, C.L., & Jacobsen, S.J. (2005). Psychostimulant treatment and risk for substance abuse among young adults with a history of attention-deficit/hyperactivity disorder: A population-based, birth cohort study. *Journal of Child & Adolescent Psychopharmacology, 15*, 764–776.

Kelly, A.M.C., Margulies, D.S., & Castellanos, F.X. (2007). Recent advances in structural and functional brain imaging studies of attention-deficit/hyperactivity disorder. *Current Psychiatry Reports, 9*, 401–407. doi:10.1007/s11920-007-0052-4

Khalifa, N., & van Knorring, A.L. (2005). Tourette Syndrome and other tic disorders in a total population of children: Clinical assessment and background. *Acta Paediatrica, 94*, 1608–1614. doi:10.1111/j.1651-2227.2005.tb01837.x

Kieling, C., Goncalves, R.R.F., Tannock, R., & Castellanos, F.X. (2008). Neurobiology of attention-deficit/hyperactivity disorder. *Child & Adolescent Psychiatric Clinics of North America, 17*, 285–307. doi:10.1016/j.chc.2007.11.012

Kisicki, J.C., Fiske, K., & Lyne, A. (2007). Phase 1, double-blind, randomized, placebo-controlled dose-escalation study of the effects on blood pressure of abrupt cessation versus taper down of guanfacine extended release tablets in adults aged 19 to 24 years. *Clinical Therapeutics, 29*, 1967–1979.

Klingberg, T., Fernell, E., Olesen, P.J., Johnson, M., Gustafsson, P., Dahlström, K., ... Westerberg, H. (2005). Computerized training of working memory in children with ADHD—A randomized, controlled trial. *Journal of the American Academy of Child & Adolescent Psychiatry, 44*, 177–186. doi:10.1097/00004583-200502000-00010

Konofal, E., Lecendreux, M., & Cortes, S. (2010). Sleep and ADHD. *Sleep Medicine, 11*, 652–658. doi:10.1016/j.sleep.2010.02.012

Kratochvil, C.J., Greenhill, L.L., March, J.S., Burke, W.J., & Vaughn, B.S. (2004). The role of stimulants in the treatment of preschool children with attention-deficit hyperactivity disorder. *CNS Drugs, 18*, 957–966. doi:10.2165/00023210-200418140-00001

Kratochvil, C.J., Newcorn, J.H., Arnold, L.E., Duesenberg, D., Emslie, G.J., Quintana, H., ... Biederman, J. (2005). Atomoxetine alone or combined with fluoxetine for treating ADHD with comorbid depressive or anxiety symptoms. *Journal of the American Academy of Child & Adolescent Psychiatry, 44*, 915–924. doi:10.1097/01.chi.0000169012.81536.38

Kratochvil, C.J., Wilens, T.E., Greenhill, L.L., Gao, H., Baker, K.D., Feldman, P.D., & Gelowitz, D.L. (2006). The effects of long-term atomoxetine treatment for young children with attention-deficit hyperactivity disorder. *Journal of the American Academy of Child & Adolescent Psychiatry, 45*, 919–927. doi:10.1097/01.chi.0000222788.34229.68

Kronenberger, W.G., & Dunn, D.W. (2003). Learning disorders. *Neurologic Clinics, 21*, 941–952. doi:10.1016/S0733-8619(03)00010-0

Langberg, J.M., Arnold, L.E., Flowers, A.M., Epstein, J.N., Altaye, M., Hinshaw, S.P., ... Hechtman, L. (2010). Parent-reported homework problems in the MTA study: Evidence for sustained improvement with behavioral treatment. *The Journal of Clinical Child and Adolescent Psychology, 39*, 220–233. doi:10.1080/15374410903532700

Lee, D.O., & Ousley, O.Y. (2006). Attention-deficit/hyperactivity disorder symptoms in a clinic sample of children and adolescents with pervasive developmental disorders. *Journal of Child and Adolescent Psychopharmacology, 16*, 737–746. doi:10.1089/cap.2006.16.737

Lipkin, P.H., Goldstein, I.J., & Adesman, A.R. (1994). Tics and dyskinesias associated with stimulant treatment in attention-deficit/hyperactivity disorder. *Archives of Pediatrics & Adolescent Medicine, 148*, 859–861.

List, B.A., & Barzman, D.H. (2010). Evidence-based recommendations for the treatment of aggression in pediatric patients with attention-deficit/hyperactivity disorder. *Psychiatry Quarterly, 82*(1), 33–42. doi:10.1007/s11126-010-9145-z

Lo-Castro, A., D'Agati, E., & Curatolo, P. (2010). ADHD and genetic syndromes. *Brain and Development 33*(6), 456–461. doi:10.1016/j.braindev.2010.05.011

Logemann, H.N., Lansbergen, M.M., Van Os, T.W., Böcker, K.B., & Kenemans, J.L. (2010). The effectiveness of EEG-feedback on attention, impulsivity and EEG: A sham feedback controlled study. *Neuroscience Letters, 479*, 49–53. doi:10.1016/j.neulet.2010.05.026

Lou, H.C., Rosa, P., Pryds, O., Karrebaek, H., Lunding, J., Cumming, P., & Gjedde, A. (2004). ADHD: Increased dopamine receptor availability linked to attention deficit and low neonatal blood flow. *Developmental Medicine and Child Neurology, 46*, 179–183. doi:10.1111/j.1469-8749.2004.tb00469.x

Maayan, L., Paykina, N., Fried, J., Strauss, T., Gugga, S.S., & Greenhill, L. (2009). The open-label treatment of attention-deficit/hyperactivity disorder in 4- and 5-year-old children with beaded methylphenidate. *Journal of Child & Adolescent Psychopharmacology, 19*, 147–153. doi:10.1089/cap.2008.053

Makris, N., Biederman, J., Monuteaux, M., & Seidman, L.J. (2009). Towards conceptualizing a neural-systems based anatomy of attention-deficit/hyperactivity disorder. *Developmental Neuroscience, 31*, 36–49. doi:10.1159/000207492

Mannuzza, S., Klein, R.G., Truong, N.L., Moulton, J.L., Roizen, E.R., Howell, K.H., & Castellanos, F.X. (2008). Age of methylphenidate treatment initiation in children with ADHD and later substance abuse: Prospective follow-up into adulthood. *American Journal of Psychiatry, 165*, 604–609. doi:10.1176/appi.ajp.2008.07091465

March, J., Silva, S., Petrycki, S., Curry, J., Wells, K., Fairbank, J., ... Treatment for Adolescents with Depression Study (TADS) Team. (2004). Fluoxetine, cognitive-behavioral therapy, and their combination for adolescents with depression: Treatment for adolescents with depression study (TADS) randomized controlled trial. *Journal of the American Medical Association, 292*, 807–820.

Martin, N.C., Piek, J.P., & Hay, D. (2006). DCD and ADHD: A genetic study of their shared etiology. *Human Movement Science, 25*, 110–124.

Martinussen, R., Hayden, J., Hogg-Johnson, S., & Tannock, R. (2005). A meta-analysis of working memory in children with attention-deficit/hyperactivity disorder. *Journal of the American Academy of Child and Adolescent Psychiatry, 44*, 377–384. doi:10.1097/01.chi.0000153228.72591.73

May, D.E., & Kratochvil, C.J. (2010). Attention-deficit/ hyperactivity disorder: Recent advances in pediatric pharmacotherapy. *Drugs, 70*, 15–40.

Mazaide, M., Rouleau, N., Lee, B., Rogers, A., David, L., & Dickson, R. (2009). Atomoxetine and neuro-psychological function in children with attention-deficit/hyperactivity disorder: Results of a pilot study. *Journal of Child & Adolescent Psychopharmacology, 19*, 709–718. doi:10.1089/cap.2008.0166

McBurnett, K., & Pfiffner, L.J. (2009). Treatment of aggressive ADHD in children and adolescents: Conceptualization and treatment of comorbid behavior disorders. *Postgraduate Medicine, 121*, 158–165. doi:10.3810/pgm.2009.11.2084

McCann, D., Barrett, A., Cooper, A., Crumpler,D., Dalen, L., Grimshaw, K., & Stevenson, J. (2007). Food additives and hyperactive behavior in 3-year-old and 8/9-year-old children in the community: A randomised, double-blinded, placebo-controlled trial. *Lancet, 370*, 1560–1567. doi:10.1016/S0140-6736(07)61306-3

McDougle, C.J., Scahill, L., Aman, M.G., McCracken, J.T., Tierney, E., Davies, M., & Vitiello, B. (2005). Risperidone for the core symptom domains of autism: Results from the study by the autism network of the research units on pediatric psychopharmacology. *American Journal of Psychiatry, 162*, 1142–1148. doi:10.1176/appi.ajp.162.6.1142

McInnes, A., Humphries, T., Hogg-Johnson, S., & Tannock, R. (2003). Listening comprehension and working memory are impaired in attention-deficit/hyperactivity disorder irrespective of language impairment. *Journal of Abnormal Child Psychology, 31*, 427–443.

McQuade, J.D., & Hoza, B. (2008). Peer problems in attention deficit hyperactivity disorder: Current status and future directions. *Developmental Disabilities Research Reviews, 14*, 320–324. doi:10.1002/ddrr.35

Merkel, R.L., & Kuchibhatla, A. (2009). Safety of stimulant treatment in attention deficit hyperactivity disorder: Part I. *Expert Opinion on Drug Safety, 8*, 655–668. doi:10.1517/14740330903279956

Molina, B.S.G., Hinshaw, S.P., Swanson, J.M., Arnold, L.E., Vitiello, B., Jensen, P.S., ... MTA Cooperative Group. (2009). The MTA at 8 years: Prospective follow-up of children treated for combined-type ADHD in a multisite study. *Journal of the American Academy of Child & Adolescent Psychiatry, 48*, 484–500. doi:10.1097/CHI.0b013e31819c23d0

Monastra, V.J. (2008). Quantitative electroencephalography and attention-deficit/hyperactivity disorder: Implications for clinical practice. *Current Psychiatry Reports, 10*, 432–438. doi:10.1007/s11920-008-0069-3

MTA Cooperative Group. (1999a). A 14-month randomized clinical trial of treatment strategies for attention-deficit/hyperactivity disorder. *Archive of General Psychiatry, 56*, 1073–1086.

MTA Cooperative Group. (1999b). Moderators and mediators of treatment response for children with attention-deficit/hyperactivity disorder. *Archives of General Psychiatry, 56*, 1088–1096.

MTA Cooperative Group. (2004a). National Institute of Mental Health multimodal treatment study of ADHD follow-up: 24-month outcomes of treatment strategies for attention-deficit/hyperactivity disorder. *Pediatrics, 113*, 754–761.

MTA Cooperative Group. (2004b). National Institute of Mental Health multimodal treatment study of ADHD

follow-up: Changes in effectiveness and growth after the end of treatment. *Pediatrics, 113*, 762–769.

Murphy, K., Ratey, N., Maynard, S., Sussman, S., & Wright, S.D. (2010). Coaching for ADHD. *Journal of Attention Disorders, 13*, 546–552. doi:10.1177/1087054709344186

Murray, D.W. (2010). Treatment of preschoolers with attention-deficit/hyperactivity disorder. *Current Psychiatry Reports, 12*, 374–381. doi:10.1007/s11920-010-0142-6

Murray, D.W., Arnold, L.E., Swanson, J., Wells, K., Burns, K., Jensen, P., ... Strauss, T. (2008). A clinical review of outcomes of the multimodal treatment study of children with attention-deficit/hyperactivity disorder (MTA). *Current Psychiatry Reports, 10*, 424–431. doi:10.1007/s11920-008-0068-4

Nevels, R.M., Dehon, E.E., Alexander, K., & Gontkovsky, S.T. (2010). Psychopharmacology of aggression in children and adolescents with primary neuropsychiatric disorders: A review of current and potentially promising treatment options. *Experimental & Clinical Psychopharmacology, 18*, 184–201. doi:10.1037/a0018059

Newcorn, J.H., & Donnelly, C. (2009). Cardiovascular safety of medication treatments for attention-deficit/ hyperactivity disorder. *Mount Sinai Journal of Medicine, 76*, 198–203. doi:10.1002/msj.20096

Newcorn, J.H., Spencer, T.J., Biederman, J., Milton, D.R., & Michelson, D. (2005). Atomoxetine treatment in children and adolescents with attention-deficit/hyperactivity disorder and comorbid oppositional defiant disorder. *Journal of the American Academy of Child & Adolescent Psychiatry, 44*, 240–248. doi:10.1097/00004583-200503000-00008

Nicolescu, R., Petcu, C., Cordeanu, A., Fabritius, K., Schlumpf, M, Krebs, R., ... Winneke, G. (2010). Environmental exposure to lead, but not other neurotoxic metals, relates to core elements of ADHD in Romanian children: Performance and questionnaire data. *Environmental Research, 110*, 476–483. doi:10.1016/j.envres.2010.04.002

Nigg, J.T. (2005). Neuropsychologic theory and findings in attention-deficit/hyperactivity disorder: The state of the field and salient changes for the coming decade. *Biological Psychiatry, 57*, 1424–1435.

Nijmeijer, J.S., Minderaa, R.B., Buitelaar, J.K., Mulligan, A., Hartman, C., & Hoekstra, P.J. (2007). Attention-deficit/hyperactivity disorder and social dysfunctioning. *Clinical Psychology Review, 28*, 692–708. doi:10.1016/j.cpr.2007.10.003

Nikolas, M.A., & Burt, S.A. (2010). Genetic and environmental influences on ADHD symptom dimensions of inattention and hyperactivity: A meta-analysis. *Journal of Abnormal Psychology, 119*, 1–17. doi:10.1037/a0018010

Olfson, M., Crystal, S., Huang, C., & Gerhard, T. (2010). Trends in antipsychotic drug use by very young, privately insured children. *Journal of the American Academy of Child & Adolescent Psychiatry, 49*, 13–23. doi:10.1097/00004583-201001000-00005

Owens, J.A. (2005). The ADHD and sleep conundrum: A review. *Journal of Developmental & Behavioral Pediatrics, 26*, 312–322.

Owens, J.S., Goldfine, M.E., Evangelista, N.M., Hoza, B., & Kaiser, N.M. (2007). A critical review of self-perceptions and the positive illusory bias in children with ADHD. *Clinical Child & Family Psychology Review, 10*, 335–351. doi:10.1007/s10567-007-0027-3

Ozdag, M.F., Yorbik, O., Ulas, U.H., Hamamcioglu, K., & Vural, O. (2004). Effect of methylphenidate on auditory event related potentials in boys with attention deficit hyperacivity disorder. *International Journal of Pediatric Otorhinolaryngology, 68*, 1267–1272. doi:10.1016/j.ijporl.2004.04.023

Palumbo, D., Spencer, T., Lynch, J., CoChien, H., & Faraone, S.V. (2004). Emergence of tics in children with ADHD: Impact of once-daily OROS methylphenidate therapy. *Journal of Child & Adolescent Psychopharmacology, 14*, 185–194. doi:10.1089/1044546041649138

Pelham, W.E., & Fabiano, G.A. (2008). Evidence-based psychosocial treatments for attention-deficit/hyperactivity disorder. *Journal of Clinical Child & Adolescent Psychology, 37*, 184–214. doi:10.1080/15374410701818681

Pelham, W.E., Fabiano, G.A., & Massetti, G.M. (2005). Evidence-based assessment of attention-deficit/hyperactivity disorder in children and adolescents. *Journal of Clinical Child and Adolescent Psychology, 34*, 449–476. doi:10.1207/s15374424jccp3403_5

Pelsser, L.M.J., Frankena, K., Toorman, J., Savelkoul, H.F.J., Pereira, R.R., & Buitelar, J.K. (2009). A randomized controlled trial into the effects of food on ADHD. *European Journal of Child & Adolescent Psychiatry, 18*, 12–19.

Piek, J.P., & Dyck, M.J. (2004). Sensory-motor deficits in children with developmental coordination disorder, attention-deficit/hyperactivity disorder and autistic disorder. *Human Movement Science, 23*, 475–488. doi:10.1016/j.humov.2004.08.019

Pliszka, S.R. (2000). Patterns of psychiatric comorbidity with attention deficit hyperactivity disorder. *Child & Adolescent Psychiatric Clinics of North America, 9*, 525–540.

Pliszka, S.R., Crismon, M.L., Hughes, C.W., Corners, C.K., Emslie, G.J., Jensen, P.S., … Lopez, M. (2006). The Texas children's medication algorithm project: Revision of the algorithm for pharmacotherapy of attention-deficit/hyperactivity disorder. *Journal of the American Academy of Child & Adolescent Psychiatry, 45*, 642–657. doi:10.1097/01.chi.0000215326.51175.eb

Polanzyck, G., de Lima, M.S., Horta, B.L., Beiderman, J., & Rohde, L.A. (2007). The worldwide prevalence of ADHD: A systematic review and meta-regression analysis. *American Journal of Psychiatry, 164*, 942–948.

Pollak, Y., Benarroch, F., Kanengisser, L., Shilon, Y., Benpazi, H., Shalev, R.S., & Gross-Tsur, V. (2009). Tourette syndrome-associated psychopathology: Roles of comorbid attention-deficit/hyperactivity disorder and obsessive compulsive disorder. *Journal of Developmental & Behavioral Pediatrics, 30*, 413–419. doi:10.1097/DBP.0b013e3181ba0f89

Popper, C.W. (2000). Pharmocologic alternatives to psychostimulants for the treatment of attention-deficit/hyperactivity disorder. *Child & Adolescent Psychiatric Clinics of North America, 9*, 605–646.

Posey, D.J., Aman, M.G., McCracken. J.T., Scahill, L., Tierney, E., Arnold, L.E., … McDougle, C.J. (2007). Positive effects of methylphenidate on inattention and hyperactivity in pervasive developmental disorders: An analysis of secondary measures. *Biological Psychiatry, 61*, 538–544. doi:10.1016/j.biopsych.2006.09.028

Posey, D.J., Stigler, K.A., Erickson, C.A., & McDougle, C.J. (2008). Antipsychotics in the treatment of autism. *Journal of Clinical Investigation, 118*, 6–14. doi:10.1172/JCI32483

Powers, R.L., Marks, D.J., Miller, C.J., Newcorn, J.H., & Halperin, J.M. (2008). Stimulant treatment in children with attention-deficit/hyperactivity disorder moderates adolescent academic outcome. *Journal of Child & Adolescent Psychopharmacology, 18*, 449–459. doi:10.1089/cap.2008.021

Quinn, P.O. (2008). Attention-deficit/hyperactivity disorder and its comorbidities in women and girls: An evolving picture. *Current Psychiatry Reports, 10*, 419–423. doi:10.1007/s11920-008-0067-5

Rabiner, D.L., Murray, D.W., Skinner, A.T., & Malone, P.S. (2010). A randomized trial of two promising computer-based interventions for students with attention difficulties. *Journal of Abnormal Child Psychology, 38*, 131–142. doi:10.1007/s10802-009-9353-x

Raggi, V.L., & Chronis, A.M. (2006). Interventions to address the academic impairment of children and adolescents with ADHD. *Clinical Child and Family Psychology Review, 9*, 85–111. doi:10.1007/s10567-006-0006-0

Rapaport, J., Buchsbaum, M., Zahn, T.P., Weingartner, H., Ludlow, C., & Mikkelsen, E.J. (1978). Dextroamphetamine: Cognitive and behavioral effects in normal prepubertal boys. *Science, 199*, 560–563. doi:10.1126/science.341313

Raz, R., & Gabis, L. (2009). Essential fatty acids and attention-deficit/hyperactivity disorder: A systematic review. *Developmental Medicine & Child Neurology, 51*, 580–592. doi:10.1111/j.1469-8749.2009.03351.x

Rehabilitation Act of 1973, PL 93-112 29 U.S.C. §§791 et seq.

Reyes, M., Croonenberghs, J., Augustyns, I., & Eerdekens, M. (2006). Long-term use of risperidone in children with disruptive behavior disorders and subaverage intelligence: Efficacy, safety, and tolerability. *Journal of Child & Adolescent Psychopharmacology, 16*, 260–272. doi:10.1089/cap.2006.16.260

Richardson, A.J., & Montgomery, P. (2005). The Oxford-Durham study: A randomized, controlled trial of dietary supplementation with fatty acids in children with developmental coordination disorder. *Pediatrics, 115*, 1360–1366. doi:10.1542/peds.2004-2164

Ritz, B.W., & Lord, R.S. (2005). Case study: The effectiveness of a dietary supplement regimen in reducing IgG-mediated food sensitivity in ADHD. *Alternative Therapies, 11*, 72–75.

Robin, A.L. (2008). Family intervention for home-based problems of adolescents with attention-deficit/hyperactivity disorder. *Adolescent Medicine, 19*, 268–277.

Rubia, K., Halari, R., Cubillo, A., Mohammad, A.M., Brammer, M., & Taylor, E. (2009). Methylphenidate normalises activation and functional connectivity deficits in attention and motivation networks in medication-naive children with ADHD during a rewarded continuous performance. *Neuropharmacology, 57*, 640–652. doi:10.1016/j.neuropharm.2009.08.013

Rucklidge, J.J. (2010). Gender differences in ADHD. *Psychiatric Clinics of North America, 33*, 357–373.

Rucklidge, J.J., Gately, D., & Kaplan, B.J. (2010). Database analysis of children and adolescents with bipolar disorder consuming a micronutrient formula. *BMC Psychiatry, 10*, 74. doi:10.1186/1471-244X-10-74

Rucklidge, J.J., Johnstone, J., & Kaplan, B.J. (2009). Nutrient supplementation approaches in the treatment of ADHD. *Expert Reviews of Neurotherapeutics, 9*, 461–476. doi:10.1586/ern.09.7

Rucklidge, J.J., Taylor, M., & Whitehead, K. (2010). Effect of micronutrients on behavior and mood in adults with ADHD: Evidence from an 8-week open label trial with natural extension. *Journal of Attention Disorders, 15*, 79–91. doi:10.1177/1087054709356173

Rushton, J.L., Fant, K.E., & Clark, S.J. (2004). Use of practice guidelines in the primary care of children with attention-deficit/hyperactivity disorder. *Pediatrics, 114*, e23–e28. doi:10.1542/peds.114.1.e23

Safren, S.A., Sprich, S., Mimiaga, M.J., Surman, C., Knouse, L., Groves, M., & Otto, M.W. (2010). Cognitive behavioral therapy vs. relaxation with educational support for medication-treated adults with ADHD and persistent symptoms: A randomized controlled trial. *Journal of the American Medical Association, 304*, 875–880. doi:10.1001/jama.2010.1192

Sallee, F.R. (2010). The role of alpha2-adrenergic agonists in attention-deficit/hyperactivity disorder. *Postgraduate Medicine, 122*, 78–87. doi:10.3810/pgm.2010.09.2204

Sallee, F.R., Lyne, A., Wigal, T., & McGough, J.J. (2009). Long-term safety and efficacy of guanfacine extended release in children and adolescents with attention-deficit/hyperactivity disorder. *Journal of Child & Adolescent Psychopharmacology, 19*, 215–226. doi:10.1089/cap.2008.0080

Sallee, F.R., McGough, J., Wigal, T., Donahue, J., Lyne, A., & Biederman, J. (2009). Guanfacine extended release in children and adolescents with attention-deficit/hyperactivity disorder: A placebo-controlled trial. *Journal of the American Academy of Child & Adolescent Psychiatry, 48*, 155–165. doi:10.1097/CHI.0b013e318191769e

Schab, D.W., & Trinh, N.T. (2004). Do artificial food colors promote hyperactivity in children with hyperactive syndromes? A meta-analysis of double-blind placebo-controlled trials. *Journal of Developmental & Behavioral Pediatrics, 25*, 423–4334. doi:10.1097/00004703-200412000-00007

Schatz, D.B., & Rostain A.L. (2006). ADHD with comorbid anxiety: A review of the literature. *Journal of Attention Disorders, 10*, 141–149. doi:10.1177/1087054706286698

Scheffler, R.M., Hinshaw, S.P., Modrek, S., & Levine, P. (2007). The global market for ADHD medications. *Health Affairs, 26*, 450–457. doi:10.1377/hlthaff.26.2.450

Schmidt, M.H., Möcks, P., Lay, B., Eisert, H-G., Fojkar, R., Fritz-Sigmund, D., ... Musaeus, B. (1997). Does oligoantigenic diet influence hyperactive/conduct-disordered children—A controlled trial. *European Child & Adolescent Psychiatry, 6*, 88–95. doi:10.1007/BF00566671

Schubiner, H. (2005). Substance abuse in patients with attention-deficit/hyperactivity disorder: Therapeutic implications. *CNS Drugs, 19*, 643–655.

Scott, N.G., Ripperger-Suhler, J., Rajab, M.H., & Kjar, D. (2010). Factors associated with atomoxetine efficacy for treatment of attention-deficit/hyperactivity disorder in children and adolescents. *Journal of Child & Adolescent Psychopharmacology, 20*, 197–203. doi:10.1089/cap.2009.0104

Setlik, J., Bond, G.R., & Ho, M. (2009). Adolescent prescription ADHD medication abuse is rising along with prescriptions for these medications. *Pediatrics, 124*, 875–880. doi:10.1542/peds.2008-0931

Shalev, L., Tsal, Y., & Mevorach, C. (2007). Computerized progressive attentional training (CPAT) program: Effective direct intervention for children with ADHD. *Child Neuropsychology, 13*, 382–388. doi:10.1080/09297040600770787

Sharp, S.I., McQuillen, A., & Gurling, H.M.D. (2009). Genetics of attention-deficit hyperactivity disorder (ADHD). *Neuropharmacology, 57*, 590–600. doi:10.1016/j.neuropharm.2009.08.011

Shaw, P., & Rabin, C. (2009). New insights into attention-deficit/hyperactivity disorder using structural neuroimaging. *Current Psychiatry Reports, 11*, 393–398. doi:10.1007/s11920-009-0059-0

Shillingford, A.J., Glanzman, M., Ittenbach, R., Clancy, R.R., Gaynor, J.W., & Wernovsky, G. (2009). Inattention, hyperactivity and school performance in a population of school-age children with complex congenital heart disease. *Pediatrics, 121*, e759–e767. doi:10.1542/peds.2007-1066

Silva, R.R., Skimming, J.W., & Muniz, R. (2010). Cardiovascular safety of stimulant medications for pediatric attention-deficit hyperactivity disorder. *Clinical Pediatrics, 49*, 840–851.

Simon, V., Czobor, P., Balint, S., Meszaros, A., & Bitter, I. (2009). Prevalence and correlates of adult attention-deficit hyperactivity disorder: Meta-analysis. *British Journal of Psychiatry, 194*, 204–211. doi:10.1192/bjp.bp.107.048827

Singer, H.S. (2005). Tourette syndrome: From behavior to biology. *Lancet (Neurology), 4*, 149–159. doi:10.1016/S1474-4422(05)70018-1

Sinn, N., & Bryan, J. (2007). Effect of supplementation with polyunsaturated fatty acids and micronutrients on learning and behavior problems associated with child ADHD. *Journal of Developmental & Behavioral Pediatrics, 28*, 82–91. doi:10.1097/01.DBP.0000267558.88457.a5

Sobel, L.J., Bansal, R., Maia, T.V., Sanchez, J., Mazzone, L., Durkin, K., & Peterson, B.S. (2010). Basal ganglia surface morphology and the effects of stimulant medications in youth with attention deficit hyperactivity disorder. *American Journal of Psychiatry, 167*, 977–986. doi:10.1176/appi.ajp.2010.09091259

Solanto, M.V., Marks, D.J., Wasserstein, J., Mitchell, K., Abikoff, H., Alvir, J., & Kofman, M.D. (2010). Efficacy of meta-cognitive therapy for adult ADHD. *American Journal of Psychiatry, 167*, 958–968. doi:10.1176/appi.ajp.2009.09081123

Solanto, M.V., Newcorn, J., Vail. L., Gilbert, S., Ivanov, I., & Lara, R. (2009). Stimulant drug response in the predominantly inattentive and combined subtypes of attention-deficit/hyperactivity disorder. *Journal of Child and Adolescent Psychopharmacology, 19*, 663–671. doi:10.1089/cap.2009.0033

Sonuga-Barke, E.J., & Halperin, J.M. (2010). Developmental phenotypes and causal pathways in attention-deficit/hyperactivity disorder: Potential targets for early interventions? *Journal of Child Psychology & Psychiatry, 51*, 368–389. doi:10.1111/j.1469-7610.2009.02195.x

Spencer, T.J. (2009). Issues in the management of patients with complex attention-deficit/hyperactivity disorder symptoms. *CNS Drugs, 23*(Suppl. 1), 9–20. doi:10.2165/00023210-200923000-00003

Spencer, T.J., Biederman, J., & Mick, E. (2007). Attention-deficit/hyperactivity disorder: Diagnosis, lifespan, comorbidities and neurobiology. *Journal of Pediatric Psychology, 32*, 631–642. doi:10.1093/jpepsy/jsm005

Spencer, T.J., Greenbaum, M., Ginsberg, L.D., & Murphy, W.R. (2009). Safety and effectiveness of coadministration of guanfacine extended release and psychostimulants in children and adolescents with attention-deficit/hyperactivity disorder. *Journal of Child & Adolescent Psychopharmacology*, *19*, 501–510. doi:10.1089/cap.2008.0152

Spencer, T.J., Kratochvil, C.J., Sangal, R.B., Saylor, K.E., Bailey, C.E., Dunn, D.W., ... Allen, A.J. (2007). Effects of atomoxetine on growth in children with attention-deficit/hyperactivity disorder following up to five years of treatment. *Journal of Child & Adolescent Psychopharmacology*, *17*, 689–700. doi:10.1089/cap.2006.0100

Sprich-Buckminster S., Biederman J., Milberger S., Faraone S.V., & Lehman B.K. (1993). Are prenatal complications relevant to the manifestations of ADD? Issues of comorbidity and familiality. *Journal of the American Academy of Child and Adolescent Psychiatry*, *32*, 1032–1037.

Stefanatos, G.A., & Baron, I.S. (2007). Attention-deficit/hyperactivity disorder: A neuropsychological perspective towards *DSM-V*. *Neuropsychology Review*, *17*, 5–38. doi:10.1007/s11065-007-9020-3

Stevenson, J., Sonuga-Barke, E., McCann, D., Grimshaw, K., Parker, K.M., Rose-Zerilli, M.J., ... Warner, J.O. (2010). The role of histamine degradation gene polymorphisms in moderating the effects of food additives on children's ADHD symptoms. *American Journal of Psychiatry*, *167*, 1108–1115. doi:10.1176/appi.ajp.2010.09101529

Swanson, J., Arnold, L.E., Kraemer, H., Hechtman, L., Molina, B., Hinshaw, S., & Wigel, T. (2008). Evidence, interpretation, and qualification from multiple reports of long-term outcomes in the multimodal treatment study of children with ADHD (MTA): Part I: Executive summary. *Journal of Attention Disorders*, *12*, 4–14. doi:10.1177/1087054708319345

Swanson, J., Greenhill, L., Wigal, T., Kollins, S., Steheli, A., Davies, M., & Wigel, S. (2006). Stimulant-related reductions of growth rates in the PATS. *Journal of the American Academy of Child & Adolescent Psychiatry*, *45*, 1304–1313. doi:10.1097/01.chi.0000235075.25038.5a

Swanson, J.M., Elliott, G.R., Greenhill, L.L., Wigal, T., Arnold, L.E., Vitiello, B., ... Volkow, N.D. (2007). Effects of stimulants on growth rates across 3 years in the MTA follow-up. *Journal of the American Academy of Child & Adolescent Psychiatry*, *46*, 1015–1027. doi:10.1097/chi.0b013e3180686d7e

ter Laak, M.A., Temmink, A.H., Koeken, A., van't Veer, N.E., Van Hattum, P.R., & Cobbaert, C.M. (2010). Recognition of impaired atomoxetine metabolism because of low CYP2D6 activity. *Pediatric Neurology*, *43*, 159–162. doi:10.1016/j.pediatrneurol.2010.04.004

Ter-Stepanian, M., Grizenko, N., Zappitelli, M., & Joober, R. (2010). Clinical response to methylphenidate in children diagnosed with attention-deficit/hyperactivity disorder and comorbid psychiatric disorders. *Canadian Journal of Psychiatry*, *55*, 305–312.

Thompson, A., Maltezos, S., Paliokosta, E., & Xenitidis, K. (2009). Risperidone for attention-deficit hyperactivity disorder in people with intellectual disabilities. *Cochrane Database of Systematic Reviews*, *2*, CD007011.

Tripp, G., & Wickens, J.R. (2009). Neurobiology of ADHD. *Neuropharmacology*, *57*, 579–589. doi:10.1016/j.neuropharm.2009.07.026

Tsai, M.H., & Huang, Y.S. (2010). Attention-deficit/hyperactivity disorder and sleep disorders in children. *Medical Clinics of North America*, *94*, 615–632. doi:10.1016/j.mcna.2010.03.008

Turgay, A. (2009). Psychopharmacological treatment of oppositional defiant disorder. *CNS Drugs*, *23*, 1–17. doi:10.2165/0023210-200923010-00001

Upadhyaya, H.P. (2007). Managing attention-deficit/hyperactivity disorder in the presence of substance use disorder. *Journal of Clinical Psychiatry*, *68*(Supp. 11), 23–30.

van den Hoofdakker, B.J., Nauta, M.H., van der Veen-Mulders, L., Syteme, S., Emmelkamp, P.M.G., Minderaa, R.B., & Hoekstra, P.J. (2010). Behavioral parent training as an adjunct to routine care in children with attention-deficit/hyperactivity disorder: Moderators of treatment response. *Journal of Pediatric Psychology*, *35*, 317–326. doi:10.1093/jpepsy/jsp060

Verbeeck, W., Tuinier, S., & Bekkering, G.E. (2009). Antidepressants in the treatment of adult attention-deficit/hyperactivity disorder: A systematic review. *Advances in Therapy*, *26*, 170–184. doi:10.1007/s12325-009-0008-7

Vetter, V.L., Elia, J., Erickson, C., Berger, S., Blum, N., Uzark, K., & Webb, C. (2008). Cardiovascular monitoring of children and adolescents with heart disease receiving stimulant drugs. A scientific statement from the American Heart Association Council on Cardiovascular Disease in the Young Congenital Cardiac Defects Committee, American Heart Association Council on Cardiovascular Nursing. *Circulation*, *117*, 2407–2423.

Visser, S.N., Lesesne, C.A., & Perou, R. (2007). National estimates and factors associated with medication treatment for childhood attention-deficit/hyperactivity disorder. *Pediatrics*, *119*, S99–S106. doi:10.1542/peds.2006-2089O

Vitiello, B., Abikoff, H.B., Chuang, S.Z., Kollins, S.H., McCracken, J.T., Riddle, M.A., ... Greenhill, L.L. (2007). Effectiveness of methylphenidate in the 10-month continuation phase of the preschoolers with ADHD treatment study (PATS). *Journal of Child & Adolescent Psychopharmacology*, *17*, 593–603. doi:10.1089/cap.2007.0058

Volkow, N.D., & Swanson, J.M. (2003). Variables that affect the clinical use and abuse of methylphenidate in the treatment of ADHD. *American Journal of Psychiatry*, *160*, 1909–1918. doi:10.1176/appi.ajp.160.11.1909

Warren, A.E., Hamilton, R.M., Belanger, S.A., Gray, C., Gow, R.M., Sanatani, S., ... Schachar, R. (2009). Cardiac risk assessment before the use of stimulant medications in children and youth: A joint position statement by the Canadian Pediatric Society, the Canadian Cardiovascular Society, and the Canadian Academy of Child and Adolescent Psychiatry. *Canadian Journal of Cardiology*, *25*, 625–630. doi:10.1016/S0828-282X(09)70157-6

Wehmeier, P.M., Schacht, A., & Barkley, R.A. (2010). Social and emotional impairment in children and adolescents with ADHD and the impact on quality of life. *Journal of Adolescent Health*, *46*, 209–217. doi:10.1016/j.jadohealth.2009.09.009

Weiss, M., Panagiotopoulis, C., Giles, L., Gibbins, C., Kuzeljevic, B., Davidson, J., & Harrison, R. (2009). A naturalistic study of predictors and risks of atypical antipsychotic use in an attention-deficit/hyperactivity disorder clinic. *Journal of Child & Adolescent Psychopharmacology*, *19*, 575–582. doi:10.1089/cap.2009.0050

Wernicke, J.F., Adler, L., Spencer, T., West, S.A., Allen, A.J., Heiligenstein, J., ... Michelson, D. (2004). Changes in symptoms and adverse events after discontinuation of atomoxetine in children and adults with attention-deficit/hyperactivity disorder: A prospective, placebo-controlled assessment. *Journal of Clinical Psychopharmacology, 24,* 30–35.

Weyandt, L.L. (2005). Executive function in children, adolescents and adults with attention-deficit/hyperactivity disorder: An introduction to the special issue. *Developmental Neuropsychology, 27,* 1–10. doi:10.1207/s15326942dn2701_1

Wigal, S.B. (2009). Efficacy and safety limitations of attention-deficit/hyperactivity disorder pharmacotherapy in children and adults. *CNS Drugs, 23*(Supplement 1), 21–31. doi:10.2165/00023210-200923000-00004

Wigal, T., Greenhill, L., Chuang, S., McGough, J., Vitiello, B., Skrobala, A., & Stehli, A.-M. (2006). Safety and tolerability of methylphenidate in preschool children with ADHD. *Journal of the American Academy of Child & Adolescent Psychiatry, 45,* 1294–1303. doi:10.1097/01.chi.0000235082.63156.27

Wilens, T.E., Adamson, J., Sgambati, S., Whitley, J., Santry, A., Monuteaux, M.C., & Biederman, J. (2007). Do individuals with ADHD self medicate with cigarettes and substances of abuse? Results from a controlled family study of ADHD. *American Journal on Addictions, 16*(Suppl. 1), 14–21. doi:10.1080/10550490601082742

Wilens, T.E., Haight, B.R., Horrigan, J.P., Hudziak, J.J., Rosenthal, N.E., Connor, D.F., ... Modell, J.G. (2005). Bupropion XL in adults with attention-deficit/hyperactivity disorder: A randomized, placebo-controlled study. *Biological Psychiatry, 57,* 793–801. doi:10.1016/j.biopsych.2005.01.027

Wilens, T.E., Hammerness, P., Utzinger, L., Schillinger, M., Georgiopoulos, A., Doyle, R.L., ... Brodziak, K. (2008). An open study of adjunct OROS-methylphenidate in children and adolescents who are atomoxetine partial responders: I. Effectiveness. *Journal of Child & Adolescent Psychopharmacology, 19,* 485–492. doi:10.1089/cap.2008.0125

Willcutt, E.G., Doyle, A.E., Nigg, J.T., Faraone, S.V, & Pennington, B.F. (2005).Validity of the executive function theory of attention-deficit/hyperactivity disorder: A meta-analytic review. *Biological Psychiatry, 57,* 1336-1346. doi:10.1016/j.biopsych.2005.02.006

Willcut, E.G., Pennington, B.F., Olson, R.K., Chabildas, N., & Huslander, J. (2005). Neuropsychological analysis of comorbidity between reading disability and attention-deficit/hyperactivity disorder: In search of the common deficit. *Developmental Neuropsychology, 27,* 35–78. doi:10.1207/s15326942dn2701_3

Wilson, J.J. (2007). ADHD and substance use disorders: Developmental aspects and the impact of stimulant treatment. *American Journal on Addictions, 161,* 5–11. doi:10.1080/10550490601082734

Wolraich, M.L., Wilson, D.B., & White, J.W. (1995). The effect of sugar on behavior or cognition in children. *Journal of the American Medical Association, 274,* 1617–1621. doi:10.1001/jama.274.20.1617

Wood, A.C., Rijsdijk, F., Asherson, P., & Kuntsi, J. (2009). Hyperactive-impulsive symptoms scores and oppositional behaviors reflect alternate manifestations of a single liability. *Behavior Genetics, 39,* 447–460. doi:10.1007/s10519-009-9290-z

Yeates, K.O., Armstrong, K., Janusz, J., Taylor, H.G., Wade, S., Stancin, T., & Drotar, D. (2005). Long-term attention problems in children with traumatic brain injury. *Journal of the American Academy of Child & Adolescent Psychiatry, 44,* 574–584. doi:10.1097/01.chi.0000159947.50523.64

Young, S., & Amarasinghe, M. (2010). Practitioner review: Non-pharmacological treatments for ADHD: A lifespan approach. *The Journal of Child Psychology and Psychiatry, 51,* 116–133. doi:10.1111/j.1469-7610.2009.02191.x

Zimmer, L. (2009). Positron emission tomography neuroimaging for a better understanding of the biology of ADHD. *Neuropharmacology, 57,* 601–607. doi:10.1016/j.neuropharm.2009.08.001

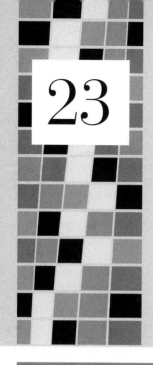

23

Specific Learning Disabilities

M.E.B. Lewis, Bruce K. Shapiro, and Robin P. Church

Upon completion of this chapter, the reader will

- Know the definition and implication of the term *learning disorder*

- Be aware of impairments associated with learning disorders and the connection to other disorders

- Know how assessment of learning disorders is done and how results are used

- Be aware of some intervention strategies

- Know the range of outcomes for children and adolescents with learning disorders

---

A great deal of learning involves processing a visual representation of concepts, attaching that perception to language in order to communicate understanding, and demonstrating that understanding with oral or written products. When a child struggles with these subtle and complex perceptual skills, their disabilities in understanding what they are encountering in the classroom impacts their ability to build a "toolbox" for more and more complex learning. This chapter focuses on those children, who represent more than a third of the students identified with disabilities in the United States (National Center for Education Statistics, 2011).

As proposed in the forthcoming *Diagnostic Statistical Manual of Mental Disorders, 5th edition (DSM-5)*, the definition of a **learning disorder** (referred to in IDEA 2004 as a specific learning disability) is a condition that interferes with the acquisition and use of one or more of the following academic skills: oral language, reading, written language, mathematics (Clay, 2011). This impairment causes serious difficulties in daily progress through the general education curriculum at all grade levels. These disorders affect individuals who otherwise demonstrate at least average abilities essential for thinking or reasoning. Thus, although intellectual disability, cerebral palsy, seizure disorders, receptive and expressive language disorders, traumatic brain injury, and hearing and vision impairments all can interfere with learning, they are not classified as primary learning disorders.

This chapter focuses on primary learning disorders. Specific reading disability (SRD), or dyslexia, is the learning disorder that is the most fully described, as it is both the most commonly recognized learning disorder and the one about which the most is known. Research and interventions related to writing and math disorders will also be discussed.

■ ■ ■ DONALD

Donald developed typically as a young child and seemed as bright and alert as his sisters, although he began to talk somewhat later than they had. In kindergarten, on a test of early reading skills, he scored well below average in knowledge of the alphabet, phonemic awareness, and early word recognition skills, although his math skills fell within the average range. In first grade, Donald entered a general education class and soon began to fail. He could not learn phonics, and his spelling was erratic, with no pattern of error or any connection of sound to symbol. He learned to add and subtract easily, however. Donald went through a battery of tests that identified SRD in the presence of his average intellectual functioning, a fact that is not atypical among students with learning difficulties—his full-scale IQ score on the Wechsler Intelligence Scale for Children–Fourth Edition (WISC-IV) was 110.

The school support team decided to keep Donald in a general education class, with an itinerant special education teacher providing extra help. This approach was not effective, however, and Donald fell further behind his peers in language arts. He started misbehaving in class and avoiding going to school, using headaches as an excuse. At the end of first grade, his reading was more than 1 year delayed, whereas his arithmetic skills were well above age-level.

When he entered second grade, Donald was anxious and unhappy. During that year, the school team recommended that he remain in a general education class but receive pullout services in reading daily for 45 minutes. Donald and three other students worked with a reading specialist who used a structured phonics approach. Donald also worked with a speech-language specialist who focused on phonological skills. His parents also worked with him at night. He remained a poor reader, but he could feel the excitement of gaining new knowledge as his class explored new concepts and procedures with teacher demonstration or by being read to by others. He started developing friendships with peers, although his less sensitive schoolmates continued to tease him.

At the end of second grade, Donald was retested and found to have made substantial progress during the prior school year.

His decoding skills had accelerated to a low-average range, but his fluency remained slow and methodical. He remained a little more than a year behind in reading, but his rate of learning had accelerated. The school team recommended that he receive extra reading services daily for another year. By this time, he excelled in mathematics, which helped to offset any feelings of inferiority or lack of engagement in learning that his difficulty with reading and spelling might have brought about. He still found school difficult, but he stopped avoiding it and saw success in learning some subjects. His behavior problems also faded. With the continued support of his teachers and parents, Donald is likely to have a good outcome.

DEFINING LEARNING DISORDERS

After a decade of intense review of research, the American Psychiatric Association will change its current organization of the *Diagnostic and Statistical Manual* in its coming fifth edition *(DSM-5)* and will place dyslexia, *dyscalculia* (impairment in the ability to solve mathematical problems), and disorders of written expression under the descriptor "learning disorders," as noted previously.

The Individuals with Disabilities Education Improvement Act of 2004 (IDEA 2004; PL 108-446) defines specific learning disability (SLD) as: "A disorder in one or more of the basic psychological processes involved in understanding or in using language, spoken or written, which disorder may manifest in imperfect ability to listen, think, speak, read, write, spell, or do mathematical calculations" (§ 602[26][a]). The term excludes learning problems that are the result of visual, hearing, or motor disabilities; of intellectual disability; of emotional disturbance; or of environmental, cultural, or economic disadvantage.

This definition is problematic because it fails to define the core features or origins of SLD. The definition does not identify the "basic psychological processes" of learning or how marked an "imperfect ability" to learn must be in order to constitute a disability. It is a definition of exclusion; all other causes for the learning problems must be eliminated. SLDs can coexist with other conditions, most notably attention-deficit/hyperactivity disorder (ADHD; McNamara, Vervaeke, & Willoughby, 2008; see Chapter 22). Other disabilities identified in IDEA are excluded from the definition in order to prevent "double dipping" from existing federal programs that deal with those issues. It is clear, however, that a child with SLD may also have other conditions that affect learning.

The common approach for diagnosing SLD has been to document a severe discrepancy between ability and achievement by demonstrating a significant difference between the child's potential to learn, often expressed as an IQ score, and his or her actual educational achievement (Gregg & Scott, 2000). Evidence now suggests, however, that this discrepancy approach has poor sensitivity and specificity in discriminating students with specific reading disability from those with low IQ scores and poor reading (Francis et al., 2005). In one study, this approach correctly identified less than half of individuals who were receiving special education services. Discrepancy formulas have also shown poor validity in projecting the child's later school performance in reading. Of the individuals classified as having SRD in first grade on the basis of a discrepancy between ability and achievement, only 17% remained in this classification by sixth grade. Studies suggest that the discrepancy formula was no better in identifying SLD than simply applying a criterion of low achievement (Fletcher et al., 1994). In addition, the discrepancy model incorrectly assumes that IQ scores measure the basic skills involved in the various learning disorders (Francis et al., 2005). For all of these reasons, there is serious doubt about the utility and validity of the discrepancy concept for specific reading disability. One alternative is to use the Component Model of Reading approach, which is an elaboration of the simple view of reading that focuses on the literacy skills necessary in each component of learning to read (Aaron, Joshi, Gooden, & Bentum, 2008).

IDEA 2004 also makes educators pause to consider the appropriateness of relying entirely on the discrepancy model (Council for Exceptional Children, 2005). Although the discrepancy model is not abandoned under this legislation, a variety of other tools and assessment strategies may be used to determine eligibility. IDEA 2004 states that "a local education agency shall not be required to take into consideration whether a child has a severe discrepancy between achievement and intellectual ability." It further states that "in determining whether a child has a specific learning disability, a local educational agency may use a process that determines if the child responds to scientific, research-based intervention" (sec 614b,

6, B page 60). This approach is often called a response to intervention (RTI) model (see also Chapter 31).

RESPONSE TO INTERVENTION

Vaughn and Fuchs (2003) advocated redefining learning disability as an inadequate response to instruction (RTI). This RTI approach has been touted as a promising alternative to traditional testing methods for identifying students with specific learning disabilities. Important benefits of such an approach include 1) identification of students using an at-risk rather than a deficit model, 2) earlier identification and intervention, 3) reduction of identification bias, and 4) a strong focus on student outcome. RTI involves the provision of intensive, systematic instruction for a defined period of time to very small groups of students who are at risk for academic failure. The initial step of RTI involves students receiving instruction in their general education classroom with their progress being carefully and regularly monitored. Those students who do not progress then receive additional services from a learning or reading specialist. Again, their progress is carefully and regularly monitored. Those who still fail to progress are referred for a special education evaluation (Fuchs, Mock, Morgan, & Young, 2003; Olitsky & Nelson, 2003).

Intensive instruction provided daily in a very small group setting is fiscally demanding in that it may impose a staffing burden in a classroom; however, those who make progress at the end of the prescribed time (usually 12–16 weeks) are then returned to the general education program, reducing needless referral of students for evaluation and potential placement in separate, special learning environments. Those who do not made adequate gains receive a second round of intensive intervention (Gortmaker, Daly, McCurdy, Persampieri, & Hergenrader, 2007; Hay, Elias, Fielding-Barnsley, Homel, & Freibery, 2007). Students who remain unresponsive to such intensive intervention are then referred for comprehensive evaluation. Despite widespread support for RTI, potential issues remain. These include relying on the instructional environment, ensuring instructional validity, defining intensive instruction, personnel preparation, and availability of trained teachers. By using scientifically derived interventions for early instructional support, however, the potential for maintaining those students in the general education environment increases. This is in contrast to the discrepancy model, which is a "wait to fail" model, in which the student may struggle with learning activities while the discrepancy emerges.

This tiered approach has reduced the numbers of students referred to pullout or special education services (Berkeley, Bender, Peaster, & Saunders, 2009). In research centers around the nation, studies continue to determine how to more effectively implement the model (Deshler, Mellard, Tollefson, & Byrd, 2005; Kennedy & Deshler, 2010; Moss, Lapp, & O'Shea, 2011; Pullen, Tuckwiller, Konod, Maynard, & Coyne, 2010; Ramaswami, 2010). Although most often described as a three-tier model, some schools identify a fourth, or "specialized" tier, which may provide intervention closer to that provided in special education classes without the express referral for a determination of eligibility for special education. Kavale and Spaulding (2008) reviewed the policy implications for these new regulations and concluded that both RTI and psychometric evaluation are appropriate for the identification of learning disorders.

The diagnosis of SLD is difficult in students identified as English language learners (ELL) or having limited English proficiency (LEP). Some of these students may be experiencing difficulty because of their lack of familiarity with English in its academic and/or social use. Alternatively, some may, in fact, have disabilities in learning in both the native language and English (Barrera, 2006; Blanchett, Klingner, & Harry, 2009; Liu, Ortiz, Wilkinson, Robertson, & Kushner, 2008). Although teacher preparation for serving students with SLD has expanded, the preparation of teachers to address the needs of students who may have both a learning disorder and English language proficiency issues needs to be improved (Paneque & Barbetta, 2006).

PREVALENCE

The U.S. Department of Education, National Center for Education Statistics (2011), reported that of the more than 6.6 million students receiving special education services during the 2007–2008 school year, approximately 2.5 million were classified as having SLD. This represents approximately 5% of the total school-age population. The size of this category has nearly doubled since its original creation in 1977, with a particular acceleration in the 1990s. Although this expansion may represent early or improved

diagnosis, it also may be a consequence of a certain amount of overdiagnosis or of inclusion of individuals with more subtle learning problems in a category previously reserved for students with more obvious disabilities (Litt, Taylor, Klein, & Hack, 2005). It should be emphasized, too, that prevalence figures depend on the definition of disability. Because of the problematic definition of SLD, it follows that prevalence figures may be unreliable and vary from author to author or study to study. These statistics represent only those students who are served in the public schools and not those who may be served in private or nonpublic schools. It also omits the 1.5 million students who are home schooled and whose status of disability is not identified.

In addition, reporting differences among school districts and states affect the prevalence of SLD. Individual school districts exercise considerable autonomy in defining, describing, and coding disabilities at the time services are determined. Districts in the same state may not code or assign services for SLD in the same way. In districts in which families are persistent in seeking special educational services and actively involved in the process of attaining those services, the correct and discrete identification of a child's disability is more certain. In districts in which some disabilities are not specified completely, or include other aspects that contribute to learning difficulties, such as attention or behavior problems, an overembracing term such as *multiple disabilities* may be used. This inexact term camouflages the exact nature of a child's problems with learning and may distort the design of an effective and useful education program, but without a wider range of descriptors in the law, such terms are often used by school teams. Needless to say, the accuracy of exact numbers of students identified as having SLD can be affected by these factors. In addition, the growing number of individuals identified as being on the autism spectrum is influencing the overall numbers of individuals identified as being in need of special education. Many of the higher functioning students with autism spectrum disorders (ASD) were formerly classified as having learning disabilities. The overlap of severe learning disorders and higher functioning autism has long been recommended for further study to examine potential links between the two conditions (Williams, Goldstein, Kojkowski, & Minshew, 2008). As of 2011, little has been studied or published to see if the disabilities may be connected.

SPECIFIC READING DISABILITY

Mechanisms of Specific Reading Disability

Specific reading disability (SRD), also called developmental dyslexia, is by far the most commonly recognized form of learning disability, accounting for nearly half of the special education population (National Association of Special Education Teachers [NASET], 2007). Theoretically, any defect in the processing or interpretation of written words can lead to SRD. Efficient reading depends on rapidly, accurately, and fluently decoding and recognizing the phonemes (speech sounds) of single words (Talcott et al., 2000; Wolf, Bowers, & Biddle, 2000). Phonological awareness includes 1) phoneme awareness (the understanding that speech is made up of discrete sounds), 2) a metacognitive understanding of word boundaries within spoken sentences, 3) a recognition of syllable boundaries within spoken words, and 4) an ability to isolate these phonemes and establish their location within syllables and words. Phonological awareness manifests in the ability to analyze and manipulate sounds within syllables (e.g., to count, delete, reorder them). If a child does not realize that syllables and words are composed of phonemes and that these segments can be divided according to their acoustic boundaries, reading will be slow, labored, and inaccurate; in addition, comprehension will be poor. A second possible mechanism may be a defect in phonetic representation in working memory, wherein the child can understand the syntactic structure of a sentence but is unable to maintain it in working memory long enough to comprehend the meaning (Kamil, Pearson, Moje, & Afflerbach, 2010; Mann, 1994).

Poor reading has been linked to phonological processing impairments, but these impairments alone are not sufficient to explain SRD. Wolf and Bowers (1999) proposed three underlying types of specific reading disability: 1) phonological impairment; 2) disrupted orthographic processing, which results from slow naming speed; and 3) a combination of both impairments. Individuals who manifest the double impairment, phonological impairments and naming speed impairments, are the poorest readers. This hypothesis has not been universally accepted. Some researchers failed to find a phonological impairment in the absence of a naming-speed impairment and noted that the double-impairment groupings identified individuals with different neuropsychological profiles (Cirino, Israelian, Morris, & Morris, 2005; Waber, Forbes, Wolff, & Weiler, 2004). Others have reviewed the topic and found little support for the theory that underlies the double-impairment hypothesis, namely that rapid serial processing and temporal integration of letter identities are the primary means by which orthographic codes are formed (Ritchey & Goeke, 2006; Vellutino, Fletcher, Snowling, & Scanlon, 2004; Vukovic & Siegel, 2006). They also question the independence of phonological and rapid naming skills and the specificity of impairments in rapid naming for reading.

Taking these findings into account, a biologically based definition of specific reading disability was proposed by Lyon, Shaywitz, and Shaywitz (2003):

> Dyslexia is a specific learning disability that is neurobiological in origin. It is characterized by difficulties with accurate and/or fluent word recognition and by poor spelling and decoding abilities. These difficulties typically result from a deficit in the phonological component of language that is often unexpected in relation to other cognitive abilities and the provision of effective classroom instruction. Secondary consequences may include problems in reading comprehension and reduced reading experience that can impede growth of vocabulary and background knowledge. (2003, p. 2)

Genetics

Since the turn of the 20th century, it has been hypothesized that reading disabilities are heritable. Often several members of a family have a SRD, and the underlying phonological processing impairments in this disorder appear to be highly heritable (Natale et al., 2008). Genetic studies using linkage and association techniques have shown a relationship among SRD and loci on chromosomes 1, 2, 3, 6, 15, and 18 (Scerri & Schulte-Körne, 2010).

Individuals with certain genetic syndromes also may have an increased risk of manifesting a particular type of learning disability. Research into these syndromes has revealed that girls with Turner syndrome and fragile X syndrome and boys with Klinefelter syndrome tend to have visual-perceptual learning disabilities (Mazzocco, 2001), whereas individuals with neurofibromatosis, type I, have both visual-perceptual and language-based learning disabilities (Cutting, Koth, & Denckla, 2000). Casey, Cohen, Schuerholz, Singer, and Denckia (2000) studied parents of individuals with Tourette syndrome and found that they showed language-based learning problems as well. Each of these syndromes is discussed further in Appendix B.

Neural Substrates of Reading

Reading is a dynamic process that develops with age and experience. It encompasses a wide variety of skills that develops at varying times. Early instruction focuses on learning to read and targets decoding. Later instruction uses reading to learn, and the focus shifts to comprehension. Beginning inexperienced readers employ a "bottom-up" approach that uses analytic and synthetic processes. Experienced readers use a "top-down" approach that results in faster, more efficient reading. Top-down, or conceptual, approaches assume that the path from text to meaning extends from prior knowledge that is applied to the process of acquiring the sound–symbol connection of reading.

Compensated poor readers recruit additional brain areas to read. Neuroimaging studies in individuals with dyslexia show reduced engagement of the left temporo-parietal cortex for phonological processing of print, altered white-matter connectivity, and functional plasticity associated with effective intervention (Fisher & DeFries, 2002; Gabrieli, 2009). Posterior systems predominate during early reading acquisition (Simos et al., 2002; Turkeltaub, Gareau, Flowers, Zeffiro, & Eden, 2003). As individuals become older and are more skilled at reading, they begin to engage parietal and superior temporal areas, with anterior regions coming on line last. Individuals who are identified as having dyslexia do not increase activation of the word form area, even after repeated trials of word exposure. As they grow older, they show the opposite—activation of the anterior system. Anterior activation is not the sole processing difference, however, as individuals with dyslexia also activate their right anterior inferior frontal gyrus as well as the right posterior occipital-temporal region (Sandak, Menel, Frost, & Pugh, 2004).

Shaywitz and colleagues (2004) have underscored the importance of dysfunction of the left hemisphere brain systems in SRD. They provided a year of intensive reading remediation to a group of individuals with SRD. After the intervention, the individuals made gains in reading fluency, and neuroimaging studies showed increased activation of the anterior and dorsal systems. A study in adults with a lifetime history of SRD demonstrated that reading remediation in older individuals

might be different. This study showed increases in both left and right hemisphere activation following successful reading intervention (Eden et al., 2004).

SPECIFIC MATHEMATICS DISABILITY

Three to six percent of individuals have performance on tests of mathematical ability that is discrepant from their IQ scores (Mazzocco, 2007; Shalev & Gross-Tsur, 2001). This percentage may be higher than the true frequency of a learning disorder in mathematics. Poor performance may be due to a lack of adequate instruction in areas that are covered by the assessment measures. Another reason for discrepant performance on math tests may relate to impairments in reading or executive function rather than mathematics (Dirks, Spyer, van Lieshout, & de Sonnerville, 2008; Donlan, 2007; Jordan, 2007). A math learning disorder commonly is seen in the presence of other learning disorders and cognitive disorders. Of individuals with a math learning disorder, approximately 17% had coexisting SRD and 26% had ADHD (Gersten, Jordan, & Flojo, 2005; Shalev & Gross-Tsur, 2001). Of kindergarteners with developmental language disorders, 26% had significantly impaired arithmetic skills (Manor, Shalev, Joseph, & Gross-Tsur, 2001). Marshall, Schafer, O'Donnell, Elliott, and Handwerk (1999) found that inattention exerts a specific and deleterious effect on the acquisition of arithmetic computation skills. This has led some to defer the diagnosis of math learning disorder in the presence of ADHD until the ADHD is properly managed (Shalev & Gross-Tsur, 2001). Finally, assessment of mathematics encompasses a variety of skills and neuropsychological processes, some of which may be impaired whereas others are relatively spared.

Difficulty with mathematics may manifest in different ways. Counting, basic calculation, problem solving, place values (base-10 concepts), equivalence, measurement, time, relations (as in algebra), and geometry are but some of the ways that mathematics is expressed. Despite the wide range of expression, math learning disorder is defined by deficiencies in fact mastery and calculation fluency (Jordan, Hanich, & Kaplan, 2003). Some of the difficulties that children encounter in mathematics evolve from their earliest encounters with numbers; that is, their number sense and early numeracy. The intuitive understanding of numbers and related concepts such as how numbers grow and diminish with calculation may be viewed as having a parallel to the initial reading skill of phonemic awareness, which includes the earliest awareness of how words are made up of discrete sounds. Research has shown that this initial "gut sense" about numbers may be significant in identifying the origins of math learning disorder (Mazzocco, Feigenson, & Halberda, 2011).

Math learning disorder evolves over time. Early presentations exhibit difficulty with retrieval of basic math facts and in computing arithmetic exercises. These have been related to immature counting skills. Older individuals have difficulty in learning arithmetic tables and comprehending the algorithms of adding, subtracting, multiplying, and dividing. These manifest as misuse of signs, forgetting to carry, misplacing digits, or approaching problems from left to right (Shalev, 2004). Ten- to eleven-year-olds with math learning disorder showed persistently poor math performance on reexamination six years later (Shalev, Manor, & Gross-Tsur, 2005).

Neurobiology of Math

Neurobiological evidence of math learning disorder is still evolving, and the exact mechanism remains to be delineated. Evidence derived from clinical syndromes, neuroimaging, and genetics suggest a number of brain-based impairments. Although the clinical syndromes point to a major role of the parietal lobe in dyscalculia, the relationship is not simple. Different types of mathematic skills require coordination of different brain functions and, by extension, activation of different brain areas. Complicating this is the finding that people who have difficulty with math will recruit other brain areas and use other psychological mechanisms to compensate for the impairment in brain function.

There is a paucity of studies that focus on the genetics of math learning disorder. Yet, familial occurrences of the disorder have been described. Shalev and Gross-Tsur (2001) found that approximately half of siblings of individuals with developmental dyscalculia also had dyscalculia. In a study of twins, one of whom had math learning disorder, significantly higher rates of dyscalculia were found in identical twins than in fraternal twins (Cohen Kadosh & Walsh, 2007).

Several psychological mechanisms have been proposed for math learning disorder. In early research, Rourke and Finlayson (1978) found that individuals with dyscalculia showed poor nonverbal skills (visual-spatial and tactile-perceptual), whereas individuals with combined math learning disorder and SRD showed poorer verbal skills (verbal and auditory-perceptual). Geary (2004) posits three subtypes of math learning disorder based on memory and cognitive impairments: 1) procedural subtype, 2) semantic memory subtype, and 3) visuospatial subtype. Others have associated dyscalculia with executive function and working memory impairments (McLean & Hitch, 1999). Dehaene and Cohen (1995) advocated a "triple-code model" wherein simple arithmetic operations are processed by the verbal system within the left hemisphere and more complex arithmetic procedures that require *subitization* (the ability to perceive at a glance the number of items presented), *cardinality* (the ability to perceive the number of elements in a set or other grouping), and visual representations are bilaterally localized.

IMPAIRMENTS ASSOCIATED WITH SPECIFIC LEARNING DISABILITIES

Donald's case is unusual in that he has an isolated SRD that responded to the interventions provided, allowing him to continue in an inclusive educational setting. One quarter to one half of individuals with learning disorders have additional impairments that interfere with school functioning. These may include executive function impairments, ADHD, social cognition impairments, and emotional and behavior disorders. These behavior and emotional problems may be externalizing (e.g., aggression, oppositional-defiant disorder, conduct disorder) or internalizing (e.g., shyness, depression, anxiety). Failure to detect and treat these additional impairments is a common reason for failed intervention programs. As comorbid conditions may adversely affect outcome, it may be most appropriate to categorize individuals not only on the basis of their learning impairments but also according to comorbid conditions.

Memory Impairments

Impairments in the ability to listen, remember, and repeat auditory stimuli have been associated with reading disability. The holding of information in immediate and working memory is essential in learning to read. A number of studies comparing individuals with equivalent IQ scores but low or high reading abilities have reported impairments in the poor readers on the Digit Span subtest of the Wechsler

Intelligence Scale for Children–Fourth Edition (D'Angiulli & Siegel, 2003; Wechsler, 2003). Executive dysfunction coupled with memory impairments may adversely affect the student's ability to choose the appropriate strategy for solving a problem. Working memory, the area of the prefrontal cortex concerned with short term management of memory and attention, has also been studied and found to be of particular interest (Schuchardt, Maehler, & Hasselhorn, 2008). As a result, the student's ability to use cognitive behavioral techniques may be limited because he or she cannot remember a sequence of problem-solving steps.

Impairments in Executive Functions

According to Pennington (1991), executive functions involve the ability to maintain an appropriate problem-solving set of procedures for attaining a future goal. This includes the ability to 1) inhibit or defer a response; 2) formulate a sequential, strategic plan of action; and 3) encode relevant information in memory for future use. These metacognitive abilities are necessary for organizational skills, planning, future-oriented behavior, maintaining an appropriate problem-solving set of procedures, impulse control, selective attention, vigilance, inhibition, and creativity in thinking. These abilities involve an awareness of what skills, strategies, and resources are needed to perform a task effectively. They also require the ability to use self-regulatory mechanisms to ensure the successful completion of a task. Yet students with learning disorders are often impulsive rather than reflective when presented with a problem-solving task. This failure to consider alternative solutions often results in errors or a poor quality solution. Executive functions become essential in middle school in order to complete homework and long-term projects, to sustain attention during lectures, and to set future goals. Disruption in this organization and control of behavior often manifests as disruption in the classroom. Executive function impairments are also a key feature in ADHD.

Attention-Deficit/ Hyperactivity Disorder

Approximately one third of individuals with learning disorders, in fact, have attention-deficit/hyperactivity disorder (ADHD), making this the most common comorbid diagnosis. Studies have found that the prevalence of ADHD in individuals with learning disorders is higher than the prevalence of learning disorders in individuals with ADHD (see Schulte, Conners, & Osborne, 1999). The symptoms typically include inattention, impulsivity, and hyperactivity (see Chapter 22).

Impairments in Social Cognition

Impairments in social cognition are noted often in individuals with learning disorders (Bauminger, Edelsztein, & Morash, 2005; Bauminger & Kimhi-Kind, 2008). Such individuals have difficulty understanding complex emotions, tend to be socially isolated, may have few close friends, and/or infrequently participate in social activities. In turn, they are often overlooked or rejected by their peers because of their odd behavior and poor school and/or athletic performance. Teachers tend to rate these individuals as having social adjustment difficulties and being easily led. There may be many reasons for these problems, including poor social comprehension, inability to take the perspective of others, poor pragmatic language skills, an inability to recognize facial expressions, and misinterpretation of body language. This awareness of the intent or perspective of others is called Theory of Mind (see Chapter 21) and sheds light on how individuals develop the means to understand the social cues sent by others so that they may develop their own awareness of social situations and form appropriate responses (Bloom & Heath, 2010; Schneider, 2008). The child who has a combination of a learning disorder, poor pragmatic language skills, executive function impairments, and impairments in social cognition may be difficult to distinguish from a child who falls on the autism spectrum. It is likely that these conditions will be more closely linked in the future.

Emotional and Behavior Disorders

Although associated emotional and behavioral impairments may represent endogenous biological conditions, they also may result from the child's experiences of school failure. Individuals with learning disorders can exhibit conduct disorders, withdrawal, poor self-esteem, and depression, but there is no connection of these social/emotional disorders to the provision of services for students with a specific learning disability as mandated in federal law. These individuals are less likely to take pride in their successes and more likely to be overcome by their failures. More than one third of students with learning disorders receive a failing grade in one or more courses each school year. These individuals often exhibit chronic frustration and anxiety as they attempt to meet the demands of skill-based tasks, such as phonological decoding, comprehension, spelling, and math. This school failure, combined with social skills impairments, may lead to peer rejection, poor self-image, and withdrawal from participation in school activities (Maag & Reid, 2006). Eventually, these individuals may avoid going to school all together or act out in class in order to obtain the attention they do not receive through good grades. The overall dropout rate of individuals with specific learning disabilities is twice that found in the general population (U.S. Department of Education, Office of Special Education Programs, 2009).

HEALTH PROBLEMS SIMULATING SPECIFIC LEARNING DISABILITIES

Some individuals who do not have learning disorders may demonstrate learning differences in school as a consequence of another developmental disability, a chronic illness, or psychosocial problems. If these individuals are misdiagnosed as having a specific learning disability, efforts directed solely at treating the learning problem will have limited success. Instead, the underlying problem must be identified and addressed. Once this problem has been treated, the learning problem may well improve or disappear.

For example, if a child has an unidentified sensory impairment, learning is likely to be impaired. The provision of hearing aids to a child with hearing loss or of glasses to the child with a refractive error may lead to a significant improvement in school performance. Individuals with epilepsy (see Chapter 27) also may have problems in school resulting either from poorly controlled seizures or from side effects of antiepileptic medication. Modifying the drug regimen may significantly improve both attention and learning. Individuals with psychiatric disorders (see Chapter 29) also may fail in school. The use of psychotropic drugs and psychotherapy often leads to significantly improved school performance, although some of these drugs can have an adverse effect on attention. (For specific information on medication side effects, see Appendix C.)

An increased incidence of learning problems also has been described in individuals with such chronic illnesses as diabetes, HIV infection, sickle-cell disease, cancer, and chronic kidney and liver disease (see Chapter 28). In these situations, a learning disability may exist, but learning difficulties also may result from other causes such as physiological derangement, excessive school absences, attention impairments, or depression. A secondary learning problem rather than a learning disability is suggested if learning improves once the medical condition is brought under control (Sexson & Madan-Swain, 1993).

Individuals who were born prematurely have an increased incidence of learning disorders. Acute disorders such as meningitis, encephalitis, and traumatic brain injury (TBI) also can result in the subsequent development of learning problems. TBI is the most common of these and is an increasingly recognized cause of behavior and learning problems in individuals (see Chapter 26). The injury may result in either temporary or permanent neurological impairments. Affected individuals present special challenges in the classroom as a result of the evolving nature of their recovery (Carney & Porter, 2009). During the acute phase, disorders of attention and other executive functions, higher language skills, and behavior are common. Because of this, TBI has been identified as a separate category of disability under IDEA 2004 (see Chapter 31) to distinguish it from specific learning disabilities and other related disorders. When recovery is completed, some individuals with TBI may have a residual learning disorder.

Finally, psychosocial influences may affect the child's ability to learn. A child who is hungry cannot pay attention or learn well. A child who comes from a home that does not value learning rarely achieves well in school. And, a home beset with family problems or abuse is a poor setting in which to encourage the child's school performance. Improvement in these psychosocial areas would likely result in improved school performance but has proven difficult to achieve. Until a complete picture of why students in a particular school are identified as having profiles of underachievement—and until the role of factors such as poverty, prematurity, nutrition, and environmental threats (e.g., lead poisoning and other environmental toxins) are fully understood and accommodated—educators will continue to struggle to reconcile cognitive disabilities and effective instructional practices.

What is vital to the improvement of this state of affairs is greater attention to how school teams obtain and use information that identifies learning disabilities and the resources available to treat the disability in the school, school district, and community. All existing information should be used in the educational process. Medical or educational assessments by qualified examiners, combined with the assessment data developed by the school, serve as the foundation for developing an effective educational program, and optimizes the use of related services (see Chapter 31).

ASSESSMENT PROCEDURES

The assessments used to identify students with a specific learning disability are individually administered tests designed to reveal both the strengths and the challenges of the child so that comprehensive recommendations can be made to support the student. A school team, including the parent and student (when appropriate) reviews all assessments and determines the appropriate level of services needed to accommodate the student's learning needs. These recommendations are written into the individual education program (IEP) with explicit, measurable goals and objectives, as well as the clear description of how progress will be evaluated (see Chapter 31). Recommendations may include specific programmatic interventions in reading, writing or mathematics, grouping strategies, or even additional therapeutic interventions from specialists (Fletcher, Lyon, Fuchs & Barnes, 2007).

The No Child Left Behind Act of 2001 (PL107-110) requires another, ongoing kind of assessment of all students, including those with learning disorders. These assessments are viewed as vital indicators of the success of the school in demonstrating student achievement and effective instruction. Although accommodations in those assessments such as increased time may be permitted, they must be specified clearly in the IEP, and not all students with specific learning disabilities will be granted these accommodations.

Psychological, language, and educational tests are the mainstay of assessment in school-age individuals (see Chapter 16). However, a complete medical, behavioral, educational, and social history also should be taken in order to consider confounding variables that may simulate or worsen a learning disorder (Francis et al., 2005; Lyon, Shaywitz, & Shaywitz, 2005). Simply looking at the discrepancy between potential and actual achievement can lead to misclassification of the students' needs. Evaluators need to use procedures for assessment that provide more information than a simple statistic as an indicator of a student's abilities (Grigorenko, 2009). The global standardized assessment tools, such as IQ tests, are not sensitive enough to allow the instructional program to be tailored

to ensure the student's academic growth. Standardized proficiency testing must be combined with authentic assessment, norm-referenced as well as criterion-referenced tests, informal assessment, and portfolio assessment to obtain the full picture of how the student is progressing. This permits connecting and applying this information to the content the student is learning. If this does not occur, inappropriate treatment recommendations can result. Labeling a test-taker as a "low achiever" does no service to the student. Well-documented strengths and challenges lead to a more serviceable IEP.

Continued periodic assessment of progress in the class is also required. This periodic "snapshot" of achievement allows the effectiveness of the program to be evaluated and the instructional program to be adjusted. Periodic reassessment of cognitive and executive functions is warranted if the student is failing to progress. In addition, annual assessment of academic subjects is important to determine the progress the child has made and the effectiveness of the program. This aligns with the purpose of response to intervention as well as the federal mandates of No Child Left Behind.

INTERVENTION STRATEGIES

The primary goal of intervention is to facilitate the acquisition and expression of the knowledge needed for effective performance in school and then in the workplace. The objectives are to achieve academic competence, treat associated impairments, and prevent adverse mental health outcomes. This requires the cooperation of educators, health care professionals, and families. If individuals with SRD are not provided with an intervention program composed of instruction in phonological awareness, sound–symbol relations, and contextual reading skills before the third grade, at least three quarters of these individuals will show little improvement in reading throughout their later school years (Shaywitz & Shaywitz, 2005). If given intensive remediation, however, improvement can occur (Lovett & Steinbach, 1997).

In addition to treating the core learning disorder, intervention strategies need to focus on associated cognitive, attention, language, perceptual, and sensory impairments. Immaturity, lack of motivation, and poor impulse control also must be considered in determining the child's needs for remediation (Bakker, Van Strien, Licht, & Smit-Glaude, 2007). Intervention must recognize the developmental changes that occur as the student gets older. It must be sensitive to the changing demands of the curriculum, the typical developmental challenges faced by the child, and the effects of maturation and intervention on the academic abilities of the student. In addition, successful interventions must not be withdrawn prematurely.

Professionals continue to debate the most effective intervention strategies. A major consideration is whether to teach to the child's abilities (i.e., compensation/circumvention strategies) or the disabilities (i.e., remedial strategies). Little evidence supports the superiority of one approach over the other. It is generally agreed, however, that there must be a combination of instructional and cognitive interventions (Alexander & Slinger-Constant, 2004).

Instructional and Other Types of Interventions

The following is a review of some interventions in reading, writing, mathematics, and other areas.

Reading

In 2000, the National Reading Panel released its report on research-based reading instruction (National Institute of Child Health and Human Development, 2000). The panel identified the following six essential components to a sound reading program: 1) phonemic awareness; 2) phonics skills; 3) fluency, accuracy, speed, and expression; 4) reading comprehension strategies to enhance understanding; 5) teacher education; and 6) computer technology. Once decoding is unlocked, students are able to use these skills to build fluency. The focus can then shift to interventions that support and develop the expansion of a vocabulary (for general communication, usage, and technical use) and enhance the student's ability to comprehend the message of the text they are reading.

Reading proficiency depends on phonological processing and alphabetical mapping. Phonics instruction, however, is different from phonological awareness training (Shaywitz, 2005). Clark and Uhry (1995) defined phonics as a low level of rote knowledge of the association between letters and sounds. Phonological awareness, on the other hand, includes higher-level metacognitive understandings of word boundaries within spoken sentences, of syllable boundaries in spoken words, and of how to isolate the phonemes and establish their location within syllables and words. Regardless of the method chosen, the major goal of reading instruction is to improve phonological awareness (the sublexical aspect of reading) so that there is effective word recognition and comprehension of meaning (the lexical aspect of reading). Reading activities focus on helping the child gain print awareness and become attuned to the sound characteristics of language (phoneme awareness) and letter–sound relationships (the alphabetic principle).

In elementary school, reading instruction includes methods designed to increase skills in acquiring vocabulary, using syntax, and understanding meaning (Alexander & Slinger-Constant, 2004; Schatschneider & Torgesen, 2004). Many different approaches are proposed for the teaching of reading. Table 23.1 lists some of the techniques and the aspect of reading upon which they focus. No single model suffices for all individuals. In the final analysis, semantic (the meaning of words), syntactic (the rules

Table 23.1. Focuses and techniques for reading instruction

Focus	Examples
Explicit phonics training	Alphabetic Phonics (Cox, 1985)
	Orton-Gillingham (Gillingham & Stillman, 1997; Orton, 1937; Sheffield, 1991)
	Recipe for Reading (Traub & Bloom, 2000)
	Wilson Reading System (Wilson, 1988)
Sounds (oral-motor characteristics of speech)	Lindamood Phoneme Sequencing Program for Reading, Spelling, and Speech (LiPS; Lindamood & Lindamood, 1998)
Overlearning basic skills to increase skill level	Reading mastery
Comprehension	Project READ (Calfee & Henry, 1986)
Oral reading to increase comprehension by focusing on miscues and errors	Retrospective Miscue Analysis (Goodman & Marek, 1996)
	Word Study (Bear et al., 1996)
At-risk children	Reading Recovery (Clay, 1985)
	Success for All (Slavin et al., 1990)

that govern the ways words combine to form phrases), and graphophonemic (using combined letters and sounds to decode words) systems must be united for successful reading.

Along with knowledge of phonics, efficient reading requires a rapid sight vocabulary (words recognized on sight, without sounding them out phonetically). Different word recognition strategies include analysis of sound (phonics or phonetics), analysis for structure (visual configuration), and use of memory skills to recognize words as total entities (whole-word approach). Comprehension strategies center on developing the ability to draw meaning from text, often using a sequence of books that introduces words and concepts in a gradual progression.

Many students with a reading disability need an adjustment in the curriculum. Some methods of teaching reading, such as Orton-Gillingham, Wilson, and Lindamood Bell, employ multisensory approaches (Birsh, 2005; Ritchey & Goeke, 2006) for the remediation of difficulties in efficient sound–symbol processing. Other approaches include 1) whole language (reinforcing a spectrum of language arts); 2) thematics (utilizing content areas conceptually); 3) literature-based methods (using trade books to build on basal program skills); 4) individualized reading programs (using trade books and alternative literature forms to build personal reading); 5) language experience (having students generate their own reading material); and 6) functional skills (involving the use of materials involved in daily living—e.g., forms, notices, directions).

Teachers at all levels and in all types of classrooms can give students with SRD tools such as 1) graphic organizers (a visual representation of the material a student is learning that assists the student in brainstorming and/or organizing information to make it easier to understand how ideas connect); 2) anticipation guides ("a study guide that prepares students to identify the major themes and concepts of a written work through a series of statements that address the concepts, rather than the story," www.education.com, n.d.); 3) question/answer strategies; 4) think-alouds ("a form of explicit modeling in which teachers give an oral description of the cognitive processes they go through as they read with their students so that students can understand how a successful reader approaches a text," www.education.com, n.d.); 5) charting and outlining; and 6) induced imagery (mental imagery that we experience while reading induced by instruction that has powerful effects on comprehension, memory, and appreciation for the text).

These schemata all help students retain the messages they get through their reading. The intent of these strategic reading methods is to provide the reader with ways to chunk or otherwise partition their reading material into segments that they can "digest" as they read in order to expand the reading "diet." The goal of such instructional interventions is movement toward higher levels of critical thinking. By attaining these skills, the student can compete with peers in academic tasks that connect reading to other skills, such as writing and oral discussion.

Middle School and High School

The mandates of No Child Left Behind, as well as the requirements of school districts for the acquisition of credits toward graduation, have raised the bar for the attainment of a diploma. In addition, a diploma is not acquired by passing courses alone. High school students must demonstrate the ability to pass statewide-standardized measures of mastery of core subjects as well. The path toward independent adulthood, higher education, and continued training for skills needed for employment has a distinct "turn" as students move into middle school and then into high school.

The demands of middle school and the pressures of high school programs can be very trying for students with learning disorders. As individuals move from the structure of elementary school to middle and high school, the demands of content reading become an additional burden. The discrete skills of content reading and the related study skills needed for success in secondary education are divided into two approaches. One is a direct instructional approach that separates skills from content, and the other is a functional approach that embeds reading and study skills into the content.

In middle and high school, the reading process must connect with other skills needed for mastering content-related matter in subjects such as social studies, geography, higher-level mathematics, and sciences. Study, organizational, and problem-solving skills must blend with the processing skills involved in obtaining meaning from words, sentences, charts, maps, books, poetry, and dramatic or narrative literature. Meaning is easier to teach in the elementary and middle grades than in high school, when it may become buried in nuances of language, such as humor, sarcasm, and metaphor.

The expertise of general educators in middle and high schools is in the content they teach and not in the instructional mechanisms that help students organize, retrieve, and explain text related to that content. In addition, secondary school requires learning multiple content areas in discrete settings with several different teachers. Consequently, the student with SRD may become a "cumulative deficit" reader who makes progress but at a rate that is too slow to maintain adequate academic achievement. The content teacher, therefore, needs to understand not only the demands and organization of his or her content but also how students must organize that content from lessons so that they can use it in the many forms that secondary school demands (e.g., exams, research papers, debates).

Writing

As much as reading dominates the instructional day of students with SRD, students with dysgraphia have specific disabilities in processing and reporting information in written form. Writing is firmly connected to reading and spelling because comprehension and exposition of these skills are demonstrated through production of written symbols as indicators of understanding (Berninger & Wolf, 2009; Mason & Graham, 2008). Although writing is a representation of oral language, it also must convey meaning without the benefit of vocal intonation or stress. This makes additional demands on the writer.

Problems in writing may result from either an inability to manipulate a pen and paper to produce a legible representation of ideas or an inability to express oneself on paper. Word processors can assist individuals who have disabilities related to the manipulation of the writing implements (Bain, Bailet, & Moats, 2001; MacArthur, 2009). Remedial and instructional techniques that are helpful with problems of written expression include the use of 1) open-ended sentences; 2) probable passages (a strategy used to draw on a student's prior knowledge of a topic while incorporating writing into a basic reading lesson); 3) journal keeping; 4) modified writing systems, using rebuses or other symbols; and 5) newspapers and other print media to demonstrate various writing styles and organizational models.

Not to be forgotten is the connection of spelling to writing. The developmental stages of spelling need to be explored as teachers approach instruction that connects what is read to the written response of students. These stages include prephonemic, phonemic, transitional, and conventional spelling (Bear & Templeton, 1998). The International Reading Association and the National Association for the Education

of Young Children (1998) issued a joint position statement that advocated a developmental approach to teaching writing as an outgrowth of the reading process. Their position is that students should be moved from the initial, prephonemic, and phonemic attempts at spelling toward correct, conventional spelling of English words. The process, however, should reflect an understanding of the developmental level and needs of the individual student.

Content area literacy calls for connections between reading and writing and the development of study skills and organization of written materials so that they are retrievable for later use. Interventions in this area may call for students to share their writing with peers and to examine the writing styles of others. Among the research-based strategies that assist the student with writing disabilities is self-regulated strategy development (SRSD), a six-step cognitive strategy model designed to make the writing process complete, automatic, and flexible for all subjects (Graham & Harris, 1989; Harris & Pressley, 1991; Read, 2005).

Writing is also a socio-cultural endeavor, representing a cognitive process learned through dialogic interactions, expressing the social and cultural perspectives of the student (Englert, 1992). The difficulties that a student with a learning disorder may have with social perception and awareness of cultural aspects of personal development may influence the written product as well as the writing process.

Mathematics

Students with a math learning disorder have an impaired ability to perform basic math operations (i.e., addition, subtraction, multiplication, division) and/or to apply those operations to daily situations (Mazzocco, 2007; Raghubar et al., 2009). Often, however, the problem is in understanding the abstract concepts of mathematical usage (Mabbott & Bisanz, 2008). When students with dyscalculia have only written math problems to solve, the concepts remain vague. When functional applications (e.g., involving money, time) and manipulatives are used, however, the student can connect the concepts to their practical applications and demonstrate greater understanding. For some individuals with this disorder, a calculator may prove helpful. Thus, teaching may focus on the use of money in fast-food restaurants (e.g., making change), grocery shopping (e.g., comparing prices per unit of weight), banking (e.g., balancing a checkbook, calculating interest), cooking (e.g., measurement), and transportation (e.g., reading, keeping to schedules).

The language aspects of instructing students with a math disability, especially those who also have SRD, have been studied to determine how the reading process influences performance in numeric problem solving (Anderson & Lyxell, 2007; Fuchs & Fuchs, 2002; Powell, Fuchs, Fuchs, Cirino, & Fletcher, 2009). For students with both reading and math disabilities, problems requiring addition were easier to solve than problems requiring subtraction; and problems requiring making change were also more difficult to solve than those requiring addition. Powell and colleagues (2009) investigated how much the format of word problems connects to numeric ability. They discovered that students with math disability demonstrated an improved ability to solve word problems in math by using diagramming as an intervention (Van Garderen, 2007) to incorporate visuospatial reasoning.

The importance of adequate assessment tools in the determination of math disability was discussed by Lembke and Foegen (2009), whose research in early numeracy (the ability to understand and work with numbers) posited the relationship of number sense to phonemic awareness in reading. As indicators of math performance among primary grade students, they identified the skills of quantity discrimination, number identification, and missing number identification as three strong predictors of early mathematical success. Assessment and determination of the possibility of other disabling conditions that might affect learning was also the concern of researchers, especially the combined impact of reading and math disabilities (Dirks, Spyer, van Lieshout, & de Sonneville, 2008). Limited study has been done on this combined disability effect, and Dirks and colleagues estimated that more than 7% of students have both SRD and math disabilities.

Powell et al. (2009) demonstrated the effectiveness of an approach that emphasizes problem type for solving mathematical word problems and complex operations (e.g., multiplication). Another approach, emphasizing executive function, involves rehearsal, practice, and mastery of math skills in combination with corrective and positive feedback throughout the process of instruction. A metacognitive approach can give students with dyscalculia hope for greater success and facility in progressing to higher and more complex mathematical operations (Desoete, Roeyers, & Buysse, 2001; Keeler & Swanson, 2001).

The concepts, principles, and procedures that are part of mathematics instruction increase in difficulty through the grades, and so the identification of a math disability may follow the student throughout his or her school career. Geary and Hoard (2005) described the executive functions that are disrupted, namely regulation of attention and the ability to distinguish between relevant and irrelevant numeric associations in solving problems.

For many students with mathematical disabilities, the more abstract levels of mathematics, such as algebra, geometry, and calculus, may remain mysteries forever; however, these students can still gain facility with basic mathematical facts used in daily life (Mercer & Pullen, 2004). Many schools teach students how and when to use calculators so that more complex problems can be simplified or homework checked for accuracy. In addition, computer-assisted instruction in mathematics may provide opportunities for practice and reinforcement.

Training in Social Cognition

The maintenance of self-esteem and the development of social cognition are very important in preventing adverse mental health outcomes in a child such as Donald with SLD (Erlbaum & Vaughn, 2003; Gans, Kenny, & Ghany, 2003). The teacher can encourage this by giving the child special jobs in the classroom and by supporting participation in extracurricular activities such as sports, scouting, music, drama, arts and crafts, and so forth. Social skills training also can be provided in a group setting (using role-play techniques) and in summer camp programs.

Counseling

Counseling may be required to treat underlying mental health issues in children with a learning disorder. This can be provided individually or in groups. Family-centered counseling also may be appropriate. Issues to be discussed may include homework, behavior management techniques, parental expectations, and the child's self-esteem. Families also should be provided a source of information about learning disorders, support groups, and their legal rights and responsibilities in the education of their child. In addition to support for families as they get help for their child with learning disorders, these families, especially parents, may need help in addressing their own feelings of grief or powerlessness in assisting their child toward independence in adulthood, higher education, and employment.

Medication

Although learning disorders cannot be "cured" through the use of medication, certain associated impairments that affect learning, such as ADHD (see Chapter 22) and behavior and emotional disorders (see Chapter 29), can be improved with the use of psychoactive drugs. If such drugs are used, their effectiveness must be monitored carefully. Medication should never be a substitute for sound educational programming.

Homework

The home and school should be able to function in partnership so that homework does not lead to tension among family members or misunderstanding of the teacher's intent in providing the home assignment. This may require assisting the parent to set up a workable system and schedule at home. Students with learning disorders often feel that homework is an imposition, providing no personal fulfillment or advancement (Nicholls, McKenzie, & Shufro, 1994), so individualization and creative use of assignments is essential for homework to fulfill its reinforcing purpose. Homework should supplement material that was taught during the day (Alvermann & Phelps, 2005). Techniques to facilitate homework performance include parents' reading and reviewing difficult material with the child and teachers, minimizing the need for rote exercises such as copying. Homework should be limited to a specific time allotment; for example, 10–20 minutes per day for individuals in kindergarten through second grade and 30–60 minutes per day for individuals in Grades 3–6. Ideally, homework should be completed in a specific area of the home that is quiet, organized, and stocked with needed supplies. Children with learning disabilities may also not bring homework assignments home either to avoid doing them or because they forgot, so communication with the teacher is essential. Some schools now post homework assignments on the Internet or through e-mails to parents.

Periodic Reevaluations

The treatment programs for students with learning disabilities are complex, and many potential gaps exist. Furthermore, the child is a developing organism whose needs and abilities change from year to year. Therefore, ongoing monitoring is essential. The goal of periodic reassessments is to evaluate academic progress, psychosocial issues, and parent–child relationships. Reassessment is also an opportunity to convey new information to the family and ensure that it is obtaining appropriate resources. Finally, it is a time for retesting the child and revising the educational program. These reevaluations should occur yearly, usually in the spring, so that planning for the next school year can occur.

OUTCOME

Academic preparation of students with learning disorders is permitting more and more students to pursue postsecondary education. However, the average college student with SRD reads only at about a tenth-grade level (Hughes & Smith, 1990; Mason & Mason, 2005). These students also read more slowly, make more spelling errors, and acquire less information from texts. They tend to have difficulty in writing essays, completing heavy reading assignments, scoring well on timed tests, and learning foreign languages (Denckla, 1993; Duquette & Fullarton, 2009; Murray & Wren, 2003). Many colleges now offer adjustments to program loads and schedules as well as tutorial and other support services, which have permitted students with learning disorders to complete college at an increasing rate (Jones, Long, & Finlay, 2007).

The National Center on Educational Statistics reports that in the 4-year period after leaving high school, 25% of students with learning disorders participate in postsecondary education, with nearly 9% attending 4-year institutions, slightly more than 13% attending 2-year institutions, and slightly more than 6% participating in vocational or technical training programs (Seo, Abbott & Hawkins, 2008). In addition, more than 77% of these individuals are competitively employed (U.S. Department of Education, 2008).

Career education should be an objective of educational programming beginning in the primary grades. Such training for students with learning disabilities begins with realistic counseling resulting from a comprehensive assessment of abilities and aptitudes. Without appropriately directed training, students may be unable to support themselves in an independent manner as adults; also, if vocational rehabilitative services are delayed until adulthood, they are less likely to be effective. The design of these programs becomes part of the student's IEP (see Chapters 31 and 40).

Career planning and training, which usually begins in high school, consists of counseling, assessment, and training in the hands-on skills that future jobs require. The

U.S. Department of Labor (1992) published competencies that have been determined to be necessary for employment. These reports by the Secretary's Commission on Achieving Necessary Skills (SCANS) have been translated into curriculum areas that deemphasize specific job-related tasks while teaching general competencies that cross all job markets.

Even as adults, some individuals with learning disorders have poor retention of verbal instructions and other problems that may interfere with effectiveness in their jobs. They also may be hesitant to ask questions and seek assistance. Social immaturity, clumsiness, and poor judgment may make social interactions more difficult. The skills taught in career education are those required to overcome these impairments and enhance success in the work environment, be it the classroom or the adult job market. Cooperation, respect, responsibility, teamwork, organization, and ways to seek information to solve one's problems are all part of career education (U.S. Department of Labor, 1992).

Long-term outcomes appear to depend less on the specific method used to help the student than on the amount of time spent on remediation/practice, the severity of the learning disorder, the age at diagnosis and intervention, the IQ score, the presence of a comorbid condition, the socioeconomic status of the family, the child's motivation to learn, and the family support system (Satz, Buka, Lippsett, & Seldman, 1998). For example, individuals with comorbid conditions such as ADHD have a less optimistic outcome than individuals with an isolated learning disorder. By middle and secondary school, students with comorbid conditions may have acquired "learned helplessness," lacking confidence in their own ability to solve learning and social problems independently (Bryan, 1986). They also are at greater risk for making poor choices in their postsecondary education, employment, and independent living.

According to the NCES report mentioned above (U.S. Department of Education, 2008), in the 4 years after leaving secondary school, although over 75% of students with learning disabilities hold jobs in competitive employment situations, only slightly more than 30% live independently. This cannot be judged too critically, however, in light of national trends in employment and living arrangements that might be influenced by economic downturns that affect all potential workers leaving high school.

SUMMARY

A specific learning disability is a developmental disorder in which a healthy child with typical intelligence fails to learn adequately in one or more school subjects. The underlying cause of these disorders is aberrant brain function, such as impaired phonological decoding in SRD. Neuroimaging, genetic, and neuropsychological studies are providing insight into how the brain guides learning. Early detection of learning disorders is important because, if untreated, the child may develop secondary emotional and behavior problems that hinder progress. If a learning disorder is suspected, a psychoeducational evaluation should be performed to identify areas of strengths and challenge. Then the education team can develop an IEP and appropriate changes in curriculum and supports can be made. No single treatment method is ideal for all individuals, so an empiric approach may be needed to find the most useful method. Studies also suggest that the amount of time spent in remediation/practice is very important. Career and vocational education should be included into the general educational curriculum and included as an individualized transition plan within the IEP. Although the individual with SLD usually carries his or her learning impairment into adulthood, outcome is often good.

REFERENCES

Aaron, P.G., Joshi, R.M., Gooden, R., & Bentum, K.E. (2008). Diagnosis and treatment of reading disabilities based on the Component Model of Reading: An alternative to the discrepancy model of LD. *Journal of Learning Disabilities, 41,* 67–84. doi:10.1177/0022219407310838

Alexander, A.W., & Slinger-Constant, A.M. (2004). Current status of treatments for dyslexia: Critical review. *Journal of Child Neurology, 19,* 744–758.

Alvermann, D.E., & Phelps, S.F. (2005). *Content reading and literacy: Succeeding in today's diverse classrooms* (4th ed.). Boston, MA: Allyn & Bacon.

Andersson, U., & Lyxell, R. (2007). Working memory, deficit in children with mathematical difficulties: A general or specific deficit? *Journal of Experimental Child Psychology, 96,* 197–228. doi:10.1016/j.jecp.2006.10.001

Bain, A., Baillet, L.L., & Moats, L.C. (2001). *Written language disorders: Theory in to practice* (2nd ed.). Austin, TX: PRO-ED.

Bakker, D., Van Strien, J.W., Licht, R., & Smit-Glaude, S.W.D. (2007). Cognitive brain potentials in kindergarten children with subtyped risks of reading retardation. *Annals of Dyslexia, 57*(1), 99–111. doi:10.1007/s11881-007-0005-y

Barrera, M. (2006). Roles of definitional and assessment models in the identification of new or second language learners of English for special education. *Journal of Learning Disabilities, 39,* 142–156. doi:10.1177/00222194060390020301

Bauminger, N., Edelsztein, H.S., & Morash, J. (2005). Social information processing and emotional understanding in children with LD. *Journal of Learning Disabilities, 38,* 45–61. doi:10.1177/0022219405038001040

Bauminger, N., & Kimhi-Kind, I. (2008). Social information processing, security of attachment, and emotion regulation in children with learning disabilities. *Journal of Learning Disabilities, 41,* 315–332. doi:10.1177/0022219408316095

Bear, D.R., & Templeton, S. (1998). Explorations in developmental spelling: Foundations for learning and teaching phonics, spelling and vocabulary. *The Reading Teacher, 52,* 222–242.

Berkeley, S., Bender, W.N., Peaster, L.G., & Saunders, L. (2009). Implementation of response to intervention—A snapshot of progress. *Journal of Learning Disabilties, 42,* 85–95. doi:10.1177/0022219408326214

Berninger, V.W., & Wolf, B.J. (2009). *Teaching students with dyslexia and dysgraphia: Lessons from teaching and science.* Baltimore, MD: Paul H. Brookes Publishing Co.

Birsh, J.R. (Ed.). (2005). *Multisensory teaching of basic language skills* (2nd ed.). Baltimore, MD: Paul H. Brookes Publishing Co.

Blanchett, W.J., Klingner, J.K., & Harry, B. (2009). The intersection of race, culture, language and disability: Implications for urban education. *Urban Education 44*(4), 389–409. doi:10.1177/0042085909338686

Bloom, E., & Heath, N. (2010). Recognition, expression, and understanding facial expressions of emotion in adolescents with nonverbal and general learning disabilities. *Journal of Learning Disabilities, 43,* 180–192. doi:10.1177/0022219409345014

Bryan, T.H. (1986). Self-concept and attributions of the learning disabled. *Learning Disability Focus, 1,* 82–89.

Carney J., & Porter P. (2009). School reentry for children with acquired central nervous systems injuries. *Developmental Disabilities Research Reviews, 15*(2), 152–158. doi:10.1002/ddrr.57

Casey, M.B., Cohen, M., Schuerholz, L.J., Singer, H.S., & Denckia, M.B. (2000). Language-based cognitive functioning in parents of offspring with ADHD comorbid for Tourette syndrome or learning disability. *Developmental Neuropsychology, 17,* 85–110. doi:10.1207/S15326942DN1701_06

Cirino, P.T., Israelian, M.K., Morris, M.K., & Morris, R.D. (2005). Evaluation of the double-deficit hypothesis in college students referred for learning difficulties. *Journal of Learning Disabilities, 38,* 29–44. doi:10.1177/00222194050380010301

Clark, D.B., & Uhry, J.K. (1995). *Dyslexia: Theory and practice of remedial instruction* (2nd ed.). Timonium, MD: York Press.

Clay, R.A. (2011). Revising the DSM. *Monitor on Psychology, 42,* 1, 54.

Cohen Kadosh, R., & Walsh, V. (2007). Dyscalculia. *Current Biology, 17*(22), R946–R947. doi:10.1016/j.cub.2007.08.038

Council for Exceptional Children. (2005, August). *CEC's Update on IDEA reauthorization.* Retrieved December 12, 2011, from http://www.cec.sped.org/content/Navigation Menu/Policy/Advocacy/IDEA Resources/IDEA Reauthorization Timeline.

Cutting, L.E., Koth, L.W., & Denckla, M.B. (2000). How children with neurofibromatosis Type I differ from "typical" learning disability clinic attenders: Nonverbal learning disability revisited. *Developmental Neuropsychology, 17,* 29–47.

Dehaene, S., & Cohen, L. (1995). Toward an anatomical and functional model of number processing. *Math Cognition, 1,* 83–120.

Denckla, M.B. (1993). The child with developmental disabilities grown up: Adult residua of childhood disorders. *Neurology Clinics, 11,* 105–125.

Deshler, D.D., Mellard, D.F., Tollefson, J.M., & Byrd, S.E. (2005). Research topics in Responsiveness to intervention: Introduction to the special series. *Journal of Learning Disabilities, 38,* 483–484. doi:10.1177/0022219405038006010

Desoete, A., Roeyers, H., & Buysse, A. (2001). Metacognition and mathematical problem solving in grade 3. *Journal of Learning Disabilities, 34,* 435–449. doi:10.1177/002221940103400505

Dirks, E., Spyer, G., van Lieshout, E.C.D.M., & de Sonneville, L. (2008). Prevalence of combined reading and arithmetic disabilities. *Journal of Learning Disabilities, 41,* 460–473.

Donlan, C. (2007). Mathematical development in children with specific language impairments. In D.B. Berch & M.M.M. Mazzocco (Eds.), *Why is math so hard for some children?: The nature and origins of mathematical learning difficulties and disabilities* (pp. 151–172). Baltimore, MD: Paul H. Brookes Publishing Co.

Duquette, C., & Fullarton, S. (2009). "With an LD you're always mediocre and expect to be mediocre": Perceptions of adults recently diagnosed with learning disabilities. *Exceptionality Education International, 19*(1), 55–71.

Eden, G.F., Jones, K.M., Cappell, K., Gareau, L., Wood, F.B., Zeffiro, T.A., & Flowers, D.L. (2004). Neural changes following remediation in adult developmental dyslexia. *Neuron, 44,* 411–422.

Englert, C.S. (1992). Writing instruction from a sociocultural perspective: The holistic, dialogic, and social enterprise of writing. *Journal of Learning Disabilities, 25,* 153–172. doi:10.1177/002221949202500303

Erlbaum, B., & Vaughn, S. (2003). For which students with learning disabilities are self-concept interventions effective? *Journal of Learning Disabilities, 36,* 101–108.

Fisher, S.E., & DeFries, J.C. (2002). Developmental dyslexia: Genetic dissection of a complex cognitive trait. *Nature Reviews Neuroscience, 3,* 767–780. doi:10.1038/nrn936

Fletcher, J.M., Lyon, G.R., Fuchs, L.S., & Barnes, M.A. (2007). *Learning disabilities: From identification to intervention.* New York, NY: Guilford Press.

Fletcher, J.M., Shaywitz, S.E., Shankweiler, D., Katz, L., Liberman, I., Stuebing, K.K., … Shaywitz, B.A. (1994). Cognitive profiles of reading disability: Comparisons of discrepancy and low achievement definitions. *Journal of Educational Psychology, 86,* 6–23. doi:10.1037//0022-0663.86.1.6

Francis, D.J., Fletcher, J.M., Stuebing, K.K., Lyon, G.R., Shaywitz, B.A., & Shaywitz, S.E. (2005). Psychometric approaches to the identification of LD: IQ and achievement scores are not sufficient. *Journal of Learning Disabilities, 38,* 98–108. doi:10.1177/0022219405038002010

Fuchs, L.S., & Fuchs, D. (2002). Mathematical problem-solving profiles of students with mathematical disabilities with and without comorbid reading difficulties. *Journal of Learning Disabilities, 35,* 563–573.

Fuchs, D., Mock, D., Morgan, P.L., & Young, C.L. (2003). Responsiveness-to-intervention: Definitions, evidence, and implications for the learning disabilities construct. *Learning Disabilities Research and Practice, 18*, 157–171. doi:10.1111/1540-5826.00072

Gabrieli, J.D. (2009). Dyslexia: A new synergy between education and cognitive neuroscience. *Science, 325*(5938), 280–283. doi:10.1126/science.1171999

Gans, A.M., Kenny, M.C., & Ghany, D.L. (2003). Comparing the self-concept of students with and without learning disabilities. *Journal of Learning Disabilities, 36*, 287–295. doi:10.1177/002221940303600307

Geary, D.C. (2004). Mathematics and learning disabilities. *Journal of Learning Disabilities, 37*, 4–15.

Geary, D.C., & Hoard, M.K. (2005). Learning disabilities in arithmetic and mathematics: Theoretical and empirical perspectives. In J.I.D. Campbell (Ed.), *Handbook of mathematical cognition* (pp. 253–267). New York, NY: Psychology Press.

Gersten, R., Jordan, N.C., & Flojo, J.R. (2005). Early identification and interventions for students with mathematics difficulties. *Journal of Learning Disabilities, 38*, 293–304. doi:10.1177/00222194050380040301

Gillingham, A., & Stillman, B.W. (1997). *The Gillingham manual: Remedial training for children with specific disabilities in reading, spelling, and penmanship* (8th ed.). Cambridge, MA: Educators Publishing Service.

Gortmaker. V.J., Daly, E.J., McCurdy, M., Persampieri, M.J., & Hergenrader, M. (2007). Improving reading outcomes for children with learning disabilities using brief experimental analysis to develop parent-tutoring interventions. *Journal of Applied Behavior Analysis, 40*, 203–221. doi:10.1901/jaba.2007.105-05

Graham, S., & Harris, K.R. (1989). Components analysis of cognitive strategy instruction: Effects on learning disabled students' compositions and self-efficacy. *Journal of Educational Psychology, 81*(3) 353–361. doi:10.1037//0022-0663.81.3.353

Gregg, N., & Scott, S.S. (2000). Definition and documentation: Theory, measurement, and the courts. *Journal of Learning Disabilities, 33*, 5–13. doi:10.1177/002221940003300104

Grigorenko, E.L. (2009). Dynamic assessment and response to intervention: Two sides of one coin. *Journal of Learning Disabilities, 42*, 111–132. doi:10.1177/0022219408326207

Harris, K.R., & Pressley, M. (1991). The nature of cognitive strategy instruction: Interactive strategy construction. *Exceptional Children, (57)*, 392–404.

Hay, I., Elias, G., Fielding-Barnsley, R., Homel, R., & Freibery, K. (2007). Language delays, reading delays, and learning difficulties: Interactive elements requiring multidimensional programming. *Journal of Learning Disabilities, 40*, 400–409. doi:10.1177/00222194070400050301

Hughes, C.A., & Smith, J.O. (1990). Cognitive and academic performance of college students with learning disabilities: A synthesis of the literature. *Learning Disabilities Quarterly, 13*, 66–79. doi:10.2307/1510393

Individuals with Disabilities Education Act Amendments of 1997, PL 105-17, 20 U.S.C. §§1400 *et seq*

Individuals with Disabilities Education Improvement Act of 2004, PL 108-446, 20 U.S.C. §§1400 *et seq.*

International Reading Association & National Association for the Education of Young Children. (1998). Learning to read and write: Developmentally appropriate practices for young children. *Young Children, 53*, 30–46.

Jones, F.W., Long, K., & Finlay, W.M.L. (2007). Symbols can improve the reading comprehension of adults with learning disabilities. *Journal of Intellectual Disability Research, 51*(7), 545–550. doi:10.1111/j.1365-2788.2006.00926.x

Jordan, N.C. (2007). Do words count? Connections between mathematics and reading difficulties. In D.B. Berch & M.M.M. Mazzocco (Eds.), *Why is math so hard for some children?: The nature and origins of mathematical learning difficulties and disabilities.* (pp. 107–120). Baltimore, MD: Paul H. Brookes Publishing Co.

Jordan, N.C., Hanich, L.B., & Kaplan, D. (2003). A longitudinal study of mathematical competencies in children with specific mathematics difficulties versus children with comorbid mathematics and reading difficulties. *Child Development, 74*, 834–850. doi:10.1111/1467-8624.00571

Kamil, M.L., Pearson, P.D., Moje, E.B., & Afflerbach, P. (Eds.). (2010). *Handbook of reading research: Vol. IV.* New York, NY: Routledge.

Kavale, K.A. & Spaulding, L.S. (2008). Is response to intervention good policy for specific learning disability? *Learning Disabilities Research & Practice, 23*, 169–179. doi:10.1111/j.1540-5826.2008.00274.x

Keeler, M.K., & Swanson, H.L. (2001). Does strategy knowledge influence working memory in children with math disabilities? *Journal of Learning Disabilities, 34*, 418–434.

Kennedy, M.J., & Deshler, D.D. (2010). Literacy instruction, technology, and students with learning disabilities: Research we have, research we need. *Learning Disabilities Quarterly, 33*, 4, 289-98.

Lembke, E., & Foegen, A. (2009). Identifying early numeracy indicators for kindergarten and first grade students. *Learning Disabilities Research and Practice, 24*, 12–20. doi:10.1111/j.1540-5826.2008.01273.x

Lindamood, P., & Lindamood, P.C. (1998). *Lindamood phoneme sequencing program for reading, spelling, and speech.* Austin, TX: PRO-ED.

Litt, J., Taylor, H.G., Klein, N., & Hack, M. (2005). Learning disabilities in children with very low birthweight: Prevalence, neuropsychological correlates, and educational interventions. *Journal of Learning Disabilities, 38*, 130–141. doi:10.1177/00222194050380020301

Liu, Y., Ortiz, A.A., Wilkinson, C.Y., Robertson, P., & Kushner, M.I. (2008). From early childhood special education to special education resource rooms: Identification, assessment, and eligibility determinations for English language learners with reading-related disabilities. *Assessment for Effective Intervention, 33*, 177–187. doi:10.1177/1534508407313247

Lovett, M.W., & Steinbach, K.A. (1997). The effectiveness of remedial programs for reading disabled children of different ages: Does the benefit decrease for older children? *Learning Disability Quarterly, 20*, 189–210. doi:10.2307/1511308

Lyon, G.R., Shaywitz, S.E., & Shaywitz, B.A. (2003). A definition of dyslexia. *Annals of Dyslexia, 53*, 1–14. doi:10.1007/s11881-003-0001-9

Maag, J.W., & Reid, R. (2006). Depression among students with learning disabilities: Assessing the risk. *Journal of Learning Disabilities, 39*, 3–10. doi:10.1177/00222194060390010201

Mabbott, D.J., & Bisanz, J. (2008). Computational skills, working memory, and conceptual knowledge in older children with mathematics learning disabilities. *Journal of Learning Disabilities, 41*, 15–28. doi:10.1177/0022219407311003

MacArthur, C.A. (2009). Reflections on research on writing and technology for struggling writers. *Learning Disabilities Research & Practice. 24*(2), 93–103. doi:10.1111/j.1540-5826.2009.00283.x

Mann, V. (1994). Phonological skills and the prediction of early reading problems. In N.C. Jordan & J. Goldsmith-Phillips (Eds.), *Learning disabilities: New directions for assessment and intervention* (pp. 67–84). Needham Heights, MA: Allyn & Bacon.

Manor, O., Shalev, R., Joseph, A., & Gross-Tsur, V. (2001). Arithmetic skills in kindergarten children with developmental language disorders. *European Pediatric Neurology Society, 5*, 71–77. doi:10.1053/ejpn.2001.0468

Marshall, R.M., Schafer, V.A., O'Donnell, L., Elliott, J., & Handwerk, M.L. (1999). Arithmetic disabilities and ADHD subtypes: Implications for *DSM-IV. Journal of Learning Disabilities, 32*, 239–247.

Mason, L.H., & Graham, S. (2008). Writing instruction for adolescents with learning disabilities: Programs of intervention research. *Learning Disabilities Research and Practice, 23*, 103–112. doi:10.1111/j.1540-5826.2008.00268.x

Mason, A., & Mason, M. (2005). Understanding college students with learning disabilities. *Pediatric Clinics of North America, 52*, 61–70. doi:10.1016/j.pcl.2004.11.001

Mazzocco, M.M.M. (2001). Math learning disability and math LD subtypes: Evidence from studies of Turner syndrome, fragile X syndrome, and Neurofibromatosis type 1. *Journal of Learning Disabilities, 34*, 520–533. doi:10.1177/002221940103400605

Mazzocco, M.M.M. (2007). Defining and differentiating mathematical learning disabilities and difficulties. In D.B. Berch & M.M.M. Mazzocco (Eds.), *Why is math so hard for some children?* (pp. 29–48). Baltimore, MD: Paul H. Brookes Publishing Co.

Mazzocco, M.M.M., Feigenson, L., & Halberda, J. (2011). Impaired acuity of the approximate number system underlies mathematical learning disability (dyscalculia). *Child Development, 82*, 1224–1237. doi:10.1111/j.1467-8624.2011.01608.x

McLean, J.F., & Hitch, G.J. (1999). Working memory impairments in children with specific arithmetic learning difficulties. *Journal of Experimental Child Psychology, 74*(3), 240–260. doi:10.1006/jecp.1999.2516

McNamara, J., Vervaeke, S.L., & Willoughby, T. (2008). Learning disabilities and risk-taking behavior in adolescents: A comparison of those with and without comorbid attention-deficit/hyperactivity disorder. *Journal of Learning Disabilities, 41*, 561–574. doi:10.1177/0022219408326096

Mercer, C.D., & Pullen P.C. (2004). *Students with learning disabilities* (6th ed.). Upper Saddle River, NJ: Merrill.

Moss, B., Lapp, D., & O'Shea, M. (2011). Tiered texts: Supporting knowledge and language learning for English learners and struggling readers. *English Journal, 100*, 54–60.

Murray, C., & Wren, C.T. (2003). Cognitive, academic, and attitudinal predictors of the grade point averages of college students. *Journal of Learning Disabilities, 36*, 407–415. doi:10.1177/00222194030360050201

Natale, K., Aunola, K., Nurmi, J.-E., Poikkeus, A.-M., Lyytinen, P., & Lyytinen, H. (2008). Mothers' causal attributions concerning the reading achievement of their children with and without familial risk for dyslexia. *Journal of Learning Disabilities, 41*, 274–285. doi:10.1177/0022219408316094

National Association of Special Education Teachers. (2007). *LD report: Introduction to learning disabilities.* Retrieved July 26, 2011, from http://www.naset.org/2522.0.html

National Center for Educational Statistics. (2010). *The condition of education: Number and percentage distribution of 3- to 21-year-olds served under the Individuals with Disabilities Act (IDEA), Part B, and number served as a percentage of total public school enrollment, by type of disability: Selected school years, 1980-81 through 200809.* Retrieved December 12, 2011, from http://nces.ed.gov/programs/coe/tables/table-cwd-1asp.

National Institute of Child Health and Human Development. (2000). *Report of the National Reading Panel: Teaching children to read. An evidence-based assessment of the scientific research literature on reading and its implications for reading instruction.* Retrieved January 8, 2002, from http://nationalreadingpanel.org/publications.htm.

Nicholls, J.G., McKenzie, M., & Shufro, J. (1994). Schoolwork, homework, life's work: The experience of students with and without learning disabilities. *Journal of Learning Disabilities, 27*, 562–569. doi:10.1177/002221949402700903

No Child Left Behind Act of 2001, PL 107-110. Washington DC: 115 Stat. 1425.

Olitsky, S.E., & Nelson, L.B. (2003). Reading disorders in children. *Pediatric Clinics of North America, 50*, 213–224. doi:10.1016/S0031-3955(02)00104-9

Paneque, O.M., & Barbetta, P.M. (2006). A study of teacher efficacy of special education teachers of English language learners with disabilities. *Bilingual Research Journal, 30*, 171–193. doi:10.1080/15235882.2006.10162871

Pennington, B.F. (1991). Genetics of learning disabilities. *Seminars in Neurology, 11*, 28–34. doi:10.1055/s-2008-1041202

Powell, S.R., Fuchs, L.S., Fuchs, D., Cirino, P.T., & Fletcher, J.M. (2009). Do word-problem features differentially affect problem difficulty as a function of students' mathematics difficulty with without reading difficulty? *Journal of Learning Disabilities, 42*, 99–110. doi:10.1177/0022219408326211

Pullen, P.C., Tuckwiller, E.D., Konod, T.R., Maynard, K., & Coyne, M.D. (2010). A tiered intervention model for early vocabulary insuruction: The effects of tiered instruction for young student at risk for learning disabilities. *Learning Disabilities Research & Practice, 25*, 3, 110–123.

Raghubar, K., Cirino, P., Barnes, M., Ewing-Cobbs, L., Fletcher, J., & Fuchs, L. (2009). Errors in multi-digit arithmetic and behavioral inattention in children with math difficulties. *Journal of Learning Disabilities, 42*, 356–371.

Ramaswami, R. (2010). Reshaping RTI: Building a better triangle. *T.H.E. Journal, 37*(8), 34-35.

Reid, B. (2005). *Cognitive strategy instruction.* UNL, University of Nebraska. Retrieved on December 12, 2011, from http//www.unl.edu/csi/Teaching Strategy.shtml.

Reschly, D.J. (2008). Learning disabilities identification: Primary intervention, secondary intervention, and then what? *Journal of Learning Disabilities, 38*, 510–515. doi:10.1177/0022219405380060601

Ritchey, K.D., & Goeke, J.L. (2006). Orton-Gillingham and Orton-Gillingham based reading instruction: A review of the literature. *The Journal of Special Education, 40*(3), 171–183. doi:10.1177/00224669060400030501

Rourke, B.P., & Finlayson, M.A.J. (1978). Neuropsychological significance of variations in patterns of academic performance: Verbal and visual-spatial abilities. *Journal of Abnormal Child Psychology, 6*, 121–133. doi:10.1007/BF00915788

Sandak R., Mencl, W.E., Frost, S.J., & Pugh, K.R. (2004). The neurobiological basis of skilled and impaired reading: Recent findings and new directions. *Scientific Studies of Reading, 8*, 273–292. doi:10.1207/s1532799xssr0803_6

Satz, P., Buka, S., Lipsitt, L., Seldman, L. 1998). The long-term prognosis of learning disabled children. In B.K. Shapiro, P.J. Accardo, & A.J. Capute (Eds.), *Specific reading disability: A view of the spectrum* (pp. 223–250). Timonium, MD: York Press.

Scerri, T.S., & Schulte-Körne, G. (2010). Genetics of developmental dyslexia. *European Child & Adolescent Psychiatry, 19*(3), 179–197. doi:10.1007/s00787-009-0081-0

Schatschneider, C., & Torgesen, J. (2004). Using our current understanding of dyslexia to support early identification and intervention. *Journal of Child Neurology, 19*, 759–765.

Schuchardt, K., Maehler, C., & Hasselhorn, M. (2008). Working memory deficits in children with specific learning disorders. *Journal of Learning Disabilities, 41*, 514–523. doi:10.1177/0022219408317856

Schneider, W. (2008). The development of metacognitive knowledge in children and adolescents: Major trends and implications for education. *Mind, Brain, and Education, 2*(3), 114–121. doi:10.1111/j.1751-228X.2008.00041.x

Schulte, A.C., Conners, C.K., & Osborne, S.S. (1999). Linkages between attention deficit disorders and reading disability. In D.D. Duane (Ed.), *Reading and attention disorders: Neurobiological correlates* (pp. 161–184). Timonium, MD: York Press.

Seo, Y., Abbott, R.D., & Hawkins, J.D. (2008). Outcome status of students with learning disabilities at ages 21 and 24. *Journal of Learning Disabilities, 41*, 300–314. doi:10.1177/0022219407311308

Sexson, S.B., & Madan-Swain, A. (1993). School reentry for the child with chronic illness. *Journal of Learning Disabilities, 26*, 115–137. doi:10.1177/002221949302600204

Shalev, R.S. (2004). Developmental dyscalculia. *Journal of Child Neurology, 19*, 765–771.

Shalev, R.S., & Gross-Tsur, V. (2001). Developmental dyscalculia. *Pediatric Neurology, 24*, 337–342.

Shalev, R.S., Manor, O., & Gross-Tsur, V. (2005). Developmental dyscalculia: A prospective six-year study. *Developmental Medicine and Child Neurology, 47*, 121–125.

Shaywitz, B.A., Shaywitz, S.E., Blachman, B.A., Pugh, K.R., Fulbright, R.K., Skudlarski, P., … Gore, J.C. (2004). Development of left occipitotemporal systems for skilled reading in children after a phonologically based intervention. *Biological Psychiatry, 55*, 926–933. doi:10.1016/j.biopsych.2003.12.019

Shaywitz, S.E. (2005). *Overcoming dyslexia: A new and complete science-based program for reading problems at any level*. New York, NY: Vintage. doi:10.1056/NEJM199201163260301

Shaywitz, S.E., & Shaywitz, B.A. (2005). Dyslexia (specific reading disability). *Biological Psychiatry, 57*, 1301–1309. doi:10.1016/j.biopsych.2005.01.043

Simos, P.G., Fletcher, J.M., Foorman, B.R., Francis, D.J., Castillo, E.M., Davis, R.N., … Papanicolaou, A.C. (2002). Brain activation profiles during the early stages of reading acquisition. *Journal of Child Neurology, 17*, 159–163. doi:10.1177/08830738020170030 1

Talcott, J.B., Witton, C., McLean, M.F., Hansen, P.C., Rees, A., Green, G.G.R., & Stein, J.F. (2000). From the cover: Dynamic sensory sensitivity and children's word decoding skills. *Proceedings of the National Academy of Sciences of the United States of America, 97*, 2952–2957. doi:10.1073/pnas.040546597

Turkeltaub, P.E., Gareau, L., Flowers D.L., Zeffiro, T.A., & Eden, G.F. (2003). Development of neural mechanisms for reading. *Nature Neuroscience, 6*, 767–773. doi:10.1038/nn1065

U.S. Department of Education, National Center for Education Statistics. (2008). *Table 390—Current postsecondary education and employment status, wages earned, and living arrangements of special education students out of secondary school up to 4 years, by type of disability*: 2005. Retrieved from http://nces.ed.gov/progams/digest/d08/tables/dt08_390.asp

U.S. Department of Labor, Secretary's Commission on Achieving Necessary Skills (SCANS). (1992). *Learning a living: A blueprint for high performance. A SCANS report for AMERICA 2000*. Washington, DC: U.S. Government Printing Office.

Van Garderen, D. (2007). Teaching students with LD to use diagrams to solve mathematical word problems. *Journal of Learning Disabilities, 40*(6), 540–556. doi:10.1177/00222194070400060501

Vaughn, S., & Fuchs, L.S. (2003). Redefining learning disabilities as inadequate response to instruction: The promise and potential problems. *Learning Disabilities Research & Practice, 18*, 137–146. doi:10.1111/1540-5826.00070

Vellutino, F.R., Fletcher, J.M., Snowling, M.J., & Scanlon, D.M. (2004). Specific reading disability (dyslexia): What have we learned in the past four decades? *Journal of Child Psychology and Psychiatry, 45*, 2–40. doi:10.1046/j.0021-9630.2003.00305.x

Vukovic, R.K., & Siegel, L.S. (2006). The double-deficit hypothesis: A comprehensive analysis of the evidence. *Journal of Learning Disabilities, 39*, 25–47. doi:10.1177/00222194060390010401

Waber, D.P., Forbes, P.W., Wolff, P.H., & Weiler, M.D. (2004). Neurodevelopmental characteristics of children with learning impairments classified according to the double-deficit hypothesis. *Journal of Learning Disabilities 37*(5), 451–461. doi:10.1177/00222194040370050701

Wechsler, D. (2003). *Wechsler Intelligence Scale for Children–Fourth Edition (WISC-IV)*. San Antonio, TX: Pearson.

Williams, D.L., Goldstein, G., Kojkowski, N., & Minshew, N.J. (2008). Do individuals with higher functioning autism have the IQ profile associated with nonverbal learning disabilities? *Research in Autism Spectrum Disorders, 2*(2), 353–361.

Wolf, M., & Bowers, P.G. (1999). The double-deficit hypothesis for the developmental dyslexias. *Journal of Educational Psychology, 91*, 415–438. doi:10.1037//0022-0663.91.3.415

Wolf, M., Bowers, P., & Biddle, K. (2000). Naming-speed processes, timing, and reading: A conceptual review. *Journal of Learning Disabilities, 33*, 387–407. doi:10.1177/002221940003300409

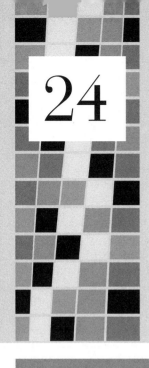

24

Cerebral Palsy

Alexander H. Hoon, Jr., and Frances Tolley

Upon completion of this chapter, the reader will

- Understand the definition and causes of cerebral palsy
- Understand how cerebral palsy is diagnosed
- Know the clinical characteristics of the various forms of cerebral palsy
- Know the sensory, cognitive, and medical problems commonly associated with cerebral palsy
- Understand the range of management options available to help children with cerebral palsy reach their full potential
- Be knowledgeable about the medical and functional prognoses for cerebral palsy

Many children with cerebral palsy (CP) first come to professional attention because of delayed motor milestones, particularly walking. Most parents know that children begin walking at about 1 year of age, and there is an implicit understanding that a child's first steps mark the transition from infancy to toddlerhood. When a young child does not reach this transition at the expected time, alarm bells sound.

■ ■ ■ JAMAL

Jamal is a 15-month-old boy seen by his pediatrician for a routine well-child checkup. His mother expressed her worry that Jamal was not yet walking. His pediatrician had previously documented mild delays in motor development at the 12-month office visit. This was attributed to the fact that he was born at 28 weeks' gestation, with a birth weight of 900 grams, following spontaneous labor associated with maternal chorioamnionitis (an infection of the membranes surrounding the fetus). In the neonatal intensive care unit (NICU), he required ventilatory support for 5 days. At 2 weeks of age, a cranial ultrasound study suggested an abnormality of brain white matter (see Chapter 7).

At his 12-month well-child checkup, his mother noted that Jamal had been sitting for about 2 months. His pediatrician explained to his mother that based on age adjustment for prematurity (9 months corrected age), he was only mildly delayed compared with chronological age expectations. Jamal's leg muscles were a little stiff, but his pediatrician knew that many premature infants have mild, temporary abnormalities of muscle tone that often resolve by 15–18 months of age.

On examination at 15 months, Jamal could crawl stiffly on all fours but was not yet pulling up to a standing position. He showed a pronounced tendency to keep his legs stiffly extended with his toes pointed and his feet crossed at the ankles (scissoring). At this point, his pediatrician expressed concern that he had CP.

WHAT IS CEREBRAL PALSY?

CP describes a group of chronic childhood motor impairment disorders defined by specific functional characteristics rather than by the underlying cause. The hallmarks of CP are limitations in mobility and hand use in association with signs of neurological dysfunction. CP is characterized by impaired control of movement and posture that appears early in life (Jacobsson et al., 2008). There is variability in overall motor function, with commonly associated nonmotor impairments in sensation, cognition, communication, and behavior. There are also commonly associated medical conditions, including strabismus and epilepsy (Bax et al., 2005).

The clinical features of CP are the result of developmental disturbances that occur during early brain development, leading to brain malformation or injury. These disorders most often occur during fetal development or in the perinatal period, but they may also arise during the first years of life. Prematurity, low birth weight, multiple-gestation pregnancy, infection/inflammation, hypoxia-ischemia, and a variety of genetic factors can underlie the development of CP (Pakula, Van Naarden Braun, & Yeargin-Allsopp, 2009).

Although CP is considered a static (nonprogressive) insult, its functional manifestations can "progress" in several different ways. For example, children with early hypotonia associated with birth asphyxia may develop spasticity or dystonia years later (Scott & Jankovic, 1996). This may be of the result of maladaptive plasticity (Johnston, 2009), wherein brain rewiring is faulty. As another example, adults with dyskinetic forms of CP (see Subtypes of Cerebral Palsy) are prone to develop secondary spinal cord compression from long-term abnormal repetitive head and cervical spine movements. This leads to progressive weakness and loss of function (see Figure 24.1). Finally, there may be progressive orthopedic deformities secondary to spasticity, chronic muscle shortening, and joint dislocations.

WHAT CAUSES CEREBRAL PALSY?

The underlying causes and risk factors leading to the development of CP disrupt the development of neuronal networks in cortical and subcortical pathways that control movement. A key concept in understanding the causes of CP is **selective vulnerability** (Johnston, 1998). This term refers to a susceptibility of specific regions and cells to injury during specific time periods in brain development. Between 24–34 weeks of gestation, immature oligodendrocytes

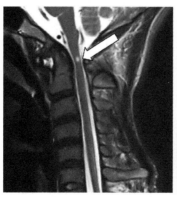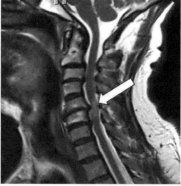

Figure 24.1. The white arrows point to areas of injury in the cervical spinal cord of two adults with dyskinetic (extrapyramidal) cerebral palsy as a result of cord compression from the chronic stress placed on the cervical spine (C-spine) from repetitive movement. These findings require emergent spinal fusion to stabilize the neck and to prevent the development of acute paralysis. Adults with cerebral palsy and new neurological findings should have a brain magnetic resonance imaging (MRI) and C-spine MRI.

(white matter cells that wrap myelin around axons) are susceptible to injury. This contrasts with full-term infants, where the vulnerability lies in deep grey matter neurons in the basal ganglia and thalamus. In children born preterm with spastic forms of CP, periventricular white matter injury, or periventricular leukomalacia (PVL), is linked to oligodendrocyte injury. In term infants with asphyxia (perinatal hypoxic-ischemic encephalopathy, HIE) or kernicterus (resulting from markedly elevated bilirubin levels), the injury in deep grey matter structures is often linked with dyskinetic (dystonic) forms of CP (see Figure 24.2). The recognition of selective vulnerability has led to new treatment approaches in the NICU setting, including the use of hypothermia (lowering body temperature) to ameliorate brain injury in term infants with HIE (Barks, 2008).

A common misconception is that most cases of CP result from birth asphyxia (HIE; see Chapter 6). HIE is defined as a disruption of blood flow (ischemia) and oxygen supply (hypoxia) to the brain as a consequence of problems encountered at the time of birth (MacLennan, Nelson, Hankins, & Speer, 2010). It is now clear that birth asphyxia is the cause of CP in only 10%–20% of affected children (Hankins & Speer, 2003; Nelson & Grether, 1999; Pschirrer & Yeomans, 2000).

A key concept in addressing CP is the recognition that understanding the underlying cause improves overall management. Approaching diagnosis with a full appreciation of the wide range of genetic etiologies promotes the identification of certain rare but often treatable disorders, such as dopa-responsive dystonia, which is treatable with levodopa (Mink, 2003), mitochondrial disorders (Koene & Smeitink, 2009), and organic acidemias (Seashore, 2009), treatable with metabolic therapies. Etiologic diagnosis is also of benefit in establishing both prognosis and recurrence risk in future pregnancies (Hemminki, Li, Sundquist, & Sundquist, 2007).

EPIDEMIOLOGY

In the developed world, CP affects about 2 in 1,000 children (Himmelmann, Hagberg, & Uvebrant, 2010). In developed countries, CP is most commonly associated with prematurity and low birth weight. Approximately 50,000 very low birth weight (less than 1,500 grams) infants are born in the United States each year, of whom 10%–15% develop spastic CP and 20%–50% develop disorders of higher cortical function, including learning disabilities and intellectual disability (Volpe, 2005). The incidence of CP increases with decreasing gestation and may occur in up to 20% of infants born before 28 weeks of gestation (Ancel et al., 2006). Despite advances in perinatal management over the last 20–30 years, the incidence of CP in term infants has not changed. This is consistent with the understanding that CP in full-term infants most commonly results from prenatal insults or genetic conditions that are independent of factors associated with delivery (Nelson & Ellenberg, 1986).

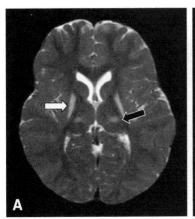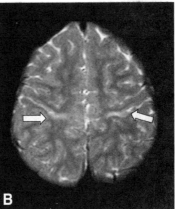

Figure 24.2. These images demonstrate the selective vulnerability of specific regions in the brain in infants born at term with asphyxia. A) The white arrow points to injury in the putamen; the black arrow points to injury in the thalamus. B) The white arrows point to injury in the motor cortex. This pattern of injury often leads to dyskinetic (dystonic) cerebral palsy, with limitations in speech and hand use.

RISK FACTORS

Infection

Both indirect (passed from the mother) and direct infection of the fetus and/or newborn infant have been shown to be associated with CP (Bale, 2009). In term and preterm infants, direct infection of the fetus by viruses such as cytomegalovirus and rubella (Lombardi, Garofoli, & Stronati, 2010) and other infectious agents (e.g., toxoplasmosis, a parasitic infection) has long been a recognized cause of CP. Bacterial meningitis in the newborn also remains a significant cause of CP (Galiza & Heath, 2009).

There has been increasing recognition that chorioamnionitis may play a key role in the genesis of CP in preterm infants (Shatrov et al., 2010). Chorioamnionitis predisposes to premature delivery and may also have direct adverse effects on the fetal brain (Jacobsson, 2004; Yoon, Park, & Chaiworapongsa, 2003). Complex relationships exist between chorioamnionitis, fetal cytokines (proteins that regulate the immune response), and other factors that can lead to white matter injury in children born preterm.

In the term infant there is an association between maternal infection, fever, and CP (Nelson & Chang, 2008). Infection during pregnancy may also promote blood hypercoagulation, leading to stroke-like events in the fetus (Leviton & Dammann, 2004; Nelson & Lynch, 2004). Finally, placental infection may contribute to the development of HIE (Wu, 2002).

Prematurity-Related Cerebral Palsy

Premature infants, especially those born prior to 28–32 weeks of gestation or with a birth weight less than 1,500 grams, represent almost half of all individuals with CP (Hagberg, Hagberg, Beckung, & Ubrevant, 2001; Marlow, Wolke, Bracewell, & Samara, 2005; O'Shea, 2002; Reddihough & Collins, 2003; Vohret et al., 2005; Winter, Autry, Boyle, & Yeargin-Allsopp, 2002). The increased risk of CP in premature infants is related to complex interrelations between destructive and developmental mechanisms (Volpe, 2009). In premature infants, the two most common types of injury are PVL (see Figure 24.3) and intraventricular hemorrhage, or IVH (see Chapter 7). Immaturity of brain development predisposes premature infants to both of these conditions. In the late 1970s to early 1980s, cranial ultrasound and computed tomography linked CP with brain hemorrhage. In the later 1980s to early 1990s, the advent of magnetic resonance imaging (MRI) revealed that the major injury was in cerebral white matter. In the last decade, more advanced MRI modalities have shown that the white matter injury is accompanied by diffuse, variable injury in cortical, subcortical, and cerebellar gray matter (Kusters, Chen, Follett, & Dammann, 2009).

Volpe (2005) demonstrated that the abnormalities in neurons and axons are the result of changes in the normal developmental trajectory of brain development, often initiated by hypoxic-ischemic or infectious/inflammatory cascades of injury. These disturbances may explain the complex patterns of motor, learning, intellectual, and neurobehavioral impairments encountered in affected children.

Finally, in children such as Jamal, there is evidence, using the advanced MRI imaging technique diffusion tensor imaging, which shows white matter tracks, that functional impairment may result from injury to both

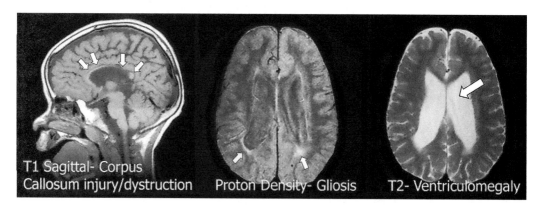

T1 Sagittal- Corpus Callosum injury/dystruction   Proton Density- Gliosis   T2- Ventriculomegaly

Figure 24.3. This MRI was taken in childhood from a child with PVL who had spastic quadriplegia. The arrows point to areas of injury or destruction of brain white matter (wiring). The enlarged ventricles (ventriculomegaly) are secondary to loss of surrounding brain tissue. (From Hoon, A.H., & Melhem, E.R. [2000]. Neuroimaging: Applications in disorders of early brain development. *Journal of Developmental and Behavioral Pediatrics, 21,* 291–302; reprinted by permission.)

sensory and motor cortical pathways (Hoon et al., 2009; Nagae et al., 2007; Figure 24.4).

Cerebral Palsy in Full-Term Infants

A wide variety of prenatal, perinatal, and genetic factors are linked with CP in full-term infants. These include birth asphyxia, congenital brain malformations, coagulation abnormalities, complications related to multiple-gestation pregnancies, and intrauterine infection/inflammation (Jacobsson et al., 2008; Nelson, 2008). Compared with those born prematurely, children born at term who subsequently develop CP are more often small for gestational age or have malformations inside and outside of the central nervous system (CNS), suggesting problems in early brain development (Krägeloh-Mann et al., 1995).

In full-term infants with severe birth asphyxia, who often develop dyskinetic (athetoid or dystonic) CP, the injury is often in the basal ganglia located deep in the center of the brain (Himmelmann et al., 2009). In the past, high bilirubin levels in the immediate postnatal period resulted in kernicterus, which led to choreoathetoid CP and to hearing impairment. Although kernicterus is rare now in developed countries, more subtle bilirubin-induced neurologic dysfunction (BIND) continues to be a concern (Shapiro, 2005).

DIAGNOSIS

CP is diagnosed clinically, based on the presence of delays in motor development and distinct abnormalities on the neurological examination. Although newborns may have known risk factors for CP (e.g., PVL, HIE), CP cannot be diagnosed at birth because the classic diagnostic signs are not apparent this early. Children with severe forms of CP are usually diagnosed in the first year of life, while those with less severe forms are usually diagnosed during the second year (Aneja, 2004; Palmer, 2004; Russman & Ashwal, 2004).

One of the key features of CP is the persistence of primitive reflexes. All infants are born with primitive reflexes. They are called "primitive" because they are present in early life (in some cases, during intrauterine development)

posterior thalamic radiation

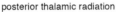

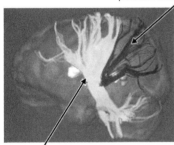

fibers penetrating
the posterior limb
of internal capsule

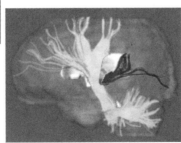

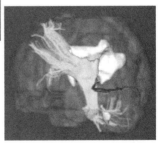

Figure 24.4. In this figure using diffusion tensor imaging and special software, three dimensional tracts of descending motor pathways (light gray fibers) and thalamocortical sensory tracts (black fibers) are shown in a typically developing child (left panel) and in two children with spastic cerebral palsy in association with preterm birth (middle and right panels). In the children with cerebral palsy, the primary injury is in the blackfibers corresponding to sensory pathways. (From Nagae, L.M., Hoon, Jr., A.H., Stashinko, E., Lin, D., Zhang, W., Levey, E., ... Mori, S. [2007]. Diffusion tensor imaging in children with periventricular leukomalacia: Variability of injuries to white matter tracts. *AJNR: American Journal of Neuroradiology, 28*[7], pp. 1213–1222; adapted by permission.)

and are thought to be controlled by the primitive regions of the nervous system (the spinal cord, the labyrinths of the inner ear, and the brain stem). Familiar examples of primitive reflexes include the suckling reflex and the hand-grasp reflex in the newborn. As the cortex matures, these reflexes are gradually suppressed and integrated into voluntary movement patterns (see Figure 24.5). The process of integration is usually complete by 12 months of age. In CP, however, these primitive reflex patterns tend to persist beyond early infancy. Among the primitive reflexes, the **asymmetric tonic neck reflex** (Figure 24.6) and the **tonic labyrinthine response** (Figure 24.7) are particularly helpful in the diagnosis of CP.

As primitive reflexes disappear in the typically developing child, **postural reactions** (also known as **automatic movement reactions**) emerge (Figure 24.8). Some of the more important of these reactions are the righting, equilibrium, and protective reactions which enable the child to develop more complex voluntary movement and better control of posture. These automatic movement responses serve as a precursor for the development of specific motor milestones, such as rolling over and sitting. In typically developing children, a protective reaction called the parachute response develops by 10–12 months of age. This reaction is manifested by forward extension of the arms when falling forward. Many children with CP have delayed or absent development of postural reactions, including this response, which makes walking inherently unsafe. CP may be viewed as the persistence of primitive reflexes combined with the lack of cortical maturation of postural reactions.

Upper Motor Neuron Dysfunction in Cerebral Palsy

The motor impairments in children with CP are secondary to injury in the upper motor neuron (UMN). The UMN system is not a discrete anatomical entity but refers collectively to the motor control systems based in the brain and spinal cord. The UMN system is distinguished from the lower motor neuron (LMN) system, which refers collectively to the peripheral nerves and the innervated muscles (Figure 24.9; see Chapter 12). The primary components of the UMN system are the **pyramidal tract** (also called the **corticospinal pathways**) and the extrapyramidal system (see Figure 24.10). These systems are differentially affected by disturbances to the developing brain.

UMN dysfunction is characterized by positive and negative signs. Positive signs include spasticity, **hyperreflexia** (increased deep tendon

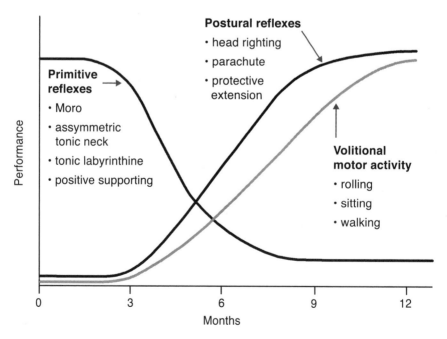

Figure 24.5. This figure illustrates the time course of primitive reflexes, postural reflexes, and volitional motor activity in typical motor development. (From Capute, A.J., Accardo, P.J., Vining, E.P.G., Rubenstein, J.E., & Harryman S. [1978]. *Primitive reflex profile*. Baltimore, MD: University Park Press; reprinted by permission.)

Full-term Infant Resting Position

Asymmetrical Tonic Neck Reflex

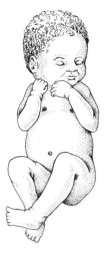
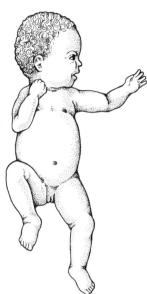
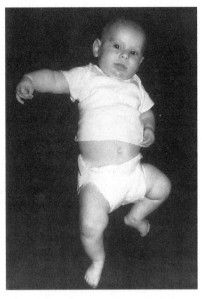

Figure 24.6. The asymmetric tonic neck reflex. In the typical newborn infant, when the head is actively or passively turned to the side, the arm and leg on the same side will extend and the arm and leg on the opposite side will flex, resulting in a "fencing" posture. The opposite pattern occurs when the head is turned to the other side. In typically developing infants, the reflex fades (is integrated) by about 6 months of age and is never obligatory (the infant can break through the pattern with spontaneous movement, even in the newborn period). In children with cerebral palsy, the reflex tends to be more pronounced, persists beyond the expected age, and may be obligatory.

reflexes, e.g., the knee jerk), **clonus** (alternate involuntary muscular contraction and relaxation in rapid succession), **flexor and extensor spasms** (spasms of bending of a limb toward or away from the body), and a positive **Babinski sign** (upgoing toe when the sole of the foot is stroked firmly). Negative signs include muscle weakness, loss of manual dexterity, and fatigability. The profile of positive signs tends to vary more from child to child and contributes to the classification of the subtypes of CP. It is the negative signs, however, that more directly impede motor function.

Walking

When a child is diagnosed with CP, one of the first questions parents pose is: "Will he or she walk?" In addressing this question, it is important to recognize that "walking" can refer to several levels of ability. A child may be able to walk independently or may need crutches or a walker. A child may be able to walk long distances (community ambulation), short distances only (household ambulation), or solely in the context of therapy (exercise ambulation). In general, children with better motor skills at a

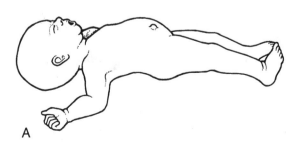
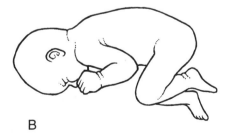

A   B

Figure 24.7. The tonic labyrinthine reflex. A) When the child is in the supine position with the head slightly extended, retraction of the shoulders and extension of the legs is observed. B) The opposite occurs when the infant is in the prone position with the head slightly flexed. In typically developing infants, the reflex pattern is barely evident in the newborn period; in children with cerebral palsy, the pattern may dominate posture and movement and may persist throughout life.

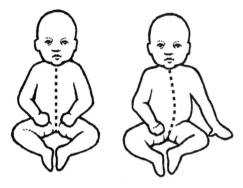

Figure 24.8. Automatic movement responses: the lateral prop reaction. At about 6 months of age, typically developing infants have already developed good postural control of the head and trunk (righting or equilibrium responses) and can stop themselves from falling forward when placed in the sitting position by extending their arms in front of them (forward prop response). By 6 months of age, most infants can also catch themselves when falling to the side by extending the arm on the same side (lateral prop response). This automatic movement reaction is critical for independent sitting and may be delayed or absent in children with cerebral palsy. (From Pellegrino, L., & Dormans, J.P. [1998]. Making the diagnosis of cerebral palsy. In J.P. Dormans & L. Pellegrino [Eds.], *Caring for children with cerebral palsy: A team approach* [p. 39; portion of Figure 2.4]. Baltimore, MD: Paul H. Brookes Publishing Co., Inc.; reprinted by permission.)

younger age (e.g., being able to sit and pull-to-stand before 2 years of age) have a better prognosis for walking than those with less well-developed skills.

The Gross Motor Function Classification System (GMFCS) can be used to estimate prognosis for walking (Rosenbaum et al., 2002; Wood & Rosenbaum, 2000). Children at any level within the classification scheme tend to stay at that level. In general, children at GMFCS Levels I or II will have a good prognosis for some degree of independent ambulation. Children at Levels III and IV will have a variable prognosis for walking with some form of assistance, and children at Level V have a poor prognosis for any type of walking. Precise probability curves for ambulation have been published and allow even more exact predictions of ambulatory potential based on motor functioning at 2½ years of age (Wu, Day, Strauss, & Shavelle, 2004). For example, using these curves it can be predicted that a child who is able to roll, sit independently, and pull-to-stand at 2½ years of age has a greater than 70% probability of being able to engage in some form of

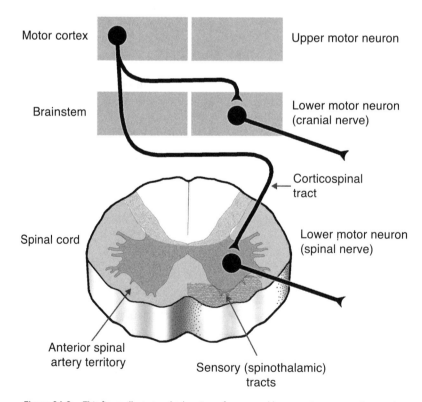

Figure 24.9. This figure illustrates the location of upper and lower motor neurons. Low motor neuron dysfunction is associated with peripheral neuropathies. (From Shrestha, S. [2010]. Lesions of upper motor neurons and lower motor neurons. *Medchrome Online Medical Magazine*, July 25, 2010. Retrieved from http://medchrome.com/basic-science/anatomy/lesions-of-upper-motor-neurons-and-lower-motor-neurons; reprinted by permission.)

ambulation by age 7 years. By contrast, a child who can roll but cannot sit or pull-to-stand at 2½ years has only a 25% chance of walking and would most likely do this with the help of an assistive device.

To walk, a child must be able to maintain an upright posture, move forward in a smoothly coordinated manner, and demonstrate protective responses for safety when falling. Even a child with mild CP has difficulty with the neurologic motor control required for ambulation. Common, treatable problems affecting gait include scissoring and equinus position of the feet. Scissoring occurs because of increased tone in the muscles that control adduction (movement toward the mid-line) and internal

rotation of the hips. Toe walking results from an equinus position of the feet (Figure 24.11) and increased extensor tone in the legs.

SUBTYPES OF CEREBRAL PALSY

CP is often divided into specific **phenotypes** (physical appearances) according to the neurological findings and body limbs that are predominately affected (Koman, Smith, & Shilt, 2004; Table 24.1; Figure 24.12). A recognized classification system divides the phenotypes into bilateral (both sides of the body affected) and unilateral (one side affected). This distinction is useful both in evaluating the underlying cause as well as directing management of CP.

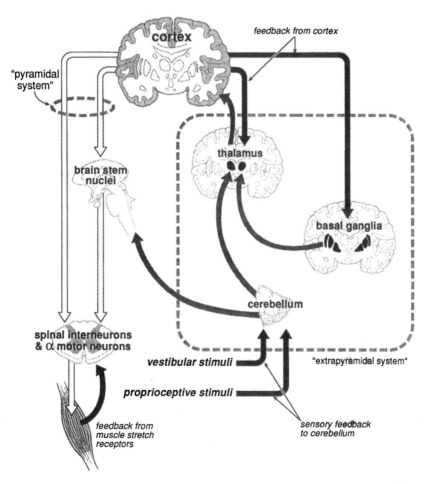

Figure 24.10. The motor control system. The upper motor neuron (UMN) system consists of the pyramidal and extrapyramidal systems. The pyramidal system connects the motor control center of the cortex to the brainstem and spinal cord and is responsible for the direct control of movement and muscle tone. The extrapyramidal system consists of deep brain structures (especially the basal ganglia and cerebellum) and works primarily by modifying and refining the output of the pyramidal system. The lower motor neuron (LMN) system consists of the muscles and the nerves that connect the muscles and the spinal cord, including the nerves that comprise the stretch reflex mechanism. (From Pellegrino, L., & Dormans, J.P. [1998]. Definitions, etiology, and epidemiology of cerebral palsy. In J.P. Dormans & L. Pellegrino [Eds.], *Caring for children with cerebral palsy: A team approach* [p. 10]. Baltimore, MD: Paul H. Brookes Publishing Co., Inc.; reprinted by permission.)

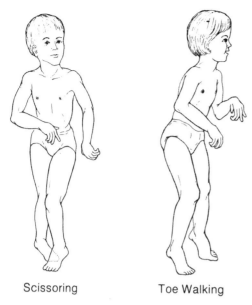

Scissoring   Toe Walking

Figure 24.11. Scissoring results from increased tone in the muscles on the inner aspect of the thigh that tend to pull the legs together and turn the legs inward. Toe walking is due to tightness of the calf muscles and Achilles tendon and increased extensor tone in the legs.

Spastic Cerebral Palsy

Spasticity is the abnormal increase in muscle tone resulting from an increased resistance to muscle stretch and lengthening. It restricts voluntary movement and, over time, leads to contractures (Barnes & Johnson, 2008). Spasticity is believed to arise from disruption of the descending pathways involved in motor control, including both pyramidal and parapyramidal pathways. The pyramidal system is composed of neurons (nerve cells) that extend from the motor cortex to the brain stem and spinal cord, the corticospinal tracks. These pathways directly control movement and influence muscle tone and deep tendon reflexes by inhibiting spinal cord mechanisms that direct these processes. In the absence of normal corticospinal inhibition, the spinal cord influences predominate, resulting in spasticity and a positive Babinski sign, two of the hallmarks of spastic CP. The parapyramidal fibers from

premotor cortex also contribute to spasticity and UMN signs.

Spastic CP is the most common type of CP (Krägeloh-Mann & Cans, 2009). It is further categorized according to the distribution of limbs involved. In **spastic diplegia**, the legs are more affected than the arms. This is the type of CP most frequently associated with prematurity. In **spastic quadriplegia**, all four limbs and usually the trunk and muscles that control the mouth, tongue, and pharynx are affected. The severity of the motor impairment in spastic quadriplegia implies wider cerebral dysfunction and a poorer outcome than for the other forms of spastic CP. Individuals with spastic quadriplegia often have intellectual disability, seizures, sensory impairments, and other medical problems. In **spastic hemiplegia**, one side of the body is more affected than the other; usually, the arm is more affected than the leg. Because the motor neurons that control one side of the body are located in the opposite cerebral cortex, a right-sided hemiplegia implies injury to the left side of the brain, and vice versa.

Dyskinetic Cerebral Palsy

Children who have CP as a consequence of disturbances in the extrapyramidal system exhibit atypical movements known as **dyskinesias** (We Move, 2010).These include chorea, athetosis, choreoathetosis and dystonia. Rapid, random, jerky movements are known as **chorea**; slow, writhing movements which appear to flow into one another are called **athetosis**. When seen together, these movements are called **choreoathetosis**. **Dystonia** refers to repetitive, twisting movements and distorted postures.

Dyskinetic CP (also known as extrapyramidal CP) is characterized by abnormalities in muscle tone that involve the whole body. Changing patterns of tone from hour to hour and day to day are common. These children exhibit increased muscle tone, especially during attempted movement, and normal or decreased tone while asleep. The term athetoid CP characterizes a form of dyskinetic CP that has been associated with kernicterus. Dystonic CP is

Table 24.1. Cerebral palsy phenotypes

Bilateral spasticity	Dyskinetic ("extrapyramidal")	Ataxic	Unilateral spasticity
Spastic diplegia	Dystonia	Hypotonic	Spastic hemiplegia
Spastic quadriplegia (tetraplegia)	Chorea (choreathetosis)	Spastic	
	Athetosis		
	Hemiballismus		

associated with asphyxia as well as with a wide range of genetic disorders. Chorea is the least common form of dyskinetic CP.

Ataxic Cerebral Palsy

Ataxia results from an abnormality in the cerebellum and manifests as the inability to maintain typical postures and perform typical movements. As a result, movements are jerky and uncoordinated, without the smooth flow of typical motion (We Move, 2010). Ataxic CP is characterized by impairments of voluntary movement, involving balance and position of the trunk and limbs in space. For children who can walk, this is manifested as a wide-based, unsteady gait. Difficulties with controlling the hand and arm during reaching (causing overshooting or past-pointing) and difficulties with the timing of motor movements are also seen. Ataxic CP may be associated with increased or decreased muscle tone.

Mixed Cerebral Palsy

The term *mixed cerebral palsy* is used when more than one type of motor pattern is present and when one pattern does not clearly predominate over another. The term *total body cerebral palsy* is sometimes used to emphasize that certain types of CP (dyskinetic, ataxic, mixed, and spastic quadriplegia) involve the entire musculoskeletal system, whereas other forms of spastic CP (diplegia, hemiplegia) are localized to a particular region of the body.

Although there is some clinical utility in classifying CP on the basis of neuromotor characteristics (e.g., spasticity, dyskinesias), there tends to be a great deal of functional variability within specific subtypes. For example, some children with spastic diplegia may be able to walk independently, whereas others depend on a wheelchair for mobility. A number of functional assessment systems have been developed to address this issue (Oeffinger et al., 2004; Palisano et al., 1997; see Table 24.2). The GMFCS (Palisano, Cameron, Rosenbaum, Walter, & Russell, 2006) is often helpful for planning therapeutic interventions and establishing goals for habilitation. It is more predictive of long-term functional outcome than traditional, impairment-focused classification schemes (Palisano et al., 2009).

ESTABLISHING THE ETIOLOGY (CAUSE) OF CEREBRAL PALSY

In CP, diagnostic evaluation often is done in parallel with the assessment that establishes the disability or functional diagnosis (Ashwal et al., 2004). Establishing the underlying etiology can have important implications for designing

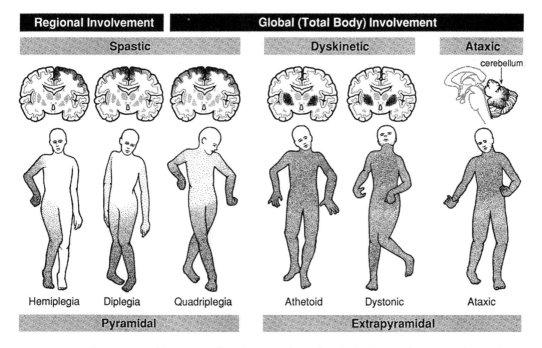

Figure 24.12. Different regions of the brain are affected in various forms of cerebral palsy. In this figure, the darker the shading, the more severe the involvement.

treatment and for understanding prognosis and recurrence risk in future children. It also can affect the parental feelings of guilt and responsibility. Information from the medical history and physical examination is critical in establishing an etiology. For example, knowing that a child was born prematurely and has signs of spastic diplegia strongly suggests cerebral white matter injury. Similarly, dystonic CP in the presence of a normal birth history may be associated with a neurogenetic disorder.

With regard to specialized diagnostic testing, brain imaging is especially helpful (Accardo, Kammann, & Hoon, 2004; Ancel et al., 2006). Seventy to ninety percent of children with CP will have significant diagnostic findings on neuroimaging. Cranial ultrasound, an inexpensive, noninvasive imaging modality, has utility both in diagnosis and management of the high-risk neonate. Ultrasonography is used for fetal and neonatal screening; it can distinguish large malformations of the brain from abnormalities related to brain hemorrhage or injury (i.e., IVH, PVL). Brain anatomic MRI, however, has been of greatest benefit in the determination of causation of CP (Vermeulen, Wilke, Horber, & Krägeloh-Mann, 2007). Based on an understanding of normal brain development, careful interpretation of MRI studies can show patterns of selective vulnerability in brain structures

Table 24.2. Summary of Gross Motor Function Classification System (GMFCS)

Level	Age			
	< 2 years	2–4 years	4–6 years	6–12 years
I: Walks without restrictions	Sits well (hands free to play), crawls and pulls-to-stand; walks between 18 and 24 months without a device	Gets up and down from floor to standing without help; walking is preferred method of mobility	Walks indoors and outdoors; climbs stairs; starting to run/jump	Independent walking, running, jumping, but speed, balance, and coordination reduced
II: Walks without device; restricted community mobility	Sits but may need hands for balance; may creep or crawl; may pull-to-stand or cruise	Floor sits, but hard to keep both hands free; mobility by crawling, cruising, or walking with assistive device	Transfers with arm assist; walks without device at home, short distances outside; climbs stairs with railing; no running or jumping	Independent walking but limitations in challenging circumstances; minimal running, jumping
III: Walks with assistive device; limited community mobility	Sits with low back support; rolls and creeps	Floor sits, often W-sitting, needs help getting to sit; creeping and crawling primary means of mobility; limited assisted standing/walking	Sits in regular chair with pelvic support to allow free hands; walks with device on level surface; transported for long distances	Walks indoors or outdoors with assistive device; wheelchair mobility or transport for long distances
IV: Limited self-mobility; power mobility	Has head control, but needs trunk support for sitting; rolls to back; may roll to front	Needs hands to maintain sitting; adaptive equipment for sitting/standing; floor mobility only (rolling, creeping, or crawling without reciprocal leg movements)	Adaptive seating needed for maximum hand function; needs assistance for transfers; walks short distances with assistance; power mobility for long distances	Maintains function achieved by ages 4–6 or relies more on power wheelchair for self-mobility
V: Self-mobility severely limited even with assistive devices	Limited voluntary control of movement; head and trunk control minimal; needs help to roll	Limited control of movement and posture; all areas of motor function are limited; adaptive equipment does not fully compensate functional limitations for sitting and standing; no independent mobility (requires transport); some children achieve very limited power mobility with extensive adaptations		

Source: Palisano, Rosenbaum, Walter, Russell, Wood, & Galuppi (1997).

characteristic of the nature of the insult, gestational timing, and severity (Barkovich, 2005). It should be noted that even a normal MRI can be of benefit, as it may lead to consideration of a potentially treatable metabolic disorder, such as dopa-responsive dystonia (Mink, 2003). In certain circumstances, enhanced MRI techniques such as diffusion weighted imaging (DWI), diffusion tensor imaging (DTI), MR spectroscopy (MRS), and functional MRI (fMRI) can be used (see Chapter 12). They provide information about brain metabolic function and white matter tracks, which in some cases are abnormal even when brain structure appears to be normal (Davidson, Thomas, & Casey, 2003; Mohan, Chugani, & Chugani, 1999; Nagae et al., 2007; Watts, Liston, Niogi, & Uluğ, 2003).

ASSOCIATED IMPAIRMENTS IN CEREBRAL PALSY

Many children with CP have associated impairments. The most common are intellectual disability, visual impairments, hearing impairments, speech-language disorders, seizures, feeding and growth impairments, and behavior-emotional disorders.

Assessment of intellectual functioning in children with CP may be difficult because most tests of cognition require both motor and verbal responses. Even taking these limitations into account, approximately one half of children with CP have intellectual disability, and many of those with typical intelligence exhibit some degree of learning disability (Nordmark, Hägglund, & Lagergren, 2001). Children with the more severe types of CP are at a greater risk for more significant intellectual disability.

Visual impairments are common and diverse in children with CP. They may be both ocular (e.g., strabismus) and central (i.e., cortical visual impairment; Guzzetta, Mercuri, & Cioni, 2001; see Chapter 11). The premature infant may have severe visual impairment caused by retinopathy of prematurity. Nystagmus, or involuntary oscillating eye movements, may be present in the child with ataxia. Children with hemiplegia may present with homonomous hemianopsia, a condition causing loss of one part of the visual field (Jacobson, Rydberg, Eliasson, Kits, & Flodmark, 2010). Strabismus, or squint, is seen in many children with CP. Finally, children with CP are more prone to hyperopia (farsightedness) than typically developing children (Sobrado, Suarez, & Garcia-Sanchez, 1999).

Hearing, speech, and language impairments are also common, occurring in about 30% of children with CP. Children whose CP is caused by congenital cytomegalovirus or other intrauterine viral infections often have hearing loss (see Chapter 10). Dyskinetic CP resulting from basal ganglia/thalamus injury is associated with articulation problems because these structures influence tongue and vocal cord movement. In children with CP and typical cognitive development, expressive or receptive language disorders may be present and evolve into a specific reading disability (see Chapter 23).

Approximately 40% of children with CP develop seizures (Nordmark et al., 2001). Children with more severe intellectual and physical disability are more prone to generalized seizures (Carlsson, Hagberg, & Olsson, 2003). Children whose CP is a consequence of brain malformation, infection, or severe gray matter injury are also at greater risk for generalized seizures (see Chapter 27).

Feeding and growth difficulties also are often present (Samson-Fang et al., 2002). They may be secondary to a variety of problems, including hypotonia, weak suck, poor coordination of the swallowing mechanism, tonic bite reflex, hyperactive gag reflex, and exaggerated tongue thrust. These problems may lead to poor nutrition and, in some cases, require the use of alternative feeding methods, such as tube feeding (see Chapter 9). Medical problems related to poor gastrointestinal motility (including gastroesophageal reflux and constipation) may add to these difficulties.

The combination of poor nutrition and lack of weight-bearing activities also leads to osteopenia (weak bones related to reduced bone mineral density). This places children with CP at increased risk for fractures. Bisphosphonates (drugs used to treat osteoporosis in older adults) also have been shown to be effective in treating osteopenia in CP (Hough, Boyd, & Keating, 2010).

These associated disorders contribute significantly to the issue of quality of life in individuals with CP (Liptak & Accardo, 2004; Samson-Fang et al., 2002). A comprehensive health plan implemented in the context of a well-defined medical home is a critical component to assuring that the health needs of children with CP are adequately addressed (Cooley & American Academy of Pediatrics Committee on Children with Disabilities, 2004; see Chapter 41).

COMPREHENSIVE MANAGEMENT FOR INDIVIDUALS WITH CEREBRAL PALSY

Neuroplasticity

A key starting point for discussing management of CP is based on an understanding of neuroplasticity. The human brain grows rapidly from conception through early childhood. During this time, connections between the brain and white matter pathways are forming. During childhood, approximately one half of these connections are retained as a result of stimulation through brain activity, while the other half are eliminated or pruned because of disuse. The concept of neuroplasticity is based on this selective pruning of connections, called synapses. It is characterized by the ability of the brain to adapt to environmental changes, to store information in memory (associated with learning), and to recover from brain and spinal cord injury (Johnston, 2009). There is a great deal of information in adults, especially following stroke, supporting the efficacy of neurorehabilitation directed at the **plasticity** (the ability to change in response to environmental stimulation) of the CNS (Wittenberg, 2009).

The child's brain has greater plasticity than the adult brain (Cramer et al., 2011). In CP, as well as in other childhood neurodevelopmental disabilities, the overarching question concerning plasticity involves the nature of the relationship between amount and timing of intervention and resultant outcome (Delgado et al., 2010; Vargus-Adams, 2009).

Overview of Management

Comprehensive management for children with CP includes both accurate diagnosis and effective treatment strategies. Management is based on the recognition that each child requires a unique combination of medical and rehabilitative interventions that are developed though a team approach and tailored to the family structure and goals (Pellegrino, 1995). Specialists in orthopedics, neurosurgery, genetics, ophthalmology, gastroenterology, neurology, physical medicine and rehabilitation, psychiatry, and neurodevelopmental pediatrics are all integral to developing a comprehensive medical-surgical treatment plan. Physical and occupational therapists, speech-language pathologists, audiologists, clinical and behavioral psychologists, special education consultants, and social workers are critical to developing the rehabilitation and educational plan. An interdisciplinary

setting is the ideal approach to management of the child with CP.

It is very important that clinicians and families agree on specific treatments as well as overall management goals. Recognized goals include improvements in function, communication, ease of care, and pain management. Including the child in the decision-making process to the greatest extent possible is critical to successful implementation. Treatment should be integrated into the lifestyles and other activities and commitments of individual families. Other practical considerations in optimizing management include

1. The recognition that a specific medical treatment or therapy may be embraced by one family but rejected by another, even when the overall clinical findings are similar

2. The need for effective care coordination, and providing a medical home (Figure 24.13)

Principles of Management

Management may be divided into rehabilitative, medical, and surgical components (Papavasiliou, 2009). Rehabilitative interventions include conventional therapeutic approaches (physical therapy and occupational therapy), serial casting, orthotic bracing, strength training, aquatherapy, hippotherapy (therapeutic horseback riding), and technology systems such

Figure 24.13. What is a family-centered medical home?

A family-centered medical home is *not* a building, house, hospital, or home health care service, but rather an approach to providing comprehensive primary care.

In a family-centered medical home the pediatric care team works in partnership with a child and a child's family to assure that all of the medical and nonmedical needs of the child are met.

Through this partnership the pediatric care team can help the family and child access, coordinate, and understand specialty care, educational services, out-of-home care, family support, and other public and private community services that are important for the overall health of the child and family.

The American Academy of Pediatrics (AAP) developed the medical home model for delivering primary care that is accessible, continuous, comprehensive, family-centered, coordinated, compassionate, and culturally effective to *all* children and youth, including those with special health care needs.

From National Center for Medical Home Implementation, American Academy of Pediatrics. (n.d.). *What is a family-centered medical home?* Elk Grove Village, IL: Author. Retrieved from http://medicalhomeinfo.org; reprinted by permission.

as augmentative communication and power mobility. The focus in physiotherapy has shifted from traditional physical and occupational therapy to approaches combining principles of motor learning and strength and fitness training. In addition to these physical approaches, specialists in social work and psychology who are aware of the effects of motor disability on other aspects of childhood development may be of great benefit in fostering social/emotional growth and active participation of the child in the rehabilitation efforts.

In terms of medication, the most commonly used drugs for spasticity and rigidity include baclofen, diazepam, and botulinum toxin (see Appendix C). Carbidopa-levodopa and trihexyphenidyl have been found to be helpful for some children with dystonic CP. Tetrabenazine has been used successfully in selected patients with dyskinetic CP. The purpose of all these medications is to improve motor tone, enabling more physical activity and/or lessening pain. Orthopedic surgical interventions include tenotomies, tendon transfers, and osteotomies (see Chapter 13). Neurosurgical procedures, including intrathecal baclofen, selective dorsal rhizotomy (SDR), and deep brain stimulation (DBS), may be of benefit in carefully selected patients (Lynn, Turner, & Chambers, 2009).

Early Intervention and Education

For most children with CP, the process of rehabilitation begins in the home environment under the Infant and Toddlers program within IDEA (the Individuals with Disabilities Education Improvement Act of 2004, PL 108-446; see Chapter 31), emphasizing involvement of parents so that they can learn effective methods of working with their child (Guralnick, 1998). Programs are individualized according to the specific needs of the child and the family. While emphasizing home-based services, they may also provide consultative and center-based interventions (see Chapter 30). For many children with CP, entry into preschool represents the first major step into the wider community. Difficulties in accommodating the physical, nutritional, and medical needs of these children must be addressed. For school-age children, concerns regarding motor function and medical needs continue, but increased attention is focused on learning disabilities, attention and behavior difficulties, intellectual disability, and sensory impairments. For many children, these associated conditions, rather than the motor disability, place them at greatest disadvantage relative

to their typically developing peers. Children with CP have traditionally been segregated into classrooms with designations such as "multiply disabled" and "orthopedically impaired," sometimes without proper regard for their intellectual needs. Inclusion is mandated by federal law (IDEA) in general education classrooms, in the least restrictive environment. Inclusive environments, however, require significant collaboration between the general and special education models and work best when a team of educators and paraprofessionals is associated with each classroom (see Chapter 31).

Specific Rehabilitative Techniques

For children with CP, therapy may come in many different forms. Most children receive traditional forms of physical, occupational, and speech therapy. The most common method of motor therapy for the young child is neurodevelopmental therapy (NDT), an approach employed by both occupational and physical therapists. It is designed to provide the child with sensorimotor experiences that enhance the development of more typical movement patterns (Campbell, 2000; see Chapter 33). NDT is an individualized program of positioning, therapeutic handling, and play. Goals include the normalization of tone and improved control of movement during functional activities.

A promising technique known as constraint-induced therapy, or forced-use therapy, has been introduced to help children with hemiplegic CP (Taub, Ramey, DeLuca, & Echols, 2004; Willis, Morello, Davie, Rice, & Bennett, 2002). The technique involves constraining the more functional arm or hand to force use of the less functional upper extremity. Randomized controlled trials suggest that this technique may be of significant benefit over traditional therapy alone in the short run (Aarts, Jongerius, Geerdink, van Limbeek, & Geurts, 2010), but whether benefits persist over the long term remains to be determined.

Physical exercise is important to strengthen muscles and bones, enhance motor skills, and prevent contractures. In addition, the social and recreational aspects of organized physical activities can be highly beneficial (see Chapter 34). Many popular activities, including swimming, dancing, and horseback riding, can be modified so that children with CP can participate (Meregillano, 2004).

The Special Olympics has enabled thousands of children and young adults with intellectual disabilities and CP to take part in various sporting events. The rewards of engaging in competitive sports are invaluable for enhancing self-esteem and providing a sense of belonging to a peer group. Parents and professionals should encourage all children to participate in whatever physical activities their interests, motivation, and capabilities allow (see Chapter 34).

Bracing, Splinting, and Positioning

Therapists make frequent use of braces and splints (collectively referred to as **orthotic** devices) and positioning (seating) devices as aids in the pursuit of functional goals for children with CP. These devices are employed to maintain adequate range of motion, prevent contractures at specific joints, provide stability, and control involuntary movements that interfere with function. For the legs, one of the most commonly prescribed orthotics is a short leg brace, known as an **ankle-foot orthosis** (AFO). The AFO stabilizes the position of the foot and provides a consistent stretch to the Achilles tendon (see Chapter 33). A variety of splints can be used to improve hand function. For example, the resting hand splint is commonly used to hold the thumb in an abducted (away from the mid-line) position and the wrist in a neutral or slightly extended position. This helps the child keep his or her hand open and works to prevent the development of hand deformities. Trunk and body bracing, called a body splint, is made of a flexible, porous material. It controls abnormal tone and involuntary movements by stabilizing the trunk and limbs. Most pediatric braces and splints are custom-made from plastics that are molded directly on the child, so they must be monitored closely and modified as the child grows or changes abilities.

Positioning devices are used to promote skeletal alignment, to compensate for atypical postures, or to prepare the child for independent mobility. Proper positioning geared to the age and functional status of the child is often a key intervention in addressing the tone and movement impairments associated with CP. For children who must sit for extended periods of time or who use a wheelchair for mobility, a carefully designed seating system becomes an all-important component of their rehabilitation. Careful attention to functional seating may also have long-term benefits in the prevention of contractures and joint deformities resulting from spasticity (Myhr, von Wendt, Norrlin, & Radell, 1995).

Adaptive Equipment

A wide variety of devices is available to aid mobility. For children who are ambulatory, the use of crutches, walkers, and canes can help in the attainment of walking or in improvement of the quality and range of ambulation. The forearm, or Lofstrand, crutch is used in preference to the familiar under-the-arm crutch. A posterior walker (i.e., the child is positioned in front of the walker, rather than behind) with wheels is used in preference to a standard forward-position walker without wheels. Canes are used less commonly.

For children with limited walking skills, wheelchairs are essential for maximizing mobility and function. A wheelchair with a solid seat and back is usually recommended. Some children, however, have difficulty using this type of chair unless modifications are made. The addition of head and trunk supports or a tray may be needed for the child who lacks postural control due to abnormalities in tone. The child with limited head control, feeding difficulties, or low tone may benefit from a high-backed chair that can be tilted back 10–15 degrees (Figure 24.14A). This helps to maintain the child's body and head in proper alignment. Special seating cushions or custom-molded inserts that conform to the contours of the body can offer necessary support for the child with orthopedic deformities such as scoliosis.

Motorized (power) wheelchairs can enhance the independence of children who are able to use them. They may be manipulated by hand control, head control, or mouth mechanisms for controlling both speed and direction (Figure 24.14B). These wheelchairs can include leg elevation and tilt-in-space options. They can provide increased independence for individuals otherwise dependent for pressure relief, self-positioning, and lower extremity stretching.

Special supportive strollers are an alternative to wheelchairs for mobility within the community, or for the young child whose potential for ambulation has yet to be determined. These are lightweight and collapsible, yet support the back and keep the hips properly aligned (Figure 24.14C).

Car seats are essential to the safety of all children who ride in automobiles. Several manufacturers offer adapted car seats that meet federal safety guidelines as well as provide proper support for the child with CP. Often these models include a base that allows the seat to be used as a stroller or a positioning chair outside of the

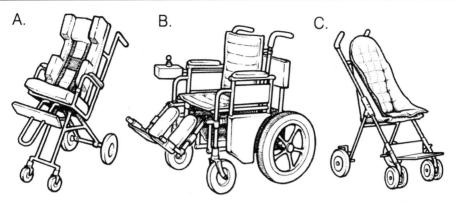

Figure 24.14. Three types of wheelchairs. A) High-backed, tilting chair with lateral inserts and head supports. B) Motorized wheelchair with joystick control. C) Supportive collapsible stroller.

car. Car beds and special straps are also available for children who have more severe disabilities or who require these special adaptations temporarily (e.g., following surgery).

Assistive Technology

Assistive technology devices are often an important part of the rehabilitation plan for children with CP (see Chapter 36). The technology involved may be as simple as Velcro or as complex as a computer chip. Although it is often true that the simplest intervention is the best, the computer is seen as the future of assistive technology. Computers can be used to control the environment, provide a lifeline with the outside world, enable a person to work at home, facilitate artificial speech and sight, and provide entertainment. The real potential of these new technologies to improve the quality of life for children with disabilities is just beginning to be appreciated. Recently, there has been a lot of enthusiasm for devices such as the iPad and the Wii for individuals with disabilities, chronic illness, and other impairments, due to the relatively low cost, the ease of the interface, graphics, and applications.

Neurocognitive Prosthetics

There is an evolving interest in neurocognitive prostheses, which can modulate neural function using implanted electrodes (Serruya & Kahana, 2008). Two currently utilized applications are cochlear implants (see Chapter 10) and DBS. Other noninvasive techniques under development include transcranial magnetic stimulation (TMS) and transcranial direct current stimulation (tDCS). It is hoped that further advances in neurocognitive prosthetics will improve both communication and mobility for individuals with a wide range of disorders, including CP.

Managing Spasticity and Dystonia

Spasticity and dystonia represent important targets for intervention in CP. The primary goals are to improve function, to prevent or postpone the musculoskeletal complications attendant to these conditions, and to ease the care of the child with significant muscle tightness.

Different treatment modalities work at different levels of brain and spine circuitry (Figure 24.15). Interventions may be employed singly, sequentially, or simultaneously depending on the specific clinical circumstance. As dystonia is caused by disturbances in the extrapyramidal motor control system, pharmacological interventions primarily target the brain and spinal cord. By contrast, the mechanisms that generate spasticity may be affected from the brain to the muscle itself. Therefore, a wider variety of therapeutic modalities are available to modulate the effects of spasticity. A potential pitfall in treatment revolves around the relationship between impairment (spasticity or dystonia) and disability. For some children, it is possible to significantly reduce spasticity or dystonia without improving (and in some cases even worsening) functional outcome. Therefore, consultation with experienced professionals who are intimately familiar with a child's particular pattern of skills and impairments is critical to the proper selection of specific interventions.

Casting

Tone-reducing, or inhibitive, casts are used in some centers as an adjunct to more traditional methods of managing spasticity (Law et al., 1991). The casts are made for arms or legs and can be either designed for use in immobilization or during weight-bearing activities. Benefits of inhibitive casting include improved gait and weight bearing, increased range of motion,

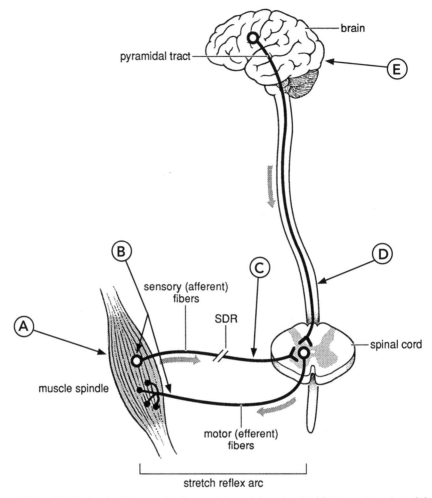

Figure 24.15. Levels of intervention for spasticity and dystonia. A) Inhibitive casting, physical therapy, exercise, and medications such as dantrolene directly affect tone at the muscle level. B) Nerve blocks, motor point blocks, and botulinum toxin work at the level of muscle and nerve entry into muscle. C) Selective dorsal rhizotomy reduces spasticity by interrupting the sensory component of the stretch reflex arc. D) Medications such as baclofen reduce spasticity at the level of the spinal cord. E) Medications for spasticity, such as diazepam, and medications for dystonia work at the level of the brain. (From Pellegrino, L., & Dormans, J.P. [1998]. Definitions, etiology, and epidemiology of cerebral palsy. In J.P. Dormans & L. Pellegrino [Eds.], *Caring for children with cerebral palsy: A team approach* [p. 46]. Baltimore, MD: Paul H. Brookes Publishing Co., Inc.; adapted by permission.)

and improved functional hand use. Casts position the limbs so that spastic muscles are in lengthened positions, being gently stretched. Serial application of casts (serial casting) can allow the therapist to increase range of motion gradually in the presence of contractures. After maximal range and position have been achieved, a cast is worn intermittently to maintain the improvement. Casting is now most often used in conjunction with other therapeutic modalities, especially following injection of **botulinum toxin**, sold under the brand name Botox (Glanzman, Kim, Swaminathan, & Beck, 2004; Kay, Rethlefsen, Fern-Buneo, Wren, & Skaggs, 2004; Wasiak, Hoare, & Wallen, 2004).

Nerve Blocks, Motor Point Blocks, and Botulinum Toxin

Several injectable agents are available that can be used to target spasticity in particular muscle groups. Certain chemical agents such as diluted alcohol or phenol, which denature muscle and nerve protein at the point of injection, can produce a decrease in muscle tone for months. A **motor point block** with these agents effectively interrupts the nerve supply at the entry site to a spastic muscle without compromising sensation. The main side effect of the procedure is localized pain that may persist for a few days after the injection. Inhibition of spasticity lasts for 4–6 months, and the procedure can be repeated after the initial effect has worn off. This temporary reduction of spasticity allows for more effective application of physical therapy to improve range of motion and function, and to potentially postpone orthopedic surgery.

Injectable botulinum toxin was introduced as an alternative to motor point blocks in the past decade and has largely supplanted alcohol and phenol (Jefferson, 2004; Mooney, Koman, & Smith, 2003; Morton, Hankinson, & Nicholson, 2004; Pidcock, 2004). Botulinum toxin is produced by the bacterium that causes botulism and is among the most potent neurotoxins known. It works by blocking the nerve-muscle junction. Small quantities can be safely injected directly into spastic muscles without significant spread of the toxin into the bloodstream. The injection results in weakening of the muscle and reduction of spasticity for 3–6 months (the anti-spasticity effects of the injections dissipate over time). Although botulinum toxin is used mainly to treat spasticity in muscles of the limbs and trunk, novel uses have been developed, such as injection of the salivary glands to reduce drooling (Jongerius et al., 2004). Although clarification is still needed regarding the definition of clinical indications and outcomes (Hoare et al., 2010), the use of injectable botulinum toxin has become a mainstay in the management of spasticity in CP and has also found applications for specific types of dystonia (Gordon, 1999; Jefferson, 2004; Mooney et al., 2003). Side effects, including weakness and mild flu-like symptoms, are usually mild and transient. It should be noted, however, that there are very rare reports in which botulism-like clinical pictures, including death, have been reported.

Oral Medication

A variety of orally administered medications have been used to improve muscle tone in children with spasticity and rigidity (Krach, 2001; Tilton, 2006; see Appendix C).

Several medications used in Parkinson's disease in adults, including carbidopa-levodopa (Sinemet) and trihexyphenidyl (Artane), have been found to be beneficial for some children with dyskinetic forms of CP (Mink & Zinner, 2009).

Although some specialists prefer trihexyphenidyl, others have reported benefits with levodopa. The medications most commonly used to control spasticity and rigidity are diazepam (Valium), baclofen, and dantrolene (Dantrium). Diazepam and its derivative compounds, lorazepam (Ativan) and clonazepam (Klonopin), affect brain control of muscle tone, beginning within half an hour after ingestion and lasting about 4 hours. Withdrawal of these drugs should be gradual, as physical dependency can develop. Side effects include drowsiness and excessive drooling, which may interfere with feeding and speech. As a result of these side effects, they are less commonly used than oral baclofen.

Baclofen, a GABA B receptor agonist, was initially used to treat adults with multiple sclerosis and traumatic damage to the spinal cord. It is now commonly used in CP clinics around the world. In children with CP, the most common side effects of the oral form of the medication are drowsiness, nausea, headache, and low blood pressure. About 10% of children treated with baclofen experience side effects that are unpleasant enough to necessitate discontinuation of the medication. Care must be taken when stopping the medication to gradually taper it, as rapid withdrawal can lead to severe side effects, including hallucinations.

Dantrolene works on muscle cells directly, as a calcium channel blocker, to inhibit their contraction. Side effects include drowsiness, muscle weakness, and increased drooling. A rare adverse effect of this drug is severe liver damage, so liver function tests should be performed periodically.

Although a discussion of the range of side effects associated with oral medications is beyond the scope of this chapter, several generalizations can be made. Some medications have easily recognizable side effects, such as sedation from diazepam and seizures from acute baclofen withdrawal. Others may be more subtle, such as cognitive or personality changes with trihexyphenidyl (Carranza-del Rio, Clegg, Moore, & Delgado, 2011).

Periodic drug "holidays" should be considered to determine whether benefits are persistent. As always, clinicians should listen carefully to parental or caregiver concerns about any changes in their children after medication initiation.

Neurosurgical Procedures

Intrathecal baclofen is a therapeutic modality that allows for the direct delivery of baclofen into the spinal fluid (i.e., intrathecal) space, where it can inhibit motor nerve conduction at the level of the spinal cord (Disabato & Ritchie, 2003; Fitzgerald, Tsegaye, & Vloeberghs, 2004; Tilton, 2004). A disk-shaped pump is placed under the skin of the abdomen, and a catheter is tunneled below the skin around to the back, where it is inserted through the lumbar spine into the intrathecal space. Baclofen is stored in a reservoir in the disk that can be refilled, and the medication is delivered at a continuous rate that is computer controlled and adjustable. Because the drug is delivered directly to its site of action (the cerebrospinal fluid), a much lower dosage can be used, with a resultant reduced risk of side effects. Improvements in ease of care and comfort are commonly reported. Although functional gains in lower extremity, upper extremity, and even oral/motor function have been observed (Fitzgerald et al., 2004), clear improvements in ambulant individuals has not been demonstrated (Pin, McCartney, Lewis, & Waugh, 2011). The main disadvantages of intrathecal baclofen are hypotonia (low muscle tone), increased seizures in individuals with known epilepsy, sleepiness, and nausea/vomiting (Gilmartin et al., 2000). Complications related to mechanical failures and infection, and the need for intensive and reliable medical follow-up, are also significant considerations (Murphy, Irwin, & Hoff, 2002).

Selective Dorsal Rhizotomy

This procedure reduces spasticity by interrupting the sensory component of the deep tendon reflex, which is exaggerated in children with spastic forms of CP. The surgery reduces spasticity permanently in the legs but not in the arms, so its use is confined mainly to children with spastic diplegia who have good antigravity strength. Although uncertainty exists in regard to long-term functional outcomes in children who undergo this procedure (Koman et al., 2004; Tedroff, Löwing, Jacobson, & Åströmn, 2011), other recent reports have been more

encouraging in this regard (Engsberg, Ross, Collins, & Park, 2006; Langerak et al., 2009).

Another neurosurgical procedure currently under investigation, DBS, has been proposed as a method to reduce choreoathetosis and dystonia associated with some forms of extrapyramidal CP. Recent results are promising, but this procedure is still in its infancy (Vidailhet et al., 2009).

Orthopedic Procedures

Because of the abnormal or asymmetrical distribution of muscle tone, children with CP are susceptible to the development of joint deformities. The most common of these result from permanent shortening or contracture of one or more groups of muscles around a joint, which limits joint mobility. Orthopedic surgery is done to increase the range of motion by lengthening a tendon, cutting through muscle or tendon (release), or moving the point of attachment of a tendon on bone. For example, a partial release or transfer of hyperactive hip adductor muscles (which cause scissoring of the legs) may improve the child's ability to sit and walk, and may lessen the chances of a hip dislocation (Hägglund et al., 2005; Stott, Piedrahita, & American Academy for Cerebral Palsy and Developmental Medicine, 2004). A partial hamstring release, involving the lengthening or transfer of muscles around the knee, also may facilitate sitting and walking. A lengthening of the Achilles tendon at the ankle improves toe walking (Figure 24.16).

More complicated orthopedic procedures may be required for correction of a dislocated hip. If this is diagnosed when there is a partial dislocation (called subluxation), release of the hip adductor muscles alone can be effective

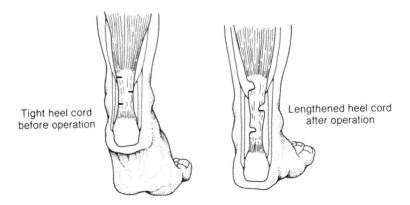

Figure 24.16.   Achilles tendon lengthening operation. When the heel cord is tight, the child walks on his or her toes. Surgery lengthens the heel cord and permits a more flat-footed gait.

(Figure 24.17). If the head of the femur (the thigh bone) is dislocated more than one third to one half of the way out of a hip joint socket, a more complex procedure called a varus derotational osteotomy may be necessary. In this operation, the angle of the femur is changed surgically to place the head of the femur back into the hip socket (Figure 24.18). In some cases, the hip socket also must be reshaped to ensure that the hip joint remains functional.

Sometimes muscle releases or lengthening are performed at the same time as these procedures.

For ambulatory children with CP, deciding which type of surgery is most likely to improve function is a complex issue. Computerized gait analysis conducted prior to surgical intervention has become increasingly common as an aid in the decision-making process. Precise measurements obtained through motion analysis, force plates, and electromyography

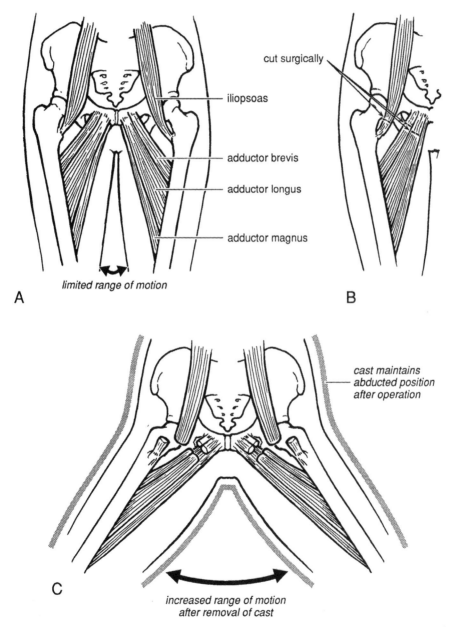

Figure 24.17. Adductor tenotomy. This operation is done to improve scissoring (Figure 24.11) and to prevent hip dislocation caused by contractures of the adductor muscles in the thigh. A) In this procedure, the iliopsoas, adductor brevis, and adductor longus muscles are cut, leaving the adductor magnus intact. B) The child is then placed in a cast for 6–8 weeks to maintain a more open (abducted) position. C) The muscles eventually grow together in a lengthened position, allowing improved sitting and/or walking.

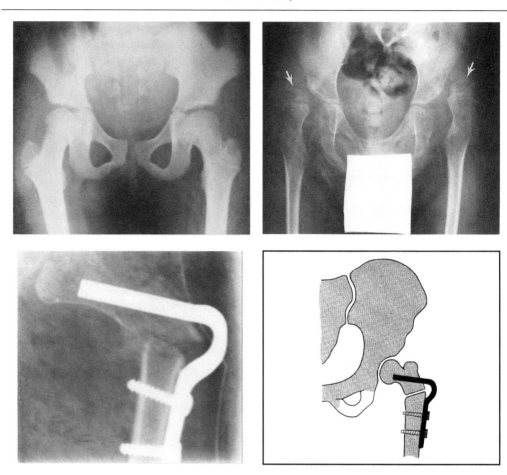

Figure 24.18. Dislocation of the hip. The upper x rays (frontal view) show a normal hip (left x ray) and a hip dislocated on both sides (right x ray). The arrows indicate the points of dislocation. The lower pictures show the results of a varus derotational osteotomy to correct the left-hip dislocation. The femur has been cut and realigned so that it now fits into the hip socket. Pins, which are later removed, hold the bone in place until it heals.

offer detailed information relating to specific abnormalities at each lower extremity joint as well as the muscle activity that controls motion through all phases of the gait (Cook, Schneider, Hazlewood, Hillman, & Robb, 2003). Preoperative gait analysis helps to determine exactly which procedures are likely to be successful. Postoperative analysis can provide an objective measure of outcome.

In addition to treating contractures and dislocations, orthopedic surgeons are involved in the treatment of scoliosis. If untreated, a spinal curvature can interfere with sitting, walking, and self-care skills. If severe enough, it also can affect lung capacity and respiratory efforts. Treatment of significant scoliosis ranges from a molded plastic jacket or a chair insert to surgery that straightens the spine as much as possible. This surgery involves using rods and wires to hold the spine in an improved alignment while

bone graft material fuses the spine in position (Figure 24.19).

Complementary and Alternative Therapies

When conventional approaches do not lead to the anticipated improvements, families may explore other treatment options, including complementary and alternative medicine (CAM; Oppenheim, 2009; see Chapter 38).

CAM includes acupuncture, craniosacral therapy, myofascial release, therapeutic taping, diet and herbal remedies, electrical stimulation, chiropractic treatments, massage, and hyperbaric oxygen therapy (HBOT). Although there are individual reports and testimonials of dramatic improvements with various alternative therapies, some carry significant risks. Furthermore, rigorous studies have not been conducted

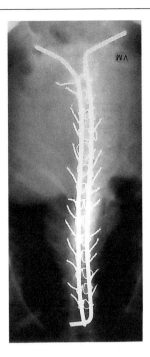

Figure 24.19. Treatment of scoliosis may require spinal fusion. This x ray shows improved scoliosis following a Luque procedure. During this surgery, the position of the spine is improved using metal hooks, rods, and wires while bone graft material fuses the spine in position.

to assess efficacy. As with any treatment, families and clinicians should consider cost, efficacy, and potential side effects before embarking on one of these approaches.

Transition into Adulthood

Adolescence is a critical time in life for all individuals, but for teenagers with CP there are additional challenges (Wood, Kantor, Edwards, & James, 2008). There is the need to transition from pediatric health care providers to those who manage CP in adults, and there are job training, employment, social, recreation, housing, and insurance considerations that require careful planning.

Adult Outcome

Adults with CP are living longer and more independent lives than in the past as a result of new treatment options. However, they face challenges, including medical care, accessibility, and vocational opportunities (Tosi, Maher, Moore, Goldstein, & Aisen, 2009; Watson, Parr, Joyce, May, & Le Couteur, 2011).

Although medical care is well established for children with CP, it is more fragmented for adults (Turk, 2009). Adults with CP should look for practitioners who are experienced in the care

of chronic disorders and who can provide the additional time that may be required for evaluation. They also need to recognize the importance of preventive care and report any changes in neurological function, as this may represent new impairments secondary to the underlying motor disorder. Adults with CP identify pain as a significant problem and should be encouraged to seek medical care in this circumstance (Vogtle, 2009).

Mobility and the ability to perform activities of daily living should be carefully monitored because some adults experience slow declines over time. Individuals should be provided with instruction in practical matters, such as hiring quality personal aides and caregivers, as well as in self-advocacy and seeking employment opportunities when able.

Although most children with CP will live to adulthood, their projected life expectancy may be less than that of the general population (Hemming, Hutton, Colver, & Platt, 2005; Katz, 2003). For example, an individual with hemiplegic CP probably will have a typical life span, whereas a person with spastic quadriplegia may not live beyond age 40 because of respiratory and nutritional issues (Strauss & Shavelle, 2001). Children with very severe impairments, measured in terms of functional characteristics, have the poorest outcome. Children who cannot lift their heads and are fed via gastrostomy tube may not survive to adulthood (Strauss, Shavelle, & Anderson, 1998).

Excess mortality for people with CP may also be related to comorbid risks such as seizures and aspiration, as well as an increased risk for breast cancer, brain tumors, and circulatory and digestive diseases, most likely related to inadequate medical screening (Murphy, 2010). Unintentional injury rates (e.g., falls) for people with CP are also higher than in the general population (Cooley & American Academy of Pediatrics, 2004; Strauss, Cable, & Shavelle, 1999).

Motor skills and mobility may not be the primary determinant of societal independence; personal characteristics, health status, and environmental factors will also factor into outcome (Liptak & Accardo, 2004). In fact, the ability to successfully participate in society may be more strongly related to intellectual and interpersonal strengths than to physical abilities. Although approximately one half of individuals with CP have normal intelligence, most still have difficulty leading completely typical lives. This may result from factors ranging from family support and quality of educational programs to availability of community-based training and technical support (Murphy, Molnar, & Lankasky, 1995; Russman & Gage, 1989). In one study of young adults with CP (van der Dussen, Nieuwstraten, Roebroeck, & Stam, 2001), 53% of individuals had some form of secondary education, but only 36% subsequently engaged in paid employment. It is hoped that these figures will improve as a result of federal mandates (e.g., the Americans with Disabilities Act [ADA] of 1990, PL 101–336), which define the rights of people with disabilities and are gradually making inroads into societal perceptions of disability. Ultimately, strengthening support to families (Raina et al., 2005), providing ready access to quality medical care, improving special education services, increasing opportunities for employment, and changing attitudes about disabilities in society at large may do as much for children with CP as traditional therapeutic and medical interventions.

SUMMARY

Cerebral palsy represents a group of chronic motor disorders that result from malformation or injury of the developing brain. The impairments associated with CP are variable and nonprogressive but permanent. Varying degrees of disability related to functional mobility, daily living skills, and communication-socialization skills result from these impairments. Effective management requires an interdisciplinary strategy that seeks to maximize function and opportunity. Efforts founded on the principles articulated in federal legislation will create new opportunities for greater participation and enhanced quality of life for people with CP. New treatment modalities offer improved quality of life and educational opportunities. The challenge is to provide these opportunities in a changing medical environment, where a premium is not always placed on coordination of care.

REFERENCES

Aarts, P.B., Jongerius, P.H., Geerdink, Y.A., van Limbeek, J., & Geurts, A.C. (2010). Effectiveness of modified constraint-induced movement therapy in children with unilateral spastic cerebral palsy: a randomized controlled trial. *Neurorehabilitation and Neural Repair, 24*(6), 509–518.

Aarts, P.B., Jongerius, P.H., Geerdink, Y.A., van Limbeek, J., & Geurts, A.C. (2011). Modified constraint-induced movement therapy combined with bimanual training (mCIMT-BiT) in children with unilateral spastic cerebral palsy: How are improvements in arm-hand use established? *Research in Developmental Disabilities, 32*(1), 271–279.

Accardo, J., Kammann, H., & Hoon, A.H., Jr. (2004). Neuroimaging in cerebral palsy. *The Journal of Pediatrics, 145*(2, Suppl.), S19–S27.

Accardo, P.J. (2008). *Capute & Accardo's neurodevelopmental disabilities in infancy and childhood* (3rd ed.). Baltimore, MD: Paul H. Brookes Publishing Co.

Americans with Disabilities Act (ADA) of 1990, 42 U.S.C. §§ 12101 *et seq.*

Ancel, P.Y., Livinec, F., Larroque, B., Marret, S., Arnaud, C., Pierrat, V., ... the EPIPAGE Study Group. (2006). Cerebral palsy among very preterm children in relation to gestational age and neonatal ultrasound abnormalities: The EPIPAGE cohort study. *Pediatrics, 117*(3), 828–835.

Aneja, S. (2004). Evaluation of a child with cerebral palsy. *Indian Journal of Pediatrics, 71*(7), 627–634.

Ashwal, S., Russman, B.S., Blasco, P.A., Miller, G., Sandler, A., Shevell, M., & Stevenson, R. (2004). Practice parameter: Diagnostic assessment of the child with cerebral palsy: Report of the Quality Standards Subcommittee of the American Academy of Neurology and the Practice Committee of the Child Neurology Society. *Neurology, 62*(6), 851–863.

Bale, J.F. (2009). Fetal infections and brain development. *Clinical Perinatology, 36*(3), 639–653.

Barkovich, J.A. (2005). *Pediatric neuroimaging* (4th ed.). Philadelphia, PA: Lippincott Williams &Wilkins.

Barks, J.D. (2008). Current controversies in hypothermic protection. *Seminars in Fetal and Neonatal Medicine, 13*(1), 30–34.

Barnes, M.P., & Johnson, G.R. (2008). *Upper motor neurone syndrome and spasticity.* Cambridge, England: Cambridge University Press.

Bax, M., Goldstein, M., Rosenbaum, P., Leviton, A., Paneth, N., Dan, B., ... Executive Committee for the Definition of Cerebral Palsy. (2005). Proposed definition and classification of cerebral palsy, April 2005. *Developmental Medicine and Child Neurology, 47*(8), 571–576.

Campbell, S. (Ed.). (2000). *Physical therapy for children* (2nd ed.). Philadelphia, PA: W.B. Saunders.

Carlsson, M., Hagberg, G., & Olsson, I. (2003). Clinical and aetiological aspects of epilepsy in children with cerebral palsy. *Developmental Medicine and Child Neurology, 45*(6), 371–376.

Carranza-del Rio, J., Clegg, N.J., Moore, A., & Delgado, M.R. (2011). Use of trihexyphenidyl in children with cerebral palsy. *Pediatric Neurology, 44*(3), 202–206.

Cook, R.E., Schneider, I., Hazlewood, M.E., Hillman, S.J., & Robb, J.E. (2003). Gait analysis alters decision-making in cerebral palsy. *Journal of Pediatric Orthopedics, 23*(3), 292–295.

Cooley, W.C., & American Academy of Pediatrics Committee on Children with Disabilities. (2004). Providing a primary care medical home for children and youth with cerebral palsy. *Pediatrics, 114*(4), 1106–1113.

Cramer, S.C., Sur, M., Dobkin, B.H., O'Brien, C., Sanger, T.D., Trojanowski, J.Q., ... Vinogradov, S. (2011). Harnessing neuroplasticity for clinical applications. *Brain, 134*(Pt. 6), 1591–1609.

Davidson, M.C., Thomas, K.M., & Casey, B.J. (2003). Imaging the developing brain with fMRI. *Mental Retardation and Developmental Disabilities Research Reviews, 9*(3), 161–167.

Delgado, M.R., Hirtz, D., Aisen, M., Ashwal, S., Fehlings, D.L., McLaughlin, J., ... Vargus-Adams, J. (2010). Practice parameter: Pharmacologic treatment of spasticity in children and adolescents with cerebral palsy (an evidence-based review): Report of the Quality Standards Subcommittee of the American Academy of Neurology and the Practice Committee of the Child Neurology Society. *Neurology, 7*(4), 336–343.

Disabato, J., & Ritchie, A. (2003). Intrathecal baclofen for the treatment of spasticity of cerebral origin. *Journal for Specialists in Pediatric Nursing, 8*(1), 31–34.

Engsberg, J.R., Ross, S.A., Collins, D.R., & Park, T.S. (2006). Effect of selective dorsal rhizotomy in the treatment of children with cerebral palsy. *Journal of Neurosurgery, 105*(1 Suppl.), 8–15.

Fitzgerald, J.J., Tsegaye, M., & Vloeberghs, M.H. (2004). Treatment of childhood spasticity of cerebral origin with intrathecal baclofen: A series of 52 cases. *British Journal of Neurosurgery, 18*(3), 240–245.

Galiza, E.P., & Heath, P.T. (2009). Improving the outcome of neonatal meningitis. *Current Opinion in Infectious Disease, 22*(3), 229–234.

Gilmartin, R., Bruce, D., Storrs, B.B., Abbott, R., Krach, L., Ward, J., ... Nadell, J. (2000). Intrathecal baclofen for management of spastic cerebral palsy: multicenter trial. *Journal of Child Neurology, 15*(2), 71–77.

Glanzman, A.M., Kim, H., Swaminathan, K., & Beck, T. (2004). Efficacy of botulinum toxin A, serial casting, and combined treatment for spastic equinus: A retrospective analysis. *Developmental Medicine and Child Neurology, 46*(12), 807–811.

Gordon, N. (1999). The role of botulinum toxin type A in treatment—with special reference to children. *Brain & Development, 21*(3), 147–151.

Guralnick, M.J. (1998). Effectiveness of early intervention for vulnerable children: A developmental perspective. *American Journal on Mental Retardation, 102*(4), 319–345.

Guzzetta, A., Mercuri, E., & Cioni, G. (2001). Visual disorders in children with brain lesions: 2. Visual impairment associated with cerebral palsy. *European Journal of Paediatric Neurology, 5*(3), 115–119.

Hagberg, B., Hagberg, G., Beckung, E., & Ubrevant, P. (2001). Changing panorama of cerebral palsy in Sweden. VIII. Prevalence and origin in the birth-year period 1991–94. *Acta Paediatrica, 90*(3), 271–277.

Hägglund, G., Andersson, S., Düppe, H., Lauge-Pedersen, H., Nordmark, E., & Westbom, L. (2005). Prevention of dislocation of the hip in children with cerebral palsy: The first ten years of a population-based prevention programme. *The Journal of Bone and Joint Surgery: British Volume, 87*(1), 95–101.

Hankins, G.D., & Speer, M. (2003). Defining the pathogenesis and pathophysiology of neonatal encephalopathy and cerebral palsy. *Obstetrics & Gynecology, 102*(3), 628–636.

Hemming, K., Hutton, J.L., Colver, A., & Platt, M.J. (2005). Regional variation in survival of people with cerebral palsy in the United Kingdom. *Pediatrics, 116*(6), 1383–1390.

Hemminki, K., Li, X., Sundquist, K., & Sundquist, J. (2007). High familial risks for cerebral palsy implicate partial heritable aetiology. *Pediatric Perinatal Epidemiology, 21*(3), 235–241.

Himmelmann, K., Hagberg, G., & Uvebrant, P. (2010). The changing panorama of cerebral palsy in Sweden. X. Prevalence and origin in the birth-year period 1999–2002. *Acta Paediatrica, 99*(9), 1337–1343.

Himmelmann, K., McManus, V., Hagberg, G., Uvebrant, P., Krägeloh-Mann, I., Cans, C., SCPE collaboration. (2009). Dyskinetic cerebral palsy in Europe: Trends in prevalence and severity. *Archives of Disease in Childhood, 94*(12), 921–926.

Hoare, B.J., Wallen, M.A., Imms, C., Villanueva, E., Rawicki, H.B., & Carey, L. (2010). Botulinum toxin A as an adjunct to treatment in the management of the upper limb in children with spastic cerebral palsy (UPDATE). *Cochrane Database of Systematic Reviews,* January 20;(1):CD003469.

Hoon, Jr., A.H., Belsito, K.M., & Nagae-Poetscher, L.M. (2003). Neuroimaging in spasticity and movement disorders. *Journal of Child Neurology, 18*(Suppl. 1), 25–39.

Hoon, Jr., A.H., Stashinko, E.E., Nagae, L.M., Lin, D.D., Keller, J., Bastian, A., ... Johnston, M.V. (2009). Sensory and motor deficits in children with cerebral palsy born preterm correlate with diffusion tensor imaging abnormalities in thalamocortical pathways. *Developmental Medicine and Child Neurology, 51*(9), 697–704.

Hough, J.P., Boyd, R.N., & Keating, J.L. (2010). Systematic review of interventions for low bone mineral density in children with cerebral palsy. *Pediatrics, 125*(3), e670–678.

Individuals with Disabilities Education Improvement Act (IDEA) of 2004, 20 U.S.C. §§ 1400 *et seq.*

Jacobson, L., Rydberg, A., Eliasson, A.C., Kits, A., & Flodmark, O. (2010). Visual field function in school-aged children with spastic unilateral cerebral palsy related to different patterns of brain damage. *Developmental Medicine and Child Neurology, 52*(8), e184–e187.

Jacobsson, B. (2004). Infectious and inflammatory mechanisms in preterm birth and cerebral palsy. *European Journal of Obstetrics, Gynecology, and Reproductive Biology, 115*(2), 159–160.

Jacobsson, B., Ahlin, K., Francis, A., Hagberg, G., Hagberg, H., & Gardosi, J. (2008). Cerebral palsy and restricted growth status at birth: Population-based case-control study. *BJOG: An International Journal of Obstetrics and Gynaecology, 115*(10), 1250–1255.

Jefferson, R.J. (2004). Botulinum toxin in the management of cerebral palsy. *Developmental Medicine and Child Neurology, 46*(7), 491–499.

Johnston, M.V. (1998). Selective vulnerability in the neonatal brain. *Annals of Neurology, 44*(2), 155–156.

Johnston, M.V. (2009). Plasticity in the developing brain: Implications for rehabilitation. *Developmental Disabilities Research Reviews, 15*(2), 94–101.

Jongerius, P.H., van den Hoogen, F.J.A., van Limbeek, J., Gabreëls, F.J., van Hulst, K., & Rotteveel, J.J. (2004). Effect of botulinum toxin in the treatment of drooling: A controlled clinical trial. *Pediatrics, 114*(3), 620–627.

Katz, R.T. (2003). Life expectancy for children with cerebral palsy and mental retardation: Implications for life care planning. *Neurorehabilitation, 18*(3), 261–270.

Kay, R.M., Rethlefsen, S.A., Fern-Buneo, A., Wren, T.A.L., & Skaggs, D.L. (2004). Botulinum toxin as an adjunct to serial casting treatment in children with cerebral palsy. *The Journal of Bone and Joint Surgery: American Volume, 86*-A(11), 2377–2384.

Koene, S., & Smeitink, J. (2009). Mitochondrial medicine: Entering the era of treatment. *The Journal of Internal Medicine, 265*(2), 193–209.

Koman, L.A., Smith, B.P., & Shilt, J.S. (2004). Cerebral palsy. *The Lancet, 363*(9421), 1619–1631.

Krach, L.E. (2001). Pharmacotherapy of spasticity: Oral medications and intrathecal baclofen. *Journal of Child Neurology, 16*(1), 31–36.

Krägeloh-Mann, I., & Cans, C. (2009). Cerebral palsy update. *Brain & Development, 31*(7), 537–544.

Krägeloh-Mann, I., & Horber, V. (2007). The role of magnetic resonance imaging in elucidating the pathogenesis of cerebral palsy: A systematic review. *Developmental Medicine and Child Neurology, 49*(2), 144–151.

Krägeloh-Mann, I., Petersen, D., Hagberg, G., Vollmer, B., Hagberg, B., & Michaelis, R. (1995). Bilateral spastic cerebral palsy—MRI pathology and origin. Analysis from a representative series of 56 cases. *Developmental Medicine and Child Neurology, 37*(5), 379–397.

Krauss, J.K., Loher, T.J., Weigel, R., Capelle, H.H., Weber, S., & Burgunder, J.M. (2003). Chronic stimulation of the globus pallidus internus for treatment of non-dYT1 generalized dystonia and choreoathetosis: 2-year follow up. *Journal of Neurosurgery, 98*(4), 785–792.

Kusters, C.D., Chen, M.L., Follett, P.L., & Dammann, O. (2009). "Intraventricular" hemorrhage and cystic periventricular leukomalacia in preterm infants: How are they related? *Journal of Child Neurology, 24*(9), 1158–1170.

Langerak, N.G., Lamberts, R.P., Fieggen, A.G., Peter, J.C., Peacock, W.J., & Vaughan, C.L. (2009). Functional status of patients with cerebral palsy according to the International Classification of Functioning, Disability and Health model: A 20-year follow-up study after selective dorsal rhizotomy. *Archives of Physical Medicine and Rehabilitation, 90*(6), 994–1003.

Law, M., Cadman, D., Rosenbaum, P., Walter, S., Russell, D., & DeMatteo, C. (1991). Neurodevelopmental therapy and upper-extremity inhibitive casting for children with cerebral palsy. *Developmental Medicine and Child Neurology, 33*(5), 379–387.

Leviton, A., & Dammann, O. (2004). Coagulation, inflammation, and the risk of neonatal white matter damage. *Pediatric Research, 55*(4), 541–545.

Liptak, G.S., & Accardo, P.J. (2004). Health and social outcomes of children with cerebral palsy. *The Journal of Pediatrics, 145*(2, Suppl.), S36–S41.

Lombardi, G., Garofoli, F., & Stronati, M. (2010). Congenital cytomegalovirus infection: Treatment, sequelae and follow-up. *The Journal of Maternal-Fetal and Neonatal Medicine, 23*(Suppl. 3), 45–48.

Lynn, A.K., Turner, M., & Chambers, H.G. (2009). Surgical management of spasticity in persons with cerebral palsy. *Physical Medicine and Rehabilitation, 1*(9), 834–838.

MacLennan, A., Nelson, K.B., Hankins, G., & Speer, M. (2010). Who will deliver our grandchildren? Implications of cerebral palsy litigation. *JAMA: The Journal of the American Medical Association, 294*(13), 1688–1690.

Magalhães, L.C., Missiuna, C., & Wong, S. (2006). Terminology used in research reports of developmental coordination disorder. *Developmental Medicine and Child Neurology, 48*(11), 937–941.

Marlow, N., Wolke, D., Bracewell, M.A., & Samara, M. (2005). Neurologic and developmental disability at six years of age after extremely preterm birth. *The New England Journal of Medicine, 352*(1), 9–19.

Meregillano, G. (2004). Hippotherapy. *Physical Medicine and Rehabilitation Clinics of North America, 15*(4), 843–854.

Mink, J.W. (2003). Dopa-responsive dystonia in children. *Current Treatment Options in Neurology, 5*(4), 279–282.

Mink, J.W., & Zinner, S.H. (2009). Movement disorders II: Chorea, dystonia, myoclonus, and tremor. *Pediatrics in Review, 31*(7), 287–294.

Mohan, K.K., Chugani, D.C., & Chugani, H.T. (1999). Positron emission tomography in pediatric neurology. *Seminars in Pediatric Neurology, 6*(2), 111–119.

Mooney, J.F., Koman, L.A., & Smith, B.P. (2003). Pharmacologic management of spasticity in cerebral palsy. *Journal of Pediatric Orthopedics, 23*(5), 679–686.

Morton, R.E., Hankinson, J., & Nicholson, J. (2004). Botulinum toxin for cerebral palsy: Where are we now? *Archives of Disease in Childhood, 89*(12), 1133–1137.

Murphy, K. (2010). The adult with cerebral palsy. *Orthopedic Clinics of North America, 41*(4), 595–605.

Murphy, N.A., Irwin, M.C., & Hoff, C. (2002). Intrathecal baclofen therapy in children with cerebral palsy: Efficacy and complications. *Archives of Physical Medicine and Rehabilitation, 83*(12), 1721–1725.

Murphy, K., Molnar, G., & Lankasky, K. (1995). Medical and functional status of adults with cerebral palsy. *Developmental Medicine and Child Neurology, 37*(12), 1075–1084.

Myhr, U., von Wendt, L., Norrlin, S., & Radell, U. (1995). Five-year follow-up of functional sitting position in children with cerebral palsy. *Developmental Medicine and Child Neurology, 37*(7), 587–596.

Nagae, L.M., Hoon, Jr., A.H., Stashinko, E., Lin, D., Zhang, W., Levey, E., … Mori, S. (2007). Diffusion tensor imaging in children with periventricular leukomalacia: Variability of injuries to white matter tracts. *AJNR: American Journal of Neuroradiology, 28*(7), 1213–1222.

Nelson, K.B. (2008). Causative factors in cerebral palsy. *Clinical Obstetrics and Gynecology, 51*(4), 749–762.

Nelson, K.B., & Chang, T. (2008). Is cerebral palsy preventable? *Current Opinions in Neurology, 21*(2), 129–135.

Nelson, K.B., & Ellenberg, J.H. (1986). Antecedents of cerebral palsy. Multivariate analysis of risk. *The New England Journal of Medicine, 315*(2), 81–86.

Nelson, K.B., & Grether, J.K. (1999). Causes of cerebral palsy. *Current Opinion in Pediatrics, 11*(6), 487–491.

Nelson, K.B., & Lynch, J.K. (2004). Stroke in newborn infants. *The Lancet Neurology, 3*(3), 150–158.

Nordmark, E., Hägglund, G., & Lagergren, J. (2001). Cerebral palsy in southern Sweden. II. Gross motor function and disabilities. *Acta Paediatrica, 90*(11), 1277–1282.

Oeffinger, D.J., Tylkowski, C.M., Rayens, M.K., Davis, R.F., Gorton III, G.E., D'Astous, J., … Luan, J. (2004). Gross Motor Function Classification System and outcome tools for assessing ambulatory cerebral palsy: A multicenter study. *Developmental Medicine and Child Neurology, 46*(5), 311–319.

Oppenheim, W.L. (2009). Complementary and alternative methods in cerebral palsy. *Developmental Medicine and Child Neurology, 51*(Suppl. 4), 122–129.

O'Shea, T.M. (2002). Cerebral palsy in very preterm infants: New epidemiological insights. *Mental Retardation and Developmental Disabilities Research Reviews, 8*(3), 135–145.

Pakula, A.T., Van Naarden Braun, K., & Yeargin-Allsopp, M. (2009). Cerebral palsy: Classification and epidemiology. *Physical Medicine and Rehabilitation Clinics of North America, 20*(3), 425–452.

Palisano, R.J., Cameron, D., Rosenbaum, P.L., Walter, S.D., & Russell, D. (2006). Stability of the Gross Motor Function Classification System. *Developmental Medicine and Child Neurology, 48*(6), 424–428.

Palisano, R., Rosenbaum, P., Walter, S., Russell, D., Wood, E., & Galuppi, B. (1997). Development and reliability of a system to classify gross motor function in children with cerebral palsy. *Developmental Medicine and Child Neurology, 39*(4), 214–223.

Palmer, F.B. (2004). Strategies for the early diagnosis of cerebral palsy. *The Journal of Pediatrics, 145*(2, Suppl.), S8–S11.

Papavasiliou, A.S. (2009). Management of motor problems in cerebral palsy: A critical update for the clinician. *European Journal of Paediatric Neurology, 13*(5), 387–396.

Pellegrino, L. (1995). Cerebral palsy: A paradigm for developmental disabilities. *Developmental Medicine and Child Neurology, 37*(9), 834–839.

Pidcock, F.S. (2004). The emerging role of therapeutic botulinum toxin in the treatment of cerebral palsy. *The Journal of Pediatrics, 145*(2, Suppl.), S33–35.

Pin, T.W., McCartney, L., Lewis, J., & Waugh, M.C. (2011). Use of intrathecal baclofen therapy in ambulant children and adolescents with spasticity and dystonia of cerebral origin: A systematic review. *Developmental Medicine and Child Neurology, 53*(10), 885–895.

Pschirrer, E.R., & Yeomans, E.R. (2000). Does asphyxia cause cerebral palsy? *Seminars in Perinatology, 24*(3), 215–220.

Raina, P., O'Donnell, M., Rosenbaum, P., Brehaut, J., Walter, S.D., Russell, D., ... Wood, E. (2005). The health and well-being of caregivers of children with cerebral palsy. *Pediatrics, 115*(6), e626–e636.

Reddihough, D.S., & Collins, K.J. (2003). The epidemiology and causes of cerebral palsy. *Australian Journal of Physiotherapy, 49*(1), 7–12.

Rosenbaum, P.L., Walter, S.D., Hanna, S.E., Palisano, R.J., Russell, D.J., Raina, P., ... Galuppi, B.E. (2002). Prognosis for gross motor function in cerebral palsy: creation of motor development curves. *JAMA: The Journal of the American Medical Association, 288*(11), 1357–1363.

Russman, B.S., & Ashwal, S. (2004). Evaluation of the child with cerebral palsy. *Seminars in Pediatric Neurology, 11*(1), 47–57.

Russman, B., & Gage, J. (1989). Cerebral palsy. *Current Problems in Pediatrics, 19*(2), 65–111.

Samson-Fang, L., Fung, E., Stallings, V.A., Conaway, M., Worley, G., Rosenbaum, P., ... Stevenson, R.D. (2002). Relationship of nutritional status to health and societal participation in children with cerebral palsy. *The Journal of Pediatrics, 141*(5), 637–643.

Scott, B.L., & Jankovic, J. (1996). Delayed-onset progressive movement disorders after static brain lesions. *Neurology, 46*(1), 68–74.

Seashore, M.R. (2009). The organic acidemias: An overview. *GeneReviews,* 1993–2001. Retrieved from http://www.ncbi.nlm.nih.gov/sites/GeneTests/query.

Serruya, M.D., & Kahana, M.J. (2008). Techniques and devices to restore cognition. *Behavioral Brain Research, 192*(2), 149–165.

Shapiro, S.M. (2005). Definition of the clinical spectrum of kernicterus and bilirubin-induced neurologic dysfunction (BIND). *Journal of Perinatology, 25*(1), 54–59.

Shatrov, J.G., Birch, S.C., Lam, L.T., Quinlivan, J.A., McIntyre, S., & Mendz, G.L. (2010). Chorioamnionitis and cerebral palsy: A meta-analysis. *Obstetrics & Gynecology, 116*(2), 387–392.

Shrestha, S. (2010). Lesions of upper motor neurons and lower motor neurons. *Medchrome Online Medical Magazine,* July 25, 2010. Retrieved from http://medchrome.com/basic-science/anatomy/lesions-of-upper-motor-neurons-and-lower-motor-neurons/.

Sobrado, P., Suarez, J., & Garcia-Sanchez, F.A. (1999). Refractive errors in children with cerebral palsy, psychomotor retardation, and other non-cerebral palsy neuromotor disabilities. *Developmental Medicine and Child Neurology, 41*(6), 396–403.

Stott, N.S., Piedrahita, L., & American Academy for Cerebral Palsy and Developmental Medicine. (2004). Effects of surgical adductor releases for hip subluxation in cerebral palsy: An AACPDM evidence report. *Developmental Medicine and Child Neurology, 46*(9), 628–645.

Strauss, D., & Shavelle, R. (2001). Life expectancy in cerebral palsy. *Archives of Disease in Childhood, 85*(5), 442.

Strauss, D., Cable, W., & Shavelle, R. (1999). Causes of excess mortality in cerebral palsy. *Developmental Medicine and Child Neurology, 41*(9), 580–585.

Strauss, D.J., Shavelle, R.M., & Anderson, T.W. (1998). Life expectancy of children with cerebral palsy. *Pediatric Neurology, 18*(2), 143–149.

Taub, E., Ramey, S.L., DeLuca, S., & Echols, K. (2004). Efficacy of constraint-induced movement therapy for children with cerebral palsy with asymmetric motor impairment. *Pediatrics, 113*(2), 305–312.

Tedroff, K., Löwing, K., Jacobson, D.N., & Åström, E. (2011). Does loss of spasticity matter? A 10-year follow-up after selective dorsal rhizotomy in cerebral palsy. *Developmental Medicine and Child Neurology, 53*(8), 724–729.

Tilton, A.H. (2004). Management of spasticity in children with cerebral palsy. *Seminars in Pediatric Neurology, 11*(1), 58–65.

Tilton, A.H. (2006). Therapeutic interventions for tone abnormalities in cerebral palsy. *NeuroRx, 3*(2), 217–224.

Tosi, L.L., Maher, N., Moore, D.W., Goldstein, M., & Aisen, M.L. (2009). Adults with cerebral palsy: A workshop to define the challenges of treating and preventing secondary musculoskeletal and neuromuscular complications in this rapidly growing population. *Developmental Medicine and Child Neurology, 51*(Suppl. 4), 2–11.

Turk, M.A. (2009). Health, mortality, and wellness issues in adults with cerebral palsy. *Developmental Medicine and Child Neurology, 51*(Suppl. 4), 24–29.

van der Dussen, L., Nieuwstraten, W., Roebroeck, M., & Stam, H.J. (2001). Functional level of young adults with cerebral palsy. *Clinical Rehabilitation, 15*(1), 84–91.

Vargus-Adams, J. (2009). Understanding function and other outcomes in cerebral palsy. *Physical Medicine and Rehabilitation Clinics of North America, 20*(3), 567–575.

Vermeulen, R.J., Wilke, M., Horber, V., & Krägeloh-Mann, I. (2010). Microcephaly with simplified gyral pattern: MRI classification. *Neurology, 74*(5), 386–391.

Vidailhet, M., Yelnik, J., Lagrange, C., Fraix, V., Grabli, D., Thobois, S., ... French SPIDY-2 Study Group. (2009). Bilateral pallidal deep brain stimulation for the treatment of patients with dystonia-choreoathetosis cerebral palsy: A prospective pilot study. *The Lancet Neurology, 8*(8), 709–717.

Vogtle, L.K. (2009). Pain in adults with cerebral palsy: Impact and solutions. *Developmental Medicine and Child Neurology, 51*(Suppl. 4), 113–121.

Vohr, B.R., Msall, M.E., Wilson, D., Wright, L.L., McDonald, S., & Poole, W.K. (2005). Spectrum of gross motor function in extremely low birth weight children with cerebral palsy at 18 months of age. *Pediatrics, 116*(1), 123–129.

Volpe, J.J. (2005). Encephalopathy of prematurity includes neuronal abnormalities. *Pediatrics, 116*(1), 221–225.

Volpe, J.J. (2009). The encephalopathy of prematurity—brain injury and impaired brain development inextricably intertwined. *Seminars in Pediatric Neurology, 14*(4), 167–178.

Wasiak, J., Hoare, B., & Wallen, M. (2004). Botulinum toxin A as an adjunct to treatment in the management of the upper limb in children with spastic cerebral palsy. *Cochrane Database of Systematic Reviews, 4*, CD003469.

Watson, R., Parr, J.R., Joyce, C., May, C., & Le Couteur, A.S. (2011). Models of transitional care for young people with complex health needs: A scoping review. *Child Care, Health & Development, 37*(6), 780–791.

Watts, R., Liston, C., Niogi, S., & Uluğ, A.M. (2003). Fiber tracking using magnetic resonance diffusion tensor imaging and its applications to human brain development. *Mental Retardation and Developmental Disabilities Research Reviews, 9*(3), 168–177.

We Move: Worldwide Education and Awareness for Movement Disorders. (2012). Retrieved from http://www.wemove.org.

Willis, J.K., Morello, A., Davie, A., Rice, J.C., & Bennett, J.T. (2002). Forced use treatment of childhood hemiparesis. *Pediatrics, 110*(1, Pt. 1), 94–96.

Winter, S., Autry, A., Boyle, C., & Yeargin-Allsopp, M. (2002). Trends in the prevalence of cerebral palsy in a population-based study. *Pediatrics, 110*(6), 1220–1225.

Wittenberg, G.F. (2009). Neural plasticity and treatment across the lifespan for motor deficits in cerebral palsy. *Developmental Medicine and Child Neurology, 51*(Suppl. 4), 130–133.

Wood, D.L., Kantor, D., Edwards, L., & James, H. (2008). Health care transition for youth with cerebral palsy. *Northeast Florida Medicine, 59*(4), 4447.

Wood, E., & Rosenbaum, P. (2000). The gross motor function classification system for cerebral palsy: A study of reliability and stability over time. *Developmental Medicine and Child Neurology, 42*(5), 292–296.

Wu, Y.W. (2002). Systematic review of chorioamnionitis and palsy. *Mental Retardation and Developmental Disabilities Research Reviews, 8*(1), 25–29.

Wu, Y.W., Day, S.M., Strauss, D.J., & Shavelle, R.M. (2004). Prognosis for ambulation in cerebral palsy: A population-based study. *Pediatrics, 114*(5), 1264–1271.

Yoon, B.H., Park, C.W., & Chaiworapongsa, T. (2003). Intrauterine infection and the development of cerebral palsy. *BJOG: An International Journal of Obstetrics and Gynaecology, 110*(Suppl. 20), 124–127.

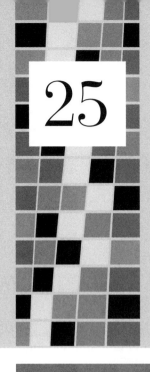

25 Neural Tube Defects

Gregory S. Liptak

Upon completion of this chapter, the reader will

- Be able to define the term *neural tube defects* and its various subtypes

- Know the occurrence and factors associated with the development of neural tube defects

- Understand the impact of meningomyelocele on body structures, on functions, and on the child's activities and participation

- Understand strategies for intervention, the need for multidisciplinary care, and goals for independence

Neural tube defects (NTDs) are a group of malformations of the spinal cord, brain, and vertebrae. The three major NTDs are encephalocele, anencephaly, and spina bifida. **Encephalocele** is a malformation of the skull that allows a portion of the brain, which is usually malformed, to protrude in a sac. The vast majority of encephaloceles occur in the occipital, or back, region of the brain. Affected children often have intellectual disability, **hydrocephalus** (excess fluid in the cavities of the brain), spastic legs, and/or seizures. Encephaloceles also occur in the frontal area, usually as a mass in the forehead, but in some cases in the nose or orbit (eye socket). The following factors are associated with better outcomes in children with encephaloceles: 1) no associated abnormalities of the brain (e.g., hydrocephalus, abnormal cell migration), 2) no other physical abnormalities, 3) frontal rather than occipital location, 4) head circumference in the typical range (rather than too small or too large),

and 5) less brain tissue in the sac. **Anencephaly** is an even more severe congenital malformation of the skull and brain in which no neural development occurs above the brainstem (the most primitive part of the brain). About half of fetuses with anencephaly are spontaneously aborted; those who are live born rarely survive infancy.

The most common NTD is **spina bifida**, which is a split of the vertebral arches. This split may be isolated to the bone or occur with a protruding meningeal sac that may contain a portion of the spinal cord. The most common form of spina bifida, spina bifida occulta, is also the most benign. Approximately 10% of the general population has this hidden separation of the vertebral arches. Individuals with spina bifida occulta do not have 1) abnormalities visible on their back, 2) a sac or protruding spinal cord, or 3) any symptoms.

A form of spina bifida not to be confused with spina bifida occulta is occult spinal dysraphism (OSD). In this condition, the infant is born with a visible abnormality on the lower back (Figure 25.1). This may be a birthmark (especially a reddish area called a **hemangioma** or a flame nevus; Drolet et al., 2010), tufts of hair, a **dermal sinus** (opening in the skin), or a small lump containing a fatty benign tumor, called a **lipoma** (Guggisberg et al., 2004; Muthukumar, 2009). A dimple that is not in the middle, is above the sacral region, is large, or does not have a visible bottom, may be associated with OSD. In OSD, the underlying spinal cord may be connected to the surface through a sinus that exposes it to bacteria, thereby increasing the risk of infection, especially **meningitis** (infection of the brain lining). The spinal cord itself may be **tethered** (tied down) to surrounding tissue, or it may be split, called diastematomyelia or diplomyelia (Kumar, Bansal, & Chhabra, 2002). These defects can lead to subsequent neurological damage as the child grows. Therefore, infants who have these signs (i.e., hemangioma, hair tufts, or lipoma) should have an evaluation of the underlying soft tissue and spinal cord. This can be accomplished by ultrasound or magnetic resonance imaging (MRI) scan. Most clinicians believe that surgical treatment to correct the OSD should be performed early, even in asymptomatic infants, to prevent progressive neurological damage (Drolet et al., 2010; Oi et al., 2009).

Some individuals are born with an exposed membranous sac covering the spinal cord, called a **meningocele**. In this form of spina bifida, the spinal cord itself is not entrapped, and these children usually have no symptoms. When the sac is associated with the presence of a malformed spinal cord, the condition is called **meningomyelocele** (or myelomeningocele). This disorder, often simply referred to as spina bifida, is associated with a complex array of symptoms that can include complete or partial paralysis, sensory loss below the lesion

of the spinal abnormality, Chiari type II malformation (see Origin of Neural Tube Defects section) with hydrocephalus, and **neurogenic** (absence of innervation to) bowel and bladder. Most meningomyeloceles are open, and a portion of the spinal cord is visible at birth as an open sac overlying part of the vertebral column. Children with meningomyelocele typically have associated abnormalities of the brain, including abnormal migration of neurons during the development of the brain (Bartonek & Saraste, 2001). These abnormalities may manifest clinically as learning disabilities. Because of its profound effects on multiple body systems, meningomyelocele has been called the most complex congenital malformation compatible with life.

This chapter focuses on meningomyelocele. It discusses 1) the effects of the condition on medical, physical, psychosocial, and cognitive development; 2) approaches to treatment; and 3) the psychological and economic impacts that can affect families of children with this disorder.

■ ■ ■ LUCITA

Lucita is a 7-year-old girl who illustrates the complexity involved in caring for a child with meningomyelocele. She has a low lumbar level meningomyelocele, which was diagnosed prenatally. She was delivered by cesarean section at an academic medical center and started on antibiotics. Her back lesion was repaired 20 hours after her birth. A cranial MRI scan showed a Chiari type II malformation. Serial cranial ultrasounds showed increasing ventricular size, so on Day 7 she had surgical placement of a **ventriculoperitoneal (VP) shunt** that drained the excess ventricular fluid into her abdominal cavity. Renal and bladder ultrasound were unremarkable. At birth she had mild clubbed feet which were treated with a cast placed when she was 10 days old.

At 6 months of age, **urodynamics** (a test that assesses how the bladder and urethra are performing their job of storing and releasing urine) revealed elevated pressure in her bladder, so clean intermittent catheterization (CIC) was started. She was also referred to an early intervention program and received physical therapy (PT), occupational therapy (OT), and early childhood education services until entry into kindergarten, when she began receiving special education services through an individualized education program (IEP).

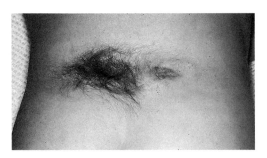

Figure 25.1. Occult spina dysraphism showing hairy patch and hyperpigmentation (gray area at right) associated with underlying abnormalities of the spine and spinal cord.

She was started on a timed toileting program and a high-fiber diet when she was 3 years of age. At 4 years of age, she developed headaches, vomiting, and lethargy. A cranial computed tomography (CT) scan showed increased ventricular size indicating malfunction of her VP shunt, so it was revised surgically.

She now attends a general education second grade class and has mild learning disabilities but is generally doing well academically. She continues to receive PT and OT at school, as well as adapted physical education; she is pulled out for special education reading services 3 times a week. She has friends and generally is cheerful.

She uses knee-ankle-foot orthoses (KAFOs) and Lofstrand crutches for mobility. She has a 20-degree thoracolumbar scoliosis, which is being monitored by her orthopedic surgeon. She has not developed skin sores. Despite her family's best efforts, however, Lucita continues to have fecal accidents. As a result, her family would like more information about the antegrade (forward-flowing) colonic enema (ACE) procedure to improve her encopresis. She has had occasional urinary tract infections that were easily treated. Repeated evaluations have shown that her kidneys are growing and functioning normally.

PREVALENCE OF NEURAL TUBE DEFECTS

The prevalence of NTDs varies among countries. In the United States, the birth prevalence of all forms of spina bifida in the years 2003–2004 was approximately 3 per 10,000; for anencephaly it was 2 per 10,000, giving a total of 5 per 10,000 (Boulet et al., 2008). These numbers do not include terminated pregnancies. In Wales and Ireland, the prevalence is 3–4 times higher; in Africa it is much lower (Rankin, Glinianaia, Brown, & Renwick, 2000). This variability is likely a reflection of genetic influences in certain ethnic groups, as well as environmental factors.

Females are affected 3–7 times as frequently as males, except for sacral-level NTDs, in which the occurrence is equal (Hall et al., 1988). The birth prevalence also increases with maternal age and with lower socioeconomic status.

The prevalence of NTDs is falling worldwide as a result of a number of factors. Many countries use maternal serum testing to screen prenatally for NTDs. More than 50% of couples, upon learning that they are carrying an affected fetus, choose to terminate the pregnancy (Aguilera, Soothill, Denbow, & Pople, 2009), although this varies according to religion and ethnic background (Forrester & Merz, 2000). A number of countries, including the United States, now enrich flour with folic acid, and obstetricians generally recommend folic acid supplementation during pregnancy because of its association with a decreased risk of NTDs. At the same time that prevalence at birth has decreased, survival has increased as a result of improved medical care. This has led to an increased population of adolescents and adults with meningomyelocele (Davis et al., 2005). Thus, improving the transition of these individuals from adolescence to adulthood and ensuring the availability of adult services has become more important.

THE ORIGIN OF NEURAL TUBE DEFECTS

The malformation causing NTDs occurs by 26 days after fertilization of the egg during the period of neurulation (Figure 25.2; Copp, Fleming, & Greene, 1998), which is the first step in the formation of the central nervous system (CNS; see Chapter 2). During this period, the neural groove folds over to become the neural tube, which develops into the spinal cord and vertebral arches. If a portion of the neural groove does not close completely during this process, an NTD results, and the spinal cord is malformed. Although the mechanism of neural tube closure is not fully understood, it does not simply work like a zipper, but has multiple sites of closure. Each of these sites may be under separate genetic control, and there may be differential sensitivity to genetic and environmental factors (Copp & Greene, 2010).

The causes of NTDs remain uncertain. Both environmental and genetic factors play a role, and they interact with each other in complex ways (Hall & Solehdin, 1998). A few candidate genes that increase the risk of NTDs have been identified in human studies (Copp & Greene, 2010). As one example, a deficiency of 5,10-methylene tetrahydrofolate reductase (MTHFR) resulting from a mutation in the gene for this enzyme involved in the metabolism of folic acid, predisposes humans to NTDs. Supplementation with its cofactor, folic acid (also called folate), reduces the risk of NTDs in affected families (Charles et al., 2005; Shurtleff, 2004). Apart from MTHFR, very few

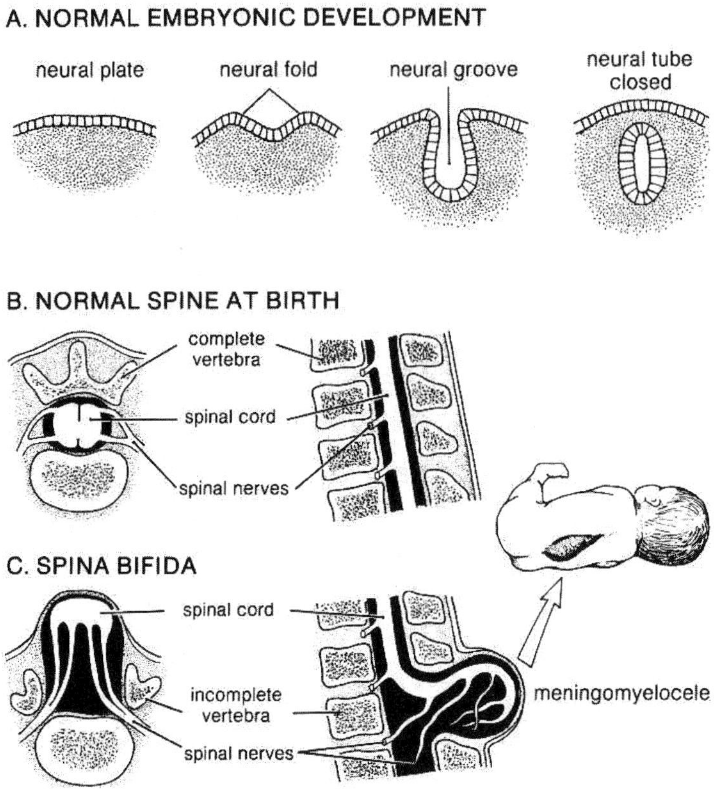

A. NORMAL EMBRYONIC DEVELOPMENT

neural plate   neural fold   neural groove   neural tube
                                                            closed

B. NORMAL SPINE AT BIRTH

complete vertebra

spinal cord

spinal nerves

C. SPINA BIFIDA

spinal cord

incomplete vertebra

spinal nerves

meningomyelocele

Figure 25.2. Normal neural tube development compared to spina bifida with meningomyelocele. A) The typical formation of the neural tube (i.e., the precursor of the spinal column) during the first month of gestation. B) Complete closure of the neural groove has occurred; the vertebral column and spinal cord appear normal in the cross-section on the left and in the longitudinal section on the right. C) Incomplete closure of an area of the spine is called spina bifida and may be accompanied by a meningomyelocele, a sac-like abnormality of the spinal cord. Because nerves do not normally form below this malformation, the child is paralyzed below (or caudal to) that point.

other candidate genes for causing NTDs have been identified. Also, abnormalities in all the candidate genes identified account for only a small percentage of NTDs in humans (Copp & Greene, 2010). Other conditions that have been associated with the development of NTDs include 1) chromosomal disorders (especially trisomy 13 and 18 and certain deletions and duplications; Lynch, 2005; see Appendix B), 2) maternal exposure to the antiepileptic drugs valproic acid (Depakene, Depakote) and carbamazepine (Tegretol) and to the acne medication isotretinoin (Accutane; Ornoy, 2006), 3) maternal alcohol abuse, 4) maternal exposure to hyperthermia (e.g., the use of saunas, high fever; Suarez, Felkner, & Hendricks, 2004), and 5) maternal diabetes (Chen, 2005). Maternal obesity has also been associated with the development of NTDs in offspring. For example, the risk of having a child with spina bifida is doubled if the body mass index (BMI; see

Chapter 8) is greater than 29 kg/m² (kilograms per meters squared; normal is less than 25). Risks have also been found to vary by ethnicity and gender of the child. For example, obese Latina women who have daughters are 8 times more likely to have a child with meningomyelocele than nonobese Caucasian women who have sons (Shaw et al., 2003).

It is controversial as to whether the neural damage in NTDs results simply from the malformed spinal cord or from a combination of malformation and the inflammatory effects of chronic exposure of the open cord to amniotic fluid. Studies in sheep (Meuli et al., 1995) suggest that closing an open lesion in the back results in less neural damage. Experimental trials of prenatal surgery have been performed in human fetuses that were diagnosed prenatally with meningomyelocele (National Institute of Child Health and Human Development, 2004). Infants born after prenatal surgery had less severe Chiari type II malformations (hindbrain herniation, i.e., the downward displacement of the back of the brain) and resultant hydrocephalus. As a result, they had less need for ventricular shunting (Bruner & Tulipan, 2005; Sutton & Adzick, 2004). They also were more likely to be walking independently than those who had surgery after birth. Overall, they had better motor function than what would be expected based on the level of the NTD. No difference was found in intelligence between the two groups. Results on urological function were not reported. In the prenatally treated group, however, mothers and children were more likely to have adverse events related to the surgery, including premature delivery, pregnancy complications, and tethered spinal cord (Adzick et al., 2011). The risks and benefits of prenatal surgery have not been sufficiently evaluated to consider it to be standard medical practice at the writing of this chapter (Adzick, Thom, Spong, & Brock, 2011).

PREVENTION OF NEURAL TUBE DEFECTS USING FOLIC ACID SUPPLEMENTATION

Although this chapter focuses on the treatment of children with meningomyelocele, it is important to recognize that prevention is possible based on the strong link between NTDs and folic acid deficiency. Couples who have had one child with an NTD have a recurrence risk that is about 30 times higher (i.e., 3 in 100) than that of the general population. If these women take 4 mg (milligrams) of folic acid per day at or before conception and continue this supplementation during the first trimester (12 weeks) of the pregnancy, their recurrence risk is reduced by 70% (Medical Research Council Vitamin Study Research Group, 1991). Women who have an NTD or have a first-degree relative with an NTD also should take 4 mg per day of folic acid from the time they are considering becoming pregnant.

Studies also have shown that daily supplemental doses of folic acid can reduce the occurrence of new cases of NTDs in the general population by 50% or more (Gucciardi et al., 2002; Martinez et al., 2002; Persad, Van den Hof, Dubé, & Zimmer, 2002). As a result, it is now recommended that all women who are contemplating a pregnancy take 0.4 mg (400 micrograms) of supplemental folic acid per day while they are trying to conceive and during the first trimester of pregnancy (American Academy of Pediatrics, Committee on Genetics, 1999; Manning, Jennings, & Madsen, 2000). Supplementation with folate can also decrease the occurrence of cleft lip and palate (van Rooij et al., 2004). Yet, only about one third of women who are planning a pregnancy were found to take folic acid around the time of conception (Schader & Corwin, 1999); in addition, half of all pregnancies in the United States are unplanned (Centers for Disease Control and Prevention, 2000). To address this problem, since 1998 certain food staples in the United States (e.g., bread, flour) have been made with grain fortified with folic acid (Honein, Paulozzi, Mathews, Erickson, & Wong, 2001).

The birth incidence of NTDs in the United States in 1995–1996 (including prenatal occurrences), prior to supplementation, was 6.4 per 100,000; in 1999–2000, after supplementation, it was 4.1 per 100,000 (Centers for Disease Control and Prevention, 2004). However, the amount of folic acid in a typical diet, even with this fortification, is not optimal to prevent NTDs; therefore, individual supplements are important in women of childbearing age. From 1999–2005, the prevalence of spina bifida in the United States declined from 2.04 to 1.90 per 10,000 live births (Centers for Disease Control and Prevention, 2009), with greater reductions observed among Hispanic and non-Hispanic white women than among non-Hispanic black women (Williams, Rasmussen, Flores, Kirby, & Edmonds, 2005). Folic acid supplementation has little effect on certain types of NTDs, however, including lipomyelomeningocele (McNeely & Howes, 2004). In some animals, inositol (a type of sugar) can prevent NTDs in those resistant to folic acid. Whether or not this treatment will be effective in humans remains to be investigated (Shaw, 2008).

PRENATAL DIAGNOSIS

NTDs can be diagnosed prenatally by several methods (see Chapter 4; Main & Mennuti, 1986). Most obstetricians first measure levels of **alpha-fetoprotein** (AFP) in the mother's serum during the 16th–18th week of pregnancy (Bahado-Singh & Sutton-Riley, 2004). AFP is a chemical typically found in the fetal spinal fluid, brain, and spinal cord. In the presence of an open meningomyelocele, encephalocele, or anencephaly, AFP leaks from the open spine into the amniotic fluid, then into the maternal circulation, where it can be detected in minute amounts. Because other conditions in both mother and fetus can lead to elevated AFP levels, maternal serum AFP (MSAFP) is used only as a screening test for NTDs. After a positive AFP screen has been obtained, a high-resolution ultrasound is used to detect specific abnormalities of the fetal head and back that have been found with an NTD (Babcock, 1995; Norem et al., 2005). Correct interpretation of the ultrasound depends a great deal on the training and experience of the radiologist conducting the study (Bruner et al., 2004).

If an NTD is suspected after the ultrasound, amniocentesis is performed. The levels of two substances in the amniotic fluid, AFP and an enzyme specific for NTDs called acetylcholinesterase (ACH), are measured. The combination of elevated levels of AFP and ACH with abnormal ultrasonographic findings makes the diagnosis of an NTD in the fetus quite certain. Chromosomal analysis of the amniotic fluid is also performed to rule out specific chromosomal disorders (e.g., trisomy 13 and 18) that are associated with NTDs. In some centers, fetal MRI or 3-D ultrasonography may be performed rather than amniocentesis.

Even if a family is not considering termination of the pregnancy if an NTD is detected, obtaining a prenatal diagnosis can help the parents plan for the special needs of their child. For example, they may opt to deliver their child via cesarean section at a center with a neonatal intensive care unit (NICU) and to have the back lesion closed early by an experienced surgeon, precautions that some believe may decrease the severity of paralysis (Liu, Shurtleff, Ellenbogen, Loeser, & Kropp, 1999).

TREATMENT OF MENINGOMYELOCELE IN THE NEWBORN PERIOD

When an infant is born with meningomyelocele, the first two priorities are to prevent spinal cord infection (meningitis) and to protect exposed spinal nerves and associated structures from physical injury. Both of these goals can be accomplished by the surgical closure of the defect within the first few days of life. In addition, a ventricular shunting procedure is often required shortly after the back closure to prevent cerebrospinal fluid (CSF), which can no longer leak from an open meningomyelocele, from accumulating and causing progressive hydrocephalus and potential brain injury (Tuli, Drake, & Lamberti-Pasculli, 2003).

PRIMARY NEUROLOGICAL IMPAIRMENTS IN CHILDREN WITH MENINGOMYELOCELE

The malformation leading to meningomyelocele affects the entire CNS (Dahl et al., 1995). Table 25.1 lists some of the brain abnormalities commonly found in children with meningomyelocele. These include 1) multiple disorders of the cranial nerve nuclei (e.g., the visual gaze centers of the brain can be affected, leading to strabismus); 2) abnormalities of the corpus callosum (the major bridge between the right and left sides of the brain); 3) excessive fluid or splitting of the spinal cord above the primary lesion, resulting in additional motor impairment; and 4) scattered changes in the brain's cortex from migration defects that are associated with cognitive impairments. The primary neurological abnormalities, however, are paralysis, loss of sensation, learning disabilities, and the Chiari type II malformation with associated hydrocephalus.

Paralysis and Loss of Sensation

The extent of motor paralysis and sensory loss in meningomyelocele depends on the location of the defect in the spinal cord (Figures 25.3 and 25.4), as sensory and motor function below that point are typically impaired. All individuals with meningomyelocele experience some loss of sensation. The loss of motor and sensory function is not always symmetrical; one side may have better motor function or sensation than the other (Figure 25.5).

Chiari Malformation and Hydrocephalus

Almost all children with meningomyelocele above the **sacral** (pelvic) level have a **Chiari**

Table 25.1. Malformations of the brain frequently seen in children with meningomyelocele

Malformation	Prevalence (%)
Dysplasia of cerebral cortex	92
Displaced nerve cells	44
Small gyri with abnormal layers	40
Abnormalities of layers	24
Profound primitive development	24
Small gyri with normal layers	12
Malformations of the brainstem	76
Malformations of the cerebellum	72

Source: Gilbert, Jones, Rorke, Chernoff, & James (1986).

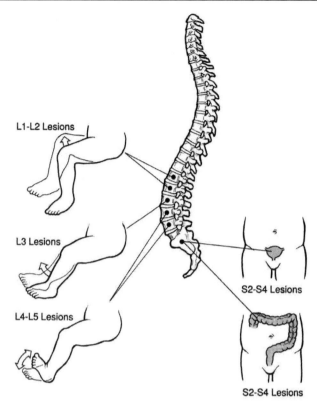

Figure 25.3. This figure shows where movement, sensation, and bladder and bowel function are usually controlled in the spinal cord. Meningomyelocele (lesions) at these levels usually prevents typical functioning at and below the levels shown.

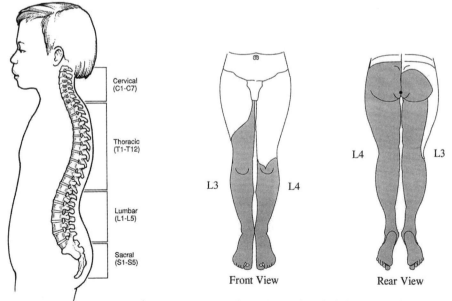

Figure 25.4. The vertebral column is divided into seven neck (cervical), 12 chest (thoracic), five back (lumbar), and five lower back (sacral) vertebrae. Meningomyelocele most commonly affects the thoracolumbar region.

Figure 25.5. Sensory loss (shaded areas) in a child with L3- to L4-level meningomyelocele. The back of the legs has more loss than the front. Asymmetry of sensory or motor loss is common; sensory loss may not completely correlate with loss of motor function.

type II malformation of the brain (Stevenson, 2004). In this abnormality, the brainstem and part of the cerebellum are displaced downward toward the neck, rather than remaining within the skull (Figure 25.6). Symptoms and signs of brainstem and spinal cord compression from the malformation include difficulty swallowing, choking, hoarseness, breath-holding spells, apnea (periodic brief respiratory arrests), disordered breathing during sleep, stiffness in the arms, and **opisthotonos** (arching of the head backward). If symptoms of compression develop, they can be treated surgically by a decompression procedure, in which a portion of the occipital region of the skull and the arches of some of the **cervical** (neck) vertebral bodies are removed to provide additional space for the brainstem. This provides short-term benefit, but the long-term effectiveness remains uncertain. Children with more severe symptoms (e.g., vocal cord paralysis) and children who have been symptomatic for a longer period (e.g., months) have worse outcomes following decompressive surgery.

Disordered breathing during sleep occurs frequently in individuals with meningomyelocele and has been called the "missed diagnosis." It may be the result of obstructive **sleep apnea** (brief episodes of respiratory arrest occurring during sleep and resulting from a temporary anatomical obstruction), central apnea (respiratory arrest during awake or sleep periods resulting from impaired brain control of respiration), or **central hypoventilation** (shallow breathing leading to low oxygen level resulting from disordered cerebral control of respiration; Kirk, Morielli, & Brouillette, 1999). Disordered sleep can cause children to be tired during the day, interfering with their ability to function in school. A formal sleep study can help differentiate among the various problems that can cause this disordered breathing. The treatment depends on the nature of the breathing disorder identified by this study. For example, **adenotonsillectomy** (surgical removal of adenoids and tonsils) may help if the upper airway is obstructed. If there is underlying central apnea, surgery to provide posterior fossa decompression of the Chiari type II malformation may be performed, although this is not always effective. A significant proportion of children with severe breathing disorders who do not respond to the above measures will require assisted ventilation through continuous positive airway pressure (CPAP) or bilevel positive airway pressure (BiPAP) during sleep. The BiPAP machine fits over the child's face and monitors the child's breathing electronically, providing a higher pressure during inhalation and a lower pressure during exhalation. If these approaches are not effective, a tracheostomy with mechanical ventilation may be required.

Hydrocephalus occurs in 60%–95% of children with meningomyelocele and is most common in **thoracolumbar** (lower chest) lesions (Tuli et al., 2003). Hydrocephalus develops as a result of an abnormal CSF flow pattern, leading to an enlargement of the ventricular system of the brain. It can be diagnosed by neuroimaging studies: ultrasound in the prenatal period and in infancy, and CT or MRI in older children.

Hydrocephalus is treated with a surgically implanted shunt. Shunting diverts CSF from the enlarged ventricular system to another place in the body where it can be better absorbed. The most common type, a VP shunt, drains fluid into the child's abdominal cavity (Figure 25.7). Shunts to the pleural space (surrounding the lungs) are less commonly used as an alternative. Neither of these types of shunts necessitates prophylactic antibiotics prior to dental procedures. However, another approach involving a shunt to the atrium of the heart does require antibiotic prophylaxis and can result in inflammation of the kidney (nephritis) and chronic embolization to the lungs. As a result, ventriculoatrial shunts are rarely used. In infants, a **ventriculo-subgaleal** (ventricle to

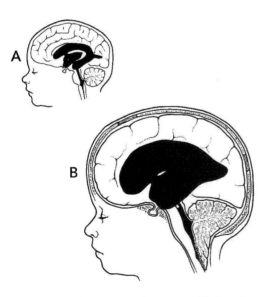

Figure 25.6. Chiari type II malformation and hydrocephalus. A) The typical brain, with ventricles of normal size (shaded area). B) In the Chiari type II malformation and hydrocephalus (shaded area), the brainstem and part of the cerebellum are displaced downward toward the neck region, which can cause symptoms such as difficulty swallowing and hoarseness.

scalp) shunt may be implanted as a temporary measure (Tubbs et al., 2003).

Shunts can become blocked or infected, especially during the first year of life. By 2–3 years of age, approximately half of the shunts inserted have failed and been replaced surgically (Tuli et al., 2003). In infants, signs of a blocked shunt include excessive head growth and a tense anterior fontanel ("soft spot") on the forehead. In all children, a blocked shunt may result in symptoms of lethargy, headache, vomiting, and irritability. The increased intracranial pressure can also lead to paralysis of the sixth cranial nerve (VI), with resultant strabismus and double vision, or to paralysis of upward gaze. A child with an infected shunt can display symptoms similar to those seen in shunt blockage but will also have a fever and an elevated white blood cell count. Signs and symptoms of a blocked shunt can mimic those of a tethered cord or Chiari type II malformation. Therefore, whenever a child with meningomyelocele develops new neurological symptoms,

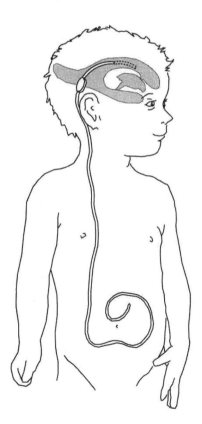

Figure 25.7. A ventriculoperitoneal shunt, which has been placed for hydrocephalus. A plastic tube is inserted into one of the lateral ventricles and connected to a one-way valve. Another tube runs under the skin from the valve to the abdominal cavity. Enough extra tubing is left in the abdomen to uncoil as the child grows.

especially deterioration of physical or cognitive function, a blocked or infected shunt should be investigated. More subtle symptoms of a partial shunt failure include a change in personality, decline in school performance, or weakness of the arms or legs (Matson, Mahone, & Zabel, 2005).

Early recognition of shunt failure or infection is critical, as both complications can be life threatening. A child who develops new neurological symptoms should be evaluated immediately for shunt failure. If a blocked shunt is suspected, the physician may order a neuroimaging study (CT or MRI) to determine if the ventricles have increased in size, as well as radiographs of the shunt system to determine if the tubing is broken or kinked. If the shunt is found to be obstructed, the blocked portion will be replaced surgically with a new catheter (tube) and/or valve.

If the shunt is infected, the child also needs to receive intravenous antibiotics. In addition, it may be necessary to remove the infected shunt surgically and, after antibiotic treatment, replace it with a new one. It is important to emphasize that the individual with hydrocephalus almost always requires a working shunt throughout his or her life. In some children, however, a new surgical procedure called endoscopic third ventriculostomy may obviate the need for ventricular shunts. This technique involves placing a hole in the floor of one of the ventricles to drain CSF within the brain. Its safety and effectiveness in the treatment of children with hydrocephalus associated with NTDs is still uncertain (Marlin, 2004; Warf et al., 2009).

ASSOCIATED IMPAIRMENTS AND MEDICAL COMPLICATIONS

Meningomyelocele, hydrocephalus, and the associated malformations of the brain lead to developmental disabilities and place the child at risk for a number of medical complications (Verhoef et al., 2004). These associated disabilities include mobility impairment, cognitive impairments, seizure disorders, fine motor impairments, and visual impairment. Medical complications include musculoskeletal abnormalities, spinal curvatures and humps, urinary and bowel dysfunction, skin sores, disordered breathing, atypical weight and stature, sexual issues (such as dysfunction and precocious puberty), and allergy to latex. Many of these disabilities and medical complications can be prevented, or their impact lessened, by meticulous clinical care and monitoring by the family, the child, and health care professionals.

Mobility Impairments

The higher the level of the meningomyelocele and the greater the muscle weakness, the more ambulation will be impaired. Even children with low-level lesions (L4 and below), however, are likely to have significant impairment in mobility. Many infants with meningomyelocele have delayed rolling, sitting, and walking skills.

Children with sacral lesions generally learn to walk well by 2 or 3 years of age with bracing at the ankles or no bracing at all (Table 25.2). Children with low lumbar level lesions can usually walk with short leg braces and forearm crutches. Children with high lumbar-thoracic lesions may stand upright and walk for short distances, but often with support of the hips, knees, and ankles. This support may be provided by extensive bracing and/or mobility devices, such as a **parapodium** (an adjustable standing brace), a reciprocal gait orthosis (RGO), or a hip-knee-ankle-foot orthosis (HKAFO) used in combination with crutches or a walker. By early adolescence, most use a wheelchair for primary mobility.

As children with low lumbar level lesions approach adolescence, and their center of gravity and relative strength changes, most will rely increasingly on wheelchairs for mobility (Norrlin, Strinnholm, Carlsson, & Dahl, 2003; van den Berg-Emons et al., 2001). Because most children with meningomyelocele will not become effective community ambulators, the supplemental or primary use of a wheelchair should be considered at least by early adolescence, as it offers the advantages of speed, efficiency, and attractiveness.

Intellectual Impairments

Approximately three quarters of children with meningomyelocele have intelligence quotient (IQ) scores that fall within the typical range (IQ > 70; Barf et al., 2004). Most of the remaining one quarter have mild intellectual disability (IQ 55–70). Children with meningomyelocele but without hydrocephalus have higher IQs, better memory, and better executive function than those with hydrocephalus (Lindquist, Uvebrant, Rehn, & Carlsson, 2009). In one study, half of the adolescents with spina bifida plus hydrocephalus required special intervention for secondary education, compared with only 8% for those with spina bifida without hydrocephalus (Barf et al., 2004). The few children with meningomyelocele who have severe intellectual disability usually have sustained secondary brain injury resulting from severe prenatal hydrocephalus or a complicating brain infection resulting from an infected shunt.

Although the majority of children with meningomyelocele have average intellectual function, they often have impairments in perceptual skills, organizational abilities, attention span, speed of motor response, memory, pragmatic language, and hand function (Norrlin, Dahl, & Rosblad, 2004). By school age, many children with meningomyelocele and hydrocephalus are diagnosed with a nonverbal learning disability (see Chapter 23). These children typically have better reading than math skills. In addition to the learning disability, they often have impairments in executive function that have an impact on education, social, and self-help skills. Executive function skills include the ability to plan, initiate, sequence, sustain, inhibit competing responses, and pace work (Burmeister et al., 2005). For example, the child may know the steps involved in self-catheterization but may have difficulty planning and carrying out the process. Also, disorders of the cerebellum have been associated with intellectual impairments, including impairments in executive function, visual-spatial function, expressive language, verbal memory, and modulation of affect (Barnes, Dennis, & Hetherington, 2004; Iddon, Morgan, Loveday, Sahakian, & Pickard, 2004; Simos et al., 2011). Many children with meningomyelocele have attention-deficit/hyperactivity disorder (ADHD), but only about one third of them respond to stimulant medication (Burmeister et al., 2005; see Chapter 22).

Table 25.2. Functional levels in children with meningomyelocele and implications for mobility

Level	Mobility
High lumbar-thoracic	Can walk for short distances using long leg (high) braces. By early adolescence most use wheelchair for mobility.
Low lumbar	Can walk with short leg braces and forearm crutches.
High sacral	Can walk with a gluteal lurch using braces to stabilize the ankle and foot. Walking ability is usually retained through adolescence.

Because children with meningomyelocele are at increased risk for multiple developmental disabilities, they should be referred to an early intervention program during infancy (see Chapter 30). This should be followed by a formal psychoeducational evaluation prior to school entry to identify strengths and weaknesses and to develop an IEP (see Chapter 31).

Seizure Disorders

Approximately 15% of individuals with meningomyelocele develop a seizure disorder (Battaglia et al., 2004). The seizures usually are generalized **tonic-clonic** and respond well to antiepileptic medication (see Chapter 27). If a new type of seizure develops or if seizure frequency increases, however, a blocked shunt or shunt infection should be suspected and investigated.

Visual Impairments

Strabismus (lazy eye) is present in about 20% of children with meningomyelocele and often requires surgical correction (Verhoef et al., 2004). Visual impairments can result from abnormalities of the visual gaze center in the brain or from increased intracranial pressure caused by a malfunctioning ventricular shunt (see Chapter 11). All children with meningomyelocele should see an ophthalmologist at least once prior to starting school.

Musculoskeletal Abnormalities

With partial or total paralysis, muscle imbalances and lack of mobility may lead to deformities around joints (Dias, 2004). This can occur even prior to birth. For example, children with meningomyelocele may be born with a calcaneus deformity (clubfoot) as a result of the foot being pressed against the uterine wall and becoming stuck in one position. Treatment of clubfoot typically involves serial casting during the first 3–4 months of life to gradually straighten the deformity. Corrective surgery, if needed, can then follow at 4 months to 1 year of age (Flynn et al., 2004). Other ankle and foot deformities may require surgical intervention to facilitate proper foot placement in shoes. Bracing is used to help maintain proper positioning of joints and should be monitored to minimize the occurrence of skin breakdown over bony prominences (e.g., decubitus ulcers of the ankle or buttocks).

Muscle imbalance and lack of movement also can lead to hip deformities. Surgical correction is controversial and may be appropriate only for those children with low lumbar paralysis who have the potential for functional ambulation (Lorente, Molto, & Martinez, 2005). The goals of orthopedic treatment are to maintain alignment and range of motion, stabilize the spine and extremities, maximize function, provide comfort, and protect the skin. Loss of muscle strength and inactivity predispose affected children to fractures (Dosa, Eckrich, Katz, Turk, & Liptak, 2007). These pathological fractures may also occur after orthopedic surgery, especially following prolonged casting. All individuals with spina bifida should receive adequate calcium and vitamin D in order to minimize osteoporosis and the susceptibility to pathological fractures. This is especially true if the child is taking antiepileptic drugs that interfere with calcium and vitamin D metabolism. In addition, weight-bearing activities should be encouraged whenever possible. Following surgical procedures, steps should be taken to prevent deep vein thrombosis, which predisposes the individual to pulmonary emboli. Lastly, as individuals with spina bifida age, they may develop arthritis of the hips or knees secondary to abnormal sensation and gait (Nagarkatti, Banta, & Thomson, 2000).

Spinal Curvatures and Humps

Almost 90% of children with a meningomyelocele above the sacral level have spinal curvatures and/or humps (Trivedi et al., 2002). These deformities include **scoliosis** (a spinal curvature), **kyphosis** (a spinal hump; see Figure 25.8), and **kyphoscoliosis** (a combination of both conditions). Scoliosis and kyphosis may be present before birth (congenital) or develop later in childhood (acquired). If untreated, spinal deformities may eventually interfere with sitting and walking and even decrease lung capacity.

Scoliosis greater than 25 degrees is treated with an orthotic support, a molded plastic shieldlike orthotic jacket called a thoracolumbosacral orthosis (TLSO). Despite this, the curvature often progresses, and surgery may be necessary (Parisini, Greggi, Di Silvestre, Giardina, & Bakaloudis, 2002). Surgical correction involves a spinal fusion with bone grafts. This often requires two surgical procedures, one through the front and one from the back. The procedures use metal rods (internal fixation) and wires (Luque procedure; see Chapter 24, Figure 24.19) for stabilization of the spinal

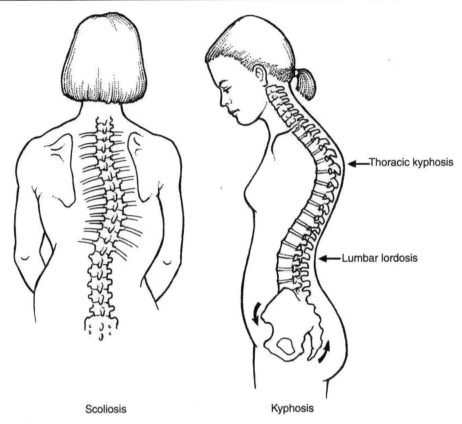

Scoliosis   Kyphosis

Figure 25.8.   Common spinal deformities associated with meningomyelocele.

column. The two-stage procedure has been successfully replaced by a single frontal (anterior) approach in some children whose curve is less than 75 degrees in the absence of abnormalities of the spinal cord. A new device, the vertebral expandable prosthetic titanium rib (or growing rod) has been used with success in the treatment of scoliosis in some children who have spina bifida (Flynn et al., 2011). Children with congenital rather than developmental scoliosis or kyphosis generally respond poorly to orthotic treatment and require spinal fusion at younger ages.

Kyphosis is usually located in the thoracic spine and may measure as much as 80–90 degrees at birth. The hump on the spine may be rigid and may worsen over time. Surgical removal of the deformity is accomplished by an operation called a kyphectomy. This procedure has a high rate of complications and recurrences in infancy, but when performed in school-age children it has been quite effective (Niall, Dowling, Fogarty, Moore, & Goldberg, 2004).

Some evidence indicates that tethering of the spinal cord (discussed later) may lead to rapidly progressive scoliosis. Surgery to untether the cord may halt or even reverse the progression of the curve in individuals whose curves are less than 50 degrees at the time of surgery (Pierz, Banta, Thomson, Gahm, & Hartford, 2000). In addition, a significant number of individuals with spina bifida will have an abnormal fluid collection in the spinal cord or even thinning (hypoplasia) of the cord (Moskowitz, Shurtleff, Weinberger, Loeser, & Ellenbogen, 1998). Because spinal surgery fuses the bones of the spine, making subsequent neurological surgery especially challenging, many centers obtain an MRI scan of the spine on all individuals prior to surgery for kyphosis or scoliosis. In this way, they can identify tethering or cavities in the spinal cord that might require surgery prior to the orthopedic procedure. Following scoliosis surgery, some children benefit in seating; however, overall physical functioning and quality of life are not improved significantly. Major complication rates following scoliosis surgery exceed 50% (Mercado, Alman, & Wright, 2007; Wright, 2010).

Urinary Dysfunction

Because the bladder, **urethra** (urinary outlet), and rectum are all controlled by nerves that leave the spinal cord in the lower sacrum (see Figure 25.3), bladder and bowel dysfunction are present in virtually all children with meningomyelocele. Even children with sacral lesions and normal leg movement typically have bladder and bowel problems. In addition, children with meningomyelocele have a higher incidence of malformations of the kidneys, such as a horseshoe kidney and an absent kidney.

The bladder has two major functions: 1) to store urine that has been produced by the kidneys, and 2) to empty the urine once the bladder is full. Children with meningomyelocele often have difficulty with both functions and are consequently incontinent. In addition, the inability to completely empty the bladder of urine may predispose the child to infections of the bladder and/or kidneys. The combination of a tight bladder outlet and increased tone in the bladder also may produce kidney damage over time (Hopps & Kropp, 2003; Snodgrass & Adams, 2004).

To detect early structural damage, the urinary tract is imaged using ultrasound at regular intervals beginning in infancy. It also permits detection of malformations and abnormal functioning of the bladder and urinary outlet. Bladder function additionally may be evaluated using a **cystometrogram**, a procedure in which fluid is injected into the bladder and pressure is measured. If elevated pressure is found, it must be reduced to avoid permanent kidney damage.

Reducing bladder pressure (and achieving continence) is accomplished by using daily CIC (Hopps & Kropp, 2003). In CIC, the child or his or her parents are taught to insert a clean, but not sterile, catheter through the urethra and into the bladder. This commonly is done at least four times per day to drain urine. When CIC is performed correctly, urine does not accumulate, become infected, or flow back into the kidneys. In some infants, however, this is not successful and a surgical procedure called a **vesicostomy** is performed. In this procedure, an opening through the abdominal wall and into the bladder is created, allowing urine to drain directly into the diaper. When the child is older, the vesicostomy typically is closed surgically and he or she begins a CIC program.

In addition to assessing bladder pressure, the infant is monitored for urinary infections, which occur in at least half of individuals with meningomyelocele. If these happen frequently, long-term prophylactic oral antibiotics such as cephalexin (Keflex) or trimethoprim/sulfamethoxazole (Bactrim, Septra) may be given to prevent infections. Alternatively, antibiotics can be instilled directly into the bladder through the catheter. Neither of these procedures has been validated with scientific research.

Attempts to achieve urinary continence are generally begun at 3–4 years of age. In addition, medications may be used. Oxybutynin chloride (Ditropan) can be given orally or instilled into the bladder to diminish bladder wall contractions; newer agents such as propiverine (Detrunorm) may be better tolerated (Madersbacher et al., 2009). Pseudoephedrine (Sudafed) or imipramine (Tofranil) may be given orally to enhance storage of urine. About 70% of children who receive a combination of CIC and medications achieve continence during elementary school.

If CIC and medication are unsuccessful in producing continence, a surgical intervention may be undertaken. In the past, a silicone-like material was injected around the urethra using an endoscope; however, its long-term effectiveness has been questioned (Block, Cooper, & Hawtrey, 2003; Dean, Kirsch, Packer, Scherz, & Zaontz, 2007; Halachmi et al., 2004). Another approach is a bladder augmentation procedure, in which the bladder capacity is increased using a flap of bowel or stomach. A third procedure is an appendicovesicostomy (Mitrofanoff procedure), in which the appendix is used to connect the bladder to the abdominal wall, permitting catheterization through the appendix. These approaches may be used in combination. A new experimental surgical procedure (Xiao, 2006) that disconnects sensory nerves from the spinal cord and connects them to the bladder nerves has been touted as being extremely successful in partially restoring bladder function but these results need to be replicated.

"Volitional" voiding is also possible using an artificial urinary sphincter that surrounds the urethra and stays closed to prevent leakage of urine. A bulb mechanism is placed in the scrotum or labia majora; when it is squeezed, fluid flows out of the artificial sphincter allowing urine to drain from the bladder. However, complications are common with this procedure, including erosion of the skin around the bulb and poor adherence leading to overdistension of the bladder with resultant kidney damage (Kryger, Spencer Barthold, Fleming, & Gonzalez, 1999). Yet, for a select group of highly motivated individuals, the artificial sphincter can permit volitional voiding. In the past 5 years, botulinum toxin (Botox) has been injected into the bladder muscles of children with neurogenic bladder; the goal is to relax the muscle and increase bladder capacity. Preliminary studies show improvement in bladder capacity and continence (Deshpande, Sampang, & Smith, 2010). Finally, because the risk of bladder cancer is increased, adults with meningomyelocele should be monitored annually with endoscopy of the bladder and cytological analysis of the cells from the urine (Gamé et al., 2006).

Bowel Dysfunction

Bowel problems in children with meningomyelocele are related to uncoordinated propulsive action of the intestines, ineffectual function of the anus, and lack of rectal sensation. Constipation is common and may be interspersed with periods of overflow diarrhea. Lack of sensation and failure of anal function also lead to soiling that can be socially devastating. In individuals with typical bowel function, the rectal sampling reflex can discriminate between gas, liquid stool, and solid stool. Absence of this reflex in children with meningomyelocele worsens continence.

Attempts at bowel management can begin as soon as the child starts eating solids, by encouraging the consumption of foods that are high in fiber. Between 2½ and 4 years of age, timed potty sitting can be tried after every meal to take advantage of the postfeeding gastrocolic (propulsive) reflex. If bowel control has not been achieved after several months, parents may be instructed to administer one or more of the following medications that will facilitate more complete bowel emptying: 1) a daily laxative such as lactulose (a complex sugar), MiraLAX (an agent that keeps water in the stool), or senna (e.g., Senokot); 2) a fiber supplement such as psyllium (e.g., Metamucil); or 3) a nightly rectal suppository such as bisacodyl (e.g., Dulcolax), or daily saline enemas. These may be used in combination.

Two surgical procedures, one that connects the appendix to the colon (Malone procedure) and another that provides a direct connection between the abdominal wall and the colon (cecostomy), allow irrigation of the colon on a regular basis (ACE procedure). The cecostomy can be performed either in the operating room or in an interventional radiology suite. These approaches have been shown to be successful in children for whom more conventional bowel techniques have failed (Aksnes et al., 2002; Leibold, Ekmark, & Adams, 2000). In one study,

about 60% of individuals were still using their ACE 5 years after the surgery (Yardley et al., 2009). There is a newer ACE procedure in which a surgical hole is placed on the left side of the abdomen; irrigation fluids can be inserted into the descending colon, allowing more rapid washout of stool (Ahn, Han, & Choi, 2004; Kim, Han, & Choi, 2006). Its long-term effectiveness, however, has not been established.

For a select group of older children with low-level (sacral) meningomyeloceles who have rectal sensation, biofeedback training may be used to improve rectal function (Aslan & Kogan, 2002). In this training technique, children use a balloon pressure transducer connected to a visible pressure monitor to optimize rectal function, including coordinating efforts to expulse stool.

Skin Sores

Skin sores, or **decubitus ulcers**, frequently occur in children with meningomyelocele, whose weight-bearing surfaces (e.g., feet, buttocks) are not sensitive to pain. These children may sustain injuries that they do not feel, often resulting in a skin sore. This problem becomes more common during adolescence and, if not caught early, the decubitus ulcer may require prolonged hospitalizations for **debridement** (removal of dead tissue), plastic surgery, and intravenous antibiotics. Therefore, the best treatment is prevention. Certain reasonable rules should be followed: 1) examine insensate skin regularly to detect small sores, 2) replace tight-fitting shoes or braces with looser-fitting ones, 3) avoid hot baths, 4) give the child protective foot covering for swimming, 5) do not let the young child crawl about on rough or hot surfaces, and 6) ensure that wheelchair cushions continue to be protective.

For children in wheelchairs, pressure sores on the buttocks or coccyx (tail bone) can be prevented by modifying the wheelchair with an adaptive seating system. Individuals can minimize prolonged pressure by performing regular wheelchair push-ups to relieve pressure and by frequently changing position (Samaniego, 2002). Small skin sores should be treated by alleviating pressure and using saline-soaked dressings or artificial skin preparations, such as Tegaderm or Vigilon. If ulcers do not heal in a reasonable time, an underlying infection may be present, requiring surgical debridement and intravenous antibiotic treatment. Many new coverings and techniques, such as vacuum-assisted closure, have been tried to heal pressure ulcers. The most important rule, however, is that the only thing that should not be placed on a pressure sore is the child!

Weight and Stature Abnormalities

Children with meningomyelocele, particularly those with thoracic to L2 lumbar lesions, are at increased risk for obesity (Dosa, Foley, Eckrich, Woodall-Ruff, & Liptak, 2009). About two thirds of these children are significantly overweight. Attention should be directed at increasing involvement in physical activities such as aerobic conditioning (e.g., wheelchair sports) and strength training, such as lifting free weights (Buffart, van den Berg-Emons, van Meeteren, Stam, & Roebroeck, 2009; Widman, McDonald, & Abresch, 2006). Exercise should be combined with dietary restrictions of sweets and fats, especially because children who have paraplegia need fewer calories to grow and maintain typical weight. Affected children also are likely to have short stature. This results from a combination of failure of growth of the legs, spinal curves, and, occasionally, a deficiency of growth hormone (Hochhaus, Butenandt, & Ring-Mrozik, 1999). Long-term treatment of select individuals with recombinant human growth hormone may lead to more typical final adult stature (Rotenstein & Bass, 2004; Trollmann, Bakker, Lundberg, & Dorr, 2006).

Sexual Issues

Although three quarters of adult males with meningomyelocele can have erections, most do not have control of them (Gamé et al., 2006). Penile implants, injection, or application of prostaglandin prior to coitus (Kim & McVary, 1995); vacuum devices (Chen, Godschalk, Katz, & Mulligan, 1995); and sildenafil (Viagra; Palmer, Kaplan, & Firlit, 1999) can help males achieve volitional erections that allow intercourse. There may be the additional problem of retrograde ejaculation, in which the semen is discharged into the bladder. Despite this, two thirds of males with spina bifida have sufficient sperm in their ejaculate to permit fatherhood using artificial insemination or in vitro fertilization (Hultling, Levi, Amark, & Sjöblom, 2000). Although there are many sexual and reproductive health issues relating to meningomyelocele, in a survey of young adults with spina bifida, 95% stated that they had inadequate knowledge about these issues (Sawyer & Roberts, 1999). In a recent study, adults with the highest chance of finding a partner and engaging in sexual activity were those with the lowest (least severe) lesion

levels (Gatti et al., 2009). It should be noted that because of the high risk of latex allergy in spina bifida, nonlatex condoms should be used.

Females with meningomyelocele have normal fertility and, if sexually active, should use the same precautions to avoid pregnancy and sexually transmitted diseases as the general population. Although many of these women are able to experience orgasm during sexual intercourse, they usually have decreased genital sensation and less sexually stimulated lubrication. As a result, frequent intercourse without adequate lubrication can lead to vaginal sores. Precocious puberty (breast development, menarche, and other sexual changes 2 or more years before average) is a common occurrence in females who have meningomyelocele with hydrocephalus due to a disorder of the hypothalamus (a part of the brain that controls certain endocrine hormones). This can be treated with leuprolide (Lupron), a synthetic sex hormone that can slow sexual development (Trollmann, Strehl, & Dorr, 1998). Women with meningomyelocele who become pregnant benefit from close monitoring during gestation. Problems such as recurrent urinary tract infections, persistent decubitus ulcers, back pain or slipped disk, and difficult vaginal delivery secondary to hip contractures may occur. Although these are concerns, it is important to note that most women with meningomyelocele have good pregnancy outcomes with relatively few complications (Arata, Grover, Dunne, & Bryan, 2000). Sexual abuse of women and female teenagers who have spina bifida appears to be more common than that found in the general population (Woodhouse, 2005).

Allergy to Latex

Between 1990 and 2000, more than half of all children with meningomyelocele developed an allergy to latex in childhood (Cremer, Kleine-Diepenbruck, Hering, & Holschneider, 2002). Although the reason for this is unclear, the allergy seems to be more common in children who have had frequent surgical procedures. The risk of allergy increases as the child gets older (Mazon et al., 2000). This allergic reaction can be life threatening. Latex allergy can be diagnosed by a clear history of an allergic reaction to latex, by skin testing, or by immunoassay blood testing (Nieto, Mazon, Estornell, Reig, & Garcia-Ibarra, 2000). As a result of the high prevalence of allergy to latex in these children, all surgical procedures, including dental procedures, should occur in latex-free settings.

Early contact of the infant to latex should be avoided, if possible, in an effort to prevent the development of allergy. Catheterization should be performed with nonlatex catheters, and nonlatex gloves should be used during care. Toys that contain significant amounts of latex, such as balloons and rubber balls, should be avoided, as should latex products that come into contact with the skin, such as Band-Aids and Ace wraps. Since the 1990s, latex-avoidance programs have been implemented around the country. Lower rates of latex sensitization have been found in children born after the avoidance programs have been instituted (Blumchen et al., 2010).

Neurological Deterioration

If a child's strength, bowel and bladder function, or daily living skills deteriorate, a cause must be sought. The origin of the deterioration may be a malfunctioning or blocked ventricular shunt, a tethered spinal cord, or, rarely, swelling in (syrinx, syringomyelia, or hydromyelia) or splitting of (diastematomyelia or diplomyelia) the spinal cord. A tethered spinal cord may result from 1) scarring at the site of the initial surgery to close the back, 2) scoliosis, or 3) the pressure of a lipoma. Pressure or stretch on the tethered cord leads to poor circulation and diminished motor functioning. The Chiari type II malformation may become symptomatic, too, leading to difficulty with swallowing, hoarseness, weakness of the arms, or difficulty with respiration.

All children who present with neurological deterioration should be evaluated for structure and function of the ventricular shunt. This involves imaging of the head (e.g., CT, MRI) with or without plain radiographic imaging of the shunt from head to abdomen (to look for a break in the tubing). In addition, the posterior fossa and spinal cord should be evaluated by head MRI with flow (to look for Chiari type II malformation and for tethered, swollen, or split cord, respectively; Levy, 1999) and by spinal MRI. If identified early, each of these problems can be addressed successfully. A blocked shunt can be replaced, a tethered cord released, a lipoma removed, and a posterior fossa decompressed. Treatment of a split or swollen cord, however, is more controversial and often less rewarding (Piatt, 2004).

EDUCATIONAL PROGRAMS

Referral to an early intervention program should occur by 6 months of age (see Chapter 30). Sensorimotor assessment during the child's first year should include evaluations of range of joint motion, muscle tone, strength and bulk, sensation, movement skills, postural control, and sensory integration skills. Treatment should focus on maintaining range of motion, enhancing strength, and moving toward standing and ambulation. Because of the considerable variability in the degree of motor delay among these children, individualized intervention plans must be developed. Adaptive equipment should be provided as needed (see Chapter 36).

As the child moves toward school entry, it is important to perform psychoeducational testing. This permits the identification of the child's cognitive and learning strengths and challenges, the development of realistic expectations that will optimize the child's learning, and the planning of an IEP for school. PT should be provided as part of the school program. Yearly reassessments will permit modification of the program based on the child's changing needs (Thompson, 1997; see Chapter 31).

PSYCHOSOCIAL ISSUES FOR THE CHILD

During the preschool years, the achievement of independence may be thwarted by difficulties with mobility and bladder and bowel control. A sense of industry that develops in the school-age child may be reduced by the child's executive function impairments, as well as by his or her inability to compete with peers in physical activities and sports. Difficulty in the school environment may exacerbate a preexisting poor self-image that many of these children have as a result of their physical disabilities. The feeling of being different can impair the establishment of peer relationships in both school and community. The child's self-esteem also may be lowered if he or she must continue to wear diapers or care for an ostomy bag (Moore, Kogan, & Parekh, 2004).

Teenagers with spina bifida tend to be more socially immature and passive, more socially isolated, less independent, and less physically active (Holmbeck et al., 2003). During adolescence, lower self-esteem may relate to a poor body image and difficulty in dealing with sexual changes and feelings. Positive self-image has been linked to factors such as higher socioeconomic status (Holmbeck et al., 2003) and the presence of social supports (Antle, 2004). Issues for the young adult with meningomyelocele may include increased social isolation, a realization that the disability is permanent, and sexual dysfunction. Achieving good social outcomes as adults, including living independently, attending college, being employed, and establishing social relationships (romantic and platonic), have been associated with the adolescent's level of executive function, socioeconomic status, intrinsic motivation, and parental support (Zukerman, Devine, & Holmbeck, 2010). Behavior problems do not necessarily relate to the severity of physical impairment but are correlated with functional status, such as scholastic achievement (Hommeyer, Holmbeck, Wills, & Coers, 1999). Several programs, such as the New York State Institute for Health Transition Training for Youth with Developmental Disabilities, and Spina Bifida University (Spina Bifida Association, 2010) are available to help adolescents with spina bifida transition to independence successfully as they enter adulthood.

Some studies have found a higher than expected rate of depression in individuals with meningomyelocele compared to age peers (Bellin et al., 2010). However, medical problems, such as an adverse reaction to medication, problems with the ventricular shunt, and infections, can cause similar symptoms to depression and must be ruled out. Many individuals with meningomyelocele develop learned helplessness; they behave in a helpless pattern, even when the opportunity to avoid or address a negative circumstance is present. This contributes to depressive feelings. Depression should be recognized and brought to the attention of an appropriate health care professional. A multimodal approach including counseling, exercise programs, and medications, especially selective serotonin reuptake inhibitors such as fluoxetine (Prozac), is usually effective.

INTERDISCIPLINARY MANAGEMENT

The goals of therapy are to improve functioning and independence and to prevent or correct secondary physical or emotional impairments. This generally involves surgical interventions, adaptive equipment, special education services, and psychosocial support for the child and family (see Chapter 37). As a result of the complexity of the resultant disabilities, an interdisciplinary approach to treating the child with meningomyelocele is essential (McDonald, 1995). The team of health care professionals should include a physician (e.g., neurodevelopmental pediatrician, pediatric neurologist, physiatrist) with particular interest and expertise in the

care of meningomyelocele; a nurse specialist; physical and occupational therapists; a social worker; consulting orthopedic, urological, and neurosurgeons; and an orthotist. Other team members or consultants may include a psychologist, plastic surgeon, dentist, special educator, speech-language pathologist, genetic counselor, and financial counselor. The services that the child needs and receives should be coordinated by a designated service coordinator. Efforts should be made to empower the child and family by involving them in the design of a management plan that is both appropriate and realistic.

The successful development of the child with meningomyelocele is largely dependent on how well the family is able to meet the child's needs. This requires emotional and behavioral supports, realistic expectations, special education services, and coordinated community services. The care of a child with meningomyelocele is expensive, with lifetime cost of illness estimated to be $635,000 (in 2002 dollars; Case & Canfield, 2009). Therefore, one of the priorities of care is to provide financial counseling to families.

OUTCOME

The survival rate of children with meningomyelocele improved dramatically between 1950 and 1970. For instance, in the 1950s survival to adulthood was less than 10% (Dunne & Shurtleff, 1986); in the 1990s, about 85% of children with meningomyelocele survived to adulthood (Davis et al., 2005). This improved survival has resulted from many factors, including the use of VP shunts to control hydrocephalus and the prevention of kidney damage by CIC and urological surgery. However, survival remains well below that of the general population. In a 40-year follow-up, Oakeshott, Hunt, Poulton, and Reid (2010) found that mortality rates between the ages of 5 and 40 years were almost 10 times higher than the national average; more than half of the deaths of individuals over the age of 5 were described as sudden and unexpected.

Outcome data for adults are incomplete, and the population is quite heterogeneous. One center found that half the individuals with meningomyelocele were able to walk 50 yards or more in adulthood (Hunt, 1990; Hunt, 1999; Hunt & Oakeshott, 2003). Half were also able to maintain urinary and bowel continence. Overall, 12% had minimal disabilities, with average IQ scores, community ambulation, and well-managed continence; 52% had moderate disability with borderline IQ scores, the ability to attend to toilet needs independently, and the ability to use and transfer from a wheelchair. Severe disability involving intellectual disability, incontinence, and dependence for most self-help skills was found in 37% of the individuals and was most often related to a history of shunt infections or shunt failure. Adults with hydrocephalus have persistent learning disabilities, including difficulties with executive function (Barnes et al., 2004; Iddon et al., 2004). Verhoef et al. (2004) found that pain was common in adults with spina bifida; males frequently had problems with sexual function. About 15% of adults in that study had problems with pressure sores.

SUMMARY

In meningomyelocele, which is a form of NTD, an overlying sac protruding from the spine contains a malformed spinal cord; this leads to the most complex birth defect compatible with life. Paralysis and loss of sensation occur below the level of the spinal cord defect, usually associated with hydrocephalus. Numerous disabilities arise as a consequence of this condition, including paralysis, musculoskeletal abnormalities, bowel and bladder incontinence, impotence, obesity, and cognitive impairments, including nonverbal learning disorders. Meningomyelocele, however, should be considered a nonprogressive condition, and any deterioration in function should lead to a search for a treatable cause, such as a blocked ventricular shunt or a tethered spinal cord. Advances in surgical and medical care have enhanced the survival and physical well-being of individuals with meningomyelocele but have not completely corrected the associated impairments. To help a child with meningomyelocele reach his or her potential, professionals must advocate for the child and family in the areas of education and psychosocial adjustment while providing integrated, high-quality health care.

REFERENCES

Adzick, N.S., Thom, E.A., Spong, C.Y., Brock, J.W. III, Burrows, P.K., Johnson, M.P., ... Farmer, D.L. (2011). A randomized trial of prenatal versus postnatal repair of myelomeningocele. New England Journal of Medicine, 364, 993–1004.

Aguilera, S., Soothill, P., Denbow, M., & Pople, I. (2009). Prognosis of spina bifida in the era of prenatal diagnosis and termination of pregnancy. Fetal Diagnostic Therapy, 26, 68–74.

Ahn, S.M., Han, S.W., & Choi, S.H. (2004). The results of antegrade continence enema using a retubularized sigmoidostomy. Pediatric Surgery International, 20, 488–491.

Aksnes, G., Diseth, T.H., Helseth, A., Edwin, B., Stange, M., Aafos, G., & Emblem, R. (2002). Appendicostomy for antegrade enema: Effects on somatic and psychosocial functioning in children with meningomyelocele. Pediatrics, 109(3), 484–489.

American Academy of Pediatrics, Committee on Genetics. (1999). Folic acid for the prevention of neural tube defects. Pediatrics, 104, 325–327.

Antle, B.J. (2004). Factors associated with self-worth in young people with physical disabilities. Health & Social Work, 29(3), 167–175.

Arata, M., Grover, S., Dunne, K., & Bryan, D. (2000). Pregnancy outcome and complications in women with spina bifida. The Journal of Reproductive Medicine, 45(9), 743–748.

Aslan, A.R., & Kogan, B.A. (2002). Conservative management in neurogenic bladder dysfunction. Current Opinion in Urology, 12, 473–477.

Babcock, C.J. (1995). Ultrasound evaluation of prenatal and neonatal spina bifida. Neurosurgery Clinics of North America, 6, 203–218.

Bahado-Singh, R.O., & Sutton-Riley, J. (2004). Biochemical screening for congenital defects. Obstetrics and Gynecology Clinics of North America, 31, 857–872, xi.

Barf, H.A., Verhoef, M., Post, M.W., Jennekens-Schinkel, A., Gooskens, R.H., Mullaart, R.A., & Prevo, A.J. (2004). Educational career and predictors of type of education in young adults with spina bifida. International Journal of Rehabilitation Research, 27(1), 45–52.

Barnes, M., Dennis, M., & Hetherington, R. (2004). Reading and writing skills in young adults with spina bifida and hydrocephalus. Journal of the International Neuropsychological Society, 10(5), 655–663.

Bartonek, A., & Saraste, H. (2001). Factors influencing ambulation in myelomeningocele: A cross-sectional study. Developmental Medicine and Child Neurology, 43, 253–260.

Bellin, M.H., Zabel, T.A., Dicianno, B.E., Levey, E., Garver, K., Linroth, R., & Braun, P. (2010). Correlates of depressive and anxiety symptoms in young adults with spina bifida. Journal of Pediatric Psychology, 35(7), 778–789.

Block, C.A., Cooper, C.S., & Hawtrey, C.E. (2003). Long-term efficacy of periurethral collagen injection for the treatment of urinary incontinence secondary to myelomeningocele. The Journal of Urology, 169(1), 327–329.

Blumchen, K., Bayer, P., Buck, D., Michael, T., Cremer, R., Fricke, C., ... Niggemann, B. (2010). Effects of latex avoidance on latex sensitization, atopy and allergic diseases in patients with spina bifida. Allergy, 65(12), 1585–1593.

Boulet, S.L., Yang, Q., Mai, C., Kirby, R.S., Collins, J.S., Robbins, J.M., ... National Birth Defects Prevention Network. (2008). Trends in the postfortification prevalence of spina bifida and anencephaly in the United States. Birth Defects Research. Part A, Clinical and Molecular Teratology, 82(7), 527–532.

Bruner, J.P., & Tulipan, N. (2005). Intrauterine repair of spina bifida. Clinics in Obstetrics and Gynecology, 48, 942–955.

Bruner, J.P., Tulipan, N., Dabrowiak, M.E., Luker, K.S., Walters, K., Burns, P., & Reed, G. (2004). Upper level of the spina bifida defect: How good are we? Ultrasound in Obstetrics & Gynecology, 24(6), 612–617.

Buffart, L.M., van den Berg-Emons, R.J., van Meeteren, J., Stam, H.J., & Roebroeck, M.E. (2009). Lifestyle, participation, and health-related quality of life in adolescents and young adults with myelomeningocele. *Developmental Medicine and Child Neurology, 51,* 886–894.

Burmeister, R., Hannay, H.J., Copeland, K., Fletcher, J.M., Boudousquie, A., & Dennis, M. (2005). Attention problems and executive functions in children with spina bifida and hydrocephalus. *Child Neuropsychology: A Journal on Normal and Abnormal Development in Childhood and Adolescence, 11*(3), 265–283.

Case, A.P., & Canfield, M.A. (2009). Methods for developing useful estimates of the costs associated with birth defects. *Birth Defects Research. Part A, Clinical and Molecular Teratology, 85,* 920–924.

Centers for Disease Control and Prevention. (2000). Folate status in women of childbearing age—United States, 1999. *Morbidity and Mortality Weekly Report, 49*(42), 962–965.

Centers for Disease Control and Prevention. (2004). Spina bifida and anencephaly before and after folic acid mandate—United States, 1995–1996 and 1999–2000. *Morbidity and Mortality Weekly Report, 53*(17), 362–365.

Centers for Disease Control and Prevention. (2009). Racial/ethnic differences in the birth prevalence of spina bifida—United States, 1995–2005. *Morbidity and Mortality Weekly Report, 57,* 1409–1413.

Charles, D.H., Ness, A.R., Campbell, D., Smith, G.D., Whitley, E., & Hall, M.H. (2005). Folic acid supplements in pregnancy and birth outcome: Re-analysis of a large randomised controlled trial and update of Cochrane review. *Paediatric and Perinatal Epidemiology, 19*(2), 112–124.

Chen, C.P. (2005). Maternal diabetes and neural tube defects: Prenatal diagnosis of lumbosacral myelomeningocele, ventriculomegaly, Arnold-Chiari malformation and foot deformities in a pregnancy with poor maternal metabolic control, and review of the literature. *Genetic Counseling, 16,* 313–316.

Chen, J., Godschalk, M.F., Katz, P.G., & Mulligan, T. (1995). Combining intracavernous injection and external vacuum as treatment for erectile dysfunction. *The Journal of Urology, 153*(5), 1476–1477.

Copp, A.J., & Greene, N.D. (2010). Genetics and development of neural tube defects. *Journal of Pathology, 220,* 217–230.

Copp, A.J., Fleming, A., & Greene, N.D.E. (1998). Embryonic mechanisms underlying the prevention of neural tube defects. *Mental Retardation and Developmental Disabilities Research Reviews, 4,* 264–268.

Cremer, R., Kleine-Diepenbruck, U., Hering, F., & Holschneider, A.M. (2002). Reduction of latex sensitisation in spina bifida patients by a primary prophylaxis programme (five years experience). *European Journal of Pediatric Surgery, 12*(Suppl. 1), S19–S21.

Dahl, M., Ahlsten, G., Carlson, H., Ronne-Engström, E., Lagerkvist, B., Magnusson, G., ... Thuomas, K.A. (1995). Neurological dysfunction above cele level in children with spina bifida cystica: A prospective study to three years. *Developmental Medicine and Child Neurology, 37*(1), 30–40.

Davis, B.E., Daley, C.M., Shurtleff, D.B., Duquay, S., Seidel, K., Loeser, J.D., & Ellenbogen, R.G. (2005). Long-term survival of patients with myelomeningocele. *Pediatric Neurosurgery, 41*(4), 186–191.

Dean, G. E., Kirsch, A.J., Packer, M.G., Scherz, H.C., & Zaontz, M.R. (2007). Antegrade and retrograde endoscopic dextranomer/hyaluronic acid bladder neck bulking for pediatric incontinence. *The Journal of Urology, 178,* 652–655.

Deshpande, A.V., Sampang, R., & Smith, G.H. (2010). Study of botulinum toxin A in neurogenic bladder due to spina bifida in children. *ANZ Journal of Surgery, 80,* 250–253.

Dias, L. (2004). Orthopaedic care in spina bifida: Past, present, and future. *Developmental Medicine and Child Neurology, 46,* 579.

Dosa, N.P., Eckrich, M., Katz, D.A., Turk, M., & Liptak, G.S. (2007). Incidence, prevalence, and characteristics of fractures in children, adolescents, and adults with spina bifida. *Journal of Spinal Cord Medicine, 30*(Suppl. 1), S5–S9.

Dosa, N.P., Foley, J.T., Eckrich, M., Woodall-Ruff, D., & Liptak, G.S. (2009). Obesity across the lifespan among persons with spina bifida. *Disability Rehabilitation, 31,* 914–920.

Drolet, B.A., Chamlin, S.L., Garzon, M.C., Adams, D., Baselga, E., Haggstrom, A.N., ... Frieden, I.J. (2010). Prospective study of spinal anomalies in children with infantile hemangiomas of the lumbosacral skin. *Journal of Pediatrics, 157*(5), 789–794.

Dunne, K.B., & Shurtleff, D.B. (1986). The adult with meningomyelocele: A preliminary report. In R.L. McLaurin (Ed.), *Spina bifida* (pp. 38–51). New York, NY: Praeger.

Flynn, J.M., Herrera-Soto, J.A., Ramirez, N.F., Fernandez-Feliberti, R., Vilella, F., & Guzman, J. (2004). Clubfoot release in myelodysplasia. *Journal of Pediatric Orthopaedics, Part B, 13*(4), 259–262.

Flynn, J.M., Ramirez, N., Emans, J.B., Smith, J.T., Mulcahey, M.J., & Betz, R.R. (2011). Is the vertebral expandable prosthetic titanium rib a surgical alternative in patients with spina bifida? *Clinical Orthopaedics and Related Research, 469,* 1291–1296.

Forrester, M.B., & Merz, R.D. (2000). Prenatal diagnosis and elective termination of neural tube defects in Hawaii, 1986–1997. *Fetal Diagnosis and Therapy, 15,* 146–151.

Gamé, X., Moscovici, J., Gamé, L., Sarramon, J.P., Rischmann, P., & Malavaud, B. (2006). Evaluation of sexual function in young men with spina bifida and myelomeningocele using the International Index of Erectile Function. *Urology, 67*(3), 566–570.

Gatti, C., Del Rossi, R.C., Ferrari, A., Casolari, E., Casadio, G., & Scire, G. (2009). Predictors of successful sexual partnering of adults with spina bifida. *The Journal of Urology, 182*(4 Suppl.), 1911–1916.

Gilbert, J.N., Jones, K.L., Rorke, L.B., Chernoff, G.F., & James, H.E. (1986). Central nervous system anomalies associated with meningomyelocele, hydrocephalus, and the Arnold-Chiari malformation: Reappraisal of theories regarding the pathogenesis of posterior neural tube closure defects. *Neurosurgery, 18*(5), 559–564.

Gucciardi, E., Pietrusiak, M.A., Reynolds, D.L., & Rouleau, J. (2002). Incidence of neural tube defects in Ontario, 1986–1999. *Canadian Medical Association Journal, 167*(3), 237–240.

Guggisberg, D., Hadj-Rabia, S., Viney, C., Bodemer, C., Brunelle, F., Zerah, M., ... Hamel-Teillac, D. (2004). Skin markers of occult spinal dysraphism in children: A review of 54 cases. *Archives of Dermatology, 140*(9), 1109–1115.

Halachmi, S., Farhat, W., Metcalfe, P., Bagli, D.J., McLorie, G.A., & Khoury, A.E. (2004). Efficacy of polydimethylsiloxane injection to the bladder neck and leaking diverting stoma for urinary continence. *The Journal of Urology, 171*(3), 1287–1290.

Hall, J.G., & Solehdin, F. (1998). Genetics of neural tube defects. *Mental Retardation and Developmental Disabilities Research Reviews, 4*, 269–281.

Hall, J.G., Friedman, J.M., Kenna, B.A., Popkin, J., Jawanda, M., & Arnold, W. (1988). Clinical, genetic, and epidemiological factors in neural tube defects. *American Journal of Human Genetics, 43*(6), 827–837.

Hochhaus, F., Butenandt, O., & Ring-Mrozik, E.J. (1999). One-year treatment with recombinant human growth hormone of children with meningomyelocele and growth hormone deficiency: A comparison of supine length and arm span. *Journal of Pediatric Endocrinology and Metabolism, 12*, 153–159.

Holmbeck, G.N., Westhoven, V.C., Phillips, W.S., Bowers, R., Gruse, C., Nikolopoulos, T., ... Davison, K. (2003). A multimethod, multi-informant, and multidimensional perspective on psychosocial adjustment in preadolescents with spina bifida. *Journal of Consulting and Clinical Psychology, 71*(4), 782–796.

Hommeyer, J.S., Holmbeck, G.N., Wills, K.E., & Coers, S. (1999). Condition severity and psychosocial functioning in pre-adolescents with spina bifida: Disentangling proximal functional status and distal adjustment outcomes. *Journal of Pediatric Psychology, 24*(6), 499–509.

Honein, M.A., Paulozzi, L.J., Mathews, T.J., Erickson, J.D., & Wong, L.Y. (2001). Impact of folic acid fortification of the US food supply on the occurrence of neural tube defects. *JAMA: The Journal of the American Medical Association, 285*(23), 2981–2986.

Hopps, C.V., & Kropp, K.A. (2003). Preservation of renal function in children with myelomeningocele managed with basic newborn evaluation and close follow up. *The Journal of Urology, 169*, 305–308.

Hultling, C., Levi, R., Amark, P., & Sjöblom, P. (2000). Semen retrieval and analysis in men with myelomeningocele. *Developmental Medicine and Child Neurology, 42*(10), 681–684.

Hunt, G.M. (1990). Open spina bifida: Outcome for a complete cohort treated unselectively and followed into adulthood. *Developmental Medicine and Child Neurology, 32*, 108–118.

Hunt, G.M. (1999). The Casey Holter lecture: Nonselective intervention in newborn babies with open spina bifida: The outcome 30 years on for the complete cohort. *European Journal of Pediatric Surgery, 9*(Suppl. 1), 5–8.

Hunt, G.M., & Oakeshott, P. (2003). Outcome in people with spina bifida at age 35: Prospective community based cohort study. *BMJ, 326*, 1365–1366.

Iddon, J.L., Morgan, D.J., Loveday, C., Sahakian, B., & Pickard, J. (2004). Neuropsychological profile of young adults with spina bifida with or without hydrocephalus. *Journal of Neurology, Neurosurgery, and Psychiatry, 75*(8), 1112–1118.

Kim, E.D., & McVary, K.T. (1995). Topical prostaglandin E1 for the treatment of erectile dysfunction. *The Journal of Urology, 153*, 1828–1830.

Kim, S.M., Han, S.W., & Choi, S.H. (2006). Left colonic antegrade continence enema: Experience gained from 19 cases. *Journal of Pediatric Surgery, 41*, 1750–1754.

Kirk, V.G., Morielli, A., & Brouillette, R.T. (1999). Sleep-disordered breathing in patients with myelomeningocele: The missed diagnosis. *Developmental Medicine and Child Neurology, 41*, 40–43.

Kryger, J.V., Spencer Barthold, J., Fleming, P., & Gonzalez, R. (1999). The outcome of artificial urinary sphincter placement after a mean 15-year follow-up in a paediatric population. *British Journal of Urology International, 83*(9), 1026–1031.

Kumar, R., Bansal, K.K., & Chhabra, D.K. (2002). Occurrence of split cord malformation in meningomyelocele: Complex spina bifida. *Pediatric Neurosurgery, 36*, 119–127.

Leibold, S., Ekmark, E., & Adams, R.C. (2000). Decision-making for a successful bowel continence program. *European Journal of Pediatric Surgery, 10*(Suppl. 1), 26–30.

Levy, L.M. (1999). MR imaging of cerebrospinal fluid flow and spinal cord motion in neurologic disorders of the spine. *Magnetic Resonance Imaging Clinics of North America, 7*, 573–587.

Lindquist, B., Uvebrant, P., Rehn, E., & Carlsson, G. (2009). Cognitive functions in children with myelomeningocele without hydrocephalus. *Child's Nervous System, 25*(8), 969–975.

Liu, S.L., Shurtleff, D.B., Ellenbogen, R.G., Loeser, J.D., & Kropp, R. (1999). 19-year follow-up of fetal myelomeningocele brought to term. *European Journal of Pediatric Surgery, 9*(Suppl. 1), 12–14.

Lorente Molto, F.J., & Martinez, G.I. (2005). Retrospective review of L3 myelomeningocele in three age groups: Should posterolateral iliopsoas transfer still be indicated to stabilize the hip? *Journal of Pediatric Orthopaedics, Part B, 14*, 177–184.

Madersbacher, H., Mürtz, G., Alloussi, S., Domurath, B., Henne, T., Körner, I., ... Strugala, G. (2009). Propiverine vs. oxybutynin for treating neurogenic detrusor overactivity in children and adolescents: Results of a multicentre observational cohort study. *British Journal of Urology International, 103*(6), 776–781.

Main, D.M., & Mennuti, M.T. (1986). Neural tube defects: Issues in prenatal diagnosis and counselling. *Obstetrics and Gynecology, 67*, 1–16.

Manning, S.M., Jennings, R., & Madsen, J.R. (2000). Pathophysiology, prevention and potential treatment of neural tube defects. *Mental Retardation and Developmental Disabilities Research Reviews, 6*, 6–14.

Marlin, A.E. (2004). Management of hydrocephalus in the patient with myelomeningocele: An argument against third ventriculostomy. *Neurosurgical Focus, 16*(2), e4.

Martinez de Villarreal, L.M., Perez, J.Z., Vasquez, P.A., Herrera, R.H., Campos Mdel, R., Lopez, R.A., ... Castro, R.N. (2002). Decline of neural tube defects after a folic acid campaign in Neuvo Leon, Mexico. *Teratology, 66*(5), 249–256.

Matson, M.A., Mahone, E.M., & Zabel, T.A. (2005). Serial neuropsychological assessment and evidence of shunt malfunction in spina bifida: A longitudinal case study. *Child Neuropsychology, 11*, 315–332.

Mazon, A., Nieto, A., Linana, J.J., Montoro, J., Estornell, F., & Garcia-Ibarra, F. (2000). Latex sensitization in children with spina bifida: Follow-up comparative study after two years. *Annals of Allergy, Asthma and Immunology, 84*(2), 207–210.

McDonald, C.M. (1995). Rehabilitation of children with spinal dysraphism. *Neurosurgery Clinics of North America, 6*, 393.

McNeely, P.D., & Howes, W.J. (2004). Ineffectiveness of dietary folic acid supplementation on the incidence of lipomyelomeningocele: Pathogenetic implications. *Journal of Neurosurgery, 100*(2 Suppl. Pediatrics), 98–100.

Medical Research Council Vitamin Study Research Group. (1991). Prevention of neural tube defects:

Results of the Medical Research Council Vitamin Study. *The Lancet, 338*, 131–137.

Mercado, E., Alman, B., & Wright, J.G. (2007). Does spinal fusion influence quality of life in neuromuscular scoliosis? *Spine, 32*(19 Suppl.), S120–S125.

Meuli, M., Meuli-Simmen, C., Hutchins, G.M., Yingling, C.D., McBiles Hoffman, K., Harrison, M.R., & Adzick, N.S. (1995). In utero surgery rescues neurological function at birth in sheep with spina bifida. *Nature Medicine, 1*, 142–147.

Moore, C., Kogan, B.A., & Parekh, A. (2004). Impact of urinary incontinence on self-concept in children with spina bifida. *The Journal of Urology, 171*(4), 1659–1662.

Moskowitz, D., Shurtleff, D.B., Weinberger, E., Loeser, J., & Ellenbogen, R. (1998). Anatomy of the spinal cord in patients with meningomyelocele with and without hypoplasia or hydromyelia. *European Journal of Pediatric Surgery, 8*(Suppl. 1), 18–21.

Muthukumar, N. (2009). Congenital spinal lipomatous malformations: Part I—classification. *Acta Neurochirurgica, 151*, 179–188.

Nagarkatti, D.G., Banta, J.V., & Thomson, J.D. (2000). Charcot arthropathy in spina bifida. *Journal of Pediatric Orthopaedics, 20*, 82–87.

National Institute of Child Health and Human Development. (2004). *Management of Myelomeningocele Study (MOMS)*. Retrieved from http://www.spinabifidamoms.com/english/overview.html

New York State Institute for Health Transition Training for Youth with Developmental Disabilities. (2010). Retrieved from http://healthtransitionsny.org/

Niall, D.M., Dowling, F.E., Fogarty, E.E., Moore, D.P., & Goldberg, C. (2004). Kyphectomy in children with myelomeningocele: A long-term outcome study. *Journal of Pediatric Orthopaedics, 24*(1), 37–44.

Nieto, A., Mazon, A., Estornell, F., Reig, C., & Garcia-Ibarra, F. (2000). The search of latex sensitization in spina bifida: Diagnostic approach. *Clinical and Experimental Allergy, 30*(2), 264–269.

Norem, C.T., Schoen, E.J., Walton, D.L., Krieger, R.C., O'Keefe, J., To, T.T., & Ray, G.T. (2005). Routine ultrasonography compared with maternal serum alpha-fetoprotein for neural tube defect screening. *Obstetrics and Gynecology, 106*(4), 747–752.

Norrlin, S., Dahl, M., & Rosblad, B. (2004). Control of reaching movements in children and young adults with myelomeningocele. *Developmental Medicine and Child Neurology, 46*, 28–33.

Norrlin, S., Strinnholm, M., Carlsson, M., & Dahl, M. (2003). Factors of significance for mobility in children with myelomeningocele. *Acta Paediatrica, 92*(2), 204–210.

Oakeshott, P., Hunt, G.M., Poulton, A., & Reid, F. (2010). Expectation of life and unexpected death in open spina bifida: A 40-year complete, non-selective, longitudinal cohort study. *Developmental Medicine and Child Neurology, 52*, 749–753.

Oi, S., Nomura, S., Nagasaka, M., Arai, H., Shirane, R., Yamanouchi, Y. ... Date, H. (2009). Embryopathogenetic surgicoanatomical classification of dysraphism and surgical outcome of spinal lipoma: A nationwide multicenter cooperative study in Japan. *Journal of Neurosurgery: Pediatrics, 3*(5), 412–419.

Ornoy, A. (2006). Neuroteratogens in man: An overview with special emphasis on the teratogenicity of antiepileptic drugs in pregnancy. *Reproductive Toxicology, 22*, 214–226.

Palmer, J.S., Kaplan, W.E., & Firlit, C.F. (1999). Erectile dysfunction in spina bifida is treatable. *The Lancet, 354*, 125–126.

Parisini, P., Greggi, T., Di Silvestre, M., Giardina, F., & Bakaloudis, G. (2002). Surgical treatment of scoliosis in myelomeningocele. *Studies in Health Technology and Informatics, 91*, 442–447.

Persad, V.L., Van den Hof, M.C., Dubé, J.M., & Zimmer, P. (2002). Incidence of open neural tube defects in Nova Scotia after folic acid fortification. *Canadian Medical Association Journal, 167*(3), 241–245.

Piatt, Jr., J.H. (2004). Syringomyelia complicating myelomeningocele: Review of the evidence. *Journal of Neurosurgery, 100*, 101–109.

Pierz, K., Banta, J., Thomson, J., Gahm, N., & Hartford, J. (2000). The effect of tethered cord release on scoliosis in myelomeningocele. *Journal of Pediatric Orthopaedics, 20*(3), 362–365.

Rankin, J., Glinianaia, S., Brown, R., & Renwick, M. (2000). The changing prevalence of neural tube defects: A population-based study in the north of England, 1984–96. Northern Congenital Abnormality Survey Steering Group. *Paediatric and Perinatal Epidemiology, 14*(2), 104–110.

Rotenstein, D., & Bass, A.N. (2004). Treatment to near adult stature of patients with myelomeningocele with recombinant human growth hormone. *Journal of Pediatric Endocrinology & Metabolism, 17*, 1195–1200.

Sawyer, S.M., & Roberts, K.V. (1999). Sexual and reproductive health in young people with spina bifida. *Developmental Medicine and Child Neurology, 41*, 671–675.

Schader, I., & Corwin, P. (1999). How many pregnant women in Christchurch are using folic acid supplements in early pregnancy? *The New Zealand Medical Journal, 112*, 463–465.

Shaw, G. (2008). Comments on inositol supplementation in pregnancies at risk of apparently folate-resistant NTDs. *Birth Defects Research. Part A, Clinical and Molecular Teratology, 82*, 543.

Shaw, G.M., Quach, T., Nelson, V., Carmichael, S.L., Schaffer, D.M., Selvin, S., & Yang, W. (2003). Neural tube defects associated with maternal periconceptional dietary intake of simple sugars and glycemic index. *The American Journal of Clinical Nutrition, 78*, 972–978.

Shurtleff, D.B. (2004). Epidemiology of neural tube defects and folic acid. *Cerebrospinal Fluid Research, 1*, 5.

Simos, P.G., Papanicolaou, A.C., Castillo, E.M., Juranek, J., Cirino, P.T., Rezaie, R., & Fletcher, J.M. (2011). Brain mechanisms for reading and language processing in spina bifida meningomyelocele: A combined magnetic source and structural magnetic resonance imaging study. *Neuropsychology, 25*(5), 590–601.

Snodgrass, W.T., & Adams, R. (2004). Initial urologic management of myelomeningocele. *Urologic Clinics of North America, 31*, 427–434, viii.

Spina Bifida Association. (2010). Spina Bifida University. Retrieved from http://www.spinabifidaassociation.org/site/c.liKWL7PLLrF/b.6281735/k.9041/SB_University.htm

Stevenson, K.L. (2004). Chiari type II malformation: Past, present, and future. *Neurosurgical Focus, 16*, e5.

Suarez, L., Felkner, M., & Hendricks, K. (2004). The effect of fever, febrile illnesses, and heat exposures on the risk of neural tube defects in a Texas–Mexico border population. *Birth Defects Research, Part A: Clinical and Molecular Teratology, 70*, 815–819.

Sutton, L.N., & Adzick, N.S. (2004). Fetal surgery for myelomeningocele. *Clinical Neurosurgery, 51*, 155–162.

Thompson, S. (1997). *The source for nonverbal learning disorders*. East Moline, IL: LinguiSystems.

Trollmann, R., Bakker, B., Lundberg, M., & Doerr, H.G. (2006). Growth in pre-pubertal children with myelomeningocele (MMC) on growth hormone (GH): The KIGS experience. *Pediatric Rehabilitation, 9*, 144–148.

Trollmann, R., Strehl, E., & Doerr, H.G. (1998). Precocious puberty in children with myelomeningocele: Treatment with gonadotropin-releasing hormone analogues. *Developmental Medicine and Child Neurology, 40*, 38–43.

Tubbs, R.S., Smyth, M.D., Wellons, J.C. III, Blount, J.P., Grabb, P.A., & Oakes, W.J. (2003). Alternative uses for the subgaleal shunt in pediatric neurosurgery. *Pediatric Neurosurgery, 39*(1), 22–24.

Tuli, S., Drake, J., & Lamberti-Pasculli, M. (2003). Long-term outcome of hydrocephalus management in myelomeningoceles. *Child's Nervous System, 19*, 286–291.

van den Berg-Emons, H.J., Bussmann, J.B., Brobbel, A.S., Roebroeck, M.E., van Meeteren, J. & Stam, H.J. (2001). Everyday physical activity in adolescents and young adults with meningomyelocele as measured with a novel activity monitor. *Journal of Pediatrics, 139*(6), 880–886.

van Rooij, I.A., Ocké, M.C., Straatman, H., Zielhuis, G.A., Merkus, H.M., & Steegers-Theunissen, R.P. (2004). Periconceptional folate intake by supplement and food reduces the risk of nonsyndromic cleft lip with or without cleft palate. *Preventive Medicine, 39*(4), 689–694.

Verhoef, M., Barf, H.A., Post, M.W., van Asbeck, F.W., Gooskens, R.H., & Prevo, A.J. (2004). Secondary impairments in young adults with spina bifida. *Developmental Medicine and Child Neurology, 46*(6), 420–427.

Warf, B., Ondoma, S., Kulkarni, A., Donnelly, R., Ampeire, M., Akona, J., … Nsubuga, B.K. (2009). Neurocognitive outcome and ventricular volume in children with myelomeningocele treated for hydrocephalus in Uganda. *Journal of Neurosurgery Pediatrics, 4*(6), 564–570.

Widman, L.M., McDonald, C.M., & Abresch, R.T. (2006). Effectiveness of an upper extremity exercise device integrated with computer gaming for aerobic training in adolescents with spinal cord dysfunction. *Journal of Spinal Cord Medicine, 29*, 363–370.

Williams, L.J., Rasmussen, S.A., Flores, A., Kirby, R.S., & Edmonds, L.D. (2005). Decline in the prevalence of spina bifida and anencephaly by race/ethnicity: 1995–2002. *Pediatrics, 116*(3), 580–586.

Woodhouse, C.R. (2005). Myelomeningocele in young adults. *British Journal of Urology International, 95*, 223–230.

Wright, J.G. (2010). Hip and spine surgery is of questionable value in spina bifida: An evidence-based review. *Clinical Orthopaedics and Related Research, 469*(5), 1258–1264.

Xiao, C.G. (2006). Reinnervation for neurogenic bladder: Historic review and introduction of a somatic-autonomic reflex pathway procedure for patients with spinal cord injury or spina bifida. *European Urology, 49*, 22–28.

Yardley, I.E., Pauniaho, S.L., Baillie, C.T., Turnock, R.R., Coldicutt, P., Lamont, G.L., & Kenny, S.E. (2009). After the honeymoon comes divorce: Long-term use of the antegrade continence enema procedure. *Journal of Pediatric Surgery, 44*(6), 1274–1276.

Zukerman, J.M., Devine, K.A., & Holmbeck, G.N. (2010). Adolescent predictors of emerging adulthood milestones in youth with spina bifida. *Journal of Pediatric Psychology, 36*(3), 265–276.

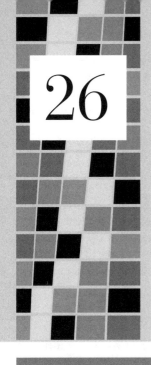

26 Traumatic Brain Injury

Melissa K. Trovato and Scott C. Schultz

Upon completion of this chapter, the reader will

- Know the incidence and causes of traumatic brain injury (TBI) in children
- Understand the types of brain injuries that can occur
- Be able to distinguish between different severities of brain injury
- Understand the treatment and rehabilitation processes associated with TBI
- Understand why a comprehensive and multidisciplinary approach is effective and sometimes necessary during TBI recovery
- Be able to determine ways to reduce the risk of TBI in children

Traumatic brain injury (TBI) is a nondegenerative, noncongenital insult to the brain resulting from an external mechanical force. After a TBI, the child will likely need to be brought to the emergency department (ED) for further evaluation and potentially acute treatment. If neurological impairments persist after the acute period, the child may need inpatient or outpatient rehabilitation. Fortunately, in most TBI cases in children the trauma is not severe and symptoms resolve within the first few weeks or months after injury. In severe TBI, however, many different cognitive and motor areas may be affected, including the ability to walk, to perform daily living skills (e.g., dressing), to swallow, and to communicate. Difficulties with attention, concentration, intellectual processing, and memory are also of concern. These impairments can cause difficulties both academically and socially when the child is interacting with peers and family in school and at home. Because TBI can cause multiple areas of damage, a comprehensive, multidisciplinary, team-oriented approach to rehabilitation is essential to identify problems and provide strategies both in the home and school environment.

◼ ◼ ◼ PAUL

Paul was 9 years old when he was involved in a motor vehicle collision. He was a belted passenger in the backseat of the family vehicle. The vehicle was hit on the driver's side by a tractor trailer while traveling on the highway. Paul was unresponsive at the scene and was noted to have an open brain injury. At the scene, Paul's Glasgow Coma Scale (GCS) score (a quantitative scale to rate or rule out coma in a neurologically impaired person) was a 5. He was intubated and transported via helicopter to the nearest trauma center. Computed tomography (CT) of the head showed an open depressed skull fracture with hemorrhage. He emergently went to the operating room for craniotomy and intracranial pressure (ICP) monitor placement. He required medications to maintain an adequate blood pressure. Paul also required a tracheostomy and a gastrostomy tube placement during his acute care hospitalization. Magnetic resonance imaging (MRI) done 1 month post injury revealed extensive injury to the left occipital lobe, right frontal lobe, and brainstem, as well as diffuse axonal injury (DAI).

Paul was admitted to an inpatient rehabilitation unit 4 weeks post injury. At that time, Paul had spontaneous eye opening and intermittent eye opening to verbal stimuli. Occasional tracking of objects was noted as well. After 16 weeks, Paul was inconsistently following simple commands and was inconsistently answering yes/no questions with a head nod/shake. Spontaneous movements of his extremities were noted, right greater than left. Paul was discharged from inpatient rehabilitation 24 weeks post injury. He required a ventilator for nighttime ventilation due to central sleep apnea and was also dependent on the gastrostomy tube for all nutrition. Paul was then admitted to a day rehabilitation program, where he continued to receive intensive physical, occupational, and speech therapy services. At 28 weeks following injury, Paul continued to be in posttraumatic amnesia (PTA), but he was consistently following commands and was able to make choices using eye gaze or reaching with the right hand. Gradually over the next 6 months, he continued to make steady gains. At time of discharge from the day program, however, his cognitive functioning was impaired in all areas. Ongoing impairments in receptive and expressive language consistent with aphasia were noted. He was able to communicate his basic wants and needs with cues, he moved all his extremities, and he was walking with a walker and bilateral forearm platforms for 200 feet with minimal assistance. Paul required the use of bilateral ankle-foot orthoses to maintain foot position and provide stability. He was able to feed himself with supervision and required minimal assistance for grooming, bathing, and dressing skills. Paul underwent a modified barium swallow and was cleared for intake of a regular diet with nectar-thickened liquids. The gastrostomy tube is currently used only for liquid supplementation.

Paul was transitioned to a Level 5 school placement. An individualized education program (IEP) was developed with the help of an educator from the day program, in coordination with the school system. At school, he continues to receive therapy services as well as outpatient physical, occupational, and speech therapy. Even though Paul's injury was over 1 year ago, he continues to make slow progress in all domains.

INCIDENCE OF TRAUMATIC BRAIN INJURY

Each year, approximately 1.7 million Americans sustain a TBI (Faul, Xu, Wald, & Coronado, 2010). Approximately 275,000 of these individuals are hospitalized and 52,000 die. In children under 14 years of age, an estimated 511,000 sustain a TBI each year. In children 17 years of age and younger, the overall rate of hospitalizations for TBI in the United States has been reported to be 119 per 100,000. The male-to-female ratio for TBI is approximately 1.4:1. TBI most commonly occurs in the seasons of spring and summer and on weekends when children and adolescents are outside participating in sports and recreation.

CAUSES OF TRAUMATIC BRAIN INJURY

The most common causes of TBI in the general population are motor vehicle accidents, falls, sports injuries (especially football, lacrosse, and hockey), recreational activities (e.g., skiing, surfing), and assault. The most common precipitants of TBI change with age. In children less than 1 year of age, physical abuse is the most common cause (e.g., shaken baby syndrome). Toddlers sustain TBI most commonly as a result of falls. In young school-age children, transportation-related injuries are common, especially bicycle crashes. In older school-age children, motor vehicle accidents and sports and recreational activities are the most common causes of TBI. During adolescence and through the mid 20s, motor vehicle accidents are the most common origin (Faul et al., 2010; Figure 26.1).

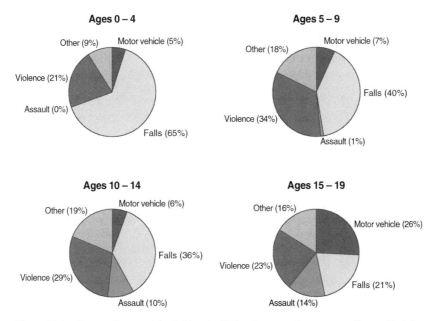

Figure 26.1. Causes of traumatic brain injury in children by age and percentage. (*Source:* Faul, Xu, Wald, & Coronado, 2010).

TYPES OF BRAIN INJURIES

Primary head injuries, which occur at the moment of impact, include brain **contusions** (a localized bruise of brain tissue), vascular injuries causing hemorrhage or hematomas (bleeding within the brain), scalp injuries, skull fractures, and cranial nerve injuries. Secondary injuries occur typically within the first 24 hours after the inciting events and include 1) brain swelling/edema; 2) elevated ICP; 3) seizures; 4) electrolyte disturbances, such as changes in sodium; and 5) **hydrocephalus** (increased fluid in the brain). Severe TBI is usually associated with DAI, an extensive injury to the white matter tracks of the brain that is caused by inertial forces at the moment of impact. During high-velocity impacts, such as motor vehicle accidents, acceleration or deceleration forces cause the brain to move about inside the skull, causing DAI. Most clinical brain injuries include both impact and inertial components.

CONCUSSIONS

The term *concussion* has received a significant amount of media attention in the last 3–4 years, especially in relation to its frequency and recurrence in professional football and the associated sequela of dementia reported by some players. Each year, there are approximately 1.6–3.8 million sports-related concussions in the United States (Langlois, Rutland-Brown, & Wald, 2006). A concussion is a closed-head type of brain injury, which may occur when the head strikes an object or when a moving object strikes the head. Common causes include motor vehicle accidents, falls, and sports injuries. A person who sustains a concussion may or may not lose consciousness. Loss of consciousness indicates a more severe injury and warrants further medical attention (i.e., an ED visit). Even brief concussions without loss of consciousness can cause both short- and long-term impairments.

Symptoms of a concussion include confusion, headache, nausea, vomiting, dizziness, hypersensitivity to lights (photophobia) or sounds (phonophobia), loss of balance, blurry vision, double vision, and loss of memory (including memories before, during, and/or after the incident). Loss of consciousness, seizures, personality changes, slurred speech, and body/facial weakness or numbness can also occur. Three validated systems exist for the rapid diagnosis of concussion: the Maddocks questions, the Standardized Assessment of Concussion (SAC), and the McGill Abbreviated Concussion Evaluation (McGill ACE). These tests, which should be completed by a physician, are used to quickly assess the individual suspected of having a concussion.

The Maddocks questions are a qualitative measure used for sideline concussion assessment in sports injuries. Any incorrect response requires removal from the field for a more comprehensive medical evaluation (Maddocks, Dicker, & Saling, 1995).

The SAC objectively documents the presence and severity of neurocognitive impairment associated with concussion. The SAC, a quantitative measure, includes measures of orientation, immediate memory, concentration, delayed recall memory, exertional maneuvers, and neurologic screening (McCrea et al., 1998).

The McGill ACE is a hybrid containing both qualitative and quantitative components. It includes measures of immediate memory, concentration, delayed memory, orientation (with some Maddocks questions), amnesia, concussion symptoms, neurologic screening, and exertional provocative tests (Johnston, Lassonde, & Ptito, 2001).

DETECTION OF TRAUMATIC BRAIN INJURY

Most head trauma is minor and does not require treatment or surgical interventions. If a child hits his or her head and is awake, alert, conversant, interactive, and otherwise asymptomatic, close observation and monitoring at home are sufficient. However, if any of the following signs or symptoms occurs, a more comprehensive evaluation is necessary and the child should be taken to the ED: 1) a change in mental status (e.g., difficulty speaking, loss of consciousness, seizures, confusion, lethargy, irritability); 2) weakness in the arms or legs; 3) complaints of severe headaches; 4) complaints of changes in hearing or vision; or 5) nausea and projectile vomiting. Any loss of consciousness should lead to an ED evaluation. In the ED, a neurological examination will be performed and a neuroimaging study may be done. CT scans are used to detect bleeding and swelling in the brain following TBI. CT is commonly used in the ED and is followed up with an MRI scan on admission, which cannot only detect bleeding and swelling but also DAI and metabolic injury (see Chapter 12). Depending on the results of the physical examination and neuroimaging studies, the child may be discharged to home with close observation and follow-up, or admitted to the hospital for further care.

SEVERITY OF TRAUMATIC BRAIN INJURY

There are two major ways to determine the severity of TBI: the GCS (Teasdale & Jennett, 1974) and duration of PTA. The GCS assesses motor response (scored from 1–6), verbal response (1–5), and eye opening (1–4) within the first 24 hours after brain injury. After assessing each category, the scores are added together, with higher scores indicating a milder brain injury. The lowest GCS score is a 3, and the highest score is a 15. Scores of 8 or below indicate a severe TBI, scores 9–12 indicate a moderate TBI, and scores 13–15 indicate a mild TBI. A person with a score below 8 is said to be comatose (Chung, Chen, & Cheng, 2006).

Duration of PTA includes the length of time in coma and the time after coma it takes the individual to remember events and store new memories. The Children's Orientation and Amnesia Test (COAT; Ewing-Cobbs, Levin, Fletcher, Minor, & Eisenberg, 1990) is a widely used tool to assess PTA. In mild TBI, duration of PTA is less than 1 hour. In moderate TBI, duration of PTA is between 1 hour and 1 day. In severe TBI, duration of PTA is longer than 1 day (Wilson, Teasdale, Hadley, Wiedmann, & Lang, 1994).

ACUTE TREATMENT OF TRAUMATIC BRAIN INJURY

Treatment of TBI begins in the ED and continues throughout any hospitalization. Initially a rapid assessment of the child's breathing ability and circulation will occur. A breathing tube may be placed in the child's airway if needed. Vital signs will be checked frequently. The head and spine will be examined and imaged for injury, and a GCS score will be assigned. The films will help determine the next step. A CT scan of the head can show bleeding, bruising, or swelling of the brain, as well as fractures of the skull. Blood pressure values and oxygen levels will be monitored. Children with more severe injuries may require a special monitor to be placed within the skull to monitor brain pressure. Pressures that are too high require further medical intervention and even surgery to help relieve the pressure.

Throughout a child's hospital course, the goal of treatment is to prevent or limit secondary brain damage. This may be achieved through ventilator management, medications to control swelling of the brain, and/or surgery (Huh & Raghupathi, 2009; Walker et al., 2009). An MRI may be obtained once the child is stabilized to provide further information on the extent of brain damage.

Seizures may occur after a TBI. If they occur within the first 24 hours, they are called immediate posttraumatic seizures; seizures within the first week are called early posttraumatic seizures; and seizures anytime after the first week are called late posttraumatic seizures. Children ages 7 and younger have a greater frequency of early seizures than do older children and adults. Older children and adults have a greater frequency of late posttraumatic seizures (Asikainen, Kaste, & Sarna, 1999; Statler, 2006). Risk factors for late seizures include skull fractures and bleeding in the brain (Annegers, Hauser, Coan, & Rocca, 1998; Asikainen et al., 1999). Antiepileptic drugs may be used for the first week after injury to prevent posttraumatic seizures (Temkin et al., 1990).

In the acute care hospital, efforts will be made to prevent the complications of "bed rest." These problems may include decreased muscle mass and strength, bone loss, skin breakdown, loss of range of motion at joints (contractures), and weight loss. Contractures and skin breakdown may be prevented by appropriate positioning and frequent repositioning. Passive range of motion should be undertaken once the child is medically stable. Nutrition plays an important role following TBI because of increased daily calorie and protein needs during the healing process (Pepe & Barba, 1999). The child may require an alternative means of nutrition, such as a nasogastric tube, to receive calories, liquids, and medication. Gastroesophageal reflux and decreased rate of stomach emptying may also be a problem. Urinary and bowel incontinence is common after moderate to severe brain injury, but there may also be urinary retention and constipation, which should be treated with medication.

The autonomic nervous system controls automatic body activity, such as breathing, heart rate, blood pressure, temperature control, sweating, and so forth. Paroxysmal autonomic instability with extensor posturing or dystonia (both terms refer to atypical positioning of limbs) may occur following severe brain injury. Symptoms can include agitation, sweating, increased temperature, hypertension, **tachycardia** (rapid heart rate), and **tachypnea** (rapid breathing). Autonomic instability can persist for weeks to months following injury. It is caused by dysfunction of the thalamus or hypothalamus (or their connections within the brain) and is treated with medication (Blackman, Patrick, Buck, & Rust, Jr., 2004).

REHABILITATION OF CHILDREN WITH TRAUMATIC BRAIN INJURY

Once a child is felt to be medically stable and ready for the next level of care, he or she may be transitioned to a rehabilitation hospital for intensive inpatient therapy or may participate in outpatient therapy services, depending on the severity of the injury and impairments. A rehabilitation facility should have the following components of care: 1) expertise in rehabilitation of children, 2) developmentally appropriate treatments, 3) family-centered care, and 4) attention to the child's education and reintegration into the school system. Many rehabilitation hospitals are accredited through the Commission on Accreditation of Rehabilitation Facilities (CARF). CARF sets standards of care for the facilities and also has specialty accreditations for brain injury programs and pediatric specialty programs.

As the child recovers from TBI, functional impairments may become apparent in the following domains: motor, sensory, communication, cognition, and behavior (Savage, DePompei, Tyler, & Lash, 2005). Rehabilitation strives to 1) prevent complications that are caused by immobilization and disuse, 2) increase the use of abilities regained, 3) teach strategies to compensate for impaired or lost function, and 4) alleviate the effect of chronic disability on the process of growth and development (Cope, 1995).

Motor Impairments

Family members will frequently ask about motor recovery and functional prognosis following TBI. Studies have shown that motor weakness tends to improve over time and that functional outcomes are good. Approximately 85% of children with a history of coma for a minimum of 1 week will regain independence with ambulation and self-care between 1–7 years after TBI (Brink, Garrett, Hale, Nickel, & Woo-Sam, 1970). Of children who are in coma for more than 24 hours, 10% are found to be physically normal at 1 year, and approximately 75% regain physical independence (Brink, Imbus, & Woo-Sam, 1980). Persistent impairments may be noted in strength, balance, speed, and coordination (Beretta et al., 2009; Katz-Leurer, Rotem, Lewitus, Keren, & Meyer, 2008). Hand function reveals decreased fine motor skills, speed, and coordination (Kuhtz-Buschbeck et al., 2003). Prognosis of motor recovery is related to duration of coma.

Significant motor recovery may occur in children who are comatose for less than 3 months (Brink et al., 1970; Brink et al., 1980).

Motor recovery is also affected by motor impairments related to movement patterns and tone, such as spasticity, dystonia, and ataxia or tremor. Medications and/or surgery may be used as treatment of these impairments. Tremor may be treated with propranolol (Inderol) or carbidopa/levodopa (Sinemet). Medications to treat spasticity and dystonia include baclofen (Lioresel), dantrolene (Dantrium), diazepam (Valium), trihexiphenadyl (Artane), and tizanidine (Zanaflex). Baclofen may be given orally or directly into the spinal fluid with an intrathecal baclofen pump (Albright & Ferson, 2006). There is, as of 2012, no medicine or surgery that is effective for ataxia.

Management of spasticity may also involve localized neuromuscular blockade with botulinum toxins or nerve blocks, such as phenol injections. The effects of botulinum toxins last several months, but repeated injections may be required (Bjornson et al., 2007; Meholjic-Fetahovic, 2007). Injections should be followed by physical or occupational therapy services to obtain the desired results. Orthopedic surgery may be necessary for treatment of contractures or bony orthopedic deformities. Surgeries may include tendon lengthening, femoral osteotomies (reconfiguring the femur to treat hip spasticity), or spinal fusion for scoliosis.

Sensory Impairments

Both vision and hearing may be affected following TBI. Visual impairments may be due to injury of the optic nerves, impaired visual processing in the brain, or limitation of eye movements resulting from cranial nerve damage. Double vision is common following TBI because of cranial nerve injury. Other impairments may include nystagmus (shaking eye movements caused by cerebellar damage), decreased visual acuity, difficulty with tracking, and visual field cuts. Traumatic injury to the optic nerve is not reversible and can cause blindness (Bodack, 2010; Cockerman, et al., 2009). Injury to the occipital lobes, leading to visual cortex damage, can cause cortical blindness (ability to see but not process visual information; see Chapter 11). Vision testing is recommended for evaluation of the above impairments.

Sensorineural hearing loss or conductive hearing loss can occur following TBI and is generally unilateral. Hearing loss may be a result of trauma to the middle (conductive) and inner (sensorineural) ear due to skull base fractures or damage to the central neuronal pathways. Sensorineural loss is more pronounced at the higher hearing frequencies (Lew, Jerger, Guillory, & Henry, 2007; Munjal, Panda, & Pathak, 2010). Audiologic evaluation is recommended following TBI. Brainstem auditory evoked responses (BAER) can be used for testing children who are unable to participate in traditional behavioral audiometric testing (Lew et al., 2004; see Chapter 10).

Feeding Disorders

Dysphagia (difficulty in swallowing) can be caused by TBI. Dysphagia affects oral nutrition and hydration. It can also have a negative impact on the child's ability to protect the airway, leading to increased risk of aspiration pneumonia (see Chapter 9). The incidence of dysphagia following TBI overall is low; however, it increases markedly with increasing severity of the TBI. The incidence of acute dysphagia associated with severe TBI is 68%–76% (Morgan, 2010; Morgan, Mageandran, & Mei, 2010). Associated impairments include atypical tongue movements, poor jaw stability, inefficient chewing, impaired lip closure, and reduced attention and impulsivity during feeding. Signs of aspiration can include coughing after a swallow, wet voice after swallowing, and delayed swallow initiation. Motor impairment is significantly associated with dysphagia (Morgan et al., 2010). A child with dysphagia may require a feeding tube to provide nutrition and hydration. The tube may be a temporary measure, such as a nasogastric tube, or a long-term option, such as a percutaneous (placed through the skin without opening the abdomen) endoscopic gastrostomy (PEG) tube. Children with a PEG tube will receive a standard concentration enteral formula to attain maximum nutrition with minimum volume (Cook, Peppard, & Magnuson, 2008).

Communication Skills Impairments

Dysarthria is a dysfunction in the motor control of the muscles used for speech. It affects articulation and intelligibility. The incidence reported ranges from 2% to 60% in children with TBI (Cahill, 2005; Morgan et al., 2010). Language impairments may be expressive or receptive (involving auditory perceptual problems). Motor impairment and dysphagia are significantly associated with dysarthria (Morgan et al., 2010). The more complex features of language processing are affected by cognitive deficits involving difficulty with judgment related to topic management, turn taking, and pause time (Fyrberg, Marchioni, & Emanuelson, 2007). Individuals with TBI are less appropriate in their use of language and style of speech and have difficulty initiating and sustaining a conversation (Dahlberg et al., 2007). Social isolation may result from these communication impairments.

Cognitive Impairments

Cognitive impairments are common following TBI. Areas affected may include attention, memory, executive function (planning, initiating, problem solving), and speed of processing (Dikmen et al., 2009). Long-term outcome is correlated with injury severity. The more severe the injury sustained, the worse the outcome across all cognitive domains. Environmental factors unrelated to the injury also have an impact on outcome. These factors include parental occupation, preinjury adaptive abilities, age of injury, and preinjury behavior (Anderson, Morse, Catroppa, Haritou, & Rosenfeld, 2004).

Preschool children with severe TBI demonstrate slower recovery with poorer cognitive outcome up to 5 years after injury compared with children less severely injured (Anderson et al., 2009; Ylvisaker & Feeney, 2007). Children who are younger at the time of injury may not show the full extent of their cognitive impairments until they reach school age, when the task complexity increases (Anderson & Catroppa, 2005; Meekes, Jennekens-Schinkel, & van Schooneveld, 2006).

Cognitive impairments are identified through evaluation by a neuropsychologist using items that measure intelligence as well as subtle impairments in cognition. The assessment is typically performed in a quiet setting with minimal distractions. It involves a set of standardized measures to assess concept formation, reasoning, problem solving, language, memory, attention, visuospatial skills, and academic performance. The results of this testing can be used during the rehabilitation stay, and to direct educational placement and accommodations as necessary (Ylvisaker et al., 2001). Additional testing may be recommended as the child reintegrates into the school and community, including parent and teacher behavior scales and educational testing. As the child ages and demands are increased, cognitive impairments may become more apparent and warrant repeat testing and monitoring.

Recovery from Mild Traumatic Brain Injury

Mild TBI is relatively common, and most of the children seen in the ED for TBI are released rather than hospitalized. Seventy-five percent of TBIs that occur each year are concussions or other forms of mild TBI (Faul et al., 2010). Recovery from mild TBI is generally complete; however, some children may continue to have symptoms consistent with a postconcussive syndrome. These symptoms include headache, fatigue, difficulties with memory and concentration, dizziness, confusion, anxiety, and vision issues (Konrad et al., 2010; Sroufe et al., 2010). The length of time that these postconcussive symptoms last is variable. Typically, symptoms decrease within the first week, but they may continue for months to years (Barlow et al., 2010; Keenan & Bratton, 2006; Sroufe et al., 2010).

OUTCOME OF MODERATE TO SEVERE TRAUMATIC BRAIN INJURY

The outcomes for children who have sustained moderate to severe TBI are variable. The more severe the injury (as documented by lower initial GCS scores), the longer the duration of intensive care unit (ICU) stay; the longer the hospital stay, the more likely is a child to have lasting impairments (Anderson & Catroppa, 2006; Campbell, Kuehn, Richards, Ventureyra, & Hutchison, 2004). Areas typically affected include receptive language, working memory, executive function, and speed of processing (Anderson & Catroppa, 2006; Anderson et al., 2004; Campbell et al., 2004). Even with these impairments, a child's preinjury academic skills and global intelligence may remain intact; it is new learning that is impaired (Ylvisaker et al., 2001).

Following severe TBI, recovery is significant over the course of the first year, with slowing over the next year (Taylor et al., 1999). Recovery is influenced not only by severity of injury but also by family factors, including socioeconomic status, resources, and support systems (Anderson & Catroppa, 2006; Keenan & Bratton, 2006). Recovery and outcome are also affected by age at the time of injury. For many years it was felt that the younger the age of injury, the better the outcome, due to the plasticity of the brain. However, it has been shown more recently that children who sustain a brain injury at an earlier age are at increased risk for lasting impairments across all areas

(Anderson et al., 2009). Stage of development at the time of injury has an impact on outcome. A child may return to the previous developmental level following injury but may have trouble progressing past that stage (Giza, Kolb, Harris, Asarnow, & Prins, 2009). This difficulty with progressing into new developmental levels or attaining new developmental milestones has been described as a neurocognitive stall (Chapman, 2007). This may be noted in all age groups and is typically a slowing or lack of further progression in the intellectual, motor, and social development of the child 1 year after injury.

Rehabilitation

The primary goals of rehabilitation for all impairments related to TBI include promotion of recovery, compensation for impairments, and identification and treatment of cognitive and behavioral issues. Following TBI, the medical team or primary care provider helps determine the level of care needed. A multidisciplinary intervention including physical therapy (PT), occupational therapy (OT), speech therapy, neuropsychology, special education, and social work may be necessary, depending on the severity of the injury and impairments.

School Reentry

One of the main goals following rehabilitation is school and community reintegration. Sustaining a TBI places a child at risk for the presence of long-term academic difficulties, especially following moderate to severe TBI. Reading and math abilities may be compromised as well as attention, concentration, and memory (Catroppa et al., 2009; Hawley, Ward, Magnay, & Mychalkiw, 2004). Educational testing as well as neuropsychological testing should be completed to obtain a comprehensive view of the child's impairments (see Chapter 16). Children injured at a younger age may not demonstrate the full effects of the injury until later, when demands and expectations are increased. Long-term follow-up studies of school-age children with TBI reveal impairments that persist or worsen as the children progress through school (Glang et al., 2008).

TBI is a special education eligibility category under the Individuals with Disabilities Education Improvement Act (IDEA) of 2004 (PL 108-446). Eligibility in most states requires medical documentation of a TBI, and physical and intellectual assessments must show a difference between preinjury and postinjury performance. If a student qualifies, an IEP will be created by a team of individuals including the parents and representatives from the school or school district (see Chapter 31). The IEP will outline modifications needed for the student to be successful in the school environment. Examples include therapy services provided by the school system, a range of classroom settings from self-contained to assistance in the classroom, focused instruction, organizational support, and increased time or strategies to address impairments in attention, organization, or memory. If a child does not qualify for an IEP because he or she is academically at or near grade level, the child may qualify to receive support and accommodations with a Section 504 plan (Rehabilitation Act of 1973, PL 93-112).

Obtaining an IEP or a Section 504 plan is an important aspect of school reintegration. Without a plan in place, educators may not recognize the impairments and needs of the student. During their training, teachers are rarely exposed to children with TBI; due to their lack of knowledge of the long-term sequelae of TBI, they may underestimate its effects on learning, memory, and behavior (Glang et al., 2008; Hawley et al., 2004; Ylvisaker et al., 2001). An IEP or Section 504 plan allows for communication across all school settings regarding the injury and the impairments (Hawley et al., 2004). Children with TBI who receive transition support from the hospital are more likely to have an IEP or Section 504 plan in place. Planning for school reentry, transition support, and education of school staff, as well as long-term monitoring, are all important for successful reintegration and school placement.

Behavioral and Social Impairments

Following TBI, changes may be noted in a child's behavioral, emotional, and social interactions. These changes may include adjustment difficulties, psychiatric disorders (including depression and anxiety), disinhibition, impulsivity, poor safety awareness, social withdrawal, and inappropriate social behavior (Anderson & Catroppa, 2006; Ylvisaker et al., 2005). Management may include medications, counseling, and/or behavioral reinforcement, all of which are tailored to the child's needs (Anderson & Catroppa, 2006; Bates, 2006; Riggio & Wong, 2009; Ylvisaker et al., 2005). Behavioral issues and social withdrawal can lead to tension within the family; social isolation not only affects the child but can lead to isolation of the entire family (Kapapa et al., 2010).

Caregivers of children with a severe TBI are also under greater stress and are at higher risk for psychological symptoms (Aitken et al., 2005; Gan & Schuller, 2002). Preinjury behavioral and family functioning is also correlated to postinjury function (Anderson et al., 2001). Coping strategies used by families may include denial and disengagement (Stancin, Wade, Walz, Yeates, & Taylor, 2008). Parents and siblings may feel guilt and remorse after the injury. Fathers are more likely to use denial, whereas mothers are more likely to use acceptance and emotionally focused strategies. These different coping styles may further exacerbate family dysfunction (Wade et al., 2010; see Chapter 37). Prolonged hospitalization may place a financial burden on the family and affect the overall finances and dynamics of the family as well.

Family support is important in all phases following a TBI, including acute hospitalization, rehabilitation, and school reintegration. Social workers, psychologists, educators, and other health professionals may work with the family to assist with resources, family coping and adjustment, discharge planning, and school reentry. Ongoing support groups in the community may be recommended and utilized (Aitken et al., 2005).

Prevention

Many types of unintentional injuries are preventable (Schnitzer, 2006). The leading causes of nonfatal injuries are falls, poisoning, burns, and motor vehicle, bicycle, and pedestrian accidents (Centers for Disease Control and Prevention, 2011). Falls are more common in younger children, bicycle and pedestrian collisions in elementary and middle school-age children, and motor vehicle collisions in adolescents (Mendelson & Fallat, 2007). The use of window guards, the use of gates at stairways, and refraining from using infant walkers are three strategies for the prevention of falls (Schnitzer, 2006). The appropriate use of car seats, boosters, and seat belts has been shown to reduce brain injury in children following a motor vehicle accident (Keenan & Bratton, 2006). The American Academy of Pediatrics (AAP) released a policy statement on child passenger safety in 2011 (Durbin & Committee on Injury, Violence, and Poison Prevention, 2011). The statement provides recommendations for best practices, including 1) rear-facing car safety seats for most infants

up to 2 years of age, 2) forward-facing car safety seats for most children through 4 years of age, 3) belt-positioning booster seats for most children through 8 years of age, and 4) lap-and-shoulder seat belts for all children who have outgrown booster seats. Children under the age of 13 years should ride in the rear seats of vehicles. Child safety seats decrease the risk of nonfatal injury by approximately 75% (Zaloshnja, Miller, & Hendrie, 2007) and the risk of fatal injury by 28% (Elliott, Kallan, Durbin, & Winston, 2006). Booster seats decrease the risk of nonfatal injury among 4- to 8-year-old children by 45% compared with seat belts (Arbogast, Jermakian, Kallan, & Durbin, 2009). The AAP also recommends that children should not ride in the flatbeds of pickup trucks; nor is it recommended for children or teenagers younger than 16 years to ride an all-terrain vehicle (ATV) or a lawn mower.

In school-age children, pedestrian injuries typically occur while the child is crossing the road. Strategies that have been utilized to improve street-crossing skills include group education and individualized behavior training. Individualized training appears to be more successful than group training (Schwebel & McClure, 2010). Programs developed to help teach pedestrian safety included the WalkSafe program. This program has been shown to improve pedestrian safety knowledge of school-age children after receiving a 3-day educational experience (Hotz et al., 2009). The Safe Kids organization was established in 1987 at Children's National Medical Center in Washington, D.C. Its goals are to change attitudes, behaviors, laws, and the environment to prevent injury to children (http://www.safekids.org).

Children ages 5–14 years have the highest rate of bicycle-related injuries. Head injury accounts for 62% of bicycle-related deaths, 33% of bicycle-related ED visits, and 67% of all bicycle-related hospital admissions (Centers for Disease Control and Prevention, 1995). Bicycle helmets are effective in decreasing head, brain, and facial injuries when used properly. The risk of TBI is reduced by 60% when wearing a bicycle helmet (Attewell, Glase, & McFadden, 2001; Lee, Schofer, & Koppelman, 2005; Thompson et al., 1999). Helmets and protective gear are also recommended for skating, skateboarding, skiing, snowboarding, scooter riding, horseback riding, motorcycle riding, and participation in contact sports such as football, hockey, and lacrosse (Dellinger & Kresnow, 2010; Jagodzinski & DeMuri, 2005; Schnitzer, 2006).

Motor vehicle collisions are the leading cause of injuries in teenagers. Prevention strategies include limiting nighttime driving, limiting driving with teenage passengers, and developing graduated licensing measures (Williams & Ferguson, 2002). As in younger children, appropriate use of seat belts is important.

Prevention should be addressed at well-child visits through parent-focused strategies and through education to teachers and community groups as well as the children themselves. The focus should be on the appropriate use of seat belts, safe pedestrian behavior, helmet use, prevention of falls, and sports injury prevention.

SUMMARY

Traumatic brain injury is a significant risk during childhood. There is a wide range of severity of injury, and the outcome may range from complete recovery to severe functional and intellectual disability. Persistent functional impairments may involve several areas, including motor, sensory, feeding, communication, cognition, and behavior. Restoration and adaptation are the goals of rehabilitation and require a multidisciplinary team including medical professionals, allied health professionals, and education specialists. Children should be followed throughout their education to provide support and accommodations as needed. Most brain injuries are preventable. Therefore, brain injury prevention programs are needed and legislation must be written and enforced to decrease the risk and long-term consequences of TBI.

REFERENCES

Aitken, M.E., Korehbandi, P., Parnell, D., Parker, J.G., Stefans, V., Tompkins, E., & Schultz, E.G. (2005). Experiences from the development of a comprehensive family support program for pediatric trauma and rehabilitation patients. *Archives of Physical Medicine and Rehabilitation, 86*, 175–179.

Albright, A.L., & Ferson, S.S. (2006). Intrathecal baclofen therapy in children. *Neurosurgery Focus, 2*(2), e3.

Anderson, V., & Catroppa, C. (2005). Recovery of executive skills following paediatric traumatic brain injury (TBI): A 2 year follow-up. *Brain Injury, 19*(6), 459–470.

Anderson, V., & Catroppa, C. (2006). Advances in post-acute rehabilitation after childhood-acquired brain injury: A focus on cognitive, behavioral, and social domains. *American Journal of Physical Medicine & Rehabilitation, 85*(9), 767–778.

Anderson, V.A., Catroppa, C., Haritou, F., Morse, S., Pentland, L., Rosenfeld, J., & Stargatt, R. (2001). Predictors of acute child and family outcome following traumatic brain injury in children. *Pediatric Neurosurgery, 34*(3), 138–148.

Anderson, V., Catroppa, C., Morse, S., Haritou, F., & Rosenfeld, J.V. (2009). Intellectual outcome from preschool traumatic brain injury: A 5-year prospective, longitudinal study. *Pediatrics, 124*(6), e1064–e1071.

Anderson, V.A., Morse, S.A., Catroppa, C., Haritou, F., & Rosenfeld, J.V. (2004). Thirty month outcome from early childhood head injury: A prospective analysis of neurobehavioural recovery. *Brain, 127*(12), 2608–2620.

Anderson, V., Spencer-Smith, M., Leventer, R., Coleman, L., Anderson, P., Williams, J., ... Jacobs, R. (2009). Childhood brain insult: Can age at insult help us predict outcome? *Brain, 132*, 45–56.

Annegers, J.F., Hauser, W.A., Coan, S.P., & Rocca, W.A. (1998). A population-based study of seizures after traumatic brain injuries. *The New England Journal of Medicine, 338*, 20–24.

Arbogast, K.B., Jermakian, J.S., Kallan, M.J., & Durbin, D.R. (2009). Effectiveness of belt positioning booster seats: An updated assessment. *Pediatrics, 124*(5), 1281–1286.

Asikainen, I., Kaste, M., & Sarna, S. (1999). Early and late posttraumatic seizures in traumatic brain injury rehabilitation patients: Brain injury factors causing late seizures and influence of seizures on long-term outcome. *Epilepsia Journal, 40*(5), 584–589.

Attewell, R.G., Glase, K., & McFadden, M. (2001). Bicycle helmet efficacy: A meta-analysis. *Accident Analysis and Prevention, 33*, 345–352.

Barlow, K.M., Crawford, S., Stevenson, A., Sandhu, S.S., Belanger, F., & Dewey, D. (2010). Epidemiology of postconcussion syndrome in pediatric mild traumatic brain injury. *Pediatrics, 126*(2), e374–e381.

Bates, G. (2006). Medication in the treatment of the behavioural sequelae of traumatic brain injury. *Developmental Medicine and Child Neurology, 48*, 697–701.

Beretta, E., Cimolin, V., Piccinini, L., Carla Turconi, A., Galbiati, S., Crivelleni, M., ... Strazzer, S. (2009). Assessment of gait recovery in children after traumatic brain injury. *Brain Injury, 23*(9), 751–759.

Bjornson, K., Hays, R., Graubert, C., Price, R., Won, F., McLaughlin, J.F., & Cohen, M. (2007). Botulinum toxin for spasticity in children with cerebral palsy: A comprehensive evaluation. *Pediatrics, 120*(1), 49–58.

Blackman, J.A., Patrick, P.D., Buck, M.L., & Rust, Jr., R.S. (2004). Paroxysmal autonomic instability with dystonia after brain injury. *Archives of Neurology, 61*, 321–328.

Bodack, M.I. (2010). Pediatric acquired brain injury. *Optometry, 81*, 516–527.

Brink, J.D., Garrett, A.L., Hale, W.R., Nickel, V.L., & Woo-Sam, J. (1970). Recovery of motor and intellectual function in children sustaining severe head injuries. *Developmental Medicine and Child Neurology, 12*(5), 565–571.

Brink, J.D., Imbus, C., & Woo-Sam, J. (1980). Physical recovery after severe closed head trauma in children and adolescents. *Journal of Pediatrics, 97*(5), 721–727.

Cahill, L.M., Murdoch, B.E., & Theodoros, D.G. (2005). Articulatory function following traumatic brain injury in childhood: A perceptual and instrumental analysis. *Brain Injury, 19*(1), 41–58.

Campbell, C.G., Kuehn, S.M., Richards, P.M., Ventureyra, E., & Hutchison, J.S. (2004). Medical and cognitive outcome in children with traumatic brain injury. *The Canadian Journal of Neurological Sciences, 31*(2), 213–219.

Carroll, L.J., Cassidy, J.D., Peloso, P.M., Borg, J., von Holst, H., Holm, L., ...WHO Collaborating Centre Task Force on Mild Traumatic Brain Injury. (2004). Prognosis for mild traumatic brain injury: Results of the WHO Collaborating Centre Task Force on Mild Traumatic Brain Injury. *Journal of Rehabilitation Medicine, 43*(Suppl.), 84–105.

Catroppa, C., Anderson, V.A., Muscara, F., Morse, S.A., Haritou, F., Rosenfeld, J.V., & Heinrich, L.M. (2009). Educational skills: Long-term outcome and predictors following paediatric traumatic brain injury. *Neuropsychological Rehabilitation, 19*(5), 716–732.

Centers for Disease Control and Prevention, National Center for Injury Prevention and Control. (1995). Injury control recommendations: Bicycle helmets. *Morbidity and Mortality Weekly Report, 44*(RR-1), 1–18. Retrieved from http://www.cdc.gov/mmwr/pdf/rr/rr4401.pdf

Centers for Disease Control and Prevention, National Center for Injury Prevention and Control (2010). *WISQARS Leading Causes of Nonfatal Injury Reports.* Retrieved from http://webappa.cdc.gov/sasweb/ncipc/nfilead.html

Chapman, S.B. (2007). Neurocognitive stall: A paradox in long term recovery from pediatric brain injury. *Brain Injury Professional, 3*(4), 10–13.

Chung, C.Y., Chen, C.L., Cheng, P.T., See, L.C., Tang, S.F., & Wong, A.M. (2006). Critical score of Glasgow Coma Scale for pediatric traumatic brain injury. *Pediatric Neurology, 34*(5), 379–387.

Cockerham, G.C., Goodrich, G.L., Weichel, E.D., Orcutt, J.C., Rizzo, J.F., Bower, K.S., & Schuchard, R.A. (2009). Eye and visual function in traumatic brain injury. *Journal of Rehabilitation Research & Development, 46*(6), 811–818.

Cook, A.M., Peppard, A., & Magnuson, B. (2008). Nutrition considerations in traumatic brain injury. *American Society for Parenteral and Enteral Nutrition, 26*(6), 608–620.

Cope, N.D. (1995). The effectiveness of traumatic brain injury rehabilitation: A review. *Brain Injury, 9*(7), 649–670.

Dahlberg, C.A., Cusick, C.P., Hawley, L.A., Newman, J.K., Morey, C.E., Harrison-Felix, C.L., & Whiteneck, G.G. (2007). Treatment efficacy of social communication skills training after traumatic brain injury: A randomized treatment and deferred treatment controlled trial. *Archives of Physical Medicine and Rehabilitation, 88*(12), 1561–1573.

Dellinger, A.M., & Kresnow, M. (2010). Bicycle helmet use among children in the United States: The effects of legislation, personal and household factors. *Journal of Safety Research, 41*, 375–380.

Dikmen, S.S., Corrigan, J.D., Levin, H.S., Machamer, J., Stiers, W., & Weisskopf, M.G. (2009). Cognitive outcome following traumatic brain injury. *Journal of Head Trauma Rehabilitation, 24*(6), 430–438.

Durbin, D.R., & Committee on Injury, Violence, and Poison Prevention. (2011). Child passenger safety. *Pediatrics, 127*(4), 788–793.

Elliott, M.R., Kallan, M.J., Durbin, D.R., & Winston, F.K. (2006). Effectiveness of child safety seats vs. seat belts in reducing risk for death in children in passenger vehicle crashes. *Archives of Pediatrics & Adolescent Medicine, 160*(6), 617–621.

Ewing-Cobbs, L., Levin, H.S., Fletcher, J.M., Miner, M.D., & Eisenberg, H.M. (1990). The Children's Orientation and Amnesia Test: Relationship to severity of acute head injury and to recovery of memory. *Neurosurgery, 27*(5), 683–691.

Faul, M., Xu, L., Wald, M.M., & Coronado, V.G. (2010). Traumatic brain injury in the United States: Emergency department visits, hospitalizations and deaths 2002–2006. *Centers for Disease Control and Prevention, National Center for Injury Prevention and Control.* Retrieved from http://www.cdc.gov/traumaticbraininjury/tbi_ed.html

Fyrberg, A., Marchioni, M., & Emanuelson, I. (2007). Severe acquired brain injury: Rehabilitation of communicative skills in children and adolescents. *International Journal of Rehabilitation Research, 30*, 153–157.

Gan, C., & Schuller, R. (2002). Family system outcome following acquired brain injury: Clinical and research perspectives. *Brain Injury, 16*(4), 311–322.

Giza, C.C., Kolb, B., Harris, N.G., Asarnow, R.F., & Prins, M.L. (2009). Hitting a moving target: Basic mechanisms of recovery from acquired developmental brain injury. *Developmental Neurorehabilitation, 12*(5), 255–268.

Glang, A., Todis, B., Thomas, C.W., Hood, D., Bedell, G., & Cockrell, J. (2008). Return to school following childhood TBI: Who gets services? *NeuroRehabilitation, 23*(6), 477–486.

Hawley, C.A., Ward, A.B., Magnay, A.R., & Mychalkiw, W. (2004). Return to school after brain injury. *Archives of Disease in Childhood, 89*, 136–142.

Hotz, F., de Marcilla, A.G., Lutfi, K., Kennedy, A., Castellon, P., & Duncan, R. (2009). The WalkSafe program: Developing and evaluating the educational component. *The Journal of Trauma Injury, Infection and Critical Care, 66*(Suppl. 3), S3–S9.

Huh, J., & Raghupathi, R. (2009). New concepts in treatment of pediatric traumatic brain injury. *Journal of Clinical Anesthesia, 27*, 213–240.

Individuals with Disabilities Education Improvement Act (IDEA) of 2004, 20 U.S.C. §§ 1400 *et seq.*

Jagodzinski, T., & DeMuri, G.P. (2005). Horse–related injuries in children: A review. *Wisconsin Medical Journal, 104*(2), 50–54.

Jennett, B., Teasdale, G., Galbraith, S., Pickard, J., Grant, H., Braakman, R., ... Kurze, T. (1977). Severe head injuries in three countries. *Journal of Neurology, Neurosurgery, and Psychiatry, 40*(3), 293.

Johnston, K.M., Lassonde, M., & Ptito, A. (2001). A contemporary neurosurgical approach to sport-related head injury: The McGill concussion protocol. *Journal of the American College of Surgeons, 192*(4), 515–524.

Kapapa, T., Pfister, U., König, K., Sasse, M., Woischneck, D., Heissler, H.E., & Rickels, E. (2010). Head trauma in children, Part 3: Clinical and psychosocial outcome after head trauma in children. *Journal of Child Neurology, 25*(4), 409–422.

Katz-Leurer, M., Rotem, H., Lewitus, H., Keren, O., & Meyer, S. (2008). Relationship between balance abilities and gait characteristics in children with post-traumatic brain injury. *Brain Injury, 22*(2), 153–159.

Keenan, H.T., & Bratton, S.L. (2006). Epidemiology and outcomes of pediatric traumatic brain injury. *Developmental Neuroscience, 28*, 256–263.

Konrad, C., Geburek, A.J., Rist, F., Blumenroth, H., Fischer, B., Husstedt, I., ... Lohmann, H. (2010). Long-term cognitive and emotional consequences of mild traumatic brain injury. *Psychological Medicine*, 1–15. Advance online publication.

Kuhtz-Buschbeck, J.P., Hoppe, B., Gölge, M., Dreesmann, M., Damm-Stünitz, U., & Ritz, A. (2003). Sensorimotor recovery in children after traumatic brain injury: Analyses of gait, gross motor, and fine motor skills. *Developmental Medicine and Child Neurology*, *45*(12), 821–828.

Langlois, J.A., Rutland-Brown, W., & Wald, M.M. (2006). The epidemiology and impact of traumatic brain injury: A brief overview. *Journal of Head Trauma Rehabilitation*, *21*(5), 375–378.

Lee, B.H., Schofer, J.L., & Koppelman, F.S. (2005). Bicycle safety helmet legislation and bicycle-related non-fatal injuries in California. *Accident Analysis and Prevention*, *37*(1), 93–102.

Lew, H.L., Jerger, J.F., Guillory, S.B., & Henry, J.A. (2007). Auditory dysfunction in traumatic brain injury. *Journal of Rehabilitation Research & Development*, *44*(7), 921–928.

Lew, H.L., Lee, E.H., Miyoshi, Y., Chang, D.G., Date, E.S., & Jerger, J.F. (2004). Brainstem auditory-evoked potentials as an objective tool for evaluating hearing dysfunction in traumatic brain injury. *American Journal of Physical Medicine & Rehabilitation*, *83*(3), 210–215.

Maddocks, D., Dicker, G.D., & Saling, M.M. (1995). The assessment of orientation following concussion in athletes. *Clinical Journal of Sport Medicine*, *5*(1), 32–35.

Mazzini, L., Campini, R., Angelino, E., Rognone, F., Pastore, I., & Oliveri, G. (2003). Posttraumatic hydrocephalus: A clinical, neuroradiologic, and neuropsychologic assessment of long-term outcome. *Archives of Physical Medicine and Rehabilitation*, *84*(11), 1637–1641.

McCrea, M., Kelly, J.P., Randolph, C., Kluge, J., Bartolic, E., Finn, G., & Baxter, B. (1998). Standardized Assessment of Concussion (SAC): On-site mental status evaluation of the athlete. *Journal of Head Trauma Rehabilitation*, *13*(2), 27–35.

Meekes, J., Jennekens-Schinkel, A., & van Schooneveld, M.M. (2006). Recovery after childhood traumatic injury: Vulnerability and plasticity. *Pediatrics*, *117*(6), 2330.

Meholjic-Fetahovic, A. (2007). Treatment of the spasticity in children with cerebral palsy. *Bosnia Journal of Basic Science*, *7*(4), 363–367.

Mendelson, K.G., & Fallat, M.E. (2007). Pediatric injuries: Prevention to resolution. *Surgical Clinics of North America*, *87*, 207–228.

Morgan, A.T. (2010). Dysphagia in childhood traumatic brain injury: A reflection on the evidence and its implications for practice. *Developmental Neurorehabilitation*, *13*(3), 192–203.

Morgan, A.T., Mageandran, S.D., & Mei, C. (2010). Incidence and clinical presentation of dysarthria and dysphagia in the acute setting following paediatric traumatic brain injury. *Child: Care, Health, and Development*, *36*(1), 44–53.

Munjal, S.K., Panda, N.K., & Pathak, A. (2010). Audiological deficits after closed head injury. *The Journal of Trauma*, *68*, 13–18.

Pepe, J.L., & Barba, C.A. (1999). The metabolic response to acute traumatic brain injury and implications for nutritional support. *Journal of Head Trauma Rehabilitation*, *14*(5), 464–474.

Rehabilitation Act of 1973, 29 U.S.C. §§ 701 *et seq.*

Riggio, S., & Wong, M. (2009). Neurobehavioral sequelae of traumatic brain injury. *Mount Sinai Journal of Medicine*, *76*, 163–172.

Safe Kids USA. (n.d.). *Safe Kids USA*. Retrieved August 4, 2011, from http://www.safekids.org

Savage, R.C., DePompei, R., Tyler, J., & Lash, M. (2005). Paediatric traumatic brain injury: A review of pertinent issues. *Pediatric Rehabilitation*, *8*(2), 92–103.

Schnitzer, P.G. (2006). Prevention of unintentional childhood injuries. *American Family Physician*, *74*, 1864–1869.

Schwebel, D.C., & McClure, L.A. (2010). Using virtual reality to train children in safe street-crossing skills. *Injury Prevention*, *16*, e1–e5.

Sroufe, N.S., Fuller, D.S., West, B.T., Singal, B.M., Warschausky, S.A., & Maio, R.F. (2010). Postconcussive symptoms and neurocognitive function after mild traumatic brain injury in children. *Pediatrics*, *125*(6), e1331–e1339.

Stancin, T., Wade, S.L., Walz, N.C., Yeates, K.O., & Taylor, H.G. (2008). Traumatic brain injuries in early childhood: Initial impact on the family. *Developmental and Behavioral Pediatrics*, *29*(4), 253–261.

Statler, K.D. (2006). Pediatric posttraumatic seizures: Epidemiology, putative mechanisms of epileptogenesis and promising investigational progress. *Developmental Neuroscience*, *28*(4–5), 354–363.

Taylor, H.G., Yeates, K.O., Wade, S.L., Drotar, D., Klein, S.K., & Stancin, T. (1999). Influences on first-year recovery from traumatic brain injury in children. *Neuropsychology*, *13*(1), 76–89.

Teasdale, G., & Jennett, B. (1974). Assessment of coma and impaired consciousness: A practical scale. *The Lancet*, *2*, 81–84.

Temkin, N.R., Dikmen, S.S., Wilensky, A.J., Keihm, J., Chabal, S., & Winn, H.R. (1990). A randomized, double-blind study of phenytoin for the prevention of post-traumatic seizures. *The New England Journal of Medicine*, *323*(8), 497–502.

Thompson, D.C., Rivara, F.P., & Thompson, R.S. (1996). Effectiveness of bicycle safety helmets in preventing head injuries: A case-control study. *JAMA: The Journal of the American Medical Association*, *276*(24), 1968–1973.

Thompson, D.C., Rivara, F.P., & Thompson, R. (1999). Helmets for preventing head and facial injuries in bicyclists. *Cochrane Database of Systematic Reviews*, *4*, CD001855.

Wade, S.L., Walz, N.C., Cassedy, A., Taylor, H.G., Stancin, T., & Yeates, K.O. (2010). Caregiver functioning following early childhood TBI: Do moms and dads respond differently? *NeuroRehabilitation*, *27*(1), 63–72.

Walker, P.A., Harting, M.T., Baumgartner, J.E., Fletcher, S., Strobel, N. & Cox, Jr., C.S. (2009). Modern approaches to pediatric brain injury therapy. *The Journal of Trauma*, *67*(2 Suppl.), S120–S127.

Williams, A.F., & Ferguson, S.A. (2002). Rationale for graduated licensing and the risks it should address. *Injury Prevention*, *8*(Suppl. 2), ii9–14.

Wilson, J.T., Teasdale, G.M., Hadley, D.M., Wiedmann, K.D., & Lang, D. (1994). Post-traumatic amnesia: Still a valuable yardstick. *Journal of Neurology, Neurosurgery, and Psychiatry*, *57*(2), 198–201.

Ylvisaker, M., Adelson, P.D., Braga, L.W., Burnett, S.M., Glang, A., Feeney, T., ...Todis, B. (2005). Rehabilitation and ongoing support after pediatric TBI: Twenty years of progress. *Journal of Head Trauma Rehabilitation*, *20*(1), 95–109.

Ylvisaker, M., & Feeney, T. (2007). Pediatric brain injury: Social, behavioral, and communication disability. *Physical Medicine and Rehabilitation Clinics of North America*, *18*(1), 133–144.

Ylvisaker, M., Todis, B., Glang, A., Urbanczyk, B., Franklin, C., DePompei, R., ... Tyler, J.S. (2001). Educating students with TBI: Themes and recommendations. *Journal of Head Trauma Rehabilitation*, *16*(1), 76–93.

Zaloshnja, E., Miller, T.R., & Hendrie, D. (2007). Effectiveness of child safety seats vs. safety belts for children aged 2 to 3 years. *Archives of Pediatrics & Adolescent Medicine*, *161*(1), 65–68.

27

Epilepsy

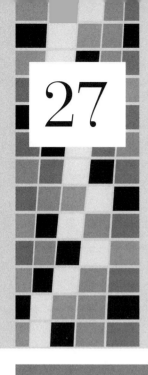

Tesfaye Getaneh Zelleke,
Dewi Frances T. Depositario-Cabacar,
and William Davis Gaillard

Upon completion of this chapter, the reader will

- Be familiar with the signs and symptoms that define epilepsy
- Understand the epidemiology and causes of epilepsy
- Understand the basic classification of epilepsy
- Be familiar with some common epilepsy syndromes
- Be knowledgeable about the evaluation and treatment of epilepsy
- Be aware of antiepileptic medications and their side effects

Seizures, also referred to as "fits" or "convulsions," are transient disturbances of brain function resulting from abnormal excessive excitation of cortical neurons. They are seen frequently in childhood. As many as 1 in 10 children will experience at least one seizure before adulthood (Hauser, 1994). The clinical signs and symptoms of a seizure vary depending on the location of the epileptic discharge in the cerebral cortex and the extent of spread of the discharge within the brain. Seizures can cause changes in motor movement (e.g., tonic or clonic movements), sensation (e.g., a tingling sensation), bodily functions (e.g., incontinence), attention (e.g., loss of attention), and awareness and behavior (e.g., loss of consciousness and/or presence of unusual behaviors such as stereotypic actions). Seizures can be provoked by an infection (e.g., meningitis, encephalitis), metabolic disturbance (e.g., hypoglycemia), toxic agent (e.g., pesticides), trauma, or other acute illness. A fever (in children ages 6 months to 6 years), an overdose of certain medications (e.g., insulin), meningitis, or a fall in which the child hits his or her head can lead to a seizure (Huang, Chang, & Wang, 1998). Most seizures are either solitary events (e.g., a single seizure following minor head trauma) or limited to a specific and narrow developmental window (e.g., febrile convulsions).

The diagnosis of epilepsy requires two unprovoked seizures that occur at least 24 hours apart. The prevalence of epilepsy in the general pediatric population is 4–10 per 1,000 (Berg, 1995). It has variable severity; the child may experience anywhere from two or three seizures to hundreds over a lifetime. Epilepsy may have a clear origin (e.g., resulting from a malformation of cortical development or a perinatal stroke) or it may not have an identifiable cause (called *idiopathic*).

Children with developmental disabilities are at a significantly increased risk for epilepsy

(Sunder, 1997). It is 5 times more common in individuals with cerebral palsy than in typically developing children (Hundozi-Hysenaj & Boshnjaku-Dallku, 2008). With intellectual disability the risk of developing epilepsy through the lifespan is 15%–20% (Besag, 2002; Forsgren, Edvinsson, Blomquist, Heijbel, & Sidenvall, 1990). In addition, if a child has comorbid conditions the risk for epilepsy is increased further. For example, autism spectrum disorders (ASD) are associated with a 2% risk of manifesting epilepsy by 5 years of age and an 8% risk by 10 years (Tuchman & Rapin, 2002); however, this risk increases to 35% at 5 years and 67% by 10 years if the child has intellectual disability associated with the ASD. In general, the more severe the cerebral pathology, the higher the risk of epilepsy (Holmes, 2002).

The control of epilepsy in children with developmental disabilities tends to be harder to achieve, and medically refractory epilepsy (> 3 seizures/year despite treatment with three standard antiepileptic drugs [AEDs]) is more common (Airaksinen et al., 2000; Alvarez, Besag, & Iivanainen, 1998). Furthermore, both epilepsy and AEDs may contribute to learning difficulties and to disruptive behavior. Children with epilepsy exhibit a higher incidence of cognitive impairments, attention-deficit/hyperactivity disorder, anxiety disorders, and depression.

▧ ▧ ▧ PATRICIA

Patricia is a 7-year-old girl who has been referred to the neurology clinic because of spells. She has been reported by her teachers at school to have staring spells and was thought to have difficulties with attention. Her teacher has noticed that she sometimes submits a written test with unfinished answers. There are also occasions when Patricia feels that she has missed a conversation and is often teased by her classmates. Her grades have also gone down. At the neurology clinic office, the pediatric neurologist had her hyperventilate, during which a typical spell was elicited. To confirm the clinical impression and establish a diagnosis, a sleep-deprived electroencephalogram (EEG) was done, which showed a generalized 3 Hz spike and wave pattern characteristic of absence seizures. She was started on ethosuximide, and although she improved, she continued to have some spells. Her medication dose was further increased, and she became asymptomatic. A follow-up EEG was normal. Her grades have also improved. She has been doing well for 2 years without any seizures and the plan is to now discontinue her medication.

EPILEPSY: DEFINITIONS AND CLASSIFICATION

Epilepsy, derived from the Greek word meaning "take hold of" or "seize" (Reynolds, 2000), is a neurologic condition in which a person experiences recurrent unprovoked seizures (Hauser, Rich, Lee, Annegers, & Anderson, 1998). For the majority of children, epilepsy resolves after several years. Thirty percent of children with epilepsy, however, will have an incomplete response to medications, and approximately 5%–10% will have intractable epilepsy (seizures that are frequent despite multiple seizure medications; Hauser, 2006).

A seizure results from an excessive discharge of a large population of cortical neurons. This usually occurs when the excitatory inputs of neurons outweighs the inhibitory components. Excessive neuronal firing continues until either excitatory neurotransmission is exhausted or the inhibitory networks extinguish it. The seizure usually stops in seconds to minutes, but it may occasionally persist, requiring acute medical intervention. When a seizure lasts more than 30 minutes, it is termed *status epilepticus*. The clinical signs and symptoms of the seizure will vary depending on the location of the epileptic discharge in the cerebral cortex and the extent of spread of the discharge in the brain.

Not everyone will have a seizure if presented with the same brain insult because structural and chemical brain interactions are modified by genetic and acquired factors (Briellmann, Jackson, Torn-Broers, & Berkovic, 2001; Frucht, Quigg, Schwaner, & Fountain, 2000). Several factors modulate a predisposition for seizures and the threshold at which they occur. For example, the age of the child and stage of brain development appear to affect the seizure threshold (Moshé, 2000). Some epilepsies are predominantly seen during particular age windows, including infantile spasms (4–16 months), childhood absence epilepsy (4–12 years), benign rolandic epilepsy (6–14 years), and juvenile myoclonic epilepsy (8–26 years). The brain undergoes global and regional structural changes over time that involve changes in cortical thickness and myelination (Gage, 2002) as well as changes in brain chemistry and metabolic rates. Changes in normal brain development, structure, or chemistry can predispose the child to epilepsy (Lowenstein & Alldredge,

1998). Repair mechanisms following some brain insults can also lead to the formation of abnormal neuronal networks that generate seizure activity (Cole, 2000). Brain maturation may explain why some children appear to grow into or out of epilepsy (Sillanpää, 2000).

Seizures are disorders of neuronal transmission and brain network interactions. Factors that predispose a child to having seizures include 1) injury to brain cells that make them dysfunctional (e.g., traumatic brain injury, stroke, and brain tumors), 2) disruption of brain cell circuits (e.g., tuberous sclerosis and malformations of cortical development), and 3) alterations in intrinsic brain cell excitability (e.g., inherited epilepsies such as severe myoclonic epilepsy and autosomal dominant nocturnal frontal lobe epilepsy).

The clinical signs and symptoms of seizures usually reflect the function of the areas from which they arise. In the 1989 classification scheme (Commission on Classification and Terminology of the International League Against Epilepsy, 1989), seizures are divided into partial (i.e., focal or localized) and generalized, depending on the origin and degree of spread of the seizure activity. Partial seizures are further divided into simple and complex, depending on whether consciousness is affected. In simple partial seizures there may be 1) a strange sensation called an aura (e.g., an epigastric sensation arising from the mesial temporal lobe), 2) unusual motor activity (e.g., a jerking of the hands, originating from the primary motor cortex of the frontal lobe), or 3) atypical dystonia-like posture (resulting from spread of the seizure through the basal ganglia). In complex partial seizures there is propagation to brain structures that alter the state of consciousness (e.g., the limbic system). As a result, there may be staring, oral automatisms (lip smacking), or fumbling with hands and clothing. When multiple parts of the brain are involved or there is spread of the electrical discharge to both cerebral hemispheres, generalized tonic-clonic activity may result. In the new classification scheme (Berg et al., 2010), seizures are described as generalized or focal, with or without loss of consciousness (replacing simple, complex, secondarily generalized, and primary generalized).

The International League Against Epilepsy (ILAE) has divided epilepsies into three categories: focal epilepsy, generalized epilepsy, and epilepsy syndromes. Epilepsy may also be divided into idiopathic, symptomatic, and cryptogenic (Commission on Classification and Terminology of the ILAE, 1989). The term *symptomatic* is used when there is a clear structural brain abnormality (e.g., tuberous sclerosis), an acquired cause of epilepsy (e.g., stroke, tumors, meningitis), or an associated neurological impairment (e.g., intellectual disability, cerebral palsy). Idiopathic epilepsies are assumed to be genetic in origin and comprise about 30% of childhood epilepsies (Hauser & Kurland, 1993). In this form of epilepsy there are no abnormal neurological or neuroimaging findings, and there may be a family history of seizures. The term *cryptogenic* has been used for epilepsies where a cause cannot be identified. More recently this classification system has been proposed to be amended to 1) genetic (replaces idiopathic), when the epilepsy is secondary to a presumed genetic defect (e.g., *SCN1A* mutation in Dravet syndrome); 2) structural (either acquired [e.g., brain tumors, stroke], or congenital central nervous system malformations) or metabolic; and 3) unknown cause (replaces cryptogenic), when the underlying cause is not identified (Berg et al., 2010).

Children with a first seizure of remote symptomatic etiology (i.e., a seizure that is removed in time following a brain insult) tend to have a higher rate of seizure recurrence: approximately 65% (Berg & Shinnar, 1991; Shinnar et al., 1996). Among those with a remote symptomatic etiology, children with static brain dysfunction since birth, such as intellectual disability or cerebral palsy, tend to have the highest rates of seizure recurrence. In contrast to children with a remote symptomatic etiology, children with a first seizure of idiopathic or cryptogenic etiology tend to have lower rates of additional seizures, with approximately a 35% chance of recurrence (Berg & Shinnar, 1991; Shinnar et al., 1996).

The causes of epilepsy vary with age. Malformations of cortical development, perinatal brain injury, and metabolic disorders are common causes of epilepsy in infancy; genetic and congenital disorders are found in early and later childhood; and hippocampal sclerosis, alcohol or drug abuse, and trauma may be present in older children and adolescents (Shorvon, 2000).

Classification of Epilepsy and Epilepsy Syndromes

The diagnosis, treatment, and prognosis of seizure disorders depend on both the correct identification of the type of seizures and its epilepsy classification. Childhood epilepsies are classified using variations of the ILAE classification system (Commission on Classification and Terminology of the ILAE, 1989).

As mentioned above, the ILAE classifies epilepsy into two major classes: generalized (seizures coming from both cerebral hemispheres simultaneously) and partial (starting in a focal area of the cerebrum), as well as a class of syndromes (see Table 27.1). Epilepsy syndromes (and recently added constellations) are classified based on the clinical appearance of the seizures, the EEG, and the age of onset. A modified classification system has been developed for some seizures (e.g., neonatal seizures, infantile seizures, status epilepticus, epilepsy surgery). Another proposed classification system is the 5-axis diagnostic scheme, which divides seizures into 1) descriptive ictal terminology, 2) seizure type, 3) syndrome, 4) etiology, and 5) impairment (Engel, 2001). Several task forces have considered providing for alternative classification schemes, and this will likely be an ongoing dynamic process (Berg et al., 2010; Engel, 2006).

Occasionally, there is difficulty in classifying epilepsy because 1) the seizure onset is not observed, 2) the focal signs may not be apparent because of the rapid spread of the seizure, or 3) the subtleties of the seizure may be missed because the observers may be too overwhelmed during the event. Fortunately, the interictal (between seizure) EEG pattern can provide some information on the seizure type in these cases (Panayiotopoulos, 1999).

Generalized Seizures

Primary generalized seizures (those without a clear focal cortical onset) account for more than one third of all pediatric epilepsy. They include absence, myoclonic, tonic, clonic, tonic-clonic, and atonic seizures. These seizures have simultaneous bilateral onset in the brain. During generalized seizures, the child may have decreased nonconvulsive motor activity (e.g., the arrest of activity and automatisms seen in absence seizures) or bilateral synchronous abnormal motor activity (e.g., myoclonic, tonic, tonic-clonic seizures).

Absence seizures, as described in the case of Patricia, are also referred to as "petit mal" and are characterized by brief episodes of impaired consciousness, usually lasting less than 30 seconds, without **postictal** (immediately following the seizure episode) confusion (Table 27.2). These seizures may occur numerous times during the day and can affect the child's learning ability by interrupting attention and vigilance. Absence seizures are mediated through the thalamus, and onset is usually between 3 and 12 years of age. The classic EEG pattern of absence seizures shows a 3 Hz spike and wave pattern, which can be precipitated by hyperventilation or photic (flickering light) stimulation (Figure 27.1). Sometimes the child may continue to perform a simple automatic activity such as walking during the seizure but is unable to continue a novel task such as reading aloud. Eye blinking or changes in head and extremity tone may accompany the behavioral arrest (e.g., abruptly stopping reading aloud). Absence seizures cannot be interrupted by verbal or tactile (touch) stimulation (Loiseau, 1992).

Myoclonic seizures are due to brief contraction of muscles often associated with cortical discharges. They often manifest as either a sudden flexion or bending backward of the upper torso and head that lasts less than a second. In

Table 27.1. Classification of seizures

Primary generalized seizures

    Absence seizures
    Myoclonic seizures
    Tonic-clonic seizures
    Atonic seizures

Partial seizures

    Simple partial seizures
    Complex partial seizures
    Partial seizures with secondary generalization

Syndromes

Unclassified

Source: Berg et al., (2010).

Table 27.2. Comparison of complex partial seizures and absence seizures

Indication	Complex partial	Absence
Incidence	Common	Uncommon
Duration	30 seconds to 5 minutes	Less than 30 seconds
Frequency of occurrence	Occasional	Multiple times daily
Aura	Yes	No
Consciousness	Partial amnesia and confusion	Immediate return to consciousness
Electroencephalogram (EEG) pattern	Focal	Generalized

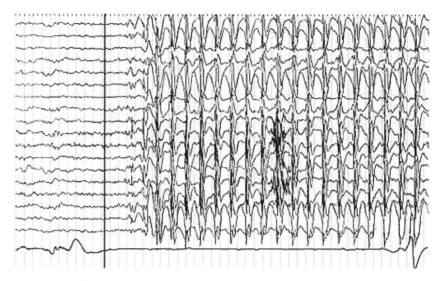

Figure 27.1. Absence seizure, generalized 3Hz spike, and wave discharge.

contrast, atonic seizures consist of a brief loss of postural tone, which may simulate a fainting spell. While the motor component of individual myoclonic and atonic seizures is brief, these seizures often cluster within a few minutes. Atonic seizures that cause an abrupt loss of postural tone are often referred to as "drop" seizures. Consciousness is usually impaired during these events, and the child makes no attempt to protect him- or herself during the fall. As a result, there is an increased risk of head injury. Brief clonic seizures may also result in falling and may be difficult to distinguish from myoclonic seizures. Children with these kinds of seizures may need to wear a protective helmet throughout the day. Following these brief seizures, the child immediately regains consciousness, often crying, seemingly not in pain but upset by the sudden disruption.

Tonic-clonic seizures are commonly referred to as "grand mal" seizures. They may originate from a focal area of the cerebral cortex (a partial seizure) that secondarily generalizes, or they may arise bilaterally (a primarily generalized seizure). Clonic motor activity involves repetitive jerking of the arms or legs at a regular rate. Tonic activity consists of sustained stiffening and/or posturing of the extremities. The seizure usually starts with a loss of consciousness followed by tonic-clonic movements. Respiration may stop briefly and cyanosis and incontinence are common. The EEG shows bilateral spike or polyspike and wave complexes.

Partial Seizures

Partial (focal) seizures start in a localized area of the cerebral cortex; they may spread in space and time, and may progress to become a generalized seizure. They may arise in areas involving motor, sensory, behavioral, autonomic, or cognitive function (see Figure 27.2). These seizures often begin with an aura and/or an abrupt and unprovoked alteration in behavior. Partial seizures are classified as simple partial, complex partial, and complex partial with secondary generalization (see 1989 ILAE classification scheme, above).

A simple partial seizure occurs when the epileptic discharge occurs in a limited region of one cerebral hemisphere and consciousness is maintained. If the event is merely sensory in nature, it is called an aura. If the seizure spreads, resulting in an alteration of consciousness, it is referred to as a complex partial seizure. As noted above, this seizure can progress to secondary generalization, resulting in a tonic-clonic motor seizure.

Complex partial seizures are usually accompanied by motor movements such as focal jerking, motor arrest, or automatisms. **Automatisms** are involuntary movements such as eye blinking, lip smacking, facial grimacing, groaning, chewing, fidgeting, and fumbling hand movements. Occasionally, as a result of impaired awareness, agitation and anxiety may occur in the confused postictal state.

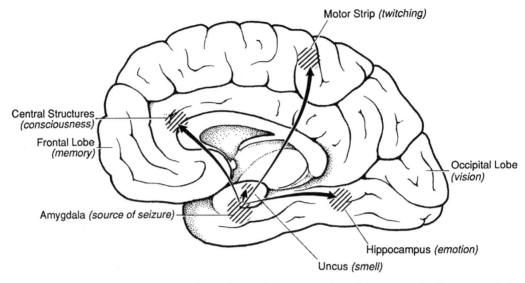

Figure 27.2. This figure shows the spread of a simple partial seizure. A simple partial seizure may begin anywhere—in this case, the amygdala of the temporal lobe. The initial feature may be the child's smelling an unusual odor. The seizure may stop there or project out to the hippocampus, which may trigger feelings of fearfulness or abdominal queasiness. Memory and visual perception may be affected if the frontal or occipital lobe is involved. The seizure might ultimately extend to the motor strip, resulting in twitching of the limb, which may spread to other limbs or to central structures (causing loss of consciousness), thus becoming a complex partial seizure. Finally, the seizure may cross the corpus callosum to the other cerebral hemisphere and thus be converted from a partial to a generalized seizure.

A focal clonic seizure may spread from one portion of the brain to a contiguous area (**Jacksonian seizure**). If there is a focal onset, occasionally tonic or clonic seizures can be followed by a reversible weakness on one side of the body, called a **Todd's paralysis**.

Epilepsy Syndromes

Epilepsy syndromes are seizure disorders that share signs and symptoms, characteristics, specific EEG features, clinical course, prognosis, response to treatment, and sometimes a common pathogenesis or genetic origin (Wolf, 1994). The epilepsy syndromes fall into two broad categories: localization-related epilepsies and generalized-onset syndromes (Table 27.3). A few of the common epilepsy syndromes are discussed below and are organized primarily by age of expression (Table 27.4).

Infantile Spasms

Infantile spasms, also known as West syndrome, are characterized by clusters of brief flexor (head, arms, and hip) or extensor (arm and trunk) contractions or spasms, typically associated with a distinctive EEG finding called **hypsarhythmia** and resulting in developmental regression or arrest (Commission on Pediatric Epilepsy of the ILAE, 1992). It is one of the most common forms of epileptic encephalopathy. The most

common onset of infantile spasms is between 3 and 7 months of age; 90% of children with this condition have onset before 12 months of age.

An underlying cause or disorder is found in over three quarters of children with infantile spasms (Transmonte & Barron, 1998), and almost half have a prenatal or congenital cause. Etiologies include neurocutaneous syndromes (especially tuberous sclerosis), metabolic syndromes (e.g., pyridoxine deficiency), genetic syndromes (e.g., Down syndrome), brain malformations of cortical development (e.g., lissencephaly, polymicrogyria, focal cortical dysplasia), and intrauterine insults (Pellock et al., 2010). The most common perinatal cause is hypoxic-ischemic encephalopathy; common postnatal causes include trauma, infection, and brain tumors (Pellock et al., 2010). Infantile spasms may evolve into Lennox-Gastaut syndrome after infancy (see the next section).

A small percentage of children with infantile spasms have a cryptogenic cause (i.e., no identifiable etiology). These children tend to respond well to therapy (Kivity et al., 2004), have normal development before the spasm onset, have a better epilepsy prognosis, and have a better developmental outcome than children with an identified etiology.

Early recognition and prompt treatment may improve outcome in infantile spasms. The goal of prompt medical therapy is to

Table 27.3. Epilepsy syndromes

Localization-related

Idiopathic with age-related onset

Benign childhood epilepsy with centrotemporal spikes

Childhood epilepsy with occipital paroxysm

Primary reading epilepsy

Symptomatic

Temporal lobe epilepsies

Frontal lobe epilepsies

Parietal lobe epilepsies

Occipital lobe epilepsies

Cryptogenic

Generalized-onset

Idiopathic with age-related onset

Benign neonatal familial convulsions

Benign neonatal convulsions

Benign myoclonic epilepsy of infancy

Absence epilepsy

Juvenile myoclonic epilepsy

Grand mal seizures

Cryptogenic or symptomatic

West syndrome (infantile spasms)

Lennox-Gastaut syndrome

Symptomatic

Undetermined

Neonatal seizures

Severe myoclonic epilepsy in infancy

Epilepsy with continuous spike-wave activity during sleep

Acquired epileptic aphasia (Landau-Kleffner syndrome)

Special syndromes

Febrile seizures

Source: Commission on Classification and Terminology of the International League Against Epilepsy (1989).

Table 27.4. Common age occurrence of various types of seizures and epilepsies

Type of seizure or epilepsy	Age of occurrence
Infantile spasms	4–16 months
Febrile seizures	6 months to 6 years
Lennox-Gastaut syndrome	1–5 years
Childhood absence epilepsy	4–12 years
Benign rolandic epilepsy	6–14 years (peak at 5–8 years)
Juvenile absence epilepsy	7–17 years (peak at 14 years)
Juvenile myoclonic epilepsy	8–26 years (peak at 17 years)

normalize the EEG pattern and to suppress the seizures. Currently, adrenocorticotropic hormones (ACTH) and vigabatrin are considered as the first line of treatment, based on limited evidence (Mackay et al., 2004); high dose prednisolone has also been used successfully (Lux et al., 2004; Pellock et al., 2010). Vigabatrin is used as a first choice for children with infantile spasms secondary to tuberous sclerosis (Wheless, Clarke, Arzimanoglou, & Carpenter, 2007). Other AEDs have also been used to treat infantile spasms, including valproate, phenobarbital, lamotrigine, topiramate, clonazepam, and pyridoxine (Vitamin B6, used to treat infantile spasms caused by pyridoxine dependency; Ito, 1998). In some instances of refractory infantile spasms initiated by partial seizures (called facilitated spasms), or when a single seizure focus is identified, epilepsy surgery may be an option (Shields et al., 1999).

Lennox-Gastaut Syndrome

Lennox-Gastaut syndrome (LGS) often evolves from infantile spasms. This syndrome is defined by a mixture of seizure types consisting of atypical absence, tonic, drop or atonic, myoclonic, tonic-clonic, and complex partial seizures. Children with LGS are at increased risk for frequent falls and injury. The EEG has characteristic features: slow background, anterior slow spike wave, and multifocal spikes. Both seizure control and resolution of EEG abnormalities appear to be necessary for improved cognitive and behavioral outcomes. Unfortunately, the seizures are difficult to control, and all affected children manifest intellectual disability.

Landau-Kleffner Syndrome

Landau-Kleffner syndrome, also called acquired epileptic aphasia, is a disorder of childhood characterized by a loss of language skills in association with EEG abnormalities. It is characterized by **auditory agnosia** (the inability to distinguish different sounds in the presence of normal hearing), language regression, and a behavioral disturbance that includes inattention. These symptoms may develop gradually over months. The EEG pattern shows continuous abnormal epileptiform activity that is activated by sleep and obscures the normal sleep pattern (Rossi et al., 1999). The goal for treatment is normalization of the EEG and control of overt clinical seizures. Several AEDs can be tried, and steroids may be useful. However, while medication may resolve the EEG abnormalities, the aphasia often persists. Prognosis is variable; some children recover some function after several years, while others are left with permanent speech impairments.

Juvenile Myoclonic Epilepsy

Juvenile myoclonic epilepsy (JME) commonly begins during adolescence and is manifested by myoclonic jerks that occur upon awakening. More commonly, these myoclonic jerks are overlooked; until a generalized tonic-clonic seizure occurs, medical attention is not sought. The seizures are exacerbated by alcohol ingestion, sleep deprivation, and photic stimulation. JME is likely to be genetically mediated, and individuals with JME have normal intelligence. In terms of treatment, AEDs that are effective for generalized rather than partial seizures are indicated, such as valproate and lamotrigine (Montalenti, Imperiale, Rovera, Bergamasco, & Benna, 2001; Wallace, 1998). Previously, individuals with JME were thought to require lifelong treatment with an AED. However, in a long-term follow-up study one third of participants experienced seizure remission over time, and lifelong AED treatment was not needed (Camfield & Camfield, 2009).

Benign Epilepsy Syndromes

The most common idiopathic benign epilepsy syndrome of childhood is called benign childhood epilepsy with centrotemporal spikes, also referred to as benign rolandic epilepsy (BRE). This syndrome usually begins between 3 and 12 years of age and causes simple partial seizures. The seizure typically starts in the region of the cortex that controls mouth and face movements; it most commonly occurs at sleep onset or at arousal and can generalize. When the seizure starts in sleep, the partial component is unobserved; therefore, children may appear to be having a generalized tonic-clonic seizure (Lerman, 1992). The characteristic EEG abnormality is epileptic spikes in the centrotemporal area (Figure 27.3). Treatment is often not needed, and these syndromes are not usually associated with long-term sequelae. Some studies, however, have found an increased incidence of language and reading disabilities in children who have BRE (Fejerman, Caraballo, & Tenembaum, 2000).

A second seizure type in this grouping is benign occipital epilepsy. It is characterized by visual disturbances and may be accompanied by vomiting, headache, eye blinking, and alteration of consciousness. At times it may be difficult to differentiate these signs from migraine headaches. Unlike BRE, one half of patients with benign occipital epilepsy will not outgrow their seizures. Panayiotopoulos syndrome, which also exhibits occipital epileptiform discharges, is characterized by brief, paroxysmal, and varying autonomic signs and symptoms.

Febrile Seizures

Febrile convulsions are the most common seizures occurring in the pediatric age group. This is not considered an epilepsy syndrome because

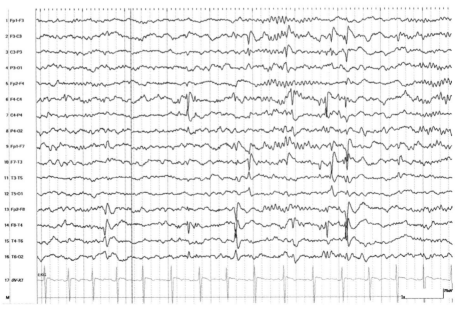

Figure 27.3. Centrotemporal spikes typical of benign rolandic epilepsy.

the seizures are provoked (by fever). Febrile seizures occur in approximately 5% of children who are between the ages of 6 months and 5 years (Nelson & Ellenberg, 1978). They generally occur with temperature elevations above 39 degrees Celsius (102 degrees Fahrenheit). Those that occur with lower temperatures are associated with an increased risk for recurrent febrile seizures (Berg, Darefsky, Holford, & Shinnar, 1998). Acute illnesses such as upper respiratory infections, middle ear infections, gastroenteritis, and viruses associated with skin rashes (e.g., roseola) are frequent causes of febrile seizures.

Febrile seizures occur in two forms: simple febrile seizures, which manifest as a single generalized tonic seizure lasting less than 15 minutes (usually much less than this) and occurring during an acute illness, and complex febrile seizures, which are prolonged, focal, and/or recurrent during a single illness (Hirtz, 1997). Febrile seizures tend to be familial and thus are postulated to have a genetic basis (Audenaert, Van Broeckhoven, & De Jonghe, 2006). In a child with a febrile seizure, the risk for a febrile seizure in a sibling is 10%; if a parent has a history of febrile seizure, the risk for that sibling increases to 50%.

In a child who presents with a febrile seizure, the risk of a subsequent febrile seizure is 30%–50%, depending on the child's age at the time of the first seizure, the presence of a family history of febrile seizures, and the degree of fever (Berg et al., 1992). After a simple febrile seizure, the risk of developing epilepsy by school age is 1%. The risk of epilepsy is 2%–3% following a complex febrile seizure (Nelson & Ellenberg, 1976). The risk of developing epilepsy later in life increases if a family history of epilepsy exists or if the child has a developmental disability such as cerebral palsy, autism, or intellectual disability (Nelson & Ellenberg, 1976). In some studies, febrile seizures with focal features or febrile status epilepticus have been associated with the development of temporal lobe epilepsy. As many as 30%–50% of adults with refractory temporal lobe epilepsy associated with mesial temporal epilepsy have a history of febrile seizures (Bower et al., 2000). In contrast, children with frequent but brief generalized febrile seizures are more likely to have a genetic cause. One example is the *SCN1A* gene mutation, which interferes with the sodium channel ionophore (an ion transporting system) that mediates neuronal firing and is the underlying cause of the syndrome known as generalized epilepsy with febrile seizures plus (GEFS+).

For prevention of febrile seizures in susceptible children, parents are taught to treat fever aggressively and promptly with **antipyretics** (medication for fever, such as acetaminophen). Prophylactic AEDs are usually not recommended because the benefit of preventing subsequent seizures does not outweigh the risks of adverse effects from long-term use. Although medications may prevent subsequent febrile seizures, AEDs do not prevent the development of future epilepsy, and they may interfere with learning and attention (Knudsen, 2000). An alternative to chronic treatment is acute management with rectal or nasal benzodiazepines at the time of the seizure, which may abort a prolonged febrile seizure or prevent clusters of febrile seizures.

Conditions that Mimic Epilepsy

There are a number of conditions that mimic seizures but are not epileptic events because they do not involve abnormal discharges of the cortical neurons (Table 27.5). In general, if a behavior can be triggered, interrupted, or modified by external stimuli, then it is probably not a seizure. A few examples are discussed below.

Most random movements seen during sleep are a part of normal sleep activity. These include random jerks of the extremities or eyes (rapid eye movements) that occur during active sleep, when the child is dreaming. Occasionally, sleep movements can be confused with seizures. Benign sleep myoclonus of infancy occurs in newborns and infants during sleep and disappears on arousal (Pachatz, Fusco, & Vigevano, 1999). It is characterized by a brief arrhythmic twitching of a limb during sleep that may be

Table 27.5.   Conditions that may mimic epilepsy

Migraine headaches

Movement disorders (tic disorders, paroxysmal kinesogenic choreoathetosis)

Breath-holding spells

Shuddering

Parasomnias and normal physiological movements in sleep

Sleep disorders (narcolepsy, cataplexy, night terrors)

Behavior disorders (rage attacks, inattentiveness, attention-deficit/hyperactivity disorder)

Panic attacks and hyperventilation

Nonepileptic seizures (previously "pseudoseizures")

Syncope and other cardiac dysrhythmias, valvular disease, or autonomic dysfunction

Hyperexplexia

Gastroesophageal reflux

mistaken for a seizure; the EEG is normal during this behavior.

Other more complex motor behaviors may occur 1–2 hours after sleep onset or occasionally upon arousal. These parasomnias include night terrors, sleep talking, sleepwalking, and teeth grinding (Laberge, Tremblay, Vitaro, & Montplaisir, 2000). Rarely, nocturnal frontal lobe seizures are misinterpreted as a parasomnia; a video EEG recording is required to distinguish between the two (Lombroso, 2000; Zucconi, Oldani, Ferini-Strambi, Bizzozero, & Smirne, 1997). During a parasomnia, the eyes are open and the child appears to be awake, but the EEG shows a normal sleep rhythm. These parasomnia episodes may last as long as 15–30 minutes, much longer than a typical seizure, and the parent may be unable to end the spell or rouse the child during this time. Rarely, treatment with medication such as diazepam is necessary if the behavior is significantly disruptive to family life.

Behavior disorders such as staring spells and rage attacks can be mistaken for seizures. Brief staring spells (daydreaming or "spacing out") are most commonly a sign of inattention but may resemble absence seizures. Staring spells, however, lack the subtle motor changes seen with absence or complex partial seizures (Bye, Kok, Ferenschild, & Vles, 2000). In temper tantrums and rage attacks, the child cries, yells, throws him- or herself on the floor, and lashes out at nearby people (Gordon, 1999). This may be associated with sweating, paleness, and dilated pupils. Although a similar **dyscontrol syndrome** (intermittent explosive disorder) has been seen following frontal or temporal lobe brain injury, ictal rage is usually unprovoked, very rare, and not directed toward a person (Pellock, 2006). After a rage attack the child resumes a normal state and may express remorse, while after an ictal event the child does not remember the episode (Pellock, 2006).

Breath-holding spells typically occur in infants 6–18 months of age and are accompanied by a loss of consciousness and a generalized convulsion. The child becomes upset and cries vigorously, followed by an arrest in breathing. If the breath holding lasts long enough, it may result in a brief loss of consciousness followed by rapid neurological recovery. In pallid infantile syncope, the child faints or convulses after a startling, often minor, injury. This presumably results from an exaggerated vasovagal reflex. Occasionally a prolonged breath-holding or syncopal (fainting) episode can be associated with brief generalized convulsions followed by lethargy (Kuhle, Tiefenthaler, Seidl, & Hauser, 2000). There is, however, no epileptic activity on the EEG during these episodes.

DIAGNOSIS AND EVALUATION

Epilepsy is defined as two or more unprovoked seizures separated by at least 24 hours. The diagnosis of epilepsy starts with the clinical history and physical examination. A detailed description of the event is crucial. The history should include mention of the presence or absence of an aura, the child's responsiveness during the event, and postictal changes, including altered mental status and transient focal neurological impairments. For example, a tongue bite and urinary or bowel incontinence during the episode suggests a seizure as a cause of the episode. Acute seizure precipitants should also be explored, including infection, trauma, and drugs (illicit or accidental ingestion).

The history helps to distinguish seizures from seizure mimics and assists in classification of seizure type. For example, an infant or young child who turns blue or pale and loses consciousness after being upset or hurt likely has a breath-holding spell rather than a seizure. The presence of an aura or a brief one-sided weakness following the convulsion suggests a partial (focal) seizure. In children who present with a generalized tonic-clonic convulsion, an initial rapid head turn or eye deviation to one side may suggest a partial seizure, with the epileptogenic focus in the **contralateral** (opposite side from the head turn) hemisphere. A staring spell that lasts for a minute or more followed by postictal altered mental status (e.g., confusion, lethargy) points to a complex partial seizure. On the other hand, brief staring spells lasting a few seconds with return to full consciousness immediately afterwards suggests an absence seizure. Staring, however, could also be a manifestation of non-epileptic events like daydreaming and inattention. About half of non-epileptic events captured on EEG monitoring are staring episodes (Uldall, Alving, Hansen, Kibæk, & Buchholt, 2006).

The physical and neurological examination may identify an acute illness or a remote neurologic disorder. Attention should be paid to head circumference, skin exam (e.g., café-au-lait spots), and focal neurological impairments (e.g., weakness on one side, as in Todd's paralysis).

Routinely performed laboratory tests such as complete blood count, electrolytes, glucose, and toxin screen are not helpful in a well child who has recovered from a brief seizure. However, electrolytes should be determined in children younger than 2 years to check for sodium, calcium, and glucose levels. Glucose should be checked in all children in status epilepticus and in those who have a history of seizures with fasting. Physicians need to individualize such tests to the specific clinical context (Hirtz et al., 2000). Similarly, lumbar puncture (spinal tap) should be reserved for febrile individuals or those with prolonged altered consciousness or in whom meningitis or encephalitis is a concern (Hirtz et al., 2000). A lumbar puncture, chemical panel, metabolic tests for inborn errors of metabolism (e.g., plasma amino acids, urine organic acids, lactate, pyruvate), imaging (computed tomography [CT]/magnetic resonance imaging [MRI]), and an EEG should be considered in children with continuing neurological impairment after a seizure.

Electroencephalogram

A sleep-deprived EEG is indicated in the workup of all children suspected of having seizures. To perform the EEG, recording electrodes (approximately 20) are placed on the scalp at set points over the frontal, central, parietal, temporal, and occipital regions bilaterally. These electrodes record voltage changes from the cortex below. The EEG displays electrical potential differences between neighboring electrodes, or an electrode and a reference point. The EEG provides information regarding 1) background electrical activity (e.g., generalized or focal slowing, which suggests diffuse or focal cerebral dysfunction, respectively), 2) the presence or absence of epileptic discharges (e.g., sharp waves or spike and wave discharges indicating cortical hyperexcitability), and 3) response to seizure-activating procedures (e.g., hyperventilation, photic stimulation, sleep deprivation). The EEG should be recorded during wakefulness and light sleep. Light sleep tends to activate epileptiform discharges and increases the yield of the EEG.

The EEG findings along with the clinical data will help to establish the diagnosis of the specific seizure type. For instance, the finding of 3 Hz generalized spike and wave discharges activated by hyperventilation is diagnostic of absence epilepsy (Figure 27.1). Centrotemporal spike and wave discharges activated in sleep suggest BRE (Figure 27.3). The EEG may also provide prognostic information. In children with a first unprovoked seizure and normal neurologic examination, the seizure recurrence risk is higher if the EEG is abnormal (Shinnar et al., 1996). In situations in which the nature of the events is unclear, continuous video EEG monitoring for 23 hours or longer may be needed to capture and characterize the events. Continuous video EEG is also required as part of the evaluation in children for whom epilepsy surgery is being considered.

Neuroimaging

Brain imaging with MRI is essential to identify structural lesions that cause seizures. In some epilepsy syndromes (BRE, childhood or juvenile absence epilepsy, and JME), the likelihood of a structural lesion is low, and routine neuroimaging is not indicated unless atypical features are present or the clinical course is unusual. In all other children with recently diagnosed localization-related (partial or focal) epilepsies or generalized epilepsies, neuroimaging is recommended (Gaillard et al., 2009; Hsieh et al., 2010). Neuroimaging should also be done in any child younger than 2 years of age with seizures that are other than benign febrile convulsions. The preferred imaging modality is brain MRI because of its higher yield and better anatomic detail than CT scan (Gaillard et al., 2009). Head CT is usually performed in the emergency department setting and may identify tumors, bleeding, and calcifications.

Functional neuroimaging studies are used to identify the location of the seizure focus when epilepsy surgery is considered and the MRI is normal. FDG-PET (a type of positron emission tomography [PET] that uses fluorodeoxyglucose [FDG], an analog of glucose) assesses interictal brain metabolism. A seizure focus tends to have low metabolism between seizures. A related technique, SPECT (single photon emission computed tomography), assesses blood flow to the brain and may identify the seizure focus. MEG (magnetoencephalography) helps in localization of the epileptiform discharges or spikes. Functional MRI is used to identify noninvasively eloquent (language) and sensory/motor areas to be spared during epilepsy surgery (O'Shaughnessy, Berl, Moore, & Gaillard, 2008). Magnetic resonance spectroscopy (MRS), which can be performed during an MRI scan, assesses the concentration of some chemicals (e.g., N-acetylaspartic acid, choline, creatine, lactate) in specific brain regions and is helpful in the workup of certain metabolic disorders (e.g., abnormal lactate peak may be seen in mitochondrial disorders).

TREATMENT

The treatment of seizures starts prior to arrival at the hospital, and parents need to be educated about prehospital care.

Prehospital Management of Acute Seizures

For children with epilepsy, the child and family must be educated about common-sense seizure precautions. These include taking a shower instead of a bath, leaving the bathroom door unlocked, avoiding climbing heights (e.g., a ladder), wearing a helmet while riding a bicycle, and swimming in clear water and only with vigilant adult supervision.

First aid measures and emergency plans during a seizure should be discussed with parents and the school nurse. During a generalized tonic-clonic convulsion (grand mal seizure) the child should be placed on a flat surface and turned to one side to prevent aspiration. Tight clothes should be loosened around the neck, but no object should be placed between the teeth. The airway should be maintained using a jaw thrust, but cardiopulmonary resuscitation is rarely required.

Seizures usually last less than 5 minutes, but if they persist longer they may continue for a prolonged period of time (status epilepticus) if there is not intervention (Shinnar, Berg, Moshé, & Shinnar, 2001). Therefore, if a seizure lasts 5 minutes or longer, rectal diazepam gel should be given at home. Intranasal or buccal midazolam (Holsti et al., 2010; Scott, Besag, & Neville, 1999) and dissolving clonazepam wafers placed between the cheeks and gum (Troester, Hastriter, & Ng, 2010) are alternatives to rectal diazepam with comparable efficacy and better ease of administration.

Antiepileptic Drugs

AEDs are the first line of treatment in almost all types of epilepsy. The ideal AED would control seizures and correct the underlying epileptogenic focus without producing adverse effects. Unfortunately, as of the publication of this book none of the currently available AEDs meet this standard. As a result, the decision to start AED treatment involves balancing the risk of potential harm caused by recurrent seizures against the adverse side effects of the medication.

In considering recurrence after a single unprovoked seizure, data indicate a risk of 40%–50% (Berg, 2008). The risk of recurrence tends to be higher in children with one of the following indicators: 1) remote symptomatic causes (i.e., occurring more than 1 week after a disorder known to precipitate a seizure, such as a head injury), 2) an abnormal EEG, 3) a history of febrile seizure, 4) Todd's paralysis, or 5) a seizure during sleep (Berg, 2008; Shinnar et al., 1996). About half of seizure recurrences occur in the first 6 months, and 88% within 2 years of the initial seizure (Shinnar et al., 1996). The seizure recurrence risk increases to 65%–79% after two unprovoked seizures (Camfield et al., 1985; Hauser et al., 1998). Postponing initiating AEDs until the second seizure does not appear to alter the ultimate prognosis, the risk of brain injury, or the efficacy of AEDs (Arts & Geerts, 2009; Hirtz et al., 2003). Thus, a child who has two or more unprovoked seizures should be considered for initiation of AED. Treatment should be individualized, however, as some children with benign epilepsy syndromes may not need AEDs even if they have two or more seizures, providing the seizures are infrequent, nocturnal, or simple partial seizures.

Mechanisms, Selection and Use of Antiepileptic Drugs

AEDs act on excitatory (glutamate) and inhibitory (gamma-aminobutyric acid, or GABA) mediated neurotransmission in cortical neurons. The specific mechanisms of action of various AEDs include 1) modulation of voltage-gated sodium channels (phenytoin, carbamazepine, felbamate, lamotrigine, topiramate, oxcarbazepine, and zonisamide), 2) modulation of calcium channels (ethosuximide, zonisamide, and valproic acid), 3) enhancing GABA action (benzodiazepines, barbiturates, tiagabine, vigabatrin), and 4) inhibiting glutamate (topiramate and felbamate). Many AEDs exert their effect through multiple mechanisms of action (Sankar & Holmes, 2004). Selection of AEDs is based primarily on seizure type (partial versus generalized), specific epilepsy syndrome, side effect profile, and comorbid conditions (Wilfong, 2007).

AEDs are broadly divided into narrow-spectrum (carbamazepine, gabapentin, lacosamide, oxcarbazepine, phenobarbital, phenytoin, tiagabine) and broad-spectrum (lamotrigine, levetiracetam, rufinamide, topiramate, valproate, and zonisamide). The narrow-spectrum drugs are effective in partial or secondarily generalized epilepsies, while broad-spectrum AEDs are effective in both partial and generalized epilepsies (Asconape, 2010). Table 27.6 shows the choice of AEDs based on seizure type. For

Table 27.6. Selection of antiepileptic drugs (AEDs) based on seizure types

Seizure type	First line AEDs
Partial or secondarily generalized epilepsy	Carbamazepine, oxcarbazepine
Generalized epilepsy	Valproate, lamotigine, topiramate
Absence seizures	Ethosuximide, lamotrigine, valproate[a]
Juvenile myoclonic epilepsy	Valproate[a], lamotrigine, topiramate
Tonic-clonic seizures	Valproate[a], lamotrigine, topiramate
Lennox-Gastaut syndrome	Valproate[a], lamotrigine, topiramate
Infantile spasms	ACTH, vigabatrin[b]

Source: Wheless, Clark, & Carpenter (2005).

[a]The risk of valproate-induced hepatic toxicity is high in children < 2 years of age.

[b]Vigabatrin is the treatment of choice in children with tuberous sclerosis.

example, carbamazepine and oxcarbazepine are first line drugs in partial seizures with or without secondary generalization, while valproate, lamotrigine, topiramate, and perhaps leviteracitam are first line drugs in generalized epilepsies (Wheless, Clarke, & Carpenter, 2005). Valproate, pregabalin, and carbamazepine are associated with weight gain while topiramate and zonisamide result in weight loss. Therefore, in children with comorbid obesity, avoiding AEDs that cause weight gain and selecting topiramate or zonisamide may be appropriate. As another example of a comorbid condition, children with migraine and epilepsy could be treated for both conditions with topiramate or valproate. Carbamazepine, lamotrigine, and valproate are appropriate choices for children with comorbid mood disorders. Phenobarbital and topiramate, on the other hand, are associated with depression and are better avoided in children with mood disorders. In terms of side effects, many parents whose children have refractory epilepsy will tolerate a few seizures if it means a more alert child with a lower AED dose or the use of fewer drugs.

AEDs should be started at a low dose and titrated steadily upward until control is achieved. Whenever possible, monotherapy is preferred to polypharmacy, which increases the risk of adverse effects and drug interactions. If two or more AEDs at appropriate doses have failed in a child with partial/focal epilepsy, other treatment modalities should be considered (e.g., surgery). For generalized seizures that are refractory to AEDs, the ketogenic diet (discussed below) may be a viable alternative. When receiving AEDs, the child should be monitored for adverse effects. In addition, AED drug levels can be useful to assess adherence to treatment, to know the individual's effective therapeutic drug level for future comparisons, to diagnose clinical toxicity, and to adjust dosage (Patsalos et al., 2008).

Antiepileptic Drugs Adverse Effects

Prior to 1993, carbamazepine, ethosuximide, phenobarbital, phenytoin, and valproate were the only commonly used AEDs. Since 1993, a number of new AEDs have been introduced: felbamate, gabapentin, lacosamide, lamotrigine, levetiracetam, oxcarbazepine, pregabalin, rufinamide, tiagabine, topiramate, zonisamide, and vigabatrin. The newer AEDs, as a group, have comparable efficacy in controlling seizures, and several have a better side effect profile overall as compared to the older AEDs.

AED adverse effects fall into three categories: dose-related adverse effects, idiosyncratic reactions, and chronic adverse effects (Perucca & Meador, 2005). Dose-related adverse effects are often related to the central nervous system and manifest as somnolence, dizziness, ataxia, and cognitive impairment. Idiosyncratic reactions include urticaria, Stevens-Johnson syndrome, hepatitis, and aplastic anemia. Chronic adverse effects include weight change, gingival hyperplasia, hair loss, and osteopenia (Perucca & Meador, 2005). When adverse effects occur, the dose of the AED should be decreased or stopped if the reaction is severe.

AED-related cognitive adverse effects are especially important in young children because they may result in long-lasting developmental impairments (Loring & Meador, 2004). AEDs predominantly affect attention and psychomotor speed (Hessen, Lossius, Reinvang, & Gjerstad, 2006; Lagac, 2006; Loring & Meador, 2004). Although all AEDs can cause cognitive adverse effects at high doses and in the presence of polypharmacy (Perucca & Meador, 2005), phenobarbital and topiramate seem to be incriminated most often (Glauser et al., 2007; Park & Kwon, 2008; Sulzbacher, Farwell, Temkin, Lu, & Hirtz, 1999). Leviteracitam is also a concern, as it has been associated with reversible deterioration in behavior and occasionally psychosis.

Drug Interactions

AEDs that induce (e.g., carbamazepine, phenytoin, and phenobarbital) or inhibit (e.g., valproate) hepatic cytochrome P450 (CYP450) enzymes may affect the levels of other concomitantly used AEDs or their metabolites, as well as different classes of drugs (Perucca, 2005). CYP450 enzyme-inducing AEDs reduce the concentration of other AEDs that are metabolized by the hepatic enzyme system, in some instances to a significant degree. Valproic acid inhibits the glucuronidation of lamotrigine and may result in higher plasma lamotrigine levels, increasing the risk of adverse effects, especially Stevens-Johnson syndrome. To prevent such adverse effects, lamotrigine should be started at a very low dose, titrated up slowly, and maintained at a lower dose in patients taking valproic acid. Other drugs could also affect the hepatic enzyme systems. Erythromycin and clarithromycin, for instance, inhibit CYP450 enzymes; children taking carbamazepine may develop toxicity if these antibiotics are used at the same time. Anticipating potential drug interactions, avoiding drug combinations that have significant interactions, adjusting doses carefully, monitoring for adverse effects, and monitoring blood levels of AEDs will all decrease the risk of drug toxicity and loss of efficacy due to drug interactions. It is also important to anticipate a significant change in the blood level of AEDs when a concomitantly administered drug that is an enzyme inducer or inhibitor is discontinued.

Antiepileptic Drugs and Bone Metabolism

Chronic use of AEDs may be associated with abnormal bone metabolism. AEDs that induce CYP450 enzymes accelerate vitamin D metabolism and may cause vitamin D deficiency (Shellhaas & Joshi, 2010). In children with prolonged AED therapy, bone metabolism should be monitored using laboratory tests (25-OH vitamin D) and imaging studies (DEXA scan). Multivitamins with calcium and vitamin D (400–800 IU) need to be considered in this group of children.

Antiepileptic Drugs in Adolescent Women

There are two major concerns in the treatment of adolescent women with epilepsy. One concern is loss of efficacy of contraception in individuals who are taking certain AEDs (carbamazepine, phenytoin, phenobarbital, and topiramate, at high dose). These drugs increase the metabolism of estrogen and increase protein binding of progesterone; therefore, increasing the estrogen dose and backup contraception may need to be considered (Zupanc, 2006). A second concern is teratogenesis (the induction of malformations in the fetus). Most AEDs are categorized as pregnancy category C (teratogenicity in experimental animals, no human studies) and the risk of congenital malformations is higher than in the general population (Asconape, 2010). Risk-benefit analysis, however, favors continuation of most AEDs during pregnancy. Valproate and phenobarbital, however, are associated with a higher incidence of congenital malformations and should be avoided during pregnancy. Valproate is associated with an increased risk of neural tube defects (see Chapter 25). In addition, a study that compared the effect of *in utero* exposure of carbamazepine, lamotrigine, phenytoin, and valproate on IQ at 3 years of age showed that valproate was associated with a substantially increased risk of cognitive impairment and perhaps autism compared with the other AEDs (Meador et al., 2010).

Discontinuing Antiepileptic Drugs

There are a number of concerns about the long-term use of AEDs. These include teratogenicity, poor self-image, adverse effects of drugs, and cost of treatment in time and money. As a result, practitioners attempt to stop AEDs after a sufficient period of seizure freedom. An EEG is performed when a decision about stopping AEDs is considered. A normal EEG is reassuring, while an abnormal EEG introduces a level of uncertainty about seizure recurrence risk. The risk of seizure recurrence after discontinuation of an AED in a child who has been seizure free for 2 years or longer is 25%–36% (Caviedes & Herranz, 1998; Shinnar et al., 1994). Children with symptomatic causes of their epilepsy or comorbid developmental disabilities have a lower rate of seizure freedom after discontinuation of AEDs (20%–50%). If a decision is made to stop AED treatment, the medication should be tapered off over several months and not abruptly discontinued, as this may precipitate a seizure or have other side effects.

Other Treatment Options

In children who failed to respond to 2 or more appropriate AEDs, the ketogenic diet and surgery are treatment options.

Ketogenic Diet

The ketogenic diet mimics the fasting state and is a high fat, low carbohydrate and low protein diet. It is restrictive and not tasty. The ketogenic diet has been used in treating a few rare inborn errors of metabolism, including glucose transporter deficiency (a condition associated with epileptic encephalopathy and resulting from impaired glucose transport to the brain; Klepper, 2008) and pyruvate dehydrogenase deficiency. More commonly, this diet has been used to treat children with a wide variety of seizure types and syndromes that have proven refractory to AEDs (Freeman, Kossoff, & Hartman, 2007). During treatment with a ketogenic diet, urine and blood ketone levels should be monitored to ensure adequate ketosis. Side effects during the initiation of this dietary therapy include metabolic acidosis, hypoglycemia (low blood sugar), gastrointestinal distress, and lethargy. Renal stones, dyslipidemia (abnormal lipid profile), and failure to thrive are late side effects (Freeman et al., 2007). The diet can be stopped after the child is seizure free for a prolonged period, in much the same way as discontinuation of AEDs.

Surgical Resection of Epileptic Focus

Surgical resection of the epileptic focus should be considered in children with partial epilepsy who have failed two or more appropriate AEDs administered at adequate dosage. After adding a third medication, the likelihood of subsequent medications working is 4%–8%. Epilepsy surgery should be considered when there is a clear focal lesion (e.g., mesial temporal sclerosis, focal cortical dysplasia, developmental tumor, vascular malformation). In these cases the likelihood of excellent outcome from surgery is 80%–85% (50%–60% seizure free, 25%–30% rare seizures). If the MRI is normal but the PET or SPECT is abnormal, then there is a 50%–60% likelihood of excellent surgical outcome. If all imaging studies are normal, surgical benefit drops to 25%–30%. Hemispherectomy (involving removal of a damaged or diseased hemisphere) is performed for hemimegalencephaly, Rasmussen's encephalitis, and occasionally for porencephaly and widespread malformations of cortical development.

Palliative Surgery

When a seizure focus cannot be identified or resected, or when there are multiple seizure foci, palliative epilepsy surgery may reduce seizure frequency or severity. These procedures rarely result in seizure freedom but may improve quality of life. Disconnecting the corpus callosum (a procedure called a corpus callosotomy)

is a treatment option for refractory epilepsy, including atonic (or drop) seizures and secondarily generalized epilepsy (Rosenfeld & Roberts, 2009). A vagus nerve stimulator (VNS) provides intermittent electrical impulse to the left vagus nerve. Approximately 30%–40% of individuals may have a 50% reduction in targeted seizures following the procedure (Mapstone, 2008). Deep brain stimulation (DBS) and direct cortical stimulation are currently being studied in adults (but not yet available for children) to control or to abort seizures (Jobst, Darcey, Thadani, & Roberts, 2010).

Nonspecific Interventions

Common seizure exacerbating or provoking factors include sleep deprivation and infection, with or without fever. Parents and children should be counseled about good sleep hygiene and the importance of prevention and treatment of infections and fever. Flashing lights provoke seizures in children with photosensitive epilepsy. Seizures may also be exacerbated around the time of ovulation or menses (catamenial epilepsy) and may respond to hormonal treatment (birth control pills). Poor adherence to medications is an important cause of breakthrough seizures, and compliance issues should be discussed with the family.

Vitamins, Minerals, and Complementary and Alternative Medicine

Folate supplementation is recommended for females of childbearing age who are taking valproate, in order to decrease the risk of neural tube defects in their fetus should they conceive while taking this AED. Pyridoxine is indicated in the treatment of a rare form of epilepsy resulting from pyridoxine dependency. Calcium and vitamin D supplementation may be helpful in preventing osteopenia and osteoporosis. Seizures resulting from certain inborn errors of metabolism may be treated with vitamins and nutritional supplements. Although some families consider alternative medicine for the treatment of epilepsy, there is no evidence that the various homeopathic and herbal remedies are effective (Danesi & Adetunji, 1994). It is also important to understand that "natural" is not necessarily harmless (see Chapter 38).

MULTIDISCIPLINARY CARE

Addressing the various needs of a child with epilepsy requires a multidisciplinary approach, preferably in a comprehensive epilepsy center. The team includes neurologists, psychiatrists, neuropsychologists, nurses, social workers, and other health professionals.

School Performance and Special Education

Children with epilepsy may have cognitive and learning difficulties. A child with absence seizures may start to do poorly in school as the seizure frequency increases. Dose change or introduction of new AEDs may cause decreased attention and somnolence, and interfere with the child's school performance. Irritability and aggression may occur as a result of medication adverse effects. Comorbidities such as attention-deficit/hyperactivity disorder may accompany epilepsy and contribute to poor school performance.

Teachers should be aware of the need for closer monitoring of school performance in children with epilepsy. A child with declining school performance needs a thorough evaluation for possible causes, including seizure exacerbation, AED adverse effects, comorbidities, learning and memory problems, and psychosocial stress. Corrective actions may include medication adjustment, treating comorbidities, and/or designing a revised individualized education program (IEP). Children with epilepsy are eligible to receive special education and related services through the Individuals with Disabilities Education Improvement Act (IDEA) of 2004 (PL 108-446) under "other health impairments."

A seizure in the classroom may be a source of anxiety and embarrassment for a child, perhaps more so when the seizure is associated with bladder or bowel incontinence. For children with seizures associated with incontinence, a towel and a fresh change of clothing can be kept in the nurse's office. Educating classmates about epilepsy and what to expect may be helpful. Parents may request a classroom discussion about seizures. The discussion does not have to identify the specific child (Coleman & Fielder, 1999). In contrast, if a child's seizures are well controlled or if he or she does not have daytime seizures, a discussion about seizures to classmates may be counterproductive.

Psychosocial Issues

Seizures affect health-related quality of life (HRQL) measures through several mechanisms. These include frequency of seizures, AED adverse effects, comorbidities (e.g., anxiety, depression,

learning disorders), the presence of an underlying neurological disorder, social stigma, and the unpredictability of seizures. Even children who have had only a single seizure or children newly diagnosed with epilepsy are more likely to report impaired HRQL, probably indicating the impact of child and parental anxiety (Modi et al., 2009). Social stigma may affect the child's self-perception, leading to low self-esteem and depression. Parents may react to seizures by overprotecting the child, which may have the unintended consequence of fostering a lifelong dependence. Seizures affect the entire family. Mothers of children with epilepsy tend to be at increased risk for depression (Ferro & Speechley, 2009). There is also a significant financial and time burden to the family. The child as well as the whole family needs to be educated about epilepsy, and support should be provided.

Children with epilepsy should generally be encouraged to participate in sports. Routine safety precautions should be applied as with any child participating in sports. However, some sport activities pose a significant danger to a person with epilepsy (e.g., scuba diving, rock climbing, parachuting, swimming in water that is not clear, and/or swimming unsupervised) and must be avoided (Fountain & May, 2003).

Family vacations and camping trips should be encouraged, but excess fatigue should be avoided. The family needs to have an adequate supply of AEDs and the doctor's and pharmacy's telephone number at hand during trips. Wearing a medical identification bracelet or necklace may be useful, if it is acceptable to parents and the child.

Independence should be encouraged as the child enters adulthood. Driving license laws vary from state to state but generally require the individual to be seizure free for between 3–12 months. Altered fertility rate and potential teratogenic effects of AEDs are issues that need to be addressed. Several organizations, such as the American Epilepsy Society, the Epilepsy Foundation, and the ILAE, advocate for acceptance of individuals with epilepsy in society.

OUTCOME

A majority of children (70%–80%) with epilepsy achieve seizure control with the first or second AED, and about two thirds can be successfully weaned off their AEDs after 2 years of being seizure free (MacDonald et al., 2000). Children who have had a single seizure exhibit intelligence scores comparable to sibling controls

(Sogawa, Masur, O'Dell, Moshé, & Shinnar, 2010). In one prospective study, about 74% of children with epilepsy had average global cognitive function, while 26% had lower cognitive function. Significant independent risk factors predisposing to cognitive impairment include young age at seizure onset, symptomatic causes, epileptic encephalopathy, and requirement for continued AED treatment (Berg et al., 2008). Children with idiopathic epilepsy have the best outcomes, followed by those with cryptogenic epilepsy, and then those with symptomatic epilepsy. Continued seizures, medication side effects, and depression are associated with poor outcomes, including reduced quality of life, undereducation and underemployment, failure to achieve independence, and failure to establish lifelong social bonds (Sillanpää, 2000).

Mortality in epilepsy is linked to accidental injury (mostly swimming related), underlying pathology (e.g., brain tumor), and sudden unexpected death in epilepsy (SUDEP; Sillanpää & Shinnar, 2010). The possible mechanisms of SUDEP are thought to be related to asphyxia, central hypoventilation, and cardiac arrhythmia associated with a seizure. Accurate data on the incidence of SUDEP is lacking, but one study reported a rate of 2 in 10,000 patient years, so it is very rare (Donner, Smith, & Snead, 2001).

SUMMARY

Epilepsy is characterized by recurrent seizures that result from abnormal electrical discharges in the brain. A seizure is classified as generalized or partial, depending on whether it involves both hemispheres at onset or starts in one hemisphere with or without subsequent spread to the other hemisphere. Most epilepsy can be controlled with a single AED, but there are other treatment options. For a child with multiple disabilities and symptomatic causes, the prognosis is more related to the disabilities and/or the underlying cause than to the epilepsy. Side effects of medications and comorbidities should be assessed in conjunction with seizure control to optimize quality of life.

REFERENCES

Airaksinen, E.M., Matilainen, R., Mononen, T., Mustonen, K., Partanen, J., Jokela, V., & Halonen, P. (2000). A population-based study on epilepsy in mentally retarded children. *Epilepsia, 41*(9), 1214–1220.

Alvarez, N., Besag, F., & Iivanainen, M. (1998). Use of antiepileptic drugs in the treatment of epilepsy in people with intellectual disability. *Journal of Intellectual Disability Research, 42*(Suppl. 1), 1–15.

American Epilepsy Society (http://www.aesnet.org).

Arts, W.F, & Geerts, A.T. (2009). When to start drug treatment for childhood epilepsy: The clinical-epidemiological evidence. *European Journal of Paediatric Neurology, 13*(2), 93–101.

Asconape, J.J. (2010). The selection of antiepileptic drugs for the treatment of epilepsy in children. *Neurology Clinics, 28*(4), 843–852.

Audenaert, D., Van Broeckhoven, C., & De Jonghe, P. (2006). Genes and loci involved in febrile seizures and related epilepsy syndromes. *Human Mutations, 27*(5), 391–401.

Berg, A.T. (1995). The epidemiology of seizures and epilepsy in children. In S. Shinnar, N. Amir, & D. Branski (Eds.), *Childhood seizures* (pp. 1–10). Basel, Switzerland: Karger.

Berg, A.T. (2008). Risk of recurrence after a first unprovoked seizure. *Epilepsia, 49*(Suppl. 1), 13–18.

Berg, A.T., & Shinnar, S. (1991). The risk of seizure recurrence following a first unprovoked seizure: A quantitative review. *Neurology, 41*(7), 965–972.

Berg, A.T., Berkovic, S.F., Brodie, M.J., Buchhalter, J., Cross, J.H., van Emde Boas, W., ... Scheffer, I.E. (2010). Revised terminology and concepts for organization of seizures and epilepsies: Report of the ILAE Commission on Classification and Terminology, 2005–2009. *Epilepsia, 51*(4), 676–685.

Berg, A.T., Darefsky, A.S., Holford, T.R., & Shinnar, S. (1998). Seizures with fever after unprovoked seizures: An analysis in children followed from the time of a first febrile seizure. *Epilepsia, 39*(1), 77–80.

Berg, A.T., Langfitt, J.T., Testa, F.M., Levy, S.R., DiMario, F., Westerveld, M., & Kulas, J. (2008). Global cognitive function in children with epilepsy: A community-based study. *Epilepsia, 49*(4), 608–614.

Berg, A.T., Shinnar, S., Hauser, W.A., Alemany, M., Shapiro, E.D., Salomon, M.E., & Crain, E.F. (1992). A prospective study of recurrent febrile seizure. *The New England Journal of Medicine, 327*(16), 1122–1127.

Besag, F.M.C. (2002). Childhood epilepsy in relation to mental handicap and behavioral disorders. *Journal of Child Psychology and Psychiatry, 43*(1), 103–131.

Briellmann, R.S., Jackson, G.D., Torn-Broers, Y., & Berkovic, S.F. (2001). Causes of epilepsies: Insights from discordant monozygous twins. *Annals of Neurology, 49*(1), 45–52.

Bye, A.M., Kok, D.J., Ferenschild, F.T., & Vles, J.S. (2000). Paroxysmal non-epileptic events in children: A retrospective study over a period of 10 years. *Journal of Paediatrics and Child Health, 36*(3), 244–248.

Camfield, C.S., & Camfield, P.R. (2009). Juvenile myoclonic epilepsy 25 years after seizure onset, a population-based study. *Neurology, 73*(13), e64–e67.

Camfield, P.R., Camfield, C.S., Dooley, J.M., Tibbles, J.A.R., Fung, T., & Garner, B. (1985). Epilepsy after a first unprovoked seizure in childhood. *Neurology, 35*(11), 1657–1660.

Caviedes, B.E., & Herranz, J.L. (1998). Seizure recurrence and risk factors after withdrawal of chronic antiepileptic therapy in children. *Seizure, 7*(2), 107–114.

Cole, A.J. (2000). Is epilepsy a progressive disease? The neurobiological consequences of epilepsy. *Epilepsia, 41*(Suppl. 2), S13–S22.

Coleman, H., & Fielder, A. (1999). Epilepsy education in schools. *Paediatric Nursing, 11*(9), 29–32.

Commission on Classification and Terminology of the International League Against Epilepsy. (1989). Proposal for revised classification of epilepsies and epileptic syndromes. *Epilepsia, 30*(4), 389–399.

Commission on Pediatric Epilepsy of the International League Against Epilepsy. (1992). Workshop on infantile spasms. *Epilepsia, 33*(1), 195.

Danesi, M.A., & Adetunji, J.B. (1994). Use of alternative medicine by patients with epilepsy: A survey of 265 epileptic patients in a developing country. *Epilepsia, 35*(2), 344–351.

Donner, E.J., Smith, C.R., & Sneed III, O.C. (2001). Sudden unexplained death in children with epilepsy. *Neurology, 57*(3), 430–434.

Engel, Jr., J. (2001). A proposed diagnostic scheme for people with epileptic seizures and with epilepsy: Report of the ILAE Task Force on Classification and Terminology. *Epilepsia, 42*(6), 796–803.

Engel, Jr., J. (2006). Report of the ILAE Classification Core Group. *Epilepsia, 47*(9), 1558–1568.

Epilepsy Foundation (http://www.epilepsyfoundation.org).

Fejerman, N., Caraballo, R., & Tenembaum, S.N., (2000). Atypical evolutions of benign localization-related epilepsies in children: Are they predictable? *Epilepsia, 41*(4), 380–390.

Ferro, M.A., & Speechley, K.N. (2009). Depressive symptoms among mothers of children with epilepsy: A review of prevalence, associated factors, and impact on children. *Epilepsia, 50*(1), 2344–2354.

Forsgren, L., Edvinsson, S.O., Blomquist, H.K., Heijbel, J., & Sidenvall, R. (1990). Epilepsy in a population of mentally retarded children and adults. *Epilepsy Research, 6*(3), 234–248.

Fountain, N.B., & May, A.C. (2003). Epilepsy and athletics. *Clinics in Sports Medicine, 22*(3), 605–616.

Freeman, J.M., Kossoff, E.H., & Hartman, A.L. (2007). The ketogenic diet: One decade later. *Pediatrics, 119*(3), 535–543.

Frucht, M.M., Quigg, M., Schwaner, C., & Fountain, N.B. (2000). Distribution of seizure precipitants among epilepsy syndromes. *Epilepsia, 41*(12), 1534–1539.

Gage, F.H. (2002). Neurogenesis in the adult brain. *The Journal of Neuroscience, 22*(3), 612–613.

Gaillard, W.D., Chiron, C., Cross, J.H, Harvey, A.S., Kuzniecky, R., Hertz-Pannier, L., & Vezina, L.G. (2009). Guidelines for imaging infants and children with recent-onset epilepsy. *Epilepsia, 50*(9), 2147–2153.

Glauser, T.A., Dlugos, D.J., Dodson, W.E., Grinspan, A., Wang, S., & Wu, S.C. (2007). Topiramate monotherapy in newly diagnosed epilepsy. *Journal of Child Neurology, 22*(6), 693–699.

Gordon, N. (1999). Episodic dyscontrol syndrome. *Developmental Medicine and Child Neurology, 41*(11), 786–788.

Hauser, W.A. (1994). The prevalence and incidence of convulsive disorders in children. *Epilepsia, 35*(Suppl. 2), S1–S6.

Hauser, W.A. (2006). The natural history of seizures. In E. Wyllie, A. Gupta, & D.K. Lachhwani (Eds.), *The treatment of epilepsy: Principles and practice* (4th ed., p. 120). Philadelphia, PA: Lippincott Williams & Wilkins.

Hauser, W.A., & Kurland, L.T. (1993). Incidence of epilepsy and unprovoked seizures in Rochester, Minnesota: 1935–1984. *Epilepsia, 34*(3), 453–468.

Hauser, W.A., Rich, S.S., Lee, J.R., Annegers, J.F., & Anderson, V.E. (1998). Risk of recurrent seizures after two unprovoked seizures. *The New England Journal of Medicine, 338*(7), 429–434.

Hessen, E., Lossius, M.I., Reinvang, I., & Gjerstad, L. (2006). Influence of major antiepileptic drugs on attention, reaction time, and speed of information processing: Results from a randomized, double-blind, placebo-controlled withdrawal study of seizure-free epilepsy patients receiving monotherapy. *Epilepsia, 47*(12), 2038–2045.

Hirtz, D.G. (1997). Febrile seizures. *Pediatrics in Review, 18*(1), 5–8.

Hirtz, D., Ashwal, S., Berg, A., Bettis, D., Camfield, C., Camfield, P., ... Shinnar, S. (2000). Practice parameter: Evaluating a first nonfebrile seizure in children: Report of the Quality Standards Subcommittee of the American Academy of Neurology, the Child Neurology Society, and the American Epilepsy Society. *Neurology, 55*(5), 616–623.

Hirtz, D., Berg, A., Bettis, D., Camfield, C., Camfield, P., Crumrine, P., ... Shinnar, S. (2003). Practice parameter: Treatment of the child with a first unprovoked seizure: Report of the Quality Standards Subcommittee of the American Academy of Neurology and the Practice Committee of the Child Neurology Society. *Neurology, 60*(2), 166–175.

Holmes, G.L. (2002). Childhood-specific epilepsies accompanied by developmental disabilities: Causes and effects. In O. Devinsky & L.E. Westbrook (Eds.), *Epilepsy and developmental disabilities* (pp. 23–40). Woburn, MA: Butterworth-Heinemann.

Holsti, M., Dudley, N., Shunk, J., Adelgais, K., Greenberg, R., Olsen, C., ... Filloux, F. (2010). Intranasal midazolam vs rectal diazepam for the home treatment of acute seizures in pediatric patients with epilepsy. *Archives of Pediatrics and Adolescent Medicine, 164*(8), 747–753.

Hsieh, D.T., Chang, T., Tsuchida, T.N., Vezina, L.G., Vanderver, A., Siedel, J., ... Gaillard, W.D. (2010). New-onset afebrile seizures in infants: Role of neuroimaging. *Neurology, 74*(2), 150–156.

Huang, C.C., Chang, Y.C., & Wang, S.T. (1998). Acute symptomatic seizure disorders in young children—a population study in southern Taiwan. *Epilepsia, 39*(9), 960–964.

Hundozi-Hysenaj, H., & Boshnjaku-Dallku, I. (2008). Epilepsy in children with cerebral palsy. *Journal of Pediatric Neurology, 6*(1), 43–46.

Individuals with Disabilities Education Improvement Act (IDEA) of 2004, PL 108–446 20 U.S.C. §§ 1400 *et seq.*

International League Against Epilepsy (http://www.ilae-epilepsy.org).

Ito, M. (1998). Antiepileptic drug treatment of West syndrome. *Epilepsia, 39*(Suppl. 5), 38–41.

Jobst, B.C., Darcey, T.M., Thadani, V.M., & Roberts, D.W. (2010). Brain stimulation for the treatment of epilepsy. *Epilepsia, 51*(Suppl. 3), 88–92.

Kivity, S., Lerman, P., Ariel, R., Danziger, Y., Mimouni, M., & Shinnar, S. (2004). Long-term cognitive outcomes of a cohort of children with cryptogenic infantile spasms treated with high-dose adrenocorticotropic hormone. *Epilepsia, 45*(3), 255–262.

Klepper, J. (2008). Glucose transporter deficiency syndrome (GLUTIDS) and the ketogenic diet. *Epilepsia, 49*(Suppl. 8), 46–49.

Knudsen, F.U. (2000). Febrile seizures: Treatment and prognosis. *Epilepsia, 41*(1), 2–9.

Kuhle, S., Tiefenthaler, M., Seidl, R., & Hauser, E. (2000). Prolonged generalized epileptic seizures triggered by breath-holding spells. *Pediatric Neurology, 23*(3), 271–273.

Laberge, L., Tremblay, R.E., Vitaro, F., & Montplaisir, J. (2000). Development of parasomnias from childhood to early adolescence. *Pediatrics, 106*(1, Pt. 1), 67–74.

Lagac, L. (2006). Cognitive side effects of anti-epileptic drugs: The relevance in childhood epilepsy. *Seizure, 15*(4), 235–241.

Lerman, P. (1992). Benign partial epilepsy with centro-temporal spikes. In J. Roger, M. Bureau, C. Dravet, P. Genton, C.A. Tassinari, & P. Wolf (Eds.), *Epileptic syndromes in infancy, childhood and adolescence* (pp. 189–200). London, England: John Libbey & Co.

Loiseau, P. (1992). Childhood absence epilepsy. In J. Roger, M. Bureau, C. Dravet, P. Genton, C.A. Tassinari, & P. Wolf (Eds.), *Epileptic syndromes in infancy, childhood and adolescence* (pp. 135–150). London, England: John Libbey & Co.

Lombroso, C.T. (2000). Pavor nocturnus of proven epileptic origin. *Epilepsia, 41*(9), 1221–1226.

Loring, D.W., & Meador, K.J. (2004). Cognitive side effects of antiepileptic drugs in children. *Neurology, 62*(6), 872–877.

Lowenstein, D.H., & Alldredge, B.K. (1998). Status epilepticus. *The New England Journal of Medicine, 338*(14), 970–976.

Lüders, H., Acharya, J., Baumgartner, C., Benbadis, S., Bleasel, A., Burgess, R., ... Wyllie, E. (1998). Semiological seizure classification. *Epilepsia, 39*(9), 1006–1013.

Lux, A.L., Edwards, S.W., Hancock, E., Johnson, A.L., Kennedy, C.R., Newton, R.W., ... Osborne, J.P. (2004). The United Kingdom Infantile Spasms Study comparing vigabatrin with prednisolone or tetracosactide at 14 days: A multicentre, randomised controlled trial. *The Lancet, 364*(9447), 1773–1778.

MacDonald, B.K., Johnson, A.L., Goodridge, D.M., Cockerell, O.C., Sander, J.W., & Shorvon, S.D. (2000). Factors predicting prognosis of epilepsy after presentation with seizures. *Archives of Disease in Childhood, 81*(3), 261–262.

Mackay, M.T., Weiss, S.K., Adams-Webber, T., Ashwal, S., Stephens, D., Ballaban-Gill, K., ... Snead, III, O.C. (2004). Practice parameter: Medical treatment of infantile spasms: Report of the American Academy of Neurology and the Child Neurology Society. *Neurology, 62*(10), 1668–1681.

Mapstone, T.B. (2008). Vagus nerve stimulation: Current concepts. *Neurosurgery Focus, 25*(3), e9.

Meador, K.J., Baker, G.A., Browning, N., Clayton-Smith, J., Combs-Cantrell, D.T., Cohen, M., ... Loring, D.W. (2010). Cognitive function at 3 years of age after fetal exposure to antiepileptic drugs. *The New England Journal of Medicine, 360*(16), 1597–1605.

Modi, A.C., King, A.S., Monahan, S.R., Koumoutsos, J.E., Morita, D.A., & Glauser, T.A. (2009). Even a single seizure negatively impacts pediatric health-related quality of life. *Epilepsia, 50*(9), 2110–2116.

Montalenti, E., Imperiale, D., Rovera, A., Bergamasco, B., & Benna, P. (2001). Clinical features, EEG findings and diagnostic pitfalls in juvenile myoclonic epilepsy: A series of 63 patients. *Journal of the Neurological Sciences, 184*(1), 65–70.

Moshé, S.L. (2000). Seizures early in life. *Neurology, 55*(5, Suppl. 1), S15–S20; discussion, S54–S58.

Nelson, K.B., & Ellenberg, J.H. (1976). Predictors of epilepsy in children who have experienced febrile seizures. *The New England Journal of Medicine, 295*(19), 1029–1033.

Nelson, K.B., & Ellenberg, J.H. (1978). Prognosis in children with febrile seizures. *Pediatrics, 61*(5), 720–727.

O'Shaughnessy, E.S., Berl, M.B., Moore, E.N., & Gaillard, W.D. (2008). Pediatric functional magnetic resonance imaging (fMRI): Issues and applications. *Journal of Child Neurology, 23*(7), 791–801.

Pachatz, C., Fusco, L., & Vigevano, F. (1999). Benign myoclonus of early infancy. *Epileptic Disorders, 1*(1), 57–61.

Panayiotopoulos, C.P. (1999). Benign childhood partial seizures and related epileptic syndromes. *Current problems in epilepsy series* (Vol. 15, pp. 13-20). London, England: John Libbey & Co.

Park, S.P., & Kwon, S.H. (2008). Cognitive effects of antiepileptic drugs. *Journal of Clinical Neurology, 4*(3), 99–106.

Patsalos, P.N., Berry, D.J., Bourgeois, B.F., Cloyd, J.C., Glauser, T.A., Johannessen, S.I., ... Perruca, E. (2008). Antiepileptic drugs—best practice guidelines for therapeutic drug monitoring: A position paper by the Subcommission on Therapeutic Drug Monitoring, ILAE Commission on Therapeutic Strategies. *Epilepsia, 49*(7), 1239–1276.

Pellock, J.M. (2006). Other nonepileptic paroxysmal disorders. In E. Wyllie, A. Gupta, & D.K. Lachhwani (Eds.), *The treatment of epilepsy: Principles and practice* (4th ed., pp. 631–642). Philadelphia, PA: Lippincott Williams & Wilkins.

Pellock, J.M., Hrachovy, R., Shinnar, S., Baram, T.Z., Bettis, D., Dlugos, D.J., ... Wheless, J.W. (2010). Infantile spasms: A U.S. consensus report. *Epilepsia, 51*(10), 2175–2189.

Perucca, E. (2005). Clinically relevant drug interactions with antiepileptic drugs. *British Journal of Clinical Pharmacology, 61*(3), 246–255.

Perucca, E., & Meador, K.J. (2005). Adverse effects of antiepileptic drugs. *Acta Neurology Scandinavia, 112*(Suppl. 181), 30–35.

Reynolds, E.H. (2000). The ILAE/IBE/WHO Global Campaign Against Epilepsy: Bringing epilepsy "out of the shadows." *Epilepsy and Behavior, 1*(4), S3–S8.

Rosenfeld, W.E., & Roberts, D.W. (2009). Tonic and atonic seizures: What's next—VNS or callosotomy? *Epilepsia, 50*(Suppl. 8), 25–30.

Rossi, P.G., Parmeggiani, A., Posar, A., Scaduto, M.C., Chiodo, S., & Vatti, G. (1999). Landau-Kleffner syndrome (LKS): Long-term follow-up and links with electrical status epilepticus during sleep (ESES). *Brain and Development, 21*(2), 90–98.

Sankar, R., & Holmes, G.L. (2004). Mechanisms of action for the commonly used antiepileptic drugs: Relevance to antiepileptic drug-associated neurobehavioral adverse effects. *Journal of Child Neurology, 19*(1), S6–S14.

Scott, R.C., Besag, F.M., & Neville, B.G. (1999). Buccal midazolam and rectal diazepam for treatment of prolonged seizures in childhood and adolescence: A randomized trial. *The Lancet, 353*(9153), 623–626.

Shellhaas, R.A., & Joshi, S.M. (2010). Vitamin D and bone health among children with epilepsy. *Pediatric Neurology, 42*(6), 385–393.

Shields, W.D., Shewmon, D.A., Peacock, W.J., LoPresti, C.M., Nakagawa, J.A., & Yudovin, S. (1999). Surgery for the treatment of medically intractable infantile spasms: A cautionary case. *Epilepsia, 40*(9), 1305–1308.

Shinnar, S., Berg, A.T., Moshé, S.L., Kang, H., O'Dell, C., Alemany, M., ... Hauser, W.A. (1994). Discontinuing antiepileptic drugs in children with epilepsy: A prospective study. *Annals of Neurology, 35*(5), 534–545.

Shinnar, S., Berg, A.T., Moshé, S.L., O'Dell, C., Alemany, M., Newstein, D., ... Hauser, W.A. (1996). The risk of seizure recurrence after a first unprovoked afebrile seizure in childhood: An extended follow-up. *Pediatrics, 98*(2), 216–225.

Shinnar, S., Berg, A.T., Moshé, S.L., & Shinnar, R. (2001). How long do new-onset seizures in children last? *Annals of Neurology, 49*(5), 659–664.

Shorvon, S. (2000). *Handbook of epilepsy treatment* (p. 18). Malden, MA: Blackwell Science.

Sillanpää, M. (2000). Long-term outcome of epilepsy. *Epileptic Disorders, 2*(2), 79–88.

Sillanpää, M., & Shinnar, S. (2010). Long-term mortality in childhood-onset epilepsy. *The New England Journal of Medicine, 363*(26), 2522–2529.

Sogawa, Y., Masur, D., O'Dell, C., Moshé, S.L., & Shinnar, S. (2010). Cognitive outcomes in children who present with a first unprovoked seizure. *Epilepsia, 51*(12), 2432–2439.

Sulzbacher, S., Farwell, J.R., Temkin, N., Lu, A.S., & Hirtz, D.G. (1999). Late cognitive effects of early treatment with phenobarbital. *Clinical Pediatrics, 38*(7), 387–394.

Sunder, T.R. (1997). Meeting the challenge of epilepsy in persons with multiple handicaps. *Journal of Child Neurology, 12*(Suppl. 1), S38–S43.

Trasmonte, J.V., & Barron, T.F. (1998). Infantile spasms: A proposal for a staged evaluation. *Pediatric Neurology, 19*(5), 368–371.

Troester, M.M., Hastriter, E.V., & Ng, Y.T. (2010). Dissolving oral clonazepam wafers in the acute treatment of prolonged seizures. *Journal of Child Neurology, 25*(12), 1468–1472.

Tuchman, R.F., & Rapin, I. (2002). Epilepsy in autism. *The Lancet Neurology, 1*(6), 352–358.

Uldall, P., Alving, J., Hansen, L.K., Kibæk, M., & Buchholt, J. (2006). The misdiagnosis of epilepsy in children admitted to a tertiary epilepsy center with paroxysmal events. *Archives of Disease in Childhood, 91*(3), 219–221.

Wallace, S.J. (1998). Myoclonus and epilepsy in childhood: A review of the treatment with valproate, ethosuximide, lamotrigine and zonisamide. *Epilepsy Research, 29*(2), 147–154.

Wheless, J.W., Clarke, D.F., Arzimanoglou, A., & Carpenter, D. (2007). Treatment of pediatric epilepsy: European expert opinion, 2007. *Epileptic Disorders, 9*(4), 353–412.

Wheless, J.W., Clarke, D.F., & Carpenter, D. (2005). Treatment of pediatric epilepsy: Expert opinion, 2005. *Journal of Child Neurology, 20*(1), S1–S56.

Wilfong, A.A. (2007). Monotherapy in children and infants. *Neurology, 69*(Suppl. 3), S17–S22.

Wolf, P. (1994). *Epileptic seizures and syndromes* (pp. 137–141). London, England: John Libbey & Co.

Zucconi, M., Oldani, A., Ferini-Strambi, L., Bizzozero, D., & Smirne, S. (1997). Nocturnal paroxysmal arousals with motor behaviors during sleep: Frontal lobe epilepsy or parasomnia? *Journal of Clinical Neurophysiology, 14*(6), 513–522.

Zupanc, M.L. (2006). Antiepileptic drugs and hormonal contraceptives in adolescent women with epilepsy. *Neurology, 66*(Suppl. 3), S37–S45.

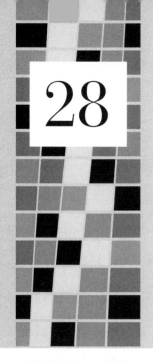

28

The New Face of Developmental Disabilities

Nancy J. Roizen and Adrienne S. Tedeschi

Upon completion of this chapter, the reader will

- Describe the effects of a silent stroke and overt stroke on children with sickle-cell disease

- Understand the role of cranial irradiation in the treatment of acute lymphocytic leukemia and brain tumors and understand irradiation's long-term effects on cognitive function

- Explain the impact of multidrug therapy and Cesarean section on the outcome in mother-to-child transmission of human immuno-deficiency virus

- Be aware of the effects of chronic kidney failure on neurodevelopment

This chapter considers a group of children with neurodevelopmental disabilities who represent a new phenemonon in that they are now surviving to adulthood with diseases that were previously fatal during childhood. These disorders include sickle-cell disease (SCD), cancer, human immunodeficiency virus (HIV) and chronic kidney failure (CKF). Affected children have been found to experience "late effects" that include significant disabilities as a consequence of their illness and/or its treatment. These late effects were previously unrecognized because of the early death of the child, and they often represent side effects of the aggressive therapy required to preserve life. Many of these comorbidities affect the central nervous system (CNS) and emerge over time, influencing developmental trajectories.

◼◼◼ KISHA

Kisha is a teenager with SCD who was diagnosed shortly after birth and treated from infancy with prophylactic penicillin, specialized immunizations, and routine well-child care. In general, her family has been able to manage the painful episodes caused by the SCD at home, but once or twice a year she has been hospitalized to control crisis-level episodes. On one occasion she was admitted to the intensive care unit with an episode of acute chest syndrome (see SCD section), but she fortunately responded well to interventions that included transfusions, antibiotics, and oxygen. She is monitored routinely using transcranial Doppler ultrasonography. So far she has had normal findings, placing her at low risk for stroke, unlike her friend Dwayne who also has SCD and suffered a stroke during early childhood. Kisha will be graduating from high school this year and plans to attend college.

SICKLE-CELL DISEASE

SCD is an autosomal recessive disorder that results in the production of an abnormal hemoglobin, called Hemoglobin S or HbS. Red blood cells that contain predominately HbS have a greatly limited life span, leading to chronic **hemolytic** (excessive breakdown of red blood cells) **anemia**. In addition, the cells become crescent or sickle-shaped in a low-oxygen environment and can cause blockage of the microvasculature, leading to severe pain in the affected limb or body organ (**vaso-occlusive episode**). The most common and severe form of SCD is homozygous sickle-cell anemia (HbSS), which comprises about two thirds of all cases (Serjeant, 1999).

SCD occurs most commonly in individuals of sub-Saharan African ancestry. Virtually all states now screen newborns for SCD, which has become the most common genetic disease identified by state screening programs. It occurs in 1 out of 2,647 births, exceeding the next highest genetic disorder, cystic fibrosis (1 out of 3,900; see Chapter 1). SCD occurs in 1 out of 396 African American births, with Asian Indians being next in frequency at 1 out of 16,000 births (DeBaun & Vichinsky, 2007).

Clinical Manifestations

SCD is a complex, chronic disorder that, as noted in the case report, is characterized by hemolysis and intermittent vascular occlusion. This results in chronic damage to multiple body organs and acute complications that can rapidly become life threatening. Acute manifestations include bacterial sepsis (blood poisoning) or meningitis, recurrent vaso-occlusive pain crises, splenic sequestration (accumulation of red and white blood cells in the spleen, leading to acute anemia and increased risk of infection), aplastic crisis (shutting down of the bone marrow which normally produces white and red blood cells), acute chest syndrome (a pneumonialike condition), and stroke. The long-term medical consequences of SCD include anemia, jaundice, splenomegaly (enlarged spleen), functional **cholelithiasis** (gall stones), restrictive lung disease, pulmonary hypertension, **avascular necrosis** (destruction of bone from microvascular occlusion) of the hip or shoulder,

retinopathy (disorder of the retina), leg ulcers, and delay in physical growth and sexual maturation (Section on Hemotology, Oncology, and Committee on Genetics, 2002).

Patients with SCD, especially infants, also have abnormal immune function which places them at risk for bacterial infections that are a leading cause of mortality and morbidity in this disorder. This is because infections can initiate the cascade of sickling of red blood cells and result in vaso-occlusive episodes with associated pain and other organ-related complications. As early as 6 months of age, and usually by 5 years of age, children with SCD have functional asplenia, increasing the risk of infection because the spleen normally helps orchestrate the body's response to infection. They are particularly at risk for infection from *Streptococcus pneumoiae* and *Haemophilus influenzae* type B. (DeBaun & Vichinsky, 2007).

Neurological complications of SCD are rather common and range from headaches to strokes. Among children with SCD, about 10% (Lopez-Vincent et al., 2010; Pegelow et al., 2002) will have **overt strokes** and almost a quarter will have silent strokes before their 18th birthday (Pegelow et al., 2002). An overt stroke involves a **focal** (localized) neurological deficit that lasts more than 24 hours. It results from an occlusion of one of the large anterior cerebral circulation vessels (DeBaun & Vichinsky, 2007). Strokes most frequently occur in the frontal lobe (59%), and usually have two or more damaged areas (77%; Gold et al., 2008). In a **silent stroke** there is evidence of a cerebral infarct on an magnetic resonance imaging (MRI) scan, but a focal neurological deficit will be absent on clinical examination. The majority of silent strokes occur in the frontal lobe (38%) and principally in one cortical area (75%; Gold et al., 2008). Strokes can occur as young as 1 year of age, but the highest incidence is between 2 and 5 years of age (Ohene-Frempong et al., 1998). Genetic factors may play a role in predisposing to stroke in SCD (DeBaun & Vichinsky, 2007).

Developmental and Behavioral Manifestations of Sickle-Cell Disease

SCD is associated with a number of biopsychosocial risk factors for neurodevelopmental deficits. Biological factors include overt and silent strokes, anemia, and insufficient oxygen and glucose delivery to CNS tissue. Children born to mothers with SCD are also at increased risk for preterm birth and perinatal problems, including infections (Schatz & McClellan, 2006). In addition, a disproportionate number of children with SCD are born into families who are in a low socioeconomic status (SES) and have fewer financial resources to assist in the care of this chronic, disabling disease.

About one quarter to one third of children with SCD have some type of developmental disability, most frequently affecting the cognitive and academic domains (Schatz & McClellan, 2006). Children with overt stroke, on average, have a 10–15 point drop in IQ scores from prestroke levels (Schatz & McClelland, 2006; Wang et al., 2001), while silent strokes impart a milder degree of cognitive impairment (Armstrong et al., 1996). But even without stroke, cognitive testing generally reveals lower overall cognitive function, with uneven abilities (Schatz et al., 2004). Although cognitive patterns are not consistent across all studies, most show that measures of attention and **executive function** (cognitive tasks related to taking in, organizing, processing, and acting on information) are adversely affected, leading to an attention-deficit/hyperactivity disorder (ADHD) picture (Schatz et al., 2001; Schatz & McClelland, 2006).

Studies demonstrate contributions to deficits in developmental functioning from both biologic and social factors. Neurocognitive functioning through the first year of life, as measured by tests of infant development, generally falls within the typical range (Thompson et al., 2002). Infants with moderate to high severity SCD, however, do show developmental delays even at this early age (Hogan et al., 2006). By 24 months of age, average scores of children with SCD in motor development are maintained, but delays become measurable on the Mental Developmental Index (MDI) of the Bayley Scales of Infant and Toddler Development. Lower MDIs are found in children with increased biomedical and parenting risk factors (Thompson et al., 2002). Meta-analysis reveals that even children with no evidence of a cerebral infarct have small but detectable decrements on IQ measures over time (4–5 point difference overall; Schatz, Finke, Kellett, & Kramer, 2002).

In measures of specific abilities, attention and executive function generally appear more sensitive to cognitive decrements than IQ scores (Schatz et al., 2002). Anemia severity predicts general cognitive ability, with a greater impact on children of higher SES (Schatz et al., 2004). When school-aged children with SCD who had not sustained silent or overt strokes were divided into high and low IQ groups and **grey matter**

was measured by MRI scans, higher IQs were found in those children with more grey matter (Chen et al., 2009).

The impact on families of having a child with SCD shares many features with families who have children with other severe neurodevelopmental disabilities. Social-environment factors related to low SES; concerns about social stigma; and recurrent, unpredictable medical complications contribute to a high level of family stress (Schatz & McClellan, 2006). Despite the increased support provided by extended family networks in the African American community (Radcliffe et al., 2006), the increased prevalence of poverty, limited access to quality health care, poor housing, lower quality schools, and undernutrition in this population can negatively affect family, parent, and child functioning (Evans 2004; McLoyd, 1998). In addition, pain, infection, and other medical complications lead to a substantial amount of school absenteeism. Children with SCD are absent from school an average of 26 days per year, compared to 16 days per year in children with other chronic diseases and fewer than 7 days per year in typical children (Eaton et al., 1995).

Behavior problems in youth with SCD are also increased. Externalizing behavior problems are increased (e.g., aggression, oppositional defiant disorder, conduct disorder), although less so in children with higher baseline IQs (Thompson et al., 2003). Additionally, depression is more common compared to physically healthy peers. Children with SCD have higher rates of moderate to severe depression symptoms (20%) compared to peers with other chronic illnesses such as diabetes mellitus (8%) and cystic fibrosis (7%), although similar to those with asthma (21%; Key et al., 2001). A longitudinal study of social function, however, revealed no significant differences in measures of friendship or social acceptance when compared with peers (Noll et al., 2010).

Treatment and Management of Sickle-Cell Disease

All newborns are now screened for SCD as part of state newborn screening programs. The results of a 15-year, multicenter natural history study of SCD have led to the use of prophylactic penicillin to prevent bacterial infections from birth. This has dramatically decreased the risk of early death from bacterial sepsis in affected children (DeBaun & Vichinsky, 2007; Falletta et al., 1995). Many new treatment options are now directed at decreasing sickling and its complications including bone marrow transplantation and hydroxyurea therapy (Iannone et al., 2003; Kratovil et al., 2006). Health maintenance includes regularly scheduled visits to the doctor, immunizations (including pneumococcal vaccines), documentation of spleen size, and baseline blood cell counts. The family needs ongoing education regarding the urgency for prompt evaluation and treatment of febrile illnesses and the acute complications that can cause morbidity and mortality. Anticipatory guidance includes a discussion of the need to avoid temperature extremes and to maintain adequate hydration. Parents also need to know initial home treatment steps for pain and **priapism** (painful and long-lasting penile erection) and the indications for urgent evaluation (Section on Hematology/Oncology and Committee on Genetics, 2002).

Effective management of painful episodes requires a collaborative management plan between the family and the multidisciplinary medical team. Pain management includes the titration (incremental increase and decrease) of potentially addicting medication. Early in the course of managing, comfort measures such as heating pads, and medications such as ibuprofen and acetaminophen, are used. This is followed by acetaminophen with codeine and short- or long-acting opiods or morphine derivatives. Severe painful episodes, however, require hospitalization and the use of intravenous morphine. Patients with multiple pain episodes requiring hospitalization within 1 year or with hospital stays of longer than 7 days should be evaluated for comorbidities and psychosocial stressors that may aggravate pain crises.

Any acute neurology symptom such as hemiparesis, aphasia, seizures, severe headache, cranial nerve palsy, stupor, or coma requires urgent evaluation for stroke. Strokes are treated acutely with oxygen and blood transfusion therapy to increase hemoglobin levels. Primary stroke prevention using **transcranial Doppler (TCD)**, which assesses blood velocity in cerebral arteries, has been shown to decrease the incidence of overt stroke by 90% (Enninful-Eghan et al., 2010). When low velocity is found, prevention of stroke is accomplished by blood transfusion therapy aimed at keeping the HbS concentration low, thereby decreasing sickling.

Outcome

As a result of early identification and the use of disease-modifying therapies, the life expectancy of children with SCD has significantly increased. Neonatal screening, penicillin prophylaxis for children, pneumococcal immunization, red cell transfusions for selected patients, hydroxyurea therapy to stimulate the production of nonsickling fetal hemoglobin, parental and patient education, and, above all, treatment at comprehensive SCD centers have all contributed to improved longevity. Earlier data reported that half of individuals with SCD did not survive beyond 20 years of age; now the vast majority (94%) of children with sickle-cell anemia and nearly all (98%) with milder forms of SCD live to become adults (Quinn, Rogers, McCavit, & Buchanan, 2010). Even with this great improvement in mortality, there are geographic discrepancies. Wang et al. (2011) have developed quality-of-care indicators to provide a starting point for quality improvement efforts.

CANCER: ACUTE LYMPHOCYTIC LEUKEMIA AND BRAIN TUMORS

About 1–2 children per 10,000 develop cancer each year in the United States. In 2001, approximately 8,600 children were diagnosed with cancer, and about 1,500 died from the disease. The most common cancers in children are **leukemias** (blood cell cancers) and central nervous system (CNS) tumors, which together account for more than half of all the new cases. Leukemia accounts for about one third of all new cases of cancer; and acute lymphocytic leukemia (ALL) accounts for approximately three quarters of all leukemia cases. CNS cancers are the second most common childhood malignancy and account for about 20% of childhood cancers (Ries et al., 2005). This chapter will limit the discussion on developmental disabilities in cancer to leukemia and brain tumors, although many of the principles apply to other cancers in children (Barrera, 2005; Bonneau et al., 2011).

Clinical Manifestations

Approximately 2,000 children under 15 years of age are diagnosed with ALL in the United States each year. ALL occurs more frequently in boys than girls and has a peak incidence between 2–6 years of age. The etiology is unknown, but it is associated with both genetic disorders (e.g., Down syndrome) and environmental factors (e.g., irradiation). The clinical presentation of ALL is usually nonspecific with anorexia, fatigue, bone pain, and irritability often associated with an intermittent, low-grade fever. The child appears listless and pale, often with **purpuric skin lesions**. The diagnosis is usually suggested by an abnormal peripheral blood count showing immature malignant blast cells, which is followed by a bone marrow aspiration to establish the definitive diagnosis (Tubergen & Bleyer, 2007)

The incidence of childhood brain tumors is highest in infants and young children (< 7 years of age), with a male predominance for **medulloblastomas** (cerebellar tumors) and **ependymomas** (tumors developing from cells that line both the hollow-cavities on the ventricles of the brain and the canal containing the spinal cord). The etiology of pediatric brain tumors is not well defined. About 5% of cases are associated with familial and hereditary syndromes (Kuttesch & Ater, 2007). The clinical presentation depends on the tumor location, tumor type, and the child's age. Subtle changes in personality, **mentation**, and speech may precede the classical symptoms of a brain tumor, which include persistent and severe headache and vomiting. Young children with open **cranial sutures** can present with irritability, lethargy, vomiting, and increased head size. Others can present with disorders of equilibrium, gait, and coordination (Kuttesch & Ater, 2007). Evaluating a child suspected to have a brain tumor is an emergency; it includes a history, physical examination, ophthalmological examination, and MRI scan of the brain (Kuttesch & Ater, 2007).

Treatment

The goal of ALL treatment is to minimize the adverse late effects, while maintaining high survival rates. Most children are treated according to a national clinical trial protocol where the initial phase involves induction of remission, achieved by eradicating leukemic cells from the bone marrow. The second phase is CNS prophylactic treatment to prevent relapses (Tubergen & Bleyer, 2007). This approach has been largely responsible for the increase in long-term survival for children with ALL because the CNS is a sanctuary for leukemic cells. Initially, cranial radiation therapy (CRT) was used to prevent relapse, but studies determined that CRT was associated with significant declines in IQ scores among survivors of childhood ALL (Cousens et al., 1988). As a result, CRT is now reserved for high-risk subgroups or for CNS relapse (Butler & Haser, 2006). CRT has largely been replaced by intrathecal chemotherapy (ITC; infusion of medication within the space surrounding the spinal cord; Butler & Haser, 2006). After remission has been induced, most children enter a maintenance phase of

chemotherapy, which lasts for 2–3 years. About 15%–20% of children have a relapse in the bone marrow and less commonly in the CNS or testes (Tubergen & Bleyer, 2007). Bone marrow transplantation may be part of the treatment regimen if there is a relapse.

Outcomes for children with brain tumors have improved with innovations in neurosurgery and radiation therapy as well as the introduction of effective chemotherapy. The foundation of treatment is complete surgical resection, if feasible, with radiation therapy and chemotherapy used depending on the diagnosis, patient age, and other factors (Kuttesch & Ater, 2007). Multidisciplinary approaches include seizure management, physical therapy, endocrine management with growth hormone and thyroid replacement, tailored educational programs, and vocational intervention, all depending on the individual needs of the child (Kuttesch & Ater, 2007).

The treatment of both ALL and brain tumors is associated with adverse effects on healthy tissue in the CNS. ITC, especially methotrexate, has been associated with acute white matter (the part of the brain with mainly nerve fibers) injury, and persisting decreased white matter volumes have been associated with IQ declines (Hudson, 1999; Janzen & Spiegler, 2008; Zhang et al., 2008). Many of the acquired neurocognitive and psychological disturbances associated with the treatment of ALL and brain tumors are similar to those found in children who suffer from ADHD and traumatic brain injury. Initial studies indicate some success using a cognitive remediation program (CRP) in which the child is guided through exercises that promote sustained, selective, divided, and executive attentional control (Butler et al., 2008; Sohlberg & Mateer, 1986). Treatment with stimulant medication has also improved performance on tests of attention and on parent and teacher reports (Butler, Copland, et al., 2008; Butler, Sahler, et al., 2008; Conklin et al., 2010; Mulhern et al., 2004; Netson et al., 2011).

Development and Behavior

Early studies of survivors of childhood ALL determined that cranial radiation therapy was associated with declines in intelligence (Cousens et al., 1988). They also reported more impairment in non dominant hemisphere functions, shortened attention spans, poor concentration, increased distractibility, and impaired school performance especially in arithmetic computation (Butler & Haser, 2006). Studies of chemotherapy-only treatment for childhood ALL also indicate a specific pattern of neuropsychological late effects. Although verbal subtests are not significantly different between the groups, perceptual reasoning skills, working memory, and processing speed are affected in the chemotherapy-only group. The result is that academic progress in both reading and math is impaired. Girls are at greater risk for these effects than boys (Peterson et al., 2008). Children who experience relapses have poorer neurocognitive outcomes, with 20% displaying IQ scores in the range of intellectual disability (Janzen & Spiegler, 2008).

Studies in children treated in the 1970s–1990s for CNS tumors with surgery and CRT reported declines in intellectual function and academic achievement (Butler & Haser, 2006). In a study of 120 children treated with surgery and CRT for medulloblastoma, 42% had a full-scale IQ of less than 80 at 5 years following treatment, and 75% had a full scale IQ of less that 80 at 10 years following treatment (Hoppe-Hirsch et al., 1990). Commonalities that emerged included deficits in all the following areas: memory, attention/concentration, sequencing, processing speed, visual perceptual ability, and language.

Children with brain tumors who require only surgical treatment can have a range of outcomes. Surgery may result in global intellectual ability remaining intact but with deficits in selected domains. This can affect a single domain motor functioning, e.g., benign cerebellar tumors; Steinlin et al., 2003), or multiple domains (cognitive, academic, social adaptive, and motor functioning, e.g., cerebellar astrocytomas; Beebe et al., 2005). In addition, more than half of children with brain tumors that are treated surgically experience some form of significant psychological adjustment problem such as depression, externalizing behaviors, and academic problems (Meyer & Kieran, 2002). In childhood survivors of both ALL and brain tumors, risk factors for increased neuropsychological dysfunction include younger age at developing the disease and being female (Butler & Haser, 2006).

Outcomes

Because of advances in treatment, the mortality rate for ALL dropped by half between 1975 and 1995. Presently, the overall survival rate for children with ALL is nearly 80% (Butler & Haser, 2006). For CNS cancers, the survival rates vary greatly depending on the tumor type; it is about 65% for a medulloblastoma and less than 10% for a brainstem glioma (Butler & Haser, 2006).

Children who have undergone cancer treatment are more likely than the general population to repeat a grade in school and/or need more learning supports and special education services. Compared to their typically developing peers, children treated for brain tumors are 4 times as likely to repeat a grade, and those receiving cerebral irradiation are 2.5 times as likely (Barrera, 2005). Other risk factors for repeating a grade include attending secondary school at the time of diagnosis, low education level of father, and requiring school-organized educational support on return to school (Bonneau et al., 2011). Compared with siblings, survivors of leukemia and CNS tumors were less likely to finish high school, but only those with CNS tumors were also less likely to complete college (Mitby et al., 2003).

Compared with healthy controls, adult survivors of childhood cancers are nearly twice as likely to be unemployed, with those with CNS or brain tumors being nearly 5 times more likely to be unemployed. Additional predictors of unemployment are younger age, lower education level or intelligence quotient, female gender, motor impairment, epilepsy, and radiotherapy (de Boer et al., 2006).

Minimizing the adverse late effects of childhood cancers while maintaining high survival rates with treatment is a goal that has been largely achieved in treatment regimens for ALL but less so for brain tumors. Improvements in therapy have greatly decreased mortality and morbidity, but more advances are needed to achieve optimal neurocognitive outcomes.

HUMAN IMMUNODEFICIENCY VIRUS

HIV is a viral infection transmitted by 1) sexual contact; 2) blood exposure from contaminated needles; 3) mucous membrane exposure to contaminated blood or bodily fluids; 4) mother-to-child transmission during pregnancy, mainly around the time of labor and delivery, or through breast feeding; and 5) contaminated blood products (Committee on Infectious Diseases, 2009). When an HIV infection manifests as a severe clinical condition, it is called AIDS (acquired immunodeficiency syndrome). In the United States, AIDS has gone from being a rapidly fatal disease for children who acquired the virus by **vertical transmission** to one in which

HIV vertical transmission is prevented in 98% of cases (Centers for Disease Control and Prevention, 2006). This has been accomplished via two ways: 1) treating HIV-infected pregnant mothers and their newborn infants with ART (antiretroviral treatment) regimens, and 2) preventing vertical transmission to infants born to HIV-infected mothers by C-section deliveries and complete avoidance of breastfeeding (Committee on Infectious Diseases, 2009). In the 100–200 children per year in the United States who do develop an HIV infection via vertical transmission, the disease is now managed as a chronic illness with survival well into late teen and early young adult years (McConnell et al., 2005). Rates of HIV infection in adolescents, however, continue to increase, primarily through sexual exposure. Fourteen percent of newly diagnosed cases of HIV infection in the United State occur among people 13 to 24 years of age (Committee on Infectious Diseases, 2009).

Clinical Manifestations

Most newborns with HIV have a normal examination despite being infected with HIV. When disease symptoms develop later in infancy they include enlargement of lymph glands, liver, and spleen; poor weight gain; diarrhea; pneumonia; and **thrush** (a fungal infection commonly involving the mucous membranes of the mouth). Symptoms found more commonly in children than in adults with AIDS include recurrent bacterial infections, chronic swelling of the **parotid** (the salivary gland beside the ear), lymphocytic interstitial pneumonia (LIP), and progressive neurologic deterioration (Yogev & Chadwick, 2007).

Development and Behavior in Children with Human Immunodeficiency Virus

There are multiple factors that determine the consequences of HIV infection including the viral load (amount of virus present in the body), the age of the child at the time of the infection, the clinical symptoms at time of diagnosis, and treatment (Armstrong & Mulhern, 1999; Corscia et al., 1997; Mintz, 1999; Mitchell, 2001; Willen, 2006). These biomedical factors are also confounded by biosocial factors including prenatal drug exposure, malnutrition, prematurity, poverty, neglect, family stress associated with death or illness of the primary caregiver, and the presence of other developmental disabilities associated with AIDS (Armstrong et al., 1993; Coscia et al., 2001).

One major medical factor affecting development in vertically infected infants and children is HIV-related encephalopathy. It can present with a number of profiles. One type, labeled **subacute progressive encephalopathy**, is characterized by a gradual and insidious loss of previously obtained cognitive and motor milestones. Although this loss of skills may stabilize for a time, usually new losses are subsequently appreciated (Armstong et al., 1993; Brouwers et al., 1994; Simpson & Berger, 1996). A second type includes children with **plateau progressive encephalopathy** who, while not progressing in their development, may not show deterioration for a lengthy time period. Nevertheless, they eventually deteriorate. A third type is **static encephalopathy** that is characterized by significantly delayed development, with new skills acquired at a slower rate than is typical. These children have cognitive skills in the low-average to impaired range (Armstrong et al., 1993; Brouwers et al., 1994). A final subset displays a relatively mild neurocognitive deficit with average overall intellectual functioning but specific learning, language, and visual-motor deficits (Armstrong et al., 1993).

Research in the cognitive development of children with HIV infection is problematic in comparability of studies (Sherr et al., 2009); however, of the 54 studies with control groups, 81% reported a detrimental effect on neurocognitive development, 3 showed no differences, and 4 had mixed findings. In a study of the development of 175 children with HIV infection (Nozyce et al., 2006), on the Wechsler Intelligence Scales for Children III, the average scores were Verbal IQ of 85, Performance IQ of 90, and Full-Scale Score of 86. In another study of 85 HIV-infected school-aged children, the mean developmental quotient (DQ) was 85, with 12% of the group having a DQ of less than 70. Of the 85% children in public schools, three quarters were in the appropriate grade level for their age, but 56% required some special education services (Mialky et al., 2001).

A large study (n = 274 children; Nozyce et al., 2006) of the behavioral and cognitive profiles of clinically and immunologically stable antiretroviral treated HIV-infected children who were 2–17 years of age revealed that over half had more than one behavior problem on the Conners Parent Rating Scale. The most common behavior problems were psychosomatic symptoms (28%), learning deficits (25%), hyperactivity (20%), impulsive-hyperactive behavior (19%), conduct disorder (16%), and anxiety (8%). In children older than 9 years of age compared with younger children, anxiety problems were more common. There was no difference in the occurrence of behavior problems in HIV-infected children and in HIV-exposed (*in utero*) children. In both groups there was no association with HIV infection or prenatal drug exposure, but biological and environmental factors were thought to be important (Mellins et al., 2003).

Children with HIV face unique challenges and barriers to care due to the stigma associated with the illness. While confidentiality rules may protect children with HIV from undue stigmatization, they may also prevent access to necessary services, particularly school-based interventions. In addition, caregivers may choose not to disclose to the child his or her HIV diagnosis. This may especially happen with vertical transmission when the mother may want to protect her own as well as her child's confidentiality (Inston, 2000; Mialky et al., 2001). Yet, studies indicate that children who are told about their HIV status generally exhibit better adjustment (Steele et al., 2007) or, at least, have no adverse change in quality of life post disclosure (Butler et al., 2009). The average age of disclosure is reported to be between 9 and 11 years of age (Mialky et al., 2001; Butler et al., 2009). Also, appropriate disclosure outside the immediate family has been found to benefit the child in psychological and physical health (Steele et al., 2007).

Treatment and Outcomes

Pizzo et al. (1988) documented the response of AIDS encephalopathy to antiretroviral therapy in children. This eventually led to the era of highly active antiretroviral therapy (HAART) or simply ART, which has greatly decreased the mortality and morbidity associated with perinatally acquired HIV infection (Gortmaker et al., 2001; de Martino et al., 2000). A good prognosis is related to sustained suppression of the blood viral load and a high CD4 lymphocyte count, a marker for immune competence to help fight the infection (Yogev & Chadwick, 2007). In infants and toddlers, those with lower neuropsychological functioning (MDI on the Bayley Scales of Infant and Toddler Development of less than 70) had a higher risk for later disease progression (56%) than did those with IQ above 90 who had a risk of progression of 18% (Pearson et al., 2000). ART has also decreased the annual mortality rate in HIV-1-infected children and adolescents in the United States from 5.3% in 1996 to 0.7% in 1999 (Gortmaker et al., 2001).

In developing countries, where most HIV-infected children are born, ART and sophisticated diagnostic testing are not available. In these countries, the prognosis is worst in children with HIV who have opportunistic infections, encephalopathy, or wasting syndrome. These children have a mortality rate of 75% before 3 years of age. Those children with persistent fever and/or oral thrush, serious bacterial infections (e.g., meningitis, pneumonia, sepsis), hepatitis, and persistent anemia and thrombocytopenia (low platelet count) also have a poor prognosis, with more than 30% dying before 3 years of age (Yogev & Chadwick, 2007).

In children treated with ART, morbidity is greatly improved. Chiriboga et al. (2005) have demonstrated a decrease in active progressive encephalopathy from 31% in 1992 to 1.6% by 2000. Of the 13 children with arrested progressive encephalopathy in his cohort of 126 perinatally infected children treated with ART, 6 out of 9 children with microcephaly had resolution, 8 out of 12 with delays in cognitive function had improved cognitive function, and of the 10 children with spastic diparesis (weakness or paralysis of lower extremities) or hypotonic diparesis, 2 improved sufficiently to no longer meet criteria for this diagnosis.

In sum, treatment with ART now prevents vertical transmission in the vast majority of cases involving HIV-infected pregnant women. For infected infants and children, ART has converted HIV from a fatal infection to a chronic condition and has markedly decreased morbidity. However, long-term survivors still have neurodevelopmental deficits that require careful follow-up and therapeutic interventions.

CHRONIC KIDNEY DISEASE

Chronic kidney disease (CKD), also known as chronic renal disease, is a progressive and irreversible loss of renal (kidney) function that occurs over a period of months to years depending on the disease's underlying cause. CKD occurs in stages based on the severity of renal function impairment, with Stage 1 representing normal glomerular filtration rate (a measure of kidney function) and Stage 5 reflecting very poor to no kidney function. Stage 5 is also referred to as kidney failure or end stage renal disease (ESRD).

There is little known about the CKD's progression in children during early stages and its effect on neurodevelopment and cognitive function. In order to answer these questions a longitudinal natural history study is being performed, the Chronic Kidney Disease in Children (CKiD) Study. This prospective, observational cohort study of 540 children aged 1–16 with mild to moderate CKD (enrollment occurred over a 2-year period beginning in 2006) are being followed annually until initiation of renal replacement therapy is required. This study was designed to 1) identify novel risk factors for CKD progression; 2) understand the impact of kidney function decline on growth, cognition, and behavior; and 3) document the evolution of cardiovascular disease risk factors (Furth et al., 2006). The longitudinal data to be collected will be used to compare the rate of decline in kidney function to changes in neurocognitive function, blood pressure, fasting lipids, and rates of growth; such data should help to improve understanding of this complex disease.

In children, CKD can result from **congenital** (present at birth) causes, acquired diseases, and genetic disorders. The incidence and prevalence of CKD in the U.S. pediatric population is unknown as epidemiological information is limited and imprecise. The 2010 Annual Data Report published by the United States Renal Data System (USRDS) reported the pediatric incident rate of ESRD to be 15 per million population, or affecting about 7,000 children ages 0–19 years in the U.S. Nearly twice as many boys as girls have CKD, the result of the higher incidence in males of congenital disorders including **obstructive uropathy** (a pathologic condition that blocks urine flow), **renal dysplasia** (small, abnormal kidneys), and **Eagle Barrett** (formerly "prune belly") **syndrome**. Eagle Barrett syndrome involves three main problems: 1) poor development of the abdominal muscles, causing the skin of the stomach area to wrinkle like a prune; 2) undescended testicles (cryptorchidism); and 3) urinary tract problems (Warady & Chadha, 2007). Compared to Caucasian children, the incidence rate of ESRD is 3.6 times higher in African American children, 1.8 times higher in Native American children, and 1.8 times higher in Hispanic children (USRDS, 2010).

Clinical Manifestations

The clinical manifestations of CKD are varied and relate to the underlying cause of the renal disease and the severity of impairment. As CKD progresses, the kidney is no longer able to balance electrolytes, filter waste products from the blood, and regulate blood pressure. Children are generally asymptomatic during the early stages of CKD (Stages 1 and 2) but become increasingly symptomatic as renal function deteriorates. Children may present with **polyuria** (excessive passage of urine), **oliguria** (decreased passage of urine), **anuria** (absence of urine), **edema** (abnormal accumulation of fluid in body tissues), **hypertension** (elevated blood pressure), **hematuria** (blood in urine), and/or **proteinuria** (protein in urine).

Children may be diagnosed prenatally via ultrasonography or postnatally through abnormalities on urinalysis or elevation in serum **creatinine** concentration (a product produced by muscle tissue and normally filtered from the blood by the kidney). Signs and symptoms of **uremia** (accumulated urinary waste products in the blood) begin to appear in some children with Stage 3 disease and become increasingly prevalent in Stages 4 and 5 ESRD. These symptoms of severe renal impairment include **anorexia** (loss of appetite), vomiting, weakness, fatigue, and deficits in neurocognitive function (Vogt & Avner, 2007).

Many complications of CKD result from impaired kidney functions. Fluid and electrolyte imbalances result when the kidney is unable to moderate sodium and water amounts in the body. Metabolic acidosis and elevations in potassium (**hyperkalemia**) occur when the kidneys are unable to remove enough acid or potassium from the blood.

The presence of acidosis results in decreased growth, as the body breaks down bone to neutralize the acid. Bone structure is further affected by **metabolic bone disease** (MBD, formerly called renal osteodystrophy), which results from abnormalities in calcium, phosphorous, vitamin D, and parathyroid hormone. Anemia results from decreased production of **erythropoietin** by the kidney and is associated with decreased exercise tolerance, weakness, and fatigue. Cardiovascular complications include hypertension, **left ventricular hypertrophy** (Mitsnefes et al., 2003), and abnormal **lipid metabolism**. Growth impairment results from metabolic acidosis, anorexia, increased caloric requirements due to chronic illness, metabolic bone disease, and abnormalities in growth hormone metabolism (Vogt & Avner, 2007).

Neurodevelopment and Behavior

Children with CKD are at increased risk for alterations and delays in neurocognitive development. Historically, the outcomes of infants and toddlers with CKD were poor, with high rates of mortality and morbidity (Gerson et al., 2006; Madden et al., 2003; Qvist et al., 2002). The aggressive treatment of malnutrition, hypertension, and anemia, plus the elimination of aluminum-containing compounds to bind phosphate in hemodialysis, are believed to have resulted in a decrease in the neurological sequelae of CKD (Gerson et al., 2006; Gipson et al., 2006); nevertheless, children with CKD remain at risk for neurodevelopmental delay (Warady et al., 1999).

Madden et al. (2003) reported on the cognitive development of 16 surviving children from a cohort of 20 who developed ESRD requiring chronic hemodialysis prior to 1 year of age. The mean IQ was 86, but with scores ranging from 50–102 (Madden et al., 2003). Gipson et al. (2006) reported similar intellectual function (mean IQ of 89) in a group of 20 children and adolescents with CKD undergoing dialysis or managed with conservative therapy. When compared to a typically developing group, Gipson's cohort demonstrated significantly lower IQ, memory difficulties, and problems with executive functioning. Duquette et al. (2007) examined the intellectual and academic functioning of 30 children and adolescents with CKD and found that the control group outperformed the CKD group on Full Scale IQ (FSIQ), Verbal IQ, Performance IQ, as well as Word Reading and Math Reasoning scores as measured by the Weschler Abbreviated Score of Intelligence (WASI) and Weschler Individual Achievement Test—Second Edition (WIAT-II). In addition, the percentage of full-scale IQ scores falling below the 25th percentile was 57% in the CKD group as compared with 15% in the control group.

While academic achievement is adversely affected by cognitive deficits and school absences, the prevalence of youth with CKD receiving special education services (6%–21%) is similar to U.S. national data (Gerson et al., 2006). Studies reporting higher numbers of children with CKD receiving special education services have included children with comorbidities (prematurity, genetic syndromes) or were conducted prior to recent improvements in medical care.

Not surprising, children with ESRD and their parents report lower health-related quality of life across all domains including physical health, psychosocial health, emotional functioning, social functioning, and school functioning when compared to their healthy peers (Goldstein et al., 2006). Gerson et al.'s (2010) study of 402 children with mild to moderate CKD reported similar findings, with parent and child reporting lower health-related quality of life and poorer physical, social, emotional, and school functioning as compared with healthy youth.

Treatment and Management

Care of the child with CKD includes efforts to slow progression of kidney failure, correction of metabolic disturbances intrinsic to CKD, provision of nutritional and hormonal support for growth failure, and preparation for renal replacement therapy (Noe & Jones, 2007). Strategies to protect the kidney (renoprotective therapy) include controlling hypertension with dietary changes (salt and fluid restriction) and pharmacotherapy (diuretics and antihypertensive medication). Correction of anemia with iron supplementation and recombinant human erythropoietin may result in decreased fatigue and increased exercise tolerance, cardiovascular improvement, and better neurocognitive outcomes (Vogt & Avner, 2007).

When a child reaches ESRD, renal replacement therapy must be initiated. The ultimate goal for the vast majority of children with ESRD is successful kidney transplantation; however, when preemptive transplantation is not an option, peritoneal dialysis or hemodialysis is chosen based on on family preference and on technical, social, and compliance issues.

Outcome

There is no cure for CKD, and the progressive loss of kidney function will generally result in the development of ESRD during childhood or early adulthood. Improvements in the treatment of CKD (including renoprotective therapies, tight control of blood pressure, improved dialysis techniques, correction of anemia and metabolic disorders, and aggressive nutrition supplementation) have resulted in improved neurocognitive function and slowed renal disease progression.

SUMMARY

Through life-saving interventions, children with SCD, cancer, HIV, and chronic renal failure are largely surviving to adulthood. These diseases that were previously considered fatal now have shifted to the level of a chronic disease. Due to rapid medical advances, children surviving with these illnesses today are very different from those who survived even 10 years ago. In addition, continued innovations are leading to improved treatment and outcomes (Table 28.1). However, all of these children remain at increased risk for the spectrum of developmental disabilities resulting from their primary disease and/or complications and side effects of treatment. Interventions for their developmental problems as well as for their chronic diseases can enable them to lead productive lives.

REFERENCES

Armstrong, F.D., & Mulhern, R.K. (1999). *Acute lymphoblastic leukemia and brain tumors.* (pp. 47–77). New York, NY: Guilford Press.

Armstrong, F.D., Seidel, J.F., & Swales, T.P. (1993). Pediatric HIV infection: A neuropsychological and educational challenge. *Journal of Learning Disabilities, 26,* 92–103.

Table 28.1. Innovations in treatment

Disease/frequency	Neuro/developmental problems	Recent interventions will improve outcomes
Sickle cell disease 1: 2,647 births; 1: 396 African American births	Strokes, biopsychosocial risk, attention-deficit/ hyperactivity disorder, executive function	1) Hydroxyurea treatment (Rx)—has changed the face of this disease, daily oral nontoxic Rx yields dramatic decreases in occurrence of pain, acute chest syndrome, and hospitalizations 2) Transcranial doppler ultrasound screening of cerebral vessels beginning at age 2–3—identifies subgroup at high risk for stroke—leading to chronic transfusion Rx which yields a dramatic decrease in stroke occurrence 3) Bone marrow transplant—curative
Acute lymphocytic leukemia (ALL) annual incidence: 3.5: 100,000	Perceptual reasoning skills, working memory, processing speed, intellectual disability (20%)	1) Escalating-dose intravenous methotrexate has improved the event-free survival of children with ALL 2) High-dose intravenous methotrexate was superior to intermediate dose for children with high-risk ALL
Brain tumors annual incidence: 28: 1,000,000	Deficits in memory, sequencing, processing speed, visual perceptual ability, language skills	1) Improvements in neuroimaging and neurosurgical techniques have resulted in better staging of patients and better outcomes for some types of tumors 2) Creation of multidisciplinary neuro-oncology centers 3) Institution of and improvement in multi-institutional, cooperative group clinical research trial design and implementation allows for the definition of "standard of care" therapy via evidence based data. 4) An explosion of basic research identifying molecular fingerprints for various types of pediatric brain tumors hopefully will change approaches and improve outcomes
Human immunodeficiency virus (HIV) 100–200 births/year in USA	Patterns of developmental progressions: gradual loss of milestones, plateauing of development, developmental delays with static encephalopathy, mild neurocognitive delays	1) Recognition of the role of heightened inflammation and immune activation in HIV and their key role in HIV comorbidities (cardiovascular disease and malignancies) and mortality 2) Recognition of the high prevalence of persistent central nervous system infection with HIV and low grade dementia 3) Potent HIV cocktail regimens leading to maintenance of virologic suppression for more than a decade and decrease in mortality and morbidity
Chronic kidney disease (CKD) annual incidence: 15: 1,000,000	Memory difficulties, executive function deficits, full scale IQ <25th percentile in 57% of children	1) Recognition of the presence of masked hypertension and provision of more aggressive treatment 2) Recognition of the role of vitamin D in bone and cardiovascular health with improved interventions and outcomes 3) Recognition of the early development of atherosclerosis and the need to institute measures to control calcium and phosphorous balance

Armstrong, F.C., Thompson, R.J., Wang, W.C., Zimmerman, R., Pegelow, C.H., Miller, S., ... Vass, K. (1996). Cognitive functioning and brain magnetic resonance imaging in children with sickle cell disease. *Pediatrics, 97,* 864–70.

Barrera, M. (2005). Educational and social late effects of childhood cancer and related clinical, personal and familial characteristics. *American Cancer Society, 104,* 1751–1760.

Beebe, D.W., Ris, D., Armstrong, F.D., Fontanesi, J., Mulhern, R., Holmes, E., & Wisoff, J.H. (2005). Cognitive and adaptive outcome in low-grade pediatric cerebellar astrocytomas: Evidence of diminished cognitive and adaptive functioning in national collaborative research studies. (CCG 9891/POG 9130). *Journal of Clinical Oncology, 23,* 5198–5204.

Bonneau, J., Lebreton, J., Taque, S., Chappe, C., Bayart, S., Edan, C., Gandemer, V. (2011). School performance of childhood cancer survivors: Mind the teenagers! *The Journal of Pediatrics, 158,* 135–41.

Brouwers, P., Belman, A.L., & Epstein, L.G. (1994). CNS involvement: Manifestations, evaluation, and pathogenesis. In P.A. Pizzo, C.M. Wilfert (Eds.), *Pediatric AIDS: The challenge of HIV infection in infants, children, and adolescents* (pp. 433–455). Baltimore, MD: Williams and Wilkins.

Butler, R.W., Copeland, D.R., Fairclough, D.L., Mulhern, R.K., Katz, E.R., Kazak, A.E., ... Sahler, O.J. (2008). A multicenter, randomized clinical trial of a cognitive remediation program for childhood survivors of a pediatric malignancy. *Journal of Consulting and Clinical Psychology, 76,* 367–378.

Butler, R.W., & Haser, J.K. (2006). Neurocognitive effects of treatment for childhood cancer. *Mental Retardation and Developmental Disabilities Research Reviews, 12,* 184–191.

Butler, R.W., Sahler, O.J.Z., Askins, M.A., Alderfer, M.A., Katz, E.R., Phipps, S., & Noll, R.B. (2008). Interventions to improve neuropsychological functioning in childhood cancer survivors. *Developmental Disabilities Research Reviews, 14,* 251–258.

Butler, A.M., Williams, P.L., Howland, L.C., Storm, D., Seage, G.R., III, & Pediatric AIDS Clincial Trials Group 219C Study Team. (2009). Impact of disclosure of HIV infection on health-related quality of life among children and adolescents with HIV infection. *Pediatrics, 123,* 935–943.

Centers for Disease Control and Prevention. (2006). Achievements in public health. Reduction in perinatal transmission of HIV infection-United States, 1985-2005. *Morbidity Mortality Weekly Report, 55,* 592–597.

Chen, R., Pawlak, M.A., Flynn, T.B., Krejza, J., Herskovits, E.H., & Melhem, E.R. (2009). Brain morphometry and intelligence quotient measurements in children with sickle cell disease. *Journal of Developmental-Behavioral Pediatrics, 30,* 509–517.

Chiriboga, C.A., Fleishman, S., Champion, S., Gaye-Robinson, L., & Abrams, E.J. (2005). Incidence and prevalence of HIV encephalopathy in children with HIV infection receiving highly active antiretroviral therapy (HAART). *The Journal of Pediatrics 146,* 402–407.

Committee on Infectious Diseases of the American Academy of Pediatrics. (2009). Summaries of infectious diseases. In L.K. Pickering, C.J. Baker, D.W. Kimberlin, & S.S. Long (Eds.), *Red Book 2009 Report of the Committee on Infectious Diseases* (28th ed., pp. 203–739). Elk Grove Village, IL: American Academy of Pediatrics.

Conklin, H.M., Reddick, W.E., Ashford, J., Ogg, S., Howard, S.C., Morris, E.B., ... Khan, R.B. (2010). Long-term efficacy of methylphenidate in enhancing attention regulation, social skills, and academic abilities of childhood cancer survivors. *Journal of Clinical Oncology, 28,* 4465–4472.

Coscia, J.M., Christensen, B.K., & Henry, R.R. (1997). Risk and resilience in the cognitive functioning of children born to HIV-1-infected mothers: A preliminary report. *Pediatric AIDS and HIV Infection, 8,* 108–113.

Coscia, J.M., Christensen, B.K., Henry, R.R., Wallston, K., Radclife, J., & Rutstein, R. (2001). Effects of home environment, socioeconomic status, and health status on cognitive functioning in children with HIV-1 infection. *Journal of Pediatric Psychology, 26,* 321–329.

Cousens, P., Waters, B., Said, J., & Stevens, M. (1988). Cognitive effects of cranial irradiation of leukaemia: A survey and meta-analysis. *Journal of Child Psychology and Psychiatry, 29,* 839–852.

DeBaun, M.R., & Vichinsky, E. (2007). Hemoglobinopathies. In R.M. Kliegman, R.E. Behrman, H.B. Jenson, & B.F. Stanton (Eds.), *Nelson textbook of pediatrics* (18th ed., pp. 2025–2038). Philadelphia, PA: Saunders Elsevier.

De Boer, A.G.E.M., Verbeek, J.H.A.M., & van Dijk, F.J.H. (2006). Adult survivors of childhood cancer and unemployment a metaanalysis. *Cancer, 107,* 1–11.

de Martino, M., Tovo, P.A., Balducci, M., Galli, L., Gabiano, C., Rezza, G., & Pezzott, P. (2000). Reduction in mortality with availability of antiretroviral therapy for children with perinatal HIV-1 infection. *Journal of the American Medical Association, 284,* 190–197.

Duquette, P.J., Hooper, S.R., Wetherington, C.E., Icard, P.F., & Gipson, D.S. (2007). Brief report: Intellectual and academic functioning in pediatric chronic kidney disease. *Journal of Pediatric Psychology, 32,* 1011–1017.

Eaton, M.L., Haye, J.S., Armstrong, F.D., Pegelow, C.H., & Thomas, M. (1995). Hospitalizations for painful episodes: Association with school absenteeism and academic performance in children and adolescents with sickle cell anemia. *Issues in Comprehensive Pediatric Nursing, 18,* 1–9.

Enninful-Eghan, H., Moore, R.H., Ichord, R., Smith-Whitley, K., & Kwiakowski, J.L. (2010). Transcranial Doppler ultrasonography and prophylactic transfusion program is effective in preventing overt stroke in children with sickle cell disease. *The Journal of Pediatrics, 157,* 479–484.

Evans, G.W. (2004). The environment of childhood poverty. *American Psychology, 59,* 77–92.

Falletta, J.M., Woods, G.M., Verter, J.I., Buchanan, G.R., Pegelow, C.H., Iyer, R.V. ... Reid, C. (1995). Discontinuing penicillin prophylaxis in children with sickle cell anemia. Prophylactic Penicillin Study II. *Disability Rehabilitation, 127,* 685–690.

Furth, S.L., Cole, S.R., Moxey-Mims, M., Kaskel, F., Mak, R., Schwartz, G., ... Warady, B.A. (2006). Design and methods of the chronic kidney disease in children (CKiD) Prospective Cohort Study. *Clinical Journal of the American Society of Nephrology, 1,* 1006–1015.

Gerson, A.C., Butler, R., Moxey-Mims, M., Wentz, A., Shinnar, S., Lande, M.B., ... Hooper, S.R. (2006). Neurocognitive outcomes in children with chronic kidney disease: Current findings and contemporary endeavors. *Mental Retardation and Developmental Disabilities Research Reviews, 12,* 208–215.

Gerson, A.C., Wentz, A., Abraham, A.G., Mendley, S.R., Hooper, S.R., Butler, R.W., ... Furth, S.L. (2010). Health-related quality of life of children with mild to moderate chronic kidney disease. *Pediatrics, 125,* e349–e357.

Gipson, D.S., Hooper, S.R., Duquette, P.J., Wetherington, C.E., Stellwagen, K.K., Jenkins, T.L., & Ferris, M.E. (2006). Memory and executive functions in pediatric chronic kidney disease. *Child Neuropsychology, 12,* 391–405.

Gold J.I., Johnson, C.B., Treadwell, M.J., Hans, N., Vichinsky, E. (2008). Detection and assessment of stroke in patients with sickle cell disease: Neuropsychological functioning and magnetic resonance imaging. *Pediatric Hematology and Oncology, 25,* 409–421.

Goldstein, S.L., Graham, N., Burwinkle, T., Warady, B., Farrah, R., & Varni, J.W. (2006). Health-related quality of life in pediatric patients with ESRD. *Pediatric Nephrology, 21,* 846–850.

Gortmaker, S., Hughes, M., Cervia, J., Brady, M., Johnson, G.M., Seage, G.R., III, ... Pediatric AIDS Clinical Trials Group Protocol 219 Team. (2001). Effect of combination therapy including protease inhibitors on mortality among children and adolescents infected with HIV-1. *New England Journal of Medicine, 345,* 1522–1528.

Greenbaum, L.A., Warady, B.A., & Furth, S.L. (2009). Current advances in chronic kidney disease in children: Growth, cardiovascular, and neurocognitive risk factors. *Seminars in Nephrology, 29,* 425–434.

Hogan, A.M., Kirkham, F.J., Prengler, M., Telfer, P., Lane, R., Vargha-Khadem, F., & Haan, M. (2006). An exploratory study of physiological correlates of neurodevelopmental delay in infants with sickle cell anaemia. *British Journal of Haematology, 132,* 99–107.

Hoppe-Hirsch, E., Renier, D., Lellouch-Tubiana, A, Sainte-Rose, C., Pierre-Kahn, A., & Hirsch, J.F. (1990). Medulloblastoma in childhood: Progressive intellectual deterioration. *Childs Nervous System, 6,* 60–65.

Hudson, M. (1999). Late complications after leukemia therapy. In C.H. Pui (Ed.), *Childhood Leukemias* (pp. 463–481). Cambridge, MA: Cambridge University Press.

Iannone, R., Casella, J.F., Fuchs, E.J., Chen, A.R., Woolfrey, A., Amylon, M., ... Walters, M.C. (2003). Results of minimally toxic nonmyeloablative transplantation in patients with sickle cell anemia and beta-thalassemia. *Biology, Blood, & Marrow Transplantation, 9,* 519–528.

Instone, S.L. (2000). Perceptions of children with HIV infection when not told for so long: Implications for diagnosis disclosure. *Journal of Pediatric Health Care, 14,* 235–243.

Janzen, L.A., & Spiegler, B.J. (2008). Neurodevelopmental sequelae of pediatric acute lymphoblastic leukemia and its treatment. *Developmental Disabilities Research Reviews, 14,* 185–195.

Key, J.D., Brown, R.T., Marsh, L.D., Spratt, E.G., & Recknor, J.C. (2001). Depressive symptoms in adolescents with a chronic illness. *Children's Health Care, 30,* 283–292.

Kratovil, T., Bulas, D., Driscoll, M.C., Speller-Brown, B., McCarter, R., & Minniti, C.P. (2006). Hydroxyurea therapy lowers TCD velocities in children with sickle cell disease. *Pediatric Blood Cancer, 47,* 894–900.

Kuttesch, J.F. & Ater, J.L. (2007). Brain tumors in childhood. In R.M. Kliegman, R.E. Behrman, H.B.

Jenson, & B.F. Stanton (Eds.), *Nelson textbook of pediatrics* (18th ed., pp. 2128–2137). Philadelphia, PA: Saunders Elsevier.

Lopez-Vincente, M., Ortega-Gutierrez, S., Amlie-Lefond, C., & Torbey, M.T. (2010). Diagnosis and management of pediatric arterial ischemic stroke. *Journal of Stroke and Cerebralvascular Diseases, 19,* 175–183.

Madden, S.J., Ledermann, S.E., Guerrero-Blanco, M., Bruce, M., & Trompeter, R.S. (2003). Cognitive and psychosocial outcome of infants dialysed in infancy. *Child: Care, Health & Development, 29,* 55–61.

McConnell, M.S., Byers, R.H., Frederick, T., Peters, V.B., Dominguez, K.L., Sukalac, T., ... Pediatric Spectrum of HIV Disease Consortium. (2005). Trends in antiretroviral therapy use and survival rates for a large cohort of HIV-infected children and adolescents in the United States, 1989–2001. *Journal of Acquired Immune Deficiency Syndrome, 38,* 488–494.

McLoyd, V.C. (1998). Socioeconomic disadvantage and child development. *American Psychology, 53,* 185–204.

Mellins, C.A., Smith, R., O'Driscill, P., Magder, L.S., Brouwers, P., Chase, C., ... Matzen, E. (2003). High rates of behavioral problems in perinatally HIV-infected children are not linked to HIV disease. *Pediatrics, 111,* 384–393.

Mialky, E., Vagnoni, J., & Rutstein, R. (2001). School-age children with perinatally acquired HIV infection: Medical and psychosocial issues in a Philadelphia cohort. *Aids Patient Care and other Sexually Transmitted Diseases, 15,* 575–579.

Meyer, E.A., & Kieran, M.W. (2002). Psychological adjustment of 'surgery-only' pediatric neuro-oncology patients: A retrospective analysis. *Psycho-oncology, 11,* 74–79.

Mintz, M. (1999). Clinical features and treatment interventions for human immunodeficiency virus-associated neurologic disease in children. *Seminars in Neurology, 19,* 165–176.

Mitby, P.A., Borinson, L.L., Whitton, J.A. Zevon, M.A., Gibbs, I.C., Tersak, J.M., ... Childhood Cancer Survivor Study Steering Committee. (2003). Utilization of special education services and educational attainment among long-term survivors of childhood cancer: A report from the Childhood Cancer Survivor Study. *Cancer, 97,* 1115–1126.

Mitchell, W. (2001). Neurological and developmental effects of HIV and AIDS in children and adolescents. *Mental Retardation and Developmental Disabilities Research Reviews 7,* 211–216.

Mitsnefes, M.M., Kimball, T.R., Witt, S.A., Glascock, B.J., Khoury, P.R., & Daniels, S.R. (2003). Left ventricular mass and systolic performance in pediatric patients with chronic renal failure. *Circulation, 107,* 864–868.

Mulhern, R.K., Kahn, R.B., Kaplan, S., Helton, S., Christensen, R., Bonner, M., ... Reddick, W. (2004). Short-term efficacy of methylphenidates: A randomized, double-blind, placebo controlled trial among survivors of childhood cancer. *Journal of Clinical Oncology, 22,* 4795–4803.

Netson, K.L., Conklin, H.M., Ashford, J.M., Kahalley, L.S., Wu, S., & Xiong, X. (2011). Parent and teacher ratings of attention during a year-long methylphenidate trial in children treated for cancer. *Journal of Pediatric Psychology, 36,* 438–450.

Noe, H.N. & Jones, D.P. (2007). Care of the child with chronic renal insufficiency and end-stage renal disease. In Wein, A.J. (Ed.), *Campbell-Walsh urology* (9th ed., pp. 3230–3232). Philadelphia, PA: Saunders Elsevier.

Noll, R.B., Kiska, R., Reiter-Purtill, J., Gerhardt, C.A., & Vannatta, K. (2010). A controlled, longitudinal study of the social functioning of youth with sickle cell disease. *Pediatrics, 125*, e1453–1459.

Nozyce, M.L., Lee, S.S., Wiznia, A., Nachman, S., Mofenson, L.M., Smith, M.E., ...Pelton, S. (2006). A behavioral and cognitive profile of clinically stable HIV-infected children. *Pediatrics, 117*, 763–770.

Ohene-Frempong, K., Weinher, S.J., Sleeper, L.A., Miller, S.T., Embury, S., Moohr, J.W., ... Gill, F.M. (1998). Cerebrovascular accidents in sickle cell disease: Rates and risk factors. *Blood, 91*, 288–294.

Pearson, D.A., McGrath, N.M., Nozyce, M., Nichols, S.L., Raskino, C., Brouwers, P., ... Englund, J.A. (2000). Predicting HIV disease progression in children using measures of neuropsychological and neurological functioning. *Pediatrics, 106*(6), E76.

Peterson, C.C., Johnson, C.E.,Ramirez, L.Y. Huestis, S., Pai, A.L., Demaree, H.A., & Drotar, D. (2008). A meta-analysis of the neuropsychological sequelae of chemotherapy-only treatment for pediatric acute lymphoblastic leukemia. *Pediatric Blood and Cancer, 51*, 99–104.

Pegelow, C.H., Macklin, E.A. Moser, F.G., Wang, W.C., Bello, J.A., Miller, S.T., ... Kinney, T.R. (2002). Longitudinal changes in brain magnetic resonance imaging findings in children with sickle cell disease. *Blood, 99*, 3014–3018.

Pizzo, P.A., Eddy, J., Faloon, J., Balis, F.M., Murphy, R.F., Moss, H., ... Rubin, M. (1988). Effect of continuous intravenous infusion of zidovudine (AZT) in chillden with symptomatic HIV infection. *New England Journal of Medicine, 319*, 889–896.

Quinn, C.T., Rogers, Z.R., McCavit, T.L., & Buchanan, G.R. (2010). Improved survival of children and adolescents with sickle cell disease. *Blood, 115*, 3447–3452.

Qvist, E., Pihko, H., Fagerudd, P., Fagerudd, P., Valanne, L., Lamminranta, S., ... Holmberg, C. (2002). Neurodevelopmental outcome in high-risk patients after renal transplantation in early childhood. *Pediatric Transplantation, 6*, 53–62.

Radcliffe, J., Barakat, L.P., & Boyd, R.C. (2006). Family systems issues in pediatric sickle cell disease. In Brown, R.G. (Ed.), *Comprehensive handbook of childhood cancer and sickle cell disease* (pp. 469–513). New York, NY: Oxford University Press.

Ries, L.A.G., Eisner, M.P., Kosary, C.L., Hankey, B.F., Miller, B.A., Mariotto, A. ... Edwards, B.K. (Eds.). (2005). *SEER Cancer Statistics Review, 1975–2002.* Bethesda, MD: National Cancer Institute. Available at http://seer.cancer.gov/csr/1975 2002/, based on November 2004 SEER data submission, posted to the SEER web site 2005.

Schatz, J., Brown, R.T., Pascual, F.M., Hus, L., & DeBaum, M.R. (2001). Poor school and cognitive functioning with silent cerebral infarcts and sickle cell disease. *Neurology, 56*, 1109–1111.

Schatz, J., Finke, R.L., Kellett, J.M., & Kramer, J.H. (2002). Cognitive functioning in children with sickle cell disease: A meta-analysis. *Journal of Pediatric Psychology, 27*, 739–748.

Schatz, J., Finke, R., & Roberts, C.W. (2004). Interactions of biomedical and environmental risk factors for cognitive development: A preliminary study of sickle cell disease. *Journal of Developmental and Behavioral Pediatrics, 25*, 303–310.

Schatz, J., & McClellan C.B. (2006). Sickle cell disease as a neurodevelopmental disorder. *Mental Retardation and Developmental Disabilities Research Reviews, 12*, 200–207.

Section on Hematology/Oncology and Committee on Genetics. (2002). Health supervision for children with sickle cell disease. *Pediatrics, 1–9*, 526–535.

Serjeant, G.R. (1999). Sickle cell disease. In J.S. Lilleyman, I.M. Hann, & V.S. Blanchettte (Eds.), *Pediatric hematology*, pp. 219–229. London, England: Churchill Livingston.

Sherr, L., Mueller, J., & Varrall, R. (2009). A systematic review of cognitive development and child human immunodeficiency virus infection. *Psychology, Health & Medicine, 14*, 87–404.

Simpson, D.M. & Berger, J.R. (1996). Neurologic manifestations of HIV infection. *Medical Clinics of North America, 80*, 1363–1394.

Sohlberg, M.M., & Mateer, C.A. (1986). *Attention Processing Training (APT).* Puyallup, WA: Washington Association for Neuropsychological Research and Development.

Steele, R.G., Nelson, T.D., & Cole, B.P. (2007). Psychosocial functioning of children with AIDS and HIV infection: Review of the literature from a socioecological framework. *Journal of Developmental and Behavioral Pediatrics, 28*, 58–69.

Steinlin, M., Imfeld, S., Zulaft, P., Boltshauser, E., Lövblad, K.O., Ridolfi Lüthy, A., ... Kaufmann, F. (2003). Neuropsychological long-term sequelae after posterior fossa tumor resection during childhood. *Brain, 126*, 1998–2008.

Thompson, Jr., R.J., Armstrong, F.D., Link, C.L., Pegelow, C.H., Moser, F., & Wang, W.C. (2003). A prospective study of the relationship over time of behavior problems, intellectual functioning, and family functioning in children with sickle cell disease: A report from the cooperative study of sickle cell disease. *Journal of Pediatric Psychology, 28*, 59–65.

Thompson, R.J., Gustafson, K.E., Bonner, M.J., & Ware, R.E. (2002). Neurocognitive development of young children with sickle cell disease through three years of age. *Journal of Pediatric Psychology, 27*, 235–244.

Tubergen, D.G., & Bleyer, A. (2007). The leukemias. In R.M. Kliegman, R.E. Behrman, H.B. Jenson, & B.F. Stanton (Eds.), *Nelson textbook of pediatrics* (18th ed., pp. 2025–2038). Philadelphia, PA: Saunders Elsevier.

U.S. Department of Health and Human Services. (1993). Screening, diagnosis, management, and counseling in newborns and infants. *Clinical Practice Guideline* No. 6. AHCRP Pub. No. 93-05562. Rockville, MD: Agency for Health Care Policy and Research, Public Health Service.

United States Renal Data System. (2010). *USRDS 2010 annual data report: Atlas of chronic kidney disease and end-stage renal disease in the United States.* Bethesda, MD: National Institutes of Health, National Institute of Diabetes and Digestive and Kidney Diseases.

Vogt, B.A., & Avner, E.D. (2007). Chronic kidney disease. In: R.M. Kliegman, R.E. Behrman, H.B. Jenson, & B.F. Stanton (Eds.), *Nelson textbook of pediatrics* (18th ed., pp. 2210–2213). Philadelphia, PA: Saunders Elsevier.

Wang, C.J., Kavanagh, P.L., Little, A.A., Holliman, J.B., & Sprinz, P.G. (2011). Quality-of-care indicators for children with sickle cell disease. *Pediatrics, 128*, 484–493.

Wang, W., Enos, L., Gallagher, D., Thompson, R., Guarini, L., Vichinsky, E., ... Cooperative study of sickle cell disease. (2001). Neuropsychologic performance in school-aged children with sickle cell disease: A report for the cooperative study of sickle cell disease. *The Journal of Pediatrics, 139,* 391–397.

Warady, B.A., Beldon, B. & Kohaut, E. (1999). Neurodevelopmental outcome of children initiating peritoneal dialysis in early infancy. *Pediatric Nephrology, 13,* 759–765.

Warady, B.A., & Chadha, V. (2007). Chronic kidney disease in children: The global perspective. *Pediatric Nephrology, 22,* 1999–2009.

Willen, E.J. (2006). Neurocognitive outcomes in pediatric HIV. *Mental Retardation and Developmental Disabilities Research Reviews, 12,* 223–228.

Yogev, R, & Chadwick, E.G. (2007). Acquired immunodeficiency syndrome (human immunodeficiency virus). In R.M. Kliegman, R.E. Behrman, H.B. Jenson, & B.F. Stanton (Eds.), *Nelson textbook of pediatrics* (18th ed., pp. 1427–1443). Philadelphia, PA: Saunders Elsevier.

Zhang, Y., Zou, P., Mulhern, R.K., Butler, R.W., Laningham, F.H., & Ogg, R.J. (2008). Brain structural abnormalities in survivors of pediatric posterior fossa brain tumors: A voxel-based morphometry study using free-form deformation. *Neuroimaging, 42,* 218–229.

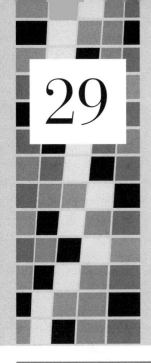

29

Behavioral and Psychiatric Disorders in Children with Disabilities

Adelaide Robb

Upon completion of this chapter, the reader will

■ Understand that individuals with developmental disabilities have a relatively high prevalence of psychiatric disorders

■ Be able to describe the types and symptoms of psychiatric disorders among people with developmental disabilities

■ Be able to discuss interventions in children who have a dual diagnosis of a developmental disability and a psychiatric disorder

Children with developmental disabilities manifest the same range of psychiatric illnesses that typically developing children do, but they may also face psychiatric illnesses specific to their disorder. The presence of a developmental disability, especially intellectual disability, often alters the symptomatic presentation of psychiatric disorders and makes accurate diagnosis more difficult. Recognition of these problems in children with "dual diagnoses" (i.e., a developmental disability and a psychiatric disorder) is crucial for caregivers. When these psychiatric disorders go unrecognized or untreated, affected children can fail in educational and social settings, be unmanageable at home, and show aggression and self-injury. These comorbid conditions may ultimately determine the child's outcome and placement. If the condition is identified early, however, treatment can be started and long-term adverse effects minimized. It is a challenge for parents and individuals working with children with developmental disabilities to be alert to the possible presence

of a psychiatric disorder and obtain early assessment, diagnosis, and treatment. This chapter addresses the identification and treatment of behavioral and psychiatric disorders in children with disabilities; it also discusses developmental transitions and their effect on behavior.

■■■■ WILLIAM

William, age 15, has Asperger's Disorder, attention-deficit/hyperactivity disorder (ADHD), and obsessive-compulsive disorder (OCD). He was in a special educational setting for high school students with Asperger's Disorder and was being treated with two **antipsychotic medications** (risperdal and **quetiapine**), a mood stabilizer (valproate), a **stimulant** (methylphenidate), and the **selective serotonin reuptake inhibitor** (SSRI; fluoxetine). He had been stable for a long period with resolution of his previous psychiatric symptoms, so the family asked that his medication regimen be simplified. In consultation with his family, the child psychiatrist began slowly tapering off the mood stabilizer, antipsychotic medications, and SSRI. Eight months into this process he was off all medications except methylphenidate. However, the school and parents were motivated to consult with the psychiatrist again after they noted that William had become withdrawn and sad for 4 weeks. He was crying at school, not eating lunch or dinner, no longer playing or reading his favorite books, not sleeping at night, and saying that he was a bad person who should be dead. The psychiatrist restarted William on a higher dose of fluoxetine (which had originally been prescribed to treat his OCD symptoms). Over the following 2 weeks, William started smiling and eating again. His sleep improved, and he was back to being himself by the end of the 6th week on fluoxetine. His "simplified" medication regimen now consists of fluoxetine and methylphenidate.

PREVALENCE OF PSYCHIATRIC DISORDERS AMONG CHILDREN WITH DEVELOPMENTAL DISABILITIES OF SPECIFIC ETIOLOGIES

In their landmark study of the epidemiology of childhood psychiatric disorders on the Isle of Wight, Rutter, Graham, and Yule (1970) found emotional disturbances in 7%–10% of typically developing children. In contrast, 30%–42% of children with intellectual disability demonstrated psychiatric disorders (Rutter et al., 1970). In a Swedish study, Gillberg et al. (1986) found that 57% of children and adolescents with mild intellectual disability and 64% with severe intellectual disability met diagnostic criteria for a psychiatric disorder. Additional studies have confirmed these results; children with intellectual disabilities have a 4–5 fold higher rate of psychiatric disorders than typically developing peers and that higher rate does not diminish as the children grow into adolescence (Calles 2008; Feinstein & Chahal 2009).

In examining specific neurodevelopmental disorders, it is apparent that patients can have different rates of psychiatric disorders (see Table 29.1). In children with velocardiofacial syndrome (*22q11.2* deletion syndrome), the most common behavioral/psychiatric disorders are ADHD (25%–46%), major depressive disorder (MDD) (12%–20%), and anxiety disorders including specific phobias (27%–61%). In

adults with *22q11.2* deletion 32% experienced psychotic symptoms and 41% had depression (Antshel et al., 2006; Arnold et al., 2001; Feinstein et al., 2002; Green, 2009). Both boys and girls with fragile X syndrome have higher rates of social anxiety than typically developing peers. Affected girls have higher rates of depression, and affected boys have higher rates of aggression (Bailey et al., 2008; Baumgardner et al., 1995; Einfeld et al., 1994). In children with fragile X syndrome, the rates of anxiety were reported to be as high as 42% when teachers were asked to rate symptoms; parents noted anxiety in 26% of the same children (Sullivan et al., 2007). In girls with fragile X syndrome, the rates of mood disorders were found to be 47%, with major depression representing half of those disorders (Freund et al., 1993). Rates of bipolar disorder, however, are lower in children with fragile X than in the general population (Hessl et al., 2001). Up to 58% of boys with fragile X syndrome can exhibit self-injurious behavior, with 72% of them biting hands and fingers (Symons et al., 2003).

Children with trisomy 21 (Down syndrome) have increased rates of behavioral disorders; 20%–40% exhibit aggression and ADHD versus 5%–8% ADHD in typically developing children. Adults are at increased risk for dementia and withdrawal depression compared to typically developing adults. In trisomy 21, conduct disorder (CD) and oppositional defiant disorder (ODD) occur at comparable rates to the general population (12%), while autism occurs in about 10% versus <1% in the general population (Dykens, 2007; Myers et al., 1995; Prasher et al., 1995; Visootsak et al., 2007; see Chapter 21).

In children with Prader-Willi syndrome, the occurrence of OCD symptoms varies according to the molecular defect. Long type I *15q* deletions have compulsive cleaning (e.g., grooming and showering); short type II *15q* deletions have academic OCD symptoms (e.g., rereading, erasing, and counting; Zarcone et al., 2007). Prader-Willi is also associated with higher rates of bipolar disorder: 15%–17%, versus 2%–5% in the typically developing; and mood disorders with psychotic features in 28% versus 0.4% in the general population (Boer et al., 2002; Vogels et al., 2004). Adolescents with Turner syndrome (XO) have high rates of social phobia and shyness, with anxiety and mood swings becoming evident in adulthood (Catinari et al., 2006; Siegel et al., 1998). Almost half of individuals with XXYY have major depression (Tartaglia et al., 2008).

Table 29.1. Percentages of mental illness by developmental disability

Population	MI	ADHD	ODD	CD	MDD	BPD	SZ/PSY	AXD	PH	GAD	SIB	ASD
General	7–10	5–8	6–10	2–9	3.3–11.2	2–5	1.1	6–25	.6–15	.4–1.0	<1	<1
DD	30–42		48									
Mild ID	57										5	
Severe ID	64											
VCF-child		25–46			12–20			27–61				
VCF-adult					41		32					
FRX								26–42				
FRX-girl					47 mood half MDD							
FRX-boy											58	
TR21		20–40	12	12								10
PWS						15–17						
TS								High SP				
XXYY					50							
FAE				50		33–35						
FAS					18	33–35			54	12		
WS	80	65										

Key: DD, developmental disability; ID, intellectual disability; VCF, velocardiofacial syndrome; FRX, fragile X; TR21, Trisomy 21; PWS, Prader-Willi syndrome; TS, Turner syndrome; FAE, fetal alcohol exposure; FAS, fetal alcohol syndrome; WS, Williams syndrome; MI, mental illness; ADHD, attention-deficit/hyperactivity disorder; ODD, oppositional defiant disorder; CD, conduct disorder; MDD, major depressive disorder; BPD, bipolar disorder; SZ/PSY, schizophrenia/psychotic disorder; AXD, anxiety disorder; PH, phobia; GAD, generalized anxiety disorder; SIB, self-injurious behavior; ASD, autism spectrum disorder; SP, social phobia.

In children who have prenatal exposure to alcohol but without features of fetal alcohol syndrome (FAS; see Chapter 3), rates of CD are as high as 50% (Burd et al., 2003). For children with FAS, both suicide and depression rates are elevated. Up to half attempt suicide, and major depression is found in approximately 18% of those exposed to alcohol *in utero* (Burd et al., 2003; O'Connor et al., 2002). For those with fetal alcohol spectrum disorder (including both FAS and prenatal alcohol exposure), rates of bipolar disorder range from 33%–35% (O'Connor et al., 2002).

In a comprehensive study of children with Williams syndrome, 80% were found to have one or more psychiatric disorders, the most common being ADHD (65%), followed by specific phobia (54%), and then generalized anxiety disorder (12%; Leyfer, 2006). As one example, a young adult with Williams syndrome was described in the literature as having a severe eating disorder which resulted from his thoughts of eating leading to constipation (Young, 2009).

CAUSES OF PSYCHIATRIC DISORDERS IN DEVELOPMENTAL DISABILITIES

Children with developmental disabilities are at risk for the same types of psychiatric disorders as typically developing children. In addition, certain maladaptive behavior disorders are found principally among individuals with severe to profound levels of intellectual disability. These behaviors include stereotypic movement disorder (i.e., repetitive, self-stimulating, nonfunctional motor behavior, which may include self-injurious behavior [SIB]) and pica (i.e., the persistent ingesting of nonfood items).

In some cases, the cause of a psychiatric disorder in individuals with developmental disabilities is the direct result of a biochemical abnormality. For example, in the inborn error of metabolism Lesch-Nyhan syndrome (see Appendix B), an abnormality in the dopamine neurotransmitter system causes affected individuals to exhibit a compulsive form of SIB (Zimmerman, Jinnah, & Lockhart, 1998). In other cases, conditions that affect the developing brain are risk factors for a psychiatric disorder. In addition to fetal alcohol exposure described above, congenital infections such as rubella (which is associated with autism spectrum disorders [ASDs]), and perinatal or neonatal hypoxic ischemic encephalopathy (brain disorders due to lack of oxygen or blood flow)

are associated with memory and language disorders (see Chapter 24). The increased risk of psychiatric disturbance due to neurobiological disorders may be attributable to factors such as irritability, affective instability, distractibility, and communication impairments (Feinstein & Reiss, 1996). Risk may also increase in the presence of conditions such as epilepsy, developmental language disorders, and sensory impairments, which are independently associated with an increased incidence of psychiatric disorders.

The cause of most psychiatric disorders among children with developmental disabilities is likely, however, to be a complex interaction among biological (including genetic), environmental, medical, and psychosocial factors. For example, a young man who has sustained a significant traumatic brain injury (see Chapter 26) with resulting cognitive impairment may regularly become depressed because of a combination of neurotransmitter changes due to brain injury, a familial predisposition to depression, his parents' grief, and his own despair over loss of previous abilities. Children with severe intellectual disability may develop SIB in response to an ear infection or constipation as they cannot verbally express feeling discomfort.

PSYCHIATRIC DISORDERS OF CHILDHOOD AND ADOLESCENCE

The following sections cover a number of psychiatric disorders; however, two important disorders, ASDs and ADHD, are not discussed here because separate chapters are devoted to them (see Chapters 21 and 22). It should be noted that in the *Diagnostic and Statistic Manual—Fifth Edition* (*DSM-5*; www.dsm-5.org) the American Psychiatric Association (APA) has proposed several criteria changes for diagnosing a number of disorders covered in this section. These are described as follows: Posttraumatic stress disorder (PTSD) in children will need only two symptoms of negative alterations in cognition and mood and two symptoms in arousal and reactivity. The trauma can be the loss of a parent and can be manifest as nonspecific frightening dreams, themes of trauma in play, or reenactment of the trauma. In pediatric eating disorders, less emphasis is placed on the strict diagnostic requirement of being < 85% of ideal body weight and having amenorrhea. The criteria now focus on previous weight and growth patterns and the impact of starvation on multiple organ systems, not just the reproductive system. A new disorder in children under consideration in *DSM-5* is temper dysregulation with dysphoria which is considered a milder condition than the classic combined oppositional defiant disorder and bipolar disorder. This proposed disorder describes children with persistent negative mood who have outbursts of rage.

Changes to other disorders will be described in each section.

Oppositional Defiant and Conduct Disorders

In order for a child to be diagnosed with oppositional defiant disorder (ODD), there must be a pattern of negative, hostile, and defiant behaviors (APA, 2011). Children must have angry/irritable moods, defiant/headstrong behaviors, and vindictiveness. In terms of the persistence and frequency used to differentiate normative and symptomatic behavior, there are different standards for under-5 and over-5 children. Under-5 children should show these behavior problems most days for at least 6 months, while over-5 children should show such problems at least once a week for at least 6 months. Developmental level, gender, and culture must also be considered in making the diagnosis, and these behaviors must occur outside of a psychotic or mood disorder. They must cause impairments in social, educational, or vocational activities and may occur in one or multiple settings. This diagnosis is usually given to preadolescent children.

To be diagnosed with a conduct disorder (CD), an individual must demonstrate a pattern of callous and unemotional behavior in which other people's rights are violated, norms are ignored, or rules are broken, and it must have continued for at least 12 months. The four main problem areas are 1) aggression toward people and animals, 2) destruction of property, 3) deceitfulness or theft, and 4) serious violation of rules. Some examples of aggression include bullying and threatening, starting physical fights, using a weapon in fights, being physically cruel to people or animals, stealing while confronting a victim, and forcing someone into unwanted sexual activity. Destruction includes deliberate fire-setting or vandalism or destruction of property. Deceitfulness or theft includes breaking into a house or car, lying to obtain goods or services, and stealing or shoplifting. Serious violation of rules includes staying out at night (but not overnight) before age 13, running away from home overnight at least twice, and frequent truancy from school before age 13. CDs are rarely diagnosed in preadolescent children. If a child meets criteria for CD, he or she does not receive a concurrent diagnosis of ODD. Both ODD and CD occur at higher rates in children with developmental disabilities than in typically developing children, 48% versus 6%–10% ODD and 2%–9% CD in nonclinical populations (Hardan et al., 1997).

Both of these disorders are often associated with ADHD, and the treatment for one may improve the condition of the other (Kutcher et al., 2004). Treatment of both CD and ODD includes the same behavior management techniques useful in ADHD. Similarly, both disorders may benefit from stimulant and other ADHD medications (Connor, Barkley, & Davis, 2000). Among the latter medications are 1) atomoxetine (Strattera), a norepinephrine reuptake inhibitor that is effective at higher doses for children and adolescents with ADHD comorbid with ODD or CD (Newcorn et al., 2005); and 2) long-acting guanfacine (Intuniv), an α-2 receptor antagonist, which also helps control ADHD with comorbid ODD/CD (Connor et al., 2010). A long-acting form of clonidine (Kapvay), another α-2 receptor antagonist, is now approved for ADHD monotherapy in 6–17 year olds (Jan 2011).

Although all categories of ADHD medication (stimulants, norepinephrine reuptake inhibitors, and α-2 receptor agonists), can help when ADHD is comorbid with ODD/CD, behavioral therapy is the preferred treatment for ODD and CD. Behavioral therapy involves setting consistent limits, behavioral expectations, and consequences (see Chapter 32). This intervention must be consistent at home and school so that the child knows that the rules and expectations are in force in all settings. For younger children, a positive reinforcement system employing stickers and/or a behavior chart, targeting being respectful and following directions, can cover most daily rules and activities. For older children and adolescents, tokens are commonly used to reinforce appropriate behavior. These can be traded for desired activities, such as an extra 30 minutes of television or free computer time. In this way, adolescents earn and pay for their privileges in the same way that adults earn money to buy what they need or want.

Impulse Control Disorders

These disorders include intermittent explosive disorder and hair-pulling disorder. Intermittent explosive disorder is diagnosed after several discrete episodes of failure to resist aggressive impulses, with resultant assaults or destruction of property. The severity of the assault must be out of proportion to the precipitating psychosocial stressor. An example might be a child who is told that he cannot have cake until he has finished his lunch. The child then throws his plate across the room, breaks his chair, and starts kicking his little sister over the incident. Treatment of intermittent explosive disorder in adults includes the use of beta-blockers such as propranolol, certain antiepileptic/mood stabilizing drugs (e.g., valproic acid [Depakote]), and novel antipsychotics (e.g., risperidone [Risperdal]; Hässler & Reis, 2010). Children with mild to moderate intellectual disability are more likely to have this disorder than their typically developing peers.

An individual fits the profile for hair pulling disorder, historically called trichotillomania, when it results in noticeable hair loss; this can be anywhere on the body. It should not be associated with an underlying skin or physical condition causing hair loss. Consultation with a dermatologist to rule out skin problems such as tinea capitis (ringworm), which can cause hair loss, may be appropriate. A child with this disorder feels tension that makes the child pull out the hair, which is followed by a sense of relief after doing it. Children who have hair pulling disorder may eat the hair, which can cause bezoars (hair balls) in the stomach or gastrointestinal track that need to be surgically or endoscopically removed. In children with hair loss, it is important to ask the parent and child if the child is pulling out and eating hair. Treatment of this disorder is similar to that for OCD, with the use of SSRIs (e.g., fluoxetine) and cognitive-behavioral therapy. This hair pulling is seen on the spectrum of OCD in contrast to other forms of self-mutilation, such as self-cutting seen in teenagers, which fall on the mood and personality disorder spectrums.

Anxiety Disorders

Anxiety disorders include the *DSM-IV-TR* classifications generalized anxiety disorder, panic disorder, social anxiety disorder, OCD, and PTSD. In *DSM-5* skin-picking disorder has been added (APA, 2011). Anxiety disorders not discussed in this section include separation anxiety, where children become anxious when away from family or the home, and simple phobias such as being frightened of needle sticks or the dark.

Generalized Anxiety Disorder

The diagnosis of generalized anxiety disorder requires at least 3 months of excessive anxiety and worry most days about two or more of family, health, finances, and school or work (APA, 2011). The child has difficulty controlling the worry and has accompanying symptoms including restlessness or feeling keyed up, quick fatigue, problems concentrating, irritability, muscle tension, and disturbed sleep. The child also shows marked avoidance of, or marked time and effort spent, preparing for situations with potentially negative outcomes. In addition, the child procrastinates in behavior or decision-making due to worries and needs repeated reassurances. The child has problems at home or school because of the anxiety and the anxiety is unrelated to another psychiatric or medical illness. Treatment includes cognitive-behavioral therapy to reduce worry and at times medication such as SSRIs. Several studies have shown that medications are effective for pediatric anxiety including sertraline for generalized anxiety disorder in children (Rynn, Siqueland, & Rickels, 2001) and fluvoxamine (Luvox) for generalized anxiety disorder, social phobia, and separation anxiety disorder (Walkup et al., 2001). More recently, a large NIMH study demonstrated that a combination of sertraline and cognitive-behavioral therapy had the best outcome in treating anxiety disorders found in children (Walkup et al., 2008).

Panic Disorder

To meet diagnostic criteria for panic disorder a person must have one or more panic attacks that include at least four of the symptoms listed in Table 29.2. People with panic disorder have panic attacks that recur, are unexpected, and combine with worry about having more panic attacks, worry about the consequence of an attack (e.g., that the child might die or go crazy), or a significant change in behavior due to the attacks (e.g., stopping exercising because of a fast heartbeat, rapid breathing, and sweating—feeling like a heart attack). Because panic attack symptoms can mimic other disorders such as heart problems, stomach disorders, seizures, and asthma, appropriate treatment is often delayed while other medical causes are ruled out. In patients with panic disorder, other family members also have or have had a history of anxiety disorder or panic attacks.

Panic attacks do not usually begin until puberty. Adolescents with panic disorder may begin to avoid certain places or situations such as crowds, public transportation, and other places where a panic attack could occur. This maladaptive change in behavior can lead to

Table 29.2. Symptoms of panic disorder

1. Rapid or racing heartbeat
2. Sweating, trembling, or shaking
3. Feeling short of breath or as if being smothered
4. Feeling as if choking
5. Chest pain or discomfort
6. Nausea or abdominal distress
7. Feeling dizzy, lightheaded, or faint
8. Feeling of unreality or detachment (like floating or in a dream)
9. Fear of losing control or going crazy
10. Fear of dying
11. Numbness and tingling
12. Hot flashes or chills

Note: At least four symptoms need to be present during an attack for a diagnosis of panic disorder.

avoiding exercise or unfamiliar situations or, in extreme cases, to comorbid agoraphobia (fear of leaving the house). Patients with panic disorder can be treated with high-potency benzodiazepines such as alprazolam (Xanax) and clonazepam (Klonopin) alone or in combination with SSRIs. Patients with panic disorder can also be helped through cognitive-behavioral therapy to develop a list of things that are least to most likely to cause a panic attack. Patients then work their way through the list, facing the different issues that cause the attacks. The therapist helps the adolescent devise strategies to temper or overcome the attacks in real time and observes how the anxiety decreases over time.

Social Anxiety Disorder

A phobia particularly relevant to children is social anxiety disorder, which includes school phobia. In this disorder there is an intense fear (phobia) of acting in a way or showing anxiety symptoms that will be negatively evaluated. The fear is out of proportion to the actual danger posed by the social situation. For children, social anxiety disorder may result in not only making excuses to avoid school but also practicing *selective mutism* in which the child does not speak at all in school but speaks normally in other situations.

Social phobia involves a marked and persistent fear of one or more social or performance situations in which a person is exposed to strangers or to scrutiny by others and worries about possibly doing something embarrassing. A diagnosis for this disorder involves a child having appropriate relationships with family members and friends but being afraid of other peers and adults. Exposure to the social situation (e.g., a birthday party) provokes anxiety and the child may cry, have a tantrum, freeze, or shrink from situations with unfamiliar people. The child may not be aware that the fear is unreasonable, and the fear must impair social functioning. Social phobia is classified as generalized if it takes place in multiple settings, and the symptoms must last for more than 6 months. Treatment includes cognitive-behavioral therapy to reduce anxiety in social situations, speech-making and acting classes for people with performance anxieties, and the use of SSRIs. Children with extreme cases of social phobia are too frightened to speak in the classroom, eat in the cafeteria, or use the restroom at school. This can markedly impair school performance and should not be dismissed as simple shyness. Some children with a variant of social phobia may, like children with social anxiety disorder, have selective mutism, in which they refuse to speak to unfamiliar people or children; SSRIs may be helpful in this case (Black & Udhe, 1994). Girls with fragile X syndrome have been found to have severe shyness that may be a manifestation of social phobia (Hagerman et al., 1992).

Obsessive-Compulsive Disorder

A child with OCD has obsessions, compulsions, or both. Obsessions are recurrent thoughts, images, or impulses that are experienced as intrusive and inappropriate and cause anxiety or distress. The obsessions are not excessive worries about real-life problems (as in generalized anxiety), and individuals attempt to ignore, suppress, or neutralize the obsessions. Children may not be aware that the obsessions and compulsions are unreasonable; furthermore, children with a developmental disability may not realize that the obsessions are a product of the mind. Compulsions are repetitive behaviors (e.g., hand washing) or mental acts (e.g., praying, counting) that are done to neutralize an obsession or as part of following rigid rules. A child with obsessions about germs would have washing compulsions to neutralize the germs. The compulsions are designed to reduce distress or to prevent some dreaded act. For example, a child might refuse to step on green tiles in the school corridor because the child believes his or her mother might die if the child stepped on green tiles. Children, especially younger ones, are more likely to have compulsions without the accompanying obsessions; thus, a child might have an elaborate 2-hour bedtime ritual without self-awareness regarding why their bedtime ritual is that certain way.

Some children develop the rapid onset of OCD after a streptococcal skin or throat infection referred to as PANDAS. Pediatric autoimmune neuropsychiatric disorders associated with *Streptococcus* infections (PANDAS; Swedo et al., 1998) describes a subset of childhood OCDs and tic disorders triggered by group-A beta-hemolytic *Streptococcus pyogenes* infection. Like adult OCD, PANDAS is associated with basal ganglia dysfunction.

Common compulsions in children include ordering and arranging, counting, tapping, touching, and collecting/hoarding. Since nearly all children exhibit some or all of such behaviors during development, in order to meet criteria for the diagnosis, the obsessions and compulsions must consume more than 1 hour per day and interfere with functioning.

The definition also includes a level of insight by the child for the irrationality of the OCD. Individuals with chronic tic disorder may exhibit OCD symptoms, and children with ASD may exhibit OCD-like rigidity and repetitive, compulsive behaviors (see Chapter 21).

Treatment of OCD in children and adolescents includes cognitive-behavioral therapy, which is aimed at experiencing the obsessive thought without carrying out the compulsion designed to reduce the anxiety. This form of cognitive-behavioral therapy is called exposure-and-response prevention. A child with fear of germs would be asked to touch a doorknob but then be forbidden to wash his or her hands. Children have weekly assignments in this therapy. Several medications are also approved for the treatment of OCD in children including clomipramine (Anafranil), sertraline (Zoloft), fluoxetine (Prozac), and fluvoxamine (Luvox) (DeVaugh-Geiss et al., 1992; Geller et al., 2001; March et al., 1998; Riddle et al., 2001). One paper in the literature described the difference in outcome among children with OCD who were treated with one of four treatments sertraline, placebo, cognitive-behavioral therapy, or a combination of medication and therapy (POTS Team, 2004); of those, combination therapy helped the most children, followed by cognitive-behavioral therapy alone, then sertraline, and placebo. OCD can be comorbid with other developmental disabilities, especially ADHD and ASDs.

Posttraumatic Stress Disorder

PTSD is an anxiety disorder that occurs after exposure to a traumatic event in which the person experiences or witnesses an actual or threatened death, serious injury, or (in the case of a child) the loss of a parent or other attachment figure. In children with developmental disabilities, PTSD may occur after physical abuse or after the injury that caused the disability. Children with intellectual disability are particularly at risk for PTSD, as they have more limited coping skills. The child responds to the inciting event with intense fear, helplessness, or horror and may have disorganized or agitated behavior. A child with diagnosis of PTSD must have symptoms for at least one month and have impaired functioning. The symptoms are broken down into three categories 1) reexperiencing the trauma, 2) avoidance and numbing, and 3) increased arousal. Reexperiencing behavior includes recurrent recollections of the event (in children, this may manifest as a repetitive theme in play), dreams of the event (children may have distressing dreams that are not trauma-specific), flashbacks of the event (children may reenact the trauma), intense mental distress at physical or mental cues that remind the child of the event, and physiological reactivity on exposure to cues that remind the child of the event. Avoidance behavior includes efforts to avoid thoughts or feelings associated with the trauma, efforts to avoid people and places associated with the trauma, inability to recall important aspects of the trauma, decreased interest or participation in activities, feelings of detachment or estrangement, restricted range of feelings, and a sense of a shortened future. Symptoms of increased arousal include difficulty sleeping, irritability or angry outbursts, difficulty concentrating, hypervigilance, and an exaggerated startle response. PTSD is characterized by duration, either acute (3 months or less) or chronic (more than 3 months), and by delayed onset (starts 6 months after the trauma).

Treatment of PTSD has included both psychotherapy and SSRIs (March et al., 1998). The largest controlled trial of the SSRI sertraline in PTSD failed to show that medication was superior to placebo (Robb et al., 2010). Other studies have shown that trauma-focused cognitive-behavioral therapy shows the best efficacy in youth with PTSD (Smith et al., 2007). Patients must practice talking through the thoughts and events that remind them of the incident that elicited the PTSD. Play therapy, in which a child has a chance to relive and triumph over the trauma, may also help work through the loss. Therapy must be based on the cognitive level of the child.

Skin Picking Disorder

In this anxiety disorder, skin picking results in actual skin lesions. It also causes clinically significant distress or impairment in social, occupation, or other important areas of function. Medical afflictions (e.g., scabies) and other psychiatric disorders (e.g., psychosis) must be eliminated from consideration to make this diagnosis.

Mood Disorders

Major Depression

Children carrying a diagnosis of major depression must have a 2-week period with at least five of the following symptoms that represent a change from previous functioning: 1) depressed mood by subjective report or as observed by others (children and adolescents may have an irritable mood), 2) decreased interest or pleasure in most activities, 3) significant change in weight or appetite (children may fail to make expected weight gains), 4) insomnia or hypersomnia (excessive sleep), 5) psychomotor agitation or retardation, 6) fatigue or loss of energy, 7) feelings of worthlessness or guilt, 8) decreased concentration or indecisiveness, and 9) recurrent thoughts of death and dying. Symptoms must not be due to bereavement and must cause impairment in the child's daily function.

A study of individuals with trisomy 21 and depression showed they were more likely to have crying, depressed appearance, hallucinations, vegetative symptoms (loss of sleep energy and appetite), mutism, and psychomotor retardation (Myers et al., 1995). Children with major depression can be treated with medication or psychotherapy or a combination of both. Studies have shown that several SSRIs are superior to a placebo in the treatment of depression (Emslie et al., 2002; Wagner et al., 2003; Wagner et al., 2004). A National Institute of Mental Health (NIMH) study found that for adolescents with major depression, placebo, and cognitive-behavioral therapy alone were similar in improvement, whereas fluoxetine was better, and fluoxetine plus cognitive-behavioral therapy had the best outcome (TADS Team, 2004).

Bipolar Disorder

Bipolar disorder consists of swings between depression and **mania/hypomania**. A manic episode consists of a distinct period of abnormally and persistently elevated, expansive, or irritable mood lasting at least 1 week. The mood disturbance must have three of the following symptoms if happy and four if irritable: 1) inflated self-esteem or grandiosity, 2) decreased need for sleep, 3) more talkative or pressured speech or vocalizations (in nonverbal children), 4) flight of ideas (idea moves from topic to topic) or racing thoughts, 5) distractibility, 6) increased goal-directed activity or psychomotor agitation, and 7) excessive involvement in pleasurable activities that have a high potential for painful consequences (e.g., sexual touching of self and others, drug use, spending sprees). Hypomania is a less severe set of symptoms than mania. A patient with hypomania would not need to be hospitalized, would have symptoms for less than 7 days, would only have two of the manic symptoms, or continue to do well at school and home despite silly goofy behavior.

Individuals with bipolar disorder are treated with mood stabilizers such as lithium or valproic acid (Depakote, which is also used as an antiepileptic drug; it is not approved for the treatment of bipolar disorder in children or adolescents). They may also benefit from antipsychotic medication such as risperidone (Risperdal), aripiprazole (Abilify), olanzapine (Zyprexa), quetiapine (Seroquel), and ziprasidone (Geodon) in conjunction with mood stabilizers or as monotherapy (use of antipsychotics alone rather than in combination with a primary mood stabilizer such as lithium or valproic acid). All of these medications except ziprasidone are FDA-approved for the treatment of bipolar disorder mixed or manic episodes in older children and teenagers. Children with bipolar disorder must have consistent bedtimes and routines so that lack of sleep does not precipitate either a manic or mixed episode.

Psychotic Disorders

Psychotic disorders (sometimes called "psychosis") consist of alterations in thinking or perceptions that are not connected with reality. The primary psychotic disorder is **schizophrenia**. The diagnosis of schizophrenia requires the presence of one or more of the following three symptoms for at least 6 months, with active symptoms for 1 month or less if treated:

1) **delusions** (fixed idiosyncratic false belief; e.g., that someone is following the person), 2) **hallucinations** (sensory perception without an environmental stimulus; e.g., hearing a voice when no one else is present), and 3) disorganized speech (APA, 2011). In children there will be an associated failure to achieve expected levels of interpersonal relationships and academic achievement.

Patients with a mood disorder or an ASD may have psychotic symptoms that are confused with the formal diagnosis of schizophrenia. An individual with ASD must have prominent delusions or hallucinations to meet the schizophrenia diagnosis in addition to ASD. Other medical conditions that can mimic schizophrenia include epilepsy, effects of an illegal drug, and brain tumors. Once the diagnosis of schizophrenia has been confirmed, treatment with antipsychotic drugs will reduce the delusions and hallucinations, thereby improving psychosocial functioning. Five atypical antipsychotic medications for schizophrenia are approved for adolescents 13 and up: aripiprazole, olanzapine (second line due to metabolic issues), quetiapine, paliperidone (Invega), and risperidone. Trials of ziprasidone for adolescent schizophrenia failed to show a benefit compared to placebo.

Eating Disorders

The three important types of eating disorders that occur in children with developmental disabilities are rumination, binge eating, and pica. In rumination, infants or young children repeatedly regurgitate without nausea or gastrointestinal illness for at least 1 month. Regurgitated food may be rechewed, reswallowed, or spit out. To meet the definition of rumination in the context of intellectual disability or ASD, regurgitation should be sufficiently frequent and severe to warrant independent clinical attention because it may instead be a self-stimulatory behavior in these children. Treatment includes behavioral interventions and the use of gastrointestinal motility agents (e.g., laxatives).

The second common eating disorder is binge eating, whereby the child has recurrent episodes of eating large amounts of food during short periods of time. Binge eating episodes demonstrate at least three of the following features: 1) eating much more rapidly than normal; 2) eating until feeling uncomfortably full; 3) eating large amounts of food when not feeling physically hungry; 4) eating alone because of embarrassment over how much one is eating; and 5) feeling disgusted with oneself, depressed,

or very guilty afterwards. The binge eating episodes should not occur exclusively during the course of anorexia, bulimia, or avoidant/restrictive food intake, and they must occur on average at least once a week for 3 months (APA, 2011). It should be emphasized that children who do binge risk choking to death. In Prader-Willi syndrome, binge eating is a frequent complication and contributes to the morbid obesity seen among individuals with Prader-Willi. Children with binge eating disorder need nutritional guidance and counseling, parental and school oversight of meals, limited access to food outside of meals, and an exercise routine. For some children with a severe binge eating disorder, admission to a long-stay residential setting with strict oversight of meals and activity levels can dramatically change the child's weight and improve the underlying medical condition. Untreated ADHD, especially in girls, has been found to place them at higher risk for binge eating in adolescence and young adulthood (Biederman, 2010).

Pica, the persistent craving and ingesting of nonfood items, is a typical behavior of toddlers. When a child older than 2 years displays pica, however, professionals should explore the possibility that the child has a psychiatric disorder or a nutritional deficiency. Also, pica in older children can also be a typical behavior of individuals with severe to profound intellectual disability. Pica from any cause described above can seriously affect a child's well-being. It can result in toxicity from ingested materials such as medications or lead-containing plaster or paint chips, and can physically damage the gastrointestinal tract. Behavior management techniques (see Chapter 32) have been found to be the most effective intervention for pica (McAdam et al., 2004).

Adjustment Disorders

These disorders involve the development of emotional or behavioral symptoms in response to an identifiable stressor and occur within 3 months of the onset of that stressor. The symptoms or behaviors are clinically significant and cause marked distress, in excess of what would be expected from exposure to the stressor, and are accompanied by significantly impaired social or occupational (academic) functioning. With the exception of an ASD, individuals with adjustment disorders do not have another major psychiatric disorder. Once the stressor ends, the symptoms do not persist for more than 6 months. Adjustment disorder with anxiety has symptoms such as nervousness, worry, or jitteriness or, in children, separation anxiety focused on parents. Adjustment disorder with depressed mood includes depression, tearfulness, or hopelessness as the predominant symptoms. Adjustment disorder with disturbances of conduct presents with significant problematic behaviors such as truancy, vandalism, reckless driving, or fighting. Finally, adjustment disorder with mixed disturbance of emotions and conduct includes anxiety or depression plus conduct symptoms.

Children with developmental disabilities may be at higher risk for adjustment disorders because they have limited coping skills and frequently have medical illnesses or require procedures that produce stress. When children with developmental disabilities enter the hospital for a medical procedure or illness, parents, caregivers, and health care providers must be prepared for exaggerated emotional and behavioral responses to being in the hospital and kept away from their normal routine. Children may cry, have tantrums, or act out; they may alternatively become quiet and withdrawn, refusing to eat or cooperate with staff. Patience and reassurance will generally help the child navigate the stressful situation and return to his or her baseline emotional and behavioral functioning. Interventions to help prevent and treat these adjustment disorders include allowing parents to stay overnight in the hospital and allowing the child to bring special bedding, pillows, transitional objects (e.g., security blankets), stuffed animals, or favorite books or games to improve the child's comfort in the hospital. Visits to the hospital or treatment center ahead of an admission may also help provide familiarity with new places and people, and thus diminish fear.

Maladaptive Behavior Disorders

Some individuals with severe to profound levels of intellectual disability develop behavioral symptoms that are qualitatively different from those seen in people without developmental disabilities. These symptoms, which include repetitive self-stimulating behavior and self-injurious behavior (SIB), rarely occur in typically developing children (Hardan et al., 1997).

Individuals who engage in SIB typically display a specific pattern for producing injury. They may bang their heads, bite their hands, pick at their skin, hit themselves with their fists, or poke their eyes. They may do this once or twice a day in association with tantrums, or as often as several hundred times an hour.

Tissue destruction, infection, internal injury, loss of vision, and even death may result. These behaviors may be accompanied by additional repetitive, stereotyped behaviors, such as hand waving and body rocking. When these repetitive behaviors interfere with activities of daily living or result in significant injury to the individual, a diagnosis of *stereotypic movement disorder* with SIB is made.

Although serious SIB occurs in fewer than 5% of people of all ages with intellectual disability, these behaviors cause enormous distress to the individuals and their caregivers, can result in severe bodily injury, and may lead to residential placement, separating the individual from the family and other community contacts. Some children with SIB also demonstrate severe aggressive behavior toward their caregivers or peers.

SIB is a puzzling and disturbing phenomenon that prompts asking why these individuals hurt themselves. Although no simple answer exists, there is evidence for both environmental and biological causes in the context of enormous individual variation (Buitelaar, 1993; Mace & Mauk, 1995; Schroeder et al., 1999). Some children exhibit SIB because it elicits a desired environmental outcome (i.e., **operant control**; Loschen & Osman, 1992). For example, a girl who is nonverbal but demonstrates head-banging will have that reinforced once she learns that this action captures the attention she craves. Other environmental factors that can reinforce SIB include access to desired items (e.g., food), avoidance of task demands (e.g., chores), and certain sensory effects (e.g., bright lights from eye pressing; Mace & Mauk, 1995). The inference that the sensations produced through self-induced painful stimulation may somehow be gratifying has led to the notion that SIB plays a role in regulating physiologic states such as arousal. Guess and Carr (1991) proposed a biobehavioral model in which the regulation of normal sleep, wake, and arousal patterns is delayed or disturbed in some individuals. These individuals then develop stereotypic movements and SIB as a way to self-regulate arousal in under- or overstimulating environments. There is also a relationship between SIB and pain in nonverbal children with severe cognitive impairment. They have been found to increase SIB during an ear infection, constipation, or other conditions associated with pain (Breau et al., 2003). Other biological factors are suggested by the increased prevalence of SIB in certain genetic syndromes, including de Lange syndrome, Lesch-Nyhan syndrome,

Prader-Willi syndrome, and Rett syndrome (see Appendix B). Psychiatric disorders such as ASDs, depression, mania, and schizophrenia are also risk factors for SIB. General medical conditions and medication side effects can be acute precipitants of SIB. For example, a painful middle-ear infection may lead to head banging. Evaluating any individual for the cause of SIB demands the systematic testing of a broad range of behavioral and biomedical hypotheses (Sternberg, Taylor, & Babkie, 1994).

Although the brain mechanisms underlying most forms of SIB remain unknown, several neurotransmitters are thought to be involved. These include dopamine, which mediates certain reinforcement systems in the brain; serotonin, the depletion of which is sometimes associated with violent behavior; gamma-aminobutyric acid (GABA), an inhibitory neurotransmitter; and opioids, the brain's natural painkillers (Verhoeven et al., 1999). The atypical antipsychotic risperidone has been found to be useful in treating SIB (Zarcone et al., 2001) together with applied behavior analysis. As of 2006, risperidone was FDA-approved for the treatment of violent and aggressive behavior, including SIB in individuals with autism. Also, by 2009 aripiprazole was approved for treating irritability and aggression in children and adolescents with autism (Robb et al., 2010).

VULNERABILITY

Individuals with developmental disabilities are at higher risk for psychiatric disorders than their typically developing peers for a variety of reasons, which include 1) higher rates for certain psychiatric disorders in specific syndromes (e.g., ADHD in Williams syndrome, irritability in ASD); 2) impairment in acquisition of age-dependant coping skills (e.g., some syndromes particularly affect skill development including trisomy 21, fragile X syndrome); 3) multiple hospital stays for treatment of associated medical problems (e.g., surgical releases of contractures in cerebral palsy); 4) physical differences readily seen by peers who may bully the child (e.g., facial features in trisomy 21, skin lesions in neurofibromatosis, morbid obesity in Prader-Willi syndrome); and 5) a family history of psychiatric disorders that adds to the genetic risk for mental illness in the child with developmental disability. When assessing patients with developmental disabilities for psychiatric symptoms the practitioner must also consider changes in school,

classmates, and living situations, including family members and pets; they all can be both strengths and vulnerabilities.

EVALUATION

Psychiatric needs can be met only if parents, teachers, and other staff who work with children with disabilities are aware that emotional disturbances may be present. Ideally, the referral for evaluation should be made to professionals (e.g., psychiatrists, psychologists, neurologists, developmental-behavioral pediatricians, neurodevelopmental pediatricians, social workers) with specific training, experience, and expertise in the psychiatric disorders of children with developmental disabilities. The goal of evaluation is to formulate an intervention plan based not only on the psychiatric diagnosis but also on the developmental level of the child, accompanying medical conditions, the family's strengths and challenges, and the needs and limitations of the settings where the child spends his or her time. Often this requires referral to a specialized tertiary care center with a multidisciplinary team, such as a university hospital. Less experienced mental health professionals who undertake such evaluations should have access to consultation from a specialized center.

The mental health professional first takes a detailed history of the current symptoms and problematic behaviors from parents or other caregivers. For example, recent changes in sleep pattern, appetite, or mood provide important evidence of depression. In addition, an individual and family medical history should be obtained. The family history may reveal, for example, other members with mood or anxiety disorders. A review of the individual's past medical and psychological assessments may indicate prior behavior or psychiatric problems. After taking the history, an interview is conducted posing both structured and open-ended questions to the child and parents. If impairments in communication and cognitive skills are significant, the professional can still gain important information from directly observing the child both alone and with parents (King et al., 1994). Input from the school and other care providers frequently helps clarify the diagnostic issues.

The evaluation should also focus on the social system and setting in which the psychiatric disorder occurs. Thus, the professional should evaluate the current level of family functioning by assessing 1) family members' ability to cope with the child's psychiatric disorder and therapy; 2) their current morale, problem-solving abilities, external social supports, and practical resources (e.g., finances, insurance); 3) the system of beliefs that sustains their efforts; and 4) the stability of the parents' relationship. It is important to understand how individual family members are reacting and adjusting to the child's underlying developmental disability as well as any current mental health problems (see Chapter 37).

Following the comprehensive interview, the child may be referred for psychological testing or behavioral assessment. Although standardized behavior rating scales are available, they are insufficient by themselves as diagnostic tools. A single, structured psychological testing instrument may not be able to cover the range of developmental levels and behavioral baselines exhibited by individuals with developmental disabilities. These instruments are important, however, for confirming or adding to information obtained from the history and interview. They can also be extremely helpful in measuring changes that occur during the course of intervention (Aman, Burrow, & Wolford, 1995; Demb et al., 1994; Linaker & Helle, 1994; Reiss &Valenti-Hein, 1994).

Standardized rating scales may be combined with a functional behavior analysis. This type of combined assessment is most useful regarding children with severe behavioral abnormalities for which specific family or behavior therapies are being considered. One of the more helpful rating scales, the Aberrant Behavior Checklist (ABC), can be completed by parents or caregivers, is normed on the developmentally disabled population, and tracks five subscales including irritability and hyperactivity (Aman, 1995). This scale can be given at baseline and then tracked over time to evaluate responses to interventions both pharmacologic and behavioral. Behavior analysis provides direct observation of the child in a natural setting, yielding a clear description of the abnormal behavior itself and its antecedents and consequences (see Chapter 32). Often, changes in a child's environment such as a new teacher, classmate, or bus driver or other changes in a child's routine can precipitate behavioral symptoms.

It is important to note that many symptoms of a psychiatric disorder can actually be caused by a variety of medical disorders and treatments. For example, hypothyroidism, common in individuals with Down syndrome, can cause emotional disturbances that present as anxiety or depression. In excessive (and sometimes therapeutic) dosages, drugs used to treat associated impairments such as epilepsy can cause symptoms of hyperactivity or depression (Alvarez, 1998). Careful evaluation for medical conditions or drug reactions should be a part of any assessment of new-onset behavioral or psychiatric symptoms.

After the evaluations have been completed, the professional can start formulating an intervention plan based not only on the psychiatric diagnosis but also on the child's developmental level, accompanying medical conditions, the family's strengths and challenges, and the needs and limitations of the settings where the child spends his or her time.

TREATMENT

Treatment of psychiatric illness in children and adolescents with developmental disabilities involves some or all of the modalities described in the following sections. Interventions must be tailored to each child's needs at home, at school, and with peers. The treatment modalities utilized may need to be adjusted as the child matures and individual needs change.

Educational Interventions

Educational interventions can include a variety of supports to help a child succeed in the classroom (see Chapter 31). Children may benefit from schoolwide positive-behavior interventions and supports, with an individualized behavior intervention plan being developed if necessary. The education setting can also be a form of support: children may be placed in smaller self-contained classes or included in the general education class but with extra aides or a one-to-one helper. When the child becomes upset, the aide can help calm the child, avoiding the need to leave the classroom. The child may also benefit from therapy sessions with the school counselor or behavioral psychologist. There should be close collaboration between school personnel, parents, and the child's medical team.

Rehabilitation Therapy

There is evidence that language impairments significantly contribute to the development of certain behavior problems. Some aggressive behaviors and SIBs have been linked to the inability to communicate needs, and teaching functional communication skills has been shown to decrease SIB. Thus, speech-language therapy and training in augmentative and alternative communication systems (see Chapter 20) may be an important part of the intervention program. Similarly, if the child has a physical disability, the pain from contractures, an inability to ambulate, or difficulty reaching for desired objects may lead to behavior and mood alterations. Physical and occupational therapy may improve motor function, with associated improvement in behavior and mood.

Psychotherapy

There is ample evidence that various forms of psychological or behavioral therapy (individual, group, and family) can benefit a child or adolescent with developmental disabilities and psychiatric disorders, if it is adapted to the child's developmental age and communication abilities (Brosnan, 2011; McGinnes, 2010; Plant, 2007). Table 29.3 shows different types of psychotherapy and the disorders that they are most useful in treating. Goals of therapy are to relieve symptoms and help the child understand the nature of the disability and associated feelings and to come to recognize and appreciate his or her strengths. Psychotherapy, particularly group work, can also enhance social skills and help the child deal with stigmatization, rejection, peer pressure, and attempts at exploitation (American Academy of Child and Adolescent Psychiatry, 1999). Regrettably, individuals with developmental disabilities are seriously underserved regarding psychotherapy, despite the fact that psychotherapy can provide a supportive relationship, help restore self-esteem, and enhance the child's capacity to recognize and master emotional conflicts and solve problems. Psychotherapy also can be added to behavior therapy and pharmacotherapy when these approaches have not adequately resolved symptoms or improved quality of life. Ideally, the therapist should have expertise in working with individuals with developmental disabilities.

Behavior therapy is perhaps the most widely researched psychotherapeutic intervention for children and adolescents with intellectual disabilities (see Chapter 32). Cognitive-behavioral therapy and family interventions have been successful in children with ASD. There are extensive findings supporting the effectiveness of behavioral approaches in psychiatric disorders (Benjamin, 2011; Weisz et al., 2004). When used in conjunction with comprehensive assessment, accurate medical and psychiatric diagnoses, and programmatic intervention, behavior therapy is among the most powerful available interventions. As with other forms of psychotherapy and pharmacotherapy, however, it should be implemented only under the supervision of licensed professionals who have been specifically trained in this methodology.

Pharmacotherapy

Medication can play an important role in treating the psychiatric disorders that occur in children with developmental disabilities (Efron et al., 2003). Table 29.4 lists the various medications in each of the diagnostic groups that are described next. (Additional information on uses and side effects of these medications can be found in Appendix C.) In order to minimize side effects when a child with a developmental disability is started on a psychotropic medication, it is important to begin treatment at a low dose and then slowly titrate the dose up. This is particularly important because these children are at a greater risk for side effects than are their typically developing peers. An example of this was seen in the aripiprazole pediatric trials:

Table 29.3. Types of psychotherapy and uses in different disorders

Therapy	Behavior	CBT	Social skills	Group	Individual	Supportive/ educational	Parent training
ADHD	X		X	X			X
ODD and conduct disorder	X		X	X			X
Generalized anxiety disorder		X			X	X	
Social phobia		X	X	X	X	X	X
Panic disorder		X			X	X	
PTSD		X			X	X	
OCD		X			X		
Major depression		X			X	X	
Bipolar disorder					X	X	X
ASDs	X	X	X	X		X	X
Schizophrenia		X	X		X	X	X

Key: CBT, cognitive-behavioral therapy; ADHD, attention-deficit/hyperactivity disorder; ODD, oppositional defiant disorder; PTSD, posttraumatic stress disorder; OCD, obsessive-compulsive disorder; ASDs, autism spectrum disorders.

the titration was quickest in typically developing adolescents with schizophrenia who could accept increased doses every 2 days to a maximum of 30 mg in less than two weeks (Findling et al., 2008). In contrast, for the children with irritability associated with autism when the dose was increased weekly to a maximum dose of 15 mg over 4 weeks these children with autism had higher rates of side effects despite a lower maximum dose and slower titration schedule (Robb et al., 2011). In another study, stimulants given to children with autism were associated with a higher rate of emotional lability, crying, and other side effects than were seen in typically developing preschool children with ADHD (Nickels et al., 2008).

Antidepressants

Antidepressants are used to treat major depression and anxiety disorders including OCD, generalized anxiety disorder, and separation anxiety disorder (De-Vaugh-Geiss et al., 1992; Emslie et al., 2002; Geller et al., 2001; March, et al., 1998; Riddle et al., 2001; Wagner et al., 2003; Wagner et al., 2004). The class of antidepressants most commonly used in children and adolescents is the SSRIs. In 2004, the Food and Drug Administration (FDA) required drug companies to start putting "black box" (black box warnings are the FDA's highest level of warning before removing a drug from the market) warnings on the packaging of all categories of antidepressants, as well as atomoxetine (Strattera) for ADHD, aripiprazole (Abilify) for treatment-resistant depression, and quetiapine (Seroquel) for bipolar depression. More recently the antidepressant black box warning has been revised and expanded to include all those individuals younger than 25 years. The warning states that these antidepressants may increase suicidal thoughts and actions when first started. Depression and other mental illnesses are the most important causes of suicidal thoughts and actions; some people may be at a particularly high risk of having suicidal thoughts and actions. Families should watch closely for changes in mood, behavior, and the appearance of suicidal thoughts and actions when starting a child on antidepressants, and clinicians should monitor their young patients for any change in mental state and for indications of suicidal ideas or plans. With these controls in place, antidepressants can continue to be useful in the treatment of pediatric mood and anxiety disorders and remain an important part of treatment for these illnesses (Hammad, Laughren, & Racoosin, 2006).

Antihypertensives

Beta-blockers, such as propranolol, are used to treat explosive and aggressive behavior, whereas alpha-2 adrenergic receptor agonists (e.g., clonidine [Catapres, Kapvay], guanfacine [Tenex, Intuniv]) are used to treat ADHD, tic disorder, and Tourette syndrome. These medications sedate and can also lower blood pressure; thus, they should be used cautiously, especially in children with developmental disabilities associated with comorbid cardiac disorders (Ahmed & Takeshita, 1996). Recently, the long-acting formulations Intuniv and Kapvay have both been FDA approved for the treatment of ADHD in children and adolescents as monotherapy and in combination with stimulants (Connor 2010; Jain, 2011; Kollins, 2011).

Antipsychotic Medications

Antipsychotic medications have been used primarily to treat aggression and SIB in children with intellectual disability or ASDs. There is, in fact, more safety data on risperidone in children with intellectual disability and ASDs than in their typically developing peers. In 2006, risperidone became the first antipsychotic medication approved for the treatment of aggressive behavior in individuals with autism. Aripiprazole has also been approved for the treatment of irritability and aggression in children 6–17 showing such symptoms in autism (Robb, 2010). Many of the other novel neuroleptics have also been studied in individuals with ASDs. Although novel neuroleptics are much more likely to cause weight gain, they are less likely to cause a movement disorder (Martin et al., 2004; Stigler et al., 2004).

Benzodiazepines

Benzodiazepines are helpful in reducing anxiety in the short term. Children with developmental disabilities, however, may have paradoxical reactions to these medications and may become agitated rather than calm and sleepy (Rothschild, 2000; Mancuso, 2004). Because chronic use of these agents can cause chemical and behavioral dependency and may alter seizure control, they should not be used for long-term control of anxiety symptoms.

Mood Stabilizers

Mood stabilizers include lithium and antiepileptic medication (Findling et al., 2005). They are most commonly used to treat bipolar disorder and aggressive behaviors. Lithium is effective in treating current episodes and in

Table 29.4. Medications used to treat psychiatric disorders

	Generic name	Trade name	Type	Uses	Other formulations
Antidepressants	Fluoxetine	Prozac, Sarefem	SSRI	Depression, anxiety, OCD	Liquid and weekly
	Fluvoxamine	Luvox	SSRI	OCD	None
	Sertraline	Zoloft	SSRI	Depression, anxiety, OCD	Liquid
	Paroxetine	Paxil, Paxil CR	SSRI	Depression, anxiety, OCD	Liquid (not in CR)
	Citalopram	Celexa	SSRI	Depression	Liquid
	Escitalopram	Lexapro	SSRI	Depression, anxiety	Liquid
	Venlafaxine	Effexor, Effexor XR	SNRI	Depression, anxiety	None
	Duloxetine	Cymbalta	SNRI	Depression	None
	Buproprion	Wellbutrin, Wellbutrin SR, Wellbutrin XL	Dopaminergic	Depression, ADHD	None
Antihypertensives	Propranolol	Inderal, Inderal LA	Beta blocker	Aggressive behavior	None
	Clonidine	Catapres, Catapres-TTS patch Kapvay	Alpha-2-adrenergic agonist	ADHD, tics, sleeping agent Monotherapy or with stimulant	Weekly skin patch
	Guanfacine	Tenex Intuniv	Alpha-2-adrenergic agonist	ADHD, tics Monotherapy or with stimulant	None
Antipsychotics	Clozapine	Clozaril	Atypical	Treatment-resistant schizophrenia, bipolar disorder (not FDA approved for acute bipolar mania)	None
	Risperidone	Risperdal, Risperdal M-Tab, Risperdal Consta	Atypical	Schizophrenia, bipolar disorder, aggressive behavior in children with autism spectrum disorders	Liquid, oral dissolving tablets (M-Tab), 2-week injection (Consta)
	Olanzapine	Zyprexa, Zyprexa Zydis, Zyprexa Relprev	Atypical	Schizophrenia, bipolar disorder, acute agitation	Oral dissolving tablets, 2-week injection (Relprev) requires extensive monitoring
	Ziprasidone	Geodon	Atypical	Schizophrenia, bipolar disorder, acute agitation	Daily injection
	Quetiapine	Seroquel	Atypical	Schizophrenia, bipolar disorder (acute mania and bipolar depression)	None
	Aripiprazole	Abilify, Abilify Discmelt	Atypical (plus serotonin agonist)	Schizophrenia, bipolar disorder	Liquid, oral dissolving tablets, daily injection

	Generic name	Trade name	Type	Uses	Other formulations
	Paliperidone	Invega, Invega Sustenna	Atypical	Schizophrenia	4-week injection (Sustenna)
	Haloperidol	Haldol, Haldol Decanoate	Typical	Schizophrenia, Tourette syndrome, agitation, severe behavior disorders	Liquid, daily injection, monthly injection
	Pimozide	Orap	Typical	Tourette syndrome	None
Benzodiazepines	Lorazepam	Ativan	Typical	Anxiety	Liquid, daily injection
	Alprazolam	Xanax, Xanax XR	High potency	Panic, anxiety	None
	Clonazepam	Klonopin, Klonopin Wafers	High potency	Panic, anxiety	Oral dissolving tablets
Mood stabilizers	Lithium carbonate	Lithobid, Eskalith, Eskalith-CR	Mood stabilizer	Bipolar disorder (acute mania and maintenance)	Liquid
	Valproic acid	Depakote, Depakote ER, Depacon, Depakene	Antiepileptic drug	Bipolar disorder	Liquid, intravenous, sprinkles
	Carbamazepine	Tegretol, Tegretol XR, Carbatrol, Equetro	Antiepileptic drug	Bipolar disorder	Chewable tablet, liquid
	Oxcarbazepine	Trileptal	Antiepileptic drug	Not FDA approved yet for bipolar disorder, but used	Liquid
	Lamotrigine	Lamictal	Antiepileptic drug	Bipolar maintenance	Chewable tablets
Stimulants and atomoxetine	Methylphenidate-racemic mixture	Ritalin, Ritalin LA, Metadate CD, Concerta, Daytrana	Synthetic stimulant	ADHD	Sprinkles for Ritalin LA and Metadate CD, transdermal patch (Daytrana)
	Dexmethylphenidate	Focalin, Focalin XR	Synthetic stimulant	ADHD	Sprinkles for XR
	Dextroamphetamine	Dexedrine, Dexedrine ER spansules	Stimulant	ADHD	Chewable generic tablet, ER spansule
	Mixed amphetamine salts	Adderall, Adderall XR	Stimulant	ADHD	Sprinkles for XR
	Modafinil	Provigil, Sparlon	Unknown	ADHD (not FDA approved for ADHD due to concern about Stevens-Johnson syndrome)	None
	Atomoxetine	Strattera	NRI	ADHD, maintenance 6–14 years	None

Key: SSRI, selective serotonin reuptake inhibitor; OCD, obsessive-compulsive disorder; CR, controlled release; SNRI, serotonin norepinephrine reuptake inhibitor; XR, extended release; SR, slow release; XL, extra long; ADHD, attention-deficit/hyperactivity disorder; LA, long acting; TTS, transdermal system; ER, extended release; FDA, Food and Drug Administration; CD, controlled delivery; NRI, norepinephrine reuptake inhibitor. For further information see Appendix C.

preventing future bipolar episodes. It is a salt that is excreted through the kidneys and causes increased thirst and urination. It must be used with caution in combination with certain other drugs that can lead to toxic lithium levels, including nonsteroidal anti-inflammatory drugs (e.g., ibuprofen) and certain anticonvulsants (e.g., topiramate [Topamax]) that are excreted by the kidneys. Lithium toxicity can occur with rapid onset if normal fluid intake is decreased, for example with vomiting, diarrhea, or acute illness; this in turn can result in coma, kidney failure, or the need for dialysis. No antiepileptic medications are currently approved for the treatment of bipolar disorder in children and adolescents. However, the antipsychotic aripiprazole is approved for bipolar disorder as monotherapy and in combination with both lithium and valproic acid.

Stimulants and Atomoxetine

Stimulants of both the amphetamine and methylphenidate classes are first-line treatments for ADHD (see Chapter 22). Both families of drugs now have long-acting preparations available that can improve control of ADHD symptoms throughout the day. Side effects include loss of appetite, insomnia, tics, headache, and gastrointestinal side effects (Pearson et al., 2003). The use of atomoxetine has been studied in children with ADHD (Newcorn et al., 2005) and ASDs and has been found to control hyperactive/impulsive symptoms with an effect similar to methylphenidate.

SUMMARY

Children with developmental disabilities are at higher risk then their typically developing peers of developing psychiatric and behavioral disorders at some time during their childhood or adolescence. By being aware of the possibility of psychiatric disorders that can affect a child's behavior, parents, educators, and clinicians can identify problem earlys and intervene. Early intervention leads to more rapid resolution of the difficulties and allows the child to function more effectively and happily at home, at school, and in the community.

REFERENCES

Ahmed, I., & Takeshita, J. (1996). Clonidine: A critical review of its role in the treatment of psychiatric disorders. *CNS Drugs, 6,* 53.

Alvarez, N. (1998). Barbiturates in the treatment of epilepsy in people with intellectual disability. *Journal of Intellectual Disabilities, 42*(1), 16–23.

Aman, M.G., Burrow, W.H., & Wolford, P.L. (1995). The Aberrant Behavior Checklist Community: Factor validity and effect of subject variables for adults in group homes. *American Journal on Mental Retardation, 100,* 293–294.

American Academy of Child and Adolescent Psychiatry. (1999). Practice parameters for the assessment and treatment of children, adolescents and adults with mental retardation and comorbid mental disorders. *Journal of the American Academy of Child and Adolescent Psychiatry, 38*(12), 5S–31S.

American Psychiatric Association. (2000). *Diagnostic and statistical manual of mental disorders* (4th ed., text rev.). Washington, DC: Author.

American Psychiatric Association. (2011). *DSM-5 development.* Retrieved September 2, 2011 from http://www.dsm5.org

Antshel, K.M., Fremont, W., Roizen, N., Shprintzen, R., Higgins, A.M., Dhamoon, A., & Kates, W.R. (2006). ADHD, major depressive disorder, and simple phobias are prevalent psychiatric conditions in youth with velocardiofacial syndrome. *Journal of the American Academy of Child and Adolescent Psychiatry, 45,* 593–603.

Arnold, P.D., Siegel-Bartelt, J., Cytrynbaum, C., Teshima, I., Schachar, R. (2001). Velo-cardio-facial syndrome: Implications of microdeletion 22q11 for schizophrenia and mood disorders. *American Journal of Medical Genetics, 105*(4), 354–62.

Bailey, D.B., Raspa, M., Olmsed, M., & Holiday, D.B. (2008). Co-occurring conditions associated with FMR1 gene variations: Findings from a national parent survey. *American Journal of Medical Genetics, 146A*(16), 2060–9.

Baumgardner, T., Reiss, A., Freund, L., & Abrams, M.T. (1995). Specification of the neurobehavioral phenotype in males with fragile X syndrome. *Pediatrics, 95,* 744–52.

Benjamin, C.L., Puleo, C.M., Settipani, C.A., Brodman, D.M., Edmunds, J.M., Cummings, C.M., & Kendall, P.C. (2011). History of cognitive-behavioral therapy in youth. *Child and Adolescent Psychiatric Clinics of North America, 20*(2), 179–189.

Biederman, J., Petty, C.R., Monuteaux, M.C., Fried, R., Byrne, D., Spencer, T., … Faraone, S.V. (2010). Adult psychiatric outcomes of girls with attention deficit hyperactivity disorder: 11-year follow-up in a longitudinal case-control study. *American Journal of Psychiatry, 167,* 409–417.

Black, B., & Udhe, T. (1994). Treatment of elective mutism with fluoxetine: A double-blind, placebo-controlled trial. *Journal of the American Academy of Child and Adolescent Psychiatry, 33,* 1000–1006.

Boer, H., Holland, A., Whittington, J., Butler, J., Webb, T., & Clarke, D. (2002). Psychotic illness in people with Prader-Willi syndrome due to chromosome 15 maternal uniparental disomy. *Lancet, 359*(9301), 135–6.

Breau, L.M., Camfield, C.S., Symons, F.J., Bodfish, J.W., Mackay, A., Finley, G.A., & McGrath, P.J. (2003). Relation between pain and self-injurious behavior in nonverbal children with severe cognitive impairments. *The Journal of Pediatrics, 142*(5), 498–503.

Brosnan, J. (2011). A review of behavioral interventions for the treatment of aggression in individuals with developmental disabilities. *Research in Developmental Disabilities, 32*(2), 437–46.

Buitelaar, J.K. (1993). Self-injurious behavior in retarded children: Clinical phenomena and biological mechanisms. *Acta Paedopsychiatrica, 56*, 105–111.

Burd, L., Klug, M.G., Martsolf, J.T., & Kerbeshian, J. (2003). Fetal alcohol syndrome: Neuropsychiatric phenomics. *Neurotoxicology and Teratology, 25*, 697–705.

Calles, J.L. (2008). Use of psychotropic medications in children with developmental disabilities. *Pediatric Clinics of North America, 55*, 1227–1240.

Catinari, S., Vass, A., & Heresco-Levy, U. (2006). Psychiatric manifestations in Turner Syndrome: A brief survey. *Israel Journal of Psychiatry and Related Sciecnes, 43*(4), 293–5.

Connor, D.F., Findling, R.F., Kollins, S.H., Sallee, F., Lopez, F.A., Lyne, A., & Tremblay, G. (2010). Effects of guanfacine extended release on oppositional symptoms in children aged 6–12 years with attention-deficit/hyperactivity disorder and oppositional symptoms: A randomized, double-blind, placebo-controlled trial. *CNS Drugs, 24*(9), 755–68.

Connor, D.F., Barkley, R.A., & Davis, H.T. (2000). A pilot study of methylphenidate, clonidine, or the combination in ADHD comorbid with aggressive oppositional defiant or conduct disorder. *Clinical Pediatrics, 39*(1), 15–25.

Demb, H.B., Brier, N., Huron, R., & Tomor, E. (1994). The adolescent behavior checklist: Normative data and sensitivity and specificity of a screening tool for diagnosable psychiatric disorders in adolescents with mental retardation and other development disabilities. *Research in Developmental Disabilities, 15*, 151–165.

DeVaugh-Geiss, J., Moroz, G., Biederman, J., Cantwell, D., Fontaine, R., Greist, J.H., ... Landau, P. (1992). Clomipramine hydrochloride in childhood and adolescent obsessive-compulsive disorder: A multicenter trial. *Journal of the American Academy of Child and Adolescent Psychiatry, 31*, 45–49.

Dykens, E.M. (2007). Psychiatric and behavioral disorders in persons with Down syndrome. *Mental Retardation and Developmental Disabilities Research Reviews, 13*, 272–278.

Efron, D., Hiscock, H., Sewell, J.R., Cranswick, N.E., Vance, A.L., Tyl, Y., & Luk, E.S. (2003). Prescribing of psychotropic medications for children by Australian pediatricians and child psychiatrists. *Pediatrics, 111*(2), 372–375.

Einfeld, S.L., Tonge, B.J., & Florio, T. (1994). Behavioral and emotional disturbance in fragile X syndrome. *American Journal of Medical Genetics, 51*, 386–91.

Emslie, G.J., Heiligenstein, J.H., Wagner, K.D., Hoog, S.L, Brown, E., ... Jacobson, J.G. (2002). Fluoxetine for acute treatment of depression in children and adolescents: A placebo-controlled, randomized clinical trial. *Journal of the American Academy of Child and Adolescent Psychiatry, 41*(10), 1205–1215.

Feinstein, C., & Chahal, L. (2009). Psychiatric phenotypes associated with neurogenetic disorders. *Psychiatric Clinics of North America, 32*, 15–37.

Feinstein, C., Eliez, S., Blasey, C., & Reiss, A.L. (2002). Psychiatric disorders and behavioral problems in children with velocardiofacial syndrome: Usefulness as phenotypic indicators of schizophrenia risk. *Biological Psychiatry. 51*(4), 312–8.

Feinstein, C., & Reiss, A.L. (1996). Psychiatric disorder in mentally retarded children and adolescents: The challenges of meaningful diagnosis. *Child and Adolescents Psychiatric Clinics of North America, 5*, 1031–1037.

Findling, R.L., McNamara, N.K., Youngstrom, E.A., Stansbrey, R., Gracious, B.L., Reed, M.D., & Calabrese, J.R. (2005). Double-blind 18-month trial of lithium versus divalproex maintenance treatment in pediatric bipolar disorder. *Journal of the American Academy of Child and Adolescent Psychiatry, 44*(5), 461–469.

Findling, R.L., Robb, A.S., Nyilas, M., Forbes, R.A., Jin, N., Ivanova, S., ... Carson, W.H. (2008). A multiple-center, randomized, double-blind, placebo-controlled study of oral aripiprazole for treatment of adolescents with schizophrenia. *The American Journal of Psychiatry*, advance published September 2, 2008. doi:10.1176/appi.ajp.2008.07061035

Freund, L.S., Reiss, A.L., & Abrams, M.T. (1993). Psychiatric disorders associated with fragile X in the young female. *Pediatrics, 91*(2), 321–9.

Geller, D.A., Hoog, S.L., Heiligenstein, J.H., Ricardi, R.K., Tamura, R., Kluszynski, S., ... Fluoxetine Pediatric, OCD Study Team. (2001). Fluoxetine treatment for obsessive-compulsive disorder in children and adolescents: A placebo-controlled clinical trial. *Journal of the American Academy of Child and Adolescent Psychiatry, 40*(7), 773–779.

Gillberg, C., Persson, E., Grufman, M., & Themner, U. (1986). Psychiatric disorders in mildly and severely mentally retarded urban children and adolescents: Epidemiological aspects. *British Journal of Psychiatry, 149*, 68–74.

Green, T., Gothelf, D., Glaser, B., Debbane, M., Frisch, A., Kotler, M., ... Eliez, S. (2009). Psychiatric disorders and intellectual functioning throughout development in velocardiofacial (22q11.2 deletion) syndrome. *Journal of the American Academy of Child and Adolescent Pyschiatry, 48*(11), 1060–8.

Guess, D., & Carr, E. (1991). Emergence and maintenance of stereotypy and self-injury. *American Journal on Mental Retardation, 96*, 299–320.

Hagerman, R.J., Jackson, C., Amiri, K., Silverman, A.C., O'Connor, R., & Sobesky, W. (1992). Girls with fragile X syndrome: Physical and neurocognitive status and outcome. *Pediatrics, 89*(3), 395–400.

Hammad, T.A., Laughren, T., & Racoosin, J. (2006). Suicidality in pediatric patients treated with antidepressant drugs. *Archives of General Psychiatry, 63*(3), 332–339.

Hardan, A., & Sahl, R. (1997). Psychopathology in children and adolescents with developmental disorders. *Research in Developmental Disabilities, 18*(5), 369–82.

Hässler, F., & Reis, O. (2010). Pharmacotherapy of disruptive behavior in mentally retarded subjects: A review of the current literature. *Developmental Disabilities Review, 16*(3), 265–272.

Hessl, D., Dyer-Friedman, J., Glaser, B., Wisbeck, J., Barais, R.G., Taylor, A., & Reiss, A.L. (2001). The influence of environmental and genetic factors on behavior problems and autistic symptoms in boys and girls with fragile X syndrome. *Pediatrics, 108*(5), E88.

Jain, R., Segal, S., Kollins, S.H., & Khayrallah, M. (2011). Clonidine extended-release tablets for pediatric patients with attention-deficit/hyperactivity disorder. *Journal of the American Academy of Child and Adolescent Psychiatry, 50*(2), 171–9.

King, B.H., DeAntonio, C., McCracken, J.T., Forness, S.R., & Ackerland, V. (1994). Psychiatric consultation in severe and profound mental retardation. *American Journal of Psychiatry, 151*, 1802–1808.

Kollins, S.H., Jain, R., Brams, M., Segal, S., Findling, R.L., Wigal, S.B., & Khayrallah, M. (2011). Clonidine extended-release tablets as add-on therapy to psychostimulants in children and adolescents with ADHD. *Pediatrics, 127*(6), e1406–13. Epub May 9, 2011.

Kutcher, S., Aman, M., Brooks, S.J., Buitelaar, J., van Daalen, E., Fegert, J., ... Tyano, S. (2004). International consensus statement on attention-deficit/hyperactivity disorder (ADHD) and disruptive behaviour disorders (DBDs): Clinical implications and treatment practice suggestions. *European Neuropsychopharmacology, 14*(1), 11–28.

Leyfer, O.T., Woodruff-Borden, J., Klein-Tasman, B.P., Fricke, J.S., & Mervis, C.B. (2006). Prevalence of psychiatric disorders in 4–16 year olds with Williams Syndrome. *American Journal of Medical Genetics B Neuropsychiatric Genetics, 141B*(6), 615–622.

Linaker, O.M., & Helle, J. (1994). Validity of the schizophrenia diagnosis of the Psychopathology Instrument for Mentally Retarded Adults (PIRMA): A comparison of schizophrenic patients with and without mental retardation. *Research in Developmental Disabilities, 15*, 473–486.

Loschen, E.L., & Osman, O.T. (1992). Self-injurious behavior in the developmentally disabled: Assessment techniques. *Psychopharmacology Bulletin, 28*, 433–438.

Mace, F.C., & Mauk, J.E. (1995). Bio-behavioral diagnosis and treatment of self-injury. *Mental Retardation and Developmental Disabilities Research Reviews, 1*, 104–110.

Mancuso, C.E., Tanzi, M.G., & Gabay, M. (2004). Paradoxical reactions to benzodiazepines: Literature review and treatment options. *Pharmacotherapy, 24*(9),1177–1185.

March, J.S., Amaya-Jackson, L., Murray, M.C., & Schulte, A. (1998). Cognitive-behavioral psychotherapy for children and adolescents with posttraumatic stress disorder after a single-incident stressor. *Journal of the American Academy of Child and Adolescent Psychiatry, 37*(6), 585–593.

March, J.S., Biederman, J., Wolkow, R., Safferman, A., Mardekian, J., Cook, E.H., ... Steiner, H. (1998). Sertraline in children and adolescents with obsessive-compulsive disorder: A multicenter randomized controlled trial. *Journal of the American Medical Association, 280*(20), 1752–1756.

Martin, A., Scahill, L., Anderson G.M., Aman, M., Arnold, L.E., McCracken, J., ... Vitiello, B. (2004). Weight and leptin changes among risperidone-treated youths with autism: 6-month prospective data. *The American Journal of Psychiatry, 161*(6), 1125–1127.

McAdam, D.B, Sherman, J.A., Sheldon, J.B., & Napalitano, D.A. (2004). Behavioral interventions to reduce the pica of persons with developmental disabilities. *Behavior Modification, 28*(1), 45–72.

McGinnes, M.A. (2010). Abolishing and establishing operation analyses of social attention as positive reinforcement for problem behavior. *Journal of Applied Behavioral Analysis, 43*(1), 119-23.

Myers, B.A., & Pueschel, S.M. (1995). Major depression in a small group of adults with Down syndrome. *Research in Developmental Disabilities 16*(4), 285–99.

National Institutes of Health. (1989). Treatment of destructive behaviors in persons with developmental disabilities. *NIH Consensus Development Conference Statement, 7*(9), 1–14.

Newcorn, J.H., Spencer, T.J., Biederman, J., Milton, D.R., & Michelson, D. (2005). Atomoxetine treatment in children and adolescents with attention-deficit/hyperactivity disorder and comorbid oppositional defiant disorder. *Journal of the American Academy of Child and Adolescent Psychiatry, 44*(3), 240–248.

Nickels, K., Katusic, S.K., Colligan, R.C., Weaver, A.L., Voigt, R.G., & Barbaresi, W.J. (2008). Stimulant medication treatment of target behaviors in children with autism: A population-based study. *Journal of Developmental and Behavioral Pediatrics, 29*(2), 75–81.

O'Connor, M.J., Shah, B., Whaley, S., Cronin, P., Gunderson, B., & Graham, J. (2002). Psychiatric illness in a clinical sample of children with prenatal alcohol exposure. *American Journal of Drug and Alcohol Abuse, 28*(4), 743–54.

Pearson, D.A., Santos, C.W., Roache, J.D., Casat, C.D., Loveland, K.A., Lachar, D., ... Cleveland, L.A. (2003). Treatment effects of methylphenidate on behavioral adjustment in children with intellectual disability and ADHD. *Journal of the American Academy of Child and Adolescent Psychiatry, 42*(2), 209–216.

The Pediatric OCD Treatment Study (POTS) Team. (2004). Cognitive-behavior therapy, sertraline and their combination for children and adolescents with obsessive-compulsive disorder: The pediatric OCD treatment study (POTS) randomized controlled trial. *Journal of the American Medical Association, 292*(16), 1969–1976.

Plant, K.M. (2007). Reducing problem behavior during care-giving in families of preschool-aged children with developmental disabilities. *Research in Developmental Disabilities, 28*(4), 362–85.

Prasher, V.P., & Day, S. (1995). Brief report: Obsessive-compulsive disorder in adults with Down syndrome. *Journal of Autism and Developmental Disorders, 25*(4), 453–8.

Reiss, S., & Valenti-Hein, D. (1994). Development of a psychopathology rating scale for children with mental retardation. *Journal of Consulting and Clinical Psychology, 62*, 28–33.

Riddle, M.A., Reeve, E.A., Yaryura-Tobias, J.A., Yang, H.M., Claghorn J.L., Gaffney, G., final is Walkup, JT (2001). Fluvoxamine for children and adolescents with obsessive-compulsive disorder: a randomized, controlled multicenter trial. *Journal of the American Academy of Child and Adolescent Psychiatry, 40*(2), 222–229.

Robb, A.S. (2010). Managing irritability and aggression in autism spectrum disorders in children and adolescents. *Developmental Disabilities Research Reviews, 16*(3), 258–64.

Robb, A.S., Andersson, C., Bellochio, E.E., Manos, G., Rojas-Fernandez, C., Mathews, S., ... Mankoski, R. (2011) Safety and tolerability of aripiprazole in the treatment of irritability associated with autistic disorder in pediatric subjects (6-17 years old): Results from a pooled analysis of 2 studies. *The Primary Care Companion for CNS Disorders, 13*(1),e1-e9.

Robb, A.S., Cueva, J.E., Sporn, J., Yang, R., & Vanderburg, D.G. (2010). Sertraline treatment of children and adolescents with posttraumatic stress: A double-blind, placebo-controlled trial. *Journal of Child and Adolescent Psychopharmacology, 20*(6), 1–9.

Rothschild, A.J, Shindul-Rothschild, V.A., Murray, M., & Brewster, S. (2000). Comparison of the frequency of behavioral disinhibition on alprazolam, clonazepam, or no benzodiazepine in hospitalized psychiatric patients. *Journal of Clinical Psychopharmacology, 20*(1),7–11.

Rutter, M., Graham, P., & Yule, W. (1970). *A neuropsychiatric study in childhood*. London, England: Spastics International.

Rynn, M.A., Siqueland, L., & Rickels, K. (2001). Placebo-controlled trial of sertraline in the treatment of children with generalized anxiety disorder. *American Journal of Psychiatry, 158*(12), 2008–2014.

Schroeder, S.R., Reese, R.M., Hellings, J., Loupe, P., & Tessel, R.E. (1999). The causes of self-injurious behavior and their clinical implications. In N.A. Wieseler & R.H. Hanson (Eds.), *Challenging behavior of persons with mental health disorder and severe developmental disabilities* (pp. 65–87). Washington, DC: American Association on Mental Retardation.

Siegel, P.T., Clopper, R., & Stabler, B. (1998). The psychological consequences of Turner syndrome and review of the National Cooperative Growth Study psychological substudy. *Pediatrics, 102*(2, Pt 3), 488–91.

Smith, P., Yule, W., Perrin, S., Tranah, T., Dalgleish, T., & Clark, D.M. (2007). Cognitive-behavioral therapy for PTSD in children and adolescents: A preliminary randomized controlled trial. *Journal of the American Academy of Child and Adolescent Psychiatry, 46*(8), 1051–61.

Sternberg, L., Taylor, R.L., & Babkie, A. (1994).Correlates of interventions with self-injurious behavior. *Journal of Intellectual Disability Research, 38*, 475–485.

Stigler, K.A., Potenza, M.N., Posey D.J., & McDougle, C.J. (2004). Weight gain associated with atypical antipsychotic use in children and adolescents: Prevalence, clinical relevance, and management. *Pediatric Drugs, 6*(1), 33–44.

Sullivan, K., Hooper, S., & Hatton, D. (2007). Behavioural equivalents of anxiety in children with fragile X syndrome: Parent and teacher report. *Journal of Intellectual Disability Research, 51*(1), 54–65.

Swedo S.E., Leonard H.L., Garvey M., Mittelman, B., Allen, A.J, Perlmutter, S., ... Dubbert, B.K. (1998). Pediatric autoimmune neuropsychiatric disorders associated with streptococcal infections: Clinical description of the first 50 cases. *American Journal of Psychiatry, 155*, 264–271.

Symons, F.J., Clark, R.D., Hatton, D.D., Skinner, M., Bailey, D.B. Jr. (2003).Self-injurious behavior in young boys with fragile X syndrome. *American Journal of Medical Genetics, 118*(2), 115–21.

Tartaglia, N., Davis, S., Hench, A., Nimishakavi, S., Beauregard, R., Reynolds, A., ... Hagerman, R. (A 2008). A new look at XXYY syndrome: Medical and psychological features. *American Journal of Medical Genetics, 146A*(12), 1509–22.

Treatment for Adolescents with Depression Study (TADS) Team. (2004). Fluoxetine, cognitive-behavioral therapy, and their combination for adolescents with depression: Treatment for Adolescents with Depression Study (TADS) randomized controlled trial. *Journal of the American Medical Association, 292*(7), 807–820.

Verhoeven, W.M., Tuinier, S., van den Berg, Y.W., Coppus, A.M., Fekkes, D., Pepplinkhuizen, L., & Thijssen, J.H. (1999). Stress and self-injurious behavior: Hormonal and serotonergic parameters in mentally retarded subjects. *Pharmacopsychiatry, 32*, 13–20.

Visootsak, J., & Sherman, S. (2007). Neuropsychiatric and behavioral aspects of trisomy 21. *Current Psychiatry Reports, 9*(2), 135–40.

Vogels, A., De Hert. M., Descheemaeker, M.J., Govers, V., Devriendt, K., Legius, E., ... Fryns, J.P. (2004). Psychotic disorders in Prader-Willi syndrome. *American Journal of Medical Genetics A, 127A*(3), 238–43.

Wagner, K.D., Ambrosini, P., Rynn, M., Wohlberg, C., Yang, R., Greenbaum, M.S., ... Deas, D. (2003). Efficacy of sertraline in the treatment of children and adolescents with major depressive disorder: Two randomized controlled trials. *Journal of the American Medical Association, 290*(8), 1033–1041.

Wagner, K.D., Robb, A.S., Findling, R.L., Jin, J., Gutierrez, M.M., & Heydorn, W.E. (2004). A randomized, placebo-controlled trial of citalopram for the treatment of major depression in children and adolescents. *American Journal of Psychiatry, 161*(6), 1079–1083.

Walkup, J.T., Albano, A.M., Piacentini, J., Birmaher, B., Compton, S.N., Sherrill, J.T., ... Kendall, P.C. (2008). Cognitive behavioral therapy, sertraline or a combination in childhood anxiety. *New England Journal of Medicine, 359*(26), 2753–66.

Walkup, J.T., Labellarte, M.J., Riddle, M.A., Pine, D.S., Greenhill, L., Klein, R., ... Roper, M. (2001). Fluvoxamine for the treatment of anxiety disorders in children and adolescents. *Journal of the American Medical Association, 344*(17), 1279–1285.

Weisz, J.R., Hawley, K.M., & Doss, A.J. (2004). Empirically tested psychotherapies for youth internalizing and externalizing problems and disorders. *Child and Adolescent Psychiatric Clinics of North America, 13*(4), 729-815.

Young, T., Apfeldorf, W., Knepper, J., & Yager, J. (2009). Severe eating disorder in a 28-year-old man with William's Syndrome. *American Journal of Psychiatry, 166*(1), 25–31.

Zarcone, J.R., Lindauer, S.E., Morse, P.S., Crosland, K.A., Valdovinos, M.G., McKercher, T.L., ... Schroeder, S.R. (2001). Effects of risperidone on destructive behavior of persons with developmental disabilities: III. Functional analysis. *American Journal on Mental Retardation, 109*, 310–321.

Zarcone, J., Napolitano, D., Peterson, C., Breidbord, J., Ferraioli, S., Caruso-Anderson, M., ... Thompson, T. (2007). The relationship between compulsive behaviour and academic achievement across the three genetic subtypes of Prader-Willi syndrome. *Journal of Intellectual Disabilities Research, 51*(Pt 6), 478–87.

Zimmerman, A.W., Jinnah, H.A., & Lockhardt, P.J. (1998). Behavioral neuropharmacology. *Mental Retardation and Developmental Disabilities Research Reviews, 4*, 26–35.

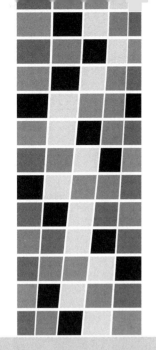

IV

Interventions, Families, and Outcomes

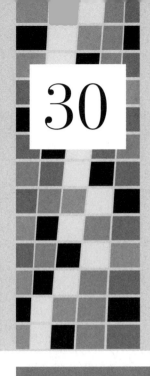

30 Early Intervention

Toby Long

Upon completion of this chapter, the reader will

- Know the rationale for early intervention services
- Understand the principles of early intervention
- Be aware of the services and supports available for early intervention
- Understand the components of federal legislation that support early intervention

The provision of early intervention services in virtually every community in the United States shows society's commitment to support infants and toddlers with developmental disabilities and their families (Guralnick, 2005a). These programs in the United States are usually provided in the context of federal early intervention legislation. Such legislation defines the structural components and principles governing state-based early intervention systems for infants and toddlers (age birth to 3 years) with disabilities. Services and supports available include habilitation therapies, family counseling, and early childhood educational services. This array of services is provided in many settings, in collaboration with a variety of agencies, and utilizes various models of service delivery.

■ ■ ■ CARL

Carl is a 6-month-old boy who was born at a gestational age of 26 weeks. After a difficult 4-month hospitalization in the neonatal intensive care unit, he was discharged home. Neurodevelopmental assessment just prior to discharge showed that his cognitive function was at a newborn level and he had markedly increased tone in his legs. Based on these significant developmental delays he was referred by his neonatologist to the local early intervention program. After a comprehensive, multidisciplinary evaluation, he was determined eligible for services, after which an intervention plan, the individualized family service plan, or IFSP, was developed. Carl attended a child care center; thus, the services he required, physical therapy and special instruction, were provided at the center on a weekly basis. Additionally, each provider arranged a home visit with Carl's parents once a month so that they could discuss family concerns and priorities. Carl's parents and Carl's early intervention staff and child care providers together have embedded creative activities and strategies into naturally occurring learning opportunities and routines. These encourage positive social relationships and help Carl develop skills to reach his full potential. As a result of these interactions, Carl's parents feel increasingly confident and competent in caring for Carl and in supporting his development.

PRINCIPLES OF EARLY INTERVENTION

The primary goals of early intervention are 1) to support families in promoting their child's optimal development, and 2) to facilitate the child's participation in family and community activities. Within those, intervention focuses on encouraging active participation of families in the intervention by embedding strategies into home routines. To meet this goal early intervention services are delivered in a manner that are

- Family centered and culturally and linguistically competent
- Developmentally supportive, strengths based, and helpful for promoting children's participation in their natural environments
- Comprehensive, coordinated, and team-based
- Individualized, flexible, and responsive to the changing needs of young children and families
- Based on the highest-quality evidence available

RESEARCH SUPPORT FOR THE VALUE OF EARLY INTERVENTION

Research over the last 25 years indicates that intervention during early childhood achieves immediate and sustained developmental benefits (Center on the Developing Child at Harvard University, 2010; Hebbler et al., 2007). Also, these benefits save money for the community and family over time (Guralnick, 2004). Much scientific evidence demonstrates that early intervention programs generate important benefits for both young children at risk for disability and for those with established disabilities (Early Childhood Outcomes Center, 2011; Ramey, Ramey, & Lanzi, 2007; Ramey, Ramey & Lanzi, 2006). Numerous studies also have identified that a decline in development can be prevented or at least mitigated through providing comprehensive early intervention programs (Guralnick, 2005b). It should be pointed out, however, that individual and subgroup responsiveness to early intervention varies, and consistent evidence for long-term benefits is limited. Current research on the effectiveness of early childhood interventions focuses on determining which program elements are most effective for which children and under which circumstances. Research also investigates how programs can produce the greatest benefits at the lowest cost.

COMPONENTS OF PART C OF THE INDIVIDUALS WITH DISABILITIES EDUCATION IMPROVEMENT ACT: THE INFANTS AND TODDLERS WITH DISABILITIES PROGRAM

Based on research indicating that services provided to young children could prevent or ameliorate biological, social, and environmental risks on development (Guralnick, 2005b), the 1986 amendments to the Individuals with Disabilities Education Act (IDEA; then called the Education of the Handicapped Children Act) included the establishment of the Infants and Toddlers Program or Early Intervention System. From its inception this part of the law was meant to be a system of cooperation and collaboration across child-serving systems to provide comprehensive services and supports to families with infants and toddlers with disabilities or delays. The purposes of the Infants and Toddlers Program, or Part C of IDEA, are stated in the supporting legislation as follows:

1. To enhance the development of infants and toddlers with disabilities, to minimize their potential for developmental delay, and to recognize the significant brain development that occurs during a child's first 3 years of life

2. To reduce the educational costs to society, including our nation's schools, by minimizing the need for special education and related services after infants and toddlers with disabilities reach school age

3. To maximize the potential for individuals with disabilities to live independently in society

4. To enhance the capacity of families to meet the special needs of their infants and toddlers with disabilities

5. To enhance the capacity of States and local agencies and service providers to identify, evaluate, and meet the needs of all children, particularly minority, low-income, inner city, and rural children, and infants and toddlers in foster care

Each state must create a system that includes 16 components (see Table 30.1). States are required to ensure that those individuals providing the services are appropriately qualified and that a central directory of providers, services, and agencies is available to help identify resources of all kinds relevant to early intervention. Other structural components are administrative in nature, addressing interagency cooperation, reimbursement, and procedural safeguards, among others. In addition to policies that regulate procedures, financing, and professional standards, five components are specific to providing services and will be discussed below. These include: 1) identification and referral, 2) determination of eligibility, 3) development of an IFSP, 4) provision of services, and 5) transition from early intervention services at age 3. Additionally, states are required to report the percentage of infants and toddlers with IFSPs who demonstrate improvement in three outcome areas: social-emotional skills, acquisition and use of knowledge and skills, and the ability to take appropriate action to meet needs.

Table 30.1. Minimum components of a statewide, comprehensive system of early intervention services to infants and toddlers with special needs

1. A rigorous definition of the term "developmental delay"
2. Appropriate early intervention services based on scientifically based research, to the extent practicable, are available to all infants and toddlers with disabilities and their families, including Native American and homeless infants and toddlers
3. Timely and comprehensive multidisciplinary evaluation of needs of children and family-directed identification of the needs of each family
4. Individualized family service plan and service coordination
5. Comprehensive child find and referral system
6. Public awareness program including the preparation and dissemination of information to be given to parents, and disseminating such information to parents
7. Central directory of services, resources, and research and demonstration projects
8. Comprehensive system of personnel development, including the training of paraprofessionals and the training of primary referral sources
9. Policies and procedures to ensure that personnel are appropriately and adequately prepared and trained
10. Single line of authority in a lead agency designated or established by the governor
11. Policy pertaining to contracting or otherwise arranging for services
12. Procedure for securing timely reimbursement of funds
13. Procedural safeguards
14. System for compiling data on the early intervention system
15. State interagency coordinating council
16. Policies and procedures to ensure that to the maximum extent appropriate, early intervention services are provided in natural environments except when early intervention cannot be achieved satisfactorily in a natural environment

Adapted from *Minimum Components Under IDEA for a Statewide, Comprehensive System of Early Intervention Services to Infants and Toddlers with Special Needs (Including American Indian and Homeless Infants and Toddlers).* National Early Childhood Technical Assistance Center. Retrieved October, 10, 2010, from http://www.nectac.org.

Identification and Referral

Under Part C regulations of The Individuals with Disabilities Education Improvement Act (IDEA) of 2004 (PL 108–446), states are required to establish programs for finding and identifying infants and toddlers who may qualify for services. These programs and procedures are referred to as Child Find. Child Find efforts (http://www.childfindidea.org/) are most effective when coordinated with other early identification programs such as Medicaid's early and periodic screening, diagnosis, and treatment (EPSDT) program. Primary care providers are in a key position to identify young children who are at risk for or who have developmental delays or disabilities (American Academy of Pediatrics, Committee on Children with Disabilities, 2010; Sand et al., 2005).

Developmental screening is often the first step in identifying and referring infants and toddlers who could benefit from early intervention services. When developmental screening occurs in the context of a well-child medical visit, it reinforces the concept that health and development are interrelated. Responding to parental concerns about a child's development has been shown to be as effective in identifying developmental delay as professional opinion and/or standardized screening (Glascoe, 2000). An infant or toddler can be referred to the local early intervention program directly by anyone (including a relative or friend) who suspects that the child has a developmental delay or disability.

Developmental screening is an option that a state may choose to include as part of its comprehensive Child Find system (IDEA, 2011). It should involve the family and other sources of information, using a process that is culturally and linguistically sensitive. It should be reliable, valid, cost effective, and time efficient. It should be seen not only as a means of early identification but also as a service that helps the family understand the child's developmental progress. Several developmental screening tests are commercially available including 1) Ages & Stages Questionnaires®, Third Edition (ASQ-3™; Squires & Bricker, 2009); 2) Denver II (Frankenburg et al., 1992); and 3) Parents' Evaluations of Developmental Status (PEDS; Glascoe, 1997).

Determining Eligibility for Early Intervention Services

According to Part C of IDEA each state is individually required to define criteria by which a child is eligible to receive early intervention services under the Part C system (note that infants and toddlers who do not meet the eligibility criteria for services under the state-run Part C program can receive services through other systems, such as directly at a clinic or through a private practitioner.)

Current federal regulations describe categories of eligibility: 1) the child demonstrates a measurable **developmental delay** as defined by each state, 2) the child has a **diagnosed physical or mental condition** that has a high probability of resulting in developmental delay (e.g., child with Down syndrome), or 3) professionals who are conducting the evaluation determine that a child demonstrates behaviors indicating atypical development and could benefit from early intervention services and supports, a process referred to as **informed clinical opinion** (e.g., a child suspected on evaluation of having autism). The federal law, IDEA, indicates that a child meets the definition of developmental delay if he or she has a "measurable delay in one or more of 5 areas (cognitive, physical, communication, social or emotional, adaptive)." States, however, decide how to define measurable delay. State-specific eligibility criteria can be found online (Shackelford, 2006).

A multidisciplinary team will conduct the eligibility evaluation to determine if a child meets the eligibility criteria. The process often begins when the family first calls the infant and toddler program for assistance. The program then makes a referral to the local agency that coordinates early intervention services, assessment, eligibility determination, and the IFSP meeting, which must be completed within 45 calendar days from the date that the family provides consent to the initial screening, evaluation, or assessment (§303.310 [b, 2]). After a family is referred, a service coordinator is assigned to partner with the family to plan and coordinate all of the steps leading to the development of a service plan, if appropriate. If the child is eligible the service coordinator will continue to assist the family in coordinating services across agency lines, serve as the single contact for parents/families to obtain needed help and services, assist families in gaining access to services identified in the IFSP, and help the family through the transition process.

The eligibility evaluation process must be timely, comprehensive, and multidisciplinary. Pertinent records relating to the child's current health status as well as medical history must be reviewed. The evaluation includes assessing the child in five areas of development: physical (including vision, hearing and gross and fine motor development), cognitive, communication, social-emotional, and adaptive. The multidisciplinary evaluation team must include a family member and two professionals representing different disciplines or may include one individual who is qualified in more than one discipline or profession (§303.24). For example, the professionals might include an early childhood special educator and a speech-language pathologist, or perhaps a motor therapist such as an occupational therapist or a physical therapist. The process must reflect the unique strengths and needs of the child. In addition, family members provide information about their concerns, priorities, and resources that may affect their child.

Development of an Individualized Family Service Plan

If the child is found eligible for services through the multidisciplinary child and family evaluation process, a multidisciplinary team, including the parents, develops an IFSP, ensuring that the diverse services are identified and coordinated and relate to the outcomes decided by the team. The array of services available in Part C includes assistive technology devices and services; audiology; family training; health services; medical services only for diagnostic or evaluation purposes; speech, physical, and occupational therapies; psychological services; service coordination services; social work services; special instruction; transportation and related costs; and vision services. This list of services is not exhaustive. The IFSP can identify other services if needed to meet the outcomes identified on the IFSP (§303.13 [d]).

Services identified in the IFSP must be provided in the natural environment, which are defined in federal regulations (Sec.303.26) as "settings that are natural or normal for an infant or toddler without a disability, may include the home." The regulations further state that early intervention services must be provided in the natural environment to the maximum extent appropriate to meet the needs of the child. However, natural environments are not limited to the home or any other place but include activities and routines that offer naturally occurring learning opportunities (DEC/NAEYC, 2009). The importance of the IFSP is evident in the law's detailed requirements regarding the plan's contents (Table 30.2).

Service Provision

According to the statement paper, Principles and Practices in Natural Environments (Hurth & Pletcher, 2007), "Part C early intervention builds upon and provides supports and resources to assist family members and caregivers to enhance children's learning and development through everyday learning opportunities." This mission is based on seven key principles that underpin family-centered services and supports (Hurth & Pletcher, 2007; Table 30.3) and act as guidelines on how early intervention services should be provided.

The principles promote a flexible system of service provision developed to respond to the team-based outcomes and not just to the diagnosis or the child's level of delay. Contemporary practice models that encompass the principles described above as well as those defined by the Division of Early Childhood (Sandall, McLean, Santos, & Smith, 2005) include routines-based intervention (McWilliam & Scott, 2001), activity-based intervention (Pretti-Frontczak & Bricker, 2004; Valvano, 2004), context-based learning opportunities (Dunst, 2001), and participation-based services (Campbell & Sawyer, 2007):

1. The critical roles of families as teachers of their children and practitioners as facilitators and teachers of both families and their children

2. The use of common activities and routines as contexts for children's learning (Chai, Zhang, & Bisberg, 2006; Stremel & Campbell, 2007)

3. The need for practice and repetition in order for learning to occur (Ulrich, 2010)

To be successful these models all require that meaningful outcomes be identified and that early-intervention professionals provide a spectrum of consultative and direct services. This approach often departs from the traditional discipline-specific model of a set frequency per week. Meaningful outcomes go beyond specific disciplinary goals to effectively address the child's participation in family and community activities and routines.

Different types of service as well as levels of service may be needed depending on the number of caregivers and the learning contexts. On the one hand, a biweekly visit with a parent and child who spend the day together at home may suffice to accomplish the desired outcome. On the other hand, a multiple-caregiver situation often requires more frequent contacts to demonstrate strategies and allow for more collaboration with key adults. A flexible model might emphasize sequential rather than simultaneous services

Table 30.2. Required elements of an individualized family service plan

1. A statement of the infant's or toddler's present levels of physical development, cognitive development, communication development, social or emotional development, and adaptive development, based on objective criteria

2. A statement of the family's resources, priorities, and concerns relating to enhancing the development of the family's infant or toddler with a disability

3. A statement of the major outcomes expected to be achieved for the infant or toddler and the family, and the criteria, procedures, and time lines used to determine the degree to which progress toward achieving the outcomes is being made and whether modifications or revisions of the outcomes or services are necessary

4. A statement of specific early intervention services necessary to meet the unique needs of the infant or toddler and the family, including the frequency, intensity, and method of delivering services

5. A statement of the natural environments in which early intervention services shall appropriately be provided, including a justification of the extent, if any, to which the services will not be provided in a natural environment

6. The projected dates for initiation of services and the anticipated duration of the services

7. The identification of the service coordinator from the professional most immediately relevant to the infant's or toddler's or family's needs (or who is otherwise qualified to carry out all applicable responsibilities under this part) who will be responsible for the implementation of the plan and coordination with other agencies and persons

8. The steps to be taken to support the transition of the toddler with a disability to preschool or other appropriate services

Source: IDEA, Part C regulations 34 CFR §§303.342–303.345.

Table 30.3.   Key principles for providing early intervention services in natural environments

1. Infants and toddlers learn best through everyday experiences and interactions with familiar people in familiar contexts.

2. All families, with the necessary supports and resources, can enhance their children's learning and development.

3. The primary role of a service provider in early intervention is to work with and support family members and caregivers in children's lives.

4. The early intervention process, from initial contacts through transition, must be dynamic and individualized to reflect the child's and family members' preferences, learning styles and cultural beliefs.

5. IFSP outcomes must be functional and based on children's and families' needs and family-identified priorities.

6. The family's priorities, needs and interests are addressed most appropriately by a primary provider who represents and receives team and community support.

7. Interventions with young children and family members must be based on explicit principles, validated practices, best available research, and relevant laws and regulations

Reprinted from Workgroup on Principles and Practices in Natural Environments. (November 2007). *Mission and principles for providing services in natural environments.* OSEP TA Community of Practice-Part C Settings. http://www.nectac.org/topics/families/families.asp

or varying levels of intensity or frequency. For example, it may be beneficial to "front-load" services, increasing the frequency of services initially and then gradually decreasing them to weekly. Each outcome should have distinct services, frequency, intensity, and location identified prior to the implementation of the IFSP. Shifting to a flexible, outcomes-guided model that is family-directed increases the likelihood that the recommendations for services will emerge from a thorough analysis of child and family priorities. This individualized, outcomes-driven model contrasts with the traditional model of providing a predetermined group of services by specific disciplines that are driven by a particular disability rather than by the specific needs, priorities, and concerns of the family (Colyvas, Sawyer, & Campbell, 2010).

Transition from Early Intervention Services

Transition is a process that children and families experience as they move from one program or setting to another. Families of young children with developmental delays and disabilities

may need to move between home and hospital or from early intervention to preschool. Under IDEA, young children will no longer be eligible to receive early intervention services at age 3. Thus, the Part C system must begin, if needed, to transition the child from the Part C system at about 2 years, 6 months to early childhood special education services, inclusive preschool or child care programs, or to other appropriate services. Careful planning and preparation can ensure that change occurs in a timely and effective manner. Transition planning may also help to alleviate parental stress. To ensure a seamless move from early intervention to other appropriate services and supports, the IFSP must include a transition plan.

STATUS OF EARLY INTERVENTION SERVICES

It has now been over 25 years since the establishment of a formal early intervention system in the United States. Judged by usual standards, this program has been successful. All 50 states and jurisdictions are participating in Part C, meaning that each of the required structural components is in place. Moreover, the number of children served continues to grow annually. Including those at risk, approximately 342,821 children, or 2.6% of the population under the age of 3, received services under Part C of IDEA in 2010 (Danaher, Goode, & Lazara, 2011).

An analysis utilizing a nationally representative sample ($N = 3,338$) from the National Early Intervention Longitudinal Study (NEILS) also suggests that Part C is achieving its intended goals. Overall, approximately 64% of children became eligible because of a developmental delay, 20% as a result of a diagnosed medical condition, and 16% due to biomedical and/or environmental risk factors (Hebbeler et al., 2007). It is also clear that the early intervention system is reaching disadvantaged groups, as 43% of children receiving services live in households with incomes less than $25,000 a year. Given the well-established association between disadvantaged status and disability (Emerson, 2007) the system's ability to enroll large numbers of these families is commendable.

Although the Part C program is serving many children, over the last 10 years 20% of the states have narrowed the eligibility criteria. Children with milder disabilities and less significant delays may actually be the ones who benefited most from early intervention services for which they are no longer eligible to receive (Hebbeler,

2010). Additionally, evidence exists to suggest that children are receiving fewer services and supports to meet IFSP outcomes (Hebbeler, Mallik, & Taylor, 2010). For example, a recent study in Texas indicated that although nationally infants and toddlers receive an average of 6.5 hours of early intervention services per month, the children in Texas receive only 2.7 hours (Hebbeler, Mallik, & Taylor, 2010). This trend may be happening in other states as well due to financial restrictions.

In many respects, the early intervention system has proven highly responsive. The NEILS study indicated that critical events in the process occurred over a 7–8 month period. The average age in which critical points occurred include: first concern about child's health or development (7.4 months), first diagnosis or identification (8.8 months), first searched-for early intervention (11.9 months) of age, first-referred early intervention (14.0 months), and age at which IFSP was developed (15.7 months; Bailey et al., 2004, 2010). Moreover, most families found an early intervention program easily, with 79% of children receiving an IFSP within 10 weeks of referral (Bailey et al., 2004). The system was not equally accessible to all families, however. Minority or low-income families were more likely to report that much effort was required to access the services (Hebbeler et al., 2010).

The NEILS data also revealed that families received numerous services offered in Part C, with 37% receiving 6 services (Hebbeler et al., 2010). Of the specific intervention services, 52% receive speech and language therapy, 43% special instruction (i.e., early childhood education), 38% occupational therapy, 37% developmental monitoring, and 37% physical therapy. The vast majority of the families receive services in their home (76%); however a sizable number (28%) receive them in either a center-based early intervention setting or clinic setting. Despite these impressive service utilization rates, the number of actual direct service hours turns out to be surprisingly quite small. NEILS data indicates that 63% of the families received 2 hours or less per week, with the average being, as noted above, 6.5 hours per month.

From the parents' perspective, the services received have been satisfactory. Although most families in the NEILS study had a positive early-intervention experience, minority or low-income families were slightly less positive. With regard to individualization of services, 61% of the families with mothers who did not graduate from high school reported that services were highly individualized compared with 69% of

those with mothers who graduated from college (Hebbeler et al., 2010).

At kindergarten, 54% of children receiving early intervention services were receiving special education services, 35% did not have a disability and thus did not receive additional services; however, 11% had a disability but were not receiving special education or related services (Hebbeler, 2010). Additionally, children who received early intervention but who were not receiving special education services were performing at peer level in reading and math skills. Teachers reported that 37% of children receiving special education services had at least average academic skills (Hebbeler, 2010).

Taken together, it is evident that a comprehensive early intervention system composed of well-defined structural components can be found in states and communities throughout the United States, providing services and supports to increasing numbers of infants and toddlers and their families. However, it is recognized that such a complex and evolving system can be substantially improved to more effectively and efficiently meet the needs of children and families (Dunst, 2007; Ramey, Ramey, & Lanzi, 2007; Tomasellio, Manning, & Dulmus, 2010).

FUTURE CONSIDERATIONS

This section will discuss some current issues that may in the future affect the effectiveness and efficiency of early intervention service delivery.

Life Course

A life course perspective (Halfon, Shonkoff, Boyce, & McEwen, 2009) posits that a complex interplay of biological, behavioral, psychological, social, and environmental factors contribute to health and developmental outcomes across the course of a person's life. This finding extends recent social science and public health literature that suggest that each life stage influences the next, and that social, economic, and physical environments interacting across the life course have a profound impact on individual and community health.

Research on the effectiveness of early intervention and early childhood practices indicate that although the impact of intervention is substantial, many children and families still do not fare well (Hebbler, 2009). This especially surfaces when families are affected by multiple stressors such as disability, poverty, substance abuse, and maternal depression (Shaw & Goode, 2008). For early intervention programs to be most successful for all children and families, a science-based approach that is responsive to variations in socio-cultural factors, health status, genetics, and neurobiology, to name a few, must be created (Halfon, Shonkoff, Boyce & McEwen, 2009). In addition, evaluation plans must surpass the child-focused developmental status to consider all factors that relate to successful adulthood, such as participation in society and health status.

System of Care Approach to Service Delivery

For implementation, the importance of coordinating services was clearly recognized in Part C and was identified as a separate and required service in the law. However, for service coordination to be most effective, simply coordinating independent services, with the potential for duplication and redundancy, may not be optimal. In such cases, the systems of care approach (Stroul & Freidman, 1986) that promote the coordination of services across agencies and providers into a network of services and supports may be more successful. Consistent with the principles of early intervention, hallmarks of systems of care include a family-centered, individualized, integrated system of supports. Collaborative consultation models that attempt to truly integrate services will achieve outcomes that will likely be more functionally valuable for the child and family (Dunst et al., 2001; Hanft & Pilkington, 2000). The increasingly diverse and complex array of services and supports required by children and families pose special challenges to the systems of care (National Research Council & Institute of Medicine, 2000). This is especially true when the services come from agencies that are not commonly part of the early intervention system, such as those related to the mental health of children and families.

Natural Environments

For infants and toddlers, Part C requires that children and families receive services in "natural environments" to the extent possible. But this has been very difficult to implement due to barriers related to financing, definitional issues, parent preferences, and provider resistance, among others (Bruder, 2001; Rabb & Dunst, 2004). Yet, contemporary practice models support intervention in the natural environment by stressing the critical roles of the family as the child's teacher and the early intervention provider as the family's educator.

Traditional service delivery is child focused; families often simply observe the service, or the professional teaches the family to execute a specific strategy (Peterson et al., 2007). Intervention strategies that assist families and other caregivers to promote the child's development within the context of naturally occurring learning opportunities are consistent with the concept of natural environments and the intent of family-centered early intervention (Bruder, 2000; Peterson et al., 2007).

By focusing intervention on activities and routines that individual families participate in rather than on locations, the provider takes advantage of natural learning opportunities and the family's role as teacher. One way to accomplish this is through participation-based early intervention (Campbell & Sawyer, 2007; Colyvas, Sawyer & Campbell, 2010), which has a primary goal of promoting a child's participation in family and community activities and routines. In a participation-based approach, early intervention professionals intervene with a child by teaching caregivers how to use two primary types of child interventions to promote the child's participation and learning: 1) adapting the environment, materials, or the activity/routine, including the use of assistive technology; and 2) embedding individualized learning strategies within family routines (Colyvas, Sawyer, & Campbell, 2010).

Other strategies, for example, activity-based intervention (Pretti-Frontczak & Bricker, 2004; Valvano & Rapport, 2006), emphasize that while intervention is within an activity, routine, and context, the *target* of intervention is the child, promoting his or her skill development. Routines-based intervention stresses the importance of engagement, independence, and social relationships within a naturally occurring child activity (McWilliam, 2010). Because intervention with infants and toddlers is a collaborative process, often including multiple caregivers, caregiver satisfaction or dissatisfaction is stressed. Caregivers must indicate dissatisfaction with the child's performance if they are going to identify functional outcomes from which they can make adaptations or embed a learning strategy. Dunst (2006) promoted the use of contextually mediated practices as an approach to promote the child's acquisition of new skills, competence, and knowledge. Contextually mediated practices use everyday family and community activities as the sources or "context" for learning.

Evidence-Based Practice

Providing services based on scientific evidence is stressed in many disciplines including medicine, therapeutic services, and education. Evidence-based practice refers to the preferential use of interventions that are supported by empirical research and describes the process of finding and using scientifically based information to guide practice. In addition to using known evidence-based strategies, evidence-based practice incorporates critical thinking in order to systematically gather and synthesize many sources of information, to help make decisions about a variety of practice and intervention questions including

- What interventions or strategies are most effective?

- How much intervention should a child receive to achieve desired outcomes?

- What is the best way to provide information and intervention to achieve the desired outcomes and support?

The process is a logical system for defining a problem and then finding the best available evidence to support decisions from research, experience, and family values about intervention, policies and practices.

Increases in scientific knowledge have been able to identify best practices and eliminate those having little validity. The early intervention field has been subject to many claims of dramatic successes that have subsequently been exposed as poorly documented (Dunst, 2007). While Part C notes that interventions should be based on peer-reviewed, scientifically based findings, this continues to be a major challenge for the early intervention field, as the research-to-practice gap is considerable (National Research Council & Institute of Medicine, 2000). A welcome addition has been the recent publication of clinical guidelines and best-practice manuals based on careful reviews of available scientific literature for screening, diagnosis, and intervention. These guidelines also support practices that promote the participation and activity-based strategies described above (National Research Council, 2001; Pretti-Frontczak, Barr, Macy, & Carter, 2003; Ramey, Ramey, & Lanzi, 2007).

SUMMARY

Infants and toddlers with disabilities and their families now have access to an early intervention system with important structural components effectively in place. Increasing numbers of children and families continue to gain access to the system and experience satisfaction with the services received. Research on the effectiveness of early intervention has demonstrated the potential for achieving important benefits for children and families. Nevertheless, fully implementing the principles that guide early intervention within a system of care that maximizes intervention effectiveness has not been achieved. As noted, this circumstance is to be expected in complex, evolving systems. Fortunately, the meaning of those critical principles is now better understood, and the interconnections among those principles is recognized. This provides clear directions to ensure that the system will continue to evolve to meet the needs of young vulnerable children and their families.

REFERENCES

American Academy of Pediatrics, Committee on Children with Disabilities. (2010). Initiatives target developmental screening services. *AAP News, 31*, 24. doi:10.1542/aapnews.2010311–24

Bailey, D., Hebbeler, K., Scarborough, A., Scarborough, A., Spiker, D., & Mallik, S. (2004). First experiences with early intervention: A national perspective. *Pediatrics, 113*, 887–896.

Bruder, M.B. (2000). Family-centered early intervention: Clarifying our values for the new millennium. *Topics in Early Childhood Special Education, 20*, 105–115.

Bruder, M.B. (2001). Inclusion of infants and toddlers: Outcomes and ecology. In M.J. Guralnick (Ed.), *Early childhood inclusion: Focus on change* (pp. 203–228). Baltimore, MD: Paul H. Brookes Publishing Co.

Campbell, P., & Sawyer, L.B. (2007). Supporting learning opportunities in natural settings through participation-based services. *Journal of Early Intervention, 29*, 287–305.

Center on the Developing Child at Harvard University. (2010). *The foundations of lifelong health are built in early childhood.* Retrieved from http://developingchild.harvard.edu/library/reports_and_working_papers/foundations-of-lifelong-health/

Chai, A.Y., Zhang, C., & Bisberg, M. (2006). Rethinking natural environment practice: Implications from examining various interpretations and approaches. *Early Childhood Education Journal, 34*, 203–208.

Colyvas, J.L., Sawyer, L.B., & Campbell, P.H. (2010). Identifying strategies early intervention occupational therapists use to teach caregivers. *American Journal of Occupational Therapy, 64*, 776–785.

Daft, R., & Lengel, R. (1998). *Fusion leadership.* San Francisco, CA: Berrett-Koehler.

DEC/NAEYC. (2009). *Early childhood inclusion: A joint position statement of the Division for Early Childhood (DEC) and the National Association for the Education of Young Children (NAEYC).* Chapel Hill, NC: The University of North Carolina, FPG Child Development Institute.

Dunst, C.J. (2001). Participation of young children with disabilities in community learning activities. In M.J. Guralnick (Ed.), *Early childhood inclusion: Focus on change* (pp. 307–333). Baltimore, MD: Paul H. Brookes Publishing Co.

Dunst, C.J. (2006). Parent-mediated everyday child learning opportunities: I. Foundations and operationalization. *CASEinPoint, 2*, 1–10.

Dunst, C.J. (2007). Early intervention for infants and toddlers with disabilities. In S.L. Odom, R.H. Horner, M.E. Snell, & J. Blacher (Eds.), *Handbook of developmental disabilities* (pp. 161–180). New York, NY: Guilford Press.

Dunst, C.J., Trivette, C.M., Humphries, T., Raab, M., & Roper, N. (2001). Contrasting approaches to natural learning environment interventions. *Infants & Young Children, 14*(2), 48–63.

Early Childhood Outcomes Center. (2011). *Summary of 2011 child outcomes data.* Retrieved from http://www.fpg.unc.edu/~eco/assets/pdfs/outcomesforchildren-final.pdf.

Emerson, E. (2007). Poverty and people with intellectual disabilities. *Mental Retardation & Developmental Disabilities Research Reviews, 13*, 107–113.

Education of the Handicapped Act Amendments of 1986, PL 99–457, 20 U.S.C. §§ 1400 et seq.

Frankenburg, W.K., Dodds, J.B., Archer, P., Bresnick, B., Maschka, P., Edelman, N., & Shapiro, H. (1992). *Denver II.* Denver, CO: Denver Developmental Materials. (Available from the publisher, Post Office Box 371075, Denver, CO 80237-5075; 800-419-4729).

Glascoe, F.P. (1997). *Parents' evaluations of developmental status (PEDS).* Nashville, TN: Ellsworth and Vandermeer Press.

Glascoe, F.P. (2000). Evidence-based approach to developmental and behavioural surveillance using parents' concerns. *Child: Care, Health and Development, 26*(2), 137–149.

Guralnick, M.J. (2004). Family investments in response to the developmental challenges of young children with disabilities. In A. Kalil & T. Deleire (Eds.), *Family investments in children's potential: Resources and parenting behaviors that promote success* (pp. 119–137). Mahwah, NJ: Lawrence Erlbaum Associates.

Guralnick, M.J. (Ed.). (2005a). *The developmental systems approach to early intervention.* Baltimore, MD: Paul H. Brookes Publishing Co.

Guralnick, M.J. (2005b). Early intervention for children with intellectual disabilities: Current knowledge and future prospects. *Journal of Applied Research in Intellectual Disabilities, 18*, 313–324.

Halfon, N., Shonkoff, J.P., Boyce, W.T., & McEwen, B.S. (2009). Neuroscience, molecular biology, and the childhood roots of health disparities: Building a new framework for health promotion and disease prevention. *Journal of the American Medical Association, 301*(21), 2252–2259.

Hanft, B.E., & Pilkington, K.O. (2000). Therapy in natural environments: The means or end goal for early intervention? *Infants & Young Children, 12*(4), 1–13.

Hebbeler, K. (2009, June). *First five years funding briefing.* Paper presented to Congressional Briefing on the Impact of Early Childhood Interventions. Washington, DC.

Hebbeler, K., Spiker, D., Bailey, D., Scarborough, A., Mallik, S., Simeonsson, R. Singer, M., & Nelson, L. (2007). *Early intervention for infants and toddlers with disabilities and their families: Participants, services, and outcomes. NEILS Final Report.* Menlo Park, CA: SRI International.

Hebbeler, K., Mallik, S. & Taylor, C. (2010). *An analysis of needs and service planning in the Texas early childhood intervention program.* Report prepared for Texas Department of Assistive and Rehabilitative Services. Menlo Park, CA: SRI International.

Hill, J.L., Brooks-Gunn, J., & Waldfogel, J. (2003). Sustained effects of high participation in an early intervention for low-birthweight premature infants. *Developmental Psychology, 39*, 730–744.

Hurth, J., & Pletcher, L. (2007). *Key principles and practices for providing early intervention services in natural environments: Reaching consensus.* Retrieved April 4, 2008, http://www.nectac.org/topics/families/families.asp

Individuals with Disabilities Education Improvement Act of 2004, PL 108–446, 20 U.S.C. §§ 1400 et seq.

McWilliam, R.A. (2010). *Routines-based early intervention: Supporting young children and their families.* Baltimore, MD: Paul H. Brookes Publishing Co.

McWilliam, R.A., & Scott, S. (2001). A support approach to early intervention: A three part framework. *Infants and Young Children, 13*, 55–66.

National Research Council. (2001). *Educating children with autism.* (Committee on Educational Interventions for Children with Autism. Division of Behavioral and Social Sciences and Education.) Washington, DC: National Academies Press.

National Research Council & Institute of Medicine (2000). *From neurons to neighborhoods: The science of early child development.* (Committee on Integrating the Science of Early Childhood Development. Jack P. Shonkoff and Deborah A. Phillips, eds. Board on Children, Youth, and Families, Commission on Behavioral and Social Sciences and Education.) Washington, DC: National Academies Press.

Peterson, C.A., Luze, G.J., Eshbaugh, E.M., Jeon, H., & Kantz, K.R. (2007). Enhancing parent–child interactions through home visiting: Promising practice or unfulfilled promise. *Journal of Early Intervention, 29*, 119–140.

Pretti-Frontczak, K., Barr, D.M., Macy, M., & Carter, A. (2003). Research and resources related to activity-based intervention, embedded learning opportunities and routines-based instruction: An annotated bibliography. *Topics in Early Childhood Special Education, 23*, 29–39.

Pretti-Frontczak, K., & Bricker, D. (2004). *An activity-based approach to early intervention* (3rd ed.). Baltimore, MD: Paul H. Brookes Publishing Co.

Rabb, M., & Dunst, C.J. (2004). Early intervention practitioner approaches to natural environment interventions. *Journal of Early Intervention, 27*, 15–26.

Ramey, S., Ramey, C., & Lanzi, R. (2007). Early intervention: Background, research findings, and future directions. In J.W. Jacobson, J.A. Mulick, & J. Rojahn (Eds.), *Handbook of intellectual and developmental disabilities* (pp. 445–463). New York, NY: Springer.

Ramey, S., Ramey, C., & Lanzi, R. (2006).Children health and education. In I. Sigel & A. Renninger (Eds.), *The handbook of child psychology.* (Vol. 4, pp. 864-892). Hoboken, NJ: Wiley & Sons.

Sand, N., Silverstein, M., Glascoe, F.P., Gupta, V.B., Tonniges, T.P., & O'Connor, K.G. (2005). Pediatricians' reported practices regarding developmental screening: Do guidelines work? Do they help? *Pediatrics, 116*, 174–179.

Sandall, S., McLean, M., Santos, R., & Smith, B. (2005). DEC's recommended practices: The context for change. In S. Sandall, M. McLean, & B. Smith (Eds.), *DEC recommended practices: A comprehensive guide for practical application in early intervention/early childhood special education* (pp. 19–26). Missoula, MT: DEC.

Scarborough, A.A., Spiker, D., Mallik, S., Hebbeler, K.M., Bailey, D.B. Jr., & Simeonsson, R.J. (2004). A national look at children and families entering early intervention. *Exceptional Children, 70*, 469–483.

Shackelford, J. (2006). *State and jurisdictional eligibility definitions for infants and toddlers with disabilities under IDEA* (NECTAC Notes, Vol. 21, pp. 1–16). Chapel Hill, NC: National Early Childhood Technical Assistance Center, The University of North Carolina.

Shaw, E., & Goode, S. (2008). *Fact Sheet: Vulnerable Young Children*. Chapel Hill, NC: National Early Childhood Technical Assistance Center.

Squires, J., & Bricker, D. (2009). *Ages & Stages Questionnaires® & Stages Questionnaires®, Third Edition (ASQ-3™): A parent-completed, child-monitoring system* (3rd ed.). Baltimore, MD: Paul H. Brookes Publishing Co.

Stremel, K., & Campbell, P. (2007). Implementation of early intervention within natural environments. *Early Childhood Services, 1*, 83–105.

Stroul, B.A., & Friedman, R.M. (1986). *A system of care for children and youth with severe emotional disturbances* (Rev. ed.) Washington, DC: Georgetown University Child Development Center, National Technical Assistance Center for Children's Mental Health.

Tomasellio, N.M., Manning, A.R., & Dulmus, C.N. (2010). Family-centered early intervention for infants and toddlers with disabilities. *Journal of Family Social Work, 13*, 163–172.

Ulrich, B. (2010). Opportunities for early intervention based on theory, basic neuroscience, and clinical science. *Physical Therapy, 91*, 1–13.

Valvano, J. (2004). Activity-focused motor interventions for children with neurological conditions. *Physical and Occupational Therapy in Pediatrics, 24*, 79–107.

Valvano, J., & Rapport, M.J. (2006). Activity-focused motor interventions for infants and young children with neurological conditions. *Infants and Young Children, 19*, 292–307.

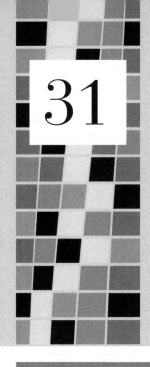

31

Special Education Services

Elissa Batshaw Clair

Upon completion of this chapter, the reader will

- Be knowledgeable about services and supports available for children with disabilities

- Understand the components of an individualized education program

- Be aware of the history of special education services

- Be familiar with the Individuals with Disabilities Education Improvement Act of 2004, The No Child Left Behind Act, and other legislation pertaining to education for children with disabilities

- Understand the roles of a special education teacher

Special education is defined by the Individuals with Disabilities Education Improvement Act of 2004 (IDEA 2004; PL 108–446) as "specially designed instruction, at no cost to parents, to meet the unique needs of a child with a disability" (§ 602[29]). Special education includes direct educational instruction by a special education teacher; related services such as language therapy, speech therapy, physical therapy, occupational therapy, or social work services; paraprofessional support; or consultation from a special education professional to the general education teacher. All special education services are individualized to provide the instruction necessary to reach each child's goals. IDEA 2004 guarantees a free appropriate public education (FAPE) for all children with disabilities ages 3–21. A zero-reject provision mandates that even students who have severe and multiple impairments have the right to a FAPE in the least restrictive environment (LRE).

Before the enactment of the Education for All Handicapped Children Act of 1975 (PL 94-142), the educational needs of millions of children with disabilities were not being fully met. They did not receive appropriate educational services, were excluded entirely from the public school system and from being educated with their peers, had undiagnosed disabilities that prevented them from having a successful educational experience, or faced a lack of adequate resources within the public school system, requiring them to find services outside of the public school system (PL 108-446 § [601][c][2]).

Since the 1970s, legislation has attempted to address each of these issues. Figure 31.1 summarizes the history of educational law prior to the current law, IDEA 2004.

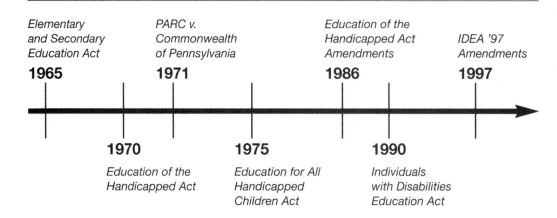

Elementary and Secondary Education Act of 1965 (PL 89-10)	Attempted to correct unequal educational opportunities that resulted from a child's economic condition
Education of the Handicapped Act (EHA) of 1970 (PL 91-230)	Amendment to earlier legislation that established a core grant program for local education agencies (LEAs) to provide services for children with disabilities
Pennsylvania Association of Retarded Citizens (PARC) v. Commonwealth of Pennsylvania (1971)	PARC proved • All children with intellectual disability are capable of benefiting from a program of education and training • Education cannot be defined as only the provision of academic experiences for children • Having undertaken to provide all children with a free appropriate public education (FAPE), the state could not deny students with intellectual disability access to FAPE • The earlier students with intellectual disability are provided education, the better the predictable learning outcomes (Yell, 1998).
Education for All Handicapped Children Act of 1975 (PL 94-142)	• Provided FAPE to all school-age children, regardless of their disability • Was a funded program • Defined the disabilities that would be covered and established guidelines for fair evaluation and assessment
Education of the Handicapped Act Amendments of 1986 (PL 99-457)	• Extended special education services to infants and preschoolers • Developed an individual family service plan (IFSP) for infants and toddlers in early intervention programs (Mercer, 1997)
Individuals with Disabilities Education Act (IDEA) of 1990 (PL 101-476)	• Used person-first language and replaced the word *handicap* with *disability* • Arranged for transition planning to occur to help students progress from high school into adulthood (Mercer, 1997) • Emphasized meeting the needs of ethnically and culturally diverse children with disabilities • Indicated early intervention programs to address the needs of children who were exposed prenatally to maternal substance abuse (Mercer, 1997)
Individuals with Disabilities Education Act Amendments of 1997 (IDEA '97; PL 105-17)	• Strengthened the role of parents • Gave increased attention to racial, ethnic, and linguistic diversity to prevent inappropriate identification and mislabeling • Ensured that schools are safe and conducive to learning • Encouraged parents and educators to work out their differences by using nonadversarial means

Figure 31.1.   History of educational law prior to the current law, the Individuals with Disabilities Education Improvement Act of 2004 (IDEA 2004; PL 108-446).

■ ■ ■ JOHN

John did not walk or speak his first word until 18 months. As a toddler, John received speech therapy in his home once per week in accordance with an individualized family service plan (IFSP) provided under Part C (Infants and Toddlers with Disabilities) of IDEA. These services were designed to help John's parents facilitate their son's communication skills. When John entered kindergarten, he was soon identified as having significant delays compared with his classmates and as needing assessment for special education services. His parents gave permission for testing, which showed him to be functioning in the range of mild intellectual disabilities. He was thus eligible for special education services.

An **individualized educational program (IEP)** was developed with input from a team consisting of a psychologist, a general education teacher, a special education teacher, a speech-language pathologist, and John's parents. The IEP identified the goals for John, the amount of time he would receive special education services, and the **related services** that would be provided to support his educational progress.

The IEP team reviewed information from his most recent evaluation as well as data collected by teachers, parental input, and IEP team discussion. The IEP team determined that the most appropriate placement for John was in an inclusive environment in a class containing children both with and without disabilities. The class was cotaught by both a general education and special education teacher working together. Ideally this class would be cotaught throughout the entire day, but it is more typical for classes to be cotaught for portions of the day, with only the general education teacher teaching other portions. The class contained children with and without disabilities. The two teachers worked together so that all children could have access to the same core curriculum, with differentiated instruction and **modifications** to the schoolwork. The team also decided that John would require related services from a speech-language pathologist. Sometimes this therapist would teach a lesson to all or part of the class; at other times, she worked with John individually.

John made good progress in this program and was reassessed regularly so that his IEP could be adjusted. When John was 16 years old, he began the transition planning process mandated by IDEA. With his input during a transition-planning inventory, a **transition IEP** was developed. John was very interested in cooking, often preparing creative meals at home. He chose to attend prevocational food service classes in addition to his academic courses. The high school offered career cluster experiences in culinary arts, and John continued taking vocational classes, honing his skills as a chef. With the help of a job coach provided by the Bureau of Vocational Rehabilitation, John secured a summer job at a local restaurant. He continued in his school program through age 21 because special education legislation offers services through this age for students with disabilities who 1) have not earned all of their credits toward graduation, 2) need additional transition services, or 3) are earning an alternative certificate rather than a general education diploma. Beginning in eleventh grade, when John was 17, he worked half days at the restaurant while continuing to attend school part-time. At 20 years old, he enrolled in culinary classes at a community college as part of his ITP. At 21, he completed his public education, receiving a diploma, and was subsequently hired full-time as an assistant chef at the restaurant.

ELIGIBILITY FOR SPECIAL EDUCATION

Eligibility for special education services is defined by IDEA 2004. Two other laws, Section 504 of the Rehabilitation Act of 1973 (PL 93-112) and the Americans with Disabilities Act (ADA) of 2008 (PL 110-325), also contribute to this concept. Another law affecting special education but not directly pertaining to eligibility, the No Child Left Behind (NCLB) Act of 2001, will be addressed later in this chapter.

Individuals with Disabilities Education Improvement Act of 2004

For a child to receive special education services, he or she must have a physical, cognitive, or behavioral impairment that interferes with the ability to benefit from instruction in the general classroom curriculum. The specific disabilities recognized by IDEA 2004 legislation (§ 602[3][a]) fall under the following categories

- Intellectual disability
- Hearing impairments (including deafness)
- Speech or language impairments
- Visual impairments (including blindness)
- Emotional disturbances
- Orthopedic impairments
- Autism
- Traumatic brain injury
- Other health impairments (including chronic diseases and attention-deficit/hyperactivity disorder [ADHD] if they impair educational performance)
- Specific learning disabilities
- Young child with a developmental delay (ages 3–9)

Autism is the fastest growing of these categories. For the 2002–2003 school year there were 137,000 students identified with autism. This accounted for 1.8% of the special education population and 0.2% of the general population. For the 2007–2008 school year there were 296,000 students identified with autism. This accounted for 4.5% of the special education population and 0.6% of the general population. (U.S. Department of Education, 2009). Students who qualify as having a disability under IDEA are provided services through an IEP.

Section 504 of the Rehabilitation Act of 1973 and the Americans with Disabilities Act Amendments Act of 2008

The basic concept of IDEA is that of zero-reject—in other words, that the public school system must accommodate or find alternate accommodations at public expense for every child with disabilities. If a child does not satisfy the IDEA 2004 criteria for disabilities, he or she may still receive special education services through Section 504 of the Rehabilitation Act of 1973 (PL 93-112) or the ADA of 2008 (PL 110-325), of which the objectives and language are very similar. These two acts are intended to establish a "level playing field" by eliminating barriers that exclude people with disabilities from participation in the community and workplace. They attempt to eliminate hurdles and discrimination that prevent or hamper participation, whether physical (e.g., steps instead of ramps) or programmatic (e.g., exclusion of a child with HIV from the classroom). The ADA

creates access to physical barriers. An example of this is mandating an elevator or lift in a school building if needed for a student with a physical disability. Section 504 of the Rehabilitation Act of 1973 creates access to programmatic needs. An example of this is requiring a place to rest and shortened assignments if needed for a student with narcolepsy.

The definition of disability is broader under Section 504 than under IDEA 2004. Although Section 504 covers the majority of students covered by IDEA 2004, the reverse is not the case. Specifically, Section 504 protects persons who have a physical or mental impairment that substantially limits one or more major life activities, have a record of such impairment, or are regarded as having such impairment. Examples of major life activities include functions such as caring for oneself, performing manual tasks, walking, seeing, hearing, speaking, breathing, learning, and working (34 C.F.R. 104.3[j][2][ii]). Congress further refined this list to include eating, sleeping, standing, lifting, bending, reading, concentrating, thinking, and communicating (US Department of Education, 2009). The following are examples of students who may be covered by Section 504 to receive special education services but not by IDEA 2004:

- Students with communicable diseases (e.g., HIV)
- Students who use alcohol
- Students with temporary disabilities resulting from accidents who may need short-term hospitalizations or homebound recovery
- Pregnant students
- Students with attention disorders without significant academic deficiencies
- Students with Tourette syndrome, epilepsy, or cancer

Attention-Deficit/Hyperactivity Disorder: IDEA or 504

Children diagnosed with ADHD may require services under IDEA in the category of Other Health Impairment, services under Section 504 of the Rehabilitation Act, or may not require any services that differ from other students at their school. Making the decision whether a child requires an IEP or a 504 plan is individual and based on a team decision after weighing that child's unique strengths and weaknesses. Examples of educational needs that may require accommodations, modifications, or instruction in students with ADHD include the following:

- Difficulty sustaining attention during instruction or when presented with long assignments
- Difficulty following multistep directions (working memory)
- Misplacing assignments/supplies
- Difficulty completing long-term assignments (organization)
- Behavior problems (impulsivity, oppositional defiant behavior)

When deciding between an IDEA diagnosis and a 504 plan, the team should consider whether the student needs accommodations, modifications, or specialized instruction to allow him or her access to the general education curriculum. For students whose needs can be served by accommodations, the team may determine that a 504 plan is the most appropriate action. Accommodations for students with ADHD may include, for example, having assignments shortened without changing the difficulty level, having multistep directions written down, or writing assignments in a daily planner. For students who need specialized instruction, the team may determine that an IEP will most appropriately address deficits in social skills, self-monitoring, accessing memory, regulating alertness, or sustaining effort. For students who require modifications such as lowering the difficulty level of assignments or shortening assignments so that integral portions are omitted, the team may develop an IEP after carefully weighing both options and considering additional factors.

Other Factors That Define Disability

Nondiscriminatory Assessment and Eligibility

Public schools are obligated to provide a nondiscriminatory evaluation for any child suspected of having a disability. This includes children enrolled in private schools and children ages 3–5 years who are not yet registered for school. Implementing this requirement varies from state to state. In addition to having access to official preschool Child Find (early intervention) programs, generally parents can bring their child to the local school district and request an evaluation. The stated purpose of the initial evaluation is to determine whether a child has a disability and, if present, to establish the child's educational needs (PL 108–446, §§ 612 [a][10][A][ii] and § 614[a] [1][A]).

Parents must consent prior to an evaluation. This consent, however, is not consent for placing the child in a special education program; this must be obtained separately. A child is usually evaluated by a multidisciplinary team consisting of a psychologist and one or more of the following education professionals: speech-language pathologist, occupational therapist, physical therapist, and/or social worker. The evaluation team should use a comprehensive assessment process to address the child's strengths, interests, goals, and needs in order to determine whether and which special education services are required. The evaluation may include tests of intelligence, academic skills, memory, visual-motor integration, adaptive behavior, reading, math, social-emotional skills, motor skills, sensory integration, and language. For children whose cognitive functioning is at a preschool level, testing focuses on communication, social, and adaptive skills.

The multidisciplinary team must follow specific guidelines during the child's evaluation. These guidelines were created in response to certain faulty evaluation practices in the past, which led to many children (especially minority children; see section called Overrepresentation) being incorrectly diagnosed and placed in special education. Many minority children who functioned appropriately outside of school were classified as "intellectually disabled" based on a single IQ test. These children became known as "6-hour retarded" children (Skiba et al., 2008). With this in mind, a number of mandates for nondiscriminatory evaluation procedures were installed as part of IDEA 2004. The key mandates are 1) that a number of tests must be used to determine whether the child has a disability, and 2) that parental input must be included (PL 108-466, § 614[a][2][A–C] and 614[b][3][A]).

With increasing concerns about the rising number of students classified as having a learning disability, IDEA 2004 prohibits eligibility decisions from being made based on a lack of instruction or as a result of limited English proficiency (PL 108-446, § 614 [b][5] [A–C]). Reevaluation of a child with a disability is required to take place no more than once per year or less than once every 3 years, unless the parent and local education agency agree that the timelines should be altered.

Overrepresentation

One of the goals of IDEA 2004 is to reduce the overrepresentation of minorities in special education. African Americans have the highest level of overrepresentation; this is most pronounced in the areas of intellectual disability and emotional disturbance. African American students make up 31% of the population with intellectual disabilities in public schools and 29% of the population with emotional disturbance, although they represent only 17% of the overall population (U.S. Department of Education, 2008). Within the population of children with disabilities, African American students are also overrepresented in the more restricted settings over a range of disabilities (Skiba et al., 2006). In 2008 African American students made up 20% of the population receiving special education services but 28% of the population spending 40% or less of the day in general education (US Department of Education, 2008). Although many posit that poverty may be the underlying cause of overrepresentation, Skiba et al. found that rates of free-lunch status was a weak predictor of overrepresentation of African American students. In fact, they found that as poverty decreases, overrepresentation increases. However, race (white) and limited classroom management skills of teachers are both strongly linked to overrepresentation of minority students (Harry & Klingner, 2006; Skiba et al., 2005).

In contrast, the Latino and Native American populations are proportionately represented in special education (20% and 20% for Latino and 1% and 1% for Native American), and Asian Americans are underrepresented in special education (2.3% in special education and 4.7% of the population; U.S. Department of Education, 2008).

Evaluation under Discrepancy Model

In the past, students were diagnosed with a specific learning disability (SLD) based on a discrepancy between their ability (IQ) and academic achievement (generally one to two standard deviations) on standardized tests. The **discrepancy model** is often called the "wait to fail" model; as a child ages, he or she will fall far enough behind to have a significant difference between his or her ability (IQ) and achievement, and the school will finally be permitted to provide special education services at that time. This delays receipt of necessary services for the student. Studies have also indicated that the discrepancy model was not applied with fidelity and that many students were identified as having SLD without having met the discrepancy criteria either because of political reasons or because of a lack of resources in general education (VanDerHeyden & Burns, 2010).

Response to Intervention

Response to intervention (RTI) represents a shift in thinking about students who have

difficulty learning at the same rate as their peers. Students with learning difficulties are provided supplementary instruction within general education, with special education being the final rung on the ladder of support. RTI also concerns the diagnosis of students with SLD. RTI was introduced by IDEA 2004 as an alternate and preferred method for diagnosing children with SLD. It is likely when IDEA is next reauthorized, RTI will be the only acceptable method for diagnosing SLD. As noted by VanDerHeyden and Burns, RTI includes

(a) quality core instruction; (b) universal screening; (c) progress monitoring for students identified with difficulties; (d) increasingly intensive interventions implemented based on student need; and (e) resulting data used to instructional, resource allocation, placement and special education identification decisions. (2010, p. 6)

The RTI model is a three-tier model. About 80% of students fall in Tier 1; these are students that respond to the research-based instruction provided in the classroom and perform near grade level or above.

About 20% of students are serviced in Tier 2; these are students performing below grade level. Tier 2 students are provided with research-based small-group instruction in deficit areas in addition to the instruction they receive in the classroom. With this additional instruction, they make progress at a rate that will allow them to catch up with their peers. Some Tier 2 students gain the requisite skills they were lacking and no longer require additional instruction; these students return to Tier 1. Some Tier 2 students make appropriate progress but require additional instruction to continue their gains; these students remain on Tier 2.

About one quarter of Tier 2 students (5% of the general population) do not progress at a rate that allows them to approximate typical student performance. These students require more intensive services and move to Tier 3. At Tier 3, students receive smaller group or individual instruction targeted to meet their unique areas of weakness in addition to the services they receive on Tiers 1 and 2 (Daly, Martens, Barnett, Witt, & Olson, 2007; Glover & DiPerna, 2007; Shinn, 2007; VanDerHeyden & Burns, 2010).

Evaluation Under the Response to Intervention Model

Within the response to intervention (RTI) model, when a student does not make adequate progress at Tier 3, he or she may be considered for a special education evaluation. Both

discrepancy and RTI evaluations are comprehensive as guaranteed by IDEA. In states or districts that use the RTI model for instruction but
not for evaluation, a discrepancy analysis evaluation will likely be used as part of the comprehensive evaluation. For states/districts that use RTI
for evaluation, a different route is taken within
the comprehensive evaluation and generally does
not involve any measure of cognition.

Dual Discrepancy Model

The most common RTI evaluation method is
called the **dual discrepancy model**. It is called a
dual discrepancy model because both a student's
level of progress and rate of progress are used
to make a SLD determination. A Tier 3 student
who continues to function at a level significantly
below his or her peers and has a rate of progress
at least one standard deviation below progress
levels of typically developing peers would qualify as a student with a SLD. An alternate RTI
evaluation method qualifies a student as having
a SLD when that student is making progress at
Tier 3 but needs a level of service that approximates special education and can no longer be
maintained using only general education services
(Shinn, 2007; VanDerHeyden & Burns, 2010).

SPECIAL EDUCATION: A DESCRIPTION

Accommodations and Modifications

Students with disabilities can be supported
within the general education curriculum in many
different ways, among which are accommodations and curriculum modifications.

Accommodations are changes in the way a
student has access to the curriculum or demonstrates learning. Accommodations provide equal
access to learning, do not substantially change
the instructional level or content, are based on
individual strengths and needs, and may vary in
intensity or degree. An example of this would
be reducing a spelling list that teaches the concept of the -*it* ending from 10 words to 5 words.
The student with a disability is responsible for
learning the same material as the students without disabilities, although with a reduced output.
Other examples include reading directions to
the student, providing extended time to complete assignments, providing study aids, giving
frequent reminders of rules, providing taped
texts, and giving note-taking assistance.

Modifications to curriculum provide material that substantially changes the general education curriculum. An example of this would be

requiring less-challenging spelling concepts. The
student is responsible for learning 5 -*it* spelling
words, such as *sit*, while his classmates are responsible for 10 -*tion* words, such as *conversation*.

Curriculum modifications in reading may
involve approximations of grade level curriculum such as Hi/Lo readers for students with mild
disabilities. Hi/Lo readers allow access to high-
content literature (e.g., *Gulliver's Travels*) at a low
reading level. Students with moderate disabilities
may access reading curriculum through activities
such as reading recipes and defining cooking
terms (Collins, Karl, Riggs, Galloway, & Hager,
2010). Cooper-Duffy, Szedia, and Hyer (2010)
propose a modified reading curriculum for students with severe disabilities that requires the
student to "stamp his name using a stamp, demonstrate awareness that a story is being read to
him, [or] go to the bookshelf to select a book he
likes" (p. 34).

Inclusion Practices

A number of practices have been developed
to accomplish the goal of inclusion. Inclusion
refers to educating persons with disabilities
alongside students without disabilities. Such
students attend neighborhood schools and general education classes with the necessary accommodations, modifications, and supplemental
supports (Williamson, McLeskey, Hoppey, &
Rentz, 2006).

Specialized Instructional Methods

One instructional method beneficial to students
with disabilities within the general education
environment is **cooperative learning**, a term
that describes a range of team-based learning strategies. Students are divided into small
teams with varying abilities and are assigned a
task that they complete together. Team members monitor, assist, and provide each other
with feedback. Methods such as direct instruction, small-group instruction, and independent
practice are combined with cooperative learning to teach skills and information. Cooperative
learning is successful in teaching both academic
and social skills (Downing, 2003; Fore, Riser, &
Boon, 2006).

Another strategy is peer tutoring, which
provides students opportunities to support each
other as they practice to attain mastery of material initially taught by the teacher. Peer tutoring
may occur as part of a classwide program such as
Peer Assisted Learning Strategies (PALS). PALS
are codified programs for a variety of subjects
with set instructional materials, routines, and

guidelines for practice. These programs allow students to master complex skills such as reading comprehension (McMaster, Fuchs, & Fuchs, 2006; Stenhoff, & Lignuaris/Kraft, 2007). Alternately, peer tutoring can be more informal, with the stronger student reviewing rote material such as spelling words or multiplication facts.

Two of the most successful instructional methods for increasing proficiency in students with disabilities are **direct instruction** (DI) and **cognitive strategy instruction** (CSI). DI is a codified approach to teacher-led instruction that provides explicit instruction with teacher modeling, extensive practice through choral response, brisk pacing, and immediate corrective feedback. The DI technique is very successful for teaching fundamental reading skills, and building reading fluency and reading comprehension (Tomas & Axelrod 2005).

CSI is beneficial when teaching more complex material involving problem solving and decision making. CSI teaches metacognitive strategies (thinking about thinking) to improve learning and performance. Montague and Dietz (2009) found that "students with learning disabilities have not acquired strategies that facilitate problem solving or may have difficulty selecting strategies" (p 285). CSI teaches students to approach problems the way that higher-achieving students solve problems. Like DI, CSI is also teacher-modeled and highly structured, with immediate corrective feedback. The CSI model has six stages, as described by Montague and Dietz (p. 286):

1. Developing and activating background knowledge
2. Discussing the strategy
3. Modeling the strategy
4. Memorizing the strategy
5. Supporting the strategy (e.g., guided practice using scaffolded instructional techniques)
6. Performing independently

POSSE (Predict, Organize, Search, Summarize, Evaluate) and SQ3R (Survey, Question, Read, Recite, Review) are commonly used CSI methods that guide struggling learners through the process of strategic reading (Jitendra, Burgess, & Gajria, 2011).

Related Services Within Special Education

In addition to the academic services provided by the teacher, children with disabilities are eligible to receive related services. The term **related services** is defined as "transportation and such developmental, corrective, and other supportive services … as may be required to assist a child with a disability to benefit from special education" (PL 108-446, § 601[26]). According to IDEA 2004 (PL 108-446, § 602[26]), these services include the following:

- Speech-language pathology and audiology services
- Psychological services
- Physical and occupational therapy
- Recreation, including therapeutic recreation
- Social work services
- Counseling services, including rehabilitation counseling
- Orientation and mobility services, including therapeutic recreation
- Medical services
- Nurse services

Table 31.1 summarizes the types of related services that may be provided for individuals by disability.

THE INDIVIDUALIZED EDUCATION PROGAM

The IEP consists of the educational services a child will receive and the expected achievement goals with the support of these services, over the course of the school year. According to IDEA 2004, these goals must be developed based on the strengths of the child; the concerns of the parents; the results of the most recent evaluation of the child; and the academic, developmental, and functional needs of the child (§ 614[d][3] [A]). A new IEP must be written at least once per year and should be modified as often as needed based on an assessment of the child's progress; however, pilot programs have been commissioned to develop an IEP that lasts up to 3 years. In addition, an IEP can now be amended when changes are necessary (as opposed to rewriting the entire IEP) if the changes are covered within the time frame of the original IEP.

Format and Content

The law is very specific about what must be included in an IEP. According to IDEA 2004, an IEP must contain the following items (PL 108-446, § 614 [d][1][A]):

- A statement of the child's present level of academic achievement and functional

Table 31.1. Examples of disabilities and typical related services provided

Disability	Services									
	Speech-language pathology	Audiology	Behavior support and counseling	Physical therapy	Occu-pational therapy	Vision (orientation and mobility)	Social work	Assistive technology	Transportation	Medical services
Vision impairment			X		X	X	X	X	X	
Hearing impairment	X	X	X				X	X	X	
Intellectual disability	X		X	X			X	X	X	
Autism	X		X		X		X	X	X	
Attention-deficit/hyperactivity disorder			X				X	X	X	
Learning disabilities			X				X	X		
Cerebral palsy	X		X	X	X	X	X	X	X	X
Traumatic brain injury	X		X	X	X		X	X	X	X

performance and how the child's disability affects participation in the general curriculum

- A statement of measurable annual goals, including academic and functional goals

- A description of how the child's progress toward the annual goals will be measured

- A statement of the special education, related services, and supplementary aids and services, based on peer-reviewed research to the extent practicable, that will be provided to the child or on behalf of the child

- A statement of modifications or supports for school personnel that will be provided for the child

- An explanation of the extent, if any, to which the child will not participate with children who do not have disabilities in the general education classroom

- A statement of any individual modifications that are needed for the child to participate in state- or districtwide assessments of student achievement

- A statement of the projected date for the beginning of the services and modifications, along with descriptions and an indication of the anticipated frequency, location, and duration of those services and modifications

- A statement for students 16 years or older of postsecondary goals based on age-appropriate transition assessments related to training, education, employment, and, when appropriate, independent living skills

Personnel

Members of an IEP team include the parent(s), the child (when appropriate), the special education teacher, representatives of related services such as therapists and social workers, the general education teacher (if the student is likely to participate in the general education environment), an interpreter if needed, a representative of the LEA (Local Educational Agency), and an individual who can interpret evaluation results (PL 108-446, § 614 [d] [1][B] [i–vii]).

Establishment of the Least Restrictive Environment

IDEA 2004 emphasizes that the general education classroom is the appropriate beginning point for planning an IEP. A more restrictive placement should be considered only when participation in the general education classroom is demonstrably not beneficial to the student. Even students with severe cognitive impairment have

benefited academically and socially from being educated in an inclusive environment (Williamson, McLeskey, Hoppey, & Rentz, 2006). IDEA clearly states that the need for modifications to the general education curriculum is by itself not a valid reason for placing a student in a more restrictive educational setting. According to the Office of Special Education and Rehabilitative Services (OSERS; 1994), appropriately placing a student is made on a case-by-case basis based on:

…that child's unique level of educational benefits available to the disabled student in a traditional classroom, supplemented with appropriate aids and services, in comparison to the educational benefits to the disabled student from a special education classroom; the non-academic benefits to the disabled student from interacting with non-disabled students; and the degree of disruption of the education of other students, resulting in the inability to meet the unique needs of the disabled student.

There has been great improvement in reducing the time students spend in separate settings for special education. Between 1989 and 2007, the percentage of students with disabilities receiving services inside of the general education environment for 80% or more of the day almost doubled, from 31%–57% (U.S. Department of Education, 2009). Table 31.2 summarizes the different approaches and environments for providing special education services and the distribution of students within these environments.

Development of Annual Goals and Benchmarks or Objectives

IDEA 2004 requires the development of measurable annual goals to enable parents and educators to determine a student's progress. These goals should address both academic and nonacademic concerns and be based on the student's current education and behavior level. Parents of children with disabilities are to be informed of their child's progress as often as are parents of children without disabilities. Therefore, if general education report cards are distributed quarterly, reports on goal progress must also be distributed quarterly. Progress toward reaching annual goals does not necessarily require a letter grade but can be performance based or criterion referenced and can be rated on a spectrum, for example, from "no progress" to "goal met." In addition to goals, students who participate in alternative assessments require benchmarks that delineate smaller steps needed to meet the goal (Federal Register, §300.320[a][2][ii]). If the

Table 31.2. Levels of educational placement, from least to most restrictive

Environment	% of all students with disabilities	Means of service provision
0%–21% of the day spent in a special education setting	All disabilities 57 Learning disabilities 59 Speech/language impairments 87 Emotional disturbance 37 Intellectual disability 16 Other health impairment 59	*General education class with consulting special education teacher or related services provider, services with or without special materials:* A special education teacher or related services provider assists the general education teacher in adapting the general education curriculum to best meet the needs of the child with a disability. The special education professional may come into the classroom to work directly with the child. The special education teacher may coteach class with the general education teacher. *Modified general education class:* The child receives services from a special education teacher and/or related services provider (e.g. physical therapist, occupational therapist, speech-language pathologist) outside of the general education setting for a small (<22%) portion of the day.
22%–60% of the day spent in a special education setting	All disabilities 22.4 Learning disabilities 30 Speech/language impairments 6 Emotional disturbance 20 Intellectual disability 27 Other health impairment 25	*General education class with resource services:* The child typically joins a small group of students in a separate classroom (21%–60% of the school day) to work on areas of need with a special education teacher or related services provider.
61%–100% of the day spent in a special education setting	All disabilities 15 Learning disabilities 9 Speech/language impairments 4.5 Emotional disturbance 24 Intellectual disability 49 Other health impairment 12	*Self-contained environment:* The child is in a separate special education class for the majority (61%–100%) of the school day but typically has lunch and nonacademic classes with peers without disabilities.
100% of the day spent in a special education setting	All disabilities 3 Multiple disabilities 20 Deaf blind 21	*Special day school:* The child attends a school that serves only children with disabilities, and he or she spends no time during the school day with children without disabilities.
	All disabilities 0.4	*Residential school:* The child attends an overnight special education program.
	All disabilities 0.4	*Hospital or home instruction:* The child is unable to attend school and is educated in the hospital during a hospital stay or receives services at home.

Sources: Mercer (1997); U.S. Department of Education, Office of Special Education and Rehabilitative Services (2009); and Ysseldyke and Algozzine (1995).

annual goal is that "David" will achieve a fifth-grade level reading score or above, as measured by the Qualitative Reading Inventory (QRI), benchmarks delineating the path to that goal may look like the following (NICHCY, 2010):

Short-Term Objectives

1. By October, when given a list of 20 unfamiliar words that contain short-vowel sounds, David will decode them with 90% accuracy on each of 5 trials.

2. By October, when given 20 unfamiliar words that contain long-vowel sounds, David will decode them with 90% accuracy on each of 5 trials.

3. By December, David will correctly pronounce 20 words with 90% accuracy on each of 5 trials to demonstrate understanding of the rule that where one vowel follows another, the first vowel is pronounced with a long sound and the second vowel is silent (ordeal, coast).

4. By December, David will correctly separate 20 words by syllables with 90% accuracy on each of 5 trials to demonstrate understanding of the [syllable-separation rule].

The Transition Individualized Educational Program

An adolescent with a disability needs to start preparing for life in the community (see Chapter 40). According to IDEA 2004, the plans for meeting this goal may include preparing for "post-secondary education, vocational training, integrated employment (including supported employment), competitive employment, continuing and adult education, adult services, independent living, or community participation" (§ 602[30][A]).

Beginning at age 16 (though it is widely recommended to start sooner), a formal transition IEP must be prepared and should be based on the individual student's needs, interests, and choices. According to the National Center for Learning Disabilities (2009), it must include

- Development of appropriate measurable post-secondary goals based upon age appropriate transition assessments related to training, education, employment, and, where appropriate, independent living skills;

- Development of a statement of the transition services (including courses of study) needed to assist the child in reaching those goals.

Carter et al. (2009) recommend that as "postsecondary goals are deeply entrenched in values and beliefs about family, community, adulthood and disability," transition IEPs should be culturally responsive. A transition IEP will map out "instruction, related services, community experiences, the development of employment and other post-school adult living objectives, and, when appropriate, acquisition of daily living skills and functional vocational evaluation" (§ 602[30][C]).

SERVICES PROVIDED BY SPECIAL EDUCATION TEACHERS

Special education teachers provide individualized instruction, supplementary aids, and support designed to meet the needs of students with disabilities. The special education teacher's mission is to instruct and support the student so he or she is able to access the curriculum, benefit from educational instruction, and be prepared for life after school. Students with disabilities receive the majority of services they need from special education teachers, with the remainder of services provided by related

service professionals (as discussed in section Related Services Within Special Education). Special education teachers spend the majority of their time directly instructing children with disabilities. The balance of time is spent creating, adapting, and modifying materials for special education students, maintaining IDEA documentation, and collaborating with general education teachers (Vannest & Hagan-Burke, 2010). As an IEP manager, the special education teacher is responsible for leading the team developing the IEP in accordance with the child's needs, interacting with families, and ensuring that the IEP is followed with integrity by general education staff, paraprofessionals, and related service providers.

Special education teachers instruct in academic, functional skills and in behavioral areas. In academics, they teach the same material or content (for moderate to severe impairments) as is taught in the general education curriculum, but with accommodations and modifications (as discussed in the previously covered section, Accommodations and Modifications) that allow the student to access the material at his or her appropriate instructional level or mode of communication. Academic material may be approximated for students with moderate to severe impairments (Browder, Wakeman, Flowers, Rickelman & Pugalee 2007; Cooper-Duffy, Szedia & Hyer, 2010). In the NCLB legislation, special education teachers who teach content, rather than support content taught by general education teachers, are required to be "highly qualified" in that content area (see section addressing No Child Left Behind). Functional skills include academic skills, social/communicative skills, recreation and leisure skills, personal care skills, vocational skills, and/or participation in the community. An example of a functional skill that approximates an academic skill is following a picture recipe instead of a written recipe in cooking class (Collins, Karl, Rigga, Galloway, & Hagar, 2010).

THE ROLE OF THE SPECIAL EDUCATION TEACHER IN THE GENERAL EDUCATION CURRICULUM

Although in the past the special educator's role in general education was to support inclusion (students who qualify for special education services during instruction in the general education classroom), that role is changing. As special education and general education services become more integrated (see section Response to Intervention), the role of the special educator becomes more complex. The responsive special educator will fill the following roles as described by Hoover and Patton (2008):

1. Data-driven decision maker
2. Implementer of evidence-based interventions
3. Differentiator of instruction
4. Implementer of socioemotional and behavioral supports
5. Collaborator

The special educator should also be prepared to supervise paraprofessionals and function as a co-teacher in the general education setting.

The Special Education Teacher as Data-based Decision Maker

Special educators serve as members of problem-solving teams for at-risk students and students with disabilities. The team interprets teacher-generated data to evaluate the amount of progress students are making. The team uses the data to make decisions about the need for instructional changes (Kovaleski & Pedersen, 2008).

The Special Education Teacher as Implementer of Evidence-Based Interventions

Evidence-based interventions are teaching methods that scientific studies have indicated are the most effective. Their use is imperative when working with students with disabilities. Students are identified with educational disabilities because they have not learned effectively when taught with typical instructional methods (Cook, Tankersley, & Landrum, 2009). Commercial evidence-based interventions can be found on the "What Works Clearinghouse" web site of the U.S. Department of Education. Information about noncommercial evidence-based practices can be found in educational research journals. As an example, publications of the Council for Exceptional Children (a professional organization for special education professionals) are valuable resources for finding evidence-based interventions.

The Special Education Teacher as Differentiator of Instruction

Differentiated instruction means that the teacher structures instruction to best fit the needs of each student. Instruction can be differentiated in the following areas (Council for Exceptional Children, 2011):

- Content (altering complexity or presentation)
- Process (altering the amount of support as necessary; e.g., determining whether teacher or peer support is most appropriate)
- Products (individual versus group projects, including varying methods of demonstrating mastery and using different scoring methods)
- Learning environment (the physical structure of the room; established learning routines and culturally inclusive materials)

The Special Education Teacher as Implementer and Facilitator of Socioemotional and Behavior Supports

Special educators provide socioemotional and behavior supports to students through social skills instruction and many other positive behavioral supports and interventions. Social skills instruction can be taught discretely with programs that break down social skills into steps and engage the students in role play. Most programs also have a homework component (the students practice the skill independently) and a self-monitoring component. Examples of such programs include Skill Streaming (McGinnis & Goldstein, 1997) and The Tough Kids Social Skills Book (Sheridan, 1995). Social skills can be taught during literacy lessons by incorporating books containing social conflicts or the use of prosocial strategies (Marchant & Womack, 2010). In addition to supporting their own students, special educators often serve on "School-Wide Positive Behavior Support teams," which provide and monitor schoolwide programs intended to decrease interfering and bullying behaviors (Simonsen, Sugai, & Negron, 2008).

The Special Education Teacher as Collaborator

As a collaborator, the special education teacher must familiarize the general education teacher with the adaptations and modifications necessary to enable the child to benefit from inclusion. The two teachers then discuss who will be responsible for each aspect of the student's instructional needs. For a student who needs only limited support, the special education teacher might provide content enhancements such as the use of graphic organizers, study guides, or visual displays

(Jitendra, Burgess, & Gajria, 2011). The special educator may create adapted tests or check on the student at the end of the day to confirm that all of the homework assignments have been written down. For a student who needs more extensive support, the special education teacher may supply modified assignments that cover the same content as the general education lesson but that are at the student's functional level (see section Accommodations and Modifications; Hoover & Patton, 2008).

The Special Education Teacher as Supervisor of Paraprofessionals

As a supervisor, the special education teacher maintains the level of service delivered to students by paraprofessionals. Teachers need to actively manage paraprofessional support by creating a job description so that expectations are clear. Paraprofessionals help provide services but should not engage in instruction, assessment, long-term planning, collaborating and consulting with general educators, or supervising other paraprofessionals. These tasks are the job of the special education teacher. The special education teacher can best maintain quality paraprofessional support by conducting frequent, brief observations with both verbal and written feedback of performance (French, 2011).

The Special Education Teacher as Coteacher

As a coteacher, the special education teacher shares the classroom with a general education teacher. The two teachers take joint responsibility for all of the students in the class, regardless of ability. Coteaching may take many forms. Although not the most effective form, the most prevalent is the "one teach, one assist" model: While one teacher teaches the entire class, the other helps any students in need. Other methods include 1) setting up stations, and 2) parallel or alternative teaching (in which students are separated into small groups based on need but not disability). In the ideal situation, teachers team-teach and both teachers share responsibilities and teaching duties equally (Scruggs, Mastropieri, & McDuffie, 2007).

GENERAL EDUCATION LEGISLATION AFFECTING SPECIAL EDUCATION TEACHERS

The No Child Left Behind Act of 2001, which is a reauthorization of the Elementary and Secondary Education Act (ESEA) of 1965 (PL 94-142), addresses IDEA in three areas: highly qualified teachers, high quality instruction, inclusion in state assessment for all children, and high-stakes testing.

Highly Qualified Teachers

"Highly qualified teachers" by NCLB regulations are teachers who hold a bachelor's degree, have full state certification, and can prove knowledge in the subject they teach. NCLB requires the special education teachers who provide direct instruction in core academic subjects to be highly qualified (see Table 31.3). New special education teachers generally prove their knowledge by taking college courses in the subjects they teach. Veteran teachers can prove that they are highly qualified by alternate methods, including a record of teaching experience or attending professional development (U.S. Department of Education, 2004, 2006, and 2007).

High-Quality Instruction

One of the most significant changes to education under NCLB is the requirement that instruction must be of "high quality," meaning proven with evidence-based research. **Evidence-based research** is defined as "research that involves the application of rigorous, systematic, and objective procedures to obtain reliable and valid knowledge relevant to education activities and programs" (U.S. Department of Education, 2007). The field of education is known for swinging from one end of the spectrum or the other when deciding policy and curriculum, (one noticeable example has been the debate between phonics instruction or whole language instruction that has has continued from the early 1980s, with an eventual recognition that both are necessary for reading progress.) Many such debates are based on beliefs about instruction rather than objective scientific processes. Additionally, many teachers (both special education and general education) engage in a personalized curriculum, combining material from many different commercial (not validated) teachers' guides. Under NCLB, idiosyncratic curricula are no longer acceptable.

High Stakes Testing

High stakes testing is one of the most controversial tenets of NCLB. Under NCLB, all students, in all schools, in all districts must take standardized assessments to determine whether they are functioning on grade level in the areas of reading/language arts, math, and science,

Table 31.3. Summary of requirements to be a highly qualified special education teacher per the Individuals with Disabilities Education Improvement Act of 2004 (PL 108-446)

Category of special education teachers	Requirements
All special education teachers—general requirements	At least a bachelor of arts degree
	Full state special education certification or equivalent licensure
	No emergency or temporary certificate
New or veteran elementary school teachers teaching one or more core academic subjects only to children with disabilities held to alternative academic standards (most severe cognitive disabilities)	In addition to the general requirements listed above, may demonstrate academic subject competence through a High, Objective, Uniform State Standard of Evaluation (HOUSSE) process
New or veteran middle or high school teachers teaching one or more core academic subjects only to children with disabilities held to alternative academic standards (most severe cognitive disabilities)	In addition to the general requirements, may demonstrate "subject matter knowledge appropriate to the level of instruction being provided, as determined by the State, needed to effectively teach to those standards"
New teachers of two or more academic subjects who are highly qualified in math, language arts, or science	In addition to the general requirements, has 2-year window in which to become highly qualified in the other core academic subjects and may do this through the HOUSSE process
Veteran teachers who teach two or more core academic subjects only to children with disabilities	In addition to the general requirements, may demonstrate academic subject competence through the HOUSSE process (including a single evaluation for all core academic subjects)
Consultative teachers and other special education teachers who do not teach core academic subjects	Only meet general requirements
Other special education teachers teaching core academic subjects	In addition to the general requirements, meet relevant requirements for new elementary school teachers, new middle or high school teachers, or veteran teachers

regardless of disability. NCLB requires states to hold schools responsible for the progress of all students. Students are ranked at four levels: below basic, basic, proficient, or advanced. Schools and districts are graded by the performance of their students. Schools and districts with significant populations of students performing at below basic or basic are labeled as "failing schools" or "failing districts."

Failing institutions are forced to pay tuition for their students who wish to go to other schools or districts. If these schools or districts continue to fail, corrective action will take place: after 4 years, they may have their staff replaced; after 5 years, districts may have their elected boards disbanded and be taken over by the state or a contracted private firm. Schools or districts with a continued history of failure can be eliminated, with their students sent to other schools or districts (Peterson, 2005). Determination of school performance depends on groups of individuals within the school, for example children with disabilities or English language learners. Each group of students must perform well on the tests. If the majority of the general education students in a

school perform well on the high stakes test but the students with disabilities do not, that school is labeled a failing school.

High Stakes Testing of Students with Disabilities

Students with disabilities are required to participate in high stakes testing because the goal of NCLB is for all students to perform on grade level. No more than 1% of students per grade level (those with significant cognitive disabilities) are assessed using alternative assessment. For example, in Missouri, alternative assessments may be used for students who "[have] limited reading, writing and or speaking, and whose primary educational priorities primarily address essential skills that will be used in adult daily living" (Missouri Department of Elementary and Secondary Education, 2010, p.10). Information regarding alternative assessment for other states is available from the National Center on Educational Outcomes.

Students with significant cognitive disabilities are required to demonstrate their competency in the general standards that are assessed by the state but on their own functional level.

The following example from Kohl, McLaughlin, and Nagle (2006; p. 114) illustrates this process:

- Reading standard (Level A): Student responds to a variety of texts.

- Benchmark (Level B): Student understands the significance of literature and its contributions to human understanding and culture.

- Indicator (Level C): Student understands diversity.

- Extended indicator: Student waves to a fellow student but shakes hands with a principal.

The majority of states make their proficiency decisions using a rubric to measure a portfolio of student work on teacher-designed activities. The portfolio represents student achievement over an extended period of time. (Kettler, Beddow, Compton & McGrath, 2010)

THE SCHOOL–PARENT CONNECTION

One of the keys to positive results for students with disabilities is the teamwork between the school and family. Educators only see one facet of a child's abilities: his or her performance at school; parents, conversely, see the whole child. For example, a parent might know of a special interest or enjoyable activity that the educator might provide as a motivator for the child's school performance. Goals and placements also need to be decided jointly by the parents and the special education team. It is encouraging to note that parent attendance at IEP meetings is strong. A federal longitudinal study (Special Education Elementary Longitudinal Study, [SEELS]) found that 90% of parents of students with disabilities attended their child's IEP meeting (SRI International, 2007).

The close partnership between special educators and parents has another direct benefit: The parents understand and appreciate the efforts being made for their children. The SEELS study found that 91% of parents believed that IEP goals were challenging and appropriate (SRI International, 2007). Additionally, The National Longitudinal Study 2 (NLTS2) Wave 4 (2007) reported that 90% of secondary school parents were satisfied with their child's special education experience.

OUTCOMES

In 2010, more than $190 billion was spent on the education of students with disabilities (CEC, 2010). As of the last census, an average of $12,474 per year was spent per student with a disability as compared with $8,080 spent per general education student. (Diskey, 2002). With this level of expenditure, it is important to evaluate outcomes. As one marker of success, 56% percent of students receiving special education services graduated with a standard diploma from high school (Realize the Dream, 2007). This rate is far from ideal, but it compares relatively favorably with the nationwide average that shows 69% of general education students graduating (Editorial Projects in Education, 2009).

Although graduation rates are an important indicator of positive educational outcomes, the outcome for many students with disabilities is more adequately represented through other means. The NLTS-2 (National Center on Secondary Education and Transition, 2009) surveyed outcomes of young adults with disabilities in many areas. As an example, 83% liked their job very much or fairly well. Unfortunately the unemployment rate for persons with disabilities is 14.5% compared to 8.4% for that of persons without disabilities (Department of Labor, 2011). One of the goals of education is to provide students with the tools they need to succeed in life; individuals who have benefited from their education should feel positively about their future. Table 31.4 represents the percent of students who feel hopeful about the future, broken down by disability. The results are positive, with over half of students with a wide range of disabilities indicating that they are hopeful about the future a lot or all of the time.

SUMMARY

Special education and related services refer to instruction and supplementary supports that are specifically designed to meet the unique educational needs of a student with a disability. These services are mandated by federal law and are provided by special education teachers and related service providers to students with defined disabilities. The scope of instruction and support for a student with a disability is documented in that student's IEP. Services are provided within the framework of LRE, which supports general education as the starting point when determining the setting most appropriate for the education of the individual student.

IDEA 2004 is federal legislation that describes diagnosis and provision of services for students with disabilities. Section 504 legislation provides coverage for the wider array of students with disabilities who do not qualify

Table 31.4. How often youth felt hopeful about the future (Item np2V2d): Overall and by primary disability category

	Total	Learning disability	Speech impairment	Mental retardation	Emotional disturbance	Hearing impairment	Visual impairment	Orthopedic impairment	Other health impairment	Autism	Traumatic brain injury	Multiple disabilities	Deaf/blindness
(1) Rarely or never	14.7%	13.7%	14.5%	22.5%	15.0%	7.2%	4.3%	8.4%	9.6%	17.1%	16.8%	20.5%	7.5%
(2) Sometimes	22.7%	19.5%	30.4%	23.5%	31.1%	23.7%	16.5%	24.3%	25.7%	26.1%	17.7%	16.8%	18.4%
(3) A lot of the time	19.3%	20.8%	19.8%	16.0%	15.4%	28.0%	29.7%	15.0%	14.9%	22.7%	24.6%	14.4%	30.1%
(4) Most or all of the time	43.3%	42.1%	41.1%	31.1%	38.6%	41.2%	49.6%	52.3%	49.8%	33.5%	41.0%	48.0%	44.0%

From National Center on Secondary Education and Transition, Institute on Community Integration. (2009). NLTS2 Wave 5 Parent/Youth Survey Youth Report of Youth Social Involvement Table 340 Estimates. Retrieved November 28, 2010, from http://www.nlts2.org/data_tables/tables/14/np5V2dfrm.html

under the stricter guidelines of IDEA. NCLB has changed the qualifications for special education teachers, required the use of research-based instruction, and caused students with disabilities to be included in high stakes testing. RTI is a recent innovation in serving struggling learners and defining SLD.

Since the advent of special education, most students with disabilities are hopeful about the future.

REFERENCES

Americans with Disabilities Act of 2008, PL 110-325.

Browder, D.M., Wakeman, S.Y., Flowers, C., Rickelman, R.J., Pugalee, D., & Karvonen, M. (2007). Creating access to the general education curriculum with links to grade-level content for students with significant cognitive disabilities: An explanation of the content. *Journal of Special Education, 41*, 2–16.

Carter, E.W., Trainor, A.A., Sun, Y., & Owens, L. (2009). Assessing the transition-related strengths and needs of adolescents with high-incidence disabilities. *Exceptional Children, 76*, 74–94.

Cedar Rapids Community School Dist. v. Garret F., 526 U.S. 66 (1999).

Collins, B.C., Karl, J., Riggs, L., Galloway, C.C., & Hager, K.D. (2010). Teaching core content with real life applications to secondary students with moderate and severe disabilities. *Teaching Exceptional Children, 43*, 52–59.

Cook, B.G., Tankersley, M., & Landrum, T.J. (2009). Determining evidence-based practices in special education. *Exceptional Children, 75*, 365–383.

Cooper-Duffy, K., Szedi, P., & Hyer, G. (2010). Teaching literacy to students with significant cognitive disabilities. *Teaching Exceptional Children, 42*, 30–39.

Council for Exceptional Children. (n.d.) News & issues: Differentiated instruction. Retrieved January 16, 2011, from http://www.cec.sped.org/AM/Template.cfm?Section=Differentiated_Instruction&Template=/TaggedPage/TaggedPageDisplay.cfm&TPLID=24&ContentID=4695

Department of Labor. (2011). *Table A-6. Employment status of the civilian population by sex, age, and disability status, not seasonally adjusted, April 2011.* Retrieved May 25, 2011, from mhtml:file://C:Documents and Settings\Teacher\Desktop\Table A-6_Employment status of the civilian population by sex, age, and disability status, not seasonally adjusted

Daly, E.J., III., Martens, B.K., Barnett, D., Witt, J.C., & Olson, S.C. (2007). Varying intervention delivery in response to intervention: Confronting and resolving challenges with measurement, instruction, and intensity. *School Psychology Review, 36*, 562–580.

Diskey & Associates LLC. (2002). Special education finance. Retrieved November 28, 2011 from www2.ed.gov/inits/commissionsboards/whspecialeducation/reports/three.html.

Downing, J.E., & Eichinger, J. (2003). Creating learning opportunities for students with severe disabilities in inclusive classrooms. *Teaching Exceptional Children, 36*, 26–31.

Editorial Projects in Education (EPE). (2009). High school graduation rates improve over the past decade: Recent decline threatens progress. *Broader Horizons, 28*. Retrieved November 28, 2010, from www.edweek.org/ew/toc/2009/06/11/index.html.

Education for All Handicapped Children Act of 1975, PL 94-142, 20 U.S.C. §§ 1400 *et seq.*

Education of the Handicapped Act Amendments of 1986, PL 99-457, 20 U.S.C. §§ 1400 *et seq.*

Education of the Handicapped Act of 1970 (EHA), PL 91-230, 84 Stat. 121-154, 20 U.S.C. §§ 1400 *et seq.*

Elementary and Secondary Education Act of 1965, PL 89-10, 20 U.S.C. §§ 241 *et seq.*

Federal Register. (2008). Title 34 Education: Subtitle B Regulations of the Offices of the Department of Education Chapter I—office for civil rights, department of education www2.ed.gov/policy/rights/reg/ocr/edlite-34cfr104.html

Federal Register. (2006). 34CFR Parts 300 and 301: Assistance to states for the education of children with disabilities and preschool grants for children with disabilities. *Federal Register Vol. 71*, No 156, 46647.

Fore, C., III., Riser, S., & Boon, R. (2006). Implications of cooperative learning and educational reform for students with mild learning disabilities. *Reading Improvement, 43*, 3–12.

French, N. (2011). *Supervising paraeducators—What every teacher should know.* Retrieved May 25, 2011, from www.cec.sped.org/AM/Template.cfm?Section=Home&CONTENTID=4543&TEMPLATE=/CM/ContentDisplay.cfm&CAT=none.

Glover, T.A., & Diperna, J.C. (2007). Service delivery for response to intervention: Core components and directions for future research. *School Psychology Review, 36*, 526–540.

Harry, B., & Klinger, J. (2006). *Why are so many minority students in special education?* New York, NY: Teachers College Press.

Hoover, J.J., & Patton, J.R. (2008). The role of special educators in a multitiered instructional system. *Intervention in School and Clinic, 43*, 195–202.

Individuals with Disabilities Education Act Amendments of 1997, PL 105-17, 20 U.S.C. §§ 1400 *et seq.*

Individuals with Disabilities Education Act (IDEA) of 1990, PL 101-476, 20 U.S.C. §§ 1400 *et seq.*

Individuals with Disabilities Education Improvement Act of 2004, PL 108-446, 20 U.S.C. §§ 1400 *et seq.*

Jitendra, A.K., Burgess, C., & Gajria, M. (2011). Cognitive strategy instruction of improving expository text comprehension of students with learning disabilities: The quality of evidence. *Exceptional Children 77*, 135–159.

Kettler, R.J., Beddow, P.A, Compton, E., & McGrath, D. (2010). What do alternative academic achievement standards measure? A multitrait-multimethod analysis. *Exceptional Children, 76*, 457–474.

Kohl, F.L, McLaughlin, M.J., & Nagle, K. (2006). Alternate achievement standards and assessments: A descriptive investigation of 16 states. *Exceptional Children, 73*, 107–123.

Kovaleski, J.F., & Pedersen, J.A. (2009). Best practices in data-analysis teaming. In A. Thomas, & J. Grimes (Eds.), *Best practices in school psychology.* Bethedsa, MD: National Association of School Psychologists.

Marchant, M., & Womack, S. (2010). Book in a bag: Blending social skills and academics. *Teaching Exceptional Children, 42*, 6–12.

McMaster, K.L., Fuchs, D., & Fuchs, L.S. (2006). Peer-assisted learning strategies: The promise and limitations of peer-mediated instruction. *Reading & Writing Quarterly, 22,* 5–25.

Missouri Department of Elementary and Secondary Education. (2010). *Missouri assessment program-alternative (MAP-A): Instructor's guide and implementation manual.* Retrieved October 1, 2010, from www.dese.mo.gov/divimprove/access/documents/2010-2011-MAP-A-Web-Instructors-Guide.pdf.

Montague, M., & Dietz, S. (2009). Evaluation the evidence base for cognitive strategy instruction and mathematical problem solving. *Exceptional Children, 75,* 285–302.

No Child Left Behind Act of 2001, PL 107-110, 115 Stat. 1425, 20 U.S.C. §§ 6301 *et seq.*

Mercer, C.D. (1997). *Students with learning disabilities.* Upper Saddle River, NJ: Prentice Hall.

National Center for Learning Disabilities. (2009). *IDEA 2004: Improving transition planning and results.* Retrieved January 16, 2011, from http://www.ncld.org/at-school/your-childs-rights/iep-aamp-504-plan/idea-2004-improving-transition-planning-and-results

National Center on Educational Outcomes. (2010). *Alternate assessments for students with disabilities.* Retrieved January 11, 2011, from www.cehd.umn.edu/NCEO/TOPICAREAS/AlternateAssessments/StatesAltAssess.htmt

NICHCY. (2010). *Benchmarks or short-term objectives.* Retrieved May 25, 2011, from http://nichcy.org/schoolage/iep/iepcontents/benchmarks.

The National Center on Secondary Education and Transition. (2009). *National Longitudinal Study 2 Wave 4, Parent/Youth Survey Satisfaction with Secondary School Experiences (Items asked of PARENT ONLY)* Table 46 Estimates. Retrieved November 26, 2010, www.nlts2.org/data_tables/tables/13/np4D6o_cfrm.html.

The National Center on Secondary Education and Transition. (2009). *National Longitudinal Study 2: Wave 5. Social involvement, young adult/ parent survey: How often does the young adult feel hopeful about the future.* Retrieved November 28, 2010, from www.nlts2.org/data_tables/tables/14/np5V2dfrm.html.

Thomas, K., & Axelrod, S. (2005). Direct instruction: An educators' guide and a plea for action. *The Behavior Analyst Today, 6,* 111–120.

Pennsylvania Association for Retarded Citizens v. Commonwealth of Pennsylvania, 334 F. Supp. 1257 (E.D. Pa. 1971).

Peterson, K. (2005). NCLB goals and penalties. *Stateline.* Retrieved November 27, 2010, from www.stateline.org/live/ViewPage.action?siteNodeld=136&langeld=l&contentld=41611.

Rehabilitation Act of 1973, PL 93-112, 29 U.S.C. §§ 701 *et seq.*

Scruggs, T.E., Mastropieri, M.A., & McDuffie, K.A. (2007). Co-teaching in inclusive classrooms: A metasynthesis of qualitative research. *Exceptional Children, 73,* 392–416.

Shinn, M.R. (2007). Identifying students at risk, monitoring performance, and determining eligibility within response to intervention: Research on educational need and benefit from academic intervention. *School Psychology Review, 36,* 601–617.

Simonsen, B., Sugai, G., & Negron, M. (2008). Schoolwide positive behavior supports. *Teaching Exceptional Children, 40,* 32–40.

Skiba, R.J., Poloni-Staudinger, L., Simmons, A.B., Feggins-Azziz, R., & Chung, C.G. (2005). Unproven links: Can poverty explain ethnic disproportionally in special education? *Journal of Special Education, 39,* 130–144.

Skiba, R.J., Poloni-Staudinger, L., Gallini, S., Simmons, A.B., & Feggins-Azziz, R. (2006). Disparate access: The disproportionally of African American students with disabilities across educational environments. *Exceptional Children, 72,* 411–424.

Skiba, R.J., Simmons, A.B., Ritter, S., Gibb, A.C., Rausch, M.K., Cuadrado, J., & Chung, C.G. (2008). Achieving equity in special education: History, status, and current challenges. *Exceptional Child 74,* 264–288.

SRI International. (2007). *Special Education Elementary Longitudinal Study (SEELS) Table 131 & 142.* Retrieved November 28, 2010, from www.seels.net

VanDerHeyden, A.M., & Burns, M.K. (2010). *Essentials of response to intervention.* Hoboken, NJ: John Wiley & Sons Inc.

Vannest, K.J., & Hagan-Burke, S.C. (2010). Teacher time use in special education. *Remedial and Special Education, 31,* 126–142.

U.S. Department of Education, Office of Special Education and Rehabilitative Services (OSERS). (1994). *Questions and answers on least restrictive environment (LRE) Requirements of the IDEA* Retrieved November 27, 2010, from www.wrightslaw.com/info/lre.osers.memo.idea.htm.

U.S. Department of Education. (2004). *Testing: Frequently asked questions.* Retrieved November 6, 2010, from www2.ed.gov/print/nclb/accountability/ayp/testing-faq-html.

U.S. Department of Education. (2006). *New No Child Left Behind flexibility: Highly qualified teachers.* Retrieved November 6, 2010, from www2.ed.gov/print/nclb/methods/teachers/hqtflexibility.html.

U.S. Department of Education. (2008). *Digest of education statistics: Table 41. Percentage distribution of enrollment in public elementary and secondary schools, by race/ethnicity and state or jurisdiction: Fall 1996 and Fall 2006.* Retrieved November 21, 2010, from nces.ed.gov/program/digest/d08/tables/dt08_041.asp.

U.S. Department of Education. (2008). *Table 1–20. Number of students ages 6 through 21 served under IDEA, Part B, by the five race/ethnicity categories and state: Fall 2008.* Retrieved November 21, 2010, from www.ideadata.org/TABLES32ND/AR_1-20.htm.

U.S. Department of Education. (2008). *Data tables for OSEP state reported data: Part B educational environments: Table 2–9.* Retrieved November 21, 2010, from www.ideadata.org/arc_toc10.asp#partbLRE.

U.S. Department of Education. (2009). *Digest of Education Statistics: Table 50, 51 Children 3–21 years old served under Individuals with Disabilities Education Act, Part B.* Retrieved November 16, 2010, from nces.ed.gov/programs/digest/d09/tables/dt09_050.aps.

U.S. Department of Education. (2009). *Office of Special Education Programs, Individuals with Disabilities Act (IDEA) database.* Retrieved November 10, 2010, from www.ideadata.org/arc_toc9.asp#partbLRE.

U.S. Department of Education Institute of Education Sciences. (2010). *Student effort and educational progress, elementary/ secondary persistence and progress.* Retrieved November 27, 2010, from nces.ed.gov/programs/coe/2010/section3/indicator18.asp

U.S. Department of Education, Office of Special Education Programs. (2007). *Alignment with the No Child Left Behind Act.* Retrieved October 21, 2010, from www2.ed.gov/policy/speced/guid/idea/tb-nclb-align.doc.

Williamson, P., McKleskey, J, Hoppy, D., & Rentz, T. (2006). Educating students with mental retardation in general education classrooms. *Exceptional Children, 72,* 347–361.

Ysseldyke, J., & Algozzine, B. (1995). *Special education: A practical approach for teachers* (3rd ed.) Boston, MA: Houghton Mifflin.

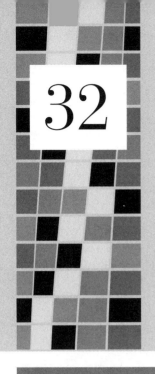

32

Behavioral Principles, Assessment, and Therapy

Michael F. Cataldo, SungWoo Kahng, Iser G. DeLeon,
Brian K. Martens, Patrick C. Friman, and Marilyn Cataldo

Upon completion of this chapter, the reader will understand

- The role of operant learning approaches in helping individuals with developmental disabilities

- Operant principles and their application to important everyday problems

- Operant learning approaches for decreasing problematic behaviors and increasing adaptive behaviors

- Intensive treatment approaches for severe behavior problems

- Principles underlying effective teaching and skill instruction

- Practical approaches for parents and teachers to address mild behavior problems and access programs

---

OPERANT LEARNING PRINCIPLES AND PRACTICES

Many of the earliest studies of behavioral principles involved groups of people with developmental disabilities. Initially, this was because people with intellectual disabilities, in general, learn more slowly, thus making it easier to study the learning process. This had two important sequelae: 1) it led to studies of clinical problems, and 2) it provided the necessary evidence for landmark court cases on the rights of those with intellectual disabilities (Levy & Rubenstein, 1996). In the late 1960s, the branch of psychology dedicated to studying operant learning began to emphasize applications (Baer, Wolf, & Risley, 1968). Since then, hundreds of studies have reported the clinical utility of operant learning principles to change behavior, both excesses and deficits.

Experts on the use of operant learning approaches generally have degrees in psychology or education, and there are several terms for their approaches, methods, procedures, and techniques. These terms include **applied behavior analysis** (ABA), **behavior analysis**, **behavior modification**, and **positive behavior intervention and supports** (PIBS). The differences in terms mainly reflect changes that have occurred during the development of this field of research and practice, both with regard to preferred terminology and to emphasis on specific techniques. For example, most recently, an emphasis has been placed on using only "positive" approaches to help people with developmental disabilities. This emphasis has validity because it lessens the likelihood of abuse resulting from the inappropriate use of operant approaches. Also, positive approaches alone are sufficient for the vast majority of people needing help.

In all instances, regardless of the term used, the approaches respond to behavioral challenges (behavioral excesses and deficits) that adversely affect the lives of people with developmental disabilities. Excesses range from common problems such as bedtime difficulties to rarer but more dramatic disorders such as **self-injurious behavior** (SIB) or **aggression**. Behavioral deficits include poor academic performance, inadequate social skills, deficient communication skills, and inability to independently complete activities of daily living. These behavioral excesses and deficits are often interrelated (e.g., children who engage in SIB and other severe forms of problem behavior often display skill deficits of various sorts; Baghdadli et al., 2003; Chadwick et al., 2000; Matson & Rivet, 2008; Murphy, Healer, & Leader, 2009). Current operant learning-based practices are grounded in a rich tradition of learning theory. Although biologic/genetic factors must be taken into account, the assumption is that typically, both appropriate and inappropriate behaviors are learned over time through their effects on the environment. Stated differently, patients change behavior based on whether it results in valuable outcomes or in escaping or avoiding unpleasant ones. This simple yet powerful functional relationship between behavior and its consequences, sometimes characterized as the **"Law of Effect,"** forms the basis for current operant learning approaches. Because behavior operates on the environment and results in differential consequences which in turn "select" future behaviors, it is termed *operant behavior*.

Reinforcement, Extinction, and Punishment

Reinforcement is fundamental to all behavior programs. Strictly defined, it is a process in which the consequences that follow a given behavior result in an increase in that behavior's future strength. Reinforcement can be formally divided into two subclasses: positive and negative (Figure 32.1). **Positive reinforcement** exists when the contingent delivery of an outcome increases the likelihood of the behavior(s) upon which it is contingent. For example, a student may receive a token, which can later be exchanged for a preferred item each time he or she correctly completes a task. This in turn would increase the likelihood that the student would complete the

task when encountering it again. **Negative reinforcement** exists when the contingent *removal* of a stimulus increases the likelihood of the behavior. For example, a teacher may provide a break from work (i.e., removal of a stimulus) after the student has completed a certain portion of the task. This would lead to an *increased* likelihood that the student would complete the task when presented again. It is important to note that reinforcement always leads to an increase in behavior and that the terms "positive" and "negative" simply refer to the action taken (i.e., a stimulus is presented or removed). Both can be used to describe the acquisition of new behaviors as well as the maintenance or reduction of problem behaviors. **Extinction** is the process through which reinforcement is withheld for a previously reinforced response, resulting in a decrease in that response's future occurrence. For example, a child in a toy store may have a tantrum if denied a toy, which in the past that child may have received. If the parent does not attend to the tantrum, tantrums should eventually decrease.

Punishment is technically defined as a process in which consequences delivered contingent upon a behavior result in decreasing the future occurrence of that behavior. Thus, its effect is opposite that of reinforcement. Punishment, too, can involve separate classes (Figure 32.1). **Positive punishment** involves the contingent delivery of a consequence (sometimes termed an **aversive stimulus**), whereas **negative punishment** involves the contingent removal of a consequence (i.e., **positive reinforcer**). An example of positive punishment is overcorrection when a child throws a toy. The teacher may order the child to pick up the toy as well as clean up the surrounding environment. This would decrease the likelihood of the child throwing the toy in the future. Common examples of negative punishment include **time-out** (the individual is removed from potential sources of

		EFFECT	
		Increases likelihood of behavior	Decreases likelihood of behavior
ACTION	Stimulus presented	Positive reinforcement	Positive punishment
	Stimulus removed	Negative reinforcement	Negative punishment

Figure 32.1. Distinction between positive and negative reinforcement and punishment.

reinforcement) and **response cost** (previously earned reinforcers, such as tokens that can be redeemed for a reward, are removed contingent on inappropriate behavior). Punishment is always defined by its effect on behavior and always decreases behavior. Punitive therapeutic arrangements have become less common over the years owing to a variety of factors, including diminished social acceptability and the increase in research on the efficacy of **reinforcement-based interventions** (Kahng, Iwata, & Lewin, 2002a; Pelios et al., 1999). Furthermore, the term *punishment* relates a basic learning principle to legal and negative associations. Yet, the facts are that regardless of the term employed, most learning cannot occur without feedback about incorrect responses. And, when feedback on incorrect responses occurs and enhances learning, it meets the technical definition of punishment. From a technical, operant learning perspective, grades in school can serve as reinforcement or as punishment.

It is important to note that punishing and reinforcing stimuli are not characterized by their outward appearance but by their effects on the behaviors upon which they are made contingent. The success of many behavior programs hinges upon the parent's, caregiver's, or teacher's ability to arrange or rearrange the relationship between behavior and its consequences. However, knowing which stimuli can be effective as consequences to increase or decrease behavior is not always intuitively obvious. For example, normally punitive consequences, such as verbal reprimands (Kodak, Northup, & Kelley, 2007) and physical restraint (Magee & Ellis, 2001) under certain circumstances actually function as reinforcers for some individuals. Thus, an important part of successful behavior management is the process of identifying stimuli that are effective consequences for each individual.

Motivation

Both behavior and response–consequence interactions are dynamic. Motivation is an important concept in understanding how the effectiveness of consequences varies across time. **Motivating operations** (MOs) play a central role in the operant learning conceptualization of motivation (Laraway, Snycerski, Michael, & Poling, 2003). An MO produces two effects: 1) a change in the value of a consequence, and 2) a corresponding change in the strength (e.g., frequency, amount) of behavior historically influenced by that consequence. For example, being lengthily deprived of attention can make

attention a stronger reinforcer and increase the frequency of behavior that has historically produced attention (McComas, Thompson, & Johnson, 2003; O'Reilly et al., 2006). Regarding human clinical problems (especially with people with developmental disabilities), examination of MOs has become increasingly prevalent in research and intervention programs. For example, the presence or absence of recurrent medical conditions (Carr & Owen-DeSchryver, 2007), medications (Crosland et al., 2003), and general states of alertness (O'Reilly & Lancioni, 2000) have all been shown to alter the effectiveness of certain consequences as reinforcers and, thus, alter the frequency of problem behaviors maintained by those reinforcers.

BEHAVIORAL ASSESSMENT OF PROBLEM BEHAVIORS

Since the early 1990s, the dominant approach to intervening with severe problem behaviors initially involves performing evaluations collectively referred to as *functional assessment*. Its basic goal is to identify the antecedent events and consequences that serve as motivational variables for a problem behavior. There are three types of functional assessment: **indirect assessment**, **descriptive analysis**, and **functional (experimental) analysis** (Iwata et al., 2000).

Indirect assessment is the simplest method of gathering information about behavioral function. Indirect assessments consist of questionnaires and rating scales (Matson & Wilkins, 2009) that are completed by caregivers (e.g., parents, teachers, school staff, child care staff). The caregivers are asked a series of questions about the problem behavior and related events (i.e., antecedent events and consequences). Typically, a score is derived from this assessment that may be suggestive of behavioral function. Indirect assessments quickly and efficiently gather preliminary information about the problem behaviors. However, it is not generally recommended that these assessments be the sole source of information about behavior because of their questionable reliability and validity.

Descriptive analyses involve the quantitative, direct observation of the individual's behaviors as well as antecedent events and consequences under naturalistic settings (Camp, Iwata, Hammond, & Bloom, 2009; Samaha et al., 2009). Conditional probability of the behavior's occurrence and the antecedents/consequences can then be determined, a process that can help identify a relationship between the problem behavior and environmental events that preceded it. Descriptive analyses are objective means of gathering more information about variables that may be maintaining a problem behavior. They permit determination of the degree of correspondence between a behavior and environmental event. However, descriptive analyses tend to be time consuming, and because they are correlational, they may not identify the variables that are maintaining the problem behavior.

The most powerful demonstration of the relationship between antecedent and consequent events on problem behaviors consists of the controlled manipulation of these events, typically called a functional analysis (Iwata et al., 1982, 1994). In this approach, the individual is exposed to a variety of antecedent conditions and consequences that may have evoked problem behaviors. The antecedent variables may include presenting demands as well as limited access to adult attention or preferred items. Consequences for problem behaviors may include a brief escape from the demand, attention, or access to preferred items. Patterns of differential responding are observed over time through repeated exposure to each of these conditions. Responses that occur more often in a particular condition (e.g., when demands are presented) leads the clinician to conclude that the problem behavior is maintained by that particular consequence (e.g., escape from demands).

FUNCTIONAL ASSESSMENT AND TREATMENT DEVELOPMENT

Interest in functional assessments as a treatment development tool has increased since the early 1980s (Iwata et al., 1982, 1994; Kahng, Iwata, & Lewin, 2002b). This interest and a corresponding body of research has resulted in government-enacted mandates in the Individuals with Disabilities Education Act Amendments of 1997 (IDEA '97; PL 105-17) and the law's 2004 reauthorization (IDEA 2004; PL 108-446) and is specifically addressed in the No Child Left Behind (NCLB) Act of 2001 (PL 107-110). Using a functional assessment, the antecedent conditions that influence a problem behavior can be identified and changed in order to reduce the likelihood of the problem behavior recurring. Once identified, the source of reinforcement for the problem behavior can be minimized or eliminated. Then, the reinforcer that maintains the behavior can be used in the behavioral intervention to reduce it. Finally,

identification of a behavioral function helps eliminate unnecessary or irrelevant components of a treatment plan.

The adoption of functional assessments has changed how behavioral interventions are developed (Mace, 1994). Prior to the advent of functional assessment, providers/clinicians attempted to change problem behaviors without consideration of the likely cause. In most cases, this resulted in a standard selection of treatment components. Functional assessment technology has led to hypothesis-based (i.e., function-based) treatment development, which has resulted in increased numbers of evidence-based treatment options and individualized treatments. When behavioral treatment fails to produce a positive outcome, functional assessment has provided information on factors responsible for the failure. Once the likely maintaining contingencies for a problem behavior have been identified, a hypothesis-driven approach to treatment development is possible. Some examples are described next.

Social-Positive Reinforcement

The most basic intervention for problem behaviors that are maintained by social-positive reinforcement is terminating the reinforcer, such as attention or access to **tangibles** (e.g., toys, TV, food). This extinction approach typically involves ignoring the problem behavior (Hagopian, Toole, Long, Bowman, & Lieving, 2004). However, extinction is sometimes associated with the problem behavior initially increasing, followed by a gradual decrease and increases in other nontargeted behaviors (Lerman & Iwata, 1996). In most instances, extinction is combined with differential reinforcement procedures, such as **differential reinforcement of other behaviors** (DRO) or **differential reinforcement of alternative behaviors** (DRA). DRO consists of the delivery of reinforcers (e.g., attention) contingent on the absence of problem behaviors. Reinforcers are typically provided after prespecified intervals of time in which the problem behavior has not occurred (Conyers et al., 2004). DRA is the delivery of the reinforcer contingent on the performance of alternative, more appropriate behaviors. Oftentimes this alternative response takes the form of appropriate communicative responses, such as requesting attention or access to the tangible item. An example is the use of functional communication training (FCT; Jarmolowicz, DeLeon, & Kuhn, 2009).

Social-Negative Reinforcement

Procedurally, extinction of problem behaviors maintained by social-negative reinforcement is different from extinction of problem behaviors maintained by social-positive reinforcement. Whereas the latter involves not giving attention (i.e., ignoring) to the problem behaviors, extinction of escape-maintained problem behaviors involves preventing escape. The aversive event (e.g., demand) is continued and NOT terminated (Kodak, Lerman, Volkert, & Trosclair, 2007). Hypothesis-based differential reinforcement procedures have also been effective in reducing escape-maintained problem behaviors. As with attention-maintained problem behaviors, DRO consists of the delivery of a brief period of escape that is contingent on absenting the problem behavior (Kodak, Miltenberger, & Romaniuk, 2003). DRA typically consists of delivering brief escape contingent on the performance of alternative behaviors, such as appropriate communication or compliance (Reed, Ringdahl, Wacker, Barretto, & Andelman, 2005).

Automatic Reinforcement

In some instances, behavior produces internal consequences that can reinforce and thus produce functional relationships that maintain problem behaviors. This has been termed *automatic reinforcement*. For example, studies have linked some forms of self-injury to releases of endogenous opiates that may relieve pain or provide pleasure. Thus, SIB in this instance can be viewed as a form of self-reinforcement. Rates of such automatically reinforced behavior have been found to decrease dramatically via the administration of an opiate antagonist (Cataldo & Harris, 1982). Although it is difficult to identify the specific source of stimulation for problem behaviors that are maintained by automatic reinforcement, the fact that responding occurs regardless of social stimulation provides useful information for treatment development. Extinction of problem behaviors that are maintained by automatic reinforcement requires the attenuation or elimination of the source of reinforcement. For SIB, this typically involves using protective equipment such as mitts or helmets that permit the occurrence of the behavior but minimize the amount of reinforcement produced (Moore, Fisher, & Pennington, 2004).

Another type of treatment focuses on providing stimuli that compete with problem behaviors. These procedures are sometimes referred to as **enriched environments** or **competing stimuli** and consist of presenting stimuli that displace the problem behavior, such as providing food or mouthing toys to children that display pica (DeLeon, Toole, Gutshall, & Bowman, 2005). Finally, some studies have attempted to replace the hypothesized source of sensory stimulation that is produced by the behavior. Although determining such sources is difficult, researchers have provided alternative sources of stimulation based on the appearance of the behavior. For example, studies have provided alternative sources of visual stimulation for individuals who demonstrate eye poking behavior (Kennedy & Souza, 1995).

PREFERENCE ASSESSMENT AND REINFORCER EVALUATION: FROM BASIC PRINCIPLE TO APPLICATION

During the early eras of applying behavioral principles to improving the lives of individuals with developmental disabilities, little attention was paid to empirically identifying reinforcers to strengthen behavior. In many cases, stimuli were arbitrarily selected and may not have functioned as reinforcers for specific behaviors. This, in turn, may have resulted in ineffective interventions.

Since the early 1980s, there has been a growing body of research that examines methods of systematically identifying stimuli that may serve as reinforcers (Hagopian, Long, & Rush, 2004). In one of the first such studies, Pace, Ivancic, Edwards, Iwata, and Page (1985) examined preference by exposing individuals with developmental disabilities to 16 stimuli to measure whether or not that individual responded to that stimulus. They identified multiple stimuli, which they later demonstrated as being reinforcers. These **preference assessments** typically expose the individual to a large number of stimuli over a relatively brief period of time. The goal of such assessments is to identify high-preference stimuli that may be potential reinforcers. More recently, research on preference and reinforcer identification has led to research that focuses more broadly on choice and its impact on behavior (Fisher & Mazur, 1997).

COMMON BEHAVIOR PROBLEMS

Research has clearly demonstrated that from these basic operant learning principles, a broad variety of applications for treatment of routine child behavior problems can be derived, a sample of which will be discussed next (Friman,

2005a; 2008). These applications are extremely effective for mild behavior problems, which if addressed early can avoid more serious and treatment resistant forms of behavior problems.

Routine Oppositional Behavior

Optimal treatment of routine oppositional behavior usually includes at least five components:

1. Establishing the clarity and simplicity of the instructions or requests that are to be followed in the program.

2. Dramatically increasing pleasant social and physical contact between the child and caregiver; this is sometimes called **time-in**. The more pleasant the circumstances at the time of oppositional behavior, the less intensive or intrusive an intervention has to be in order to produce a behavior changing aversive experience. Mere cessation of or removal from the pleasant circumstances is often highly aversive (an example of negative punishment).

3. Causing a temporary dramatic decrease in pleasant social and physical contact between child and caregiver, ceasing all preferred activity, and confining the child to a specified location, usually a chair or a bedroom; this is usually called **time-out** (the obverse of time-in). The key to effectiveness is its contiguity with and contingency upon the targeted oppositional behavior and its release criteria. Generally, release requires quiet acceptance of the time-out (which can take a while to achieve, especially in the beginning stages) and verbal or gestural assent to a query by the caregiver (i.e, asking whether the child would like to leave time-out).

4. Providing an immediate and brief but intensive practice session wherein the child is instructed to complete several small tasks (e.g., put the pencil on the desk, place the paper in the wastebasket) and is praised for compliance or sent back to time-out for noncompliance.

5. Making an ardent attempt to catch the child complying with commands or following instructions in his or her everyday life and to praise (reinforce) the performance. This is sometimes called **incidental teaching**.

Variations on this procedure have been used successfully with oppositional behavior in more children at more developmental levels than any other documented treatment.

Toileting

Toileting accidents are common in young children and continue to be present in many typically developing children through age 6 (especially boys). When achievement of developmental milestones is slowed by a developmental disability, the probability of toileting problems increases substantially and extends well past age 6. Effective treatment of toileting problems usually includes at least four components.

1. *Detection of accidents by the child and caregiver must be heightened.* Market forces in the United States are actually working against this first component through the use of diapers and pull-ups in increasingly older children. Both garments inhibit detection of accidents. The polymer structure of the garments prevents urine from dampening clothing, thus interfering with visual detection by caregivers. The structure also traps urine within the garment itself and maintains its temperature at or near body levels; thus this delays the child's sensory detection of accidents. Not surprisingly, wearing the garments inhibits developing continence (Tarbox, Williams, & Friman, 2004). As a result, achieving the first component involves removing diapers and pull-ups when and where possible (Figure 32.2).

2. *Learning trials must be increased in frequency.* This can be accomplished by increasing fluid loads, usually by providing unlimited amounts of the child's favorite beverages.

3. *Any movement associated with imminent urination should be quickly followed by a guided trip to the bathroom.* In addition, during the training period, guided trips should be scheduled at least every 2 hours.

4. *Attempts to urinate should be praised, and successes should be rewarded* (positive reinforcement). If timing is critical or if the previously listed components do not yield success, a vibrating urine alarm can be added (e.g., Wet Stop). Alarms are moisture-sensitive, and they simultaneously increase detection of accidents by child and caregiver (there is a detectable sound) and supply a mildly unpleasant consequence. This sequence teaches the child to engage the lower abdominal musculature responsible for inhibiting or forestalling urination (i.e., the muscles used to "hold it" when urination is inconvenient; Christopersen & Friman, 2010).

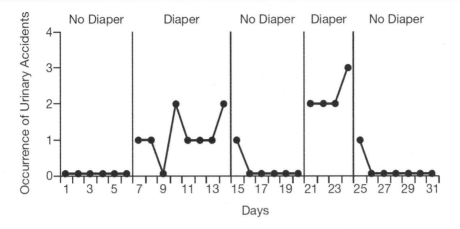

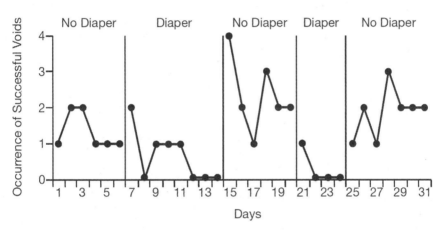

Figure 32.2. Number of toileting accidents per day are depicted in the top panel. Number of successful voids per day are depicted in the bottom panel. (From Tarbox, R., Williams, L., & Friman, P.C. [2004]. Extended diaper wearing: Effects on continence in and out of the diaper. *Journal of Applied Behavior Analysis, 37,* 99; reprinted by permission.)

Bedtime Problems

Crying, calling, and/or coming out of the bedroom after bedtime are among the most common behavior problems for young children, and this is true whether they are typically developing or have a developmental disability. The potential for bedtime problems is high because, faced with the prospect of being alone in the dark for hours, children often exhibit distress. Furthermore, any response from caregivers to the bedtime problem, pleasant or unpleasant, creates a reinforcing experience because children prefer human contact to being alone (Friman, 2005b).

Treatment involves a variation on ignoring distress calls and preventing bedroom exits, essentially an extinction procedure. The intensity and duration of the child's distress, however, frequently impedes caregiver compliance

with extinction. Fortunately, a method used to reduce disruptive behavior can be adapted to improve bedtime problems and increase parental compliance. This method involves allowing a brief period of time during which children's (appropriate) requests and demands are met, contingent upon their exhibiting the **target behaviors** (Bowman et al., 1997). The derived method involves giving children who appropriately prepare for bed (e.g., brushed teeth, put pajamas on) a "bedtime pass" (usually a laminated piece of cardboard) that they are allowed to use in exchange for the satisfaction of one (appropriate) request. The children are allowed to call out the request or get up and deliver the "pass" to the caregiver. Following satisfaction of the request, the pass is surrendered, the child is tucked in bed for the night, and all subsequent distress calls are ignored. The pass has successfully eliminated bedtime problems in children between the ages of 3 and 10 years (Moore, Friman, Fruzetti, & MacAleese, 2007) and both parents and pediatricians rate it as highly acceptable. The bedtime pass program's high success with children as young as 3 years of age suggests it could be mastered by children with disabilities whose cognitive abilities approach the 3-year level.

Common Habit Disorders

Habit disorders ("bad habits") are highly prevalent in children, especially in those with developmental disabilities. The likelihood of a behavior hardening into a habit increases along with the size and frequency of intervals between stimulating or nurturing events in the lives of children (e.g., contacts with people, absorbing social activities; Friman, Byrd, & Oksal, 2001). Thus, habits are more prevalent in industrialized societies than in developing or agrarian ones because children in nonindustrialized societies have abundantly more "skin-to-skin" contact with caregivers in the early periods of their lives (e.g., they sleep with parents for years, are swaddled with a parent throughout the day). Because of the abundance of highly stimulating contact and activities throughout the day, the pleasant but less stimulating experiential contrast provided by self-stimulatory habits is insufficient to result in their developing or continuing.

Common habits include biting fingernails, picking skin, grinding teeth, and playing with or pulling hair; however, the most prevalent habit is probably thumb-sucking and, with minor exceptions, successful treatment of it is prototypical for most habits. All of these behaviors, like other pediatric presenting problems, can be signs of underlying medical or psychiatric problems. A proper evaluation is a prerequisite for behavioral treatment. If warranted, however, a behavioral approach would proceed as follows:

1. *Aversion of time-in (as previously described) is used.* To the extent possible, the frequency and length of intervals associated with limited external stimulation is reduced by increasing the delivery of pleasant social and physical contact.

2. *Detection of the habit is increased through intensive monitoring.*

3. *The child's awareness of the habit is raised through methods that increase its recognition.* With thumb-sucking, this is achieved by applying edible but bitter-tasting substances to the thumbnail.

4. *All public exhibitions of the habit result in a brief time-out, but private practice of the habit is allowed.* The logic behind allowing private practice is that unless a child spends an inordinate amount of time alone, the likelihood that a private habit will cause social or physical problems is minimal.

5. *An incentive system is employed to reward the child when the habit is not exhibited during an established number of defined intervals.*

Variations on this form of treatment for common habits have proven highly successful in research studies, even when the habit is part of a cluster of self-stimulatory behaviors (Friman, 2003). Other variations have been used to treat a broad range of behavior problems including fingernail biting and chronic hair pulling (Woods & Miltenberger, 2001).

Obviously, the previously mentioned problems form a much abbreviated sample of common behavior problems. But those discussions so far represent the kind of problems for which operant learning-based strategies have proven effective. These techniques are evidence-based and can easily be disseminated to parents through brief well-child visits.

SEVERE PROBLEM BEHAVIORS

Problem behaviors such as **self-injurious behavior** (SIB), aggression, and property destruction cannot be dealt with in the same practical manner described in the preceding section. Although there is compelling evidence that problem behaviors (e.g., SIB) involve **neurobiological mechanisms** (Nyhan, 2002), medical approaches, such as the use of atypical **antipsychotic medicines** (i.e., risperidone), are only partially successful. Research shows that these problem behaviors also have a learned component, which influences frequency and long-term disability, and can be reduced by applying operant-learning–based approaches (Hastings & Noone, 2005; Iwata, Pace, Dorsey, et al., 1994; National Institutes of Health, 1991). For example, studies show that SIB is maintained by environmental contingencies such as negative reinforcement (escape) and positive reinforcement (attention; Carr, Newsom, & Binkoff, 1976; Lovaas et al., 1965). Numerous studies have demonstrated that other problem behaviors such as aggression and property destruction can be maintained through similar environmental contingencies (Crockett & Hagopian, 2006; Fisher, DeLeon, Rodriguez-Catter, & Keeney, 2004). Therefore, children with severe behavior problems should be referred to properly trained and credentialed behavior analysts, psychologists, or educators.

The environmental contingencies that maintain problem behavior can be categorized into three groups that were only briefly mentioned previously: social-positive reinforcement, social-negative reinforcement, and automatic reinforcement (Iwata et al., 2000). These are described in more detail next.

Social-Positive Reinforcement

Events or stimuli that follow a behavior's occurrence may function to strengthen that behavior. Oftentimes, these consequences are socially mediated (i.e., delivered by other individuals) and take the form of attention or material items (e.g., toys, food). For example, a common response by parents when their child engages in less intensive forms of SIB (or stereotypic behavior) may be to provide a verbal reprimand (e.g., saying "Don't do that") or physical comfort (e.g., hugging the child). Although these consequences may lead to a temporary decrease in the problem behavior, repeated pairing of either consequence with the problem behavior may inadvertently result in a future increase in both the frequency and intensity of this problem behavior.

Social-Negative Reinforcement

The removal of some unwanted or aversive event contingent on a behavior may also result in strengthening of that behavior and may manifest as escape or avoidance from the unwanted event. For example, a teacher may present a student with a challenging task (e.g., answering a difficult question), which may result in the child becoming aggressive. This aggressive behavior may eventually lead the teacher to terminate the task and provide the student a break so that he or she will calm down. In this situation, the escape may temporarily reduce aggression. However, the inadvertent pairing of the escape with the aggression may lead to future increases in aggression by the student when he or she is presented with similarly challenging tasks.

Automatic Reinforcement

Some forms of SIB occur independent of environmental or socially mediated consequences (Kern, Bailin, & Mauk, 2003; Long, Hagopian, DeLeon, Marhefka, & Resau, 2005). These behaviors are oftentimes said to be self-stimulatory, and a variety of biological explanations have been suggested. These include biochemical deficiencies, insensitivity to pain, and the body's response to opiate-like substances (Cataldo & Harris, 1982). These nonsocially mediated contingencies have collectively become referred to as automatic reinforcement (O'Reilly et al., 2010; Vaughan & Michael, 1982).

The Viability of Extinction and Implications from Behavioral Economics

Although extinction is clearly effective in the treatment of problem behaviors, applied behavioral researchers have increasingly acknowledged that extinction is not always possible in natural environments (Carter, 2010; Lomas, Fisher, & Kelley, 2010). For example, it may be difficult or unethical to ignore disruptive and dangerous behaviors. And, it may be impossible to persist in issuing academic demands when the learner acts aggressively towards the instructor or throws tasks materials to the floor. In each case, the behavior may result in even brief periods of escape and thus be reinforced. Considerable research has been devoted to how well interventions hold up if problem behavior continues to be reinforced (Vollmer, Roane, Ringdahl, & Marcus, 1999). A related consideration is that alternative behavior cannot always be reinforced each time it occurs. Reinforcers must sometimes be delivered intermittently (e.g., for every third or fifth appropriate response) if the procedure is to remain practical enough for caregivers to implement. Combining these considerations creates a situation in which both the problem behavior and an appropriate alternative are each reinforced only some of the time.

To address this situation, clinical research has begun to study the variables that spur choice-making behavior. Such research investigates choices when two schedules are concurrently in effect by extending findings from the field of behavioral economics. Behavior analysts have increasingly applied economic concepts to understand issues of social significance in areas including consumer choice, gambling, substance abuse, and more recently, to the treatment of problem behaviors. Behavioral economics is concerned with how reinforcers are earned when the number of responses required to produce them are increased, as in making a reinforcement schedule increasingly intermittent (DeLeon, Neidert, Anders, & Rodriguez-Catter, 2001; Roane, Falcomata, & Fisher, 2007; Shore, Iwata, DeLeon, Kahng, & Smith, 1997).

The behavioral "translation" of the economic law of demand asserts that as the number of responses required to produce a reinforcer increases, the total number of reinforcers consumed declines. How those decreases affect consumption can differ dramatically from reinforcer to reinforcer. Although two reinforcers may be consumed equally when each can be earned for a single response, they may have highly disparate "demand profiles"—one may continue to be consumed at relatively high levels while consumption of the other declines steeply—when the response requirements are increased.

Laboratory investigations involving individuals with developmental disabilities have shown that these relationships similarly remain when considering common classroom reinforcers (DeLeon, Iwata, Goh, & Worsdell, 1997; Tustin, 1994). One of the variables that influences consumption decline is related to the type of reinforcer concurrently available. Generally, consumption of a reinforcer declines more steeply when response requirements increase or when "substitute" commodities (for example, those that provide a similar kind of reinforcement) can be earned with less effort. The implication in the treatment context is that if the problem behavior continues to elicit its maintaining reinforcer while the reinforcement schedule for the alternative behavior is made increasingly intermittent, interventions relying on differential reinforcement of alternative behaviors may remain effective. This is true if the alternative behavior is reinforced with something dissimilar to what the person can gain with less effort by emitting the problem behavior. Thus, when extinction is difficult to implement and schedules must be thinned for practical reasons, reinforcing alternative behavior with a reinforcer that is distinct from that maintaining the problem behavior may be a more viable treatment option.

PRACTICAL STRATEGIES FOR THE CLASSROOM

Establishing Routines and Schedules

In order to reduce behavior problems and create an organized, predictable classroom, it is key to establish individual student and classroom schedules. Using schedules in a classroom provides students with predictability and can teach them to tolerate waiting and transitions between activities.

Several types of schedules can be used, including picture schedules, word schedules, and checklists. Choosing the appropriate schedule and its design should be influenced by each student's cognitive level, adaptive skills, and motor abilities. For example, a student with minimal reading or word identification skills may benefit most from a picture schedule (McClannahan & Krantz, 1999), with each picture corresponding to an activity or step within an activity (see Figure 32.3). During a morning routine, a child may be required to remove his or her jacket and bag, place them in a locker, collect materials for an independent activity, and then sit at a desk. Each step would be depicted by a picture that appears on a board or folder and is removed as the step is completed. For example, Miguel, Yang, Finn, and Ahearn (2009) used a match-to-sample procedure with two children with autism to transfer control

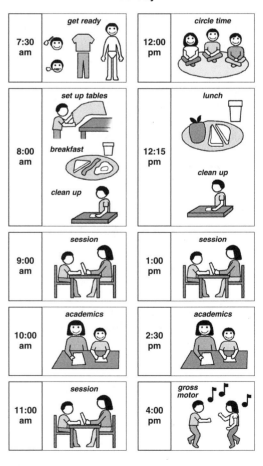

Figure 32.3. Picture schedule using line drawings and their corresponding words.

over the completion of activity schedules from photographs to printed words contained in a binder. Activities used in this study required students to retrieve items corresponding to the picture/word on each page of the binder (e.g., sorting shapes, completing a puzzle, obtaining a play set) from an array or from a bookshelf.

Arranging the Classroom for Maximum Impact

The concept of space management and positioning of staff and students can powerfully affect behavior, and it is one of the easiest variables to manipulate (see Figure 32.4). First, it may be necessary to assess the level of supervision each student requires. Some students may need to sit close to the teacher or might benefit from working one to one with a support staff person, either periodically or for extended periods. Second, the use of individual carrels, and appropriately locating them in the room, can reduce distractibility in students with attention problems. If carrels are located in high-traffic areas, it should be determined whether they can be relocated to a quieter or less-traveled section of the room. In addition, the location of group activities and lessons should be considered, and if possible, moved away from individual work stations into an area where group work will not be distracting to other students. It is critical to frequently assess auditory and visual stimulation during the day and modify as needed for students who are easily distracted.

Providing Instruction

First and foremost, readiness skills such as remaining seated, attending to materials, and listening to instructions are extremely important. If a child is unable to sit in a chair or make eye contact with an instructor, he or she will be more likely to become distracted or focused on irrelevant stimuli. A good strategy for addressing attention problems is to teach students to ready themselves. Each student can be taught a "ready position." For example, before any instruction begins, the students can be prompted to "get ready to learn," meaning that they should sit quietly in their chairs with their feet on the floor and hands on their desk, looking at the instructor and listening for instructions. For children who are very distractible, teaching these attending skills one at a time may be necessary (e.g., sitting, then keeping feet on floor, then keeping hands still, then looking at the instructor, and so forth) before beginning to address other educational objectives.

Where and how instructions are given also greatly influence providing an optimal learning environment. For some activities and students, written instructions on the board may be most effective in conjunction with verbal instructions, whereas for other activities and students recorded instructions may be necessary so that students can replay them as needed. Regardless of the activity, instructions should be determined by student ability and modified based on performance progress.

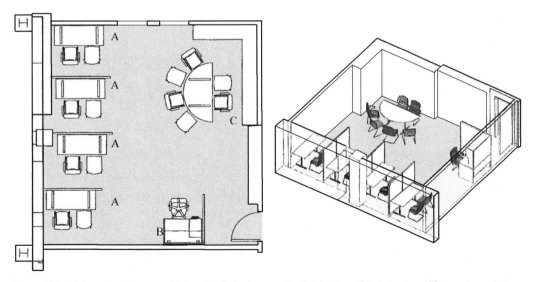

Figure 32.4. Schematic of classroom (A) Carrels to help decrease visual distraction. This design is used for one-to-one instruction or independent work (B) A computer workstation, separate from the rest of the stations with a divider to minimize distraction (C) Table for small-group instruction.

Just as instructions should be individualized based on activity and ability, the types of instructional materials chosen for each student should be individualized. These materials may need to address a number of variables including motor abilities, sight limitations, hearing deficits, attention deficits, and student interests. For instance, if a student has a hearing impairment, an FM receiver to amplify sounds may be helpful. Also materials should be visually stimulating and easily viewed from afar. By choosing materials based on these criteria, a teacher is less likely to encounter problem behaviors that arise out of boredom or frustration.

Another important variable is the appropriate arrangement of educational materials. Although choosing materials based on cognitive and motor abilities is important, the presentation of these materials is equally important. The use of easily destroyed or thrown materials with a child who has disruptive behavior will only contribute to these problems. Conversely, the use of Velcro to attach materials to a table could serve to decrease the opportunity for problem behaviors to occur, therefore maximizing the student's opportunity to learn. In addition, it is always a good idea to keep any excess materials out of reach or sight of the student. This will also reduce distractions and self-stimulatory or disruptive behaviors.

Finally, prompting procedures (both verbal and nonverbal) are critical tools for improving skill acquisition and minimizing the occurrence of maladaptive behaviors. Prompting procedures should be selected according to the students'

abilities, as some students learn best via modeling whereas others learn best from more restrictive guidance. Severe aggression might warrant use of limited physical prompting focusing mainly on verbal and gestural models. Extremely disruptive behavior, such as ripping and throwing materials, may require more intrusive physical guidance, at least initially.

These guidelines arrange space, materials, and routines, to name a few, to reduce the probability of the problem behavior and increase the occurrence of behavior that is appropriate and necessary for learning skills and academics. This attention to setting events or establishing operations, as discussed previously, decreases reliance on staff intensive behavioral programs that employ positive and negative social contingencies.

Reinforcement

Every classroom should have a system of reinforcement. Ideally, this system would include reinforcement programs for both individuals and the group as a whole. However, it is important to remember that individual students have specific preferences, and what works to reinforce appropriate behavior for one student may not work for another. In addition, a student's preferences can change, either gradually or frequently. Therefore, students should be assessed regularly and reinforcement systems changed accordingly (Deleon, Fisher, Rodriguez-Catter, Maglieri, Herman, & Marhefka, 2001; Hanley, Iwata, & Roscoe, 2006).

Some examples of reinforcement systems commonly used in the classroom are 1) token

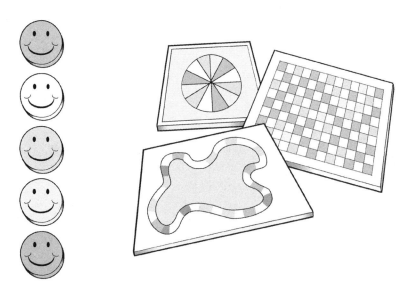

Figure 32.5.   Example of a token board. The icon on the left is the reinforcer for which the child is working.

boards and token economies, 2) sticker charts, 3) edible and tangible reinforcers (including access to self-stimulatory behaviors), 4) classroom "stores," and 5) extracurricular activities (see Figure 32.5). In addition, reinforcement may be provided for a variety of contingencies. Students may earn tokens, for instance, for the absence of a problem behavior, the completion of a specified task, or the appropriate communication of a want or need. Furthermore, the frequency at which these reinforcers should be delivered is determined by a number of factors, including the student's skill level, compliance, and motivation. It is a common practice to deliver reinforcement more frequently when a system is first initiated and then gradually thin the schedule of reinforcement as student compliance and behavior problems improve. As the frequency of reinforcement is decreased, it may be beneficial to provide visual cues (e.g., tokens, pieces of a puzzle) that indicate progress toward distribution of a reinforcer (McClannahan & Krantz, 1999).

BEHAVIORAL TEACHING STRATEGIES

Goals of Effective Teaching

Teachers are rarely satisfied if their students' accurate performance of a new skill or behavior is only done with assistance and under simplified conditions. Rather, instruction is considered effective when learners can perform newly-acquired skills independently, with accuracy and fluency, and in situations outside of training (what is termed *generalization*; Miltenberger, 2008; Stokes & Baer, 1977). Common forms of generalization include 1) performing the same skill when the stimuli that occasion it differ in some way from the training stimuli (e.g., holding up a yellow card to request attention from adults other than the therapist); 2) performing the same skill when the stimuli that occasion it are presented in different contexts (e.g., requesting attention from adults at school and at home); and 3) combining different skills in ways not trained (e.g., holding up the card and an empty glass to ask for a drink).

Stimulus control is a prerequisite to all forms of generalization and develops as the learner's response is brought under the control of certain key stimuli. Stimulus control does not happen instantly but accumulates gradually over time as learners receive multiple opportunities to respond with feedback and differential

reinforcement (i.e., practice). Notice that as practice progresses, two types of learning take place: how to perform the behavior correctly (e.g., tearing lettuce into bite-sized pieces), and when performing the behavior is likely to be reinforced (e.g., in response to the instruction, "Let's make a salad"). Key factors in developing stimulus control are 1) the ability to perform the behavior, 2) differential reinforcement of correct responding, and 3) attention to the relevant situational cues that signal that the behavior will be reinforced. Early in training, a learner's response becomes more accurate and eventually efficient as a result of corrective feedback and reinforcement. At the same time, the key features of stimuli that control responding become more salient, making them easier to detect across learning trials. Later in training, when nonessential features of the controlling stimuli are varied (e.g., font of text, person giving the command) or their context changes, stimulus control enables the learner to continue responding correctly. Stimulus control and generalization, therefore, represent two ends of a skill-training continuum linked in the middle by repeated practice opportunities in tandem with feedback and reinforcement.

Tailoring Instruction to Student Performance Levels

Whether learning to read, prepare meals, or engage in leisure or sporting activities, a student's mastery of a skill is attained through a sequence of stages referred to as the **learning/instructional hierarchy** or IH (Daly, Martens, Barnett, Witt, & Olson, 2007). The IH describes behaviors to be learned and mastered, not only by their form (e.g., single-digit addition, sums to 18), but by the proficiency level with which they are performed (e.g., at least 20 digits correct per minute two days after training has ended). Each stage of the IH (i.e., acquisition, fluency and maintenance, generalization) can be described by a different training goal and performance measure (a learning hierarchy) and an associated set of teaching strategies (an instructional hierarchy). Once the student reaches the training goal at each stage, opportunities for learning are maximized by then "shifting" the focus of instruction to the next stage.

The IH is an important teaching tool for several reasons. First, it describes how performance of a wide range of behaviors and skills improves over time with effective instruction. Second, because learning at each IH stage is promoted in different ways, knowing how well a learner performs a skill enables selection of the most effective teaching strategy for that proficiency level (Daly et al., 2007). Third, frequent performance monitoring allows for changes in instructional procedures as needed in order to maximize practice opportunities, minimize errors, and avoid escape-motivated problem behaviors. In this respect, behavioral approaches to effective teaching require educators to actively change their instructional activities, and be responsive to improvements in their students' performance.

Acquisition

The goal at the IH's first stage, acquisition, is for learners to perform a new skill or behavior accurately on repeated occasions without assistance. Performance measures during acquisition typically include the percentage of correct responses across trials, the percentage of errors, and type of assistance provided. Because learners are attempting new skills and behaviors for the first time during acquisition-level training, teaching these skills in their natural context may provide too few learning opportunities or be too difficult for some learners. For these students, learning the skill in isolation at least initially may be more effective. This requires teachers to guide students through a number of discrete learning opportunities with assistance (prompting), feedback, and reinforcement, or what are termed **complete learning trials** (Granpeesheh, Tarbox, & Dixon, 2009; Miltenberger, 2008). A complete learning trial refers to an opportunity to respond that is controlled by the trainer. Complete learning trials include several components as illustrated in the following example:

1. A task direction that includes key stimuli (saying, "Pick up the *fork*")

2. A controlling prompt (holding up another fork as a model)

3. An opportunity to respond (waiting 10 seconds)

4. Corrective feedback for incorrect responses (providing hand-over-hand guidance)

5. Reinforcement for correct responses (the child is given a bite of a preferred food item)

Although prompts may take a variety of forms (i.e., gesturing, verbal instructions, modeling, pictures, partial physical guidance, full physical guidance), controlling prompts consistently produce the correct response. Once learners can perform a skill accurately with a certain amount of assistance (i.e., prompting and error correction), the assistance is withdrawn or gradually faded until the learner can perform the skill accurately and independently. Numerous procedures for systematically **fading** prompts have been documented in previous research and include the following (Erchul & Martens, 2010):

1. *Prompt and test*, in which a set number of prompted trials are followed by unprompted test trials to assess learning

2. *Prompt and fade*, in which the prompt presented on initial trials is gradually withdrawn on later trials

3. *Most-to-least prompting*, in which successively less-intrusive prompts from a hierarchy are presented on subsequent trials after learners meet a performance criterion on previous trials

4. *Least-to-most prompting*, in which successively more intrusive prompts from a hierarchy are presented if needed after a delay on each trial

5. *Graduated guidance*, in which prompts are provided as needed

6. *Time delay* (constant or progressive), in which the controlling prompt is presented on initial trials immediately after the discriminate stimulus (0 second delay), with presentation delayed on subsequent trials

Promoting the acquisition of new, more adaptive forms of behavior (e.g., imitation, receptive language, appropriate play) is particularly important for children with autism spectrum disorders (ASDs), who often fail to learn such skills on their own. For these children, complete learning trials form the basis of a comprehensive training package known as **discrete trial training** (DTT). With DTT, children may receive up to several hours of complete learning trials a day with breaks in between each session or block of trials (Lovaas, 1987; Smith, 2001). During each session, data are taken on the percentage of correct trials as well as the level of prompting required to produce a correct response. Because DTT takes learning out of context, it allows for more individualized training (e.g., type of controlling prompt, preferred reinforcers) and more frequent opportunities to respond. Moreover, the careful use and gradual withdrawal of prompts during DTT enables accuracy goals to be reached with few or no errors, promotes positive interactions between teachers and learners as well as high rates of reinforcement, reduces problem behaviors that are motivated by escape or avoidance, and decreases the chances of practicing errors. Once stimulus control has been established with DTT, instruction can shift to teaching the skill in the natural environment through techniques such as incidental teaching or activity schedules, discussed previously in the chapter. DTT has shown effectiveness at teaching children with ASD a wide variety of behaviors including initiating conversations with peers (Krantz & McClannahan, 1993) and functional communication using Picture Exchange Communication System (PECS) cards (Charlop-Christy, Carpenter, Le, LeBlanc, & Kellet, 2002).

Fluency and Maintenance

During fluency building, the goal is to perform an already acquired skill accurately but at higher rates as indexed by the frequency of correct responses during brief timings (e.g., words read correctly per minute; McDowell & Keenan, 2001; Shinn, 1989). Productive practice time should include 1) tasks and/or materials to which the learner can respond with high accuracy and minimal assistance (i.e., instructionally-matched materials); 2) brief, repeated practice opportunities with feedback and reinforcement; 3) monitoring and charting of performance; and 4) performance criteria for changing to more difficult material (Chard, Vaughn, & Tyler, 2002; Martens et al., 2007). Implicit in these requirements is the need to assemble a large enough pool of materials, sequenced by difficulty and with sufficient variety, in order to allow for repeated practice opportunities over time. Students are initially assigned material to which they can respond with high accuracy but minimum fluency (e.g., at least 90% accuracy and between 50 and 70 words correct per minute in reading). When students reach the performance goal on material at this level (e.g., 100 words correct per minute on first-grade passages), practice begins again using more difficult material (e.g., second-grade passages), and the sequence is repeated (Martens et al., 2007). Two aspects of this sequence are noteworthy. First, fluency building is a dynamic process that requires periodic changes in practice material to ensure that it matches the student's proficiency level. Second, when using instructionally-matched material, students require less assistance to respond correctly. This means that practice can still be productive minus direct teacher involvement.

Because fluency building occurs gradually and involves a variety of tasks and materials, students are inevitably exposed to both programmed variations (e.g., different types of clothing and fasteners when learning to dress) and naturally occurring variations (e.g., interruptions by staff, dropped clothing items) in the stimulus conditions surrounding performance. Under such conditions, practice to high levels of fluency can also help promote the generalization of responding. First, as performance becomes more efficient and even automatic, it becomes easier to execute at different times and in different contexts, and this ease of execution itself can be reinforcing as students notice it (Martens & Collier, 2011). Second, when correct performance is reinforced under different practice conditions and with different materials, relevant dimensions of the key stimuli that control behavior become more easily recognized. From this perspective, the benefits of fluency building result, not only from increases in response rate per se (Doughty, Chase, & O'Shields, 2004) but also from the strengthening of stimulus control and stimulus generalization of prolonged practice under varying conditions.

In order to prepare both typically developing children and children with disabilities for testing that was mandated in 2001 by the No Child Left Behind Act (NCLB; PL 107-110) public educators have emphasized the training of **complex composite skills** (e.g., reading a word problem in math, executing the relevant computations, graphing or writing a narrative of the answer) instead of **basic component skills** (e.g., fluency with multiplication facts). Fluency researchers advocate the opposite approach and have found an interesting, albeit counterintuitive, benefit of devoting time to building fluency in basic skills. As learners develop basic component skills to higher levels of fluency, less instruction and assistance is needed to combine these skills in the performance of more difficult, composite tasks (Johnson & Layng, 1996).

Generalization

The goal of generalization training is accurate and rapid performance of behavior in the natural environment or in situations that differ from training. Generalization is best promoted by reinforcing the correct use and application of skills with diverse materials, people, or contexts (Daly et al., 2007). By varying practice conditions, learners gain experience in responding to key stimuli in different contexts (e.g., identifying the symbol for men on bathroom doors in different public locations) and responding to key stimuli that differ in nonessential ways (e.g., identifying the symbol for men when it appears in different sizes, colors, or with other features).

Based on the principle of stimulus control, a rule of thumb for promoting generalization is that skills trained in one condition will transfer to another condition to the extent that the two conditions are similar (i.e., contain the same key stimuli or reinforce the same behaviors in the same way). In order to promote generalization, this can be accomplished by training in the natural environment or training under conditions that are made to resemble the natural environment in terms of stimuli, behaviors, or reinforcers. Common stimuli might involve having the same people present or highlighting common parts of words, training in multiple and varied settings, using multiple trainers, or using a range of stimulus examples (Mesmer et al., 2010; Silber & Martens, 2010). Focusing on behaviors that are trained in order to promote generalization has included 1) training to high levels of fluency as discussed previously (Codding, Archer, & Connell, 2010); 2) training behaviors that are useful in a variety of settings (e.g., functional communication training; Charlop-Christy et al., 2002); and 3) training behaviors that remind the child of what to do (e.g., self-instruction training; Mithaug & Mithaug, 2003). Finally, focusing on common reinforcers has involved using reinforcers from the natural environment during training trials, providing reinforcement on an irregular schedule and thereby encouraging persistence, and teaching children to recruit reinforcement (Cammilleri, Tiger, & Hanley, 2008).

BEHAVIORAL INSTRUCTION PROGRAMS

Direct instruction (DI) is a behavioral instruction program based on the IH that uses scripted routines to promote the development of student skills (Adams & Engelmann, 1996; Carnine, Silbert, & Kameenui, 1997). DI lessons are characterized by clear instructions and materials, frequent opportunities to respond to both examples and nonexamples, and consistent consequences for correct responding (Daly et al., 1996). Results of Project Follow Through, a large-scale comparison of instructional programs, suggested that students receiving DI outperformed those receiving all other instructional programs on basic skill, comprehension,

and affective measures (Adams & Engelmann, 1996; Watkins, 1997).

Precision teaching (PT) is a behavioral instruction and monitoring program, also based on the IH, that emphasizes practicing skills to high levels of fluency and charting of performance (Binder, 1996). PT involves daily, timed practices of basic skills (e.g., writing answers to math problems or reading aloud for 1 minute) until learners reach fluency levels high enough to promote maintenance and application (i.e., Retention, Endurance, Stability, Application, and Adduction [RESAA] fluency aims). Performance frequencies during these brief, timed practices (e.g., 50 words correct per minute) are displayed on charts that easily illustrate changes in learning rate. The charts, in turn, are used to evaluate the effectiveness of instruction and to make changes as needed. Students in PT classrooms have been shown to gain between two and three grade levels per year on group-administered achievement tests (Johnson & Layng, 1992).

SUMMARY

The decades since the 1950s have seen dynamic advancement in society's support to individuals with developmental disabilities. Behavioral research, based on operant learning theory, has resulted in innovative and effective approaches that have led to significant improvements in the lives of individuals with developmental disabilities. Much of this research has focused on making socially significant changes to harmful behaviors, as well as improvements in skills necessary for success in everyday community living.

REFERENCES

Adams, G.L., & Engelmann, S. (1996). *Research on direct instruction: 25 years beyond DISTAR*. Seattle, WA: Educational Achievement Systems.

Baer, D.M., Wolf, M.M., & Risley, T.R. (1968). Some current dimensions of applied behavior analysis. *Journal of Applied Behavior Analysis, 1*, 91–97.

Baghdadli, A., Pascal, C., Grisi, S., & Aussilloux, C. (2003). Risk factors for self-injurious behaviours among 222 young children with autistic disorders. *Journal of Intellectual Disability Research, 47*, 622.

Begeny, J.C., & Martens, B.K. (2006). Assessing preservice teachers' training in empirically-validated behavioral instruction practices. *School Psychology Quarterly, 21*, 262–285.

Binder, C. (1996). Behavioral fluency: Evolution of a new paradigm. *The Behavior Analyst, 19*, 163–197.

Bowman, L.G., Fisher, W.W., Thompson, R.H., & Piazza, C.C. (1997). On the relation of mands and the function of destructive behavior. *Journal of Applied Behavior Analysis, 30*, 251–266.

Cammilleri, A.P., Tiger, J.H., & Hanley, G.P. (2008). Developing stimulus control of young children's requests to teachers: Classwide applications of multiple schedules. *Journal of Applies Behavior Analysis, 41,* 299–303.

Camp, E.M., Iwata, B.A., Hammond, J.L., & Bloom, S.E. (2009). Antecedent versus consequent events as predictors of problem behavior. *Journal of Applied Behavior Analysis, 42,* 469–483.

Carnine, D., Silbert, J., & Kameenui, E. (1997). *Direct instruction reading* (3rd ed.). Upper Saddle River, NJ: Prentice Hall.

Carr, E.G., Newsom, C.D., & Binkoff, J.A. (1976). Stimulus control of self-destructive behavior in a psychotic child. *Journal of Abnormal Child Psychology, 4,* 139–153.

Carr, E.G., & Owen-DeSchryver, J.S. (2007). Physical illness, pain, and problem behavior in minimally verbal people with developmental disabilities. *Journal of Autism and Developmental Disorders, 37,* 413–424.

Carter, S.L. (2010). A comparison of various forms of reinforcement with and without extinction as treatment for escape-maintained problem behavior. *Journal of Applied Behavior Analysis,* 543–546.

Cataldo, M.F., & Harris, J. (1982). The biological basis for self-injury in the mentally retarded. *Analysis and Intervention in Developmental Disabilities, 2,* 21–39.

Chadwick, O., Piroth, N., Walker, J., Bernard, S., & Taylor, E. (2000). Factors affecting the risk of behavior problems in children with severe intellectual disability. *Journal of Intellectual Disability Research, 44,* 108–123.

Chard, D.J., Vaughn, S., & Tyler, B.J. (2002). A synthesis of research on effective interventions for building reading fluency with elementary students with learning disabilities. *Journal of Learning Disabilities, 35,* 386–406.

Charlop-Christy, M.H., Carpenter, M., Le, L., LeBlanc, L., & Kellet, K. (2002). Using the Picture Exchange Communication System (PECS) with children with autism: Assessment of PECS acquisition, speech, social-communicative behavior, and problem behavior. *Journal of Applied Behavior Analysis, 35,* 213–231.

Christophersen, E.R., & Friman, P.C. (2010). *Encopresis and enuresis.* Cambridge, MA.

Codding, R.S., Archer, J., & Connell, J. (2010). A systematic replication and extension of using incremental rehearsal to improve multiplication skills: An investigation of generalization. *Journal of Behavioral Education, 19,* 93–105.

Conyers, C., Miltenberger, R., Maki, A., Barenz, R., Jurgens, M., Sailer, A., … & Kopp, B. (2004). A comparison of response cost and differential reinforcement of other behavior to reduce disruptive behavior in a preschool classroom. *Journal of Applied Behavior Analysis, 37,* 411–415.

Crockett, J.L., & Hagopian, L.P. (2006). Prompting procedures as establishing operations for escaped-maintained behavior. *Behavioral Interventions, 21,* 65–71.

Crosland, K.A., Zarcone, J.R., Lindauer, S.E., Valdovinos, M.G., Zarcone, T.J., Hellings, J.A., & Schroeder, S.R. (2003). Use of functional analysis methodology in the evaluation of medication effects. *Journal of Autism and Developmental Disorders, 33,* 271–279.

Daly, E.J., Lentz, F.E., & Boyer, J. (1996). The instructional hierarchy: A conceptual model for understanding the effective components of reading interventions. *School Psychology Quarterly, 11,* 369–386.

Daly, E.J., Martens, B.K., Barnett, D., Witt, J.C., & Olson, S.C. (2007). Varying intervention delivery in response-to-intervention: Confronting and resolving challenges with measurement, instruction, and intensity. *School Psychology Review, 36,* 562–581.

DeLeon, I.G., Fisher, W.W., Rodriguez-Catter, V., Maglieri, K., Herman, K., & Marhefka, J. (2001). Examination of relative reinforcement effects of stimuli identified through pretreatment and daily brief preference assessments. *Journal of Applied Behavior Analysis, 34,* 463–473.

DeLeon, I.G., Iwata, B.A., Goh, H., & Worsdell, A.S. (1997). Emergence of reinforcer preference as a function of schedule requirements and stimulus similarity. *Journal of Applied Behavior Analysis, 30,* 439–449.

DeLeon, I.G., Neidert, P.L., Anders, B.M., & Rodriguez-Catter, V. (2001). Choices between positive and negative reinforcement during treatment for escape-maintained behavior. *Journal of Applied Behavior Analysis, 34,* 521–525.

DeLeon, I.G., Toole, L.M., Gutshall, K.A., & Bowman, L.G. (2005). Individualized sampling parameters for behavioral observations: Enhancing the predictive validity of competing stimulus assessments. *Research in Developmental Disabilities, 46,* 440–455.

Doughty, S.S., Chase, P.N., & O'Shields, E.M. (2004). Effects of rate building on fluent performance: A review and commentary. *The Behavior Analyst, 27,* 7–23.

Erchul, W.P., & Martens, B.K. (2010). *School consultation: Conceptual and empirical bases of practice* (3rd ed.). New York, NY: Springer.

Fisher, W.W., DeLeon, I.G., Rodriguez-Catter, V., & Keeney, K.M. (2004). Enhancing the effects of extinction on attention-maintained behavior through noncontingent delivery of attention or stimuli identified via a competing stimulus assessment. *Journal of Applied Behavior Analysis, 37,* 171–184.

Fisher, W.W., & Mazur, J.E. (1997). Basic and applied research on choice responding. *Journal of Applied Behavior Analysis, 30,* 387–410.

Friman, P.C. (2003). Finger sucking. In T. Ollendick and C. Schroeder (Eds), *Encyclopedia of pediatric and child psychology* (pp. 398–340). New York, NY: Kluwer.

Friman, P.C. (2005). Behavioral pediatrics. In M. Hersen (Ed.), *Encyclopedia of behavior modification and therapy* (Vol. II, pp. 731–739). Thousand Oaks, CA: Sage Publications.

Friman, P.C. (2005). *Good night, we love you we will miss you, now go to bed and go to sleep: Managing sleep problems in young children.* Boys Town, NE: Girls and Boys Town Press.

Friman, P.C. (2008). Primary care behavioral pediatrics. In M. Hersen, & A. Gross, (Eds.), *Handbook of Clinical Psychology* (Vol. II, pp. 728–758). New York, NY: John Wiley.

Friman, P.C., Byrd, M.R., & Oksol, E.M. (2001). Oral digital habits: Demographics, phenomenology, causes, functions, and clinical associations. In D.W. Woods & R. Miltenberger (Eds.), *Tic disorders, trichotillomania, and other repetitive behavior disorders: Behavioral approaches to analysis and treatment* (pp. 197–222). New York, NY: Kluwer Academic/Plenum Publishers.

Granpeeshen, D., Tarbox, J., & Dixon, D.R. (2009). Applied behavior analytic interventions for children with autism: A description and review of treatment research. *Annals of Clinical Psychiatry, 21,* 162–173.

Greer, D.R. (2002). *Designing teaching strategies: An applied behavior analysis systems approach.* San Diego, CA: Academic Press.

Hagopian, L.P., Long, E.S., & Rush, K.S. (2004). Preference assessment procedures for individuals with developmental disabilities. *Behavior Modification, 28,* 668–677.

Hagopian, L.P., Toole, L.M., Long, E.S., Bowman, L.G., & Lieving, G.A. (2004). A comparison of dense-to-lean and fixed lean schedules of alternative reinforcement and extinction. *Journal of Applied Behavior Analysis, 37,* 323–337.

Hanley, G.P., Iwata, B.A., & Roscoe, E.M. (2006). Some determinants of changes in preference over time. *Journal of Applied Behavior Analysis, 39,* 189–202.

Hastings, R.P., & Noone, S.J. (2005). Self-injurious behavior and functional analysis: Ethics and evidence. *Education and Training in Developmental Disabilities, 40,* 335–342.

Individuals with Disabilities Education Act Amendments of 1997, PL 105-17, 20 U.S.C. §§ 1400 *et seq.*

Individuals with Disabilities Education Improvement Act of 2004, PL 108-446, 20 U.S.C. §§ 1400 *et seq.*

Iwata, B.A., Dorsey, M.F., Slifer, K.J., Bauman, K. E., & Richman, G. S. (1994). Toward a functional analysis of self-injury. *Journal of Applied Behavior Analysis, 27,* 197–209. (Reprinted from *Analysis and Intervention in Developmental Disabilities, 2,* 3–20, 1982)

Iwata, B.A., Pace, G.M., Dorsey, M.F., Zarcone, J.R., Vollmer, T.R., Smith R. G., .Willis, K.D. (1994). The functions of self-injurious behavior: An experimental-epidemiological analysis. *Journal of Applied Behavior Analysis, 27,* 215–240.

Iwata, B.A., Kahng, S., Wallace, M.D., & Lindberg, J.S. (2000). Functional analysis of behavior disorders. In J. Austin & J.E. Carr (Eds.), *Handbook of applied behavior analysis* (pp. 61–89). Reno, NV: Context Press.

Jarmolowicz, D.P., DeLeon, I.G., & Kuhn, S.C. (2009). Functional communication during signaled reinforcement and/or extinction. *Behavioral Interventions, 24,* 265–273.

Johnson, K.R., & Layng, T.V.J. (1992). Breaking the structuralist barrier: Literacy and numeracy with fluency. *American Psychologist, 47,* 1475–1490.

Johnson, K.R., & Layng, T.V.J. (1996). On terms and procedures: Fluency. *The Behavior Analyst, 19,* 281–288.

Johnson, L., McComas, J., Thompson, A., & Symons, F.J. (2004). Obtained versus programmed reinforcement: Practical considerations in the treatment of escape-reinforced aggression. *Journal of Applied Behavior Analysis, 37,* 239–242.

Kahng, S., Iwata, B.A., & Lewin, A. (2002a). Behavioral treatment of self-injury, 1964 to 2000. *American Journal on Mental Retardation, 107,* 212–221.

Kahng, S., Iwata, B.A., & Lewin, A. (2002). The impact of functional assessment on the treatment of self-injurious behavior. In S. Schroeder, M.L. Oster-Granite, & T. Thompson (Eds.), *Self-injurious behavior: Gene-brain-behavior relationships* (pp. 119–131). Washington, DC: American Psychological Association.

Kern, L., Bailin, D., & Mauk, J.E. (2003). Effects of a topical anesthetic on non-socially maintained self-injurious behavior. *Developmental Medicine and Child Neurology, 45,* 769–771.

Kennedy, C.H., & Souza, G. (1995). Functional analysis and treatment of eye poking. *Journal of Applied Behavior Analysis, 28,* 27–37.

Kodak, T., Lerman, D.C., Volkert, V.M., & Trosclair, N. (2007). Further examination of factors that influence preference for positive versus negative reinforcement. *Journal of Applied Behavior Analysis, 40,* 25–44.

Kodak, T., Miltenberger, R.G., & Romaniuk, C. (2003). A comparison of differential reinforcement and noncontingent reinforcement for the treatment of a child's multiply controlled problem behavior. *Behavioral Interventions, 18,* 267–278.

Kodak, T., Northup, J., & Kelley, M.E. (2007). An evaluation of the types of attention that maintain problem behavior. *Journal of Applied Behavior Analysis, 40,* 167–171.

Krantz, P.J., & McClannahan, L.E. (1993). Teaching children with autism to initiate to peers: Effects of a script-fading procedure. *Journal of Applied Behavior Analysis, 35,* 213–231.

Laraway, S., Snycerski, S., Michael, J., & Poling, A. (2003). Motivating operations and terms to describe them: Some further refinements. *Journal of Applied Behavior Analysis, 36,* 407–414.

Lerman, D.C., & Iwata, B.A. (1996). Developing a technology for the use of operant extinction in clinical settings: An examination of basic and applied research. *Journal of Applied Behavior Analysis, 29,* 345–382.

Lerman, D.C., Kelley, M.E., Vorndran, C.M., Kuhn, S.A.C., & LaRue, R.H., Jr. (2002). Reinforcement magnitude and responding during treatment with differential reinforcement. *Journal of Applied Behavior Analysis, 35,* 29–48.

Levy, R.M., & Rubenstein, L.S. (1996). *The rights of people with mental disabilities: The authoritative ACLU guide to the rights of people with mental illness and intellectual disability.* Carbondale, IL: Southern Illinois University.

Lomas, J.E., Fisher, W.W., & Kelley, M.E. (2010). The effects of variable-time delivery of food items and praise on problem behavior reinforced by escape. *Journal of Applied Behavior Analysis, 43,* 425–435.

Long, E.S., Hagopian, L.P., DeLeon, I.G., Marhefka, J.M., & Resau, D. (2005). Competing stimuli in the treatment of multiply controlled problem behavior occurring during hygiene routines. *Research in Developmental Disabilities, 26,* 57–69.

Lovaas, O.I. (1987). Behavioral treatment and normal educational and intellectual functioning in young autistic children. *Journal of Consulting and Clinical Psychology, 55,* 3–9.

Lovaas, O.I., Freitag, G., Gold, V.J., & Kassorla, I.C. (1965). Experimental studies in childhood schizophrenia: Analysis of self-destructive behavior. *Journal of Experimental Child Psychology, 2,* 67–84.

Mace, F.C. (1994). The significance and future of functional analysis methodologies. *Journal of Applied Behavior Analysis, 27,* 385–384.

Magee, S.K., & Ellis, J. (2001). The detrimental effects of physical restraint as a consequence for inappropriate classroom behavior. *Journal of Applied Behavior Analysis, 34,* 501–504.

Martens, B.K., Eckert, T.L., Begeny, J.C., Lewandowski, L.J., DiGennaro, F., Montarello, S., Fiese, B.H. (2007). Effects of a fluency-building program on the reading performance of low-achieving second and third grade students. *Journal of Behavioral Education, 16,* 39–54.

Martens, B.K., Martens, B.K., & Collier, S.R. (in press). Developing fluent, efficient, and automatic repertoires of athletic performance. In J.K. Luiselli & D.R. Reed (Eds.), *Behavioral sport psychology: Evidence-based approaches to performance enhancement.* New York, NY: Springer.

Matson, J.L., & Rivet, T.T. (2008). Characteristics of challenging behaviours in adults with autistic disorder, PDD-NOS, and intellectual disability. *Journal of Intellectual and Developmental Disability, 33,* 323–329.

Matson, J.L., & Wilkins, J. (2009). Factors associated with the Questions About Behavioral Function for functional assessment of low and high rate challenging behaviors in adults with intellectual disability. *Behavior Modification, 33,* 207–219.

McClannahan, L.E, & Krantz, P.J. (1999). *Activity schedules for children with autism: Teaching independent behavior.* Bethesda, MD: Woodbine House.

McComas, J.J., Thompson, A., & Johnson, L. (2003). The effects of presession attention on problem behavior maintained by different reinforcers. *Journal of Applied Behavior Analysis, 36,* 297–307.

Mesmer, E.M., Duhon, G.J., Hogan, K., Newry, B., Hommema, S., Fletcher, C., & Boso, M. (2010). Generalization of sight word accuracy using a common stimulus procedure: A preliminary investigation. *Journal of Behavioral Education, 19,* 47–61

Miguel, C.F., Yang, H.G., Finn, H.E., & Ahearn, W.H. (2009) Establishing derived textual control in activity schedules with children with autism. *Journal of Applied Behavior Analysis, 42,* 703–709

Miltenberger, R.G. (2008). *Behavior modification: Principles and procedures* (4th ed.). Belmont, CA: Thomson Wadsworth.

Mithaug, D.K., & Mithaug, D.E. (2003). Effects of teacher-directed versus student-directed instruction on self-management of young children with disabilities. *Journal of Applied Behavior Analysis, 36,* 133–136.

Moore, J.W., Fisher, W.W., & Pennington, A. (2004). Systematic application and removal of protective equipment in the assessment of multiple topographies of self-injury. *Journal of Applied Behavior Analysis, 37,* 73–77.

Moore, B., Friman, P.C., Fruzetti, A.E., & MacAleese, K. (2007). Brief report: Evaluating the bedtime pass program for child resistance to bedtime: A randomized controlled trial. *Journal of Pediatric Psychology, 32,* 283–287.

Murphy, O., Healy, O., & Leader, G., (2009). Risk factors for challenging behaviour for 157 children with autism spectrum disorder in Ireland. *Research in Autism Spectrum Disorders, 3,* 474–482.

National Institutes of Health. (1991). *Treatment of destructive behaviors in persons with developmental disabilities.* Washington, DC: U.S. Department of Health and Human Services.

No Child Left Behind Act of 2001, PL 107–110, 115 Stat. 1425, 20 U.S.C. §§ 6301 *et seq.*

Nyhan, W.L. (2002). Lessons from Lesch-Nyhan Syndrome. In S. Schroeder, M.L. Oster-Granite, & T. Thompson (Eds.), *Self-injurious behavior: Gene-brain-behavior relationships* (pp. 251–267). Washington, DC: American Psychological Association.

O'Reilly, M.F., & Lancioni, G. (2000). Response covariation of escape-maintained aberrant behavior correlated with sleep deprivation. *Research in Developmental Disabilities, 21,* 125–136.

O'Reilly, M., Rispoli, M., Davis, T., Machalicek, W., Lang, R., Sigafoos, J., .Didden, R. (2010). Functional analysis of challenging behavior in children with autism spectrum disorders: A summary of 10 cases. *Research in Autism Spectrum Disorders, 4,* 1–10.

O'Reilly, M., Sigafoos, J., Edrisinha, C., Lancioni, G., Cannella, H., Choi, H.Y., & Barretto, A. (2006). A preliminary examination of the evocative effects of the establishing operation. *Journal of Applied Behavior Analysis, 39,* 239–242.

Pace, G.M., Ivancic, M.T., Edwards, G.L., Iwata, B.A., & Page, T.J. (1985). Assessment of stimulus preference and reinforcer value with profoundly retarded individuals. *Journal of Applied Behavior Analysis, 18,* 249–255.

Pelios, L., Morren, J., Tesch, D., & Axelrod, S. (1999). The impact of functional analysis methodology on treatment choice for self-injurious and aggressive behavior. *Journal of Applied Behavior Analysis, 32,* 185–195.

Roane, H.S., Falcomata, T.S., & Fisher, W.W. (2007). Applying the behavioral economics principle of unit price to DRO schedule thinning. *Journal of Applied Behavior Analysis, 40,* 529–534.

Samaha, A.L., Vollmer, T.R., Borrero, C., Sloman, K., St. Peter Pipkin, C., & Bourret, J. (2009). Analyses of response–stimulus sequences in descriptive observations. *Journal of Applied Behavior Analysis, 42,* 447–468.

Shinn, M.R. (1989). *Curriculum-based measurement: Assessing special children.* New York, NY: Guilford.

Shore, B.A., Iwata, B.A., DeLeon, I.G., Kahng, S., & Smith, R.G. (1997). An analysis of reinforcer substitutability using object manipulation and self-injury as competing responses. *Journal of Applied Behavior Analysis, 30,* 21–40.

Silber, J.M., & Martens, B.K. (2010). Programming for the generalization of oral reasing fluency: Repeated readings of entire text versus multiple exemplars. *Journal of Behavioral Education, 19,* 30–46

Smith, T. (2001). Discrete trail training in the treatment of autism. *Focus on Autism and Other Developmental Disabilities, 16,* 86–92.

Stokes, T.F., & Baer, D.M. (1977). An implicit technology of generalization. *Journal of Applied Behavior Analysis, 10,* 349–367.

Tarbox, R., Williams, L., & Friman, P.C. (2004). Extended diaper wearing: Effects on continence in and out of the diaper. *Journal of Applied Behavior Analysis, 37,* 97–101.

Tustin, R.D. (1994). Preference for reinforcers under varying schedule arrangements: A behavioral economic analysis. *Journal of Applied Behavior Analysis, 27,* 597–606.

Twyman, J.S. (1998). The Fred S. Keller School. *Journal of Applied Behavior Analysis, 31,* 695–701.

Vaughan, M.E., & Michael, J. (1982). Automatic reinforcement: An important but ignored concept. *Behaviorism, 10,* 217–227.

Vollmer, T.R, Roane, H.S, Ringdahl, J.E, & Marcus B.A. (1999). Evaluating treatment challenges with differential reinforcement of alternative behavior. *Journal of Applied Behavior Analysis, 32,* 9–23.

Watkins, C.L. (1997). *Project Follow Through: A case study of contingencies influencing instructional practices of the educational establishment.* Concord, MA: Cambridge Center for Behavioral Studies.

Woods, D.W., & Miltenberger, R. (2001). *Tic disorders, trichotillomania, and other repetitive behavior disorders: Behavioral approaches to analysis and treatment.* New York, NY: Kluwer Academic/Plenum Publishers.

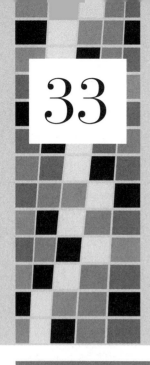

33

Occupational and Physical Therapy

Philippa Campbell

Upon completion of this chapter, the reader will

■ Understand the role(s) that occupational therapists and physical therapists may play in supporting families and helping children with disabilities to achieve their full potential

■ Become familiar with common intervention frameworks and how they are applied to children of different ages and disabilities

■ Identify intervention strategies used by pediatric therapists to enhance children's skill development and to increase participation in everyday activities and routines

Children with disabilities may experience a wide range of impairments in body structure and function, limitations in participation in daily life activities, and restrictions in their ability to be an active part of their community (World Health Organization [WHO], 2001). Occupational therapy and physical therapy are commonly recommended to enhance participation in everyday activities and routines, teach new skills, improve physical function, and prevent any possible future physical limitation. Pediatric therapists frequently work with children's families and other disciplines in a team approach and provide services in a variety of settings including homes, schools, and hospitals or clinics. Both occupational and physical therapists work with children who have experienced delays in learning various skills. They also assist children with physical dysfunctions, such as cerebral palsy and other neuromotor or neuromuscular disorders, to acquire skills

and improve physical areas such as increasing strength or range or motion. Occupational therapists also work with children whose performance may be affected by differences in sensory processing often associated with **autism spectrum disorders** (ASD), intellectual disability, and learning disabilities.

Experienced pediatric therapists are knowledgeable about strategies to promote children's learning across developmental areas. In terms of skill development, occupational therapy practice usually focuses more on upper extremity and fine motor skills (i.e., play and self-care) while physical therapists more frequently center on lower extremity or gross motor skills (i.e., mobility). Most therapists select play activities for young children as a context for providing specific interventions. Depending upon the individual child's needs, these interventions may include exercise, physical agents, splinting or casting, adaptive aids and equipment, adaptations and assistive technology, and behavioral training (American Occupational Therapy Association [AOTA], 2002; American Physical Therapy Association [APTA], 2001). Overlap in the roles of physical and occupational therapists exists for several reasons. Both professions require similar educational backgrounds in human development, anatomy and physiology, the scope and nature of disabilities, and a general approach to habilitation (teaching skills not yet learned) and rehabilitation (teaching skills lost through illness or injury). Postgraduate continuing education allows therapists from both disciplines to develop advanced skills in selected interventions, such as splinting, application of assistive technology, and other specialized therapy approaches. The interests and talents of individual therapists, along with the philosophy and needs of the workplace, often dictate the exact nature of a therapist's role in that setting.

While important, both skill learning and improving physical function are not the only areas addressed by occupational or physical therapists. Both disciplines recognize the importance of meaningful life outcomes as a goal of therapy services. These functional child outcomes relate to children's successful participation in the everyday activities and routines at home, in school, and in community settings. For example, satisfactory family mealtimes may occur when a child independently eats and drinks. The fact that mealtimes go well may be more important than whether or not the child actually performs the skills of bringing the cup or spoon to his or her mouth. A child may be independent at mealtimes by using a straw to drink from a cup that is fastened to the table. Similarly the utensils and dishes may be modified so that the child is able to hold the spoon and get it to the mouth independently.

■ ■ ■ AMEENA: LIFELONG IMPACT OF PHYSICAL DISABILITY

Ameena was born prematurely and was diagnosed with periventricular leukomalacia (a cause of cerebral palsy; see Chapter 7) shortly after birth. Physical therapy intervention began in the neonatal intensive care unit (NICU). The physical therapist met with Ameena's parents and taught them ways of positioning her and changing her position so that she would have opportunities to develop postural control and maintain a quiet, alert state during her waking hours. By 6 months of age, Ameena was actively engaged with both people and objects in her environment. She was, however, unable to sit without support, and the muscle tone in her legs had increased compared with the tone in her arms. A diagnosis of spastic diplegic cerebral palsy was made during a visit to the Neonatal Follow-Up Program, and she was referred for early intervention services.

An early intervention physical therapist made weekly home visits and learned about how Ameena participated in typical family activities and routines and the extent to which her motor disability affected her participation. At 6 months of age, her motor disability primarily affected playtime activities and influenced functional skills, such as exploring her environment. As she got older, other motor skills such as walking were affected by the high muscle tone in her legs. This, in turn, affected how often she had to be carried and her positioning for mobility, for example, in a stroller. The therapist arranged for Ameena to be fitted for bilateral foot orthoses and showed her parents how to use them. She and Ameena's mother explored a variety of off-the-shelf chairs, strollers, and walking devices and selected ones that allowed Ameena to be independent. The physical therapist also taught the mother a variety of strategies to use within typical activities and routines to provide opportunities for Ameena to sit, crawl, and walk. By 3 years of age, Ameena was able to walk with canes and was enrolled in a preschool program where she was provided with adaptations and assistive technology devices that allowed her to participate in classroom activities with the other children. Occupational and physical therapy consultations with the preschool staff allowed for design and use of supports to enable Ameena to be successful in a variety of activities, such as using the bathroom. Upon entering kindergarten, Ameena was eligible to continue receiving consultative physical therapy and occupational therapy services under the provisions of Section 504 of the Rehabilitation Act of 1973 (PL 93–112).

At age 6, Ameena underwent orthopedic surgery to lengthen her lower extremity muscles, followed by a period of intensive physical therapy to improve her hip and knee control. This allowed her to continue to walk for fairly long distances in her community with only the support of canes, although she preferred a manual wheelchair for extended trips. By third grade,

Ameena was falling behind in schoolwork due to handwriting difficulties. Her occupational therapist recommended classroom modifications that included provision of a word processor with accompanying instruction so that she completed classroom assignments more efficiently. As she continues to progress through school and participates in more extracurricular activities, Ameena may not need continual or regularly scheduled occupational or physical therapy sessions. However, occupational and physical therapists will be available throughout her school career to provide consultation when needed to address specific situations that may occur or limit her participation in home, school, or community activities and routines.

THERAPY TYPES AND PURPOSES

Occupational and physical therapy have two different purposes when provided to children with disabilities. The first purpose is rehabilitation. Here therapy services are provided to increase functional or developmental abilities or to reduce limitations that may be present in physical or sensory areas (e.g., muscle strength or tactile sensitivity). Therapy may help achieve increased range of motion or decreased sensory defensiveness. It may also support learning a particular skill such as walking, reaching, grasping, or talking. A second purpose is to achieve full participation or inclusion. When the purpose is participation, services may be directed less at addressing a child's physical or skill limitations than at enhancing participation in activities and routines that occur in the home, school, or other community settings (Campbell, 2004; Jung, 2003; Rogers, 2010.)

Therapy outcomes may include successful completion of, for example, participation in home routines such as getting up in the morning, bathing, going to bed at night, and going on family errands like grocery shopping. It also includes active participation in school activities such as circle time, language arts, or after-school activities (Campbell, 2011b; Dunst & Bruder, 1999; McWilliam, 2010). Participation is not necessarily tied to improvements in physical limitations or increases in skill learning; it may result from environmental changes or the use of adaptations including assistive technology (AT; Campbell, Milbourne, & Wilcox, 2005; Jones & Gray, 2005a; Jones & Gray, 2005b; Milbourne & Campbell, 2007; Sadao & Robinson, 2010; Chapter 36). For example, a child with a physical disability may be independent in visiting a neighborhood friend's house with the use of a power chair and curb cuts in neighborhood streets. A young child may participate in bath time by using a bath seat, foam soap, and a washcloth mitt, even when he or she is unable to sit independently or demonstrate grasp and release functionality.

INTERVENTION FRAMEWORKS USED BY PHYSICAL AND OCCUPATIONAL THERAPISTS

The types of interventions used by occupational or physical therapists when working with children of varying age levels or disabilities are guided generally by one of two frameworks: a rehabilitation/traditional framework or a participation-based framework. While many interventions are used within both disciplines, there are instances, particularly within the rehabilitation/traditional framework, where the expertise of a particular discipline is better matched to a specific situation. For example, a physical therapist would be more likely than an occupational therapist to provide therapy designed to teach a child with a physical disability such as myelomeningocele to walk, while an occupational therapist would be the more likely discipline to provide intervention for a child with autism who has a sensory processing deficit.

The Rehabilitation or Traditional Framework

Occupational and physical therapy are often delivered via a traditional framework when rehabilitation is the purpose (Campbell & Sawyer, 2007; Dunst, Trivette, Humphries, Raab, & Roper, 2001). In a traditional service framework, also referred to as the "medical model," individual disciplines focus on identifying deficits (or areas of need) and then provide intervention to improve functioning in deficient areas. Physical therapists using a rehabilitation/traditional framework might provide exercises to increase a child's muscle strength or design activities to improve endurance. When a child's grasp has been identified as deficient, occupational therapists might create opportunities for a child to hold and manipulate toys to eventually achieve independent play skills.

In pediatrics, traditional services are more frequently provided in acute care or rehabilitation hospitals or clinics than in early intervention or school-based settings. Therefore physicians and other medically-based personnel may be more familiar and comfortable with a traditional than with a participation-based framework. Figure 33.1 illustrates a "traditional service" process. In general, a physician or other professional refers a child for evaluation from which the OT or PT makes recommendations and plans for intervention, follows through on the recommended plan, and discontinues services when the child has either achieved goals or made as many gains as are likely in the short term.

The Participation-Based Framework

From birth through the early young adult years, a majority of children with disabilities who receive occupational or physical therapy services do so through publicly-supported early intervention or school programs, although additional therapy services may be provided privately. The emphasis in early intervention therapy is shifting from a rehabilitation focus to a broader perspective where therapy outcomes are expected to enhance infants' and toddlers' participation in natural environments. In older children the focus is on inclusion and participation in typical school settings including their access to the general education curriculum (e.g., Campbell, 2004; Dunst, 2001; Law et al., 2006; Rogers, 2010; Coster & Khetani, 2010).

Participation frameworks are tied directly to the World Health Organization's Classification of Functioning, Disability and Health (ICF, 2001), which considers disability as an *interaction* among a number of components that may limit or promote functioning including disease, structure, activity (i.e., skill performance), environment, and participation. The WHO interactive perspective allows therapists not just to provide exercises or activities to remediate structural or activity limitations; the interactive perspective also recommends strategies to support participation by addressing the social and physical characteristics of the environments where the person with a disability spends time. This model expands the focus of both occupational and physical therapy beyond structure and activity (i.e., skills) to encompass environmental and participation components. A physical therapist addresses environment and participation components, for example, by evaluating a child's home and/or school environment and making recommendations to install a

Steps In Providing Traditional Occupational or Physical Therapy Service

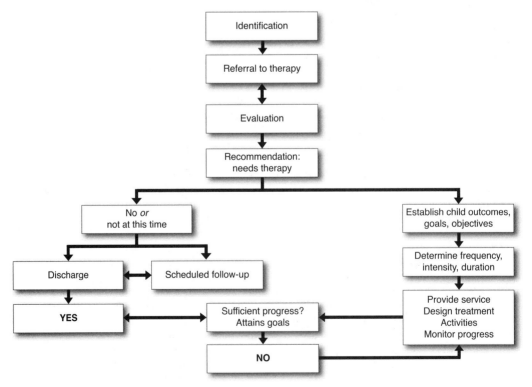

Figure 33.1. An illustration of a traditional service process.

ramp or arrange classroom furniture so that a child may move independently in a wheelchair or safely when using crutches or a walker.

In work with infants and young children, participation has been interpreted through models such as routines-based intervention (McWilliam, 2000, 2010; Stremel & Campbell, 2007), activity-based physical therapy (Valvano & Rapport, 2006), participation-based services (Campbell, 2004, 2011a; Campbell & Sawyer, 2007, 2009) and coaching other professionals (Buysee & Wesley, 2007) and caregivers (Hanft, Rush, & Shelden, 2004; Rush & Shelden, 2011). In school settings, the term *inclusion* is used to represent children's participation in school settings and activities. An important purpose of school-based therapy is to enable children to access the general education curriculum and participate in social activities (Dunn, 2011; Effgen, 2005, 2006).

A common element across both early intervention and school-based therapy is to embed the child's goals and interventions into family or classroom activities and routines (Dunn, 2007; Pretti-Frontzcak & Bricker, 2004; Sandall & Swartz, 2008; Wilson, Mott, & Batman, 2004). One approach has been developed that encompasses 1) assessment of the child's participation in activities and routines, 2) embedding the child's intervention strategies in daily activities, 3) collaborating with and training caregivers and teachers, and 4) monitoring the child's progress (Campbell, 2010; Campbell, Milbourne, & Kennedy, 2012). In this approach, activities and routines provide a context for embedding two distinct categories of intervention strategies: 1) adult-provided intervention strategies; and 2) adaptations including environmental modifications, assistive technology (AT), and visual supports. Because therapists are unlikely to be with a child during all typical daily activities and routines, other adults who spend time with the child such as parents, child care workers, relatives, and professionals of various disciplines, are taught how to embed the intervention strategies within typical activities and routines.

TEAM STRUCTURES AND THERAPIST ROLES

Traditionally, therapists' roles have focused on evaluating performance and providing hands-on intervention to help children improve physical functioning or acquire identified skills. Therapists have played this direct service provider role to children across many settings (i.e., school, home, clinic), age levels (i.e., infant to adolescent), and developmental disabilities (e.g.,

autism, cerebral palsy, learning disabilities). Occupational and physical therapists work with a child and family as part of a team of professionals; they seldom work in isolation. Many different structures have been described to delineate various types of teams and to outline team member roles. Teams are described using labels such as multidisciplinary, interdisciplinary, transdisciplinary, integrated, collaborative or single service provider. They may also be labeled by the service plan title (e.g., IEP team). The array of structures defines different ways that professionals interact with children, families and each other, and describe how services are coordinated.

Different team structures inherently entail roles for both families and professionals. For example, in an interdisciplinary team, a professional from each discipline conducts an evaluation separately, meets with the team to discuss findings, and then makes recommendations for services to the family. In contrast members of a multidisciplinary team might conduct an arena evaluation, where all team members evaluate and discuss the child's needs at the same time. Families are acknowledged as members of most teams, but in reality families may or may not be substantively included in decision making or implementation of interventions. For example, a caregiver may not truly be an equal team member when all therapy is provided in a school setting and the parent and the therapist(s) communicate little outside of the annual IEP meeting.

In services provided to children, the most commonly used team structures are transdisciplinary, integrated, collaborative, or single service provider, all of which describe fairly similar team structures. The common feature across these approaches is the central role of professional team members as consultants to and teachers of families and other team members rather than as hands-on providers of therapy for children (King, Stracham, Tucker, Duwyn, Desserud, & Shillington, 2009). In these structures, team members such as occupational and physical therapists spend considerable time consulting with and teaching caregivers, teachers, or other health care professionals (e.g., speech and language pathologist). When therapy services are provided in traditional ways, the OT or PT might teach specific activities or strategies to use with a child in a home or follow-up program. But when services are provided from a participation-based framework, teaching is explicit and focuses on embedding intervention strategies within existing activities and routines. Even though therapists may have willingness to teach others, recent data suggest that many of them lack experience teaching other adults and thus lack confidence to do so (Campbell, Milbourne, Chiarello, & Wilcox, 2009). Other data show positive outcomes when therapists teach others. For example, parents report increased confidence and competence when taught about interventions such as adaptations and assistive technology (Kling, Campbell, & Wilcox, 2010).

FEATURES OF PEDIATRIC THERAPY SERVICES AND THE ROLE OF THERAPISTS

Although the emphasis of therapy is different within traditional and participation-based frameworks, evaluation/assessment, intervention planning, implementation, and progress monitoring are common components of both frameworks. Each component, however, may be implemented differently (Table 33.1) and is discussed next.

Evaluation and Assessment

Therapists select different evaluation and assessment instruments dependent on the age of the child being evaluated and the therapy framework being used. The evaluation process typically depends on using formal tests or instruments to assess the child's skill in developmental or physical areas and to identify areas where performance does not meet a particular standard such as chronological age, speed, or efficiency (Bagnato, Neisworth, & Pretti-Fronczak, 2010; Chiarello & Kolobe, 2007; Dunn, Nickelson, Cox, Pope, & Rinner, 20011; Effgen, 2006). A physical therapist evaluating an infant or young toddler is likely to select instruments to determine a child's abilities

in gross motor developmental skills such as sitting, crawling, or walking. As the child gets older the therapist may examine functional mobility in the school or neighborhood or even when using public transportation. In a traditional framework, when deficits or delays are identified, therapists design special activities to provide opportunities for the child to acquire or master skills (Campbell, Vanderlinden, Palisano, 2006; Dunn, 2011; Effgen, 2005). The underlying philosophy is that when improvements are noted in skill performance, children will be able to participate in a variety of tasks, activities, or routines. For example, if a child is unable to dress or undress independently because fine motor skills are not performed well enough to manage fastenings, the child must improve his or her fine motor skills before becoming independent in the task of dressing, improvements in fine motor skills will be necessary before the child will be independent in the task of dressing or in morning routines.

Therapists also assess areas related to motor skill performance such as endurance, efficiency, or speed, and determine the level of functioning in body structures such as joints, muscles, or sensory systems (e.g. vision, hearing). Occupational therapists, for example, may use family- or teacher-completed checklists or questionnaires to gather information about areas such as sensory processing, temperament, or behavior. If an occupational therapist's role on a team is to be responsible for the child's eating, other adaptive/self-care, and fine motor skills, then formal instruments or informal assessments are used to measure baseline performance in these tasks. Physical therapists may use instruments to measure gross motor skills such as walking, jumping,

Table 33.1. Features of traditional and participation-based frameworks

Feature	Traditional service framework	Participation-based framework
Evaluation/assessment	Standard evaluation measures and clinical judgment to determine functioning in comparison to a norm	Assessment of participation in typical activities/routines via interview, survey, observation; evaluation measures/clinical judgment of functioning
Intervention planning	Identify goals and outcomes based on areas where deficits are identified (e.g., skills; physical structure)	Identify goals and outcomes based on activities/routines going well or not going well
Implementation	Direct intervention by the therapist with the child; caregiver or other adult may observe and carry-over using home program suggestions	Adult-administered, environmental or adaptation intervention strategies embedded into activities and routines; collaboration/teaching for people who will use the interventions
Progress monitoring	Track client progress by review of performance of goals and objectives	Track client abilities to participate in activities/routines successfully

or balance, and use observation or clinical judgment to assess strength, range of motion, and endurance. Evaluation results provide information to support recommendations for therapy services and provide a basis for establishing therapy goals and objectives and measuring change over time.

The same skill performance evaluations and assessments of physical functioning are implemented when therapy is provided within a participation-based framework. Additionally, the therapist collects information about activities and routines that are part of settings where children spend time. Therapists may gather this information by observing a child, interviewing those who spend time with the child, or using surveys or checklists to find out about settings, activities and routines. Before children are able to clearly explain their own experiences, parents or other caregivers provide information about what happens in typical family routines, such as at bath or meal time (Campbell, 2011; McWilliam, Casey, & Sims, 2009; Woods & Lineman, 2008). Occupational or physical therapists might select instruments such as the Routines-Based Interview (RBI; McWilliam, 2010) or the Assessment of Family Activities and Routines (Campbell, 2005, 2011). When children are older, therapists may directly observe participation in structured settings such as child care, school activities, or routines, or may use interviews or checklists to gather information from teachers (Campbell, Milbourne, & Kennedy, 2012; Milbourne & Campbell, 2007; Sandall & Schwartz, 2008). These formats are designed for intervention planning and to help identify therapy goals. Therapists may intervene to "fix" activities or routines that are not going well or to embed learning opportunities and therapy intervention strategies into activities or routines that are going well.

Because encouraging the child's participation in daily activities is an emerging focus in pediatric therapy, ways of assessing participation is an emerging area of test development. New instruments are being designed and tested so that participation may be measured over time (Coster & Khetani, 2010). Evaluation instruments such as the School Function Assessment (SFA; Coster, Deeney, Haltiwanger, & Haley, 1998) are designed to assess the child's participation in elementary school activities and routines over time so that progress can be assessed through readministrations of the instrument. Participation is evaluated in activities or routines that occur in settings such as the classroom, cafeteria, bathroom, or hallways (for transition from one class or activity to another). Student performance is assessed in terms of the number and type of supports required to achieve independence). The focus of this type of assessment is on identifying areas where performance may be enhanced so that the child is more successful in environments such as schools. This has a distinctly different purpose than evaluation measures designed to assess skill performance or physical functioning in order to identify deficits.

Other newly developed instruments such as the Children's Assessment of Participation and Enjoyment (CAPE; King, Law, King, Hurley, Hanna, & Kertoy, 2004) or similar instruments for use with preschoolers (Kemps, Siebes, Gorter, & Ketelaar, 2011; Petrenchik, Law, King, Hurley, Forhan, & Kertoy, 2006) assess participation based on parental or client report. Information is provided about a child's preference or interest in particular activities as well as the frequency and intensity of participation in recreation, leisure, and other related activities. These instruments are used to assess interest and participation in extracurricular or non-school activities so that therapists may support families to expand opportunities for their children with disabilities and provide supports for child engagement and success.

When disability is viewed from the perspective of the International Classification of Functioning, Disability, & Health (ICF, 2001) it is clear that far more instruments are available to assess the dimension of activity (i.e., skill performance) than to assess environment or participation dimensions (Bagnato, Neisworth, & Pretti-Fronczak, 2010). Some instruments have been published that measure structural factors such as muscle strength or the sensory systems, but more often structure is assessed through indirect and informal clinical judgment-based procedures. With the exception of the SFA, rarely do available instruments consider the environments in which the child needs to function.

Intervention Planning

All disciplines and programs use an intervention plan of some sort to define outcomes or goals. Most plans include essentially the same features but may differ based on the service setting or funding source. In early intervention programs funded through Part C of IDEA or through Early Head Start, individualized family service plans (IFSP) are used. For school-aged children individualized education programs (IEPs) or 504 plans define goals while services for children in residential settings are generally described in individual habilitation plans

(IHPs). In hospitals, rehabilitation centers, or outpatient programs, children's therapy services generally also require treatment plans with similar information to that written on documents such as the IEP, IFSP, or IHP.

Optimally, the evaluation/assessment information of one discipline is integrated with data from other disciplines and then goals are identified in collaboration with the child and family. When intervention is remedial in focus, goals are based on evaluation data about structure and skill performance. Goals target what needs to be fixed (e.g., increase range of motion) or improved (e.g., pick up small objects using a pincher grasp; walk 10 steps without assistance). Therapists then design treatment and home program activities to provide opportunities for improvements in these skills. For example, an OT might suggest a tabletop play activity where small toys are provided so that opportunities to use and practice a pincher grasp occur. Or, a physical therapist might use an activity where a child's parent stands away from but leaning toward the child, encouraging independent steps.

When services aim to promote the child's participation in activities/routines, goals are based on assessment data about the child's participation in combination with information about any structural or skill performance limitations. Integrating assessment information from all three sources (i.e., skill, structure, participation) helps support goals that emphasize reducing the negative impact of structural, skill, or environmental limitations on the child's participation. For example, if a child with difficulties grasping small objects is unable to participate in play activities with other children at child care, a goal may be to increase playtime participation by using environmentally based interventions. This could include adaptations and assistive technology, such as correctly-sized toys so that the child is able to participate regardless of having the fine motor skills to manipulate small objects/toys. The emphasis in a participation framework is on using existing activities/routines rather than creating therapist-designed activities.

Implementation

Traditional services can take place anywhere: a hospital, therapy clinic, child care program or school, or home. Participation-based services are more likely to be implemented in typical settings (e.g., child care, home, school classroom or other areas, community settings) than in hospitals or clinics. However, physical location where services are provided is not the distinguishing factor between the two service frameworks. Rather, the primary distinguishing features are 1) the activity/routine that is used for intervention, and 2) the ways in which the actual intervention strategies are delivered. In traditional services, the therapist plans and selects the activity through which therapeutic opportunities will be provided and, via hands-on interaction with the child, functions as the implementer of both the activity and the intervention. The therapist may also design programs for the caregiver to do with the child outside of the therapy session. This may involve writing up or illustrating program directions or modeling the therapy for parents, caregivers, or teachers.

In contrast, natural activities that occur in home, child care/school, or community settings are therapeutic opportunities when participation is the goal. Intervention strategies are not delivered directly as they are in providing traditional services but are embedded into activities/routines and implemented by the person who spends time with the child in that setting. Therapists collaborate with parents, caregivers, and teachers and explicitly teach them both how to create learning opportunities and implement therapeutic interventions by embedding them within these naturally occurring routines/activities (Colyvas, Sawyer, & Campbell, 2010; Spagnoia & Fiese, 2007; Woods, Kashinath, & Goldstein, 2004).

The responsibilities of the therapist in traditional services are to 1) identify the areas in which a child needs to develop; 2) design activities such that learning opportunities are present; and 3) show parents, caregivers, or teachers activities they can use to support learning between therapy sessions. In contrast, the responsibilities of the therapist providing participation-based services are to 1) learn about activities/routines that are going well or not going well for the child as well as areas in which a child needs to develop; 2) collaboratively create plans for embedding learning opportunities and intervention strategies into existing activities/routines; and 3) teach parents, caregivers, and teachers how to create learning opportunities and use intervention strategies.

Progress Monitoring

Tracking the child's performance and the outcomes of occupational or physical therapy services is important irrespective of whether a traditional rehabilitation or participation-based framework is employed, where the therapy is being provided, or what sources of funding are being provided (Case-Smith & O'Brien, 2010; Dunn, 2011; Effgen, 2005). Monitoring the child's progress allows therapists to determine if implemented intervention strategies are working or should be changed and to determine when goals are achieved. Progress monitoring also provides objective data to inform adjustments in the frequency or duration of therapy services, including discontinuing therapy when goals have been achieved to the satisfaction of the child or caregiver or when therapy is no longer of benefit to the child or family.

INTERVENTION STRATEGIES

Both occupational and physical therapists employ a variety of intervention strategies that enable the child to learn and practice new skills and participate successfully in activities and routines across many settings. Intervention strategies may be divided into two basic categories (Campbell, 2010; Campbell, Milbourne, & Wilcox, 2008). The first category is strategies requiring an adult to implement them with a child. For example, physical guidance is an intervention strategy used by both occupational and physical therapists to guide a movement pattern so that the child is able to perform a particular skill. A therapist might physically guide the hand and arm so that the child moves a spoon to the mouth, sometimes called hand-over-hand feeding. In a situation like this, a child is being taught how to eat using a spoon. The strategy provides passive practice and experience of the movement pattern.

A second intervention category is labeled as environmental strategies and includes adaptations and AT interventions. These do not require another person and, in fact, are designed to allow a child to be independent without any greater amount of adult assistance than would be appropriate for the child's chronological age.

In order to help a child eat independently, a therapist might carefully consider how the child is positioned and then use an adapted spoon, a special bowl or plate, or even a feeding device so that the child is able to eat independently and without adult assistance. In this situation, the therapist promotes participation and independence via the use of adaptations and AT devices. This contrasts with the use of a hand-over-hand feeding strategy where the required motor pattern is potentially taught through movement experience and practice. The two types of intervention strategies are not necessarily mutually exclusive and are frequently combined. For example, a therapist might consider 1) positioning, 2) providing the child with an adapted spoon and dish, and 3) using the adult-aided intervention strategy of hand-over-hand feeding.

Each of the these two intervention categories are further subdivided into levels: 1) *universal*, used with all same-aged children; 2) *specialized*, used with some but not all same-aged children; and 3) *customized*, used only in very specific circumstances. Table 33.2 provides examples of strategies for each of these levels.

Universal Intervention Strategies

Strategies are labeled as universal because of their use with all children, whether they have disabilities or delays or are, in fact, developing typically. Universal strategies are not linked to a particular discipline and, because anyone may use these strategies with children, few require specific training or expertise. Any strategy that supports child learning and participation and

Table 33.2. Examples of categories and levels of intervention strategies

	Category	
	Require another person to use with child	Environment, adaptation, & assistive technology
Universal	Physical prompting or cueing; labeling; expanded language; selection of age-appropriate toys; opportunity to use or do; opportunity to practice; feedback for correct performance or behavior	High chair; bath seat; computerized toys; special spoons and bowls; choice making with pictures; picture schedule boards
Specialized	Physical guidance; specially designed reinforcers; time delay; specially designed access and practice (e.g., treadmill)	Picture communication board; personal picture schedule; if-then board, social story book; bath seat for 4-year-old; use of off-the-shelf battery-operated car for mobility
Custom	Craniosacral therapy; neurodevelopmental therapy	Power chairs; computerized communication devices; access to and specialized computers; architecturally (universally) designed bathroom for wheelchair accessibility

may be used by parents, teachers, child care-givers, therapists, and other professionals is included in this category.

Occupational and physical therapists use universal strategies such as opportunity, practice, and consequences to promote the child's acquisition of sensory or motor skills and to further their participation in activities or routines. A primary universal strategy is *opportunity*. Children need opportunities to perform a particular skill in order to learn how to use the skill. A child who is never placed on the floor may lack the opportunity to perform motor skills, such as rolling or crawling. Similarly, a child who is dressed by her parents lacks opportunities to learn dressing skills. All children also need opportunities to participate in activities or routines. Any infant or young child can be placed in a bath seat to increase the child's opportunities to participate safely in bath time. Similarly, children's opportunities to participate in playtime are structured by the types of toys provided. A 6-month-old's toys are different from those that would be safe or of interest to a 4-year-old. Both the bath seat and the types of toys are examples of universal-adaptation/AT-intervention strategies.

Another strategy that supports all children's learning is *practice*—a strategy that goes hand in hand with opportunity. The child is afforded opportunities to use a particular skill, to participate in a specific activity, or to routinely practice these skills by virtue of having repeated opportunities to use them. Practice is a primary learning strategy for refining skills and performing them competently for functional use. A child who engages in outdoor play many times will be better at using equipment and interacting with other children than when first spending time at the playground.

A third universal strategy is broadly termed *consequences*. This strategy describes outcomes that follow the child's actions either by design or naturally as part of the environment. For example, a child may crawl not just for the sake of moving around but for the purpose of obtaining a toy or to be picked up by a caregiver. The natural consequences to crawling, in this example, include playing with a toy or being cuddled by a caregiver. A physical therapist who wants a child to crawl may place a preferred toy distant from the child, creating an opportunity for the child to crawl, and then may encourage the child by drawing attention to the consequence of crawling (e.g., being able to play with the toy). Self-feeding with a spoon is likely to be acquired more rapidly when the consequence of moving the spoon to the mouth is the ability to eat a highly preferred (as opposed to a disliked) food. One of the consequences of activating a computer-based toy may be to hear sounds. A consequence of being positioned in a car seat is to see the environment from a different perspective than when lying on the floor at home.

Occupational and physical therapists help children achieve skill acquisition and successful participation in activities or routines by using universal intervention strategies. For example, therapists who use strategies to support the child's sensory processing may suggest adaptations that any caregiver might perform. Examples include cutting tags out of the back of shirts so that they don't bother the child, and providing play opportunities such as finding objects "hidden" in wet sand to give tactile learning experiences (Dunn, 2007). Many of the motor learning strategies used by therapists to promote a child's acquisition of motor skills are based on opportunity, practice, and consequences (Hickman, Westcott, Long, & Rauh, 2011; Valvano & Rapport, 2006). Occupational and physical therapists are likely to have more knowledge of these universal strategies (as used in sensory or motor skill situations) than most parents, caregivers, or teachers.

Specialized Intervention Strategies

Universal strategies that are used longer than would be typical for children or are individualized to reflect unique needs are included in the category of specialized intervention strategies. These strategies are more carefully designed than are universal strategies. For example, most children under 9–18 months of age would sit in a bath seat if being bathed in an adult bathtub, but most children older than 18–24 months do not require this adaptation as their sitting balance allows them to participate safely. Bath seats are a specialized-adaptation/AT-intervention strategy that might be suggested so that an older child without sufficient sitting balance may participate safely in bath time. Similarly, permitting logical consequences to an action is a universal strategy used with all children. When a specific consequence is selected and used, for example, to motivate a child to move, the intervention is now specialized because it has become individualized to a particular child's unique characteristics.

When a child is initially taught self-feeding only by feeding herself ice cream, a food that she really likes, the consequence of bringing the spoon to the mouth has been individualized to match this particular child's preferences and to promote learning to eat with a spoon independently. Infant- or preschool-sized treadmills are another example of a specialized intervention strategy to promote acquisition of walking skills by providing maximum opportunities for practicing taking steps (Angulo-Barroso, Burghardt, Lloyd, & Ulrich, 2008; Ulrich, Lloyd, Tiernan, Looper, & Angulo-Barroso, 2008). A picture schedule board posted on the wall is likely to be used by a child care or preschool teacher so that all the children know what is happening throughout the day. When an individualized picture schedule board is made for a child who has difficulty with concepts of time or knowing what will happen next, this universal strategy has been individualized and used in a specialized way (Kluth & Danaher, 2010; Milbourne & Campbell, 2007; Sandall & Swartz, 2008; Schwarz & Kluth, 2007).

Both occupational and physical therapists may design a variety of specialized strategies that require involvement of another person, are adaptations or AT, or are a combination of both adult-directed and adaptation interventions. Although therapists design specialized strategies, they are not likely to be the only people who will implement these strategies with the child. When specialized strategies are embedded into the child's activities/routines, other adults, or peers who spend time with the child, become the implementers.

Custom Intervention Strategies

These interventions are used most often with children who have diagnoses such as sensory impairment, motor disability, autism, severe health conditions, sensory processing disorders, or specific language disorders or some combination of these conditions. Children with diagnoses such as these are often labeled as "low incidence" within the population of children with special needs. They are the children, however, most likely to benefit from customized occupational or physical therapy interventions. Use of these customized strategies may require specialized training, certification, or other credentials. For example, occupational and physical therapists complete specific requirements to become certified to practice **neurodevelopmental treatment** (NDT), an intervention approach used with children with neurologically based motor disabilities such as cerebral palsy. Therapists may need advanced training to use other custom interventions such as craniosacral therapy or myofascial release (MFR). Additional training and certification to administer and interpret tests is also needed by therapists working within the area of sensory integration. Certification in design and use of positioning equipment and assistive technology is also available for therapists who wish to acquire expertise in designing positioning devices such as adaptive seating including power chairs. Occupational and physical therapists also may pursue pediatric specialization within their disciplines by acquiring postgraduate knowledge, training, and skills specific to pediatric practice. There are many other specialized techniques such as constraint-induced therapy or specific handwriting approaches that may not require certification but are best used by therapists who have completed training in the particular custom strategy.

EVIDENCE-BASED INTERVENTION

Use of all intervention strategies but especially specialized and custom strategies should be based on evidence of their appropriateness and effectiveness. Optimally, this evidence should be the result of well-designed research studies that have tested the intervention systematically (Law, 2002a; Palisano, Campbell, & Harris, 2006). A body of research evidence about the use and effects of therapeutic interventions is just emerging in both the occupational and physical therapy fields. Availability of well-designed studies of almost any practice or intervention strategy is limited although some studies have examined the effectiveness of strategies such as using weighted vests (Fertel-Daly, Bedell, & Hinojosa, 2001), providing treadmill training (Dieruf, Burtner, Provost, Phillips, Bernitsky-Beddington, & Sullivan, 2009), and teaching power mobility (Ragonesi, Chen, Agrawal, & Galloway, 2010).

A well-established research base for a particular practice or intervention strategy is only one source of evidence. Data about potential appropriateness or effectiveness may be gathered from other sources such as policy or experiential knowledge (Winton, Buysse, Epstein, & Lim, n.d.; Law, Baum, & Dunn, 2005). A first step in searching for various types of evidence is to define the practice (e.g., intervention strategy) operationally so that the practice that is being investigated will be understood across people and situations. For example, an operational definition of the category of adaptation and AT intervention strategies might be worded as

Assistive technology (AT) interventions involve a range of strategies to promote a child's access to learning opportunities, from making simple changes to the environment and materials to helping a child use special equipment. Combining AT with effective teaching promotes the child's participation in learning and relating to others. (CONNECT, 2012)

The operational definition forms a basis for using literature-based search engines such as PubMed or ERIC to identify peer-reviewed research reports but also provides structure for Internet searches to identify a wider range of evidence including policy or best-practice documents. Both the American Occupational Therapy Association (AOTA) and the American Physical Therapy Association (APTA) provide a number of publications that discuss best practice for therapists working in pediatrics. These documents give guidance about the extent to which an intervention is appropriate for a particular age group or type of disability or is within the scope of practice for the profession. Therapists make decisions about intervention approaches by using policy and best-practice documents as a source for determining the appropriateness of an intervention practice.

A third source of evidence is experiential knowledge, a source that is used by many clinicians to judge both appropriateness and effectiveness of intervention practices. Within this category is a therapist's own personal experience as well as the experiences of the recipients of the practice. For example, testimonials from a group of people about effectiveness or their own personal satisfaction with a practice are widespread and easily accessed via the Internet and social networking or video websites. Experiential knowledge is an important source of evidence but needs to be balanced with other evidence sources and considered objectively. In highly clinical fields such as occupational or physical therapy, intervention strategies originating from clinical practice situations may eventually be found to be effective (or not). In other words, a therapist may try something out with a child and find it successful and then try it out with other children, thus creating an experiential data base about a practice that may inform future decisions about its appropriateness and effectiveness.

SUMMARY

Both the occupational and physical therapy disciplines are integral in supporting families and their children with limitations in structural, activity (i.e., skill), or participation areas. In pediatric practice the differences between these occupational and physical therapy professionals may not always be distinct especially among experienced therapists. Many factors differentiate how therapists work and what they do in their discipline. Therapists focus on children's skill acquisition and use, and on their participation in everyday activities and routines.

Therapists may do things differently depending on whether they use a traditional or participation-based framework, the settings in which they practice, and the ages and disabilities of children with whom they work. When using a traditional framework, therapists are likely to create activities to provide learning opportunities, work directly with the child, and create follow-through programs to be used by other people (e.g., parents, teachers). Therapists practicing from a participation-based framework will embed learning opportunities and intervention strategies within existing activities or routines and teach others how to implement the strategies. Therapists who practice in school settings may collaborate more with children themselves or their teachers than with children's parents but, when working with infants, are likely to work more with families. Practice may also look different depending on the age of the child as well as limitations in the child's performance or participation. As with other professionals, occupational and physical therapists are likely to use what they know about and what matches their cultural values, childrearing perspectives, and other personal factors. Strategies used by therapists may be based more often on experiential or policy/best-practice evidence, although there are emerging databases documenting the effectiveness of particular therapy strategies. In the future, these data may provide therapists with a more robust basis for making decisions about the appropriateness and effectiveness of both occupational and physical therapy intervention strategies used with children.

REFERENCES

Angulo-Barroso, R., Burghardt, A.R., Lloyd, M., Ulrich, D.A. (2008). Physical activity in infants with Down syndrome receiving a treadmill intervention. *Infant Behavior and Development, 31*(2), 255–69.

Bagnato, S., Neisworth, J., & Pretti-Frontczak, K. (2010). *Linking authentic assessment & early childhood intervention: Best measures for best practices* (2nd ed). Baltimore, MD: Paul H. Brookes Publishing Co.

Basu, S., Salisbury, C.L., Thorkildsen, T.A. (2010). Measuring collaborative consultation practices in natural environments. *Journal of Early Intervention, 32*, 127–150.

Buysse, V. & Wesley, P.W. (2007). *Consultation in early childhood settings*. Baltimore, MD: Paul H. Brookes Publishing Co.

Campbell, P.H. (2011a). Addressing motor disabilities. In M. Snell & F. Brown, *Instruction of students with severe disabilities* (7th ed., pp 340–376). Upper Saddle River, NJ: Pearson Education.

Campbell, P.H. (2011b). Using the assessment of family activities and routines to develop embedded programming. *Young Exceptional Children Monograph Series*, No. 13, 64–78.

Campbell, P.H. (2010). *Participation-based services*. Retrieved December 3, 2010 from http://jeffline.jefferson.edu/cfsrp/pbs.html.

Campbell, P.H. (2009). *Caregiver Assessment of Activities & Routines: Revised*. Philadelphia, PA: Child & Family Studies Research Programs, Thomas Jefferson University. Retrieved from http://jeffline.jefferson.edu/cfsrp/pbs.html.

Campbell, P.H. (2004). Participation-based services: Promoting children's participation in natural settings. *Young Exceptional Child*, 8(1), 20–29.

Campbell, P.H., Milbourne, S., Chiarello, L., Wilcox, M.J. (2009). Preparing related services personnel for work in early intervention. *Infants and Young Children*, 22(1), 21–31.

Campbell, P.H., Milbourne, S., & Kennedy, A. (2012). *Cara's kit for toddlers: Creating adaptations for routines and activities*. Baltimore, MD: Paul H. Brookes Publishing Co.

Campbell, P.H., Milbourne, S. & Wilcox, M.J. (2008). Adaptation interventions to promote participation in natural settings. *Infants and Young Children*, 21(2), 94–106.

Campbell, P.H. & Sawyer, L.B. (2007). Supporting learning opportunities in natural settings through participation-based services. *Journal of Early Intervention*, 29(4), 287–305.

Campbell, P.H. & Sawyer, L.B. (2009). Changing early intervention providers' home visiting skills through participation in professional development. *Topics in Early Childhood Special Education*, 28(4), 219–234.

Campbell, P.H., Sawyer, L.B., & Muhlenhaupt, M. (2009). Parent and professional views of natural environment services. *Infants and Young Children*, 22(4), 264–278.

Case-Smith, J., & O'Brien, J. (2010). *Occupational therapy for children* (6th ed.). Maryland Heights, MO: Mosby.

Chiarello, L., & Kolobe, T.H.A. (2006). Early intervention services. In S.K. Campbell, D.W. Vander Linden, & R.J. Palisano, *Physical therapy for children*, (3rd ed., pp. 933–954). St. Louis, MO: Saunders/Elsevier.

Colyvas, J.L., Sawyer, B.E., & Campbell, P.H. (2010). Identifying strategies early intervention occupational therapists use to teach caregivers. *American Journal of Occupational Therapy*, 64, 776–785.

CONNECT: The Center to Mobilize Early Childhood Knowledge. (2012). *Module 5: Assistive technology interventions*. Retrieved from http://community.fpg.unc.edu/sites/community.fpg.unc.edu/files/imce/documents/CONNECT-Module-Descriptions.pdf

Coster, W., Deeney, T., Haltiwanger, T., & Haley, S. (1998). *School function assessment*. San Antonio, TX: Pearson Educational.

Coster, W., Deeney, T., Haltiwanger, T., & Haley, S. (2008). *Technical report: School function assessment*. Retrieved September 30, 2011, from http://www.pearsonassessments.com/NR/rdonlyres/D50E4125-86EE-43BE-8001-2A4001B603DF/0/SFA_TR_Web.pdf.

Coster, W., & Khetani, M.A. (2008). Measuring participation of children with disabilities: Issues and challenges. *Disability and Rehabilitation;* 30(8), 639–648.

Dieruf, K., Burtner, P.A., Provost, B., Phillips, J., Bernitsky-Beddington, A., Sullivan, K. (2009). A pilot study of the quality of life in children with cerebral palsy after intensive body weight-supported treadmill training. *Pediatric Physical Therapy*, 21(1), 45–52.

Dunn, W.W. (2007). Supporting children to participate successfully in everyday life by using sensory processing knowledge. *Infants and Young Children*, 20(2), 84–101

Dunn, W.W. (2011). *Best practice occupational therapy for children and families in community settings* (2nd ed.). Thorofare, NJ: Slack.

Dunn, W.W., Nickelson, B., Cox, J.A., Pope, E., & Rinner, L.A. (2011). Best practice occupational therapy evaluation. In W.W. Dunn, *Best practice occupational therapy for children and families in community settings* (2nd ed.). Thorofare, NJ: Slack.

Dunst, C.J. (2001). Participation of young children with disabilities in community learning activities. In M.J. Guralnick (Ed.), *Early childhood inclusion: Focus on change* (pp. 307–333). Baltimore, MD: Paul H. Brookes Publishing Co.

Dunst, C.J., & Bruder, M.B. (1999). Family and community activity settings, natural learning environments, and children's learning opportunities. *Children's Learning Opportunity Report*, 1(2), 1–2.

Dunst, C.J., Trivette, C.M., Humphries, T., Raab, M., & Roper, N. (2001). Contrasting approaches to natural learning environment interventions. *Infants and Young Children*, 14(2), 48–63.

Effgen, S.K., (Ed.). (2005). *Meeting the physical therapy needs of children*. Philadelphia, PA: FA Davis Co.

Effgen, S.K (2006). The educational environment. In S.K. Campbell, D.W. Vander Linden, & R.J. Palisano, *Physical therapy of children*, (3rd e.d., pp. 955–982). St. Louis, MO: Saunders/Elsevier.

Fertel-Daly, D., Bedell, G., & Hinojosa, J. (2001). Effects of a weighted vest on attention to task and self-stimulatory behaviors in preschoolers with pervasive developmental disorders. *American Journal of Occupational Therapy*, 55(6), 629–40

Hanft, B., Rush, D., & Shelden, M. (2004). *Coaching families and colleagues in early childhood*. Baltimore, MD: Paul H. Brookes Publishing Co.

Hickman, R. Westcott, S., Long, T., & Rauh, M.J. (2011). Applying contemporary developmental and movement science theories and evidence to early intervention practice. *Infants and Young Children*, 24(1), 29–41.

Jung, L.A. (2003). More is better: Maximizing natural learning opportunities. *Young Exceptional Children*, 6(3), 21–27.

Jones, M.A., & Gray, S. (2005). Assistive technology: Augmentative communication and other technologies. In S. K. Effgen (Ed.), *Meeting the physical therapy needs of children* (pp 455–474). Philadelphia, PA: FA Davis Co.

Jones, M.A., & Gray, S. (2005). Assistive technology: Positioning and mobility. In S.K. Effgen (Ed.), *Meeting the physical therapy needs of children* (pp 475–487). Philadelphia, PA: FA Davis, Co.

Kemps, R.J.K., Siebes, R.C., Gorter, J.W., & Ketelaar, M. (2011). Parental perceptions of participation of preschool children with and without mobility limitations: Validity and reliability of the PART. *Disability and Rehabilitation*, 33(15–16), 1421–1423.

King, G., Law, M., King, S., Hurley, P., Rosenbaum, P., Hanna, S., ... Young, N. (2004). *Children's Assessment of Participation and Enjoyment (CAPE) and Preferences for activities for Children (PAC)*. San Antonio, TX: Pearson Education.

King, G., Stracham, D., Tucker, M., Duwyn, B., Desserud, S., & Shillington, M. (2009). The application of a transdisciplinary model for early intervention services. *Infants and Young Children, 22*(3), 211–223.

Kling, A., Campbell, P.H., & Wilcox, M.J. (2010). Young children with physical disabilities: Caregiver perspectives about assistive technology. *Infants and Young Children, 23*(3), 169–183.

Kluth, P., & Danaher, S. (2010). *From tutor scripts to talking sticks: 100 Ways to differentiate instruction in K-12 classrooms*. Baltimore, MD: Paul H. Brookes Publishing Co.

Law, M. (2002a). Building evidence in practice. In Law, M. (Ed.), *Evidence-based rehabilitation: A guide to practice* (pp 185–194). Thorofare, NJ: Slack.

Law, M. (Ed.) (2002b). *Evidence-based rehabilitation: A guide to practice*. Thorofare, NJ: Slack.

Law, M., Baum, C., & Dunn, W.W. (2005). *Measuring occupational performance: Supporting best practice in occupational therapy* (2nd ed). Thorofare, NJ: Slack.

Law, M., King, G., King, S., Kurtoy, M., Hurley, P., Rosenbaum, P., ... Petrickick, T. (2006). *Patterns and predictions of recreational and leisure participation for children with physical disabilities*. CanChild Centre for Childhood Disability Research. Retrieved November 30, 2010, from http://www.canchild.ca/en/canchildresources/patternsandpredictors.asp.

McWilliam, R.A. (2000). It's only natural—to have early intervention in the environments where it is needed. *Young Exceptional Children Monograph Series, 2*, 17–26.

McWilliam, R.A. (2010). *Routines-based early intervention: Supporting young children and their families*. Baltimore: Paul H. Brookes Publishing Co.

McWilliam, R.A., Casey, A.M., & Sims, J. (2009). The routines-based interview: A method for gathering information and assessing needs. *Infants and Young Children, 22*(3), 224–233.

Milbourne, S.A., & Campbell, P.H. (2007). *CARA's kit: Creating adaptations for routines and activities*. Missoula, MT: Division for Early Childhood (DEC).

Palisano, R.J., Campbell, S.K., & Harris, S.R. (2006). Evidence-based decision making in pediatric physical therapy. In S.K. Campbell, D.W. Vander Linden, & R.J. Palisano (Eds.), *Physical Therapy of Children* (3rd ed., pp. 3–32). St. Louis, MO: Saunders/Elsevier.

Pretti-Frontczak, K., & Bricker, D. (2004). *An activity-based approach to early intervention* (3rd ed). Baltimore, MD: Paul H. Brookes Publishing Co.

Ragonesi, C.B., Chen, Xi, Agrawal, S., Galloway, J.C. (2010). Power mobility and socialization in preschool: A case study of a child with cerebral palsy. *Pediatric Physical Therapy, 22*(3), 322–329.

Rogers, S.L. (2010). Common conditions that influence children's participation. In J. Case-Smith & J. O'Brien, *Occupational therapy for children* (6th ed.). Maryland Heights, MO: Mosby.

Rush, D., & Shelden, M. (2011). *The early childhood coaching handbook*. Baltimore, MD: Paul H. Brookes Publishing Co.

Rush, D., Shelden, M., & Hanft, B. (2003). Coaching families and colleagues: A process for collaboration in natural settings. *Infants and Young Children, 16*(1), 33–47.

Sadao, K.C. & Robinson, N.B. (2010). *Assistive technology for young children: Creating inclusive learning environments*. Baltimore, MD: Paul H. Brookes Publishing Co.

Sandall, S., & Schwartz, I. (2008). *Building blocks for teaching preschoolers with special needs*. (2nd ed.) Baltimore, MD: Paul H Brookes Publishing Co.

Schwarz, P., & Kluth, P. (2007) *You're welcome: 30 innovative ideas for the inclusive classroom*. Portsmouth, NH: Heinemann.

Spagnoia, M., & Fiese, B.H. (2007). Family routines and rituals: A context for development in the lives of children. *Infants and Young Children, 20*(4), 284–299.

Stremel, K., & Campbell, P.H. (2007). Implementation of early intervention within natural environments. *Early Childhood Services, 1*(2), 83–105.

Ulrich, D.A., Lloyd, M.C., Tiernan, C.W., Looper, J.E., & Angulo-Barroso, R.M. (2008). Effects of intensity of treadmill training on developmental outcomes and stepping in infants with Down syndrome: A randomized trial. *Physical Therapy, 88*(1), 114–22.

Valvano, J.A., & Rapport, M.J. (2006). Activity-focused motor interventions for infants and young children with neurological conditions. *Infants & Young Children, 19*(4), 292–307.

Wilson, L., Mott, D.W., & Batman, D. (2004). The asset-based context matrix: A tool for assessing children's learning opportunities and participation in natural environments. *Topics in Early Childhood Special Education, 24*, 110–120.

Winton, P.J., Buysse, V.M., Epstein, D.J., Lim, C. (n.d.). Frank Porter Graham Child Development Institute. In CONNECT: The Center to Mobilize Early Childhood Knowledge. Retrieved from http://www.fpg.unc.edu/projects/connect-center-mobilize-early-childhood-

Woods, J.A., & Lindeman, D. (2008). Gathering and giving information with families. *Infants and Young Children, 21*(4), 272–284.

Woods, J., Kashinath, S., & Goldstein, H. (2004). Effects of embedding caregiver-implemented teaching strategies in daily routines on children's communication outcomes. *Journal of Early Intervention, 26*(3), 195–193.

World Health Organization. (2001). *International classification of functioning, disability, & health* (ICF). Geneva, Switzerland: World Health Organization.

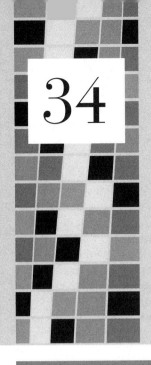

34 Physical Activity, Exercise, and Sports

Donna Bernhardt Bainbridge and James Gleason

Upon completion of this chapter, the reader will

- Be familiar with the specific benefits of exercise for the child with developmental disabilities

- Be aware of the laws regarding the inclusion of children with physical and cognitive disabilities in physical education and community programs

- Understand how to incorporate physical education adaptations into a child's individualized education program (IEP) based on his or her abilities

- Be aware of community sports and recreation programs available to children with special needs

- Know about the pre-participation evaluation for children and adolescents with disabilities

- Have knowledge of the types of injuries encountered in athletes with disabilities

Physical activity is important for all children as it promotes general and cardiovascular health (Faulkner, Lurbe, & Schaefer, 2010), weight management (Kitzman-Ulrich et al., 2010), and development of strong muscles (Katz et al., 2010) and bone (McKay, Liu, Egeli, Boyd, & Burrows, 2010; Nikander et al., 2010). Physical activity is especially important for children with developmental disabilities, in whom the risks of inactivity are increased. In 2010, the Centers for Disease Control and Prevention (CDC) recommended that children should engage in 60 minutes of moderate to vigorous physical activity per day, including muscle- and bone-strengthening exercises 3 times per week. Not only is physical activity necessary for health of the body, but it also promotes psychological health and well-being. In a recent study by Parfitt, Pavey and Rowlands (2009), children with higher levels of vigorously intense activity were found to be less anxious and reported higher perceptions of self-worth than children with high levels of light activity but low vigorous activity. Despite these recommendations, the Healthy People 2010 mid-course review (2006) indicated that only 64% of adolescents have regular physical activity and only 8% of middle and high schools' curricula require students to engage in daily physical activity (CDC and President's Council on Physical Fitness and Sports, 2006). This data suggests greater opportunity is needed for participation in physical activity, as well as improved understanding of strategies that are effective in increasing children's physical activity (Baruth et al., 2010). Recent reports indicate that the number of minutes per day children spend in moderate to vigorous physical activity decreases significantly from 180 minutes at age 9 to less than 50 minutes by age 15 (Nader, Bradley, Houts, McRitchie, & O'Brien, 2008). This problem of inadequate physical activity is accentuated in children with developmental disabilities. A recent report by the American Academy of Pediatrics' (AAP) Council on Children with Disabilities (COCWD) encourages physicians to 1) counsel children and families on the importance of physical activity; 2) encourage schools to include interventions that enhance motor skill development and provide instruction geared toward the individual skills and needs of the child; 3) encourage communities to develop safe and accessible environments for outdoor activities, including playgrounds and parks; and 4) support walking and biking to school (Keeton & Kennedy, 2009).

▪ ▪ ▪ JAMIE

Jamie is a 14-year-old boy with Down syndrome who is interested in playing on a Special Olympics basketball team. He became interested in the Special Olympics because one of his classmates plays in a local league. In preparation for his participation, Jamie visited his pediatrician, who noted that Jamie has not had many of the medical complications associated with Down syndrome. Jamie's pediatrician first asked about symptoms suggestive of atlantoaxial subluxation (see Chapter 18), including neck pain, stiff neck, torticollis (wry neck, a condition in which contracted or spastic neck muscles cause the head lean or twist to one side), progressive loss of bowel or bladder control, change in strength or sensation in any of his limbs, or change in gait pattern. Jamie's mother reported that Jamie had not had any of these symptoms. The pediatrician then examined Jamie and concluded that he was mildly overweight and had mild to moderate ligamentous laxity (hyperflexible, flat feet) but had no neurologic signs or symptoms suggestive of atlantoaxial subluxation.

After discussing the findings with Jamie's family, the pediatrician decided to obtain special cervical spine (neck) x rays to screen for atlantoaxial subluxation; these were found to be normal. As a result of the examination, the pediatrician signed the form permitting Jamie's

participation in sports activities without specific limitations. She also told the family that this activity could be helpful to Jamie in a number of ways. It could aid in weight control, which is often an issue for people with Down syndrome. It could also support Jamie's emerging social skills and self-esteem. The pediatrician, however, counseled the family about certain injuries that Jamie was at higher risk to sustain as a result of his generalized ligamentous laxity. To avoid these, she suggested that he perform particular warm-up exercises and avoid certain sustained activities that would predispose him to injury. She also recommended a generalized strengthening program, explaining that stronger muscles help to stabilize and protect joints from injury.

HEALTH RISKS OF CHILDREN WITH DISABILITIES RELATED TO A LACK OF PHYSICAL ACTIVITY

Special concerns related to exercise and physical activity exist for children and youth with developmental and related disabilities. Some of these concerns relate to community access and barriers that hamper including children with disabilities, and some relate to specific needs of individual children. Participation of children with disabilities in routine physical activity may be less than what is reported in typically developing children and youth (Emck, Bosscher, Wieringen, Doreleijers, & Beek, 2010; Frey, Stanish, & Temple, 2009; Maher, Williams, Olds, & Lane, 2007; Pan, 2008; Schott, Alof, Hultsch, & Meerman, 2007). In addition, compared to children with typical development, children with disabilities are at greater risk for adverse health consequences including the potential for secondary conditions and loss of functional skills as they grow older due to lack of physical activity. Levels of obesity in 2010 were reported at 17% in children ages 2–19 years of age (CDC, 2010) with potentially higher risk for overweight in children with physical disabilities (50.9% versus 30.6%) and learning disorders (35.1% versus 31.1%) when compared to children without disability (Bandini, Curtin, Hamad, Tybor, & Must, 2005). In a national study of youth in Grades 9–12 just 35% of children with disabilities reported meeting current physical activity recommendations according to self-report using the CDC data set of the Youth Risk Behavior Survey (Everett Jones & Lollar, 2008). Maher et al. (2007) found children with cerebral palsy had less physical activity than typical peers, their activity level declined with age, and children with greater functional limitations on the Gross Motor Function Classification System (GMFCS) engaged in less physical activity. Shields, Dodd, and Abblitt (2009) found a similar pattern of declining physical activity with increasing age in children with Down syndrome, with 8 of 19 children achieving 60 minutes per day of moderate to vigorous physical activity.

Children with disabilities encounter many potential barriers to physical activity including less opportunity for in- and after-school exercise, inaccessible facilities and playgrounds, attitudinal barriers of coaches, physical education instructors and teachers, and in many sports and competitive activities, an emphasis on winning rather than participation (Rimmer & Rowland, 2008). Parents of youth with disabilities may be reluctant to encourage their child's participation in activities where there is potential for physical harm or verbal abuse. Additionally, concern is warranted in relation to children with intellectual disability (ID) regarding lack of knowledge of the importance of physical activity and its contribution to health, and lack of understanding of long-term health consequences (Rimmer, Rowland, & Yamaki, 2007). Many communities do not offer adequate opportunities for children with disabilities to participate in physical activity on a regular basis. At the same time, parents of children with disabilities are seeking out and identifying appropriate and interesting activities for their child in the hopes of finding fun and engaging activities that encourage movement. An array of options that promote physical activity and movement within each child's capabilities and interests must be explored. Incorporating behavioral techniques into program planning and intervention, and family-based strategies to promote healthy life styles and physical activity, may be crucial to achieving effective behavioral change in children, particularly children with intellectual disability (Fleming et al., 2008).

Parents must observe carefully when starting any new physical activity to ensure that staff and facilities provide appropriate programs for their child's individual needs. Parents must consider many factors: the needs, desires and enjoyment of the individual child; the experience, training and expertise of staff and volunteers; supervision of these providers, and the degree to which there may be established protocols, interventions strategies, or curricula. Organizations such as the National Center on Physical Activity

and Disability (NCPAD; http://www.ncpad.org/) can assist children with special needs, their parents, caregivers, and health professionals in understanding disability-specific needs, options, and resources and can facilitate greater participation of children with disabilities in community activities, sports and recreation.

CONSIDERATIONS FOR SPECIFIC DISABILITIES

Recent research that has focused on children with specific developmental conditions related to exercise and activity participation provides important insight into their intervention needs and strategies. The following examples are not exhaustive but include studies on children with **autism spectrum disorders** (ASD), Down syndrome, intellectual disability and **cerebral palsy** as a basis for principles that might apply to other developmental conditions or disabilities. For additional information the National Center on Physical Activity and Disability (NCPAD) web site provides excellent resources and information. As a general principle, the needs of children with disabilities are not unlike any other child; they need opportunities to participate, to be active and to exercise, as well as the benefits these bestow in terms of physical health and psychological well-being.

Autism

Children with autism spectrum disorders (ASD) have been described as having a range of movement difficulties including, among others, low scores on tests of motor skill and coordination (Green et al., 2009), unevenness of developmental milestone acquisition (Baranek, 2002), atypical features of motor function including low muscle tone, oral-motor difficulties, repetitive movement and dyspraxia (Klim, Volkman, & Sparrow, 1992), and motor planning difficulties and dyspraxia (Baranek, 2002; Rinehart et al., 2001). These studies suggest that while children with ASD are at significant risk for motor impairments, the type and severity of motor difficulty varies from child to child with no consistent pattern across the population; indeed some children with ASD are found to have good motor abilities (Pan, Tsai, & Chu, 2009). Pan (2007) measured recess time activity in children with ASD in Taiwan using accelerometry, an instrument that uses motion sensing to record movement, and noted that these children did not achieve a target of 40% of school recess time in physical activity. Pan and

Frey (2006) found that youth with ASD are less active than their peers without ASD and that activity level of children with ASD declines with increasing age. Interventions to improve strength and aerobic fitness in children with ASD have demonstrated attainable improvements (Lochbaum & Crews, 2003; Pitetti, Rendoff, Grover, & Beets, 2007) in strength, aerobic fitness, several parameters of treadmill walking including speed, elevation, frequency of use, and body mass index (BMI; Pitetti et al., 2007; see Chapter 8). Some medications used to treat behavioral symptoms in children with ASD have been found to contribute to weight gain and movement difficulty (McPheeters et al., 2011); additional research on the role of physical activity in helping to manage these complications is needed (Hellings et al., 2001).

Programming for persons with ASDs has also identified that moderate and vigorous levels of physical activity can be beneficial in reducing undesirable behavior. Elliot, Dobbin, Rose, and Soper (1994) studied vigorous aerobic exercise engaged in prior to a community-based vocational task and found that compared to general motor training activities, maladaptive and stereotypic behaviors (during the vocational task) were reduced in 6 adults with ASD and ID when they participated in vigorous activity prior to vocational tasks. In addition, a study by Fragala-Pinkham et al. (2005) of children with a range of disability including ASD found that a group program was much more effective than individualized home programs in achieving fitness goals and consistent participation. Studies of physical activity programming indicate that with appropriate training and supervision of staff, participation by children with ASD in physical activity can increase and have a positive impact on their health and well-being (Todd & Reid, 2006). Strategies such as visual displays for self-monitoring, daily activity logs, social stories, social reinforcement and other behavioral reinforcement are all useful in encouraging and sustaining participation.

Down Syndrome and Intellectual Disabilities

Children with ID can also benefit from exercise and physical activity. In one study, adolescents with ID 16–22 years of age (members of Special Olympics) who participated in a structured strengthening program for 3 months, twice per week demonstrated improvements in the force generated by one repetition in several muscle groups (Machek et al., 2008; Tamse et al., 2010).

In another study, Fragala-Pinkham, Haley and O'Neil (2008) reported about an aquatic program that emphasized aerobic and strength training for ambulatory children with a range of disabilities (ASD, myelomingocele, cerebral palsy, Down syndrome and developmental delay), and found improvements in cardiorespiratory endurance on a half-mile run/walk test. Many of these programs identify not only improvements in the target measures of strength or aerobic conditioning, but suggest improvements in functional skills, vocational performance, and athletic performance (Tamse et al., 2010). Exercise interventions indicate that adults and adolescents with Down syndrome have the capacity to improve muscle strength and speed of climbing stairs as a result of resistance training (Crowley et al., 2011), and significantly improve cardiovascular fitness (Dodd & Shield, 2005). Mondonca et al. (2010) have extensively evaluated the exercise capacity in adults with Down syndrome, pointing out that no studies exist that include adequate follow-up to evaluate the long-term impact of exercise in this population. They strongly encourage physical activity and exercise programs early in life for children with Down syndrome in in order to improve the potential for better health and physical capacity throughout life. These authors have identified specific concerns related to the exercise capacity of people with Down syndrome including chronotropic incompetence, or inability of the heart to increase rate appropriately in response to increased activity or metabolism, and low strength, which affects their ability to achieve and sustain vigorous activity and points to the need for continued attention to evaluating and understanding the exercise needs and the impact of strength and conditioning on children with Down syndrome and other disabilities (Mondonca et al., 2010).

Children with Special Health Care Needs

In addition to children with identified or known developmental disabilities, other children who at some point can be identified as children with special health care needs (CSHCN) may be at risk for decreased participation in physical activity. For example, a recent study (Burns et al., 2008) found that children weighing less than 1,000 grams at birth, termed extremely low birth weight (ELBW; see Chapter 7), were found to have significant motor coordination difficulties (on the Movement Assessment Battery for Children—MABC) at 11–13 years of age. Roberts et al. (2010) found that 16% of children in their sample of 132 children with a history of extreme prematurity or extremely low birth weight were identified as having developmental coordination disorder, including poor coordination and clumsiness, at 8 years of age. Similarly, Emck et al. (2010) found that a significant number of children with psychiatric disorders including emotional, behavioral, and pervasive developmental disorders also had motor impairments and poorer neuromotor and aerobic fitness than their peers. In this context the findings of Wrotniak et al. (2006) are useful, in that they identified a clear relationship between motor proficiency and participation in physical activity or sedentary behaviors in a study of 10- to 13-year-old children (without disabilities). Children who rated in the 75th percentile on the Bruninks-Oseretski Test of Motor Proficiency, First Edition, had significantly higher levels of physical activity and a higher percentage of time in moderate to vigorous physical activity than all other children (Wrotniak et al., 2006). Attention to improving motor skill and proficiency in children at risk for even mild motor impairments may have significant implications in health-promoting physical activity in childhood and beyond.

Palisano et al. (2010) have identified a range of factors that impact the ability of a child with cerebral palsy to participate in recreation and leisure time activities. These factors include the child's preferences, other family members' interest and participation levels, and family cohesion and relationships; they all impact the types of activities a child participates in. Rimmer and Rowland (2008) provide important guidance for understanding the lack of participation of youth with disability in physical activity, recreation and sport, and provide an important conceptual framework described as the Pep-for-Youth physical activity intervention model. This model assists families and service providers with understanding individual preferences and desires that are relevant to participating in activities and evaluating individual needs, opportunities for, and barriers to, community-based participation. Key concepts in this approach are a clear understanding of the individual child's interests and experiences, careful assessment of community resources, setting realistic goals, offering routine support guidance to reassess where necessary, and offering positive reinforcement for the successes achieved.

COMMUNITY PROGRAMS

Community sports programs help many children develop sports skills and enthusiasm, as well as improve health. Parents may consult a physician, therapist, or other health professional to decide which physical activities or programs are best for their children. Some activities may be physically demanding, stressful, or demand particular expertise, behavioral support, or specific coaching skills. Some may need to be monitored or provided by licensed or certified practitioners or health professionals. As the exertion level, competition, or challenge increases, the league or sponsoring organization may require physical examinations.

Soccer, basketball, baseball, and other youth sports may include children with disabilities when possible, and properly trained coaches can facilitate meaningful inclusion. Children with relatively minor impairments and good physical abilities can continue competing in such programs into high school. Although it is uncommon, some children with disabilities may be able to participate in varsity level sports, and examples are becoming more frequent of children with autism on basketball teams and children with Down syndrome on swimming teams (among others).

Specialized sports associations and programs provide meaningful physical activity, competitive participation, and social recreation. Special Olympics and the International Sports Federation for Persons with Intellectual Disability (INAS-FID) promote sports and competition for those with intellectual and developmental disability, while Paralympics, Disabled USA, and Blaze Sports provide sports programs for anyone with a physical disability. The President's Council on Fitness, Sports, & Nutrition has a Presidential Active Lifestyle Award (PALA) for people with disability. Other programs with local programming include Little League Baseball's Challenger Division, Wheelchair Sports, USA, TOPSoccer, STRIDE, YMCA, and National Disability Sports Alliance. Additional resources can be found on the Educated Sports Parent (http://www.educatedsportsparent.com).

It is important to recognize that youth with disabilities may not be as active as their peers without disabilities. Programs need to encourage participation of children with disabilities at all levels. Unfortunately, even when community resources exist to support youth with disabilities, most staff are lacking in the expertise, facilities, equipment and supervision required to realize a goal of universal access, particularly for children with more significant disability or behavioral difficulties. Recent research indicates that youth with disabilities can benefit tremendously from increased participation in such activities and that lifelong health can be improved, but many barriers continue to exist.

Sample Program Models

Two types of programs, initially designed for children with disabilities, serve as models of enjoyable recreation with potential health benefits and therapeutic impact. As previously mentioned, Special Olympics, a program for children, youth and adults with intellectual and physical disabilities, provides sports activities and competitions worldwide with over 3 million participants (Special Olympics, 2010). It offers coaches' training, sport-specific instruction manuals, weekly practices and seasonal competitions. Special Olympics uses a "divisioning" system to ensure that athletes and teams compete against others with similar abilities. In another venue, Unified Sports, typically developing youth of similar age compete on a team with Special Olympics athletes. Competitions are organized at every level: local, state, regional, national, and even international. Additionally, Special Olympics offers health screenings and health promotion advice at many events.

For many years, horseback riding centers have developed expertise in providing horseback riding therapy, therapeutic riding, or **hippotherapy** (Sterba, 2007; Sterba, Rogers, France, & Vokes, 2002). Children with a broad range of disabilities, including significant multiple impairments, can participate (Murphy, Kahn-D'Angelo, & Gleason, 2005). These programs can provide integrated activities or programs to address specific developmental, therapeutic, and functional skills of these children. National organizations have emerged to promote dissemination of information and intervention strategies, and education and certification programs for instructors and therapists (NAHRA; American Hippotherapy Association, 2010). Research evaluating the impact of these interventions on function has been modest, but physicians, therapists, and parents advocate for the importance of riding therapies for recreational reasons at minimum (Dirienza, Dirienzo, & Baceski, 2007; Dunst,& Rolandelli, 2003; Sterba, 2007).

POLICIES AFFECTING PARTICIPATION IN PHYSICAL ACTIVITY

School-based physical education (PE) requirements vary from state to state (http://www. ncsl.org/default.aspx?tabid=14027). In 2010, only five states required PE in every grade K–12, with only one state aligning with national recommendations for physical activity time (National Association for Sport and Physical Education, 2010). As a consequence of increased awareness regarding high rates of overweight and obesity in all children, many communities have advocated for increased access to PE. In this context parents, teachers and advocates need to understand state education requirements for PE and whether the IEP for a child with a disability needs to contain specific recommendations related to PE, physical activity, and exercise. The web site of the National Association for Sport and Physical Education (http://www.aahperd.org/naspe/standards/stateStandards/) provides links to current state standards. Individual schools and local education agencies (LEAs) may provide PE as part of a routine education curriculum on a weekly basis. In terms of an individual child's need, parents need to understand the PE program's contents, and their duration and frequency in the child's schedule, to evaluate whether the school provides enough physical activity. Parents also need to evaluate what after-school and weekend activities need to be planned so the child may achieve recommended levels of physical activity for fitness and strength development. Even if PE is a regular part of the school curriculum, the frequency, duration and consistency of PE throughout the school year may vary according to how the school system schedules courses and content delivery, especially at the high school level. For example, block scheduling approaches may provide significant amounts of access to PE during some months or quarters of the school year and minimal PE during other periods.

Where necessary parents should consider including specific objectives in the child's IEP that provide access to PE, adapted PE, or physical therapy or other related services offering consistent opportunity to be physically active, and also to learn necessary life skills. In addition to strength and fitness goals, some individuals may benefit from the inclusion of exercise or moderate to vigorous activity as part of the IEP in order to enhance behavioral interventions. Both IEP planning and Section 504 plans (see Chapter 31) can be used to ensure necessary levels of access and the child's inclusion into the appropriate type of class or programming.

Transition planning beginning at age 16 should also emphasize the range of life skills that need to be learned in preparation for adulthood and independent living, including health- and wellness-related objectives that help youth understand the importance of physical activity, what types of activities they enjoy, and what skills are needed in order to ensure that physical activity will become a routine part of their adult life (see Chapter 40 for further details on transition planning).

Research shows that levels of physical activity decline as individuals with disabilities age. In recent interviews of adults living with cerebral palsy, participants noted a noticeable decline in physical ability with increasing age in their 30s and 40s; related to this decline were symptoms of fatigue, pain, decline in ability to work a full work day, and loss of flexibility, strength and balance (Horsman et al., 2010). A key recommendation resulting from this and related research is that children and adolescents need to develop a clear understanding of their condition or disability, plus the potential course of their condition over their lifetime. They also need to have access to key information on how to plan for adulthood and prevent loss of function or adverse health consequences throughout life. Children with disabilities need this awareness prior to leaving school and fostering such awareness should be part of the transition planning process beginning at age 16 or earlier.

Both within the school, and when considering access to community-based recreation and fitness opportunities, the Americans with Disabilities Act (ADA; Title II) of 1990 with 2008 amendments (PL 110-325) and the Architectural Barriers Act of 1968 (90-480, 82 Stat. 718) are important laws to be aware of. All new construction must comply with these laws, providing physical access and accommodation for people with disabilities. When evaluating the potential barriers, certainly physical access to the facility is necessary, but the programs, instructors, equipment, and interior facility areas where desired activities must be held barrier-free. For example, some equipment or classes may be located in an area lacking ramped or elevator access; or equipment such as weight machines may not be useable by an individual in a wheelchair. Several equipment manufacturers now produce exercise equipment that is more accessible and safer for use by people with disabilities including swivel seats for easier transfer, covered weight stacks to prevent finger or other injuries, and other modifications. Exercise trainers and health facility staff can be an important resource for learning specific exercise routines, and in many places physical

therapists and other health consultants are available to provide guidance, instruction and accommodation (Heller, Marks, & Ailey, 2001).

CHOICE AND PREPARATION FOR PHYSICAL ACTIVITY, EXERCISE, OR SPORTS

Most physical activity is experienced, chosen, and repeated by the child based on his or her interests and desires. However, families can facilitate exposure to additional activities after consulting health professionals or other families who have children with disabilities. Physicians performing pre-participation examinations (PPE) examinations can assist in suggesting suitable sports. Several questions can help frame the relevant issues when choosing physical activity:

- *What are the child's interests?*
- *What activities are readily available to the family?* This question includes proximity, cost, coaches/support personnel, and access.
- *What activities could the child be most successful in?* For example, children with spastic cerebral palsy may succeed in horseback riding, wheelchair racing, or field events. Likewise, children with spina bifida might excel in swimming, track-and-field, or archery. A wide continuum of physical activity and sport options combined with proper evaluation and response monitoring will be the most appropriate approach for assuring ongoing and successful participation.

Key components of an exercise program (for all children) should include warm-up activities, aerobic activities, balance activities, strength training, and cool-down activities. The warm-up and cool-down activities can be 5–10 minutes each with the majority of exercise/activity time spent on aerobic, balance, and strength-training, activities. For many people just beginning a program, exercise duration can be fairly short, with successful participation being the initial goal. With consistent participation, the duration and intensity of exercise can be increased based on individual response and need. A total exercise period including warm-up and cool-down is usually 60–75 minutes.

Pre-participation Examinations

Medical examination prior to sport or exercise participation is designed to ensure safety and manage injury risk. PPEs are typically mandated to meet legal or insurance requirements in junior high or high school. Currently, 49 of 50 states and the District of Columbia require some form of physical evaluation before high school sport participation (Saglimbeni, 2010). Physical exams for younger children and preadolescents, while not mandatory, should be encouraged to promote engagement in physical activity; assess developmental and medical suitability to participate; and match physical, social, and cognitive maturity with appropriate activities (Kurowski & Chandran, 2000; Lyznicki, Nielsen, & Schneider, 2000; Maron et al., 2007).

Although frequency of PPE is debated, the American Medical Association Guidelines for Adolescent Preventive Services recommends evaluation at least every other year during adolescence. The American Academy of Pediatrics (AAP) recommends that adolescents involved in strenuous activity have an examination prior to entering high school, followed by a limited annual reevaluation (Saglimbeni, 2010). Desired outcomes of a PPE are to 1) define general health status and detect conditions that cause risk, 2) identify medical contraindications to participation, 3) assess physical maturity and readiness, 4) identify safe sports, and 5) educate the child and family about risks and benefits of participation in PA.

The *Preparticipation Physical Evaluation (PPE)*, Fourth Edition (Bernhardt & Roberts, 2010) is the definitive guide for implementing PPE and expands evaluation to athletes with special needs. It includes a medical history, physical examination, and clearance form. In addition to screening for potentially catastrophic conditions, the PPE, Fourth Edition also screens for conditions that predispose to injury or illness. Areas that require attention for all participants include exercise-induced syncope or asthma; family history of heart disease or sudden death; personal history of heart symptoms, loss of consciousness, concussion, neurological problems; heat stroke or hypothermia, musculoskeletal dysfunction; allergies, surgery, or hospitalization; and absence or loss of a paired organ (see Table 34.1).

Table 34.1. Components of the Preparticipation Examination (Bernhardt & Roberts, 2010)

Variable assessed	Normative values	Source	Cautions
Height and weight	Standard growth charts	Centers for Disease Control and Prevention	
Blood pressure	Gender and Ht percentiles	National Heart, Lung and Blood Institute	BP > 95% requires further evaluation before clearance
Heart sounds	Normal rhythm and rate	Stethoscope	Assess any murmur in supine and standing; further evaluation needed if change in murmur
Organs	Assess tenderness and size	Auscultation	Note any missing organs with cautions for participation in certain sports
Vision	—	Snelling Charts or Lea Chart for those with intellectual disability	Vision should be correctable to 20/40; note pupil inequality in size or reactivity for baseline
Skin	Visual and sensation exam	—	Defer participation if communicable skin disease
Musculoskeletal			
Posture	—	Visual assessment	—
Spinal symmetry	—	Visual assessment	—
Leg lengths	—	Tape measure	—
Gait	Walk and run	Visual assessment	—
Joint mobility	Standards range of motion	Goniometry	Caution with instability in Down syndrome
			Consider ROM requirements of sport
Muscle strength	Grade 5/5	Manual muscle testing	Note weakness or muscle atrophy
Muscle tone	Normal, hypo-, or hypertonic	—	May restrict certain sports like archery
Balance	—	Berg Balance Test	May limit certain sports like skiing
Equipment	Fit, function, safety	—	Equipment must conform to the sport and the sport regulations

As children with special needs may be at risk for additional injury or illness secondary to their disability, the *Supplemental History for the Athlete with Special Needs* further defines the nature of the disability, assistive devices used for it, history of autonomic dysreflexia, seizures or urinary tract infections, and specific disability-related impairments. In addition, the physician may assist with functional classification of the athlete based on physical ability and type or severity of impairment. The physician must be aware of national and international classification systems for competition such as those developed by the International Paralympics Committee.

The PPE's outcome will determine clearance level for participation, defined as

- Unrestricted for any sport
- Unrestricted with recommendation for further evaluation or treatment
- Not cleared pending further evaluation for any sports, or for certain sports

If the physician's recommendation is "no clearance for certain sports," the physician must specify which sports are prohibited and why. The AAP Committee on Sports Medicine and Fitness wrote a policy statement, "Medical Conditions and Sports Participation" (2001), with an excellent sports classification system (contact or physical touching, collision or violent, direct impact, limited contact, or noncontact) that is used in defining sports recommendations. The committee also developed participation recommendations for children with various medical conditions to assist physicians in decision making (Rice, 2008).

INJURY RISK IN CHILDREN

Three questions arise when discussing risks for injury in children with disabilities.

- What are the major reasons for injury risk to children with disabilities?
- What injuries are specific to children with disabilities?
- Do children with disabilities receive similar injuries as other children?

Although injuries such as fractures can result from a single trauma, repetitive **microtrauma** (or overuse) causes many injuries in children (Adirim & Cheng, 2003; Bainbridge, 2006; Oeppen & Jaramillo, 2003). Several factors predispose to overuse injury (Cassas & Cassettari-Wayhs, 2006; Hogan & Gross, 2003).

Training Errors

Sudden transitions from unregulated play to increased hours of participation can increase the incidence of overuse. Repetitive demands of activity or sport may result in **muscle** or **tendon imbalances** unless the child is on a well-designed training plan. For example, a swimmer might develop shoulder problems from a loose anterior and tight posterior joint capsule (Chen et al., 2005). Repetitive running increases strength only in the anterior thigh muscles, so increasing stride length could stress the weaker posterior muscles.

Developmental Conditions

Poor posture and joint limitation or deformity, frequent issues in children with disability, can cause injury if the body cannot compensate under sport-caused demands. Increased curvature of the lower spine or excess extension of the knee can cause abnormal joint loading and pain. Flat feet can increase stress on the inside of the knee, and cause the body weight to land on a flexible instead of rigid foot.

The major cause of overuse injury in children is growth. Bones grow primarily in length with secondary lengthening of soft tissues. During periods of rapid bone growth, or "spurts," the **muscle and tendon structures** tighten and lose flexibility. Recent studies have documented an increase in overuse injuries during such spurts (Soprano, 2005). Also, as bone matures, it stiffens and loses resistance to impact. Sudden overload may cause the bone to bow or buckle. The growth area in long bones is most susceptible to shear or fracture, potentially impacting bone growth. Likewise, growing cartilage offers low resistance to repetitive loading, resulting in **microtrauma** to the cartilage or the underlying growth plate. Damage may result in growth asymmetry or **osteoarthritis** (Caine, DiFiori, & Maffulli, 2006).

Injuries in Children with Disabilities

Minimal information exists on incidence and type of activity-related injuries in individuals with disabilities. Studies use small sample sizes and select groups of individuals with specific disabilities.

Several studies indicate a lower injury rate in students with disability. A study was conducted of 210 athletes (including children with ID, emotional disturbance, learning disability, multiple disability [including traumatic brain injury], and autism) in 8 special education high schools that participate in interscholastic sports (basketball, softball, soccer, and field hockey). The study's results noted 38 injuries among 512 athletes, a rate of 2.0 per 1000 athlete exposures (Ramirez et al., 2009). Soccer had the highest rate of injury (3.7 per 1000). Youth with ASD, although few in number, had the highest injury risk, five times that of athletes with other disabilities. Those with histories of seizures had injury rates >2.5 times the rate of those with no seizure history. Injuries to athletes with special needs were less severe, required less time away from the sport, and resulted in less missed school days than typically developing peers. They also had fewer sprains and strains, and no fractures or concussions.

Other studies indicate *higher injury rates* in children with disability; the authors posit that a compromised ability to perceive and manage environmental hazards may increase risk for injury. Ramirez, Peek-Asa, and Kraus (2004) studied 697 reported injuries in 6,769 school children with disability, and documented an injury rate of 4.7/100 students per year. Children with multiple disabilities had a 70% increased odds of injury compared with those with intellectual (1.7) or physical disability (1.4). Xiang, Stallones, Chen, Hostetler, and Kelleher (2005) noted injury rates of 4.2% vision disability, 3.2% mental retardation, 4.5% attention-deficit/ hyperactivity disorder, and 5.7% asthma versus 2.5% for typically developing children. Raman, Boyce, and Pickett (2007) also documented increased risk in children with disabilities compared to those without disability (67% versus 51%) for single, multiple, or serious injuries.

Disorder-Specific Injuries and Strategies for Prevention

Children with disabilities and related physical impairments have greater risk for specific injuries and may need modifications to training and participation for safety and success.

Spinal Cord Injury and Spina Bifida

A child with spinal cord injury or spina bifida may not perceive pain below their injury level, and may be at risk for soft-tissue damage from contusions or pressure. Athletes with spinal cord lesions at or above the sixth thoracic vertebra (T6) may have problems with autonomic dysreflexia, resulting in poor thermoregulation and altered blood pressure control (Klenk & Gebke, 2007). Trunk balance and stability may be compromised by lack of muscles. Strategies for safe participation include (according

to NCPAD, American College of Sports Medicine, Field, & Oates, 2001):

- Monitoring heart rate and blood pressure before and during participation for any sudden or significant changes; avoiding any breath-holding during exercise
- Padding any adaptive equipment or wheelchairs to reduce pressure
- Checking skin below the level of the injury for irritation
- Utilizing adaptive equipment such as cuffs, gloves, or Velcro straps to assist with grip
- Using wide benches and low seats for easier transfers
- Considering the need to stabilize the trunk and pelvis with strapping
- Using machines for strengthening instead of free weights
- Forbidding breath-holding during exercise—encouraging slow breathing

Cerebral Palsy

Abnormal muscle tone or inadequate muscle control in children with cerebral palsy may increase risk for ligament sprains and muscle strain. Contractures place stress on affected joints, and increased muscle tone that is exacerbated by exercise. Appropriate padding and fitting of adaptive equipment (e.g., braces, wheelchairs) is essential. Strategies for safe participation (NCPAD) include:

- Padding any adaptive equipment or wheelchairs to reduce pressure
- Utilizing adaptive equipment such as non-slip handgrips, cuffs, gloves, and Velcro straps to assist with grip
- Using wide benches and low seats for easier transfers
- Performing slow, controlled movements; using a metronome to set a pace
- Avoiding exercises that increase tone
- Strengthening muscle group opposed to spastic muscle to induce relaxation
- Slowly stretching spastic muscles; not using bouncing stretches
- Using seated exercises if standing balance is unsteady

Muscular Dystrophy

This progressive disorder results from damage to the nerves at an individual rate with episodes of exacerbation and remittance. Maintaining muscle strength slows the functional decline, but the child can be easily fatigued. Strategies for safe participation (NCPAD, American College of Sports Medicine) include

- Maintaining proper hydration
- Emptying bladder prior to exercise
- Utilizing adaptive equipment such as non-slip handgrips, cuffs, gloves, and Velcro straps to assist with grip
- Using wide benches and low seats for easier transfers
- Performing slow, controlled movements; stopping when fatigued
- Using seated exercises if standing balance is unsteady
- Demonstrating exercises near child as vision may be impaired or blurred

Down Syndrome and Intellectual Disability

Individuals with Down syndrome have specific physical concerns associated with their disability. A 10%–20% incidence of **atlanto-axial instability** (AAI) necessitates screening prior to participation in activities that put the neck at risk (e.g., gymnastics, contact sports, diving). If a child is found to have AAI by x ray, an examination should determine if the AAI is symptomatic. Research has demonstrated that only 1%–2% are symptomatic, demonstrating compression of the spinal cord (Ali, Al-Bustan, Al-Busairi, Al-Mulla, & Esbaita, 2006). If so, further consultation is necessary prior to clearance for sport (Ali et al., 2006; Down syndrome Health Issues online, 2011; Tassone & Duey-Holtz, 2008). Children with Down syndrome also have a higher incidence of orthopedic conditions including pronated feet, which may become painful with increased physical activity. Cardiac problems are prevalent in many types of ID. Fetal alcohol, Down, fragile X, and Williams syndromes are highly associated with heart or aorta defects. Experts believe the occurrence rate for the cardiac defect that underlies sudden cardiac death syndrome is 10–20 times more prevalent in the ID population (Jewell, 2011; Khan, 2009; Vaux, 2010; Vis et al., 2009). Those with ID are also more likely to be taking medications that cause abnormal heart rhythms. Seizure disorders occur in about 36% of people with ID (McBrien & Macken, 2009). Strategies for safe participation (NCPAD; American College of Sports Medicine) include

- Familiarizing child with environment and exercise protocol
- Demonstrating, then practicing all exercises one at a time
- Providing simple, short instructions and feedback; using pictures and large font
- Providing frequent reminders of good form and technique
- Checking for correct socks (wicking fabric as those with ID tend to produce more foot perspiration)
- Controlling the seizure disorder for water sports, or sports involving heights; compliance with medications should be stressed
- In children with cardiac problems, stopping exercise if they have extreme or sudden shortness of breath, leg cramps, or abnormal fatigue

Children with Impairments in Vision or Hearing

Impairments in vision or hearing can have many causes, but with children with partial or complete loss of vision or hearing can still actively participate in exercise and sports with modification for their physical limitation.

Children who are visually impaired or blind often exhibit lower levels of fitness than sighted peers (Houwen, Hartman, & Visscher, 2010; Lieberman & McHugh, 2001). Physical activity levels of children who are visually impaired and blind can be improved, bettering their economy of movement (Lieberman, Butcher, & Moak, 2001).

Those who are hard of hearing typically rely on hearing aids and other assistive listening devices to maximize residual hearing. Individuals who are deaf use modalities ranging from verbal communication to manual sign language. In some cases, the use of interpreters may be required to aid in communication. Strategies for safe participation (NCPAD; American College of Sports Medicine) include

- Always facing the child so that he or she sees supervisor's face, lips, eyes, and body
- Maintaining eye contact and speaking directly to the person, not to the interpreter
- Demonstrating in person or by video exactly what is required from beginning to end
- Using visual and tactile cues, facial expressions, body language, gestures, and common signs, such as thumbs-up or thumbs-down to communicate meaning

- Using normal enunciation and loudness
- If an individual's speech is unclear or difficult to understand, the listener not pretending at comprehension, but rather asking for clarification
- Avoiding loud, constant background noise that may cause headaches or reduce effectiveness of hearing aids
- Orienting the child to all aspects of the environment with special attention to emergency aspects (exits and fire evacuation procedures)
- Equipping facilities with strobe or visual fire alarms or other alerting devices (buddy or tapping system, very loud sounds, vibrations, colorful flags)
- Establishing and consistently using cue or feedback gestures for whatever words are necessary for activities such as "ready," "start," "ok," and "stop"
- Removing hearing aids and external cochlear implant devices before participating in water activities or those involving contact

Children Using Assistive Technologies

Children who use wheelchairs are particularly susceptible to injuries resulting from extensive use of their upper extremities in sports like road racing, basketball, track, and tennis (Barnard, Nelson, Xiang, & McKenzie, 2010). Most common injuries involve sprains, strains, and wrist and shoulder overuse (Chen, Diaz, Loebenberg et al., 2005; Finley & Rogers, 2004). Strategies for safe participation (NCPAD; American College of Sports Medicine) include

- Using appropriate equipment
- Implementing a well-designed stretching, training, and rest program
- Being aware of new or modifiable equipment designed to minimize repetitive use injuries
- Paying careful attention to blisters and lacerations
- Using straps or harnesses if needed for trunk stability
- Using brakes to stabilize chair during static activities

Low Bone Density

Low bone density (**osteopenia/osteoporosis**) occurs in many children with disability due to many causes including medications, lack of physical movement, and diet (Plotkin & Sueiro, 2007; Skrinth, Cassidy, Joiner, et al., 2010). Osteoporosis is common in the lower extremities of children in wheelchairs and can lead to increased risk of fractures, even in situations where similar force might not affect ambulatory children (Wilson, 2005). Further evaluation and management might be warranted if a child is taking medications that might induce bone loss or has a disability with a predilection for low bone density (Apkon, Fenton, & Coll, 2009; Kilpinen-Loisa et al., 2010). Strategies for safe participation (National Osteoporosis Foundation) include

- Using low-impact aerobics if child is frail or falls easily
- Avoiding full sit-ups or stretches that bend the spine forward and twist
- Avoiding extreme back extension

Equipment and Support

The use of proper equipment should be mandated and enforced for the safety of all children. Equipment must be activity-appropriate, high-quality and fit properly to function correctly. Proper footwear with adequate cushioning, rear foot control, sole flexibility for the activity (Ceroni, De Rosa, De Coulon, et al., 2007; Micheli & Jenkins, 2001), and protective padding such as shoulder and shin pads (for contact or kicking sports) should be required. Protective headgear can limit head and neck injuries that occur from contact and collision in football, baseball, and hockey; such headgear is approved by the National Operating Committee on Standards for Athletic Equipment and the American National Safety Institute.

Eye protectors should be required for racquet sports, ice hockey, baseball, basketball, and football and should cover a wide area, be made of impact-resistance material, and not reduce the visual field. All eye protectors should be approved by the American Society for Testing and Materials or the Canadian Standards Association.

Mandatory use of mouth guards has cut the rate of oral trauma. Mouth guards absorb oral and facial blows, preventing not only injury to teeth and mouth, but also fractures, dislocations, and concussions. Mouth guards should be inexpensive, strong, and easy to clean and should not interfere with speech or breathing. They can function alone in field hockey, rugby, wrestling, basketball, and similar field events, or together with face protectors in football, ice hockey, baseball, and lacrosse (Roccia, Diaspro, Nasi, et al., 2008).

Environment assessment is also vital to safety. All playing areas should be well-lit; surfaces should be smooth and obstacle free with good shock-absorbing qualities (wood as opposed to concrete). Equipment modifications shown to decrease injury (e.g., breakaway bases in baseball) should be installed. Sports equipment and playing environments should be scaled to athlete size.

Temperature and humidity should also be carefully monitored as children have greater surface area for body weight compared with adults and thus a greater rate of heat exchange. They have less ability to exercise in weather extremes, demonstrating greater heat gain on hot days and greater heat loss on cold days. Children also produce less sweat with less evaporative heat loss, so they carry a larger heat load (AAP, 2000). Children acclimatize slower and require more "exposures" (Bergeron, Laird, Marinik, et al., 2009; Bytomski & Squire, 2003; Naughton & Carlson, 2008). Since children require more fluid replacement per kilogram of body weight during exercise to prevent dehydration, it is important to drink plenty of liquid before, during, and after play; thirst is not a valid indicator of water needed (Decher, Casa, & Yeargin, 2008). Hydration recommendations include pre-activity hydration of 3–6 oz for less than 90 lbs; 6–12 oz for greater than 90 lb weight 1 hour before activity, and 3–6 oz just prior to activity. During activity, 3–5 oz for less than 90 lb; 6–9 oz for greater than 90 lb should be ingested every 10 to 20 minutes relative to temperature and humidity (Casa, Clarkson, & Roberts, 2005).

Children will generally not drink enough water to hydrate; flavor-added water often stimulates greater-volume intake (Passe et al., 2000; Rivera-Brown, Ramirez-Marrero, Wilk, et al., 2008). In addition, well-constituted sports drinks have a low-carbohydrate content that provides energy, speeds fluid absorption, and provides sodium to stimulate thirst (Davis et al., 2001; Meadows-Oliver & Ryan-Krause, 2007). As cool fluids infuse more easily, liquids should be cold or iced. Universal education about hydration, and common signs of dehydration—irritability, headache, nausea, dizziness, weakness, cramps, abdominal distress, and decreased performance—are a positive influence for compliance, problem recognition, and intervention (Casa et al., 2000).

Children with disabilities often require specialized equipment to participate. Special wheelchairs, skiing outriggers, ergonomic handles, rotation platforms, and custom prostheses are examples of technological advances that make sports more accessible. Children with spinal cord injury (SCI), who may have abnormal sensory function, can wear aqua boots in the pool to avoid pressure ulcers. Likewise, children with racing wheelchairs may require specifically placed padding to prevent skin breakdown (Wilson, 2002). The use of bells in balls can make activities more inclusive for those with visual impairments.

Proper supervision is the final ingredient to safe participation. The coach is a supervisor, educator, and motivator. Approximately 2.5 million adult volunteers with varying levels of expertise currently coach 20 million children. The AAP recommends coaches enforce warm-up procedures, require suitable protective equipment, and enforce safety rules. In addition, AAP recommends coaching certification that covers teaching techniques, basic sports skills, fitness, first aid, sportsmanship, and improving self-image and motivational skills (AAP, 2010).

Qualified officials and medical personnel at games and practices are the second level of supervision. These individuals provide game control and immediate injury containment. Medical personnel can include physicians, physical therapists, or athletic trainers certified in first aid and CPR along with their sports medicine skills (AAP, 2010).

Parents are the final level of supervision since many activities occur in the home and local community. Parents have unique knowledge of their child, but medical personnel can educate them about specific issues their child might confront when participating in activities. Parents can also provide valuable modeling and encouragement to their child, since many children with disabilities have less experience with exercise and sport.

SUMMARY

Physical activity helps maintain and promote physical health, functional capacity, and stamina for daily activities in all children. There is significant need for families, schools and health professionals to increase attention to physical activity needs of children with developmental disability. Concern is increasing in relation to health and overweight status of children because it appears that physical activity levels in general may be decreasing while more sedentary options compete for time and attention among children and youth. In many communities families have a wide range of recreational and sports program options including programs specifically designed for children with special health care needs. Unfortunately, some communities lack these resources so families need to use their own networks to identify the possibilities and determine the degree to which a desired activity may need assistance from staff, coaches, teachers or health professionals with specific expertise in working with children. Adapted physical education instructors, physical and occupational therapists and other health professionals with knowledge of children with developmental disabilities or special health care needs may be helpful in facilitating participation. All children need the opportunity to experience, explore, and pursue new and enjoyable movement experiences.

REFERENCES

Adirim, T.A., & Cheng, T.L. (2003). Overview of injuries in the young athlete. *Sports Medicine, 33*, 75–81.

Ali, F.E., Al-Bustan, M.A., Al-Busairi, W.A., Al-Mulla, F.A., & Esbaita, E.Y. (2006). Cervical spine abnormalities associated with Down syndrome. *International Orthopedics, 30*(4), 284–289. Epub 2006 Mar 7.

American Academy of Family Physicians, American Academy of Pediatrics, American College of Sports Medicine, American Medical Society for Sports Medicine, American Orthopaedic Society for Sports Medicine, & American Osteopathic Academy of Sports Medicine, Bernhardt, D., & Roberts, W., (Eds). (2010). PPE—*Preparticipation Physical Evaluation, Edition 4*. Elk Grove Village, IL: American Academy of Pediatrics.

American Academy of Pediatrics (2007). Organized athletics for children and preadolescents. *Pediatrics, 107*(6), 1459–1462. Retrieved from http://aappolicy.aappublications.org/cgi/content/full/pediatrics;107/6/1459

American Academy of Pediatrics, Committee on Sports Medicine and Fitness (2001). Climatic heat stress and the exercising child and adolescent. *Pediatrics, 106*, 158–159.

American College of Allergy, Asthma, & Immunology. (2011). *Exercising with allergies and asthma*. Retrieved from http://www.acaai.org/allergist/asthma/asthma-treatment/management/Pages/exercising-with-allergies-asthma.aspx

American College of Sports Medicine. (2010). *Exercising following a brain injury*. Retrieved from http://www.medscape.com/viewarticle/719401

American College of Sports Medicine. (2010). *Exercising with arthritis*. Retrieved from http://www.medscape.com/viewarticle/719393

American College of Sports Medicine. (2010). *Exercising with asthma*. Retrieved from http://www.medscape.com/viewarticle/719394

American College of Sports Medicine. (2010). *Exercising with cerebral palsy*. Retrieved from http://www.medscape.com/viewarticle/719531

American College of Sports Medicine. (2010). *Exercising with cystic fibrosis*. Retrieved from http://www.medscape.com/viewarticle/719536

American College of Sports Medicine. (2010). *Exercising with epilepsy*. Retrieved from http://www.medscape.com/viewarticle/719395

American College of Sports Medicine. (2010). *Exercising with hearing loss*. Retrieved from http://www.medscape.com/viewarticle/719759

American College of Sports Medicine. (2010). *Exercising with mental retardation*. Retrieved from http://www.medscape.com/viewarticle/719870

American College of Sports Medicine. (2010). *Exercising with muscular dystrophy*. Retrieved from http://www.medscape.com/viewarticle/719871

American College of Sports Medicine. (2010). *Exercising with type 2 diabetes*. Retrieved from http://www.medscape.com/viewarticle/719183

American College of Sports Medicine. (2010). *Exercising with visual impairment*. Retrieved from http://www.medscape.com/viewarticle/719878;

American Hippotherapy Association. (2010). Retrieved from http://www.americanhippotherapyassociation.org/

American Medical Association. (1997). Retrieved from http://www.ama-assn.org//resources/doc/ad-hlth/gapsmono.pdf

Apkon, S.D., Fenton, L., & Coll, J.R. (2009). Bone mineral density in children with myelomeneningocele. *Developmental Medicine and Child Neurology, 51*(1), 63–67. Epub 2008 Sep 20.

Bainbridge, D.B. (2006). Sports injuries in children. In S.K. Campbell, D.W. VanderLinden, & R.J. Palisano (Eds.), *Physical therapy for children* (3rd ed., pp. 517–556. Philadelphia, PA: W.B. Saunders.

Bandini, L.G., Curtin, C., Hamad, C., Tybor, D.J., & Must, A. (2005). Prevalence of overweight in children with developmental disorders: I. The continuous national health and nutrition examination survey (NHANES) 1999-2002. *Journal of Pediatrics, 146*(6), 738–743.

Baranek, G.T. (2002). Efficacy of sensory and motor interventions for children with autism. *Journal of Autism and Developmental Disorders, 32*(5), 397–422.

Barnard, A.M., Nelson, N.G., Xiang, H., & McKenzie, L.B. (2010). Pediatric mobility aid-related injuries treated in US emergency departments from 1991 to 2008. *Pediatrics, 125*(6), 1200–1207.

Baruth, M., Wilcox, S., Dunn, A.L., King, A.C., Marcus, B.H., Rejeski, W.J., … Blair, S.N. (2010). Psychosocial mediators of PA and fitness changes in the activity counseling trial. *Annals of Behavioral Medicine, 39*(3), 274–89. doi 10.1007/s12160-010-9178-4

Bergeron, M.F., Laird, M.D., Marinik, E.L., Brenner, J.S., & Waller, J.L. (2009). Repeated-bout exercise in the heat in young athletes: Physiological strain and perceptual responses. *Journal of Applied Physiology, 106*(2), 476–485.

Bernhardt, D.T., & Roberts, W.O. (2010). Preparticipation physical evaluation, Fourth Edition. Elk Grove Village, IL: American Academy of Pediatrics.

Burns, Y.R., Danks, M., O'Callaghan, M.J., Gray, P.H., Cooper, D., Poulsen, L., & Watter, P. (2008). Motor coordination difficulties and physical fitness of extremely-low-birthweight children. *Developmental Medicine and Child Neurology, 51*, 136–142.

Bytomski, J.R., & Squire, D.L. (2003). Heat illness in children. *Current Sports Medicine Reports, 2*(6), 320–324.

Caine, D., DiFiori, J., & Maffulli, N. (2006). Physical injuries in children's and youth sports: Reasons for concern? *British Journal of Sports Medicine, 40*(9), 749–760.

Casa, D.J., Clarkson, P.M., & Roberts, W.O. (2005). American College of Sports Medicine roundtable on hydration and physical activity: Consensus statements. *Current Sports Medicine Reports, 4*(3), 115–127.

Casa, D.J., Armstrong, L.E., Hillman, S.K., Montain, S.J., Reiff, R.V., Rich, B.S., ... Stone, J.A. (2000). National Athletic Trainers' Association position statement: fluid replacement for athletes. *Journal of Athletic Training, 35*(2), 212–224.

Cassas, K.J., & Cassettari-Wayhs, A. (2006). Childhood and adolescent sports-related overuse injuries. *American Family Physician, 73*(6), 1014–1022.

Centers for Disease Control and Prevention (2010). *National diabetes fact sheet.* Retrieved from http://www.cdc.gov/diabetes/pubs/pdf/ndfs_2011.pdf

Centers for Disease Control and Prevention (2010). *How much physical activity do children need.* Retrieved from http://www.cdc.gov/physicalactivity/everyone/guidelines/children.html

Centers for Disease Control and Prevention, & President's Council on Physical Fitness and Sports (2006). *Healthy People 2010: Midcourse Review.* Retrieved from http://www.healthypeople.gov/data/midcourse/html/focusareas/FA22TOC.htm

Ceroni, D., De Rosa, V., De Coulon, G., & Kaelin, A. (2007). The importance of proper shoe gear and safety stirrups in the prevention of equestrian foot injuries. *Journal of Foot and Ankle Surgery, 46*(1), 32–39.

Chen, F.S., Diaz, V.A., Loebenberg, M., & Rosen, J.E. (2005). Shoulder and elbow injuries in the skeletally immature athlete. *Journal of American Academy of Orthopedic Surgery, 13*(3), 172–185.

Crowley, P.M., Ploutz-Snyder, L.L., Baynard, T., Heffernan, K.S., Young Jae, S., Hsu, S., ... Fernhall, B. (2011). The effect of progressive resistance training on leg strength, aerobic capacity and functional tasks of daily living in persons with Down syndrome. *Disability Rehabilitation* [Epub ahead of print].

Dirienza, L.N., Dirienzo, L.T., & Baceski, D.A. (2007). Heart rate response to therapeutic riding in children with cerebral palsy: An exploratory study. *Pediatric Physical Therapy, 19*(2), 160–165. doi: 10.1097/PEP.0b013e31804a57a8

Dodd, K.J., & Shields, N. (2005). A systematic review of the outcomes of cardiovascular exercise programs for people with Down syndrome. *Archives of Physical Medicine and Rehabilitation, 86,* 2051–2058.

Down syndrome: Health Issues Online. (2011). Available at http://www.ds.health.com

Decher, N.R., Casa., D.J., Yeargin, S.W., Ganjo, M.S., Levreault, M.L., Dann, C.L., ... Brown, S.W. (2008). Hydration status, knowledge, and behavior in youths at summer sports camps. *International Journal of Sports Physiology Perform, 3*(3), 262–278.

Dunst, C.J., & Rolandelli, P.S. (2003). Influences of hippotherapy on the motor and socio-emotional behavior of young children with disabilities. *Bridges, 1*(9), 1–9. Retrieved from http://www.wbpress.com/index.php?main_page=product_book_info&products_id=263

Eliot, R.O., Dobbin, A.R., Rose, G.D., & Soper, H.V. (1994). Vigorous, aerobic exercise gernal motor training activities: Effects on maladaptive and stereotypic behavior of adults with both autism and mental retardation. *Journal of Autism and Developmental Disorders, 24,* 565–576.

Emck, C., Rosscher, R., Wieringen, P., Doreleijers, T., & Beek, P. (2010). Gross motor performance and physical fitness in children with psychiatric disorders. *Developmental Medicine and Child Neurology.* Advance online publication. doi: 10.1111/j.1469-8749.2010.03806.x.

Everett Jones, S., & Lollar, D.J. (2008) Relationship between physical disabilities or long-term health problems and health risk behaviors or conditions among US high school students. *Journal of School Health, 78*(5), 252–257. doi: 10.1111/j.1746-1561.2008.00297.x

Faulkner, B., Lurbe, E., & Schaefer, F. (2010). High blood pressure in children: Clinical and health policy implications. *The Journal of Clinical Hypertension, 12*(4), 261–276. doi: 10.1111/j.1751-7176.2009.00245.x

Farrell, P.A. (2003). Diabetes, exercise, and competitive sports, sports science exchange 90. *Gatorade Sports Science Institute, 16,* 3.

Field, S.J., & Oates, R.K. (2001). Sports and recreation activities and opportunities for children with spina bifida and cystic fibrosis. *Journal of Science & Medicine in Sport 4*(1), 71–76.

Finley, M.A.& Rogers, M.M. (2004). Prevalence and identification of shoulder pathology in athletic and nonathletic wheelchair users with shoulder pain: A pilot study. *Journal of Rehabilitation Research and Development, 41*(3B), 395–402.

Fleming, R.K., Stokes, E.A., Curtin, C., Bandini, L.G., Gleason, J., Scampini, R., ...Hamad, C. (2008) Behavioral health in developmental disabilities: A comprehensive program of nutrition, exercise, and weight reduction. *International Journal of Behavioral Consultation and Therapy 4*(3), 287–296. Retrieved from http://www.ncbi.nlm.nih.gov/pmc/articles/PMC2846829/?tool=pubmed

Fragala-Pinkham, M., Haley, S., & O'Neil, M.E. (2008). Group aquatic exercise for children with disabilities. *Developmental Medicine and Child Neurology, 50,* 822–827.

Fragala-Pinkham, M.A., Haley, S.M., Rabin, J., & Kharasch, V.S. (2005). A fitness program for children with disabilities. *Physical Therapy, 85,* 1182–1200.

Frey, G.C., Stanish, H.I., & Temple, V.A. (2008). Physical activity of youth with intellectual disability: review and research agenda. *Adapted Physical Activity Quarterly, 25*(2), 95-117.

Green, D., Charman, T., Pickles, A., Chandler, S., Loucas, T., Simonoff, E., & Baird, G. (2009). Impairment of movement skills of children with autism spectrum disorders. *Develomental Medicine and Child Neurology, 51,* 311–316.

Heller, T., Marks, B.A., & Ailey, S.H. (2001). *Exercise and nutrition health education curriculum for adults with developmental disabilities.* Chicago, IL: Rehabilitation Research and Training Center on Aging with Developmental Disabilities, University of Illinois at Chicago.

Hellings, J.A., Zarcone, J.R., Crandall, K., Wallace, D., & Schroeder, S.R. (2001). Weight gain in a controlled study of risperidone in children, adolescents and adults with mental retardation and autism. *Journal of Child and Adolescent Psychopharmacology, 11,* 229–238.

Hogan, K.A., & Gross, R.H. (2003). Overuse injuries in pediatric athletes. *Orthopedic Clinics of North America, 34*(3), 405–415.

Horsman, M., Suto, M., Dudgeon, B., & Harris, S. (2010). Growing older with cerebral palsy: Insiders' perspective. *Pediatric Physical Therapy, 22,* 296–303.

Houwen, S., Hartman, E., & Visscher, C. (2010). The relationship among motor proficiency, physical fitness, and body composition in children with and without visual impairments. *Research Quarterly for Exercise and Sports, 81*(3), 290–299.

Jewell, J. (2011). *Fragile X syndrome.* Retrieved from http://emedicine.medscape.com/article/943776-overview

Journal of Academy of Pediatrics. (2010). Available at: http://pediatrics.aappublications.org/cgi/content/full/103/6/1313/b

Katz, D.L., Cushman, D., Reynolds, J., Njike, V., Treu, J.A., Walker, J., ... Katz, C. (2010). Putting physical activity where it fits in the school day: Preliminary results of the ABC (Activity bursts in the classroom) for fitness program. *Preventing Chronic Disease 7*(4), 1–10. Retrieved from http://www.cdc.gov/pcd/issues/2010/jul/09_0176.htm

Keeton, V.F., & Kennedy, C. (2009). Update on physical activity including special needs populations. *Current Opinion in Pediatrics, 21*(2), 262–268. doi: 10.1097/MOP.0b013e3283292614

Kitzman-Ulrich, H., Wilson, D.K., St. George, S.M., Lawman, H., Segal, M., & Fairchild, A. (2010). The integration of a family systems approach for understanding youth obesity, physical activity, and dietary programs. *Cllinical Child and Family Psychology Review 13*(3), 231–253. doi: 10.1007/s10567-010-0073-0

Khan, A. (2009). *Williams syndrome.* Retrieved from http://emedicine.medscape.com/article/893149-overview#a0199

Kilpinen-Loisa, P., Paasio, T., Soiva, M., Ritanen, U.M., Lautala, P., Palmu, P., ... Mäkitie, O. (2010). Low bone mass in patients with motor disability: Prevalence and risk factors in 59 Finnish children. *Developmental Medicine and Child Neurolology, 52*(3), 276–82. Epub 2010 Aug 26.

Klenk, C., & Gebke, K. (2007). Practical management: Common medical problems in disabled athletes. *Clinical Journal of Sports Medicine, 17*(1), 55–60.

Klim, A., Volkmar, F.R., & Sparrow, S.S. (1992). Autistic social dysfunction: Some limitations of the theory of mind hypothesis. *Journal of Child Psychology and Psychiatry, 33*(5), 861–876

Kurowski, K., & Chandran, S. (2000). The preparticipation athletic evaluation. *American Family Physician, 61,* 2683–2690, 2696–2698.

Lieberman, L.J., Butcher, M., & Moak, S. (2001). Preferred guide-running techniques for children who are blind. *Palaestra, 17*(3), 20–26, 55.

Lieberman, L.J., & McHugh, B.E. (2001). Health related fitness of children with visual impairments. *Journal of Visual Impairment and Blindness, 95*(5), 272–286.

Lochbaum, M., & Crews, D. (2006). Viability of cardiorespiratory and muscular strength programs for adolescents with autism. *Complimentary Health Practice Review, 8,* 225–233.

Lyznicki, J.M, Nielsen, N.H., & Schneider, J.F. (2000). Cardiovascular screening of student athletes. *American Family Physician, 15,* 2332.

McKay, H., Liu, D., Egeli, D., Boyd, S., & Burrows, M. (2010). Physical activity positively predicts bone architecture and bone strength in adolescent males and females. *Acta Paediatrica.* Advance online publication. doi: 10.1111/j.1651-2227.2010.01995.x

Machek, M.A., Steopka, C.B., Tillman, M.D., Sneed, S.M., & Naugle, K.E. (2008). The effects of supervised resistance training program on Special

Olympics athletes. *Journal of Sport Rehabilitation, 17,* 372–379.

Maher, C.A., Williams, M.T., Olds, T., & Lane, A. (2007). Physical and sedentary activity in adolescents with cerebral palsy. *Developmental Medicine and Child Neurology, 49*(6), 450–457. doi: 10.1111/j.1469-8749.2007.00450.x

Malina, R.M. (2006). Weight training in youth-growth, maturation, and safety: An evidence-based review. *Clincial Journal of Sports Medicine, 16*(6), 478–487.

Maron, B.J., Thompson, P.D., Ackerman, M.J., Balady, G., Berger, S., Cohen, D., ... American Heart Association Council on Nutrition, Physical Activity, and Metabolism. (2007). Recommendations and considerations related to preparticipation screening for cardiovascular abnormalities in competitive athletes: 2007 update: A scientific statement from the American Heart Association Council on Nutrition, Physical Activity, and Metabolism: Endorsed by the American College of Cardiology Foundation. *Circulation, 115*(12), 1643–1645.

McBrien, J., & Macken, S. (2009). Meeting the health care needs of school-age children with intellectual disability. *Irish Medical Journal, 102*(8), 252–255.

McPheeters, Warren Z., Sathe, N., Bruzek, J.L., Krishnaswami, S., Jerome, R.N., & Veenstra-Vanderweele, J. (2011). A systematic review of medical treatments for children with autism spectrum disorders. *Pediatrics, 127*:e1312-21. Epub April 4, 2011.

Meadows-Oliver, M., & Ryan-Krause, P. (2007). Powering up with sports and energy drinks. *Pediatric Health Care, 21*(6), 413–416.

Micheli, L.J., & Jenkins, M. (2001) *The sports medicine bible for young athletes* (1st ed.). Naperville, IL: Sourcebooks.

Mondonca, G., Pereira, F.D., & Fernhall, B. (2010). Reduced exercise capacity in persons with Down syndrome: Cause, effect, and management. *Therapeutics and Clinical Research Management, 6,* 601–610.

Murphy, D., Kahn-D'Angelo, L., & Gleason, J. (2008). The effect of hippotherapy on functional outcomes for children with disabilities: A pilot study. *Pediatric Physical Therapy, 20*(3), 264–270. doi: 10.1097/PEP.0b013e31818256cd

Nader, P.R., Bradley, R.H., Houts, R.M., McRitchie, S.L., & O'Brien, M. (2008). Moderate-to-vigorous physical activity from ages 9 to 15 years. *Journal of the American Medical Association, 300*(3), 295–305.

Naughton, G.A., & Carlson, J.S. (2008). Reducing the risk of heat-related decrements to physical activity in young people. *Journal of Sports Science and Medicine, 11*(1), 58–65.

NARHA (2010). Retrieved from http://www.narha.org/

National Association for Sport and Physical Education (2010). Shape of the Nation Report. Retrieved from http://www.aahperd.org/naspe/publications/upload/Shape-of-the-tion-Revised2PDF.pdf

National Center on Physical Activity and Disability (NCPAD). (2010). Chicago, IL: Department of Disability and Human Movement, University of Illinois at Chicago. Retrieved from http://www.ncpad.org/

National Council of State Legislators (NCSL). (2011). *Physical education and physical activity for children: State physical education requirements.* Retrieved from http://www.ncsl.org/default.aspx?tabid=14027/

National Association for Sport and Physical Education. (2011). *Standards and position statements: State standards.* Retrieved from http://www.aahperd.org/naspe/standards/stateStandards/

National Osteoporosis Foundation. (2011). *Exercise for healthy bones.* Retrieved from http://www.nof.org/aboutosteoporosis/prevention/exercise

Nikander R., Sievänen H., Heinonen A., Daly R.M., Uusi-Rasi K., & Kannus P. (2010) Targeted exercise against osteoporosis: A systematic review and meta-analysis for optimising bone strength throughout life. *BMC Medicine, 8*(47), 1–16. Retrieved from http://www.biomedcentral.com/content/pdf/1741-7015-8-47.pdf doi:10.1186/1741-7015-8-47

Oeppen, R.S., & Jaramillo, D. (2003). Sports injuries in the young athlete. *Topics Magnetic Resonance Imaging, 14*(2), 199–208.

Palisano, R.J., Chiarello, L.A., Orlin, M., Oeffinger, D., Polansky, M., Maggs, … Children's Activity and Participation Group. (2010). Determinants of intensity of participation in leisure and recreational activities by children with cerebral palsy. *Developmental Medicine and Child Neurology, 53*(2), 142–149. doi: 10.1111/j.1469-8749.2010.03819.x.Epub 2010 Oct 21.

Pan, C.Y. (2008). Objectively measured physical activity between children with autism spectrum disorders and children without disabilities during inclusive recess settings in Taiwan. *Journal of Autism and Developmental Disorders, 38*(7), 1292–1301. doi: 10.1007/s10803-007-0518-6

Pan, C.Y., & Frey, G. (2006). Physical activity patterns in youth with autism spectrum disorders. *Journal of Autism and Developmental Disorders, 36,* 597–606.

Pan, C.Y., Tsai, C.L., & Chu, C.H. (2009). Fundamental movement skills in children diagnosed with autism spectrum disorders and attention deficit hyperactivity disorder. *Journal of Autism and Developmental Disorders, 39*(12), 1694–1705. http://dx.doi.org/10.1007/s10803-009-0813-5

Parfitt, G., Pavey, T., & Rowlands, A. (2009). Children's physical activity and psychological health: The relevance of intensity. *Acta Paediatrica, 98*(6), 1037–1043. doi: 10.1111/j.1651-2227.2009.01255.x

Passe, D., Horn, M., & Murray, R. (2000). Impact of beverage acceptability on fluid intake during exercise. *Appetite, 35,* 219–225.

Pitetti, K., Rendoff, A.D., Grover, T., & Beets, M.W. (2007). The efficacy of a 9-month treadmill walking program on the exercise capacity and weight reduction for adolescents with severe autism. *Journal of Autism and Developmental Disorders, 37,* 997–1006.

Plotkin, H., & Sueiro, R. (2007). Osteoporosis in children with neuromuscular diseases and inborn errors of metabolism. *Minerva Pediatrica, 59*(2), 129–135.

President's Council on Fitness, Sports and Nutrition (2008). *School physical education as a viable change agent to increase youth physical activity.* Retrieved from http://www.fitness.gov/resources-and-grants/council-research/

Raman, S.R., Boyce, W., & Pickett, W. (2007). Injury among 1107 Canadian students with self-identified disabilities. *Disability Rehabilitation, 29*(22), 1727–1735.

Ramirez, M., Peek-Asa, C., Kraus, J.F. (2004). Disability and risk of school related injury. *Injury Prevention, 10*(1), 21-26.

Ramiriz, M., Yang, J., Bourque, L., Javien, J., Kashani, S., Limbos, M.A., & Peek-Asa, C. (2009). Sports injuries to high school athletes with disabilities. *Pediatrics, 123*(2), 690–696. doi:10.1016/j.amepre.2004.12.006

Rice, S., & the Council on Sports Medicine and Fitness. (2008). Medical conditions affecting sports participation. *Pediatrics, 121*(4), 841–848 (doi:10.1542/peds.2008-0080)

Rimmer, J.H., & Rowland, J.L. (2008). Physical activity for youth with disabilities: A critical need in an underserved population. *Developmentl Neurorehabilitation, 11,* 141–148.

Rimmer, J.H., Rowland, J.L., & Yamaki, K. (2007). Obesity and secondary conditions in adolescents with disabilities: Addressing the needs of an underserved population. *Journal of Adolescent Health, 41,* 224–229.

Rinehart, N.J., Bradshaw, J.L., Brereton, A.V., & Tonge, B.J. (2001) Movement preparation in high-functioning autism and Asperger Disorder: A serial choice reaction time task involving motor reprogramming. *Journal of Autism and Developmental Disorders, 31,* 79–88.

Rivera-Brown, A.M., Ramirez-Marrero, F.A., Wilk, B., & Bar-Or, O. (2008). Voluntary drinking and hydration in trained, heat-acclimatized girls exercising in a hot and humid climate. *European Journal of Applied Physiology, 103*(1), 109–116.

Roberts, G., Anderson, P.J., Davis, N., De Luca, C., Cheong, J., & Doyle, L.W. (2011) Developmental coordination disorder in geographic cohorts of 8-year-old children born extremely preterm or extremely low birthweight in the 1990s. *Developmental Medicine and Child Neurology, 53,* 55–60. doi: 10.1111/j.1469-8749.2010.03779.x.

Roccia, F., Diaspro, A., Nasi, A., & Berrone, S. (2008). Management of sport-related maxillofacial injuries. *Journal of Craniofacial Surgery, 19*(2), 377–382.

Saglimbeni, A. (2010). *Sports physicals.* Retrieved from http://emedicine.medscape.com/article/88972-overview

Schott, N., Alof, V., Hultsch, D., & Meerman, D. (2007). Physical fitness in children with developmental coordination disorder. *Research Quarterly for Exercise and Sport, 78*(5), 438–450.

Shields, N., Dodd, K.J., & Abblitt, C. (2009). Do children with Down syndrome perform sufficient physical activity to maintain good health? A pilot study. *Adaptive Physical Activity Quarterly, 26*(4), 307–320.

Soprano, J.V. (2005). Musculoskeletal injuries in the pediatric and adolescent athlete. *Current Sports Medicine Reports, 4*(6), 329–334.

Special Olympics (2010). Retrieved from http://www.specialolympics.org/

Srikanth, R., Cassidy, G., Joiner, C., & Teeluckdharry, D. (2010). Osteoporosis in people with intellectual disabilities: A review and a brief study of risk factors in a community sample of people with intellectual disabilities. *Journal of Intellectual Disability Research,* doi 10.1111/j.1365-2788.2010.01346.x

Sterba, J.A. (2007). Does horseback riding therapy or therapist-directed hippotherapy rehabilitate children with cerebral palsy? *Developmental Medicine and Child Neurology, 49*(1), 68–73. doi: 10.1017/S0012162207000175.x

Sterba, J.A., Rogers, B.T., France, A., & Vokes, D.A. (2002). Horseback riding in children with cerebral palsy. *Developmental Medicine and Child Neurology, 44*(5), 301–308. doi: 10.1111/j.1469-8749.2002.tb00815.x

Tamse, T.R., Tillman, M.D., Stopka, C.B., Weimer, A.C., Abrams, G.L., & Issa, I.M. (2010). Supervised moderate intensity resistance exercise training improves strength in Special Olympic athletes. *Journal of Strength and Conditioning Research, 24,* 695–700.

Tassone, J.C., & Duey-Holtz, A. (2008). Spine concerns in the Special Olympian with Down syndrome. *Sports Medicine Arthroscopy, 16*(1), 55–60.

Todd, T., & Reid, G. (2006). Increasing physical activity in individuals with autism. *Focus on Autism and Other Developmental Disorders, 21*, 167–176.

Vaus, K. (2010). *Fetal alcohol syndrome.* Retrieved from http://emedicine.medscape.com/article/974016-overview

Vis, J.C., Duffels, M.G., Winter, M.M., Weijerman, M.E., Cobben, J.M., Jusiman, S.A., & Mulder, B.J. (2009). Down syndrome: A cardiovascular perspective. *Journal of Intellectual Disabilities Research, 53*(5), 419–425.

Wilson, P.E. (2002). Exercise and sports for children who have disabilities. *Physical Medicine and Rehabilitation Clinics of North America, 13*, 907–923.

Wrotniak, B.H., Epstein, L.H., Dorn, J.M., Jones, K.E., & Kondilis, V.A. (2006). The relationship between motor proficiency and physical activity in children. *Pediatrics, 118*(6), e e1758-e1765. doi:10.1542/peds.2006-0742

Wrotniak, B.H., Epstein, L.H., Dorn, J.M., Jones, K.E., & Kondilis, V.A. (2006). The relationship between motor proficiency and physical activity in children. *Pediatrics, 118*(6), e e1758–e1765. doi:10.1542/peds.2006-0742

Xiang, H., Stallones, L., Chen, G., Hostetler, S.G., & Kelleher, K. (2005). Nonfatal injuries among US children with disabling conditions. *American Journal Public Health, 95*(11), 1970–1975.

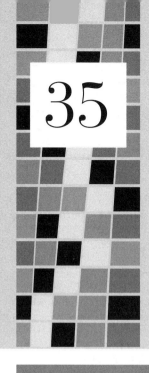

35 Oral Health Care

H. Barry Waldman, Steven P. Perlman, and George Acs

Upon completion of this chapter, the reader will

- Understand the causes of dental decay and periodontal disease and become familiar with preventive strategies and treatment
- Become aware of the special oral considerations for children with disabilities
- Appreciate the oral health needs during the transition to adulthood
- Know the needs of the medical-dental home

Providing services for individuals with intellectual/developmental disabilities includes the responsibility of community practitioners to give needed dental care. This is not always realized effectively, however, due to numerous factors. Limited training, experience, attitude, and interest of health care professionals combine to make one factor. Another factor sometimes limiting care is inadequate financial reimbursement for dental care professionals provided through the Medicaid program (Mansell et al., 2002; Waldman et al., 2001; see Chapter 41). Educators and clinicians also frequently lack knowledge about the dental needs of children with specific developmental disabilities. Such knowledge is important so they can advocate for care and prevent dental issues from interfering with learning activities. This chapter focuses on providing this information regarding dental needs of children with disabilities.

■ ■ ■ MAGGIE

Maggie is a 6-year-old girl with Down syndrome being examined by her pediatrician. She is accompanied by her parents, who have tried to prepare their daughter for this experience. However, Maggie gyrates her head and is distracted by bright lights and other stimuli in the pediatrician's office, and the clinician thus struggles to observe her face, lips, and tonsils. She concludes that everything appears to be "within normal limits." Unfortunately, all too often when it comes to the oral cavity, many pediatricians' examinations tend to be rather cursory, consisting of just a glance at the lips and throat. For most children this sort of examination would be routine and sufficient, but for children like Maggie, oral-examination procedures warrant special care and the gathering of more information than might be apparent to routine observations because of the specific risks for dental disease related to her Down syndrome.

ERUPTION OF TEETH

Although it is commonly said that the first primary tooth should erupt by 6 months of age, the age of eruption actually varies widely, with the first primary tooth coming anywhere between 4 and 17 months of age, while the full complement of primary teeth takes 2–3 years for complete eruption. The first permanent tooth typically emerges around 6 years of age, and most permanent teeth have erupted by 12–13 years of age. Third molars ("wisdom teeth") may erupt between 17–25 years of age.

When a permanent tooth erupts, a primary tooth is usually exfoliated. This does not occur with the first, second, and third molars, however, because they do not have primary teeth counterparts. As noted previously, tooth eruption tables should be evaluated cautiously, especially in children with developmental disabilities, as each child's growth and development is unique. Symmetry in eruption may be more important than development coinciding with a conventional time schedule. What occurs on the right side should occur within a few months on the left, and what occurs in the mandible should occur in the maxilla within a reasonable period of time.

PROBLEMS AFFECTING THE DEVELOPMENT OF TEETH

Many genetic syndromes associated with developmental disabilities may have characteristic developmental dental anomalies. These could include the presence of extra teeth, congenitally absent teeth, unusually shaped teeth, abnormalities in their mineralization, or delays in eruption. These abnormalities may contribute to malocclusion (i.e., an overbite) and/or to an increased risk for **dental caries** (decay; Poole & Redford-Badwal, 1991) and periodontal disease. **Anodontia** (the absence of all teeth) is rare, but **oligodontia** (the absence of one or several teeth) can be seen in children with a number of genetic syndromes including **Hallermann-Streiff syndrome**, **chondroectodermal dysplasia**, **Williams syndrome**, **Crouzon syndrome**, **achondroplasia**, **incontinentia pigmenti**, **ectodermal dysplasia**, and cleft lip and palate (see Appendix B). Disorders affecting development of teeth may also lead to enamel defects and abnormally shaped teeth or contribute to eruption difficulties as seen in **Cornelia de Lange syndrome**. Dentition anomalies also occur in children with chromosomal disorders such as Down syndrome, or in children with inborn errors of metabolism such as mucopolysaccharidoses, **Lesch-Nyhan syndrome**, and inherited disorders of bone formation such as **osteogenesis imperfecta**.

Environmental influences can also affect intrauterine tooth development. For example, nutritional deficiencies—especially of calcium; phosphorus; and vitamins A, C, and D—may result in generalized **enamel hypoplasia** (underdevelopment), resulting in defective mineralization of the teeth during their development.

Teeth developmental anomalies may also occur as a result of childhood illness or its treatment. For example, if a developing fetus or child between 4 months and 8 years of age is exposed to the antibiotic tetracycline, the primary or permanent teeth may have yellow, brown, or gray discoloration when they erupt. Traumatic injury to a tooth can cause a white or brown defect on a single tooth, whereas infectious diseases (e.g., measles, chickenpox) and chronic diseases (e.g., liver failure, congenital heart disease) can cause hypoplasia or defects in multiple teeth (Avery et al., 2004).

CONTRIBUTING FACTORS TO ORAL CONDITIONS OF INDIVIDUALS WITH DISABILITIES

It is essential to overcome the pervasive attitude that "children lose teeth anyway." While extraction is always one treatment to relieve discomfort (and is often the answer for children, whether with or without special needs), extraction is but one solution. Another approach is to emphasize the role of teeth in eating, speech, growth and development, and aesthetics. Children with or without special needs may not smile because of missing teeth, and missing teeth can negatively affect the child's physical, social, and psychological well-being as he or she develops. Various factors related to the individual child's disability, such as being able to articulate the source of oral pain, may make it more difficult to prevent, diagnose, and treat dental disease. The actual treatment may also differ because oral disease often presents at a later stage, and treatment must be adapted to the individual's physical and cognitive impairment. Therefore in examining the oral cavity in the child with a developmental disability, it is important to consider many factors.

Regurgitation

Regurgitation (rumination) is often seen in many individuals with moderate to profound intellectual disabilities. Swallowing of food, followed by regurgitation, may lead to acid reflux, indigestion, malnutrition, erosion of teeth, and possibly **gastroesophageal reflux disease** (GERD). Excessive drooling may be associated with regurgitation, pouching (accumulation of food between cheeks/lips and gums) or pocketing.

Physical Limitations

Physical limitations, as seen in cerebral palsy, for example, may affect individuals' ability to carry out personal care, including teeth brushing, rinsing, and flossing. In addition, involuntary movement may make treatment more difficult.

Prescription–Medication-Induced Decay

As the saying goes, "A little bit of sugar may help the medicine go down," but antibiotics, pain, seizure control and antihistamine medication with a high sugar concentration to mask the taste can prove to be an ideal medium for bacterial growth, acidic biofilm, and dental decay.

Altered Salivary Flow

Psychotropic medications will result in decreased salivary flow. This can cause **xerostomia** (dry mouth), salivary gland with retrograde infections, possible stone formation, and an increased rate of dental decay. In addition, reduced salivary flow is associated with increased burning/soreness of oral mucosal tissues, and with difficulty in chewing, speaking, and swallowing. These all can adversely affect food selection and dietary compliance.

"Placating" Tooth Decay

Fruit Roll-Ups, candy bars, and yes, pediatrician-dispensed lollipops may meet the immediate need to calm and soothe a child or serve as positive reinforcers for behavior, but combined with other factors, they may dramatically increase decay rates. Frequent intake of sugary snacks and sugar-coated cereals is also a potential source of tooth decay.

Fractured and Avulsed Teeth

Mutilated dentitions, particularly of anterior teeth, are often associated with poor ambulatory skills, a past history of trauma (accidental or nonaccidental as with seizures or physical abuse), pica, or self-injurious behavior. **Pica** may include chewing on hard, nonedible objects that tend to fracture teeth. Broken and/or discolored teeth can indicate potential infection and should be documented and treated. Dentists need to be aware also that the fracture of anterior teeth may be associated with physical abuse.

Soft Tissue Complications

Seizure medication (i.e., phenytoin) can cause hypertrophy or overgrowth of the gingival (gum) tissue. This can lead to difficulties in delayed exfoliation or eruption of primary and permanent teeth, masticatory and possible advanced periodontal problems.

Bruxism

This is the grinding of teeth and usually occurs while the individual is asleep. Continued grinding erodes tooth structure and may cause the need for restoration.

ORAL DISEASES

There are two basic types of oral disease: dental caries and periodontal disease. Both are usually initiated by specific bacteria and, therefore, can be considered infectious in nature. In general, they occur more commonly in children with disabilities than in their neurotypical peers.

Dental Caries

Dental caries, commonly called dental decay or cavities, occur in children and adolescents and is related to the presence of the bacteria *Streptococcus mutans* and *Lactobacillus acidophilus*. Tooth decay is a multifactorial process that involves the teeth themselves, bacteria, diet, saliva, biofilm, the immune system, biochemistry, and physiology. The "chain of decay" can be seen in Figure 35.1. Bacteria adhering to the teeth break down food, creating acid as a byproduct. The acid damages the integrity of the enamel, and cavitation begins. Tooth breakdown and possible abscess formation can occur when caries is left untreated over a period of time.

Bacteria adhere to the teeth in an organized mass called **dental plaque**. Plaque consists of bacteria, bacterial byproducts, **epithelial** cells (from the linings of the lips and mouth), and food particles (Pinkham, 2005). When plaque becomes calcified, it is called **calculus**, or tartar. Plaque, as well as unremoved tartar, can cause dental decalcification and decay, inflammation, tenderness, and swelling of the gums. This is an early phase of periodontal disease and can lead to loosening of the teeth. The process of decay

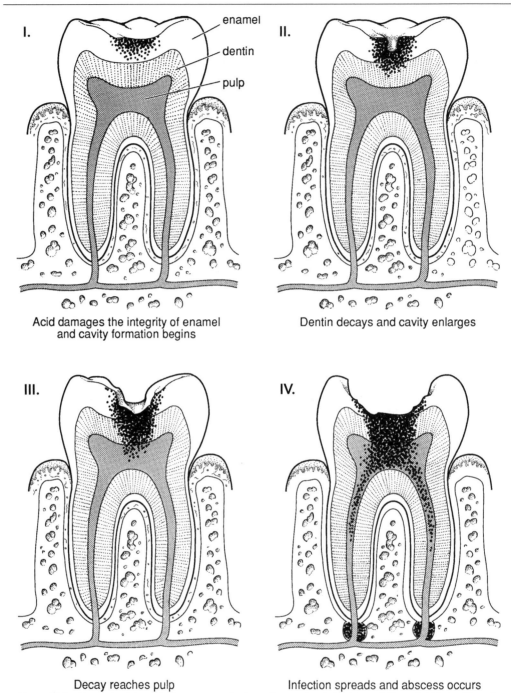

Figure 35.1. The chain of decay. In the presence of adverse factors, the chain of decay follows: Acid formed from the action of bacteria on carbohydrates damages the enamel, leading to cavity formation. If untreated, the decay eventually affects the dentin and pulp layer of the tooth and may lead to abscess formation.

is characterized by demineralization of enamel and dentin. The prevalence of dental caries has been cited in 42% of 2–11 year olds (National Health and Nutrition Examination Survey, 1999–2004).

For young children who are receiving carbohydrate-enriched diets to treat growth and development problems or who require chronic liquid medications that contain sugar, cavities may be rampant. Evidence suggests that the infant formula's impact on the development of early childhood caries depends on the specific properties of the formula. Until more definitive information is available, children should not be allowed to fall asleep with a nursing bottle containing any liquid other than water. The same principle applies to children who are breast-fed. Prolonged breast-feeding and falling asleep with the nipple in the mouth can also promote decay by acid demineralization. In addition, some cultures' practice of dipping pacifiers in sweetened solutions increases the risk of cavities.

In considering the role of bacteria in the tooth decay cycle, it is important to note that children acquire cavity-causing bacteria during the early phases of eruption of their first few teeth. They usually contract the bacteria from their primary caregiver. If that person has a high bacterial count or possesses bacteria that are more efficient in causing cavities, the child is at increased risk for future cavities. Parents can help reduce the risk of bacterial spread by themselves undergoing frequent dental cleanings and restoring carious teeth.

Periodontal Diseases

Periodontal diseases involve the gingiva and bony sockets of the teeth. Like caries, gingivitis (the most common and reversible form of periodontal disease) is associated with plaque and specific bacterial organisms (Matthewson & Primosch, 1995). The early signs of periodontal disease involve inflammation and bleeding of the gums, insidious processes whose true impact can go unrecognized for years. Advanced stages lead to loss of the alveolar bone that supports the tooth. Periodontal disease is caused by both local and systemic factors. Local factors can include dental crowding of teeth, poor oral hygiene, dry mouth, and destructive dental habits. Systemic factors include side effects of medications, hormonal alterations, and immune deficiency states. Although the exact etiology of this condition is unknown, the overgrowth is generally regarded as an exaggerated response to a local irritant. Overall, gingivitis can be found in up to half of children 4–5 years of age with disabilities (Pinkham, 2005). All too often, tooth extraction may be the inevitable solution in cases of advanced periodontal disease and extensive dental decay. Difficulties in patient behavior, the effects of the disability on teeth, and limited financial resources are some of the variables that may lead to the removal of the teeth of individuals with disabilities.

MALOCCLUSION

Malocclusion is the improper interdigitation or alignment of the teeth or jaws. It can interfere with oral functions such as speech and chewing and increase the risk of dental caries and periodontal diseases. In addition, it can create problems with facial appearance and self-image. Although most malocclusions are minor and require attention only for cosmetic reasons, others may be more severe and debilitating. The prevalence of severe malocclusion has been reported to be as high as 14% in children with disabilities; however, children with certain developmental disabilities, such as cerebral palsy, have an even higher prevalence (Avery et al., 2004). In these children, correcting malocclusion by orthodontic therapy to position the teeth properly can also ease routine oral hygiene and thus decrease the risk of dental disease.

PREVENTION OF DENTAL CARIES AND PERIODONTAL DISEASE

Perhaps the most important component of preventing dental decay begins even before a child's birth. Eliminating or reducing the transmission of cavity-causing bacteria from the mother to the child, particularly during the susceptible period of bacterial colonization as the first teeth are erupting, can have enormous benefits. Therefore, strategies such as the mother having routine professional dental cleanings, rinsing with the antimicrobial mouthwashes, or using xylitol containing products such as chewing gum or lozenges can suppress the number of cavity-forming bacteria that would ultimately be transmitted to the child (Soderling et al., 2000).

Once the child's teeth have erupted, the three most important factors in protecting the teeth from dental decay are 1) maintaining good oral hygiene, 2) limiting ingestion of carbohydrates, and 3) eliminating or reducing cavity-causing bacteria. Tools for preventive dentistry include brushing, flossing, fluoride intake, rinsing, and **dental sealants** when necessary for permanent teeth.

Brushing

Children younger than 6 years generally have not developed the manual dexterity to effectively remove plaque from their teeth. They should be encouraged to participate in their own oral hygiene; however, adults must take an active role and assume responsibility for adequately cleaning the teeth and gums. Individuals older than 6 with an intellectual disability may not understand how to take care of their own oral hygiene, and others with physical disabilities may not be able to accomplish it.

A soft, nylon bristle brush with polished, rounded ends works best. A scrubbing motion of the brush is nearly universal, and a power-assisted toothbrush can be helpful and may be advantageous for gingival health (Barnes, Weatherford, & Menaker, 1993). When brushing, a small, pea-sized amount of toothpaste with fluoride is best. If bubbles and foam from the paste cause a problem for the child or guardian performing the tooth brushing, an alternative to paste would be to use water or a fluoride-containing mouth rinse. Positioning the child in a supine (reclining) position facilitates good vision, access, and head control and will help the adult doing the brushing. The myriad of successful positions are as unique as the disability with which the child presents (Avery et al., 2004; Pinkham, 2005).

Flossing

Adults should floss for a child until he or she has demonstrated adequate dexterity to do the task, as improper flossing can harm gingival tissues. Flossing should be performed wherever teeth are in contact with each other as the toothbrush cannot clean in between the teeth. Unwaxed floss is preferred; however, any floss may be used. When dexterity or motor-coordination is a problem, floss-holding devices are available and can be used by parents and/or caregivers.

Fluoride

Whether present in the municipal water supply, taken as a daily supplement, found in toothpaste, contained in a mouth rinse, or professionally applied, fluoride treatment has been shown to significantly reduce the incidence of dental decay and is an integral part of a preventive program. Studies have demonstrated that fluoride in water can decrease the prevalence of tooth decay by up to 60% (Pinkham, 2005). Fluoride makes enamel more resistant to decay and remineralizes incipient carious lesions, making them hard again. Fluoride supplementation should be considered if fluoride is absent in the community drinking water or in the water where child care is provided. Although reverse osmosis home filtration does remove fluoride from water, other systems do not. Bottled water must disclose its fluoride content if fluoride has been added but not if it is naturally occurring. On the basis of the child's needs and abilities, specific fluoride supplements may be recommended. It should be noted that excessive systemic fluoride, however, could cause fluorosis, a condition in which permanent teeth are discolored or malformed.

Many different fluoride formulations are available, each with specifically indicated uses. For children who are capable of rinsing, low-potency over-the-counter fluoride rinses may be helpful in preventing cavities. In addition, some children may need prescribed fluoride rinses, varnish, pastes, or gels that contain higher concentrations of fluoride. Very often, these higher-concentrated products are provided to attempt to reverse the early stages of cavity formation. For patients at high risk for developing cavities, and for those for whom it may be difficult to apply daily fluoride supplements, professionally applied fluoride varnishes may help. Varnish applications may provide benefits for up to 3 months.

Dental Sealants

Sealants consist of a plastic coating that is bonded to the chewing surface of molars to prevent decay. Many children's permanent molars have deep grooves that are difficult to keep clean, but if warranted, the molars can be protected by the application of sealants. Sealants are most effective upon eruption when the molars can be isolated. Studies have shown that in the absence of sealants, two thirds of children will have a cavity on at least one of their first permanent molars (Pinkham, 2005).

Diet

Frequent feedings or snacking is common in children with poor weight gain (see Chapter 8). It also increases the total amount of time that teeth are exposed to foods or liquids that initiate the development of dental caries. To prevent caries, more frequent and intensive oral hygiene regimens are required. Similarly, children with neuromuscular disorders that result in decreased oral-motor abilities need an extended period of time to clear food from their mouths. The increased contact time between teeth and food, especially puréed carbohydrates, places these children at greater risk to develop cavities. Children with neurological impairments who have gastrostomy tubes often have poor oral hygiene and low salivary flow, which may result in greater frequency of aspiration pneumonia and significant build-up of calculus (Jawadi et al., 2004). Even for neurotypical children, the consistency, frequency, and timing of snacks contributes to the potential for decay. Snacks that are sticky (not just caramels but also foods such as sweet rolls) or oily (potato chips, fries), eaten frequently, and eaten between meals have a high potential for causing dental decay. Table

35.1 contains a list of snacks that do not compromise dental health.

PROVIDING DENTAL AND ORTHODONTIC TREATMENT

The American Academy of Pediatric Dentistry (AAPD) recommends that all children have their first dental visit by 12 months of age. At this time, parents or caregivers are educated about development issues that affect the teeth and are taught strategies to effectively prevent dental disease. The greatest benefits are derived when a combination of preventive dentistry techniques is recommended. Usually, very little if any treatment is necessary at this time (AADP, 2004–2005a).

In order to establish effective interaction among the patient, parents, medical professionals, and other health care professionals, the child's oral health needs are best served in a "dental home." The concept of a dental home is derived from the American Academy of Pediatrics' (AAP's) definition of a "medical home," which states that primary health care is best achieved when comprehensive, continuously accessible, family-centered, compassionate, and culturally effective care is delivered or supervised by qualified child health specialists (AAP, 2002). The AAPD supports the concept of a dental home for all infants, children, adolescents, and people with special health care needs (AAPD, 2004, 2005b). Family-centered care is an approach to planning, delivery, and evaluation of health care where the cornerstone is active participation between families and professionals. The patient-centered medical-dental home is modeled after this approach. Children who have a dental home are more likely to receive appropriate preventive and routine oral health care because of the ongoing monitoring they receive.

The first dental visit should be followed by regular checkups, at intervals depending on the child's risk for oral disease. During these checkups, an oral prophylaxis and topical fluoride application will be performed to help minimize the risk of caries and periodontal disease. If caries is present despite all preventive efforts, the dentist will treat this condition by removing the decay and placing a restorative material or a crown. The newer dental materials available today are able to offer combined advantages of good strength, aesthetics, and antimicrobial activity.

In terms of orthodontic care, the objectives are to realign the teeth using mechanotherapy (braces) and other techniques. Although malocclusion is the most common condition requiring orthodontic care, other aesthetic, functional, or periodontal considerations may pertain. Orthodontic care may be indicated in certain genetic syndromes associated with developmental dental abnormalities. For patients with Down syndrome, cerebral palsy, or cleft palate, for example, orthodontic therapy may be used to increase room for teeth, to shape the dental arches more appropriately, or to align teeth to fabricate a well-fitting appliance. In patients with poor oral hygiene or who have a history of high caries activity, however, deferring orthodontic treatment may be necessary until the patient improves oral hygiene or cooperation. This is necessary to protect against the development of new dental problems, which are more likely to occur if braces are worn for extended periods of time.

SPECIAL ISSUES REGARDING DENTAL CARE FOR CHILDREN WITH SPECIFIC DEVELOPMENTAL DISABILITIES

The basic principles of pediatric dental care and oral health apply to all children. There are, however, specific dental care issues related to several common developmental disabilities,

Table 35.1. Foods that are good to use as snacks to maintain dental health

Raw vegetables
  Carrot sticks
  Celery sticks
  Cauliflower bits
  Cucumber sticks
  Green pepper rings
  Lettuce wedges
  Radishes
  Tomatoes
Drinks
  Milk
  Sugar-free carbonated beverages
  Unsweetened vegetable juices
Other snacks
  Nuts
  Popcorn
  Unsweetened plain yogurt
  Unsweetened peanut butter
  Cheese
  Sugarless gum or candy

Source: American Dental Association (1983).

including Down syndrome, autism, cerebral palsy, meningomyelocele (spina bifida), and patients that have seizure.

Down Syndrome

In addition to having an intellectual disability, children with Down syndrome may have certain congenital anomalies such as a crowded dentition that place them at increased risk for oral disease. They often exhibit mid-face hypoplasia and can have extra (supernumerary), missing, or small teeth which can contribute to the development of malocclusion and periodontal disease (Cooley & Sanders, 1991). Their open-mouth posture with mouth breathing can lead to dry gum tissue. Congenital heart disease is also sometimes present, which places these children at increased risk for bacterial **endocarditis** (a severe infection of the inner lining of the heart chambers) that may require antibiotic prophylaxis prior to dental procedures.

Autism Spectrum Disorders

In autism, oral health needs are often dictated by the behavior or level of cooperation in prevention by a child with sensory integration issues, how the disorder manifests itself in the child's abilities to care for his or her own dental needs, the risk of self-injurious behavior to teeth, and the impact of restricted food preferences on dental health. Dental issues related to pica, bruxism, pocketing, and side effects of psychotropic and antiepileptic medication are of particular concern in these children. In addition, the often sugar-based food reinforcers that may be used in applied behavior analysis therapy (ABA; see Chapter 32) increase the risk of caries. Dental care in children with autism thus may require a number of strategies. Behavioral guidance approaches can prepare the child for visiting the dentist's office and can desensitize the child to preventive-practice difficulties. Limiting foods that generate caries should be a goal as well as using reinforcers that have lower carbohydrate content.

Cerebral Palsy

Poor motor control and altered muscles complicate routine dental care in children with cerebral palsy (see Chapter 24), who have specific and unique oral problems. A higher incidence of malocclusion is more likely as a consequence of the involuntary movements of the muscles of the jaws, lips, and tongue. Persistent tongue thrusting is a particular concern. As the tongue is a powerful muscle, it can reposition the teeth, leading to an anterior open bite and flared, widely spaced teeth. Poor motor control also results in a high incidence of uncontrolled drooling (Inga et al., 2001).

The predilection for falling due to gait problems, and the frequent protrusion of the maxillary incisors, also increase these children's risk for dental trauma. In addition, mouth breathing and bruxism are often present (Avery, Dean, & McDonald, 2004; Cooley & Sanders, 1991; Nowak, 1976). Furthermore, caries and periodontal disease appear more frequently because of problems in the oral clearing of food (pocketing) and difficulty in brushing and flossing. The soft, sticky, high-carbohydrate diet that may be needed to maintain adequate nutrition is also a problem. Despite receiving limited or no nutrition by mouth, children with cerebral palsy who are fed through gastrostomy tubes (see Chapter 9) are still susceptible to reflux of stomach acid as well as plaque and calculus buildup, placing them at increased risk for aspiration problems, dental caries, and periodontal disease.

A number of treatment approaches can help. Providing dental care in the child's wheelchair or using positioning supports such as pillows in the dental chair will allow the patient to be more comfortable. If brushing teeth after eating is not possible, wiping soft food debris from the mouth using a moistened face cloth or gauze pad provides benefits. In older children, an adapted toothbrush with handle modifications, an electric toothbrush, and floss holders can help maintain good oral hygiene. Involuntary movements and severe bruxism will often make restorative dentistry more difficult.

Meningomyelocele

Individuals with meningomyelocele have a caries rate similar to that found in the general population. As a result of compromised oral hygiene, however, they have a high level of periodontal disease. Because so many of these individuals have spinal curvatures and many individuals ambulate using a wheelchair, positioning and comfort are important in their dental care. The presence of hydrocephalus with a shunt may also bear on the child's dental treatment; individuals with ventricular shunts may require antibiotic prophylaxis prior to dental procedures. Also, individuals with meningomyelocele have an increased risk of developing an allergic reaction to latex (Engibous, Kittle, & Jones, 1993).

Seizure Disorders

In children with seizure disorders, the major issues are side effects from certain antiepileptic drugs (see Chapter 29), as discussed previously, and from dental trauma. Approximately half of the children receiving the antiepileptic drug phenytoin, and occasionally those receiving phenobarbital (Luminal), develop overgrown gingiva. Eliminating the medication may begin to reverse the condition, but the child may require surgical removal of the overgrown tissue. Fortunately these drugs have been largely replaced by newer antiepileptic medications that do not cause these side effects. In children with poorly controlled generalized tonic–clonic seizures, the use of a helmet throughout the day to reduce risk of dental trauma from falls may be appropriate until seizure control is achieved (Avery et al., 2004; Cooley & Sanders, 1991; Nowak, 1976).

THE CHALLENGE OF PROVIDING DENTAL SERVICES TO INDIVIDUALS WITH DISABILITIES

As of the time of this publication, no nationwide study has been conducted to determine the prevalence of dental disease or the availability of dental services among the adult populations with disabilities in the USA. As for children, the report from the *National Study of Children with Special Health Care Needs* highlighted the finding that "the service most commonly reported as needed but not received was dental care" [sic] (U.S. Department of Health and Human Behavior, 2007). Numerous local and regional reports, however, provide a general appreciation of the needs (Dao et al., 2005; Lewis et al, 2005; Ngui & Flores, 2007; Waldman & Perlman, 2006; White, 2002).

While dentistry for children was elective under the SCHIP legislation (see Chapter 41), most state programs included dental services. In 2007, the reenactment of SCHIP as the Children's Health Insurance Program (CHIP) mandated the inclusion of dental services for all children up to age 19 who are eligible in a particular state. The reality is that the Medicaid/CHIP programs provide a critical funding source for needed medical and dental services for youngsters with disabilities (Centers for Medicare and Medicaid Services, 2010b; Edelstein, 2009). Unfortunately, the reimbursement to practitioners providing this service is low and many dentists have opted out of accepting patients with this insurance.

The 2006 National Survey of Children with Special Health Care Needs (CSHCN) reported that over 81% of CSHCN were in need of routine preventive dental care and 24% needed other dental care in the past twelve months. Preventive dental care was second only to prescription medication in the frequency of needs. Overall, almost 580,000, or 9% of CSHCN who needed dental care, were unable to obtain it. Lewis (2009) noted that "dental care was the most common unmet need of CSHCN… a (statistically) significant higher proportion of CSHCN relative to children without special health care needs." In particular, 10% of teenagers with special health care needs from 13–17 (who are approaching the end of their Medicaid/CHIP eligibility years) had unmet dental care needs (Lewis, 2009).

Whether due to the financial and bureaucratic limitations of the Medicaid/CHIP programs or other factors, the reality is that general and specialist practitioners are providing only limited oral health services for children and adults with disabilities and a wide range of special needs. The facts are 1) many children, due to passing the allowed age, are out of programs that provide support for oral health care and into a virtual financial-assistance void in most states; and 2) only 10% of general dentists report that they treat children with cerebral palsy, intellectual disabilities, or medically compromising conditions often or very often (Casamassimo, 2004).

Another issue is competency to provide the services required. In the past, dental students received little to no educational experiences in caring for children and adults with disabilities. Recent changes in dental school accreditation require creating new learning experiences to prepare them to care for individuals with special needs who increasingly reside in the general community. The unresolved issue is the fact that adult Medicaid programs in many states are limited to relief of pain and infection—even for adults with disabilities. In essence, youngsters with special needs are aging out of dentistry (Waldman & Perlman).

It should also be noted that the costs of dental services are far higher than the costs of other health services for individuals with (and without) special health care needs. For families with limited financial means this may result in their seeking less dental care. In 2009, private insurance accounted for 48% of expenditures for dentist and physician services and 35% of hospital costs. By contrast, out-of-pocket payments represented 44% spending for dentist,

10% of physician and 3% of hospital expenditures. Government spending represented 8% of dental, 36% of physician, and 58% of hospital expenditures. Despite the recent enactment of national health legislation, limited changes in the comparative sources of funding are anticipated during the 2010s (Centers for Medicare and Medicaid Services, 2009). As a result of limited government support and the inability of private insurance to compensate for the void, particularly for youngsters and adults with the complications of special health needs, dental costs often are "felt" to a greater extent than the proportional total higher costs for medical services.

SUMMARY

Oral health is an important component of overall health. It contributes to wellness of the child, eliminates pain and discomfort, and enhances quality of life. Furthermore, good oral health maximizes healthy nutrition, speech, and appearance. The emphasis in oral care for the child with a developmental disability should be the same as the neurotypical developing child: prevention through home dental care and regular office checkups in the dental home.

REFERENCES

Casamassimo, P.S., Seale, N.S., & Ruchs, K. (2004). General practitioners' perceptions of educational and treatment issues affecting access to care for children with health care need. *Journal of Dental Education, 68,* 23–28.

Centers for Disease Control and Prevention. (2008a). *Adverse childhood experiences study: Welcome.* Retrieved from mhtml:file://F:ACE%20Study%20-%20Adverse%20Childhood%20Experiences.mht.

Centers for Disease Control and Prevention. (2008b). *Adverse childhood experiences study: Major findings.* Retrieved from http://www.cdc.gov/nccdphp/ACE/findings.htm.

Centers for Medicare and Medicaid Services, Office of the Actuary. (2010). *National heath expenditure projections 2009–2019.* Retrieved from http://www.cms.hhs.gov/NationalHealthExpendData/downloads/proj2009.pdf.

Centers for Medicare and Medicaid Services. (2010a). *Medicaid early periodic screening.* Retrieved from http://www4.cms.gov/MedicaidEarlyPeriodicScrn/01_Overview.asp#TopOfPage.

Centers for Medicare and Medicaid Services. (2010b). *CHIP dental coverage.* Retrieved from http://www.1.cms.gov/CHIPDentalCoverage.

Cornell University. (2008). *Disability status report: United States.* Retrieved from http://disabiltystatistics.org.

Dao, L.P., Zwetchkenbaum, S., Inglehart, M.R. (2005). General dentists and special needs patients: Does dental education matter. *Journal of Dental Education, 69,* 1107–15.

Edelstein, B.L. (2009). Putting teeth in CHIP: 1997-2009 retrospective of Congressional action on children's oral health. *Academic Pediatrics, 9,* 467–75.

Gastroesophageal Reflux Disease (GERD). (2010). Retrieved from http://www.medicinenet.com/gastroesophageal_reflux_disease_gerd/page3.htm. Retrieved November 22, 2010

Kaiser Family Foundation. (2010a). *Medicaid/CHIP.* Retrieved from http://www.kff.org/medicaid. Retrieved April 13, 2010.

Kaiser Family Foundation. (2010b). *Focus on health report.* Medicaid and Children's Health Insurance Program provisions in the new health reform law. Retrieved from http://www.kff.org/. Retrieved April 13, 2010.

Kozol, J. (1999). *Savage inequalities: Children in America's schools.* New York, NY: Harper Perennials.

Lewis, C., Robertson, A.S., & Phelps, S. (2005). Unmet dental care needs among children with special health care needs: Implications for the medical home. *Pediatrics, 116,* e426–e31.

Lewis, C.W. (2009). Dental care and children with special health care needs: A population-based perspective. *Academic Pediatrics, 9,* 420–6.

Mansell, J., Ashman, B., Macdonald, S., & Beadle-Brown, J. (2002). Residential care in the community for adults with intellectual disabilities: Needs, characteristics and services. *Journal of Intellectual Disability Research, 46,* 625–33.

Maternal and Child Health Bureau. (2007). *The national survey of children with special health care needs chartbook 2005–2006.* Rockville, MD: US Department of Health and Human Services.

Ngui, E.M., & Flores, G. (2007). Unmet needs for specialty, dental, mental, and allied health care among children with special health care needs: Are there racial/ethnic disparities? *Journal of Health Care for the Poor and Underserved, 18,* 931–49.

U.S. Census Bureau. (2010). *Statistical Abstract of the United States.* Retrieved from http://www.census.gov/compendia/statab/2010/tables/10s0010.pdf.

U.S. Department of Health and Human Services. (2007). *The national survey of children with special health care needs, chart book, 2005–2006.* Rockville, MD: US Department of Health and Human Services.

Waldman, H.B., & Perlman, S.P. (2000). Deinstitutionalization of children with mental retardation: What of dental services? *Journal of Dentistry for Children, 67,* 413–417

Waldman, H.B., & Perlman, S.P. (2005). Abuse of children with disabilities. *Environmental Protection Magazine, 35*(6), 63–68.

Waldman, H.B., & Perlman, S.P. (2006). California community residential facilities for individuals with intellectual and developmental disabilities. *Journal of the California Dental Association, 34,* 235–238.

Waldman, H.B., & Perlman, S.P. (2006). Dental needs assessment and access to care for adolescents. *Dental Clinics of North America, 50,* 1–16.

Waldman, H.B., Perlman, S.P., & Swerdloff M. (2001). Children with mental retardation/developmental disabilities: Do physicians ever consider needed dental care? *Mental Retardation, 39,* 53–56.

White, P.H. (2002). Access to health care: Health insurance considerations for young adults with special health care needs/disabilities. *Pediatrics, 110,* 1328–35.

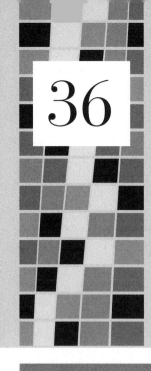

36 Assistive Technology

Larry W. Desch

Upon completion of this chapter, the reader will

■ Know the definitions of *assistive technology* and *medical assistive technology*

■ Be aware of the major types of both rehabilitative and medical assistive technology and know examples of each

■ Understand the types of conditions that frequently create a need for assistive technology.

■ Understand the basics of assessment for, acquisition of, and training for assistive technology including the principles of "universal design"

■ Be aware of issues regarding funding for assistive technology including the definition of Durable Medical Equipment (DME) and the limitations that are often put on the purchase of DME by insurance companies and other third parties.

The goal of this chapter is to provide necessary information about the major categories of currently available rehabilitative and medical technology assistance and the process for evaluating their use and effectiveness. This chapter does not address complementary, or alternative, therapies—for example, devices using unproven or disproven methodologies, such as colored lenses for treatment of dyslexia (AAP-Section on Opthalmology & Council on Children with Disabilities et al., 2009; see Chapter 38). The devices discussed in this chapter have at least some basic empirical or scientific evidence to document their effectiveness. The chapter also focuses on "mid-tech" and "high-tech" devices; many "low-tech" devices are discussed in Chapter 33.

■ ■ ■ **JEFFREY**

Jeffrey is a 10-year-old boy who, according to his mother, "has come a long way" but had a "rough beginning" to his life. Jeffrey was born 6 weeks premature and had severe hyperbilirubinemia (jaundice) due to blood group incompatibility. He spent more than a month in the neonatal intensive care unit. Jeffrey had occasional episodes of **apnea** and **bradycardia** (periodic breathing arrests accompanied by low heart rate) and was sent home on a cardiorespiratory monitor. At 6 months of age, he had severe gastroesophageal reflux (GER) that led to placement of a gastrojejunal tube. This required Jeffrey's parents to learn how to use a feeding

641

pump that would give him formula over several hours. After 2 months the manner of feeding shifted to oral, and by one year he seemed to be doing fairly well with feeding and in most other areas. At 16 months, however, he often would rock back and forth "for no reason" and his language development was delayed. Soon thereafter, Jeffrey was referred to early intervention, had an extensive evaluation by a team of developmental specialists, and was found to have an **autism spectrum disorder** (ASD). Despite intensive speech-language therapy for 9 months Jeffrey did not develop much speech and exhibited increasing frustration because of his communication difficulties. Jeffrey's speech therapist recommended, initially, a simple picture-based card system and, later, a computerized speech-generating device for Jeffrey. After nearly a year of negotiating with their insurance company and with Jeffrey's school, his parents were finally able to purchase the device. Jeffrey gradually became less irritable and after 6 months of using the speech-generating device he was beginning to say some words himself.

DEFINITIONS AND OVERVIEW

Many children with disabilities are able to function more independently, have increased opportunities, and have improved access to the world through the use of assistive, adaptive (alternative), or augmentative devices. Although definitions for these types of devices vary, there seems to be some consensus emerging (Alper & Raharinirina, 2006; Beukelman & Mirenda, 2005; Desch & Gaebler-Spira, 2008). **Assistive devices** are those that help alleviate the impact of a disability, thus reducing the functional limitations (e.g., tape-recorded lessons for students with a specific reading disability; Alper & Raharinirina, 2006). **Adaptive**, sometimes called **"alternative," technology** substitutes or makes up for the loss of function brought on by a disability (e.g., a sophisticated robotic feeding device providing more independence for people with severe spastic quadriplegia; Desch & Gaebler-Spira, 2008). **Augmentative devices** increase an area of functioning that is deficient, sometimes severely, but for which there are some residual abilities (e.g., a microchip-powered voice output augmentative device for a person with dysarthria; Beukelman & Mirenda, 2005). The term *augmentative devices* currently only refers to devices used to improve

communication. In this chapter, the term **assistive technology** is used to encompass all of these terms. The chapter uses this general term for medical devices as well. **Medical assistive technology** refers to that subset of assistive technology that is used for primarily medical or life-sustaining reasons (e.g., ventilators, feeding pumps). These devices also improve functioning but perhaps in more basic ways. Medical assistive devices are the only type of assistive technology which are regulated by a division of the FDA that deals with medical devices (http://www.fda.gov/MedicalDevices/default.htm).

There are also legal definitions for "assistive technology" described in laws of the United States. Although it is beyond the scope of this chapter to go into detail about these laws, Sadao and Robinson's book (2010, pp. 9–23) provides an excellent summary. The most recent update of special education law (Individuals with Disabilities Education Act [IDEA] of 2004) has defined assistive technological devices as "any item, piece of equipment, or product system, whether acquired commercially, off-the-shelf, modified or customized, that is used to increase, maintain, or improve the functional capabilities of a child with a disability. The term does not include a medical device that is surgically implanted, or the replacement of such a device" (IDEA, 2004, C.F.R. § 300.5).

For many years, assistive technology has often been thought of as referring only to devices containing microcomputers or other electronics (Desch, 1986). Although such complicated devices may be the only solution for a particular disability-related problem, they represent the higher end of the spectrum of assistive technology that includes low-tech, mid-tech, and high-tech categories and everything in between (Desch, 2008). Many people, even professionals working with children with disabilities, do not realize that they may themselves be using assistive technology on a daily basis. For example, a foam or rubber cushion placed over a pencil or pen to help with one's grip and prevent writer's cramp is a low-tech assistive device. However, the use of assistive technology is usually reserved for people with considerably more loss of function due to disability.

Table 36.1 provides examples of assistive devices. Some items on the table are **low-tech** assistive technology—that is, those using low-cost materials and not requiring batteries or other electric sources to operate. Examples include wheelchair ramps, gastrostomy

Table 36.1. Examples of available assistive devices

Area of disability	Types of technology		
	Low-tech	Mid-tech	High-tech
Physical	Swivel spoon (and other feeding aids)	Reciprocating gait orthoses	Electronically controlled wheelchairs
	Wheelchair ramps	Lightweight wheelchairs	Environmental control units
	Adapted playgrounds	Adapted toys	Robotic devices
	Most orthotics		Functional electric stimulation
	Grips for pencils		Voice-input and eye-gaze-input devices
Communication	Simple picture/word boards	On/off light for yes/no responses	Adapted laptops
	Eye-gaze picture boards	One to multiple digital message recorders	Commercial computerized speech generating devices (e.g. TouchTalker)
	Visual schedule/planner	Scanning light board	
Sensory	Magnifying lenses	Alerting systems (to movement/sound)	Digital hearing aids
	Large-print books	Braille typewriters	Cochlear implants
	Books on tape	FM transmitting	Kurzweil 1000 voice-output scanner
Learning	Color-coded notebooks	Talking calculators	Problem-solving software
	Post-it™ tags	Electronic spelling/dictionary	Hypertext learning programs
	Flash-cards	Tape recorders	Software for cognitive/attention rehabilitation
	Visual schedule/planner	Books on tape	
Medical assistance	Nasogastric tubes	Oxygen systems	Home ventilators
	Bladder catheters	Gastrostomy tubes	Oxygen monitors
		Indwelling intravenous tubes	Apnea monitors
			Dialysis machines

feeding tubes, and printed picture communication boards. **Mid-tech assistive technology** generally requires battery/electrical power or is more complex in its use; for example, **teletypewriter** (TTY) devices for those who are deaf, home-infusion pumps, suction machines, and sophisticated manual wheelchairs. Finally, **high-tech assistive technology** is more complicated and often expensive to own and maintain. Examples include microcomputer-enabled voice-output devices, home ventilators, cochlear implants, electronic wheelchairs, and even a robotic arm controlled by a microchip implanted into the brain (the latter recently developed by a division of the Pentagon).

Assistive devices are acquired in one of three ways: 1) direct purchase from a commercial supplier; 2) development of a custom-made device (these can be simple, handmade devices or complex, one-of-a-kind devices made by an engineer or technician for use by one person); or 3) modification of an existing device such as a desktop computer, laptop computer, or telephone (these modifications can also be commercially available

items). Some of these modified devices are constructed at rehabilitation centers at a high cost. However, the availability of microprocessing technology has increased such that the purchase of commercial devices or commercial modifications to devices is becoming the most common way to acquire even the most complex, high-tech assistive devices. Where assistive devices can be obtained also varies, from public schools and therapy providers to large university or private rehabilitation centers. Most assistive devices, excluding the medical assistive devices, can be obtained without prescriptions from physicians (but doing so usually precludes their purchase using insurance or other third party medical-related funding).

TECHNOLOGY FOR MEDICAL ASSISTANCE

The Office of Technology Assessment (OTA) defined a child who receives medical technology assistance as one "who requires a mechanical device and substantial daily skilled nursing care to avert death or further disability" (OTA, 1987, p. 8). These medical devices replace or augment a vital body function and include **respiratory technology assistance** (e.g., nasal cannulae for oxygen supplementation, mechanical ventilators, positive airway pressure devices, artificial airways such as tracheotomy tubes), monitoring and **surveillance devices** (e.g., cardiorespiratory monitors, pulse oximeters), **nutritive assistive devices** (e.g., nasogastric or gastrostomy feeding tubes), equipment for **intravenous (IV) therapy** (e.g., parenteral nutrition, medication infusion), devices to augment or protect kidney function (e.g., dialysis, urethral catheterization), and ostomies (artificial openings for feeding or for the elimination of bodily wastes; e.g., gastrostomy urostomy or colostomy). The use of medical technology assistance by infants and children is fortunately uncommon and most of these uses are temporary (e.g., premature infants on apnea monitors or home IV use). However a recent study found that about 20% of children admitted to a tertiary hospital are dependent on technological devices (Feudtner et al., 2005).

In a 1987–1990 survey of children in Massachusetts who are dependent on technology, more than half (57%) had neurological deficits, and 13% had multisystem involvement (Palfrey et al., 1994). Since then, the incidence of technological dependency does appear to be increasing especially in children younger than 3 years of age, primarily as a result of improved survival of very low birth weight infants which leads to increases in "chronic illness" (Wise, 2007). The types of medical assistive devices that are required in a number of these chronic illnesses are described next (see Table 36.1 for examples).

Respiratory Support

Infants and children who require respiratory support most often fall into one of two categories: 1) those with lung or heart problems, and 2) those with problems with neurological control of breathing and/or weakness of the muscles used to control breathing. As an example of the first category, severe damage to the lungs related to prematurity, called **bronchopulmonary dysplasia**, can lead to the prolonged need for supplemental oxygen (Bass et al., 2004; see Chapter 7). Another example is the child with **spastic quadriplegic cerebral palsy** who may develop a **severe scoliosis** (curvature of the spine), leading to rib cage distortion and stiffness (see Chapter 13). This chest wall abnormality can decrease respiratory muscle power and lung function necessitating supplemental oxygen. An example of the second category is neuromuscular disorders, including **Duchenne muscular dystrophy** and **spinal muscular atrophy** (Bush et al., 2005; Gilgoff et al., 2003; see Chapter 20).

Children who have chronic respiratory failure require medical technology assistance to maintain normal blood oxygen levels, prevent additional lung injury from recurrent infections, and promote optimal growth and development. These goals usually can be accomplished via a combination of oxygen supplementation, **continuous positive airway pressure** (CPAP), **chest physiotherapy** (CPT), suctioning, and medications (e.g., bronchodilators). When these treatments are ineffective or insufficient, however, mechanical ventilation and **tracheostomy** tube placement are considered. Equipment for monitoring the child's cardiorespiratory status may also be required (e.g., heart rate and blood oxygen monitors).

Oxygen is the single most effective agent in treating the infant or child with chronic lung disease, and supplemental oxygen may be required for months or even years. Oxygen can be administered by **nasal cannulae** (plastic prongs placed in the nose and connected to a tube that delivers an oxygen/air mixture), facemask, oxygen tent or hood, or an artificial airway (i.e., tracheostomy).

For the child with mild respiratory failure or obstructive sleep apnea, CPAP may be employed (Downey, Perkin, & MacQuarrie, 2000). CPAP can be applied to the child's natural airway (via a tight-fitting mask or nasal pillows/cannulae). For more severe conditions CPAP can be given long-term through a tracheostomy tube (Tibballs et al., 2010). If a child is on a mechanical ventilator, positive pressure can be administered between mechanical breaths, in which case the technique is referred to as **positive end expiratory pressure** (PEEP).

Children with respiratory or oral-motor problems also may produce excessive secretions (e.g., saliva) and/or be unable to cough effectively. **Chest physiotherapy** (CPT) and suctioning, which can be taught to all caregivers, help clear pulmonary secretions (Krause & Hoehn, 2000). CPT involves the repetitive manual percussion of the chest wall using cupped hands. For infants, this often involves using a vibrator. Secretions are loosened and can then be cleared by coughing or, in children with tracheostomies, by suctioning. Typically, supplemental oxygen is administered before and after suctioning to prevent hypoxia from occurring during the procedure (Flenady & Gray, 2000). Suctioning and CPT are done in response to need, which can mean several times a day. The newest modality for CPT is the use of an automatic device, the high-frequency chest compression vest. A number of recent studies attest to its effectiveness, especially in people who have cystic fibrosis (Davidson, 2002; Dosman & Jones, 2005).

A tracheostomy involves inserting a plastic tube through a surgically created incision in the trachea cartilage, just below the Adam's apple. It is secured around the neck with foam-padded strings. This open airway can then be attached to a mechanical ventilator or to a CPAP device with tubing that provides humidified air or an air/oxygen mixture. If ventilatory support or oxygen is not needed, then a humidifying device (an "artificial nose") is attached to the tracheostomy tube. A **speaking valve** (e.g., Passey-Muir valve) often is used with the tracheostomy tube to increase air through the vocal cords to allow phonation. The tracheostomy tube also allows the caregiver to have direct access to the airway, permitting suctioning of secretions or removal of other blockages. Children who have tracheostomies may spend part or all of their day connected to a mechanical ventilator that augments or replaces their own respiratory efforts (Edwards, O'Toole, & Wallis, 2004).

Monitoring and Surveillance Devices

Children with disorders that affect the heart or lungs are likely to require monitoring or surveillance devices. Although these instruments provide no direct therapeutic benefit, they warn early of potential problems and thereby improve care indirectly. The two most common types of electronic surveillance devices are pulse **oximeters** and **cardiorespiratory monitors**. They can be used individually or in combination in the hospital and at home.

To avoid giving too much or too little oxygen, oxygen saturation (the oxygen-carrying capacity of red blood cells) can be monitored using a device called a **pulse oximeter**. The pulse oximeter measures oxygen saturation in the arterial blood, using a probe that is attached with a special tape to one of the child's fingers or toes (Nadkarni, Shah, & Deshmukh, 2000). An alarm can be set to sound below a certain oxygen saturation level. This most commonly occurs when there is low oxygen delivery (e.g., kinked tubing, low oxygen level in the oxygen tank) or a change in the child's condition (e.g., an increased need for supplemental oxygen because of a respiratory infection). Because this device records how well oxygen is being delivered to vital organs, it is an important monitor; unfortunately, it is quite susceptible to false alarms resulting from probe displacement, movement of the extremity, or electrical interference.

A cardiorespiratory monitor has electrodes pasted to the child's chest to record heart and respiratory rate (Silvestri et al., 2005). An alarm is part of the system and is set off by rates that are either too high or too low. If the alarm sounds, the caregiver should examine the child's respiratory, cardiovascular, and neurological status. Like the oximeter, the cardiorespiratory monitor can produce false alarms, most commonly resulting from inadvertent detachment of the chest leads. In the very rare event that the alarm sounds because of a **cardiorespiratory arrest** (i.e., slowing or stopping of breathing and/or heart rate), **cardiopulmonary resuscitation** (CPR) and possibly the use of an **automated external defibrillator** (AED) must be instituted immediately.

Nutritional/ Gastrointestinal Fluid Assistance

Children with cerebral palsy and other chronic neurological conditions are often limited in their ability to take in nutrition by mouth. Despite often needing increased food intake as a result of their motor-control problems (e.g., dyskinesia), these children may be unable to ingest even a normal intake because of **oral-motor impairments**, gastroesophageal reflux (GER), or food refusal. In these instances, nutritional assistance devices may prove helpful. Tube feedings can be provided in a number of ways. The tube can be temporarily inserted into one nostril and passed into the stomach (**nasogastric [NG] tube**) or the second part of the intestine (**nasojejeunal tube**). When long-term feedings are required, a permanent tube can be placed directly through the skin and into the stomach (**gastrostomy [G] tube**) or intestine (**jejunostomy [J] tube**). A G-J tube combines a G tube and a J tube. The J tube portion travels through the stomach, the duodenum, and into the jejunum to prevent reflux of nutrients. If the child has GER, the intervention of choice may be the combination of a surgical antireflux procedure (e.g., fundoplication by open or laparoscopic route; see Chapter 9) and insertion of a G tube or G-J tube. Once the feeding tube is inserted, nutrition can be provided by using a commercially available formula, such as Jevity or Pediasure or foods from the family's meals that have been puréed along with fluids.

Intravenous Fluid Assistive Devices

Long-term IV therapy (months to years), generally provided through a central venous line, is most often used to provide nutrition and/or to administer medication (McInally, 2005). Total parenteral nutrition involves providing a high-calorie, high-protein solution directly into the bloodstream by intravenous administration. Prolonged intravenous access may also be needed to provide antibiotics (e.g., when a child has osteomyelitis, a deep bone infection) or for cancer chemotherapy. In these situations, a catheter (often called a central line, Hickman, or Broviac line) may be tunneled into a deep vein under radiological guidance and advanced to a more central position, near the heart. This type of catheter averts the need for repeated placement of peripheral venous lines. In addition, a central venous catheter allows the child to receive medication and/or nutrition at home rather than having to remain in the hospital. Central lines are more stable than peripheral lines and can be maintained for months or years, provided that child and caregivers strictly adhere to sterile techniques and proper care. For a medical need of a few week to months, a peripherally inserted central catheter (PICC) can be used (e.g., for short-term parenteral nutrition), and for longer-term but intermittent use (e.g., chemotherapy) a subcutaneous infusion port can be used (e.g., Mediport). Both of these catheters, however, can limit a child's movement considerably, and the subcutaneous port site needs to be prepared before use with a local anesthetic to lessen the pain of the needle insertion. However, the subcutaneous port greatly decreases the risk of site infections.

ASSISTIVE TECHNOLOGY FOR DISABILITIES— PRINCIPLES AND EXAMPLES

The past three decades have seen increasing emphasis on ways to enable children (and adults) who have disabilities to improve their functioning and participation in various activities (e.g., mobility, communication). An important methodology for assistive technology which has been actively promoted and validated is the principles of "universal design."

Universal design is defined as "the design of products and environments to be usable by all people, to the greatest extent possible, without the need for adaption or specialized design" (Center for Universal Design, accessed 3/2/12 at http://www.ncsu.edu/project/design-projects/udi/center-for-universal-design/the-principles-of-universal-design/). A common example of this is wheelchair ramps. Although originally conceived with wheelchair users in mind, anyone can use these ramps including harried parents pushing child strollers through theme parks. The exponential increase in technology has accelerated the pace of universal design and most high-tech companies have discovered the profitability of making devices suitable for the largest number of people (e.g., touch screens on tablet computers). Table 36.2 lists some other principles that have been supported by research, as defined by Sadao and Robinson (2010). Additional principles will be discussed later as they pertain more to specific types of disabilities or the assessment process.

Table 36.2. Principles for assistive technology (AT) device use with children

1. Families are involved in selecting, developing and implementing AT devices for children.
2. AT devices should be an integral part of the child's daily routines across the home, child care, school, and other settings.
3. AT devices should be easy to use and adaptable to all of the environments of the child and family.
4. Families are always able to obtain needed AT from providers or a lending library and receive directions for using the device or an activity.
5. AT assessment and interventions are always done using an interdisciplinary team-based manner with the family and child (if possible) being integral members of the decision-making team.
6. AT should be a consideration for every child during the development of the IFSP or IEP in the schools.
7. AT should always be seen as a tool to foster increased learning, functioning and independence.
8. Families and professionals should have access to ongoing opportunities for training to increase knowledge and understanding of AT use and benefits.
9. Families and professionals should have adequate knowledge about funding sources for AT devices and for the training needed for these devices.

Source: Sadao and Robinson (2010).
Key: IFSP, individualized family service plan; IEP, individualized education program.

Technology for Physical Disabilities

Children with cerebral palsy or neuromuscular disorders commonly use assistive technology, especially low-tech devices such as **ankle-foot orthoses**, **hand splints**, and **spinal braces** (see Chapters 24 and 25). Mid-tech devices include **functional electrical stimulators** (FES), which provide neural stimulation to increase mobility; treadmills with support frames to increase strength even in nonambulatory people; and dynamic braces for treatment of a hemiplegic arm (see Chapter 24). Personal computers, with the appropriate adaptations, can be very useful high-tech tools for people with physical disabilities. Transparent modifications to a computer can be made using add-on equipment and/or specialized software programs. These modifications permit most commercially available software programs (including computer games, word-processing programs, and instructional programs) to be used. Transparent modifications do not modify or interfere with either the computer or the standard software program. An example is the keyboard emulator, which is often a device such as a joystick that replaces the keyboard (Keates & Robinson, 1999). Keyboard emulators function by taking the output from a special keyboard or input device, altering it, and then translating the original signal into a different format that the computer interprets as coming from its own keyboard. Another keyboard emulator is the popular, affordable speech recognition systems, such as those known under the Dragon name, where a keyboard is not necessary (especially useful to those persons with no ability to control hands or fingers). More information about these and related devices and vendors is available from websites such as http://www.abledata.org and http://www.closingthegap.com.

In addition to multiple-use devices such as computers, many single-application devices have been designed or adapted for people with physical disabilities. Examples range from relatively simple mid-tech feeding devices to elaborate high-tech environmental control units that can turn lights and appliances on and off and can dial a telephone (See Table 36.1).

Technology for Sensory Impairments

People with sensory impairments have been helped in many ways by assistive devices. For people with visual impairments there are low-tech magnification devices and mid-tech aids such as alerting systems, laser canes, taped books or hand-held digital text-to-speech systems.

Many high-tech devices such as personal computers or e-book readers that allow extra-large type on video screens often with one-touch page-turning (helpful for those with physical limitations), have been truly life-changing. All microcomputers being made today (e.g., e-book readers like Kindle, tablets like iPads) have built-in, easily accessible ways to increase the size of the typeface on the screen or to allow for screen text-to-speech (including reading off rows and columns, such as with spreadsheets). This is another example of using the principles of universal design.

Various devices using electronic technology have also been developed for people who are blind. These include the Kurzweil 3000 reading machine that translates printed words to voice-synthesized output and refreshable braille displays (e.g., ALVA Satellite) that provide an alternative access in the form of braille to the text or content displayed on a computer monitor. See Chapter 11 for more information on assistive technology for people with visual impairments.

Since the mid-1980s, there has been an explosion in the complexity and efficacy of hearing aids for people with hearing impairment. Digital programmable hearing aids were one device to emerge, allowing improved customization for an individual's specific degree and range of hearing loss. Many mid-tech solutions are also available—for example, assistive listening devices (infrared or FM transmitters) in movie theaters and classrooms, and palm-sized telecommunication devices for use with telephones.

For the child with a profound hearing impairment, as well as for their families and others, there have been advances in methods to learn lip-reading and sign language by computer modeling programs. In addition, versions of the electronic **cochlear implant** (CI) have been gradually improving; for most individuals, this device can restore a type of hearing or at least an improved awareness of sounds (Stern et al., 2005; Zwolan et al., 2004). The surgical implantation of CI, however, is not without risks, such as meningitis, and children need careful follow-up (Rubin & Papsin, 2010). See Chapter 10 for more information on assistive technology for people with hearing impairments.

Technology for Communication Impairments

Many types of augmentative and alternative communication (AAC) devices exist to assist a person who is unable to use speech for communication (see Table 36.1). Most devices are used for persons who have physical disabilities, but AAC has recently been shown to be quite effective for children who have an autism spectrum disorder (ASDs; Schlosser & Wendt, 2010). Concerns have been raised in the past that using AAC might slow down the acquisition of verbal language, but recent research has shown that the use of AAC actually increases the development of speech (Binger et al., 2008).

Low-tech devices include various lists of words or pictures mounted on durable material. These communication cards, books or boards are used in face-to-face communication; the user points to the selected word or picture to communicate a specific message. A battery-operated scanning communication device using moving lights on pictures is an example of a mid-tech AAC device. Other mid-tech AAC devices include portable voice output storage units that require direct selection and hold only a few minutes of prerecorded sentences or phrases.

High-tech electronic communication aids, often incorporating single symbols to substitute for groups of words, are becoming more commercially available (Beuekelman & Mirenda, 2005). Building upon the principle of universal design, various software companies have started using laptop or tablet computers (e.g., the Apple iPad), which have internal speakers, as the core part of a communication system, thus increasing the versatility of these communication aids. Rather than being used only for person-to-person communication, these adapted portables can be used for all types of communication—letter-writing, telecommunications, social networking, e-mail, and tweeting. Transparent modifications to allow for simple switch controls have been developed for those persons who also have physical disabilities (see http://www.closingthegap.com for examples). These adapted computers also can be the foundation for environmental controls, safety systems, and therapeutic recreation (e.g., Internet-based, virtual-reality computer communities such as Second Life; Lange, Flynn, & Rizzo, 2009; Sigafoos et al., 2004; Weiss, Bialik, & Kizony, 2003). The aforementioned websites, http://www.abledata.org and http://www.closingthegap.com, have examples of these systems as well as lists of vendors.

Proper assessment is critical when dealing with AAC devices as communication demands change with developmental level and with the environment. There are many areas of functioning that have to be evaluated such as cognitive, attentional, and motivational demands as well as any physical limitations. An overview of the evaluation process is presented later in this chapter but resources such as the book edited by Soto and Zangari are invaluable for more complete details about AAC assessment and use with both younger and older children (Soto & Zangari, 2009).

When compared with high-tech computerized AAC technology, there are significant problems with low-tech and mid-tech devices: 1) they get the message across slowly, 2) they provide limited messages (i.e., usually only those about basic needs), and 3) they require face-to-face interaction. Spoken communication among typical individuals is normally performed at such high speed that much patience is needed for conversations between typically communicating people and those using a communication system (especially low-tech systems involving symbols, letters, or word boards). Although these methods are extremely slow, such low-tech devices should not be abandoned. They often are just as effective, if not more so, than high-tech devices in face-to-face communication. Electronic devices are often limited by their need for a power source, and most are not suitable for outdoor activities such as going to the beach or walking in the rain. Thus, low-tech solutions such as word and picture boards should always be part of an overall communication system and should be available as a backup to electronic devices. An extensive table which addresses no- and low-tech AAC interventions can be found in the recent publication by Sadao and Robinson (2010, pp. 78–81).

Technology for Cognitive, Attentional and Learning Disabilities

Children who have learning differences have been helped by various assistive technology devices and strategies (Behrmann & Schaff, 2001; Hetzroni & Shrieber, 2004). Often these strategies have been used with cognitive rehabilitation as well, such as after a traumatic brain injury (LoPresti, Mihailidis & Kirsch, 2004). Many software programs have been developed since the late 1980s that use computers to assist in reading, math, and other types of special education instruction. These programs range widely in price and utility, and only recently has enough research been performed to begin to determine their effectiveness and generalizability, especially over the long term (Edyburn, 2006; Lahm et al., 2001). Computer-based instruction, however, has several unique advantages, perhaps the most important of which is the ease of individualization. It is possible to build on children's strengths and talents and develop alternative ways of learning. Very few children in special education have their own personal teacher on a full-time basis, so using a computer can allow these children to begin to develop independent learning skills. It is crucial to first fully evaluate the educational strengths and needs of a student who has learning difficulties and then apply the assistive technology where it can best support learning in multiple environments (e.g., home, school, college). Most of the time, however, low-tech and mid-tech solutions should be considered initially. A high-tech solution is often not the best answer for a specific problem that a child is having in school (Edyburn, 2006).

The most promising examples of computer-based instructional software have been developed recently using the principles of universal design such that differing levels of need for assistance can be incorporated in the same software (i.e., text-to-speech for those children who have severe reading disabilities) and, thus, being more cost-effective for schools to purchase (Curry, Cohen, & Lightbody, 2006). The National Center on Accessible Instructional Materials has information for schools and families on assistive technology and alternate-format materials for children with disabilities (their web site is at http://aim.cast.org/learn/aim4families). For example, a child who may or may not have a math disability and requires additional work to learn a math concept might benefit from drill and practice type of software. Or a child who is having difficulty with vocabulary improvement may need additional independent practice using software that helps to create words and phrases (e.g., using a game format to enhance adherence).

"Distance education" methodologies using the Internet are another potentially cost-effective method for instruction or rehabilitation. A student can work from an interactive learning experience asynchronously at home or in a hospital at their own pace and convenience (Moisey, 2004; Sitzmann, Kraider, Stewart, & Wisher, 2006). These methods can be either a substitution for in-school instruction or in addition to that instruction and also often use universal design to improve their accessibility. Distance methods have also been used for rehabilitation purposes (which is often game-based; Lange, Flynn & Rizzo, 2009): 1) when adaptive equipment is needed (e.g., a keyboard emulator) the student doesn't need to transport this equipment to/from a school; and 2) when recovering at home from a hospitalization or orthopedic surgery (e.g., common in children who have cerebral palsy or spina bifida).

ASSESSMENT FOR ASSISTIVE TECHNOLOGY

It is important that the assessment process for and the prescribing of any assistive device be done by a knowledgeable team of individuals. Depending on the type of assistive device to be prescribed, this interdisciplinary team may include a speech-language therapist, a physical therapist, an occupational therapist, a rehabilitation engineer, a neurodevelopmental pediatrician, neurologist, a physiatrist or other physician, special educator, a social worker, and a computer specialist. Also included in the team are the child who will be using the device(s) and his or her family members, who can offer critical advice in making final device recommendations. This team approach is needed to properly evaluate the child's motor and intellectual capabilities and to narrow down the devices that may fit within the child's abilities and needs (e.g., be part of an IEP—individualized educational program). A recent Clinical Report from the American Academy of Pediatrics (AAP) is available that provides detailed information about this assessment process (Desch & Gaebler, 2008).

Figure 36.1 summarizes the assessment process. (See the functional evaluation of the individual section, which follows, for more information on the assessment tools mentioned in this figure). An important aspect of assessment is the consideration of the range of assistive technology that may be useful. The best approach is to begin with the low-tech devices and to move on to mid-tech or high-tech devices only if needed. For example, to get around the home, a child with a severe physical disability may benefit more from ramps and wider doors than from a power wheelchair. The assessment process often involves making educated guesses (based on prior experiences with other people with similar disabilities) and then having the individual try out the devices chosen. A single-subject design methodology is often used to add some objectivity to this device selection process (Zhan & Ottenbacher, 2001). The most complete evaluation possible should be undertaken prior to purchasing the equipment, including testing the device in all settings where it will be used. This avoids buying a device that is unusable or inappropriate.

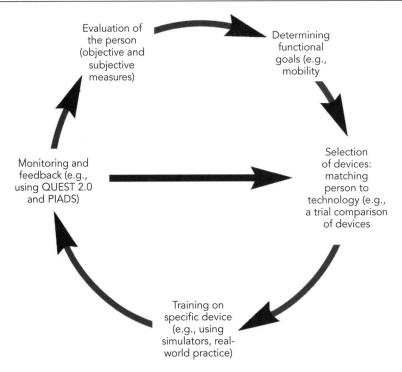

Figure 36.1. The assistive device assessment cycle. (*Key:* QUEST 2.0, Quebec User Evaluation of Satisfaction with Assistive Technology, Version 2.0 [Demers, Weiss-Lambrou, & Ska, 2000]; PIADS, Psychosocial Impact of Assistive Devices Scale [Day, Jutai, & Campbell, 2002; Routhier et al., 2001].)

Functional Evaluation of the Individual

The ultimate goal for a person using an assistive device is to achieve the highest possible level of functioning. The World Health Organization (WHO) has introduced the International Classification of Functioning, Disability and Health (ICF), a system that produces an overall picture of an individual's capabilities, rather than solely focusing on the disability (WHO, 2001). A number of other standardized instruments have been developed that can be used to evaluate the current functioning and impact of treatment or intervention, including assistive technology, on children with various types of disabilities. These include the children's version of the Functional Independence Measure (Wee-FIM; Wong et al., 2005) and the Pediatric Disability Inventory (PEDI; Ostensjo et al., 2006).

A number of studies have shown that between one third and three quarters of assistive devices are abandoned shortly after they are obtained (see Table 36.3; Day, Jutai, Woolrich & Strong, 2001; Galvin & Scherer, 2004). To improve utilization, techniques have been developed to predict the successful use of assistive devices. One approach is the Matching Persons and Technology (MPT) model (Scherer, 1998a; Scherer & Craddock, 2002). It stresses the importance of addressing environmental, personal, and technology-related issues. Environmental issues include the family structure and the work or school settings. The personal area includes recognition of functional limitations, motivation, coping skills, and personality traits (e.g., optimism exerts much influence.) The technology area includes the characteristics of the assistive device: reliability, ease of use, adaptability, and whether any discomfort or stress is caused by its use. Scherer and colleagues developed an assessment tool, the Assistive Technology Device Predisposition Assessment, which uses the MPT model to facilitate a match between the device and the person to ensure a good long-term result (Scherer, 1998b; Scherer & Craddock, 2002). Table 36.3 lists factors that are part of this model, in particular, those relating to the potential abandonment of devices. There are also assessment tools that determine the efficacy and satisfaction of the device once in place: the Quebec User Evaluation of Satisfaction with Assistive Technology (QUEST), now called QUEST 2.0 (Demers, Weiss-Lambrou, & Ska, 2002), and the Psychosocial Impact of Assistive Devices Scale (PIADS; Day, Jutai, & Campbell, 2002; Jutai et al, 2005).

Table 36.3. Factors associated with abandonment of an assistive device

Possible issues	Possible solutions/preventatives
Improper or ineffective training on the use of a device (e.g., single-session training without follow-up and feedback)	Use a multi- or interdisciplinary team approach to training with the device.
Problems or obstacles in the environment preventing use of a device (e.g., second-floor rooms inaccessible to a power wheelchair user)	Assess *all* potential environments in which the device will be used.
Faults or failures in performance of the device (e.g., assistive device that is too sensitive to movement)	Consider using a rental or loaner device to try out. Become very knowledgeable about the devices being considered.
Device size, weight, or appearance (e.g., assistive device decorated with pink roses given to a boy)	Develop connections with several vendors of devices. Be creative with individualizing the devices (e.g., put colorful stickers on).
Motivational factors in the user and/or family members (e.g., depression occurring after traumatic injuries)	Consider cultural factors. May need social work or similar evaluations of the client and the family.
Perceived lack of or minimal need for the device (e.g., decision made not to leave the house rather than to use a wheelchair)	Consider cultural factors and socioecomic factors (e.g., social work assessment)
Functional abilities that worsen or improve (e.g., progressive disorder or recovery)	Ensure appropriate medical follow-up of the underlying condition (usually with subspecialists)

Source: Scherer (1998a).

Training in the Use of the Device

The physicians, therapists, or educators who prescribe or recommend electronic assistive devices or assistive devices in general must also ensure that the child receives proper training for using the device, and then be monitored afterwards. For some devices and software, demos and simulators are available (e.g., power wheelchair controls, AAC devices), which can help with training before the actual device is ordered (Harrison et al., 2002). Simulators are especially helpful in evaluating reaction time, speed, and accuracy (Furumasu, Guerette, & Deffi, 2004).

EFFECTS OF ASSISTIVE TECHNOLOGY ON THE FAMILY AND COMMUNITY

Assistive technology compensates for or builds on the individual skills that each person already possesses. It can lead to increased feelings of success and self-worth and, it is hoped, improved functioning (Kirk & Glendinning, 2004; Wang & Barnard, 2004). For example, several studies have provided evidence for the positive effects of adapted toys on intellectual development (Besio, 2002; Brodin, 1999). Although much uncertainty remains about the earliest age at which a child can successfully use an assistive device, some pilot studies suggest children younger than 5 years of age can benefit.

For example, studies of power wheelchair use have demonstrated that a child as young as 2 years old can be quite successful manipulating one and reap considerable social benefits as well from the success (Bottos et al., 2001). One study suggests that for children with communicative disabilities, if AAC devices are not being successfully used by first grade, the child will not be an active participant in the classroom setting (Buekelman & Mirenda, 2005).

Although assistive devices can markedly improve function, medical technology can sometimes promote social isolation. In school, the child is likely to be treated differently because of the accompanying equipment and medical/nursing needs. The presence of a tracheostomy and ventilator can be particularly intimidating. This can be partially offset by educating classmates and teachers and providing psychological counseling for the child. The child and family must also learn to deal with the underlying medical problems that led to the technology dependence. It is generally easier for a child and family to cope with medical technology assistance on a short-term basis, such as when intravenous antibiotics are necessary to treat a severe infection or when a temporary ostomy is required following abdominal surgery. If the child has a severe chronic disease, however, adaptation to assistive technology is only one issue among many that the child and family must face. Studies have suggested that families fare better if the more significant type of technological assistance, such as mechanical ventilation, lasts less than 2 years (Edwards, O'Toole, & Wallis, 2004; Montagnino & Mauricio, 2004). More prolonged periods are associated with an increased risk of parental stress and depression (Montagnino & Mauricio, 2004). The provision of in-home respite care and family-to-family support systems can be extremely helpful in these situations.

Despite financial and psychosocial difficulties, children who require chronic and substantial medical technology assistance are being included in the community (Feudtner et al., 2005; O'Brien & Wegner, 2002; Rehm & Rohr, 2002). A very useful, extensive, and practical book is available from the American Academy of Pediatrics which has many recommendations that help to ensure successful home care (AAP Section on Home Health Care, 2009).

Home care, especially when ventilator assistance is required, becomes a viable option only after a number of requirements have been met (Carnevale et al., 2006; Heaton et al., 2005):

1. The family must master the child's medical and nursing care

2. The family needs to select a nursing agency if home nursing services are required

3. A durable medical equipment (DME) supplier needs to be found for equipment, disposable supplies, and in-home support (e.g., equipment maintenance and monitoring)

4. The funds to pay for all of these services must be arranged

5. Modifications to the family's home may be needed, such as changing existing electrical systems and adding ramps for wheelchair or adapted stroller accessibility

6. If mechanical ventilation is required, local electric, ambulance, and telephone companies must be notified that a person dependent on life-support technology will be living in the family's home so that the household can be placed on a priority list in the event of a power failure or a medical emergency

Medical, educational, and therapy (e.g., occupational therapy, physical therapy) services also need to be arranged before discharge from the hospital. A community pediatrician or family physician should be identified to provide general medical care. The hospital team should contact this physician prior to the child's discharge to introduce the child and encourage the community physician's active participation in the child's care. If the child requires special rehabilitation therapies after discharge, either center- or home-based providers should be arranged. Educational services also need to be identified, and the child's health care and rehabilitative plans should be written into an individualized family service plan (IFSP) for early intervention services if the child is younger than age 3, or into an IEP if the child is older (Committee on Children with Disabilities, 1999, Council on Children with Disabilities, 2007). In addition, the school nurse needs to develop an individualized health care plan as well as emergency plans for the child. A center- or school-based educational program offers the child the opportunity to interact with other children in a stimulating environment. These out-of-home experiences should be encouraged if the child's physical condition permits and if appropriate medical or nursing supports are available.

Funding Issues

Assistive technology can be very expensive, depending on the type of equipment required and the extent of the disability and the professional staffing needs of the child. For medical assistive technology, the two major issues are payment for home nursing care and DME and supplies (including technological assistance). It is sometimes easier to obtain funding for the former than for the latter; however there is a national shortage of pediatric home care nurses. The primary source of funding of both is insurance, private and public, and each has restrictions that may affect the provision of medical assistive technology (see Chapter 41). Every third-party medical payment source has documents which detail which DME will be paid for and under what circumstances. It is crucial that both the providers (e.g., physician) and the family be familiar with this "approved DME listing," as it is difficult to get funding approval for items that are not part of the contract from the insurance carrier.

For assistive technology that can be used in schools, the Individuals with Disabilities Education Improvement Act of 2004 (PL 108-446) as well as other laws (e.g., the Technology-Related Assistance for Individuals with Disabilities Act of 1988 [PL 100-407]—the "Tech Act") and legal opinions specifically indicate that funding should be provided for "technological" devices (including software) that are part of a student's IEP. Yet, finding funds to support this actually can be difficult, and insurance companies, philanthropic agencies, school systems, and parents often must cooperate. Another concern is that often schools will restrict the use of the software or device to the school program (and the student is not able to take it for use at home). However, this situation should only occur if the school paid the full amount for the device.

For some devices, such as home ventilators, suctioning, or specialized feeding equipment, insurance companies universally recognize that these are medically necessary DME and will pay for them. There continues to be controversy, however, as to whether other assistive devices are medically necessary or whether they are educationally necessary. For example, AAC devices, wheelchairs, or standing frames for children who have cerebral palsy could be used both at home and at school. If a device is shown to be primarily medically necessary, and therefore DME, it may be possible to obtain funding from medical insurance companies. If they are educationally necessary, the school system should purchase the needed devices. The Tech Act has tried to solve the problem of discriminating between medical and educational use by legally allowing Medicaid funding to be used by the school to purchase the assistive device. The Tech Act further requires that the child be permitted to take home such devices for educationally related purposes. This federal Tech Act sets a precedent for medical funding to be at least considered for the purchase of essentially all assistive devices. The Tech Act also funds lending libraries in most states, and many commercial vendors also allow opportunities for lending out devices for a short time for a "trial use."

For years, most forms of private and government medical insurance (e.g., Medicaid) have been willing to pay for the purchase of wheelchairs, and they gradually are beginning to fund other types of assistive devices. Fortunately, AAC devices are increasingly being seen as medically necessary in much the same way as wheelchairs are. Physicians are often called upon to send medical necessity letters and prescriptions to funding sources for assistive technology (Committee on Children with Disabilities, 1999; Council on Children with Disabilities, 2007; Desch et al., 2008; Sneed, May, & Stencel, 2004). This can best be done after the physician consults with the child's therapists and then summarizes current abilities and expected outcomes from using the assistive device. Many assistive devices and their related professional services are relatively

new and specialized, and they usually are not included on lists of approved products that are eligible for funding. As a result, many funding agencies need to be properly educated about these devices' potential use to improve functioning and independence for individuals with disabilities. Patience and perseverance are frequently necessary for funding to be secured. Initial denials of payment are almost automatic for some funding sources; however, these denials are usually subject to appeal and reversal. A recent Clinical Report from the AAP has additional information about the funding process, especially for AAC devices (Desch et al., 2008). Other resources are the guidelines and charts included in Sadao and Robinson (2010, pp. 17–23).

Advocacy Information

Fortunately, sources of information about assistive technology are increasingly accessible. Statewide Technological Assistance Services (Tech Act sites) are now available in all states, and information from them is becoming more widely accessible. ABLEDATA, which is funded by the National Institute for Disability and Rehabilitation Research, is an example of a large database that holds continuously updated information about assistive technology pertinent to many disabilities (http://www.abledata.org). Various organizations dealing with children who have disabilities, such as the Council for Exceptional Children (http://www.cec.sped.org), have developed user-friendly online services that can be used to obtain references and abstracts about many facets of assistive technology, especially in regard to school-related services. On the Internet, there are an increasing number of sites offering resources for people interested in assistive technology, although many of these are thinly veiled advertisements from companies or sites that propose "alternative therapies." Therefore, all web sites must be evaluated critically.

SUMMARY

Most children with disabilities who use assistive technology employ it to make their day-to-day living easier or to improve functioning. However, some children use a medical assistive device that replaces or augments a vital bodily function such as breathing. For the group using rehabilitative assistive technology (e.g., power wheelchairs, AAC, hearing and vision aids), perhaps the best way to ensure the availability of future vocational opportunities is to provide access to appropriate assistive devices at an early age—thereby allowing the children to become proficient in use of the devices by the time they are young adults. Improved access to these devices also has social implications. As children with disabilities become better able to use their assistive devices or communication devices, they likely will be less isolated and have more contact with the community as teenagers and adults.

For children who require medical assistive technology (e.g., respiratory technology devices, surveillance devices, nutritive assistive devices, ostomies, dialysis), the requirement for prolonged medical technology assistance places both financial and emotional stresses on the family. It also leads to considerable challenges for health care professionals and other caregivers. Knowing how to correctly use medical devices and having confidence in dealing with potential emergencies is important for parents, educators, and other caregivers. Training of caregivers and others in the use of medical technology assistance is best done while the child is hospitalized. Arrangement for financial, nursing, and equipment support is essential before the child goes home. Ultimately, the outcome for the child who depends on assistive technology appears to be more a function of the underlying disorder than the type or extent of technology, but the role of the family cannot be overemphasized (Fuhrer et al., 2003; AAP Section on Home Health Care, 2009).

The future of assistive technology will undoubtedly be marked with continuing change and improvements at a nearly exponential pace (just as the last 30 years have been). However, due partly to the growing influence of the principles of universal design, the children with disabilities of today will begin to experience increasing access to both the physical world and the Internet that could have only been dreamt about years ago. Because of the creative work of some dedicated researchers there are now tools and methods to better assess children with disabilities, the devices or software themselves, and most importantly, the outcomes. These tools will continue to be used and refined and new methods will continue to be developed. Thus, in coming years we will have increasing evidence which defines what is the most useful assistive technology and more specific information about how best to use assistive technology to improve the functional outcomes of all children with disabilities.

REFERENCES

Alper, S., & Raharinirina, S. (2006). Assistive technology for individuals with disabilities: A review and synthesis of the literature. *Journal of Special Education Technology, 21*(2), 47–59.

American Academy of Pediatrics: Section on Ophthalmology, Council on Children with Disabilities; American Academy of Ophthalmology; American Association for Pediatric Ophthalmology and Strabismus; & American Association of Certified Orthoptists. (2009). Joint statement—Learning disabilities, dyslexia, and vision. *Pediatrics, 124*(2), 837–844.

AAP Section on Home Health Care. (2009). In R.C. Libby & O. Imaizumi (Eds.) *Guidelines for pediatric home health care* (2nd ed.). Elk Grove, IL: American Academy of Pediatrics.

Bass, J.L., Corwin, M., Gozal, D., Moore, C., Nishida, H., Parker, S., ... Kinane, T.B. (2004). The effect of chronic or intermittent hypoxia on cognition in childhood: A review of the evidence. *Pediatrics, 114*(3), 805–816.

Behrmann, M., & Schaff, J. (2001). Assisting educators with assistive technology: Enabling children to achieve independence in living and learning. *Children and Families, 42*(3), 24–28.

Besio, S. (2002). An Italian research project to study the play of children with motor disabilities: The first year of activity. *Disability and Rehabilitation, 24*, 72–79.

Binger, C., Berens, J., Kent-Walsh, J., & Taylor, S. (2008) The effects of aided AAC interventions on AAC use, speech, and symbolic gestures. *Seminars in Speech and Language, 29*(2), 101–111.

Bottos, M., Bolcati, C., Scuito, L., Ruggeri, C., & Feliciangeli, A. (2001). Powered wheelchairs and independence in young children with tetraplegia. *Developmental Medicine and Child Neurology, 43*, 769–777.

Brodin, J. (1999). Play in children with severe multiple disabilities: Play with toys—a review. *International Journal of Disability, Development and Education, 46*, 25–34.

Buekelman, D.R., & Mirenda, P. (2005). *Augmentative and alternative communication: Supporting children and adults with complex communication needs* (3rd ed.). Baltimore, MD: Paul H. Brookes Publishing Co.

Bush, A., Fraser, J., Jardine, E., Paton, J., Simonds, A., & Wallis, C. (2005). Respiratory management of the infant with type 1 spinal muscular atrophy. *Archives of Disease in Childhood, 90*(7), 709–711.

Carnevale, F.A., Alexander, E., Davis, M., Rennick, J., & Troini, R. (2006). Daily living with distress and enrichment: The moral experience of families with ventilator-assisted children at home. *Pediatrics, 117*(1), e48–e60.

Center for Universal Design. (2008). *About UD*. Retrieved from http://www.ncsu.edu/www/ncsu/design/sod5/cud/about_ud/about_ud.htm

Committee on Children with Disabilities. (1999). The pediatrician's role in development and implementation of an individual education plan (IEP) and/or an individual family service plan (IFSP). *Pediatrics, 104*(1), 124–127

Council on Children With Disabilities. (2007). Provision of Educationally Related Services for Children and Adolescents with Chronic Diseases and Disabling Conditions. *Pediatrics, 119*, 1218–1223.

Curry, C., Cohen, L. & Lightbody, N. (2006). Universal design in science teaching. *The Science Teacher, 73*(3), 32–37.

Davidson, K.L. (2002). Airway clearance strategies for the pediatric patient. *Respiratory Care, 47*(7), 823–828.

Day, H.Y., Jutai, J., Woolrich, W., & Strong, G. (2001). The stability of impact of assistive devices. *Disability and Rehabilitation, 23*, 400–404.

Day, H., Jutai, J., & Campbell, K.A. (2002). Development of a scale to measure the psychosocial impact of assistive devices: Lessons learned and the road ahead. *Disability and Rehabilitation, 24*, 31–37.

Demers, L., Weiss-Lambrou, R., & Ska, B. (2002). The Quebec user evaluation of satisfaction with assistive technology (QUEST 2.0). *Technology and Disability, 14*, 101–105.

Desch, L.W. (1986). High technology for handicapped children: A pediatrician's viewpoint. *Pediatrics, 77*, 71–85.

Desch, L.W. (2008). The spectrum of assistive and augmentative technology for individuals with developmental disabilities. In P.J. Accardo (Ed.), *Capute and Accardo's neurodevelopmental disabilities in infancy and childhood, Third Edition* (Vol. I). Baltimore, MD: Paul H. Brookes Publishing Co.

Desch, L.W., Gaebler-Spira, D., & Council on Children With Disabilities. (2008). Prescribing assistive-technology systems: Focus on children with impaired communication. *Pediatrics, 121*(6), 1271–80.

Dosman, C.F., & Jones, R.L. (2005). High-frequency chest compression: A summary of the literature. *Canadian Respiratory Journal, 12*(1), 37–41.

Downey, R., III, Perkin, R.M., & MacQuarrie, J. (2000). Nasal continuous positive airway pressure use in children with obstructive sleep apnea younger than 2 years of age. *Chest, 117*, 1608–1612.

Edwards, E.A., O'Toole, M., & Wallis, C. (2004). Sending children home on tracheostomy dependent ventilation: Pitfalls and outcomes. *Archives of Disease in Childhood, 89*(3), 251–255.

Edyburn, D.L. (2006). Failure is not an option: Collecting, reviewing, and acting on evidence for using technology to enhance academic performance. *Learning and Leading with Technology, 34*(1), 20–23.

Feudtner, C., Villareale, N.L., Morray, B., Sharp, V., Hays, R.M., & Neff, J.M. (2005). Technology-dependency among patients discharged from a children's hospital: A retrospective cohort study. *BioMedCentral Pediatrics, 5*(1), 8.

Flenady, V.J., & Gray, P.H. (2000). Chest physiotherapy for preventing morbidity in babies being extubated from mechanical ventilation. *Cochrane Database of Systemic Reviews, 2*, CD000283.

Fuhrer, M.J., Jutai, J.W., Scherer, & DeRuyter, F. (2003). A framework for the conceptual modeling of assistive device outcomes. *Disability and Rehabilitation, 25*, 1243–1251.

Furumasu, I., Guerette, P. & Deffi, D. (2004). Relevance of the Pediatric Powered Wheelchairs Screening Test for children with cerebral palsy. *Developmental Medicine and Child Neurology, 40*, 468–474.

Galvin, J.C., & Scherer, M.J. (Eds.). (2004). *Evaluating, selecting and using appropriate assistive technology.* Austin, TX: PRO-ED.

Gilgoff, R.L., & Gilgoff, I.S. (2003). Long-term follow-up of home mechanical ventilation in young children with spinal cord injury and neuromuscular conditions. *The Journal of Pediatrics, 142*(5), 476–480.

Harrison, A., Derwent G., Enticknap, A., Rose, F.D., & Attree, E.A. (2002). The role of virtual reality technology in the assessment and training of inexperienced powered wheelchair users. *Disability and Rehabilitation, 24*, 599–607.

Heaton, J., Noyes, J., Sloper, P., & Shah, R. (2005). Families' experiences of caring for technology-dependent children: A temporal perspective. *Health and Social Care in the Community, 13*(5), 441–450.

Hetzroni, O.E., & Shrieber, B. (2004). Word processing as an assistive technology tool for enhancing academic outcomes of students with writing disabilities in the general classroom. *Journal of Learning Disabilities, 37*(2), 143–154.

Individuals with Disabilities Education Improvement Act of 2004, PL 108-446, 20 U.S.C. §§ 1400 *et seq.*

Jutai, J., Fuhrer, M.J., Demers, L., Scherer, M.J., & DeRuyter, F. (2005) Towards a taxonomy of assistive technology device outcomes. *American Journal of Physical Medicine and Rehabilitation, 84*(4), 294–302.

Keates, S., & Robinson, P. (1999). Gestures and multimodal input. *Behavior and Information Technology, 18*(1), 36–44.

Kirk, S., & Glendinning, C. (2004). Developing services to support parents caring for a technology-dependent child at home. *Child: Care, Health and Development, 30*(3), 209–218; discussion, 219.

Krause, M.F., & Hoehn, T. (2000). Chest physiotherapy in mechanically ventilated children: A review. *Critical Care Medicine, 28*, 1648–1651.

Lahm, E.A., Bausch, M.E., & Hasselbring, T.S. (2001). National assistive technology research institute. *Journal of Special Education Technology, 16*, 19–26.

Lange, B., Flynn, S.M., & Rizzo, A.A. (2009). Game-based telerehabilitation. *European Journal of Physical and Rehabilitative Medicine, 45*(1), 143–151.

LoPresti, E., Mihailidis, A., & Kirsch N. (2004). Assistive technology for cognitive rehabilitation: State of the art. *Neuropsychological Rehabilitation, 14*, 5–39.

McInally, W. (2005). Whose line is it anyway? Management of central venous catheters in children. *Pediatric Nursing, 17*(5), 14–8.

Moisey, S. (2004). Students with disabilities in distance education: Characteristics, course enrollment and completion, and support services. *Journal of Distance Education, 19*(1), 73–91.

Montagnino, B.A., & Mauricio, R.V. (2004). The child with a tracheostomy and gastrostomy: Parental stress and coping in the home—a pilot study. *Pediatric Nursing, 30*(5), 373–380, 401.

Nadkarni, U.B., Shah, A.M., & Deshmukh, C.T. (2000). Non-invasive respiratory monitoring in paediatric intensive care. *Journal of Postgraduate Medicine, 46*, 149–152.

O'Brien, M.E., & Wegner, C.B. (2002). Rearing the child who is technology dependent: Perceptions of parents and home care nurses. *Journal for Specialists in Pediatric Nursing, 7*(1), 7–15.

Office of Technology Assessment. (1987). *Technology-dependent children: Hospital versus home care: A technical memorandum* (DHHS Publication No. TM-H-38). Washington, DC: US Government Printing Office.

Østensjø, S., Bjorbaekmo, W., Carlberg, E.B., & Vøllestad, N.K. (2006). Assessment of everyday functioning in young children with disabilities: An ICF-based analysis of concepts and content of the Pediatric Evaluation of Disability Inventory (PEDI). *Disability and Rehabilitation, 28*(8), 489–504.

Palfrey, J.S., Haynie, M., Porter, S., Fenton, T., Cooperman-Vincent, P., Shaw, D., … Walker, D.K. (1994). Prevalence of medical technology assistance among children in Massachusetts in 1987 and 1990. *Public Health Reports, 109,* 226–233.

Rehm, R.S., & Rohr, J.A. (2002). Parents', nurses', and educators' perceptions of risks and benefits of school attendance by children who are medically fragile/technology-dependent. *Journal of Pediatric Nursing 17*(5), 345–353.

Routhier, F., Vincent, C., Morrissette, M.J., & Desaulniers, L. (2001). Clinical results of an investigation of paediatric upper limb myoelectric prosthesis fitting at the Quebec Rehabilitation Institute. *Prosthetics and Orthotics International, 25,* 119–131.

Rubin, L.G., & Papsin, B. (2010) Cochlear implants in children: surgical site infections and prevention and treatment of acute otitis media and meningitis. *Pediatrics, 126*(2), 381–391.

Scherer, M.J. (1998a). *Matching person and technology model and accompanying assessment forms* (3rd ed.). Webster, NY: Institute for Matching Person and Technology.

Scherer, M.J. (1998b). The impact of assistive technology on the lives of people with disabilities. In D.B. Gray, L.A. Quatrano, & M.L. Lieberman (Eds.), *Designing and using assistive technology: The human perspective* (pp. 99–115). Baltimore, MD: Paul H. Brookes Publishing Co.

Scherer, M.J., & Craddock, G. (2002). Matching person and technology (MPT) assessment process. *Technology and Disability, 14*(3), 125–131.

Schlosser, R.W., & Wendt, O. (2008). Effects of augmentative and alternative communication intervention on speech production in children with autism: A systematic review. *American Journal of Speech Language Pathology, 17*(3), 212–230.

Sigafoos, J., O'Reilly, M.F., Seely-York, S., Weru, J., Son, S.H., Green, V.A., & Lancioni, G.E. (2004). Transferring AAC intervention to the home. *Disability and Rehabilitation, 26*(21–22), 1330–1334.

Silvestri, J.M., Lister, G., Corwin, M.J., Smok-Pearsall, S.M., Baird, T.M., Crowell, D.H., ... Willinger, M. (2005). Collaborative Home Infant Monitoring Evaluation Study Group—Factors that influence use of a home cardiorespiratory monitor for infants: The collaborative home infant monitoring evaluation. *Archives of Pediatrics and Adolescent Medicine, 159*(1), 18–24.

Sitzmann, T., Kraiger, K., Stewart, D., & Wisher, R. (2006). The comparative effectiveness of web-based and classroom instruction: A meta-analysis. *Personnel Psychology, 59,* 623–664.

Sneed, R.C., May, W.L., & Stencel, C. (2004). Policy versus practice: Comparison of prescribing therapy and durable medical equipment in medical and educational settings. *Pediatrics, 114*(5), e612–e625.

Sadao, K.C., & Robinson, K.C. (2010). *Assistive technology for young children: creating inclusive learning environments.* Baltimore, MD: Paul H. Brookes Publishing Co.

Soto, G., & Zangari, C. (Eds.) (2009). *Practically speaking: Language literacy, & academic development for students with AAC Needs.* Baltimore, MD: Paul H. Brookes Publishing Co.

Stern, R.E., Yueh, B., Lewis, C., Nortin, S., & Sie, K.C. (2005). Recent epidemiology of pediatric cochlear implantation in the United States: Disparity among children of different ethnicity and socioeconomic status. *Laryngoscope, 115,* 125–131.

Technology-Related Assistance for Individuals with Disabilities Act of 1988, PL 100–407, 29 U.S.C. §§ 2201 *et seq.*

Tibballs, J., Henning, R., Robertson, C.F., Massie, J., Hochmann, M., Carter, B., ... Bryan, D. (2010) A home respiratory support programme for children by parents and layperson carers. *Journal of Paediatrics and Child Health, 46*(1–2), 57–62.

Wang, K.W., & Barnard, A. (2004). Technology-dependent children and their families: A review. *Journal of Advanced Nursing, 45*(1), 36–46.

Weiss, P.L., Bialik, P., & Kizony, R. (2003). Virtual reality provides leisure time opportunities for young adults with physical and intellectual disabilities. *CyberPsychology and Behavior, 6,* 335–343.

Wise, P. (2007). The future pediatrician: The challenge of chronic illness. Journal of Pediatrics, 151, S6–S10.

Wong, V., Au-Yeung, Y.C., & Law, P.K. (2005). Correlation of Functional Independence Measure for Children (WeeFIM) with developmental language tests in children with developmental delay. *Journal of Child Neurology, 20*(7), 613–616.

World Health Organization. (2001). *International Classification of Functioning, Disability and Health (ICF).* Geneva, Switzerland: Author.

Zhan, S., & Ottenbacher, K.J. (2001). Single subject research designs for disability research. *Disability and Rehabilitation, 23,* 1–9.

Zwolan, T.A., Ashbaugh, C.M., Alarfaj, A., Kileny, P.R., Arts, H.A., El-Kashlan, H.K., & Telian, S.A. (2004). Pediatric cochlear implant patient performance as a function of age at implantation. *Otology and Neurotology, 25,* 112–120.

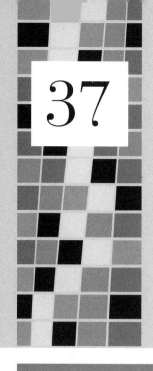

37 Caring and Coping

Helping the Family of a Child with a Disability

Michaela L. Zajicek-Farber

Upon completion of this chapter, the reader will

- Understand the impact a developmental disability has on family functioning

- Be knowledgeable about strategies and resources that can help families cope with having a child with a developmental disability

- Learn the principles of family-centered care

- Recognize the influence of societal attitudes on the outcome of children with disabilities

---

The preceding chapters have focused on the medical, rehabilitative, and educational supports for various developmental disabilities. Equally important is the impact disabilities exert on family functioning. All families are not alike and how a family handles the day-to-day needs, wants, and stresses of its members' influences to a great extent the well-being and outcome of the child with disabilities (Reichman, Corman, & Noonan, 2008). Professionals have come to realize that most families possess strengths and resiliency for guiding their own life course and for grappling with childrearing issues, regardless of the type and degree of their child's disability. In addition, professionals have also come to appreciate the importance of listening to the immediate and long-term needs of the families. This leads to building a collaborative partnership with families and other professionals to assure optimal care and quality of life for children with disabilities and their families. To be effective in working with families of these children, professionals must engage in family-centered care (Seligman & Darling, 2007). This chapter addresses issues that families face throughout their lifecycle and the approaches professionals can take to help them.

■ ■ ■ SAMANTHA

Samantha is an 8-year-old girl with Down syndrome. When Samantha was born, her parents, Monica and Sean, were excited by the prospect of having their first child. Both parents were in their mid-to-late twenties, healthy, and well connected with their extended families and friends in the community. They were diligent about prenatal care, Sean often attending prenatal visits with Monica. They were both employed full time, but Monica planned to take a 6-month maternity leave. Following a medically uneventful delivery, they were devastated to learn that Samantha had Down syndrome. As a way to cope, Monica spent several hours in her hospital room refusing to see anyone, including Sean or her baby. Sean left the hospital, trying to figure out what to do. He made calls to his and Monica's parents about the turn of events. Everyone in the family was distressed. The obstetrician convened a quick team meeting to provide assistance. By the end of the day, Monica and Sean agreed to meet with their obstetrician, the hospital social worker, and the lactation nurse. The obstetrician reviewed the health of their baby and noted that baby Samantha, although currently healthy, had a heart defect that would need to be corrected in the future. The social worker explained her role in supporting new families and provided a folder with a variety of resource information about maternal postpartum care, breastfeeding, baby care, and specific information about raising a child with Down syndrome. The nurse explained how she would provide support to Monica regarding Samantha's feeding. Both parents agreed to a follow-up meeting. Monica cried as she breastfed Samantha for the first time. In the subsequent days, the social worker and Samantha's pediatrician met together with the parents and one set of grandparents, while the out-of-town grandparents participated by a teleconference, to answer questions about Samantha's condition and care.

The whole family was overwhelmed. Monica and Sean kept asking, "What did we do wrong?" while one set of grandparents worried whether they needed to do genetic testing on everyone in their family, and the other set of grandparents worried whether Samantha would be able to attend regular school and support herself in the future. The social worker and the pediatrician answered many different kinds of questions about what the parents and extended family could do to help Samantha to develop in healthy and positive ways. This intensive meeting took over an hour and served as a precursor to many other meetings coordinated by the social worker.

Subsequently, Samantha's parents learned about available supports for families of children with developmental disabilities. They learned how to establish a medical home for Samantha through primary pediatric care that provided regular well-baby follow-ups and also coordinated her ongoing medical needs through the hospital's Down syndrome clinic. They gained information on how to access early intervention services for Samantha's early educational and developmental care, including nutrition and feeding, speech and language, and optimal ways for promoting parent–child attachment through play and regular parent–child interaction. They received information on health insurance options and future life care planning for Samantha. They were provided with connections on how to meet other families of children with Down syndrome in the community and with information on services that other families found helpful in caring for their child.

They learned how to gain emotional and mental health support for coping with ongoing distress and for respite care, and where to seek information as future needs arose. The hospital social worker continued to meet with the family each time they came for Samantha's follow-up at the Down syndrome clinic and coordinated community services. She noted that over time, the parents' coping and adaptation changed in the context of Samantha's and family members' needs. Samantha's parents' feelings of distress, sorrow, and anger were periodically triggered by life-cycle events such as when they first enrolled Samantha into a local preschool program that was unfamiliar with needs of children with Down syndrome, or when Sean became temporarily "downsized" in his employment and lost family health insurance. Such feelings were balanced by her parents' ongoing love and commitment to Samantha's well-being and care.

With time, Monica became involved with the local Down syndrome organization and a resource to other parents; Sean became involved in the Special Olympics, assisting Samantha and other children with disabilities to participate in exercise and other socialization events. Their marriage went through stressful times, and following Samantha's heart repair, they sought marriage counseling that supported their bonds. Most of the extended family has learned to realistically understand Samantha's abilities and challenges, but periodically differences in their views and lack of available services in the community create family tensions and worries about the future.

UNDERSTANDING FAMILY SYSTEMS

Families exist within the broader network of their communities and social networks. Bronfenbrenner's (1986) **ecological systems model** helps illustrate the interactive nature of family existence within a *microsystem, mesosystem, exosystem*, and *macrosystem*. The family, through its matrix of activities, roles, interpersonal relationships, and material and physical characteristics, represents the primary microsystem. The family interacts with other microsystems such as child care, schools, employment, health care, and a variety of community programs. In turn, the interactions among microsystems constitute the mesosystem. The functioning of both the micro- and mesosystems is further influenced by the exosystem and macrosystem. The exosystem represents the policy environment, and the macrosystem the broader societal and cultural beliefs and values that influence all systems.

Within the microsystem, families are viewed as interactive, interdependent, or reactive, and when something happens to one member in the family, the whole family system is affected. Families differ with regard to their membership characteristics and views. Families must be considered as configurations that include not only two-parent families but also step-families, adoptive families, foster families, and intergenerational families. Families may consist of committed persons who 1) may not be legally married, 2) have gay and lesbian partners, 3) are cohabiting or remarried heterosexual couples, 4) are widowed with children, or 5) are single parents. Families may be adversely affected by an unemployed "breadwinner," a member with a major psychosocial disorder (e.g., substance abuse, mental illness), or a deceased family member whose cultural influence continues to permeate families' thinking and behavior (Seligman & Darling, 2007).

Family membership represents a dynamic system that changes with time and throughout the lifecycle of a family. This family system transmits traditions, values, ethnic heritage, and spiritual or religious beliefs. In turn, traditions provide members with guidance, strength, comfort, and strategies for coping with the difficulties of daily life (Mackleprang & Slasgiver, 2009). Beliefs, communications, and interactions shape the family's ideological style, relationships, and functional priorities. A family's adherence to their ethnicity, culture, and religious/spiritual rituals and observances in public and private life and socio-economic and educational status—all

influence their cultural style and behavior, including their childrearing beliefs and parenting practices (Hanson & Lynch, 2004). Their beliefs can influence how much they will trust professionals, caregivers, or caregiving institutions and the manner in which the family adapts to their child's disability.

As families deal with their child's disability, they also confront their beliefs systems about who and what can influence the future course of events (Farber & Maharaj, 2005). Some families believe that this control rests in their own hands, while others believe that control rests in the hands of their religious beliefs, fate, or even pure chance (Ariel & Naseef, 2006). Family views influence the interpretation of events related to the disability, their help-seeking behavior as a response to the disability, and their approach to caregiving (Xu, 2007). Views and values also influence the family's ability to adapt, negotiate differences, manage stress, and make decisions. In turn, families' adaptability influences their ability to provide or facilitate the following: daily care, economic employment, sustenance, housing, education, vocational-skill development, socialization, community engagement, recreation, bonds of affection, and spirituality.

Children with disabilities can both positively and negatively affect these and other family functions (Durà-Vilà, Dein, & Hodes, 2010; Turnbull et al., 2006). Moving through developmental life cycle transitions can be a major source of stress and challenge for any family, particularly for those raising children with disabilities. These life cycle events begin with the parent's marriage and move through childrearing, management of child schooling and adolescence, launching of young adults, postparenting, and aging. Stress in families is inevitable, but not all family members are impaired by it (Alvard & Grados, 2005). However, accumulated stresses from unmet needs, lack of access to and use of resources, and inadequate management strategies can impair adaptation and result in a crisis in the family's functioning (McCubbin & Patterson, 1983; Xu, 2007).

HOW FAMILIES COPE WITH THE DIAGNOSIS

When families are informed of their child's disability, individual members and families as a whole differ widely in their initial responses. This may depend on 1) the severity of their child's disability, 2) their preparedness for the possibility of this occurring, 3) their prior knowledge about the disability including their own beliefs about why their child might be aflicted with a disability, 4) their experience of interacting with an individual with a similar disability, and 5) the health care professional's manner of delivery of the news (Meet et al., 2008). The timing, the words used, duration of verbal exchange, and the emotional support that professionals provide greatly influence the family's response to the news (Bartolo, 2002). The impact on the family also depends on their previous life experiences, religious and cultural backgrounds, and age of the child at diagnosis (Reichman et al., 2008; Poston & Turnbull, 2004). Other factors that may influence their reactions include family members' beliefs about individuals with disabilities, knowledge of health treatments, and receptiveness to accepting help from professionals, friends, and other family members (van der Veek, Kraaij, & Garnefski, 2009). In other families, individuals who have had previous experiences with a family member with a disability may be able to adjust more easily to the news, or they may become more distressed depending on that previous experience. Some parents, after years of searching, may be relieved to finally receive answers and help for their child, but they also express delayed anger at those who previously reassured them that their child would "grow out of it."

Parental Responses to Diagnosis and Stresses

Responding to the news that a child has a disability is unique, very personal, and often embedded in distress. The most common initial response of parents is some combination of shock, denial, disbelief, guilt, and an overwhelming sense of loss. Some parents deny their child's diagnosis and visit various professionals, hoping that the conventional wisdom to "get a second opinion" will yield a more optimistic diagnosis or prognosis (Sullivan-Bolyai et al., 2004). Based on the complexity of the child's condition, some parents experience several misdiagnoses before a correct one is given. Families have additional challenges when a child who initially develops typically later acquires a disability. They often have a difficult time accepting that prior aspirations for their child (and potentially for their family) may need to be adjusted.

When professionals withhold or create ambiguity about the diagnosis, this often enhances the parents' anxiety (Seligman &

Darling, 2007). Professionals need to deliver the diagnosis honestly, with compassion, carefully choosing their words, and responding to any questions that parents may have. However, professionals also need to understand that the questions parents ask at this juncture are likely to predominantly reflect the answers they are prepared for or emotionally able to hear (Seligman & Darling, p. 187). Professionals involved in establishing the diagnosis should provide parents with a written summary that captures the main points to be understood and schedule a follow-up meeting for review of details and answering questions.

After being informed of a diagnosis, parents usually experience a compelling need for information (Hornby, 2000). Brinthaupt (1991) suggested that in learning to understand the implications of their child's disability, parents experience various **intellectual stresses**. They may be required to integrate vast amounts of information about physiology, timing and type of treatments, rationale for treatment approaches, and potential adverse effects and their management (Roland, 2003). Families are also often faced with managing **instrumental stresses** that relate to 1) the financing of their child's needs, 2) dealing with learning about and administering unfamiliar insurance health policies, and 3) managing the division of labor for providing care for a child with special needs while accomplishing household chores and attending to the other family members' needs. Families strive to normalize their life despite the immediate demands posed by their child's disability, but they come from a wide range of circumstances that may impinge on their care. Some families are very knowledgeable about their choices and can financially afford to obtain multiple expert opinions and services. Other families do not have a good understanding of the health care and educational systems, or the means to obtain private fee-for-service programs. These problems, often combined with poverty, can directly affect the well-being of both the child and family (Park, Turnbull, & Turnbull, 2002).

Specialized medical/therapeutic services and equipment, adapted toys and clothing, and alterations to the household environment can pose substantial financial burdens, which are often overlooked until they urgently surface. Using a **family-centered care** approach in partnering with families involves educating them about their child's condition, making them aware of the resources and entitlements available, and helping them examine different treatment choices. Families who are knowledgeable about available resources and assertive in advocating for their child are usually better able to meet their child's needs (Freedman & Boyer, 2000).

Along with intellectual and instrumental stresses, families also struggle with **emotional stresses**. Uncertainty regarding the diagnosis and the prognosis is a major factor contributing to an emotional response to a disability. As the child grows, family responses are subject to periodic exacerbations tied to their child's transitions along developmental life cycle events as well as to unexpected events (e.g., surgeries, new onset seizures) that may be tied to the child's condition and health care needs. An uncertainty or ambiguity about a child's diagnosis/prognosis can compromise a parent's sense of control and create distress (Pollin, 1995). Children's ongoing manifestation of severe behavior problems (e.g., hyperactivity, self-injury, aggression) can challenge parents' patience and leave them exhausted from the need for heightened supervision and from sleep deprivation. This can place them at risk for posttraumatic stress disorder (PTSD) (Oberleitner et al., 2006). Parents of children with rare disorders may feel particularly isolated as they will not have a community of families dealing with the same condition (Dellve et al., 2006). For these families a useful resource is the "Readers' Forum" in the magazine *Exceptional Parent* where such families often share their experiences (http://www.eparent.com).

Parental Depression

It is not unusual that after the initial shock or denial subsides, some family members experience depression (Reichman et al., 2008). This can result from emotional stress combined with the physical strain (or sheer exhaustion) of following through on the many appointments, procedures, recommendations, and care requirements for their child (Ello & Donovan, 2005). Other factors contributing to depression may be parental or guardian disagreement over the meaning of the diagnosis/prognosis, assignment of blame, sorting through the choice of treatment options, and/or responsibility in caring for the child (Glidden & Schoolcraft, 2003).

Women may tend to be more at risk for depression (Singer & Floyd, 2006) than males when dealing with the news of a child's diagnosis. Symptoms of clinical depression include extreme fatigue, restlessness or irritability, insomnia, changes in appetite, and/or loss of sex drive. Professionals should screen for depression in family caregivers and refer them for further evaluation and treatment as needed (Earls et al., 2010). Parents' depression may also be accompanied by anger, which may be directed at a person, an event, their sense of divine intervention, or life in general. If directed at a person, the anger may be focused on the doctor, other professionals, the other partner, other children in the family, the child with the disability, or it may be self-directed (Heiman, 2002). Regardless of where the anger is directed, it is important to recognize that such expressions are part of a coping strategy. Anger may well be an appropriate expression of frustration when parents feel their opinions are not being heard or respected. However, it may be inappropriately directed at a "safe" target (e.g., the partner) rather than at the person for whom it is felt (i.e., the professional who communicated the diagnosis). The professional can suggest several evidence-based psychotherapeutic approaches to assist the family. The two most validated time limited therapies are **cognitive-behavioral therapy** (CBT) (Dobson, 2002) and **interpersonal psychotherapy** (IPT; Blanco, Lipsitz, & Caligor, 2001). Family therapy can also be effective (Carr, 2000). Such programs are available specifically directed at parents who struggle with domestic violence, abuse, neglect, or addictions, or live in very impoverished environments (Thomas & Zimmer-Gembeck, 2007).

Accessing support from the family and community environment is critical for family well-being (Hastings, 2002). Families who have strong interpersonal relationships are better able to meet the challenges they encounter. Sometimes, however, family or friends may be unable or ill-equipped to provide the needed support. The extended family may not accept the diagnosis or may assign blame to one of the parents, most commonly to the one unrelated to them. Friends may feel uncomfortable in the presence of the child with a disability, and as a result, they often stay away. Parents may also be embarrassed by their child's disability and rarely venture into the community. They may find it difficult to see their friends' typically developing children. All of these factors can lead to social isolation.

Family Coping

With time, most parents are able to cope with their child's disability and recognize positive outcomes from the experience. In many families, the process of raising a child with a disability increases cohesion, hardiness, and compassion among family members. For some, it even leads to a more meaningful life (Bittles & Glasson, 2004). With experience and support, parents also become experts in meeting their child's needs. They develop assertiveness in learning to ask for and obtain what is needed from professionals and agencies. Their resilience and increasing abilities not only protect but also benefit the child, who may ultimately advance more than what was originally predicted at the time of diagnosis.

For most families, the sadness lessens as they develop routines for care, gain access to early intervention and respite care services, and begin seeing progress in their child's development (Turnbull et al., 2006). The need for enhanced support and/or therapy, however, may recur at various developmental stages. Use of **telehealth** or electronic and video-based communication is rapidly expanding and can be effectively used to support families (Oberleitner et al., 2006). **Parenting networks** in which parents educate and support one another are often very powerful and may be even more effective than professional information and support in some cases (Kerr & McKintosh, 2000).

LONG-TERM EFFECTS ON THE PARENTS

Research on support to families suggests that services benefit families when they are delivered in a family-centered manner and address parent-identified and prioritized issues (King, Teplicky, King, & Rosenbaum, 2004). Dunst, Trivette, and Deal (1994) have suggested that to promote positive family functioning, service efforts need to

- Focus on family-identified needs, aspirations, and plans
- Identify and capitalize on family strengths for harnessing resources
- Strengthen existing social support networks and identify other potential sources
- Use helping behaviors that promote family competencies and strengths
- Use culturally sensitive communication strategies that convey care and empathy
- Promote collaboration in examining different treatments and service options
- Be proactive in mobilizing resources
- Respect families' decisions for making choices

Conducting an assessment of family strengths and needs is important when trying to determine how much assistance might be provided (Trute & Hiebert-Murphy, 2005). Several assessment instruments exist for this purpose including the Family Functioning Style (FFS) scale (Trivette et al., 1990) and the Parents Need Survey (PNS; Seligman & Darling, 2007).

Considering the many stresses families experience in childrearing, research has found that having a strong marital relationship, good parenting and problem-solving skills, financial stability, and supportive social networks lead to more positive outcomes (Marshak & Prezant, 2007; Risdal & Singer, 2004). Although some parental relationships are strengthened by challenges in raising a child with a disability, others deteriorate, especially if the relationship was previously troubled (Wieland & Baker, 2010). Fostering early assistance through community affiliations and providing effective behavioral interventions in the home increase family functioning (Poston & Turnbull, 2004).

Parents of children with severe developmental disabilities, chronic behavior problems, and/or medical fragility (e.g., requiring technology assistance to live and function) are at the greatest risk for caregiver burnout and impaired functioning (Ello & Donovan, 2005). Although many families with severely impaired children do well, some have difficulty finding or accepting support systems for their child (O'Brien, 2001). As a result, they continue to experience chronic stress (Wickler, Wasow, & Hatfield, 1981), which can lead to depression, physical illness, or **post-traumatic stress disorder**. When feelings of sadness or grief become chronic and interfere with the parent's ability to function, psychological intervention is indicated (Gordon, 2009). Kazak et al. (2005) contended that professionals need to explore how the family has dealt with previous stressors and whether family members emerged with a sense of competence or insecurity.

Reframing and normalizing are important intervention strategies in helping families cope. **Normalizing** involves communicating that the emotions and struggles experienced are both normal and expected (Rehm & Bradley, 2005). This approach from a professional can help reduce family members' feelings of isolation and stigma. **Reframing** means reinterpreting a behavior or its context by viewing it from a different lens-frame and focusing on the adaptive and positive aspects rather than negative ones

(Hastings & Taunt, 2002). Family-oriented approaches are particularly effective in altering the counterproductive belief that children with disabilities should be the sole focus of family concerns. When in need, the whole family should take part in the intervention, rather than the child alone (Seligman & Darling, 2007).

There is much research documentation regarding how families of children with disabilities encounter barriers to access or experience unfamiliarity with community and human services including special education services and health care (Odom et al., 2007). Such difficulties are further compounded by some families' lower socioeconomic and educational status. They may also be affected by the providers' lack of training in providing culturally sensitive services, or services to individuals with developmental disabilities. Finally, access may also be limited by a lack of acceptance of Medicaid payments by the health care providers (Reichard, Sacco, & Turnbull, 2004).

To ensure that the values, beliefs, and perspectives of families are considered when conducting assessments and in developing and implementing services, Klinger et al. (2007) recommend that professionals:

- Become knowledgeable about the impact that race, class, culture, and language have on families' access to services

- Communicate with families and their children (with or without disabilities) in their preferred language using interpreter services

- Communicate in a manner that uses common (culturally sensitive) lay words and avoids over-reliance on professional jargon

- Recognize that families may have their own individualistic ways of handling things that do not fit one "particular" culture or style

- Make sure that any printed materials are in the families' preferred language

- Whenever possible, provide services to diverse families within the inclusive context of community services

EFFECTS ON SIBLINGS

The siblings of a child with a disability have unique needs and concerns that may vary with gender, age, birth order, and temperament (Stoneman, 2005) as well as genetic predisposition and family factors (Orsmond & Seltzer, 2007, 2009). A number of years ago, Coleby (1995) found that older male siblings had an increased appreciation for children with disabilities, whereas older female siblings showed increased behavior problems perhaps because of being overburdened with child care responsibilities. The same study showed that near-age siblings had less contact with peers, and younger siblings showed increased anxiety. Sibling concerns also appeared to reflect such situational variables as whether their own needs were being met, how the parents were handling the diagnosis emotionally, what the children were being told, and how much they understood. Some more recent studies have also found an increased risk for behavior problems (Ross & Cuskelly, 2006) and social impairment (Constantino et al., 2006) in siblings, especially in the presence of demographic risks such as immigrant status and poverty (Macks & Reeve, 2007). Other studies, however, have reported siblings to be well-adjusted (Hastings, 2007).

It is important to remember that children, in general, have mixed feelings about their siblings whether they have a disability or not (Schuntermann, 2009). Children may be glad that they do not have a disability but feel simultaneously guilty about this feeling. They may worry that they will "catch" the disability or fantasize that they actually caused it by having bad thoughts about their sibling. Adolescents may question whether they will pass on a similar disability to their future children. Because of the extra care and time required by the child with a disability, the typically developing siblings may think that their parents love their brother or sister more than them. As a consequence, siblings may misbehave to get attention, or they may isolate themselves, worrying about taxing their overburdened parents (Williams, Williams, & Graff, 2003). Giallo and Gavidia-Payne (2006) found that parent and family factors were stronger predictors of sibling adjustment difficulties than siblings' own experience with stress and coping. In particular, family socioeconomic status, management of stress, degree of family time and routines, problem-solving and communication, and family hardiness influenced siblings' difficulties. Hence, care must be taken to balance parenting efforts so that both children with and without disabilities are adequately supported.

Despite these concerns, some evidence indicates that siblings of children with disabilities may demonstrate increased maturity, a sense of responsibility, a tolerance for being different, a feeling of closeness to the family, and enhanced self-confidence and independence

(Meyers & Vipond, 2005; Taeyoung & Horn, 2010). Many siblings of individuals with disabilities choose to enter helping professions (Lobato, 1990).

Siblings of children with disabilities fare best psychologically when their parents' relationship is stable and supportive, feelings are discussed openly, the disability is explained completely, and the siblings are not overburdened with child care responsibilities (Lobato & Kao, 2005). Parents must remember that children observe them closely and take their lead. Parents' approach to assuring that all family members' needs are being addressed sets the tone for the entire family.

Children should be informed at an early age about their sibling's disability so their knowledge is based on fact, not misconception. This education must be done in an age-appropriate fashion, with the siblings feeling free to ask questions at any time. By the time the typically developing siblings reach adolescence, parents need to be ready to share with them information about genetic counseling, estate planning, guardianship arrangements, wills, and so forth. It is helpful for siblings to know what resources and options exist. Some typically developing siblings may choose to have their sibling with a disability live with them as adults, while others may prefer seeking independent or assisted living arrangements or other choices for their sibling once their own parents can no longer provide the needed care (Giallo & Gavidia-Payne, 2006).

EFFECTS ON THE EXTENDED FAMILY

Having grandchildren creates strong feelings of satisfaction, fulfillment of life's purpose, joy, and comfort, but learning that a grandchild has a disability can lead to mixed feelings (Kolomer, 2008). Just like parents, grandparents can harbor guilt, assign blame, or even reject the child (Lee & Gardner, 2010). The quality of the relationship grandparents have with their own children affects their acceptance of the grandchild's disability (Kornhaber, 2002). Typically, when a grandchild is born with a disability, grandparents grieve for their own loss of a "normal grandchild" and for their child's loss. Some may experience denial more strongly than do the parents, and their reaction can interfere with the family's adaptation to the disability (Seligman & Darling, 2007). Counseling, support groups for grandparents, and/or information

given via the parents can lead them to become more supportive of the family and better able to cope with a child's disability (McCallion, Janicki, & Kolomer, 2004).

But grandparents can also be a strong source of support to the family. They may provide respite care, help out with household chores, and provide financial assistance (Trute, 2003). Other extended family members and friends also can help or hinder the parents' ability to cope. Some may have their own concerns or beliefs that interfere with their ability to be supportive; others may not know what to say or how to be supportive. In these instances, professionals can suggest ways to discuss these issues with family or friends or access other supportive social networks (e.g., advocacy groups for their child's disorder).

EFFECTS ON THE CHILD WITH A DISABILITY

Preschool Age

In early childhood, the child with a disability may not recognize that he or she is different from other children. Parents, however, closely scrutinize their child's development (Ray, Pewitt-Kinder, & George, 2009). Play serves as the early learning experience of young children (Myck-Wayne, 2010). Children's interactions with family members and peers during play serves as a preparation for future school interactions, and how parents manage those interactions is critical (Guralnick, 2005).

Parent education regarding the process and course of their child's early development and a referral to early intervention and special preschool services are very important at this stage (Noonan & McCormick, 2006; Chapter 30). Federal legislation plays a key role in providing services to young children with disabilities. Part C of the IDEA addresses the specific needs of infants and toddlers with disabilities (birth to age 3) and their families, and Part B mandates services for children ages 3–5 (Beirne-Smith, Patton, & Kim, 2006; see Chapter 30). Children with disabilities and their parents who participate in early intervention programs often benefit from accompanying services (Zajicek-Farber et al., 2011). The focus on providing early intervention leads to interactions between parents and (often) multiple professionals to set up an individualized family service plan (IFSP), setting the tone for addressing the child's disability in the home and the community. This process, however, can be overwhelming for parents, and it helps when they work closely with the designated service coordinator or social worker on the team.

School Age

By school age, most children with disabilities are aware of their abilities and challenges and may need help in dealing with feelings of being different. Obesity in young children with disabilities can present additional challenges for their immediate social participation and long-term health (Emerson & Robertson, 2010). Assessment of mood and affect in children with developmental disabilities has been a growing area of importance for their well-being (Leffert, Siperstein, & Widaman, 2010). Full acceptance of the child's abilities must first come from the home. If the child is seen as being worthwhile and capable by parents and siblings, his or her self-image is usually positive. This acceptance includes participating in family activities ranging from family events and vacations to religious services and community recreational programs, and if possible, sports or physical play. This acceptance requires that the child's abilities (or lack thereof) are discussed openly and the child is involved in these discussions in an age-appropriate fashion. Discussing and demonstrating how to handle different situations at home improves the child's ability to cope with social situations in the community. Seeking input and guidance from teachers or school staff who interact regularly with the child can help identify the child's strengths and weaknesses in social interactions (Webb, Greco, Sloper, & Beecham, 2008). In order for school and community inclusion to work well, however, teachers and school personnel and community-relevant persons must be adequately informed and trained about the specific needs of the child (Ross-Watt, 2005).

The child with disabilities gains self-confidence through participation in activities in which he or she can be successful (Diamond, 2001). The philosophy of inclusion is that children who are differently challenged can participate in general activities, provided there are appropriate adaptations or assistance. This approach, however, should not preclude participation in specific (segregated) programs, such as the Special Olympics, or camp programs for children who have varied abilities (Cross, Traub, Hutter-Pishgahi, & Shelton, 2004).

Some children with disabilities need encouragement and assistance in building social skills and developing friendships during typical social activities (Rogers, Hemmeter, & Wolery, 2010). Summer camps that welcome children with varied needs provide an avenue to develop important socialization skills and experience independence from parents (Henderson et al., 2007). Such participation encourages maturation and skill development for the child with disabilities (Smith et al., 2004). Furthermore, by participating in an inclusive environment, children and staff without disabilities learn more about tolerance, acceptance, and what it means to have a disability. In turn they become more knowledgeable and caring of people with differences and less prone to bias (Siperstein, Glick, & Parker, 2009).

Adolescence

Adolescence is a challenging period for all children and their families because many biological and social changes are taking place. It can be a particularly difficult time for adolescents with developmental disabilities and their parents (Kim & Turnbull, 2004). For parents, adolescence signals their child's proximity to adulthood and adult responsibilities. It quite naturally elicits anxieties and fears about independence, self-sufficiency, and maturity especially if the child has a disability (Mitchell & Hauser-Cram, 2010). For adolescents, this is a period of many discoveries about self and others, and many adolescents become preoccupied with comparing themselves to their peers (Orsmond, Krauss, & Seltzer, 2004). This desire for fitting in and peer approval in areas of physical and intellectual development may need to be adjusted because of limitations posed by the developmental disability. Negotiating these differences tends to be less of an issue if the adolescent with a disability has 1) at least one supportive peer friend (with or without a disability), 2) a peer group with diverse members, 3) parents who actively encourage the adolescent's participation and involvement in activities that promote independence, and/or 4) him- or herself accepted being "different" (Zajicek-Farber, 1998). For the adolescent who has just acquired a disability (e.g., from a traumatic brain injury) or has significantly impaired intellectual functioning, there is an increased risk of mood upheavals and behavior difficulties. In these cases individual, group, or family counseling and/or medication should be strongly considered (Kolaitis, 2008). Active professional vigilance is needed to screen and assess the mental health of adolescents with disabilities (Emerson, Einfeld, & Stancliffe, 2010). However, accessing mental health care that adequately treats such issues can be difficult and requires strong parental persistence, positive provider relationship, and access to financial resources (Scal & Ireland, 2005).

Adolescents with disabilities are at high risk for being excluded from typical daily activities, which in turn influences their emotional well-being. Heah, Case, McGuire, and Law (2007) found that children with disabilities enjoyed the same activities as typically developing children. Activities allowing children to experience enjoyment (perceived as "fun") have the best chance of ensuring children's engagement and participation. Parents' ability to encourage and promote the child's engagement in the activity by their attitude, emotional responses, and resources are crucial for the child's successful participation. Murphy and Carbone (2008) made similar observations regarding participation in sports and recreational physical activities.

Adolescents with disabilities who remain more isolated and parent dependent tend to have struggles reaching a more independent adulthood (Burdo-Hartman & Patel, 2008). Therefore, they need to be particularly included in mainstream health promotion activities including socializations and sex education (Maart & Jelsma, 2010). They should be provided with appropriate material about friendships and intimate relationships and encouraged to discuss issues of sexuality and emotions in a way and at a level at which they feel comfortable and can understand. Parents also need to be encouraged to give their adolescent with a disability the necessary freedom to become progressively more independent. This approach requires taking certain reasonable risks (Ankeny, Wilkins, & Spain, 2009). If parents persist in managing their child's life and the disability, they are imparting to the adolescent that he or she is not competent to manage independently. Such a well-meaning parental approach often results in poor outcomes. When youths with disabilities and their parents are encouraged and supported to become actively involved in planning for transitions, be they educational or in life, they fare better (Cobb & Alwell, 2009).

Young Adulthood

The transition to adulthood is both important and difficult for parents and adolescents with disabilities (Blomquist, 2007; Landmark, Ju, & Zhang, 2010). Brotherson, Backus, Summers, and Turnbull (1986) identified tasks that are unique to families of young adults with disabilities:

- "Adjusting to the adult implications of the disability"
- Identifying an appropriate residence
- Initiating vocational involvement
- Addressing special issues of intimacy, sexuality, and procreation
- Recognizing the need for continuing family responsibilities
- Managing health- and condition-related needs
- Managing the continued financial implications of dependency
- Dealing with limited socialization opportunities outside of the family environment
- Planning for guardianship

Although some adolescents with disabilities *do* achieve independence, many struggle, and some never attain this goal. For young adults who cannot achieve true independence a number of alternatives are available depending on where they live, their self-care abilities, employment and social/recreational activities, and finances. A young adult's ability to cope and become as independent as possible depends not only on the degree of the disability but also on the effectiveness of the family to plan and manage this transition emotionally and financially, and their ability to access community resources effectively (Wells, Sandefleur, & Hogan, 2003). However, moving into an independent living situation can become a difficult time for the family because it disrupts established structures and relationships (Albrecht & Devlieger, 1999). Turnbull and Turnbull (1993) offer useful advice to professionals and families in planning toward adulthood:

- Foster decision making and self-determination skills in children with disabilities, starting from the earliest years
- Approach transitions as generic issues by focusing on similarities among transitions at various life stages
- Focus on family services and supports throughout the life span, not just during early childhood or adolescence
- Connect children and families with different adult role models

PRINCIPLES OF FAMILY-CENTERED CARE: ROLE OF THE PROFESSIONAL

Table 37.1 lists principles of family-centered care that represent the current philosophy guiding the interaction between professionals and families of children with disabilities (Epley, Summers, & Turnbull, 2010). The goal of family-centered care is to facilitate the best possible outcomes for both children and their families. To achieve this goal, professionals must initiate a process of service delivery and support that

Table 37.1. Professional behavior using principles of family-centered care

- Demonstrate respect for the child and family in all types of interactions, including communication.
- Be knowledgeable about and recognize the importance of racial, ethnic, cultural, and socio-economic diversity and its effect on the family's experiences in seeking help and perception of care and support.
- Actively seek to indentify strengths of each child and family, and help the child and family use these strengths to promote their natural resilience and address challenging situations.
- Facilitate a partnering climate and time, and encourage the child and family to ask questions and express their choices about treatment, care, and support.
- Explore options and potential effects of different choices for treatment and care with both the child and family.
- Assist the family in obtaining interdisciplinary input and coordination of care regarding options for treatment and support services.
- Ask about barriers or challenges the child and family may be experiencing in their psychosocial adjustment to treatment, care, or receipt of support.
- Provide and share with the child and family the types of available formal and informal support services that might be helpful for ensuring healthy child and family functioning during critical and transitional developmental periods.
- Encourage the child and family input and advocacy in all forms of professional interaction and education and the development of policies for treatment and program interventions.
- Ensure flexibility in developing organizational policies and procedures and providers' practices so that all services can be individualized to the diverse needs, beliefs, and cultural values of each child and family.
- Strive to collaborate and partner with families at all levels of health care service delivery.

Sources: Johnson and Eichner (2003); National Center for Medical Home Implementation (n.d.); and National Early Childhood Technical Assistance Center (n.d.). For more information, see http://www.medicalhomeinfo.org and http://www.nectac.org.

invites and establishes a collaborative relationship based on mutual respect and open communication (Lotze, Bellin, & Oswald, 2010). When such a family-centered relationship is forged, families come to see the professionals as partners who are flexible in solving problems and in giving constructive feedback. They are also seen as being respectful of cultural diversity and able to listen to family needs with empathy and compassion (see http://www.familyvoices.org/). Through this shared focus, both families and professionals appreciate the unique expertise that each contributes.

Over time, families of children with disabilities encounter a bevy of professionals including physicians, nurses, teachers, physical and occupational therapists, psychologists, social workers, and agency or hospital administrators. Individually and as a group, professionals bear the primary responsibility for explaining the results of developmental evaluations and testing, presenting treatment options, teaching intervention and advocacy strategies, and exploring and accessing available support systems. The initial contact that families have with professionals often takes place when they are stressed, confused, and vulnerable; and how professionals respond sets the tone for future interactions (Ray, Pewitt-Kinder, & George, 2009). Wright, Heibert-Murphy, and Trute (2010) examined professional perceptions and organizational factors that support or hinder the implementation of family-centered practices. These included the organization's culture and climate (e.g., caseload size and activity, supervision, staff training), policy limitations, and availability of collateral services. All these factors can affect the successful implementation of family-centered services. Sloper, Greco, Beecham, and Webb (2006) found that when the case worker provided emotional support, information, assistance in identifying and meeting needs, advocacy, and service coordination, and when there were increased contact hours between the worker and the family, outcomes improved. Hiebert-Murphy, Trute, and Wright (2008) found that family-centeredness in coordinating services significantly decreased the family's need for additional psychosocial supports.

Professionals need to be flexible and responsive in coordinating efforts with the family and other professionals. As a result of their training, experience, and expertise, professionals often have strong opinions about what is best for the child and family. Yet, they must remember that individuals with disabilities and their families have the right to choose their own path. If a family encounters difficulties along the way, members can always turn to professionals for further assistance to accomplish their goals. Families who make their own choices are self-sustaining (Seligman & Darling, 2007). The inclusion of families as active decision-makers in clinical care is becoming more readily accepted; however, more needs to be done for their inclusion in health care policy (Goldfarb et al., 2010).

In partnering with families, the professional must take action, however, when the choices the family makes are perceived as potentially deleterious to the child's well-being. For example, it is the professional's responsibility to inform the family of the risks and benefits of validated and nonvalidated therapies, while respecting the family's autonomy. The one exception is when it is believed that the family's actions may be harmful to the child. The professional must then contact the local child welfare agency (child protective services) to report the professional's suspicion or knowledge of abuse or neglect.

THE ROLE OF SOCIETY AND COMMUNITY

The family's social context plays an important role in determining the outcome of its members. Fortunately, in today's society there is greater appreciation for people with disabilities. There are more educational, vocational, housing and support services available. Federal legislation guarantees equal opportunities for all members of society. Federal funding provides for a protection and advocacy system for people with disabilities in each state. The Individuals with Disabilities Education Improvement Act of 2004 (IDEA 2004; PL 108446) mandates free and appropriate educational and rehabilitative services for school-age children. Reaching citizens of all ages with disabilities, the Americans with Disabilities Act (ADA) of 1990 (PL 101-336) focuses on the establishment of rights regarding access to employment, transportation, telecommunications, and public accommodations. Effects of the ADA are increasingly visible through the presence of accessible city sidewalks, ramps on buildings, public transportation equipped with wheelchair lifts, accessible computers in libraries, and other universal technological advances. As a result of these efforts and other laws (e.g., Assistive Technology Act of 2004 [AT Act]), individuals with disabilities and their families are guaranteed the same civil rights as individuals without disabilities (Beirne-Smith et al., 2006).

Although laws are important, they need to be accompanied by a change in the public's perception and attitudes toward individuals with disabilities. Signs of such change seem to be emerging. Young adults who have grown up in schools with children with disabilities are more sensitive to and appreciative of their needs and abilities. More individuals with disabilities are in the workforce. They are seen in movies, on television shows, advertisements, and in the news. Adaptive and assistive technologies, including the use of universal design, are slowly removing barriers and increasing overall societal integration of individuals with diverse abilities (Burgstahler, 2005). Although society has made itself more accessible to and supportive of individuals with disabilities, the future remains challenging.

SUMMARY

As a family moves through its life cycle, its members face many challenges and changes. This journey is particularly challenging for families of children with disabilities. The child, parents, siblings, extended family members, and friends are all affected and may initially undergo periods of grieving and disappointment for their loss of a chance of a "normal life" for their child. Over time, the family's coping strategies generally improve. Parents learn to master the child's care and to advocate effectively for necessary medical, education, and other services. The child learns to cope with the disability at school and in the community and to become a self-advocate. Working closely with the parents and child in a family-centered approach, the social worker, therapists, teachers, and physicians can play a crucial role in promoting these adjustments and may be instrumental in determining the prognosis of the child and the outcome of the entire family.

REFERENCES

Americans with Disabilities Act (ADA) of 1990, PL 101336, 42 U.S.C. §§ 12101 et seq.

Albrecht, G., & Devlieger, P. (1999). The disability paradox: High quality of life against all odds. *Social Science and Medicine, 48*, 977–988.

Alvard, M., & Grdos, J. (2005). Enhancing resilience in children: A proactive approach. *Professional Psychology: Research and Practice, 36*, 238–245.

Ankeny, E., Wilkins, J., & Spain, J. (2009). Mothers' experiences of transition planning for their children with disabilities. *Teaching Exceptional Children, 41*(6), 28–36.

Ariel, C., & Naseef, R. (2006). *Voices from the spectrum.* London, UK: Jessica Kingsley.

Bartolo, P. (2002). Communicating a diagnosis of developmental disability to parents: Multiprofessional negotiation frameworks. *Child Care Health and Development, 28*(1), 65–71.

Beirne-Smith, M., Patton, J., & Kimm, S. (2006). *Mental retardation: An introduction to intellectual disabilities* (7th ed.). Pearson: Merril/Prentice Hall.

Bittles, A., & Glasson, E. (2004). Clinical, social, and ethical implications of changing life expectancy in Down syndrome. *Developmental Medicine and Child Neurology, 46,* 282–286.

Blanco, C., Lipsitz, J., & Caligor, E. (2001). Treatment of chronic depression with a 12-week program of interpersonal psychotherapy. *American Journal of Psychiatry, 158,* 371–375.

Blomquist, K.B. (2007). Health and independence of young adults with disabilities: Two years later. *Orthopedic Nursing, 26*(5), 296–309.

Brinthaupt, J. (1991). Pediatric chronic illness, cystic fibrosis, and parental adjustment. In M. Seligman (Ed.), *The family with a handicapped child* (2nd ed., pp. 295–336). Boston, MA: Allyn & Bacon.

Bronfenbrenner, U. (1986). Ecology of the family as a context for human development research perspectives. *Developmental Psychology, 22,* 723–742.

Brotherson, M., Backus, L., Summers, J.A., & Turnbull, A.P. (1986). Transition to adulthood. In J.A. Summers (Ed.), *The right to grow up: An introduction to adults with developmental disabilities* (pp. 17–44). Baltimore, MD: Paul H. Brookes Publishing Co.

Burdo-Hartman, W., & Patel, D. (2008). Medical home transitions planning for children and youth with special health care needs. *Pediatric Clinics in North America, 55*(6), 1287–1297.

Burgstahler, S. (2005). *Universal design of instruction: Definition, principles, and examples.* Retrieved from http://www.smith.edu/deanoffaculty/Burgstahler.pdf

Carr, A. (2000). Evidence-based practice in family therapy and systemic consultation I. *Journal of Family Therapy, 22,* 29–60.

Cobb, R., & Alwell, M. (2009). Transition planning/coordinating interventions for youth with disabilities: A systematic review. *Career Development for Exceptional Individuals, 32*(2), 70–81.

Cohen, D., Feurer, S., Goldfarb, F., Lalinde, P., Smith, M., Yingling, J., … Pariseau, C. (2006). *Family discipline competencies.* Silver Spring, MD: Association of University Centers on Disabilities.

Coleby, M. (1995). The school-aged siblings of children with disabilities. *Developmental Medicine and Child Neurology, 37,* 415–426.

Constantino, J., Lajonchere, C., Lutz, M., Gray, T., Abbacchi, A., McKenna, K., … Todd, R.D. (2006). Autistic social impairment in the siblings of children with pervasive developmental disorders. *American Journal of Psychiatry, 163,* 294–296.

Cross, A., Traub, E., Hutter-Pishgahi, L., & Shelton, G. (2004). Elements of successful inclusion for children with significant disabilities. *Topics in Early Childhood Special Education, 24*(3), 169–183.

Dellve, L., Samuelsson, L., Tallborn, A., Fasth, A., & Hallberg, L.R. (2006). Stress and well-being among parents of children with rare diseases: A prospective intervention study. *Journal of Advanced Nursing, 53*(4), 392–402.

Diamond, K. (2001). Relationships among young children's ideas, emotional understanding, and social contact with classmates with disabilities. *Topics in Early Childhood Special Education, 21*(2), 104.

Dobson, K. (Ed.). (2002). *Handbook of cognitive-behavioral therapies* (2nd ed.). New York, NY: Guilford.

Dunst, C.J., Trivette, C.M., & Deal, A.G. (1994). *Supporting and strengthening of families: Methods, strategies, and practices* (Vol.1). Cambridge, MA: Brookline Books.

Durà-Vilà, G., Dein, S., & Hodes, M. (2010). Children with intellectual disability: A gain not a loss: Parental beliefs and family life. *Clinical Child Psychology & Psychiatry, 15*(2), 171–184.

Earls, M.F., & The Committee on Psychosocial Aspects of Child and Family Health. (2010). Clinical Report—Incorporating recognition and management of perinatal and postpartum depression into pediatric practice. *Pediatrics, 126*(5), 1032–1039.

Ello, L.M., & Donovan, S.J. (2005). Assessment of the relationship between parenting stress and a child's ability to functionally communicate. *Research on Social Work Practice, 15*(6), 531–544.

Emerson, E., Einfeld, S., & Stancliffe, R.J. (2010). The mental health of young children with intellectual disabilities or borderline functioning. *Social Psychiatry and Psychiatric Epidemiology, 45*(5), 579–587.

Emerson, E., & Robertson, J. (2010). Obesity in young children with intellectual disabilities or borderline intellectual functioning. *International Journal on Pediatric Obesity, 5*(4), 320–326.

Epley, P., Summers, J.A., & Turnbull, A. (2010). Characteristics and trends in family-centered conceptualizations. *Journal of Family Social Work, 13*(3), 269–285.

Farber, M., & Maharaj, R. (2005). Empowering high-risk families of children with disabilities. *Research on Social Work Practice, 15*(6), 501–515.

Freedman, R.I., & Boyer, N.C. (2000). The power to choose: Supports for families caring for individuals with developmental disabilities. *Health and Social Work, 25*(1), 59–68.

Giallo, R., & Gavidia-Payne, S. (2006). Child, parent, and family factors as predictors of adjustment for siblings of children with disability. *Journal of Intellectual Disability and Research, 50,* 937–948.

Goldfarb, F., Devine, K., Yingling, J., Hill, A., Moss, J., Ogburn, E.S., … Pariseau, C. (2010). Partnering with professionals: Family-centered care from the parent perspective. *Journal of Family Social Work, 13,* 91–99.

Goldenberg, I., & Goldenberg, H. (2003). *Family therapy: An overview* (6th ed.). Pacific Grove, CA: Brooks/Cole.

Gordon, J. (2009). An evidence-based approach for supporting parents experiencing chronic sorrow. *Pediatric Nursing, 35*(2), 115–119.

Green, S.E. (2001). Grandma's hands: parental perspectives of the importance of grandparents as secondary caregivers in families of children with disabilities. *International Journal of Aging and Human Development, 53,* 11–33.

Guralnick, M. (2005). Early intervention for children with intellectual disabilities: Current knowledge and future prospects. *Journal of Applied Research in Intellectual Disabilities, 18,* 313–324.

Hanson, M.J., & Lynch, E.W. (2004). *Understanding families: Approaches to diversity, disability, and risk.* Baltimore, MD: Paul H. Brookes Publishing Co.

Hastings, R.P. (2002). Parental stress and behaviour problems of children with developmental disability. *Journal of Intellectual and Developmental Disability, 27*(3), 149–160.

Hastings, R.P. (2007). Longitudinal relationships between sibling behavioral adjustment and behavior problems of children with developmental disabilities. *Journal of Autism and Developmental Disorders, 37,* 1485–1492.

Hastings, R.P., & Taunt, H.M. (2002). Positive perceptions in families of children with developmental disabilities. *American Journal on Mental Retardation, 107,* 116–127.

Heah, T., Case, T., McGuire, B., & Law, M. (2007). Successful participation. The lived experience among children with disabilities. *The Canadian Journal of Occupational Therapy, 74*(1), 38–47.

Heiman, T. (2002). Parents of children with disabilities: Resilience, coping, and future expectations. *Journal of Developmental and Physical Disabilities, 14*(2), 159–171.

Henderson, K., Whitaker, L., Bialeschki, M., Scanlin, M., & Thurber, C. (2007). Summer camp experiences. *Journal of Family Issues, 28*(8), 987–1007.

Hiebert-Murphy, D., Trute, B., & Wright, A. (2008). Patterns of entry to community-based services for families with children with developmental disabilities: Implications for social work practice. *Child & Family Social Work, 13,* 423–432.

Hornby, G. (2000). *Improving parental involvement.* London, UK: Continuum.

Individuals with Disabilities Education Improvement Act of 2004, PL 108-446, 20 U.S.C. §§ 1400 *et seq.*

Johnson, B.H., & Eichner, J.M. (2003). Family-centered care and the pediatrician's role. *Pediatrics 112*(3), 691–696.

Kazak, A., Kassam-Adams, N., Schneider, S. Zelikovsky, N., Alderfer, M., & Rourke, M. (2005). An integrative model of pediatric medical traumatic stress. *Journal of Pediatric Psychology, 31*(4), 343–355.

Kerr, S.M., & McIntosh, J.B. (2000). Coping when a child has a disability: Exploring the impact of parent-to-parent support. Child: *Care, Health and Development, 26*(4), 259–342.

Kim, K., & Turnbull, A. (2004). Transition to adulthood for students with severe intellectual disabilities: Shifting toward person-family interdependent planning. *Research and Practice for Persons with Severe Disabilities, 29*(1), 111–124.

King, S, Teplicky, R., King, G., & Rosenbaum, P. (2004). Family-centered service for children with cerebral palsy and their families: A review of the literature. *Seminars in Pediatric Neurology 11*(1), 78–86.

Klinger, J., Blanchett, W., & Harry, B. (2007). Race, culture, and developmental disabilities. In S.L. Odom, R.H.Horner, M.E. Snell, & J. Blacher (Eds.), *Handbook of developmental disabilities* (pp. 55–75). New York, NY: Guilford.

Kolaitis, G. (2008). Young people with intellectual disabilities and mental health. *Current Opinion in Psychiatry, 21*(5), 469–473.

Kolomer, S. (2008). Grandparents as caregivers. *Journal of Geronotlogical Social Work, 50*(1), 321–344.

Kornhaber, A. (2002). *The grandparent guide.* Chicago, IL: Contemporary Books.

Landmark, L.J., Ju, S., & Zhang, D. (2010). Substantiated best practices in transition: Fifteen plus years later. *Career Development for Exceptional Individuals, 33*(3), 165–176.

Lee, M., & Gardner, J. (2010). Grandparents' involvement and support in families with children with disabilities. *Educational Gerontology, 36*(6), 467–499.

Leffert, J.S., Siperstein, G.N., & Widaman, K.F. (2010). Social perception in children with intellectual disabilities: The interpretation of benign and hostile intentions. *Journal of Intellectual Disability Research, 54*(2), 168–180.

Lobato, D.J. (1990). *Brothers, sisters, and special needs: Information and activities for helping young siblings of children with chronic illnesses and developmental disabilities.* Baltimore, MD: Paul H. Brookes Publishing Co.

Lobato, D.J., & Kao, B.T. (2005). Brief report: Family-based group intervention for young siblings of children with chronic illness and developmental disability. *Pediatric Psychology, 30*(8), 678–682.

Lotze, G.M., Bellin, M.H., & Oswald, D.P. (2010). Family-centered care for children with special health care needs: Are we moving forward? *Journal of Family Social Work, 13*(2), 100–113.

Maart, S., & Jelsma, J. (2010). The sexual behaviour of physically disabled adolescents. *Disability and Rehabilitation, 32*(6), 438–443.

Macks, R.J., & Reeve, R.E. (2007). The adjustment of non-disabled siblings of children with autism. *Journal of Autism and Developmental Disorders, 37,* 1060–1067.

Marshak, L.E., & Prezant, F. (2007). *Married with special needs children: A couple's guide to keeping connected.* Bethesda, MD: Woodbine House.

McCallion, P., Janicki, M.P., & Kolomer, S.R. (2004). Controlled evaluation of support groups for grandparent caregivers of children with developmental disabilities and delays. *American Journal of Mental Retardation, 109*(5), 352–361.

McCubbin, H.I., & Patterson, J.M. (1983). The family stress process: The double ABCX model of adjustment and adaptation. *Marriage and Family Review, 6*(1–2), 7–37.

Meyers, C., & Vipond, J. (2005). Play and social interactions between children with development disabilities and their siblings: A systematic literature review. *Physical and Occupational Therapy in Pediatrics, 25*(1–2), 81–103.

Mitchell, D.B., & Hauser-Cram, P. (2010). Early childhood predictors of mothers' and fathers' relationships with adolescents with developmental disabilities. *Journal of Intellectual Disabilities Research, 54*(6), 487–500.

Murphy, N.A., & Carbone, P.S. (2008). Promoting the participation of children with disabilities in sports, recreation, and physical activities. *Pediatrics, 121*(5), 1057-1061.

Myck-Wayne, J. (2010). In defense of play: Beginning the dialog about the power of play. *Young Exceptional Children, 13*(4), 14–23.

National Center for Medical Home Implementation. (n.d.). *Family-centered medical home overview.* Retrieved from http://www.medicalhomeinfo.org/about/medical_home

National Early Childhood Technical Assistance Center. (n.d.). *NECTAC: The National Early Childhood Technical Assistance Center.* Retrieved from http://www.nectac.org

Noonan, M.J., & McCormick, L. (2006). *Young children with disabilities in natural environments: Methods and procedures.* Baltimore, MD: Paul H. Brookes Publishing Co.

O'Brien, M.E. (2001). Living in a house of cards: Family experiences with long-term childhood technology dependence. *Journal of Pediatric Nursing, 16,* 13–22.

Oberleitner, R., Ball, J., Gillette, D., Naseef, R., & Stamm, B. H. (2006). Technologies to lessen the distress of autism. *Journal of Aggression, Maltreatment & Trauma, 12*, 221–242.

Odom, S., Horner, R., Snell, M., & Blacher, J. (Eds.). (2007). *Handbook of developmental disabilities.* New York, NY: Guilford.

Ogburn, E., Roberts, R., Pariseau, C., Levitz, B., Wagner, B., Moss, J., & Adelmann, B. (2006). *Promising practices in family mentorship: A guidebook for MCHB-LEND training programs.* Silver Spring, MD: Association of University Centers on Disabilities.

Orsmond, G., & Seltzer, M. (2007). Siblings of individuals with autism or Down syndrome: Effects on adult lives. *Journal of Intellectual Disability Research, 51*(9), 682–696.

Orsmond, G., & Seltzer, M. (2009). Adolescent siblings of individuals with an Autism Spectrum Disorder: Testing a Diathesis-Stress model of sibling well-being. *Journal of Autism and Developmental Disorders, 39*(7), 1053–1065.

Park, J., Turnbull, A.P., & Turnbull, H.R. (2002). Impacts of poverty on quality of life in families of children with disabilities. *Exceptional Children, 68*(2), 151–170.

Pollin, I. (1995). *Medical crisis counseling.* New York, NY: Norton.

Poston, D., & Turnbull, A. (2004). Role of spirituality and religion in family quality of life for families of children with disabilities. *Education and Training in Developmental Disabilities, 39*(2), 95–108.

Ray, J., Pewitt-Kinder, J., & George, S. (2009). Partnering with families of children with special needs. *Young Children, 64*(5), 16–22.

Rehm, R., & Bradely, J. (2005). Normalization in families raising a child who is medically fragile/technology dependent and developmentally delayed. *Qualitative Health Research, 15*(6), 807–820.

Reichard, A., Sacco, T.M., & Turnbull, R. (2004). Access to health care for individuals with developmental disabilities from minority backgrounds. *Mental Retardation, 42*, 459–470.

Reichman, N., Corman, H., & Noonan, K. (2008) Impact of child disability on the family. *Maternal and Child Health Journal, 12*(6), 679–683.

Risdal, D., & Singer, G. (2004). Marital adjustment in parents of children with disabilities: A historical review and meta-analysis. *Research and Practice for Persons with Severe Disabilities, 29*(2), 95–103.

Rogers, L., Hemmeter, M., & Wolery, M. (2010). Using a constant time delay procedure to teach foundational swimming skills to children with Autism. *Topics in Early Childhood Special Education, 30*(2), 102–111.

Ross P., & Cuskelly, M. (2006). Adjustment, sibling problems and coping strategies of brothers and sisters of children with autistic spectrum disorder. *Journal of Intellectual & Developmental Disability, 31*, 77–86.

Ross-Watt, F. (2005). Inclusion in the early years: From rhetoric to reality. *Child Care in Practice, 11*(2), 103-118.

Scal, P., & Ireland, M. (2005). Addressing transition to adult health care for adolescents with special health care needs. *Pediatrics, 115*(6), 1607–1612.

Schuntermann, P. (2009). Growing up with a developmentally challenged brother or sister: A model for engaging siblings based on mentalizing. *Harvard Review of Psychiatry, 17*(5), 297–314.

Seligman, M., & Darling, R.B. (2007). *Ordinary families, special children.* New York, NY: Guilford.

Singer, G., & Floyd, F. (2006). Meta-analysis of comparative studies of depression in mothers of children with and without developmental disabilities. *American Journal on Mental Retardation, 111*(3), 155–169.

Siperstein, G., Glick, G., & Parker, R. (2009). Social inclusion of children with intellectual disabilities in a recreational setting. *Intellectual and Developmental Disabilities, 47*(2), 97–107.

Sloper, P., Greco, V., Beecham, J., & Webb, R. (2006). Key worker services for disabled children: What characteristics of services lead to better outcomes for children and families? *Child: Care, Health & Development, 32*, 147–157.

Smith, R., Austin, D., Kennedy, D., Lee, Y., & Hutchison, P. (2004). *Inclusive and special recreation: Opportunities for persons with disabilities* (5th ed.). New York, NY: McGraw Hill.

Stoneman, Z. (2005). Siblings of children with disabilities: Research themes. *Mental Retardation, 43*(5), 339–350.

Sullivan-Bolyai, S., Sadler, L., Knafl, K.A., & Gilliss, C.L. (2004). Great expectations: A position description for parents as caregivers: Part II. *Pediatric Nursing, 30*(1), 52–56.

Taeyoung, K., & Horn, E. (2010). Sibling-implemented intervention for skill development with children with disabilities. *Topics in Early Childhood Special Education, 30*(2), 80–90.

Thomas, R., & Zimmer-Gembeck, M. (2007). Behavioral outcomes of parent-child interaction therapy and Triple P-Positive Parenting program: A review and meta-analysis. *Journal of Abnormal Clinical Psychology, 35*(3), 475–495.

Trivette, C., Dunst, C., Deal, A., Hamer, A., & Propst, S. (1990). Assessing family strengths and family functioning style. *Topics in Early Childhood Special Education, 10*(1), 16–35.

Trute, B. (2003). Grandparents of children with developmental disabilities: Intergenerational support and family well-being. *Families in Society, 84*, 119–126.

Trute, B., & Hiebert-Murphy, D. (2005). Predicting family adjustment and parenting stress in childhood disability services using brief assessment tools. *Journal of Intellectual and Developmental Disability, 30*(4), 217–225.

Turnbull, A.P., & Turnbull, H.R. (1993). Enhancing beneficial linkages across the lifespan. *Disability Studies Quarterly, 13*(4), 34–36.

Turnbull, A.P., Turnbull, H.R., Erwin, E. J., & Soodak, L.C. (2006). *Families, professionals, and exceptionality* (5th ed.). Upper Saddle River, NJ: Merrill/Prentice Hall.

van der Veek, S., Kraaij, V., & Garnefski, N. (2009). Down or up? Explaining positive and negative emotions in parents of children with Down syndrome: Goals, cognitive coping, and resources. *Journal of Intellectual and Developmental Disabilities, 34*(3), 216–229.

Webb, R., Greco, V., Sloper, P., & Beecham, J. (2008). Key workers and schools: Meeting the needs of children and young people with disabilities. *European Journal of Special Needs Education, 23*(3), 189–205.

Wells, T., Sandefleur, G.D., & Hogan, D.P. (2003). What happens after high school years among young persons with disabilities? *Social Forces, 82*(2), 803–832.

Wickler, L., Wasow, M., & Hatfield, E. (1981). Chronic sorrow revisited: Parent vs. professional depiction of the adjustment of parents of mentally retarded children. *American Journal of Orthopsychiatry, 51*, 63–70.

Wieland, N., & Baker, B. (2010). The role of marital quality and spousal support in behaviour problems of children with and without intellectual disability. *Journal of Intellectual Disability Research, 54*(7), 620–633.

Williams, P., Williams, A., & Graff, J. (2003). A community-based intervention for siblings and parents of children with chronic illness or disability: The ISEE study. *The Journal of Pediatrics, 143*(3), 386–393.

Wright, A., Hiebert-Murphy, D., & Trute, B. (2010). Professionals' perspectives on organizational factors that support or hinder the successful implementation of family-centered practice. *Journal of Family Social Work, 13*, 114–130.

Xu, Y. (2007). Empowering culturally diverse families of young children with disabilities: The Double ABCX model. *Early Childhood Education Journal, 34*(6), 431-437.

Zajicek-Farber, M.L. (1998). Promoting good health in adolescents with disabilities. *Health and Social Work, 23*(3), 203–213.

Zajicek-Farber, M.L., Wall, S., Kisker, E., Luze, G.J., & Summers, J.A. (2011). Comparing service use of Early Head Start families of children with and without disabilities. *Journal of Family Social Work, 14*(2), 159–178.

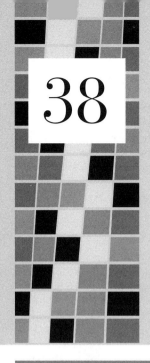

38

Complementary and Alternative Therapies

Michelle H. Zimmer

Upon completion of this chapter, the reader will

■ Be introduced to the concept of complementary and alternative medical (CAM) therapies

■ Become aware of the different types of CAM

■ Be knowledgeable about some of the more common CAM therapies and how they have been used in treating children with developmental and related disabilities

Complementary and alternative medicine (CAM) therapies have been increasingly utilized in the treatment of children with developmental disabilities, with over half of these children receiving at least one form of CAM (see below). The National Center for Complementary and Alternative Medicine (NCCAM) defines CAM as a group of diverse medical and health care systems, practices, and products that are not presently considered to be part of conventional medicine. Complementary medicine is used together with conventional Western medicine, while alternative medicine (e.g., Chinese and Indian medicine) is used in place of conventional medicine. **Integrative medicine** refers to a practice that combines conventional and types of CAM treatments for which there is evidence of safety and effectiveness (http://nccam.nih.gov).

In 2007, the Centers for Disease Control and Prevention (CDC) reported that nearly 12% of all children had participated in some form of CAM in the last 12 months, with significantly higher rates of use among patients with chronic medical conditions. When considering the group of children with developmental disabilities, estimates of CAM use are much higher than in the general pediatric population, ranging from 50%–70% (Ball, Kertesz, & Moyer-Mileur, 2005; McCann & Newell, 2006; Sanders, Davis, Duncan, Meaney, Haynes, & Barton, 2003). For specific disabilities, the prevalence of CAM use has been studied in children with attention-deficit/hyperactivity disorder (ADHD), autism spectrum disorders (ASD), cerebral palsy (CP), and Down syndrome. Reports of CAM use among children with ADHD range between 28% and 67%, depending on the definition of CAM (Gross-Tsur, 2003; Sinha & Efron, 2005). Estimates of CAM use among children with ASD are particularly high, ranging from 52%–95%. (Hansen, Kalish & Bunce, 2007; Harrington, Rosen, Garnecho,& Patrick, 2006). Data is sparse regarding the use of CAM among children with Down syndrome. The few studies that have examined the issue report rates of CAM use as high as 87% (Prussing, Sobo, Walker, Dennis, & Kurtin, 2004). Among children with cerebral palsy, Samdup, Smith, and Il Song (2006) reported that severity of CP was positively correlated with higher CAM use. Hurvitz, Leonard, Ayyangar, and Nelson (2003) studied CAM use among children with CP and estimated its prevalence at 56%.

EVIDENCE OF TREATMENT EFFICACY

NCCAM categorizes complementary and alternative medicine into four broad categories: 1) biologically based practices, which include nutrition, medicinal herbs and dietary supplements; 2) mind-body medicine, including practices such as meditation that focus on the interactions among the brain, mind, and body, to affect health and behavior; 3) manipulative and body-based practices such as massage; and 4) energy-based practices such as acupuncture (http://nccam.nih.gov).

Biologically Based Practices

Diets

Various dietary changes and restrictions have been suggested to treat symptoms of developmental disabilities, most commonly for children with ADHD and ASD. The **gluten-free—casein-free diet**, which involves removing all wheat and milk products from a child's diet has been studied in children with ASD, and although commonly used, research does not support its effectiveness (Elder, Shankar, Shuster, Theriaque, Burns, & Sherrill, 2006; Johnson, Handen, Zimmer, Mayer Costa, & Sacco, 2011). Removing milk products from the diet carries a risk of inadequate intake of vitamin D and calcium. There is some data to suggest that children on the autism spectrum have lower bone density than typically developing children (Hediger, England, Molloy, Yu, Manning-Courtney, & Mills, 2008); some have hypothesized that this is due, at least in part, to avoidance of milk products. The **Feingold diet** is a controversial diet for children with ADHD or autism. It involves removing synthetic colors, flavors, artificial preservatives, salicylates, and sweeteners from the diet. A typical Feingold diet would exclude sodas, many common snack foods, and even many fruits which are high in salicylates such as raisins, berries, and grapes. Although controversial, there is some European data suggesting that this diet reduces hyperactivity in both typical

children and children with ADHD (Kemp, 2008). No study of this diet in children with autism has been published. Sugar restriction is a common dietary change made by families of children with ADHD. The research literature, however, suggests that restricting sugar from the diet does not significantly improve symptoms of ADHD and is not necessary for the vast majority of children with this condition (Wolraich, Wilson, & White, 1995).

Vitamins/Supplements

Dietary supplements for children with disabilities are numerous and beyond the scope of this review. Many supplements, such as multivitamins and vitamin C, while having unclear health benefits, are safe and most health care workers do not discourage their use. Other supplements, such as megavitamin therapy (dosage more than 1,000 times the daily requirement), **chelation therapy** (the use of an oral, intravenous or topical medication to remove metal from the body), and antifungal treatments (prescription medications such as nystatin) carry a significant risk of side effects and potential for harm, and their use should be discouraged. **Melatonin**, a naturally occurring hormone that has been promoted as an over-the-counter remedy for jet lag, is one dietary supplement for which there is substantial evidence of efficacy for improving sleep onset in children with disabilities. Several small clinical trials demonstrated benefits in reducing time to sleep onset (also called sleep latency) in children with ASD (Andersen, Kaczmarska, McGrew, & Malow, 2008; Garstang & Wallis, 2006), developmental disabilities (Phillips & Appleton, 2004; Wasdell, Jan, Bomben, 2008), and fragile X syndrome. (Wirojanan, Jacquemont, & Diaz, 2009)

Hyperbaric Oxygen Therapy

Hyperbaric oxygen therapy (HBOT) uses compressed oxygen chambers to treat specific medical illnesses such as carbon monoxide poisoning (e.g., from the bends in rapid ascent from deep-sea diving or from a malfunctioning furnace). Hyperbaric oxygen saturates tissues with oxygen and proponents state that this higher tissue availability of oxygen can reverse neurologic damage. HBOT is available only via prescription and in some outpatient clinics of alternative medical providers. However, families have been known to purchase HBOT chambers for their personal use at the cost of thousands of dollars. Frequent hourly treatments (40 or more treatments) are recommended by their practitioners and cost between $100–250 per treatment. Use of HBOT has been reported in children with Down syndrome, ASD, and CP; however, the scientific evidence for its effectiveness in these conditions is completely lacking. Critics of this and other CAM practices also have raised concerns about the opportunity cost of spending time and money engaged in unproven therapies rather than in therapies that have proven efficacy. HBOT also has inherent risks, such as the potential of tympanic membrane rupture due to high air pressure and an increased risk of seizures (McDonagh, Morgan, Carson, & Russman, 2007). HBOT is generally discouraged by health care professionals due to its lack of demonstrated positive outcomes and potential for financial and medical harm.

Mind–Body Practices

Biofeedback/ Electroencephalogram Biofeedback

Biofeedback/Electroencephalogram (EEG) biofeedback is a mind-body therapy that provides information about physiologic processes such as heart rate, blood pressure and skin temperature, with the goal of gaining control over these processes to improve mental functioning and performance. Biofeedback equipment involves a computer screen, a finger temperature monitor, and a heart rate sensor. The goal is to induce the child's own relaxation response. As "coherence" is achieved (meaning more regular breathing, lowered pulse rate), the child receives immediate feedback on the computer monitor that he or she is succeeding in the relaxation exercise. Biofeedback/EEG biofeedback as a treatment for children with ADHD (Arns, de Ridder, Strehl, Breteler, & Coenen, 2009) and ASD (Coben & Padolsky, 2007) has been considered controversial but is gaining an evidence base for efficacy. Methodological issues exist in most of the biofeedback/EEG biofeedback studies, but the promising results of preliminary studies make this an area that warrants further investigation and consideration as a complementary therapy.

Auditory Integration Training

Auditory integration training is a therapy in which children who have a "sensory integration disorder" are screened for sound sensitivities and then delivered a tailored program of auditory input that filters out the sound frequencies to which they are sensitive. It should be noted that sensory integration disorder itself is not a recognized medical term but is often used in describing children with ASD. Auditory integration training

sessions are conducted over several months and can be rather costly. The American Academy of Pediatrics (1999) has not endorsed its use for children with ASD, and states in their literature review of this topic that significant methodological flaws exist in all studies in this area.

Music Therapy

Music therapy is delivered by a therapist who uses musical experiences to engage the child in a relationship on focused dyadic exchange surrounding rhythm tones and music tailored to the child's individual preferences. Only case reports and preexperimental designs have evaluated this therapy in children with disabilities. No study with control groups or experimental designs has assessed the utility of this therapy.

Manipulative/Body-Based Practices

Massage Therapy

Massage therapy is a body-based practice that promotes a relaxation response and tissue healing. There is abundant evidence in the adult literature for the value of massage for anxiety reduction and relief from pain. In the disability literature there is some evidence to support its utility in alleviating symptoms of ADHD (Khilnani, Field, Hernandez-Reif, Schanberg, 2003; Maddigan et al., 2003), in promoting sleep and decreasing repetitive behavior in ASD (Escalona, Field, Singer-Strunck, Cullen, Hartshorn, 2001; Silva, Schalock, Ayres, Bunse, & Budden, 2009), and improving motor function in children with CP (Macgregor, Campbell, Gladden, Tennant, & Young, 2007). In sum, massage is a safe practice that has some promise in alleviating problematic symptoms of certain developmental disabilities.

Craniosacral Therapy

Craniosacral therapy is a practice in which the therapist "senses" waves of spinal fluid and applies gentle touch to manipulate these flows. Although parents may pursue this as a treatment for their child, no controlled studies have evaluated the effectiveness of this therapy in children with disabilities. It may be that the "spa's" therapeutic environment during the session lends some relaxation benefits, but this is yet to be explored in controlled studies.

Osteopathy

Osteopathic treatments involve physical manipulation of joints, muscle, bone and fascia (connective tissue) to aid the recuperative powers of the body. Osteopathic manipulative treatment (OMT) has been reported to improve motor function and quality of life in children with cerebral palsy (Duncan, McDonough-Means, Worden, Schnyer, Andrews, & Meaney, 2008).

Chiropractic

Manipulation of the spine has been used to treat a variety of pediatric medical conditions. However, the rationale for its use in treating core symptoms of most developmental disabilities has not been established scientifically. Rare adverse events have occurred with spinal adjustments, including subarachnoid hemorrhage, quadriplegia, and vertebral dislocation (Vohra, Johnston, Cramer, & Humphreys, 2007). The cervical spine in children may be particularly vulnerable to injury. Patients with chronic motor disabilities and Down syndrome should be warned of these potential risks.

Hippotherapy

Hippotherapy or horseback-riding therapy uses the core strength as well as gross and fine motor balance and coordination skills to improve physical functioning of children with disabilities. Cherng (2004) noted improvement in gross and fine motor functioning of children with CP who engaged in a 16-week hippotherapy program.

Patterning

Patterning is a movement therapy based on the principles that brain injury can be overcome by teaching the young "plastic" brain the developmentally normal sequence of motor activities. These movements are passively facilitated by a therapist who delivers frequent intensive therapy to retrain the brain. This involves multiple people manipulating the child's limbs and positions for many hours each day. But open trials of patterning have failed to demonstrate a benefit of this therapy (James, Kolt, McConville, & Bate, 1998). The large financial and opportunity cost makes this therapy suspect, and families should be counseled about the lack of evidence to support the utility of this treatment.

Yoga

Yoga is an ancient body-based practice that combined postures, breathing work, and meditative practices to achieve a sense of well-being and physical health. There is some limited evidence to support the use of this practice for certain developmental disabilities. Uma, Nagendra, Nagarathna, Vaidehi, and Seethalakshmi (1989)

studied children with intellectual disability who engaged in regular yoga practice and found that it increased cognitive performance. Jensen and Kenney (2004) reported on a small controlled trial of yoga in ADHD children whose symptoms were stable on medication; yoga showed a positive effect on hyperactivity.

Sensory Integration Therapy

Sensory integration therapy involves exposing the child to a series of sensory-based experiences such as swinging, joint compressions, brushing, holding, and squeezing. These experiences are designed to address the observed hypo- and hyperresponsiveness to sensory stimuli often seen in children with disabilities. Although a few articles have been written about these therapies, no large double blind clinical trial exists. Although this therapy is safe, behavior problems seen in children with sensory integration problems must still be handled with appropriate behavioral reinforcement strategies and not merely attributed to their problems with handling sensory input.

Energy-Based Practices

Acupuncture

Acupuncture is an ancient energy-based therapy that restores flow of energy (called *Qi*) between meridians in the body. There is a growing literature supporting its use in chronic pain conditions. Zhang, Liu, Wang, and He, (2010) published a meta-analysis of the utility of Traditional Chinese Medicine in treatment of CP and found that there is some evidence that acupuncture increases global physical functioning in patients with CP who utilize acupuncture versus no treatment or a sham acupuncture treatment. Acupuncture is a safe therapy that could be considered as part of a comprehensive treatment plan focusing on enhancing functioning.

APPROACHES TO ADVISING FAMILIES ABOUT COMPLEMENTARY AND ALTERNATIVE MEDICINE

Given the common use of CAM therapies for children with disabilities, traditional health care providers are challenged with balancing the desire to support parents' decisions regarding their child's treatment with providing evidence-based medical advice. These challenges can be managed effectively by incorporating principles of **family-centered care** and shared medical decision making into these types of patient encounters. Family centered care is an approach to health care that is based on mutual respect which promotes optimal health outcomes and treatment adherence by encouraging shared decision making in daily patient interactions. The American Academy of Pediatrics (2001) endorses the use of shared medical decision making as a way to promote treatment adherence for children with chronic illness.

Shared medical decision making for use of CAM treatments implies that the health care provider becomes expert enough about the potential risks and benefits of the proposed treatment to participate in the decision making process as a medical expert. For many practitioners, training in CAM therapies is limited at best, and this may hinder or even prevent provider-patient communication and subsequent decision making around these issues. However, health care providers may be able to give a good deal of guidance to families regarding medical decision making around CAM treatment by advising families on how to scientifically evaluate a potential treatment. This approach does not require expertise about a particular herb, supplement, diet or therapy, but rather facilitates a discussion about the treatment.

The shared decision making approach also encourages provider-patient communication. It is well-known that families frequently do not disclose CAM use to their child's health care provider. It is also true that many families who suspect an ASD diagnosis in their child have implemented one or more alternative treatments while they are waiting for an appointment with a specialist to confirm the diagnosis (Levy, Mandell, Merhar, Ittenbach, & Pinto-Martin, 2003). Families may resent the fact that their health care provider does not provide them with information about alternative treatments when they are so readily available from other sources such as the Internet.

The provider might open the door to discussions about CAM by actively asking the following questions during the course of the medical history: Is your child taking any medications? Have you considered, or is your child currently taking any vitamins, supplements, herbs, or on any special diet restrictions? Is your child participating in any therapies in addition to conventional ones that include physical, occupational, and speech-language therapy? This might include massage, acupuncture, or sensory integrative therapy.

Receiving the responses nonjudgmentally is a good way to begin these types of discussions.

It is important to make parents aware of alternative therapies early on in the diagnosis. The practitioner should provide families with list of resources that include parent support groups, reliable web sites, and books and review articles that present balanced discussions of CAM. This can build trust in the provider-patient relationship and lead to a discussion of how to critically evaluate these treatments.

After openly listening to the family's concerns and interest in a given CAM treatment, the practitioner has a basis to transition into teaching the family about applying the principles of evidence-based medicine to evaluate the treatment. Evidence-based medicine refers to the practice of evaluating the strength of scientific evidence behind a proposed medical treatment. Many CAM therapies have no scientific evidence behind them or use anecdotal reports as evidence of efficacy. Others have some research support that has yet to be replicated or are supported by studies with significant methodological flaws that prevent the study's acceptance by the mainstream medical community. The National Institutes of Health provides parent-friendly information regarding how to evaluate the scientific validity of a particular CAM treatment at http://nccam.nih.gov.

Of great concern is the fact that some CAM websites actively discourage parents from considering evidence-based medicine in their decision making process, saying that these types of studies are only necessary for potentially harmful treatments, not natural treatments. It is important for physicians to inform families that the distinction between natural and manufactured pharmaceuticals is not so clear. Many effective medications come from natural plant sources and *all* pharmaceuticals, natural or not, have potential side effects.

SUMMARY

Despite the lack of supporting evidence, CAM therapies are used as part of the treatment regimen for the majority of children with developmental disabilities. Yet, the typical health care practitioner has received little if any training in the use of CAM modalities. Clear information about the potential benefits, the evidence base, and the potential side effect profile of the specific CAM therapy is important information to relay to families who are pursuing these sometimes time consuming and financially draining therapies. The health care practitioner should communicate this information to families in a way that is open and nonjudgmental.

Serious safety concerns or health risks of CAM approaches also must be clearly communicated. The health care practitioner must always keep the "do no harm" principle in the forefront of decision making around CAM therapies. This approach opens the lines of communication with families and it displays respect and understanding of the families' need to explore alternatives or complementary approaches to treating their child's developmental disability.

REFERENCES

American Academy of Pediatrics, Committee on Children with Disabilities. (1998). Auditory integration training and facilitated communication for autism. *Pediatrics, 102*(2,Pt1), 431–433.

American Academy of Pediatrics, Committee on Children with Disabilities. (2001). Counseling families who choose complementary and alternative medicine for their child with chronic illness or disability. *Pediatrics, 107*(3), 598–601.

Andersen, I.M., Kaczmarska, J., McGrew, S.G., & Malow, B.A. (2008). Melatonin for insomnia in children with autism spectrum disorders. *Journal of Child Neurology, 23*, 482–485.

Arns, M., de Ridder, S., Strehl, U., Breteler, M., & Coenen, A. (2009). Efficacy of neurofeedback treatment in ADHD: The effects on inattention, impulsivity and hyperactivity: A meta-analysis. *Clinical EEG and Neuroscience, 40*(3), 180–189.

Ball, S.D., Kertesz, D., & Moyer-Mileur, L.J. (2005). Dietary supplement use is prevalent among children with a chronic illness. *Journal of American Dietetic Association, 105*(1), 78–84.

Cherng, R.J., Liao, H.F., Leung, H.W.C., & Hwang, A.W. (2004). The effectiveness of therapeutic horseback riding in children with spastic cerebral palsy. *Adaptive Physical Activity Quarterly, 21*, 103–121.

Coben, R., & Myers, T.E. (2010). The relative efficacy of connectivity guided and symptom based EEG biofeedback for autistic disorders. *Applied Psychophysiological Biofeedback, 35*(1), 13–23

Duncan, B., McDonough-Means, S. Worden, K., Schnyer, R., Andrews, & Meaney, J. (2008). Effectiveness of osteopathy in the cranial field and myofascial release versus acupuncture as complementary treatment for children with spastic cerebral palsy: A pilot study. *Journal of the American Osteopathic Association, 108*(10), 559–570.

Elder, J.H., Shankar, M., Shuster, J., Theriaque, D., Burns, S., & Sherrill, L. (2006). The gluten-free, casein-free diet in autism: Results of a preliminary double blind clinical trial. *Journal of Autism Development Disorders, 36*(3), 413–420.

Escalona, A., Field, T., Singer-Strunck, R., Cullen, C., Hartshorn, K. (2001) Brief report: Improvements in the behavior of children with autism following massage therapy. *Journal of Autism Development Disorders, 31*(5), 513–516.

Field, T.M., Quintino, O., Hernandez-Reif, M., & Koslovsky, G. (1988) Adolescents with attention deficit hyperactivity disorder benefit from massage therapy. *Adolescence, 33*(129), 103–108.

Garstang, J., Wallis, M. (2006). Randomized controlled trial of melatonin for children with autistic spectrum disorders and sleep problems. *Child Care and Health Development, 32*, 585–589.

Gross-Tsur, V. (2003). Use of complementary medicine in children with ADHD and epilepsy. *Pediatric Neurology, 29*, 53–55.

Harrington, J.W., Rosen, L., Garnecho, A., & Patrick, P.A. (2006). Parental perceptions and use of complementary and alternative medicine practices for children with autistic spectrum disorders in private practice. *Journal of Developmental Behavior Pediatrics, 27*, S156–S161.

Hanson, E., Kalish, L.A., & Bunce, E., (2007). Use of complementary and alternative medicine among children diagnosed with autism spectrum disorder. *Journal of Autism Development Disorders, 37*, 628–631.

Hediger, M.L., England L.J., Molloy, C.A., Yu, K.F., Manning-Courtney, P., & Mills, J.L. (2008). Reduced bone cortical thickness in boys with autism or autism spectrum disorder. *Journal of Autism Development Disorders, 38*(5), 848–856.

Hurvitz, E.A., Leonard, C., Ayyangar, R., & Nelson,V. (2003). Complementary and alternative medicine use in families of children with cerebral palsy. *Developmental Medicine and Child Neurology, 45*(6), 364–370.

James, M., Kolt, G., McConville, J., Bate, P. (1998). The effects of Feldenkrais program and relaxation procedures on hamstring length. *Australian Physiotherapy, 44*, 49–54.

Jensen, P.S., & Kenny, D.T. (2004). The effects of yoga on the attention and behavior of boys with attention-deficit/disorder (ADHD). *Journal of Attention Disorders, 7*, 205–216.

Johnson, C.R., Handen, B.L., Zimmer, M.H., Mayer Costa, M., & Sacco, K. (2011) Effects of gluten free casein free diet on young children with autism: A pilot study. *Journal of Development and Physical Disabilities, 23*(3), 213.

Kemp, A. (2008). *Food additives and hyperactivity. BMJ, 336*(7654), 1144.

Khilnani, S., Field, T., Hernandez-Reif, M., Schanberg, S. (2003). Massage therapy improves mood and behavior of students with attention-deficit/hyperactivity disorder. *Adolescence, 38*(152), 623–638.

Levy, S.E., Mandell, D.S., Merhar, S., Ittenbach, R.F., & Pinto-Martin, J.A. (2003). Use of complementary and alternative medicine among children recently diagnosed with autistic spectrum disorder. *Journal of Developmental and Behavioral Pediatrics, 24*(6), 418–423.

Liptak, G.S. (2005). Complementary and alternative therapies for cerebral palsy. *Mental Retardation and Developmental Disabilities Research Reviews, 11*, 156–163.

Loman, D.G. (2003). The use of complementary and alternative health care practices among children. *Journal of Pediatric Health Care, 17*(2), 58–63.

Maddigan, B., Hodgson, P., Heath, S., Dick, B., St. John, K., McWilliam-Burton, T., … White, H. (2003). The effects of massage therapy & exercise therapy on children/adolescents with attention deficit hyperactivity disorder. *Canadian Child Adolescent Psychiatric Review, 12*(2), 40–43.

McCann, L.J., & Newell, S.J. (2006). Survey of paediatric complementary and alternative medicine use in health and chronic illness. *Archives of Disabled Children, 91*(2), 173–174.

McDonagh, M.S., Morgan, D., Carson, S., & Russman, B.S. (2007). Systematic review of hyperbaric oxygen therapy for cerebral palsy: The state of the evidence. *Developmental Medical Children's Neurology, 49*, 942–947.

Nickel, R.E., & Gerlach, E.K. (2001). The use of complementary and alternative therapies by the families of children with chronic conditions and disabilities. *Infants and Young Children, 14*(1), 67–78.

Phillips, L., & Appleton, R.E. (2004). Systematic review of melatonin treatment in children with neurodevelopmental disabilities and sleep impairment. *Developmental Medicine and Child Neurology, 46,* 771–775.

Prussing, E., Sobo, E.J., Walker, E., Dennis, K., & Kurtin, P.S. (2004). Communicating with pediatricians about complementary/alternative medicine: Perspectives from parents of children with Down syndrome. *Pediatrics, 488,* 494–636.

Samdup, D.Z., Smith, R.G., & Il Song, S. (2006). The use of complementary and alternative medicine in children with chronic medical conditions. *American Journal of Physical and Medical Rehabilitation, 85,* 842–846.

Sanders, H., Davis, M.F., Duncan, B., Meaney, F.J., Haynes, J., & Barton, L.L. (2003). Use of complementary and alternative medical therapies among children with special health care needs in southern Arizona. *Pediatrics, 111*(3), 584–587.

Sinha, D., & Efron, D. (2005) Complementary and alternative medicine use in children with attention deficit hyperactivity disorder. *Journal of Paediatrics and Child Health, 41*(1–2), 23–26.

Uma, K., Nagendra, H.R., Nagarathna, R., Vaidehi, S., & Seethalakshmi, R. (1989). The integrated approach of yoga: A therapeutic tool for mentally retarded children: A one-year controlled study. *Journal of Mental Deficiency Research, 33*(5), 415–421.

Vohra, S., Johnston, B., Cramer, K., & Humphreys, K. (2007). Adverse events associated with pediatric spinal manipulation: A systematic review. *Pediatrics, 119,* e275–e283

Wasdell, M.B., Jan, J.E., & Bomben, M.M., (2008). A randomized, placebo controlled trial of controlled release melatonin treatment of delayed sleep phase syndrome and impaired sleep maintenance in children with neurodevelopmental disabilities. *Journal of Pineal Research, 44,* 57–64.

Wirojanan, J., Jacquemont, S., Diaz, R., Bacalman, S., Anders, T.F., Hagerman, R.J., & Goodlin-Jones, B.L. (2009). The efficacy of melatonin for sleep problems in children with autism, fragile X syndrome, or autism and fragile X syndrome. *Journal of Clinical Sleep Medicine, 5,* 145–150.

Wolraich, M.L., Lindgren, S.D., Stumbo, P.J., Stegink, L.D., Appelbaum, M.I., & Kiritsy, M.C. (1994). Effects of diets high in sucrose or aspartame on the behavior and cognitive performance of children. *New England Journal of Medicine, 330*(5), 301–307.

Wong, H.H., & Smith, R.G. (2006). Patterns of complementary and alternative medical therapy use in children diagnosed with autism spectrum disorders. *Journal of Autism Development Disorders, 36,* 901–909.

Zhang, Y., Liu, J., Wang, J., & He, Q. (2010). Traditional Chinese Medicine for treatment of cerebral palsy in children: A systematic review of randomized clinical trials. *Journal of Alternative and Complementary Medicine, 16*(4), 375–395.

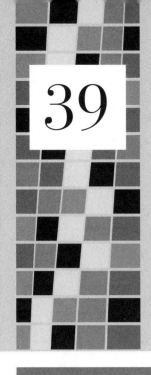

39

Ethical Considerations

Kruti Acharya, Michelle Huckaby Lewis, and Peter J. Smith

Upon completion of this chapter, the reader will

- Become familiar with medical ethical issues concerning children with disabilities, such as informed consent and assent, prenatal diagnosis, genetic testing and screening, withholding of treatment, and human subjects research

- Learn the vocabulary of pediatric ethics, including language related to parental rights and the best interest of the child

- Understand the differences and similarities between ethical decision making and legal requirements

- Be cognizant of ethics committees and the availability of ethics consultations

Given the diversity of cultures and perspectives within American society, there is an increasing need to integrate the fields of clinical care, medical research, law, and ethics with the diverse beliefs and values inherent within families and physicians regarding children with developmental disabilities. All of these fields play a role in the decision-making processes of both parents and practitioners. Many of the ethical and legal issues facing parents of children with disabilities today have resulted from significant advances in medical technology. In this chapter the ethical paradigms and dilemmas faced by physicians and families will be discussed as well as points of concern to be included in decision-making processes.

BASIC ETHICAL PRINCIPLES

The practice of medicine is not an exact science. Health professionals are faced at times with situations that highlight the conflicting values

and beliefs that may exist within families. The physician's moral obligation to families in these cases is not always clear, especially in the care of children with disabilities. Heightened emotions about a child's disability may make decision making particularly difficult. Professional codes of conduct have been developed to help guide physicians and other medical personnel in resolving these conflicts, but these codes do not provide obvious answers in all situations.

Several different ethical frameworks have been used to assist health professionals in the resolution of these ethical dilemmas. One example is the principle-based framework in which the four principles of biomedical ethics provide moral guidance to health care practitioners. These are respect for autonomy, nonmaleficence, beneficence, and justice (Beauchamp & Childress, 2001; National Commission for the Protection of Human Subjects of Biomedical and Behavioral Research, 1979).

Respect for autonomy refers to respecting the decision-making capacities of autonomous (self-determining) persons. Children are not considered autonomous persons in this regard, but their parents possess the legal and moral authority to make decisions on their behalf. Parents are required to act in the best interests of their children and are considered to be in the best position to do so. Informed consent must be obtained from a child's parent or legal guardian in order to treat a pediatric patient. This ability to grant permission for their children's care is grounded in the concept of respect for persons and should be honored in all but extraordinary circumstances (e.g., following an auto accident when the child and parent may be unconscious and unable to give consent for acutely needed treatment).

Nonmaleficence refers to the avoidance of harm, the principal behind the Hippocratic oath, which all physicians swear to observe. Inherent in this concept is the *obligation* not to harm others. This principle supports more specific rules that prohibit killing, causing pain or suffering, or causing incapacitation. This principle is often invoked in discussions regarding whether to withhold or withdraw care. It is central to the debate about distinctions between "killing someone" versus "letting them die."

Beneficence refers to providing benefits and also to balancing benefits against risks. This principle requires health professionals to take active, positive steps to help others. The principles of respect for autonomy and beneficence may be in conflict when paternalistic views affect medical decision making. Many physicians consider their primary obligation to be to their patient's medical benefit and not equally to encourage autonomous decision making by parents. This conflict can be problematic.

Justice

This concept refers to the fair distribution of benefits, risks, and costs. Issues of social justice are particularly salient with respect to the care of children with disabilities. An increasing number of infants with severe disabilities are surviving into childhood and adulthood, placing increased demands upon the resources available for their care and treatment (McCullough, 2005). Children with severe disabilities are seen by some people as being less worthy of the consumption of scarce health care resources (Savage, 1998). Health practitioners involved in the care of children with disabilities are in a position to advocate for these children's needs.

In the consideration of moral dilemmas, no single principle has priority, and no single principle may override all other moral considerations. Rather, these principles should be used to evaluate a moral dilemma, and the appropriate weight that should be given to each principle under the circumstances should be considered carefully.

THE RELATIONSHIP BETWEEN LAW AND ETHICS

While law and ethics are related, they are not synonymous. In some circumstances, consideration of whether a proposed course of action is legal may not answer the question of whether it is ethical (e.g., performing a hysterectomy on a teenager with profound intellectual disability). Conversely, a practice that may be considered ethical by some may not be within the bounds of the law (e.g., euthanasia).

Many current laws regarding bioethical issues have been enacted in response to novel bioethics issues. For example, the Baby Doe Amendment (1984) extended the federal definition of child abuse to include the withholding of medical care to seriously ill newborns unless the provision of such care would be "virtually futile." This legislation was enacted in the 1980s after the death of a baby with Down syndrome resulting from the parents' decision to decline lifesaving and fairly straightforward surgery to repair a gastrointestinal condition common to Down syndrome.

Ethical obligations typically are thought to exceed legal duties. Under this principal when health care providers believe that a law is unjust, they should work to change the law (American Medical Association, 1994). In addition, health care personnel have a responsibility to be aware of laws that govern their care of children, such as laws requiring health care providers to report suspected child abuse to the appropriate authorities and laws that may be used to intervene in parental health care decisions that could harm their child. Respect for autonomy and nonmaleficence most clearly correspond to legal duties as currently understood in modern culture. However, not all the principles are even part of legal considerations; for example, the entire principle of beneficence is usually not considered a legal duty. Also, the concept of justice, although key to a general understanding of the structure and foundation of legal duties, does not always enter into specific cases or disputes between individual parties.

Unique Aspects of Pediatric Ethics

The care of children presents health care practitioners with ethical dilemmas unique to pediatrics. Although many of the ethical issues involved in the care of children are similar to those that arise in the care of adults, pediatric care involves additional ethical questions, such as pediatric assent and issues related to the beginnings of life.

Pediatric Assent

A competent adult has the legal right to determine which medical intervention he or she will accept. In situations in which an adult patient is judged not competent to make autonomous medical decisions, the court designates a surrogate to make these decisions for the patient. In this context, significant value is placed on the previously expressed desires and/or values of the patient, if known. In contrast, in pediatric settings, the patient has never been autonomous and has never possessed legal decision-making authority. Rather, through a process known as pediatric assent, the child participates increasingly as he or she matures in the decision-making process. Yet, a child's developmental ability to participate in medical decision making is difficult to measure and will vary among children of similar chronological ages, depending upon each child's unique circumstances. For children with disabilities, the child's cognitive or physical impairments may limit his or her ability to participate in this decision-making process.

Health Care Professionals as Advocates

In general, parents are given the legal authority to make medical decisions on their child's behalf. This legal authority is based upon the premise that parents are in the position to make decisions in the best interest of their child. Parental authority is not unlimited, however. If parents do not make decisions in their child's best interest, the child's physician, therapists, educators, caregivers, and so forth have a legal and ethical obligation to advocate for the child, providing an additional safeguard for the care of the child (American Medical Association, 2008).

ETHICAL DILEMMAS

Prenatal Testing— Physician versus Parental Views

■ ■ ■ MR. AND MRS. JONES

At a routine 20-week prenatal ultrasound, Mr. and Mrs. Jones were told, "Something may be wrong with your baby, and we want to do an advanced ultrasound." Concerned by the possibility of a condition that would require immediate intervention, they agreed. The test was actually ordered by the obstetrician to exclude Down syndrome since calcifications in the baby's heart, a sign suggestive of the disorder, were noted on the initial ultrasound. The subsequent test showed no congenital heart defect, but other findings were strongly suggestive of Down syndrome. Upon learning that the test had been done principally to diagnose Down syndrome, Mr. and Mrs. Jones, who had refused first trimester screening for Down syndrome as they would not consider termination, were upset about the time, anxiety, and expense of the additional testing.

Parental decision making about prenatal testing is complex. It is based both on medical facts and moral judgments. In the above example, the physician and parents had differing value systems informing their assumptions about the treatment plan. The physician subscribed to the medical model of disability. He viewed Down syndrome as equivalent to "a medical disorder," even in the absence of congenital malformations. From his perspective, the possibility of Down syndrome required a definitive answer, warranting the additional prenatal testing. The physician believed he was acting in accordance with the principle of beneficence. For the parents, however, learning prenatally whether or not their child had Down syndrome was not a priority, unless it would influence treatment. In contrast to the medical model of disorder, they did not view having a child with Down syndrome as equivalent to having a child with a medical disorder or a challenge to their hopes for a healthy baby. Even though the physician viewed the testing as a benefit, the parents viewed the additional testing as harmful, against the principle of nonmaleficence.

Mr. and Mrs. Jones affirm the perspective of disability rights, arguing that Down syndrome, like all developmental disabilities, comprises only one aspect of an individual, and that decisions should be made about the person as a whole and not based on this one characteristic. Other parents may hold different views about disability, and for them prenatal testing would have been very important. In Mr. and Mrs. Jones case it would have been better for the physician to explain specifically his reason for doing the ultrasound and whether it would have any therapeutic implications. A discussion would have better respected parental autonomy. Any physician–patient dialogue about prenatal testing should present balanced information about the rationale for testing so that the decision is informed by the parents' religious, spiritual, or value systems (Munger, Gill, Ormond, & Kirschner, 2007).

In 2000, the Hastings Center convened a working group to determine for which conditions prenatal screening is ethical. The group's conclusions were 1) prenatal diagnosis was ethically permissible for conditions with mortality in childhood; and 2) there was no consensus on the ethical permissibility of prenatal testing for all other conditions; thus, parents could choose to pursue or reject prenatal testing based on their own values (Parens & Asch, 2007). Since 2000, however, there has been a tremendous explosion in the number and types of prenatal screening tests that are performed (see Chapter 14). There has not been a corresponding increase in resources for families to help them understand these tests, which has lead to a dramatic and unfortunate shift away from the prior consensus for balance in these discussions. The de facto experience for most families, like that of the Jones family, is that these are seen as "needed" tests for "disorders" and not the socially constructed odysseys that they truly are.

It must be acknowledged that the issue of abortion becomes important in any discussion of prenatal screening and ethics. The central question in a discussion of abortion is the definition of personhood. A detailed discussion of the abortion debate, however, is beyond the scope of this chapter. Suffice it to say that individual attitudes towards abortion are diverse and that abortion is a sensitive, politically- and religiously-charged topic.

Newborn Screening

▮ ▮ ▮ NAJAR

Before going home from the hospital, the proud parents of baby boy Najar are informed by a nursing assistant that their new baby is required to have a blood test performed. The nursing assistant tells the parents that all babies have the test before leaving the hospital, but she is unable to answer any questions about the purpose of the test. The parents are upset when their baby cries during the heel stick procedure and they don't understand why it's being done.

Newborn screening (NBS) testing is performed on virtually all of the 4 million babies born annually in the United States. Most states require mandatory newborn screening, but the public health justification of mandatory newborn screening has come into question in recent years. Originally, newborn screening testing, commonly called the "**PKU test**," was performed to prevent the devastating consequences of a few heritable metabolic conditions, such as **phenylketonuria** (PKU). Only conditions for which effective treatment was available were included (see Chapter 19).

Each state determines which disorders to include in the state's newborn screening panel. Until recently, wide variability existed amongst states regarding which disorders were included in state newborn screening panels. This state-by-state variability led to obvious disparities and to calls by parent advocacy groups to create national newborn screening standards. This became more of an issue with the recent development of tandem mass spectrometry, which permits the testing of dozens of disorders instead of just a few. As a result, in 2005, a working group convened by the American College of Medical Genetics recommended a uniform newborn screening panel. This panel included 29 core conditions and 25 secondary conditions that would be discovered incidentally in the screening for the core conditions. As of 2008, all 50 states have adopted the uniform panel (see Chapter 14).

The expanded newborn screening panel, however, has not been without controversy. Proponents of expanded screening have used a broader definition of "benefit" than that of the past. Previously, only the possibility of direct medical benefit to the child was considered in evaluating whether to include a condition in the newborn screening panel. The concept of benefit, however, has expanded now to include benefit to the family, to inform future reproductive decisions about conditions that carry an increased recurrence risk (see Chapter 1) and to prevent parental anxiety from future medical odysseys to diagnose these rare and frequently misdiagnosed conditions. In this framework, knowledge, in and of itself, is considered a benefit.

Critics of expanded NBS have argued, however, that it is inappropriate to screen infants for conditions for which no effective therapy currently exists. In addition, although the technological capacity exists to further expand NBS to screen for thousands of genetic variants by microarray technology, the ability to counsel parents about positive test results from this technology is limited, as information about a particular variant's clinical significance is limited or unknown. It also has been argued that the opportunity cost of expanding newborn screening cannot be adequately justified when there are competing underfunded health initiatives.

The retention and use of residual dried blood samples (DBS) for medical research unrelated to newborn screening is another area of controversy. Whether explicit parental permission (opt-in) is required to retain the DBS or whether the state may retain the sample unless parents object (opt-out) is a contentious issue. In Texas and Minnesota, parents sued the state Departments of Health for retaining their babies' DBS without their permission (*Bearder v. State of Minnesota, Beleno v. Texas Department of State Health Services*).

In Texas, a group of parents filed a class action lawsuit in federal court claiming the action infringed on their constitutional protection against unreasonable seizures (i.e., the DBS) and their right to privacy (14th Amendment). In response to the Texas lawsuit, the state legislature enacted a law that would require parents to be informed that DBS could be retained by the state and used for medical research (H.B. 1672, 81st Leg. Tex. 2009). Furthermore, the law states that parents be given the option to refuse to allow the state to retain their babies' DBS. The Texas lawsuit subsequently was settled, and as part of the settlement, the state agreed to destroy over 5 million DBS that had been retained prior to the new legislation's enactment. After the media reported that 800 residual dried blood samples from Texas had been given to the U.S. Armed Forces Pathology Laboratory, a second lawsuit was filed in federal court against the Texas Department of Health Services (*Higgins v. Tex. Dept. of State Health Services*). The second lawsuit was dismissed in July, 2011, based upon the court's finding that the Texas Constitution granted the Department of Health Services immunity from suit by individuals and the court's determination that since the residual dried blood spots of the plaintiffs

had been destroyed as part of the settlement from the initial case, the legal claims were moot. It is important to note that the claims regarding the legality of the state retention and use of residual newborn screening blood samples were not fully adjudicated in either case.

In Minnesota, the newborn screening lawsuit was based upon different legal claims. In *Bearder v. State of Minnesota*, nine families sued the Minnesota Department of Health in 2009 alleging that the state retention of residual newborn screening DBS violated the state genetic privacy law requirement to obtain informed consent to store genetic information (Treatment of Genetic Information Held by Government Entitites and Others, 2010). The state initially prevailed in the Minnesota lawsuit because the lower court ruled that the genetic privacy act did not supersede existing newborn screening law. The lower court's decision was upheld upon appeal. The Minnesota Court of Appeals noted that the broad authority of the Commissioner of Health to manage the newborn screening program provided authorization to retain, use, and disseminate blood specimens for newborn screening related research.

The Minnesota Supreme Court rejected these arguments. The Court held that residual newborn screening DBS are biological information subject to protection under the genetic privacy act and that the use of the residual DBS for purposes other than the screening of newborn children and for follow-up services requires written informed consent.

From a national perspective, the issue remains unsettled. As the debate continues about the future development of newborn screening programs, the public health mission of NBS needs to be balanced against parents' right to be informed and to protect the best interests of their child.

Care for Infants at Risk for Disability

▣ ▣ ▣ BABY GIRL SMITH

Baby girl Smith was born at an estimated gestational age of 25 weeks. In the delivery room she was immediately intubated and transferred to the newborn intensive care unit (NICU), where she was stabilized on moderate ventilatory support for the first 48 hours. On her third day of life, however, she was found to have a bulging **fontanel** (soft spot on the crown of the head). A head ultrasound revealed a Grade IV **intraventricular hemorrhage** (IVH), which carries significant mortality and morbidity (see Chapter 7).

For those infants surviving this event, the risk of developing cerebral palsy, intellectual disability, and/or other developmental disabilities is significant. The care team arranged for a meeting with her parents to discuss the goals of therapy and potential outcomes.

One of the greatest advancements in medical technology of the past few decades has been in the NICU care of low-birth-weight infants, resulting in improved survival of newborn infants like baby girl Smith. Although smaller and sicker infants now survive, they have a greater chance than their larger, full-term peers of having function-limiting impairments of cognitive and motor development. This is further problematic as it is often difficult to predict, even for children with known central nervous system abnormalities, the degree of future deficits or their effect on long-term personal and familial happiness. These factors combine to make important life-affecting treatment decisions of the care team and baby girl Smith's parents quite difficult. Research has shown that clinicians and therapists in the NICU are generally overly pessimistic about their predictions of cognitive and motor outcomes (Saigal, Stoskopf, Feeny, et al., 1999). This is because post-NICU factors, such as early intervention services, have been shown to have a larger influence upon long-term outcomes than most NICU teams factor into their considerations (Stephens, Tucker, & Vohr, 2010). There is currently an ethical mandate to improve the training of pediatricians, especially those who seek to become neonatologists, to improve their knowledge, skills, and attitudes about appropriately facilitating increasingly common but difficult treatment decisions regarding prematures and other at-risk neonates (McCabe, Hunt, & Serwint, 2008).

Interventional Decisions

▪ ▪ ▪ NICHOLAS

Nicholas was diagnosed with **Duchenne muscular dystrophy** (DMD) at 6 years of age. Now, at age 16, he has multiple impairments, including severe restrictive lung disease (secondary to extreme scoliosis along with his muscular weakness). He currently needs overnight pressurized oxygen delivery by a nasal canula (bi-pap) as well as multiple daily respiratory treatments. His father, who is his sole care provider, has requested a consultation with an ear, nose, and throat surgeon for possible placement of a tracheotomy for continuous mechanical ventilation.

Paralleling the increasing survival seen in the NICU has been a quiet revolution in the outpatient management of many progressive/chronic conditions that were previously fatal during childhood. These include cystic fibrosis, DMD, sickle-cell disease, congenital heart disease, and several other severe chronic diseases of childhood. One of the most dramatic improvements has been in the effective use of home mechanical ventilation to allow children like Nicholas, with DMD, to live many years longer. Helping families navigate the clinical pathways leading to decisions about whether to pursue invasive surgeries and aggressive, ongoing therapies (e.g., total parenteral [intravenous] nutrition or mechanical ventilation), or to decline them is a relatively new problem in pediatrics. These decisions should account for the adolescent patient's emerging preferences and autonomy as well as parental autonomy.

Because these medical technologies are new, their long-term risks and benefits frequently have not been well-studied. As a result, there continues to be a wide range of perspectives about their suitability for use in these populations. Questions persist regarding 1) the impact of the individual's choice on his or her own life, and on the life of the family and of the community which surrounds and supports him or her, and 2) economic factors (both positive and negative) that may need to be considered in supporting the decision. It is critical that practitioners, who are engaging in the care of individuals and families who are making these decisions, keep abreast of all these changing factors and not rely solely on past experiences or conceptions of "what can be done" or even "what should be done."

Diagnostic Categorization

▪ ▪ ▪ CLAIRE

Claire is a beautiful 3-year-old who has come to the Down syndrome clinic. She has a very mild phenotype, with developmental delays that are responding well to therapy. She is small and has some of the physical features of Down syndrome, including a transpalmer crease. It is noted that although she was diagnosed prenatally with **mosaic Trisomy 21**, she never had blood drawn after birth for karyotyping, so it is ordered at this visit. Full evaluation of all her blood cells reveals not a single one with trisomy

21. The clinician is then asked by her family, "Does she really have Down syndrome?"

Practicing clinicians are increasingly finding that the labels and diagnostic categories that once seemed clear are increasingly hard to define and use with precision in children with variant expression, such as Claire. "Does Claire have Down syndrome?" It is likely that some cell lines within her do have trisomy 21 and that it was chance that the sample of blood collected did not contain these cells. The question is, however, "Does she have it enough to qualify for governmental programs that assist individuals with known specific conditions such as Down syndrome?" Is it sufficiently present to warrant a label that may limit the expectations of others for her future achievements? Different perspectives on these questions lead to radically different answers, and it is important for all who work in this rapidly changing field to recognize that past simple categorizations fail to capture the more complicated future of variants of normal.

The Ashley "Enhancement"

▪ ▪ ▪ ASHLEY

Ashley is a young girl with a mixed picture of severe cognitive and motor impairments of unclear etiology. Her parents hope that her premature puberty might lead to a shortened stature, making her easier to care for. In order to increase the chances of a smaller adult height, they ask her doctor if she should undergo treatment with hormonal therapy to stunt her linear growth, have a **hysterectomy** (but not **oophorectomy**), and breast bud removal. The doctor asked for an ethics committee consultation as she is not sure whether to comply with parental wishes in this case. The committee that was consulted unfortunately lacked a representative from the long-term care community and lacked a clinician specializing in the care of individuals with intellectual disability. In addition, the committee, the doctors, and the hospital failed to consult or inform a representative of the legal team of the state that is mandated by federal law to monitor the treatment of individuals with intellectual impairment. Because of these oversights, the committee recommendation was that the parents' request for treatments should be respected. When Ashley's care team publicized their actions (Gunther & Diekema, 2006), however, they were found to be in violation of the law; were strongly

criticized by the leading professional organizations in the field (Board of Directors of the American Association on Intellectual & Developmental Disabilities, 2006); and were required to offer institutional changes to prevent this type of decision making from being repeated in the future at their hospital (Ostrom, 2007).

The saga of this case has been well documented, and articles both promoting and denouncing "growth attenuation therapy" continue to be written. Two points can be made from this case: 1) membership on an ethics committee does not automatically make a person an expert in all the laws (e.g., special statutes related to this population or procedure) or clinical facts (e.g., at what weight is a person not usually able to be lifted) involved in all case consultations; and 2) expertise in addressing the above issues can often be found outside the ethics committee, if time is taken to seek it out. It is incumbent upon ethics committees to seek out the expertise necessary to make recommendations about a particular course of action, particularly in the case of novel or controversial situations.

In addition, it is particularly important to have broad public discussion beyond the confines of hospital ethics committees for many of these issues. This is especially true for those medical interventions, like hysterectomy in a woman with a cognitive impairment, that have been specifically condemned by many bodies outside of medicine. Our current culture is more diverse than at any previous time in history, and care should be taken to ensure that diverse and divergent views have a voice in these discussions (MacIntyre, 1999).

End of Life Decision Making

▪ ▪ ▪ MIGUEL

Miguel was born with an **anterior encephalocele**, which was surgically removed in the first days of life to prevent a potentially life-threatening infection (see Chapter 25). After surgery, his medical difficulties were many, and he required both a gastrostomy tube for feeding and a tracheotomy to protect his airway. The abnormalities in his brain made even the basic function of maintaining a stable body temperature difficult. Most of the nurses and doctors taking care of him thought he should be allowed to die peacefully. They recommended that the goals of care should be changed from aggressive interventions to comfort alone. However, Miguel's parents disagreed;

they wanted continued aggressive interventions so he could live as long as possible.

In Greek mythology, there is the story of the two deadly monsters, Scylla and Charybdis, located in close proximity to one other; together they posed an inescapable threat to passing sailors. Avoiding Charybdis meant passing too closely to Scylla and vice versa. The phrase "between Scylla and Charybdis" has come to mean being in a state where one is between two dangers and moving away from one danger will cause you to be at risk from the other. That precisely expresses the dangers that lurk when attempting to navigate the difficult ethical dilemmas related to withdrawal of support from individuals with severe intellectual and developmental disabilities.

Charting a course between the Scylla of vitalism and the Charybdis of futility is an apt metaphor for the difficulty inherent in end-of-life decision making and lies behind the Baby Doe legislation discussed previously. Participants in these morally profound decisions generally agree that they desire to avoid both the unnecessary suffering of patients and the unwarranted prolongation of death that can sometimes accompany decisions for life-sustaining treatment options.

Similarly, discussion participants and decision makers share a desire to avoid bias and discrimination against those with intellectual and other developmental disabilities, and seek to resolve conflicts among the parties involved. The disagreements lie in their interpretations of the course that they need to navigate. The "answers" to these dilemmas are not found in textbooks, but rather through the process of honest, caring, and often lengthy deliberations between the important decision makers: clinicians and staff, family and supportive friends, clergy, and professional advisors. Unfortunately, such lengthy and balanced discussions do not always occur, due to the demands placed on care providers, hospital staff, clergy, and families. Miguel's family never came to agreement with his care team, and he died only after a prolonged attempt at resuscitation: This outcome was seen as a "good" one by his family but as a "bad" one by the care team.

INSTITUTIONAL ETHICS COMMITTEES

Recognizing the prevalence of ethical dilemmas in health care settings and the importance of achieving resolution, the Joint Commission on Accreditation of Healthcare Organizations (JCAHO) requires that every U.S. health care organization provide a mechanism to address ethical conflicts. To satisfy this requirement, most hospitals have developed institutional ethics committees (IECs) to serve three main purposes: 1) educating health care professionals about bioethics issues, 2) developing institutional policies concerning bioethics, and 3) providing clinical ethics consultation.

Through case consultations, IECs can 1) help facilitate communication between family members and the health care team, 2) identify a range of morally acceptable treatment options, and 3) assist in the resolution of conflicts about treatment decisions. It should be noted that the recommendations of IECs are advisory and not binding (Committee on Bioethics, 2001).

The American Academy of Pediatrics' (AAP) guidelines for the operation of IECs include recommendations that any patient, parent/guardian, or family member be able to initiate an ethics consult. Similarly, the guidelines recommend that any physician, nurse, or other health care provider involved in the care of the child also be allowed to initiate an ethics consult (Committee on Bioethics, 2001). The care of children with severe disabilities can result in significant moral distress for health care providers, and consultation with an IEC can provide one mechanism to ease this distress.

IEC membership should be multidisciplinary and include community representation (Lyren & Ford, 2007). The hospital attorney or risk manager may participate in the IEC (Mercurio, 2011). This member may play a crucial role in the interpretation of case law or state regulation. It should be recognized, however, that the hospital attorney or risk manager may experience a conflict of interest between the duty to protect the patient's interests and the duty to protect the institution. In these cases, participation of the attorney or risk manager should be limited to providing specific legal or administrative advice.

PROTECTION OF HUMAN SUBJECTS IN RESEARCH

In the past, the boundaries between clinical practice and biomedical research have blurred for some investigators, resulting in a lack of protection of their research participants. In response to these abuses, the U.S. government has adopted stringent guidelines to regulate research involving human subjects, especially for those in vulnerable populations including children, individuals with disabilities, and prisoners.

The Willowbrook Experiments

The Willowbrook experiments are one example of research involving children with disabilities that resulted in serious violations of ethical principles. Beginning in 1955 and continuing for 15 years, hepatitis research was conducted at Willowbrook State School, an institution for children with intellectual disability. The research protocol involved the deliberate infection of new patients with the hepatitis virus followed by the injection of protective antibodies (Education Development Center, 2009).

This research was criticized for two main reasons. First, it was not appropriate to use a vulnerable, institutionalized population of children with cognitive impairments for these experiments, particularly when no benefit to the children could result. Second, the children's parents were unduly influenced to give consent for their children's participation; that is, admission to Willowbrook was contingent upon consent to participate (Goldby, 1971).

Subsequent to the Willowbrook experiments, rigorous standards to protect human subjects in federally funded biomedical research were adopted by the U.S. government. They require Institutional Review Board (IRB) review and oversight for most categories of research. These standards involve special regulatory requirements that provide additional protection for children who may be involved in biomedical research. These regulations in the United States Federal Regulations, 45 CFR 46, Subpart (D) permit IRBs to only approve three categories of research involving children as subjects:

1. "Research not involving greater than minimal risk to the child" (§46.404).

2. "Research involving greater than minimal risk but presenting the prospect of direct benefit to the individual child subject involved in the research" (§46.405). In this category, the risk must be justified by the anticipated benefits to the research subject. In addition, the relationship of the anticipated benefit to the risk presented by the study must be at least as favorable to the subject as that provided by available alternative approaches to treatment.

3. "Research involving greater than minimal risk and with no prospect of direct benefit to the individual child subjects involved in the research, can be considered if it is likely to yield generalizable knowledge about the subject's disorder or condition" (§46.406). In this category, the risk of the research must represent a minor increase over minimal risk. In addition, the intervention must present to the child-subjects experiences that are reasonably commensurate with those inherent in their actual, or expected, medical, dental, psychological, social, or educational situations. Finally, the intervention must be likely to yield generalizable knowledge about the subject's disorder or condition which is of vital importance for understanding or ameliorating the disorder.

For all three categories, provisions must be made to elicit the assent of the children (over age 6 years) and the permission of their parents for participation in the research. Research that does not meet the above criteria is subject to a special level of review by the U.S. Department of Health and Human Services beyond that provided by local IRB.

There is another side to the issue of children's participation in research. While children need to be protected, they also need to have the opportunity to participate in clinical research. Right now over 80% of drugs used to treat children have not been rigorously tested in children to establish correct dosage. The result is an increased risk of overdose and side effects from medication. In response to concerns that children were denied fair access to medical advances due to their exclusion from medical research, in 1998 the National Institutes of Health (NIH) began requiring that children be included in all human subjects research protocols unless researchers could demonstrate a compelling reason to exclude them. This requirement's goal is to increase children's participation in research so that adequate data will be developed to support therapeutic modalities employed in the care and treatment of medical disorders in children and adults (Office of Extramural Research, 1998). The result of this mandate has been a marked increase in child participation in drug trials, and important new research information has been gained on dosage and side effects of many medications commonly used in pediatric care.

SUMMARY

The information provided in this chapter is meant to assist health care professionals in providing a framework for ethical decision making in cases involving pediatric patients. The issues raised in this chapter make it clear that physicians and other health care professionals should consider many points of view in their decision making, especially seeking out parents (or parent groups), patients (or patient advocacy organizations), experts in fields outside of medicine (including law, disability rights, and professional organizations outside of medicine), and local community members. This may lead to the development of practical steps that will allow physicians and families to come to ethical decisions regarding the care of children with disabilities, the education of trainees in these issues, and the awareness of the different perspectives required, recognizing that social constructions of the past are no longer adequate for the more complicated future.

REFERENCES

American College of Obstetrics and Gynecology (2007). ACOG practice bulletin no. 77: Screening for fetal chromosomal abnormalities. *Obstetrics and Gynecology, 109*, 217–227.

American Medical Association. (1994). *The relation of law and ethics. Code of medical ethics.* Opinion 1.02. Retrieved August 8, 2011, from http://www.ama-assn.org/ama/pub/physician-resources/medical-ethics/code-medical-ethics/opinion102.shtml.

American Medical Association. (2008). *Pediatric decision-making. Code of medical ethics.* Opinion 10.016. Retrieved August 8, 2011, from http://www.ama-assn.org/ama/pub/physician-resources/medical-ethics/code-medical-ethics/opinion10016.shtml

Beachamp, T.L, & Childress, J.F. (2001). *Principles of biomedical ethics.* New York, NY: Oxford University Press.

Bearder et al v State of Minnesota, et al. Fourth Judicial Circuit, County of Hennepin District Court; November 24, 2009. Order granting motion to dismiss court file 27-CV-09-5615

Beleno v Texas Dept. of State Health Services. Case 5:2009cv00188. U.S. District Court for the Western District of Texas in San Antonio, March 3, 2009.

Board of Directors of the American Association on Intellectual & Developmental Disabilities. (2006). *Board position statement: Growth attenuation issue.* Retrieved July 26, 2011, from http://www.aamr.org/content_173.cfm?navID=31

Committee on Bioethics, American Academy of Pediatrics. (2001). Institutional ethics committees. *Pediatrics, 107*, 205–209.

Education Development Center, Inc. (2009). Willowbrook hepatitis experiments. *Exploring bioethics, Master 5.4.* Retrieved August 8, 2011, from http://science.education.nih.gov/supplements/nih9/bioethics/guide/pdf/Master_5.4.pdf,

Goldby, S., (1971). Experiments at the Willowbrook State School. *Lancet, 297*(7702), 749.

Gunther, D.F., & Diekema, D.S. (2006). Attenuating growth in children with profound developmental disability: A new approach to an old dilemma. *Archives of Pediatric & Adolescent Medicine, 160*, 1013–1014.

H.B. 1672, 81st Texas Leg. (2009) Retrieved August 4, 2011, from http://www.legis.state.tx.us/BillLookup/Text.aspx?LegSess=81R&Bill=HB1672.

Higgins v Texas Department of Health Services, Civil Action No. SA-10-CV-990-XR. U.S. District Court for the Western District of Texas, July 7, 2011.

Lyren, A., & Ford, P.J. (2007). Special considerations for clinical ethics consultation in pediatrics: Pediatric care provider as advocate. *Clinical Pediatrics, 46*, 771–776.

MacIntyre, A. (1999, February). *Social structures and their threats to moral agency.* Annual lecture of the Royal Institute of Philosophy.

McCabe, M.E., Hunt, E.A., & Serwint, J.R., (2008). Pediatric residents' clinical and educational experiences with end-of-life care. *Pediatrics, 121*(4), e731–737.

McCullough, L.B. (2005). Neonatal ethics at the limits of viability. *Pediatrics, 116*, 1019–1021.

Mercurio, M.R. (2011). The role of a pediatric ethics committee in the newborn intensive care unit. *Journal of Perinatology, 31*, 1–9.

Munger, K.M., Gill, C.J., Ormond, K.E., & Kirschner, K.L., (2007). The next exclusion debate: Assessing technology, ethics, and intellectual disability after the human genome project. *Mental Retardation and Developmental Disabilities Research Reviews, 13*, 121–128.

National Commission for the Protection of Human Subjectsof Biomedical and Behavioral Research (1979). *Belmont report.* Retrieved August 8, 2011, from http://www.hhs.gov/ohrp/humansubjects/guidance/belmont.html

Office of Extramural Research. (1998). *Inclusion of children policy implementation.* Washington, DC: United States Department of Health and Human Services. Retrieved August 4, 2011, from http://grants.nih.gov/grants/guide/notice-files/not98-024.html

Ostrom, C.M. (2007, May 8). Children's hospital says it should have gone to court in case of disabled 6 year old. *Seattle Times.* Retrieved August 8, 2011, from http://community.seattletimes.nwsource.com/archive/?date=20070508&slug=webchildrens08m

Parens, E., & Asch, A. (2007). The disability rights critique of prenatal genetic testing: Reflections and recommendations. In E. Parens, & A. Asch (Eds.), *Prenatal testing and disability rights.* Washington, DC: Georgetown University Press.

Savage, T.A. (1998). Children with severe and profound disabilities and the issue of social justice. *Advanced Practice Nursing Quarterly, 4*(2), 53–58.

Treatment of Genetic Information Held by Government Entities and Other Persons Act, Minnesota Stat.§ 13.386 (2010). Retrieved August 4, 2011, from https://www.revisor.mn.gov/statutes/?id=13.386

U.S. Department of Health and Human Services, Code of Federal Regulations, Title 45 Public Welfare C.F.R. 46 (1991).

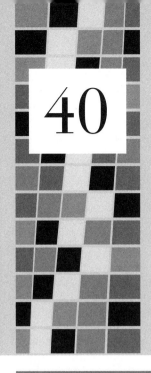

40

Future Expectations

Transition from Adolescence to Adulthood

Nienke P. Dosa, Patience H. White, and Vincent Schuyler

Upon completion of this chapter, the reader will

- Be aware of the importance of planning for the transition to adulthood for youth with disabilities

- Understand the relationship between self-determination and health outcomes and social participation

- Understand the resources and mandated laws available to assist youth with disabilities

- Know the role of employment and postsecondary education in the transition process

- Understand the role health care providers play in promoting successful transition to adulthood of youth with disabilities

---

Individuals with developmental disabilities encounter the same life transitions as typically developing people. Perhaps the most challenging is the transition to adulthood, a period of complex biological, social, and emotional change. This transition involves learning to move from 1) school to work, 2) home to community, and 3) child- to adult-oriented health care. This chapter focuses on the steps involved in the successful transition of an individual with developmental disabilities from adolescence to adulthood.

■ ■ ■ BRYAN

Bryan is a young man with cerebral palsy and intellectual disability who was born prematurely 23 years ago. He completed his public school education 2 years ago. Bryan currently works in a supported employment position at a local supermarket. He receives support and guidance from co-workers who were trained by a local job placement program to provide natural supports in the workplace. After work he participates in many recreational and leisure activities with friends. He goes to the gym and swims regularly at the advice of his physician, for general health, and to prevent obesity. With his increasing job satisfaction and financial independence, this past year Bryan expressed a desire to live on his own. He and his parents contacted the local United Cerebral Palsy Association chapter and, with assistance from the staff, found an apartment and a live-in personal-care attendant.

Bryan still goes to his parents' house for family dinners and events at least once per week and spends additional time with his two younger siblings, ages 16 and 18, who come to visit him frequently in his apartment. Bryan has recently started dating a young woman he met at his job.

GENERAL PRINCIPLES OF TRANSITION

There are three basic tenets of successful transition. First, transition is a process, not an event. Planning for transition to adulthood should begin as early as possible in adolescence on a flexible schedule that recognizes the young person's increasing autonomy and capacity for making choices (American Academy of Pediatrics, American Academy of Family Physicians, and American College of Physicians, Transitions Clinical Report Authoring Group, 2011). Second, coordination among health care, educational, vocational, and social-service systems is essential. It is particularly important to recognize the complex interplay between health and social outcomes as youth with developmental disabilities age into an employment-based health insurance system. Third, self-determination skills should be fostered throughout the transition process. Standards for transition services call for a youth-centered and asset-oriented approach that involves the person as a decision maker during the entire transition process (Pilnick, Clegg, Murphy, & Almack, 2010).

MOVING TOWARD INDEPENDENCE: SELF-DETERMINATION

Human **self-determination** is an outlook that involves a combination of attitudes and abilities that lead people to set goals for themselves, to take the initiative to reach these goals, and to realize those goals (Ryan & Deci, 2000). The capabilities needed for self-determination are learned through real-world experiences (including mistakes) and by an open and supportive acknowledgement of one's disability (Nota, Ferrari, Soresi, & Wehmeyer, 2007). Families, teachers, and other well-intentioned people often protect youth with disabilities from making mistakes and avoid discussing the ramifications of a child's disability as they help them prepare for adulthood. This can predispose the developing child to future failure or can result in learned helplessness (Peterson, Maier, & Seligman, 1995).

Teachers and other individuals providing assistance to families can and should begin preparing children with developmental disabilities for independence as early as possible. For example, young children between 3–5 years of age can begin to incorporate chores into their daily routine. Families that give children opportunities to demonstrate competence through developmentally appropriate household chores send a clear message of support and capability. By the developmental age of 6–11 years, children should begin to assume responsibility for their self-care. During adolescence, self-determination skills should be focused on identifying and meeting educational and vocational goals. In early adulthood, these skills can then be used to identify and meet goals related to independent living. Curricula, tools, and policies have been developed to enhance self-determination for students with disabilities (Calkins & Wehmeyer, 2011).

MOVING FROM SCHOOL TO WORK

The concept of transition planning originated with schools, and education policies are the driving force for almost all aspects of transition. Five pieces of legislation—the Individuals with Disabilities Education Improvement Act of 2004 (PL 108-446; IDEA 2004), the School-to-Work Opportunities Act of 1994 (PL 103-239), the Workforce Investment Act (WIA) of 1998 (PL 105-220), the Americans with Disabilities Act (ADA) of 1990 (PL 101-336), and the Higher Education Opportunity Act (HEOA; PL 110-315) outline important educational practices that lead to successful adult outcomes for students with disabilities. Certain aspects of these key laws are discussed in the following sections.

Legislation for Transition Individuals with Disabilities

The 2004 reauthorization of IDEA in particular has strengthened school-to-work transitions. This legislation established 16 years of age as a clear starting point for transition planning in the **individualized education program** (IEP). It strengthened the working definition of transition services and redefined transition planning from a statement of needed services to a set of measurable postsecondary goals based upon age-appropriate transition assessments related to training, education, employment, and, where appropriate, independent living skills. This legislation also requires schools to report progress toward meeting transition goals in the IEP. Under IDEA 2004, schools must provide a "summary of performance" to students whose special education eligibility is terminated. This new summary must include information on the student's academic achievement and functional performance and include recommendations on how to assist the student in meeting his or her postsecondary goals. While schools are not required to conduct any new assessments or evaluations in order to provide the summary, they must satisfy the disability documentation required under other federal laws such as the Americans with Disabilities Act and Section 504 of the Rehabilitation Act of 1973 (http://www.ncld.org/at-school/your-childs-rights/iep-aamp-504-plan/idea-2004-improving-transition-planning-and-results).

Vocational Rehabilitation

Linking schools with systems of care that serve adults with disabilities, including vocational rehabilitation (VR) agencies, strengthens the transition process. The School-to-Work Opportunities Act of 1994 provides workplace mentoring and skills certificates for youth with developmental disabilities. The Workforce Investment Act of 1998 links education, employment, and training services to a network of resources in local areas called One-Stop Career Centers (Barnow & King, 2005). Transition planning as mandated by IDEA 2004 stipulates that schools are responsible for bringing in representatives from other agencies, such as vocational rehabilitative services, to be part of the transition planning process. Vocational rehabilitation agencies help pay for postsecondary education for qualified young adults. These agencies may also be responsible for delivering some of the student's needed services. Should these agencies fail to provide the agreed-upon services, schools must find alternative ways to fulfill the transition objectives for the student. It is important to note that VR counselors are typically assigned to students only during their last 2 years of school but that parents and students can request their participation as early as age 14 via One-Stop Career Centers (U.S. Department of Labor, 2005) or through the school.

Unlike the entitlement based system for K–12 education, all adult services and systems are eligibility-based and require that individuals meet the established requirements, including financial eligibility criteria, to receive services. Once individuals are determined to be eligible, the VR agency can provide or arrange for a host of training, educational, medical, and other services designed to help these individuals acquire and maintain gainful employment. Similar to the IEP in the school system, all services aim to develop an individualized plan for employment (IPE; previously called an individualized written rehabilitation program [IWRP]), which is directed at meeting the needs of the young person. Although VR counselors can provide direct services, they more often refer the individual to appropriate community-based agencies. Services covered by VR may include self-advocacy training, the development of employment-readiness skills, adaptive driving evaluation and instruction, identification and procurement of assistive technology, job coaching, and so forth.

Moving Toward Postsecondary Education

Postsecondary education can take many forms. Although traditionally thought of as college, it may be any form of education or training that takes place after a young adult leaves high school, including on-the-job training, specialized coursework, or even courses through postgraduate study. Most colleges and universities have an office designated as disability support services (DSS) or, at a minimum, a staff member designated to assist students with disabilities. To receive assistance or request accommodations for disability-related needs, a student must take the lead in disclosing his or her disability, providing current documentation of the disability and identifying needed accommodations. Accommodations are established on a case-by-case basis and do not necessarily replicate those provided in the K–12 setting. Examples of accommodations that can be requested of DSS include extra time in test-taking, a sign language interpreter, a note taker, and recorded books. Postsecondary education facilities that receive federal funding are required to provide reasonable accommodations to qualified individuals with disabilities under Section 504 of the Rehabilitation Act of 1973 (PL 93-112) and under Titles II and/or III of the ADA. The Higher Education Opportunity Act (HEOA) (PL 110-315) was enacted in 2008, reauthorizing the Higher Education Act (HEA) of 1965. This law improves access to postsecondary education for students with intellectual disabilities by opening up eligibility for Pell Grants, Supplemental Educational Opportunity Grants, and Federal Work-Study Programs, and by creating model demonstration programs and

coordinating centers for students with intellectual disabilities (Smith, 2009).

Entering the Work Force

Work experience is a prerequisite for many jobs.
Unfortunately, most youth with developmental
disabilities enter the work force later than their
peers who do not have disabilities (U.S. Department of Labor, 2005; Von Shrader, 2010).
Nationwide, 41% of high school freshman and
85% of high school seniors have regular jobs
either during the school year or during summer
months (U.S. Department of Labor, 2005). In
contrast, only 26% of adolescents aged 16–20
years who have disabilities are wage earners
prior to high school graduation (Von Shrader,
2010). Among youth with developmental
disabilities, those with learning challenges,
emotional disabilities, speech impairments, or
other health impairments are most likely to be
employed. (Cameto et al., 2003). Only 15% of
youth with autism spectrum disorders; approximately 25% of youth with multiple disabilities,
deaf-blindness, or orthopedic impairments; and
about 33% of youth with intellectual disability
or visual impairments are employed during high
school (Cameto et al., 2003). The implications
of limited early job experience on work force
readiness, long-term employment, economic
status, and social functioning in adulthood are
profound. Employment rates in 2009 for the 15
million U.S. adults who have a disability (8.1%
of adults ages 18–64 years) were substantially
lower than for adults who do not have a disability (16.8% versus 74%). The correlate to this is
a poverty rate for adults who have a disability
that is substantially higher than that of the population without disabilities (28.1% versus 10%;
Von Shrader, 2010).

A plan for paid work experiences should
be written into a student's IEP starting no later
than age 16 years (IDEA, 2004). Job placement
choices should be based, when possible, on individual interests, abilities, and post-secondary
goals. For example, if a student has set comput-
ing-related career goals, an appropriate placement would be one that allows the student to
work with a computer in some fashion.

Work Options

Individuals with disabilities who are entering
the work force, like those without disabilities,
have the option of participating in competitive employment, but they also have a range of
other work alternatives available to them (Butterworth, Smith, Hall, Migliore, Winsor, 2009).

An individual engaged in competitive
employment is expected to perform essential
functions at the same level as other employees
without disabilities. Individuals with disabilities may request an accommodation under the
protections of the ADA that enables them to
perform these functions, as long as the accommodation does not fundamentally alter the
nature of the job. Accommodations covered by
ADA include adaptive seating, computer input
devices, large-print text, and so forth. To succeed in this **competitive employment** setting,
individuals with disabilities must have the same
skills requisite for any employee to succeed
in the workplace: knowledge base for the job,
appropriate social skills, effective communication skills, and motivation. Individuals with
disabilities also must have appropriate independent living skills, and the skills and abilities to
manage their disability-related needs, such as
hiring and managing personal care attendants
and transportation services.

Work-Study Employment

Work-study employment is part-time work
for students sanctioned by the school either
on or off campus. Age-appropriate transition
assessment information and the student's IEP
goals for transition should inform the appropriateness of this type of work. Persons with
disabilities are not immune from social preju-
dices and stereotypes, so it is important to avoid
employment options for adolescents who have
disabilities that reinforce these stereotypes. For
example, the number of individuals with developmental disabilities employed in food service
(19% of work-study jobs and 16% of regular
jobs) and maintenance (16% of work-study jobs
and 24% of regular jobs) far exceeds what one
would expect to be representative of the interest
level for these jobs among youth with developmental disabilities (Cameto et al., 2003).

Supported Employment

Supported employment is defined by the
Rehabilitation Act Amendments of 1986 (PL
99-506) and 1992 (PL 102-569) as employment in an inclusive setting with ongoing support services for an individual with a disability.
Supported employment programs are generally
administered through the state-level Bureaus
of Vocational Rehabilitation and state developmental disability agencies. These agencies help
people with disabilities obtain employment
by identifying supports through supervisor or
co-worker assistance (natural supports) or job

coaches. A job coach or employment consultant is a person who is hired by the individual or the placement agency; his or her duty is to provide specialized on-site training to assist the employee with a disability in learning and performing his or her job and adjusting to the work environment with the ultimate goal of full inclusion at the worksite (Degeneffe, 2000).

Customized Employment

Customized employment is a blend of services designed to increase employment options for individuals with significant disabilities such as self-employment, entrepreneurship, job carving and restructuring, personal agents and customized training (United States Department of Labor, 2009).

Enclaves

Enclaves (sheltered workshops) were once considered a viable employment option for individuals with severe disabilities (Wehman & Kregel, 1985). The enclave brings together groups of individuals with disabilities at one site with a common job coach engaged around a work task. Enclaves are seen as a cost-saving model for agencies but are controversial because individuals often are paid substandard wages and the model does not promote worksite inclusion. Placement of individuals in enclave settings is not recommended.

Volunteering

In today's competitive job market, **volunteering** is an opportunity for adolescents to gain valuable insight into the world of work, to develop skills, and to build work-related experience. It can be a positive step toward achievement of full employment or community inclusion goals in the IEP. However, volunteer experiences should not replace paid work experiences when those opportunities are also available as they may inadvertently promote cultural stereotypes about the employability of individuals with developmental disabilities (Wolf-Branigin, Schuyler, & White, 2007).

Other Options

Some youth with intellectual disabilities may not be ready to make the transition into a work-related setting immediately after exiting the school system. (Shaw et al., 2008). For these individuals, other more supportive options are available, such as day treatment/habilitation or work-readiness programs. These programs provide a more intensive level of support and focus on the development of daily living skills rather than job skills. The ultimate goal for any of these programs should remain moving the individual toward employment.

MOVING FROM HOME INTO THE COMMUNITY

There are several key financial and legal issues that need to be addressed to insure that at age 18 there is no loss of income and/or services, family assets are protected, and youth with developmental disabilities are assured suitable independent living options as they move from home to the community. Financial barriers are the most common reason youth with developmental disabilities fail to make the transition to independent living in the community (McPherson et al., 2004).

Financial Independence

Supplemental Security Income (SSI) is a monthly payment for individuals with disabilities. To qualify for SSI, individuals must meet both disability and financial eligibility requirements. SSI eligibility is generally determined using adult criteria when adolescents turn 18 years old, with the exception being youth enrolled in a Social Security Administration (SSA) work incentive program. Young people with developmental disabilities may lose their SSI at this time if they fail to meet the adult disability criteria. Conversely, some individuals with disabilities may now qualify for SSI when they had previously been ineligible because individual income, rather than household income, is used to determine income eligibility at age 18. Generally speaking, adults who receive SSI cannot have individual assets greater than $2,000 and still remain eligible. The SSA, however, does allow several important exceptions to this rule, which are referred to as work incentives (see http://www.SSA.gov/work).

Despite these incentive programs, a significant number of youth with developmental disabilities lose SSI benefits when they become adults. In 2009, adolescents in the 13–17 year age bracket represented 8.8% of SSI recipients. This dropped to 6.9% for young adults in the 18–21 year age bracket (United States Social Security Administration Annual Statistical Supplement, 2010). Youth who lose SSI benefits when eligibility is redetermined at age 18 should request a second review because more than one third of such requests result in the reinstatement of SSI benefits (American Academy of Pediatrics, 2009; Rupp, et al., 2005–2006). Some individuals who are found ineligible can continue to receive SSI benefits as long as they participate in approved VR programs. In most states, people who receive SSI automatically also qualify for Medicaid.

Social Security Disability Insurance (SSDI) is a monthly payment for individuals with disabilities. There are two ways to qualify for SSDI benefits. Workers (including those in sheltered or supported work settings) who have paid into the Social Security system are eligible for SSDI if they are no longer able to work. Monthly SSDI benefits are also paid to an adult with developmental disabilities when a parent or guardian meets disability criteria and cannot work. It is important to know that beneficiaries who receive SSDI for more than 2 years are eligible for health care coverage under Medicare.

Legal Status/Guardianship

In most states, the natural **guardianship** of parents ends when children reach age 18 years. At that point, parents no longer have the legal ability to make decisions or sign consent forms for their child unless they submit an application for guardianship at their local probate court. Two prerequisites must exist before a court appoints a guardian: 1) the child must show incompetence in at least one important area of life, such as health care decisions or financial matters; and 2) there must be a present need for the guardianship. In accord with the principles of self-determination, it is important to evaluate the extent to which an individual can participate in decisions that affect his or her own life (Buchanan & Brock, 1992; Burt, 1996). This allows probate courts to appoint someone as a guardian only over that portion of a person's life where the person both shows incompetence and has a need (e.g., health care guardianship). Making a decision about guardianship is essential to the health transition process. When a youth who has a developmental disability cannot make health care decisions independently, there are several options to consider and procedures to follow in order to obtain legal guardianship. It is important to make these decisions before the youth's 18th birthday because an 18-year-old is considered a legal adult unless actions are taken to establish guardianship. In other words, guardianship is not automatic. The process of establishing guardianship can be daunting for some families, but it is necessary for enabling caregivers to continue to advocate more effectively. Once obtained, guardianship papers should be kept in a wallet so that they can be presented at all health care encounters. Guardianship papers are as important as an insurance card when patients with developmental disabilities enter the adult health care system.

There are several alternatives to guardianship that may be preferable because they avoid legal "red tape" and are more specific to the individual's needs and rights. A representative payeeship can be useful when the only income an individual receives is his or her monthly SSI check and there are no major financial decisions. A special needs trust permits adults with developmental disabilities to inherit money, which can be used for services not covered by Medicaid or Medicare without interrupting these government benefits. A conservatorship is established when an individual is mentally competent but has a physical disability that limits his or her ability to participate in the decision-making process. Adult protective services can be ordered by a court if abuse or neglect of an adult with developmental disabilities is suspected.

In situations where legal guardianship is not indicated, support can be provided informally. A **circle of support** is a group of volunteer advocates, such as family members, friends and neighbors, who make sure that an individual with a developmental disability has a support system that meets all of his or her needs. A **microboard** is a circle of support that is incorporated to include the individual with developmental disabilities as the chairperson (Wetherow & Wetherow, 2004). Although these sorts of informal alternatives to guardianship are gaining acceptance, it should be noted that a legal guardian or a **representative payee** is often required by programs and services in order to disburse funds to an individual with developmental disabilities. The paperwork for this should be completed before age 18 to avoid interruption in benefits.

Housing

Approximately 28% of adults with developmental disabilities live in their own homes, 58% live with their families, and 15% reside in publicly funded residential settings (Lakin, Larson, Salmi, & Webster, 2010) Most new group homes are designed for 1–3 individuals and are referred to as **independent residential alternatives** (IRA), reflecting a trend away from institutional settings of 16 or more people, which was the norm a generation ago. In 2009 the average per resident expenditures per year were $203,670 in state operated IRAs (Lakin et al., 2010). Home and community-based services and programs for young adults with developmental disabilities cost substantially less, and are in high demand. However, waiting lists are the norm. An estimated total of 122,870 persons in the U.S. with intellectual and developmental disabilities were waiting for residential services in 2009 (Lakin et al., 2010).

Services and programs that assist individuals with community living have increased dramatically since the 1990s as a result of the New Freedom Initiative (Executive Order No. 13217), the ADA, and the Olmstead decision (*Olmstead v. L.C.*, 527 U.S. 581, 1999). The Olmstead decision interpreted Title II of the ADA to require states to administer their services, programs, and activities "in the most integrated setting appropriate to the needs of qualified individuals with disabilities" (*Olmstead v. L.C.*, 527 U.S. 581, 1999). State-funded programs as well as private nonprofit agencies such as The Arc of the United States, Easter Seals, and United Cerebral Palsy (UCP) provide service coordination and access to a wide array of independent living options. **Independent living centers** foster networking among people with disabilities and offer assistance in four key areas: information and referral, independent living skills and training, peer counseling, and advocacy (Seekins, Enders, & Innes, 1999).

Family Home

Many families whose grown children have developmental disabilities will choose for the individual to continue to live at home. Between 1999 and 2009, the number of adults with developmental disabilities living with family members in the United States increased from 355,152 to 599,152 (68.7%; Lakin, Larson, Salmi, & Webster, 2010). The aging of these families is an emerging concern. Approximately one quarter of home-based adults with developmental disabilities live in homes headed by elderly parents. Support systems for aging parents of adults with developmental disabilities are lacking (Heller, Caldwell, & Factor, 2007).

Group Home

The most common form of assisted living program (outside of the family home) is the group home (Lakin et al., 2010). The trend is toward smaller group homes of one to three residents

(Prouty et al., 2004). Most group homes have on-site counselors who provide supervision and support in daily living skills, employment, and recreation.

Supported Living Services

Supported living services (SLS) provide services to adults with developmental disabilities who live in homes that they own or lease in the community. SLS may include assistance with 1) selecting and moving into a home, 2) choosing personal attendants and housemates, 3) acquiring household furnishings, 4) addressing common daily living activities and emergencies, 5) becoming a participating member in community life, and 6) managing personal financial affairs (Stancliffe & Lakin, 2005)

MOVING FROM PEDIATRIC- TO ADULT-ORIENTED HEALTH CARE

As a result of advances in medical technology and dramatic improvements in the delivery of acute health care, the vast majority of children with developmental disabilities can now expect to survive to adulthood (Day, Strauss, Shavelle, & Reynolds, 2005; Hemming, Hutton, & Pharoah, 2006; Picket, Paculdo, Shavelle, & Strauss, 2006; Strauss, Shavelle, Rosenbloom, & Brooks, 2008). As life expectancy for individuals with developmental disabilities approaches that of the general population, socioeconomic factors are increasingly being recognized as important determinants of health, with quality of life and social inclusion as meaningful health outcomes (Krahn & Campbell, 2011; Nota, Ferrari, Soresi, & Wehmeyer, 2007).

The International Classification of Functioning, Disability and Health (ICF) provides a framework for understanding the impact of the social and physical environment on health for individuals with developmental disabilities (World Health Organization, 2001). This framework broadens the array of interventions to be considered as strategies for improving health and social outcomes. For example, identifying accessible recreation opportunities in the community may be one of the most effective ways to treat obesity in individuals with **meningomyelocele** (Rimmer, Riley, Wang, Rauworth, & Jurkowski, 2004).

Coincidental with the ICF's reconceptualization of functioning, disability and health is a paradigm shift in the way health care is delivered to people with developmental disabilities. Institutions and hospital-based programs are rapidly being replaced by home and community-based supports and services. This trend is reflected by the federal health care goal (in *Healthy People 2020*) that young people with developmental disabilities receive services needed to make necessary transitions to *all* aspects of adult life, including health care, work, and independent living (U.S. Department of Health and Human Services, 2010).

A major obstacle to transition to adult-oriented care is that youth often have no options (Crowley, Wolfe, Lock, & McKee, 2011; Greiner, 2007; Reiss & Gibson, 2002). Many adult health care providers lack training in the care of individuals with developmental disabilities (Peter, Forke, Ginsburg, & Schwarz, 2009). Curricula are in development to address this issue (Betz, 2004; Brin, 2008; Nehring, 2005). Some resources have already been developed. One, from the National Health Care Transition Center (http://www.gottransition.org/) offers resources and toolkits for health care providers. Specific strategies for successful transition to an adult medical home model are outlined in the joint statement on health care transition put forth in 2011 (American Academy of Pediatrics, American Academy of Family Physicians, and American College of Physicians, Transitions Clinical Report Authoring Group, 2011).

Low patient satisfaction with adult providers has been reported in terms of availability, thoroughness, respect, and privacy (McDonagh & Viner, 2006). Pediatric providers, in turn, often struggle to "let go" of their adolescent patients and fail to actively promote the transition to adult health care (Reiss, Gibson, & Walker, 2005). Studies have documented that only one out of six pediatricians routinely discusses health care transition with young adult patients who have developmental disabilities (Scal & Ireland, 2005). Lack of insurance and underinsurance are also major barriers to health care transition (see Chapter 41). In the United States, young adults have the highest uninsured rate of any age group. Nearly half (45%), or approximately 20 million young adults between the ages of 19–29, are uninsured for a part of each year (Hackett, Comeau, Hess, & Sloyer, 2010). Approximately one third (30%) of young adults who have developmental disabilities are uninsured (Callahan & Cooper, 2006). To help remedy this situation, the Patient Protection and Affordable Care Act within the American Recovery and Reinvestment Act (ARRA; PL 111-5) of 2009 now prohibits discrimination based on preexisting conditions and ends lifetime caps in coverage. ARRA guarantees continuation of insurance coverage under the parents' plans to age 26 years. It also includes long-term services and supports insurance (CLASS Act provisions) that will benefit people with developmental disabilities and their families.

An algorithm for transitioning youths with developmental disabilities to adult health care is outlined in a recent clinical report (American Academy of Pediatrics, American Academy of Family Physicians, American College of Physicians, 2011). This report underscores the importance of the patient centered medical home, which is an approach to providing comprehensive primary care that facilitates partnerships between individual patients, and their personal providers, and when appropriate, the patient's family (American Academy of Family Physicians et al., 2007). The algorithm is driven by a process that includes longitudinal assessment of transition readiness, the planning and implementation of specific transition goals, and documentation. This algorithm identifies a sequence of transition-related activities that are ideally (although not necessarily) implemented at specific ages:

Step 1: Discuss office transition policy (12–13 years)

Step 2: Initiate a transition plan jointly with parent and youth (14–15 years)

Step 3: Review and update the transition plan (16–17 years)

Step 4: Transfer care to adult provider(s) (18–21 years)

Written documentation is a key component of the actual transfer of care. The clinical report recommends that adult providers be given a copy of the transition plan as well as documentation of a youth's transition readiness, or self-care and health care navigation skills. They should also be provided with legal documentation (signed HIPAA form and/or guardianship paperwork) that clearly defines the responsible party for medical decision making. Finally, the clinical report recommends that adult providers be given a portable medical summary that includes a succinct medical history as well as 1) a list of medical providers, 2) key social service providers, 3) baseline functional and neurologic status, 4) cognitive status, including formal test results and date of administration, 5) condition-specific emergency treatment plans and contacts, and 6) the patient's health education history. The latter should also include an assessment of the individuals' understanding regarding health conditions, treatments, and prognosis with particular attention focused on entry into adult life, including procreation potential and genetic information. **Medication reconciliation**, when the medication lists are checked for accuracy and to make sure there are no adverse interactions, is recommended at both the giving and receiving end of the transfer. The report also underscores the importance of direct communication. In addition to the previously mentioned algorithm for health care transition, several clinical topics generic to adolescent health care have unique applications for youth with developmental disabilities during the transition to adulthood.

Adherence and Health Literacy

To be ready to move to the adult system, the adolescent needs to be responsible for taking medications (with supervision when appropriate); to develop the ability to understand and discuss his or her disability; and to use required adaptive equipment or appliances (American Academy of Pediatrics, American Academy of Family Physicians, and American College of Physicians, Transitions Clinical Report Authoring Group, 2011). During this process, health care professionals should consider when to start seeing the individual alone and when to develop a confidential relationship with him or her. For many adolescents this transition occurs around ages 12–13 years. Health care checklists, curricula, and tools can be found on the web site for the National Health Care Transition Center (http://www.gottransition.org/).

Health Promotion

Good nutrition and regular exercise are the basis of maintaining health. Adults with developmental disabilities have similar rates of obesity and risky behaviors (e.g., tobacco use) as people without disabilities but are less likely to participate in prevention programs or to receive periodic cancer screening (Liptak, Kennedy, & Dosa, 2010; Shireman, Reichard, Nazir, Backes, & Greiner, 2010). Adults with developmental disabilities are also at risk for preventable secondary conditions such as osteoporosis and **decubitus ulcers** (bed sores). Early and sustained participation in community-based programs is essential for adolescents to maintain healthy lifestyles beyond the school years (Bazzano, Zeldin, Diab, Garro, Allevato, & Lehrer, 2009).

Leisure activities are particularly important for young adults with developmental disabilities, who tend to become socially isolated. People with developmental disabilities requiring extensive to pervasive support (severe to profound intellectual disability) are less likely to participate in leisure activities (Van Naarden Braun, Yeargin-Allsopp, & Lollar, 2009). Therapeutic recreation programs that incorporate social skills training can help individuals with developmental disabilities hone conversation skills, maintain eye contact, use appropriate body language, and become a self-advocate (http://www.atraonline.com/displaycommon. cfm?an=1&subarticlenbr=105). Examples of therapeutic recreation programs include the Special Olympics (http://www.specialolympics. org/) and Best Buddies Programs (http://www. bestbuddies.org/). For individuals with motor impairments, there is Wheelchair and Ambulatory Sports USA (http://www.wsusa.org/). The National Center on Physical Activity and Disability (http://www.ncpad.org) is a clearinghouse for information to promote physical activity among individuals with disabilities.

Sexuality

Sexuality is a natural aspect of human development and is important to all individuals regardless of gender, orientation, or developmental level (Ailey et al., 2003). Unfortunately adolescents with developmental disabilities often do not receive information about sexuality and reproductive health. Professionals and parents either lack the awareness to consider sexuality as part of the adolescent's normal growth and development or are fearful of discussing sensitive issues and acknowledging vulnerability (Murphy, 2005; Tice & Hall, 2008). This results in an information gap that may increase the chances of sexual exploitation and unintended pregnancy. Youth with developmental disabilities are four times more likely to be sexually abused or exploited than their typically developing peers (Dixon, Bergstrom, Smith, & Tarbox, 2010; Bowman, Scotti, & Morris, 2010). Lack of knowledge of sexuality, lack of information on exploitation, cognitive deficits, poor social skills, poor self-esteem, and poor body image are some of the factors that place adolescents with developmental disabilities at increased risk (Bowman, Scotti, & Morris, 2010; Dixon, Bergstrom, Smith, & Tarbox, 2010).

Mental Health

Individuals with developmental disabilities are at a higher risk for developing mental health problems than their typically developing peers (see Chapter 29). This so-called "dual diagnosis" affects nearly 40% of children with intellectual disability, compared to 8% in the general population (Emerson, 2003). Children with autism have even higher rates of mental health disorders. Specific phobias and obsessive-compulsive disorder are very common in children with autism who are dually diagnosed (DD; Leyfer et al., 2006). Children with cerebral palsy are not reported to have increased rates of psychiatric diagnosis, compared to the general population; however, ascertainment may be problematic in this population. Boys and teens have higher rates of dual diagnosis than girls and younger children. For intellectual disability, factors associated with an increased risk of psychopathology include, in addition to age and gender, social deprivation, family composition, number of potentially stressful life events, the mental health of the child's caregiver, and family functioning (Emerson, 2003). Among adults with developmental disabilities, the prevalence of mental illness is approximately four times higher than that found in the general population (Rush et al., 2004). Substance abuse, however, affects approximately 2% of the DD population which is lower than in the general population (Slayter, 2010). The proportion of anxiety and mood disorders are similar to the general population. Rates for psychosis are higher (Deb, Thomas, & Bright, 2001).

Despite the high reported rates of dual diagnosis, the proper diagnosis of mental illness in a person with intellectual or other developmental disabilities remains a challenge. Reiss, Levitan, and Szyszko (1982) termed one major obstacle "diagnostic overshadowing." This refers to the tendency clinicians have to attribute all the behavioral and emotional problems to the developmental disability rather than to a comorbid mental illness. Another problem is that many professionals in the field of mental illness simply do not have training or experience in the field of developmental disabilities (Fletcher, Loschen, Stavrakaki, & First, 2007).

Most service systems for people with developmental disabilities are oriented to chronic care and long-term support, and provide limited, if any, services for acute mental health crises. Emergency mental health services are typically geared to the needs of the general population. Access to preventive mental services is problematic as well. Adults with developmental disabilities are seven times more likely to report inadequate emotional support, compared with adults who do not have disabilities (Havercamp et. al., 2004; see also Chapter 29). Behavioral concerns should be investigated rather than ascribed to the individual's developmental disability. It is important to question adolescents and their families about physical symptoms of anxiety and depression, such as altered sleep patterns and appetite. Professionals should also monitor excessive school absences as these may be evidence of a mental health issue.

Environmental factors should be considered as precipitants when adolescents with developmental disabilities present with challenging behaviors. For example, it is not unusual for an adolescent with developmental disabilities to experience anxiety when a long-time aide is no longer available at school or when opportunities to socialize diminish with high school graduation. Surgery, a prolonged hospitalization, or medical setbacks can also precipitate depressive episodes. It should be emphasized that behaviors that occur across all settings are more likely to be due to organic causes. Treatments can include psychological, behavioral, and/or environmental interventions along with pharmacotherapy, if needed. Quality-of-life spheres should not be overlooked. Community-based models of support combined with neuropsychiatric intervention can be a potent therapeutic approach in the management of challenging behaviors in individuals with developmental disabilities (Ferrell et al., 2004).

SUMMARY

Health care providers, educators, other professionals, and families must foster the expectation that youth with developmental disabilities will become healthy, happy, active, and productive members of their community. Youth should be provided with opportunities to learn about their strengths, abilities, skills, needs, and interests. They should also be allowed to take risks and to learn from failure. They should assume responsibility for themselves and understand the difference between the protected worlds of school and home and the worlds of work and adult life. Most of all, they must believe they are capable of success. These goals can be accomplished through comprehensive transition planning and advocacy, including self-advocacy, to promote full participation in society.

REFERENCES

Ailey, S.H., Marks, B.A., Crisp, C., & Hahn, J.E. (2003). Promoting sexuality across the life span for individuals with intellectual and developmental disabilities. *Nursing Clinics of North America, 38*(2), 229–352.

American Academy of Family Physicians (AAFP), American Academy of Pediatrics (AAP), American College of Physicians (ACP), American Osteopathic Association (AOA). (February 2007). *Joint principles of the patient centered medical home.* Retrieved March 20, 2011, from http://www.pcpcc.net/content/joint-principles-patient-centered-medical-home

American Academy of Pediatrics, Council on Children With Disabilities. (2009). Policy statement: Supplemental Security Income (SSI) for children and youth with disabilities. *Pediatrics, 124*(6), 1702–8.

American Academy of Pediatrics, American Academy of Family Physicians, & American College of Physicians–American Society of Internal Medicine. (2002). A consensus statement on health care transitions for young adults with special health care needs. *Pediatrics, 110*(6, Pt. 2), 1304–1306.

American Recovery and Reinvestment Act of 2009 (ARRA) PL. 111-5.

Americans with Disabilities Act (ADA) of 1990, PL 101336, 42 U.S.C. §§ 12101 *et seq.*

Barnow, B.S., & King, C.T. (2005). *Workforce Investment Act in eight states* (U.S. Department of Labor Employment and Training Administration Occasional Reports 2005-1 [AK-12224-01-60].) Retrieved February 10, 2007, from http://rockinst.org/publications/ federalism/wia/Rockefeller_Institute_WIA%20_Final _Report2-17-05.pdf

Bazzano, D., Zeldin, A.T., Diab, A.S., Garro, I.R., Allevato, N.A., & Lehrer, D. (2009). WRC Project Oversight Team. The Healthy Lifestyle Change Program: A pilot of a community-based health promotion intervention for adults with developmental disabilities. *American Journal of Preventive Medicine, 37*(6 Suppl 1), S201–8.

Betz, C.L. (2004). Transition of adolescents with special health care needs: Review and analysis of the literature. *Issues in Comprehensive Pediatric Nursing, 27*(3), 179–241.

Bowman, R.A., Scotti, J.R., & Morris, T.L. (2010). Sexual abuse prevention: A training program for developmental disabilities service providers. *Journal of Child Sex Abuse, 19*(2), 119–27.

Braddock, D., Emerson, E., Felce, D., & Stancliffe, R.J. (2001). Living circumstances of children and adults with mental retardation or developmental disabilities in the United States, Canada, England and Wales, and Australia. *Mental Retardation and Developmental Disabilities Research Reviews, 7,* 115–121.

Brin, A., & American Academy of Pediatrics (2008). *The State of Transitions Report American Academy of Pediatrics, National Center for Medical Home Initiatives.* Retrieved March 20, 2011, from http://www.medicalhomeinfo.org/how/care_delivery/transitions.aspx,

Buchanan, A.E., & Brock, D.W. (1992). *Deciding for others: The ethics of surrogate decision making.* Cambridge University Press.

Burt, R.A. (1996, September/October.). *The suppressed legacy of Nuremberg (Hastings Center Report).* Garrison, NY: The Hastings Center.

Butterworth, J., Smith, F.A., Hall, A.C., Migliore, A., & Winsor, J. (2009). *State Data: The National Report on Employment Services and Outcomes 2009, Institute for Community Inclusion UCEDD.* Boston, MA: University of Massachusetts.

Calkins, C., & Wehmeyer, M.L. (2011). *A National Gateway to Self-Determination Web Portal, a clearinghouse on resources, training, and information on self-determination.* Retrieved March 20, 2011, from http://www.aucd.org/ngsd/template/index.cfm.

Callahan, S.T., & Cooper, W.O. (2006). Access to health care for young adults with disabling chronic conditions. *Archives of Pediatrics & Adolescent Medicine, 160*(2), 178–182.

Cameto, R., Marder, C., Wagner, M., & Cardoso, D. (2003). Youth employment. *NLTS2 Data Brief, 2*(2). Retrieved June 16, 2005, from http://www.ncset.org/publications/ viewdesc.asp?id=1310

Casey Family Programs. (2004). *Adolescent autonomy checklists.* Seattle, WA: Author.

Crowley, R., Wolfe, I., Lock, K., & McKee, M. (2011). Improving the transition between paediatric and adult healthcare: A systematic review. *Archives of Disabled Children, 96*(6), 548–553.

Day, S.M., Strauss, D.J., Shavelle R.M., & Reynolds, R.J. (2005). Mortality and causes of death in persons with Down syndrome in California. *Developmental Medicine & Child Neurology, 47,* 171–176.

Deb, S., Thomas, M., & Bright, C. (2001). Mental disorder in adults with intellectual disability: Prevalence of functional psychiatric illness among a community-based population aged between 16 and 64 years. *Journal of Intellectual Disability Research, 45,* 495–505.

Degeneffe, C.E. (2000). Supported employment services for persons with developmental disabilities: Unmet promises and future challenges for rehabilitation counselors. *Journal of Applied Rehabilitation Counseling, 31*(2), 41–47.

Dixon, D.R., Bergstrom, R., Smith, M.N., & Tarbox, J. (2010). A review of research on procedures for teaching safety skills to persons with developmental disabilities. *Research into Developmental Disabilities, 31*(5), 985–94.

Edelman, A., Schuyler, V.E., & White, P.H. (1998). *Maximizing success for young adults with chronic health-related illnesses: Transition planning for education after high school.* Washingon, DC: HEATH Resource Center.

Emerson, E. (2003). Prevalence of psychiatric disorders in children and adolescents with and without intellectual disability. *Journal of Intellectual Disability Research, 47*(1), 51–58.

Executive Order No. 13217, 66 Federal Register 33155 (June 21, 2001).

Ferrell, R.B., Wolinsky, E.J., Kauffman, C.I., Flashman, L.A., & McAllister, T.W. (2004). Neuropsychiatric syndromes in adults with mental retardation: Issues in assessment and treatment. *Current Psychiatry Reports, 6*(5), 380–390.

Fletcher, R., Loschen, E., Stavrakaki, C., & First, M. (Eds.). (2007). *Diagnostic manual—intellectual disability (DM-ID): A textbook of diagnosis of mental disorders in persons with intellectual disability.* Kingston, NY: NADD Press.

Greiner, A. (2007). White space or black hole: What can we do to improve care transitions? *American Board of Internal Medicine Foundation, 6,* 1–4.

Hackett, P., Comeau, M., Hess, J., & Sloyer, P. (2010). *Just the facts: The 411 on health care insurance for Florida young adults 18–30.* Tallahassee, FL: Florida-HATS, Florida Department of Health. Available at www.FloridaHATS.org.

Heller, T., Caldwell, J., & Factor, A. (2007) Aging family caregivers: Policies and practices. *Mental Retardation and Developmental Disabilities Research Reviews, 13*(2), 136–42.

Hemming, K., Hutton, J.L., & Pharoah, P.O. (2006). Long-term survival for a cohort of adults with cerebral palsy. *Developmental Medicine & Child Neurology, 48,* 90–95.

Higher Education Opportunity Act of 2008, PL 110-315.

Individuals with Disabilities Education Improvement Act of 2004, PL 108-446, 20 U.S.C. §§ 1400 *et seq.*

Krahn, G., & Campbell, V.A. (2011). Evolving views of disability and public health: The roles of advocacy and public health. *Disability and Health Journal, 4*(1), 12–18.

Lakin, K.C., Larson, S.A., Salmi, P., & A. Webster. (2010). *Residential services for persons with developmental disabilities: Statues and trends through 2009.* Minneapolis: University of Minnesota, Research and Training Center on Community Living, Institute on Community Integration.

Leyfer, O.T., Folstein, S.E., Bacalman, S., Davis, N.O., Dinh, E., Morgan, J., ... Lainhart, J.E. (2006) Comorbid psychiatric disorders in children with autism: Interview development and rates of disorders. *Journal of Autism Development Disorders, 36,* 849–861.

Levey, E.B., & Murphy, N.A. (2005). Addressing transition to adulthood with special needs patients. *AAP News, 26*(2), 19.

Liptak, G.S., Kennedy, J.A., & Dosa, N.P. (2010). Youth with spina bifida and transitions: Health and social participation in a nationally represented sample. *Journal of Pediatrics, 157*(4), 584–588.

McDonagh, J., & Viner, R. (2006). Lost in transition? Between paediatric and adult services. *British Medical Journal, 332,* 435–436.

McPherson, M., Weissman, G., Strickland, B.B., van Dyck, P.C., Blumberg, S.J., & Newacheck, P.W. (2004). Implementing community-based systems of services for children and youths with special health care needs: How well are we doing? *Pediatrics, 113*(5, Suppl.), 1538–1544.

Murphy, N. (2005) Sexuality in children and adolescents with disabilities. *Developmental Medicine and Child Neurology, 47*(9), 640–4.

Nehring, W.M. (Ed.). (2005). *Core curriculum for specializing in intellectual and developmental disability: A resource for nurses and other health care professionals.* Boston, MA: Jones and Bartlett Publishers.

Nota, L., Ferrari, L., Soresi, S., & Wehmeyer, M. (2007) Self-determination, social abilities and the quality of life of people with intellectual disability. *Journal of Intellectual Disabilities Research, 51*(11), 850–65.

O'Brien, J. & Lyle O'Brien, C. (1994). More than just a new address: Images of organization for supported living agencies. In V.J. Bradley, J.W. Ashbaugh, & B.C. Blaney (Eds.), *Creating individual supports for people with developmental disabilities* (pp. 109–140). Baltimore, MD: Paul H. Brookes Publishing Co.

Olmstead v. L.C., 527 U.S. 581 (1999).

Olsen, D.G., & Swigonski, N.L. (2004). Transition to adulthood: The important role of the pediatrician. *Pediatrics, 113,* e159–e162.

Peter, N.G., Forke, C.M., Ginsburg, K.R., & Schwarz, D.F. (2009) Transition from pediatric to adult care: Internists' perspectives. *Pediatrics, 123*(2), 417–423.

Peterson, C., Maier, S.F., & Seligman, M.E.P. (1995). *Learned helplessness: A theory for the age of personal control.* New York, NY: Oxford University Press

Picket, J.A., Paculdo, D.R., Shavelle, R.M., & Strauss, D.J. (2006). 1998–2002 update on causes of death in autism. *Journal of Autism and Developmental Disorders, 36,* 287–288.

Pilnick, A., Clegg, J., Murphy, E., & Almack, K. (2010). Questioning the answer: Questioning style, choice and self-determination in interactions with young people with intellectual disabilities. *Sociology of Health and Illnesses, 32*(3), 415–436.

Rehabilitation Act Amendments of 1986, PL 99-506, 29 U.S.C. §§ 701 *et seq.*

Rehabilitation Act Amendments of 1992, PL 102-569, 29 U.S.C. §§ 701 *et seq.*

Rehabilitation Act of 1973, PL 93-112, 29 U.S.C. §§ 701 *et seq.*

Reiss, J., & Gibson, R. (2002). Health care transition: Destinations unknown. *Pediatrics, 110*(6, Pt. 2), 1307–1314.

Reiss, J.G., Gibson, R.W., & Walker, L.R. (2005). Health care transition: Youth, family, and provider perspectives. *Pediatrics, 115*(1), 112–120.

Rimmer, J.H., Riley, B., Wang, E., Rauworth, A., & Jurkowski, J. (2004). Physical activity participation among persons with disabilities barriers and facilitators. *American Journal of Preventive Medicine 26*(5), 419–425.

Reiss, S., Levitan, G.W., & Szyszko, J. (1982). Emotional disturbance and mental retardation: Diagnostic overshadowing. *American Journal of Mental Deficiency, 86*(6), 567–574.

Rupp, K., Davies, P.S., Newcomb, C., Iams, H., Becker, C., Mulpuru, S., ... Miller, B. (2005-2006). A profile of children with disabilities receiving SSI: highlights from the National Survey of SSI Children and Families. *Social Security Bulletin 2005–2006, 66*(2), 21–48.

Rush, K.S., Bowman, L.G., Eidman, S.L., Toole, L.M., & Mortenson, B.P. (2004). Assessing psychopathology in individuals with developmental disabilities. *Behavior Modification, 28*(5), 621–637.

Ryan, R.M., & Deci, E.L. (2000). Self-determination theory and the facilitation of intrinsic motivation, social development, and well-being. *American Psychologist, 55*(1), 68–78.

Scal, P., & Ireland, M. (2005). Addressing transition to adult health care for adolescents with special health care needs. *Pediatrics, 115,* 1607–1612.

Shaw, P., Kabani, N.J., Lerch, J.P., Eckstrand, K., Lenroot, R., Gogtay, N., ... Wise, S.P. (2008) Neurodevelopmental trajectories of the human cerebral cortex. *Journal of Neuroscience, 28*(14), 3586–3594.

Shireman, T.I., Reichard, A., Nazir, N., Backes, J.M., & Greiner, K.A. (2010). Quality of diabetes care for adults with developmental disabilities. *Disability and Health Journal, 3*(3), 179–85.

School-to-Work Opportunities Act of 1994, PL 103239, 20 U.S.C. 6101 *et seq.*

Section 504 of the Rehabilitation Act, 29 U.S.C. § 794d.

Seekins, T., Enders, A., & Innes, B. (1999). *Ruralfacts: Centers for independent living, rural and urban distribution.* Missoula, MT: The University of Montana, The Research and Training Center on Rural Rehabilitation Services. Retrieved October 4, 2006, from http://rtc.ruralinstitute.umt.edu/IL/Ruralfacts/RuCILfacts.htm

Seltzer, M.M., & Krauss, M.W. (2001). Quality of life of adults with mental retardation/developmental disabilities who live with family. *Mental Retardation and Developmental Disabilities Research Reviews, 7,* 105–114.

Slayter, E.M., (2010). Demographic and clinical characteristics of people with intellectual disabilities with and without substance abuse disorders in a Medicaid population. *Intellectual Developmental Disabilities, 48*(6), 417–31.

Smith, L.S. (2009). *Overview of the Federal Higher Education Opportunity Act Reauthorization. Think College Insight Brief,* Issue No. 1. Boston, MA: Institute for

Community Inclusion, University of Massachusetts Boston. Retrieved March 26, 2011, from http://www.thinkcollege.net/component/docman/cat_view/23-policy-briefs .

Stancliffe, R.J., & Lakin, K.C. (2005). *Costs and outcomes of community services for people with intellectual disabilities*. Baltimore, MD: Paul H Brookes Publishing Co.

Strauss, D.J., Shavelle, R.M., Rosenbloom, L., & Brooks, J.C. (2008). Life expectancy in cerebral palsy: An update. *Developmental Medicine & Child Neurology, 50*, 487–493.

Tice, C.J., & Hall, D.M. (2008). Sexuality education and adolescents with developmental disabilities: Assessment, policy, and advocacy. *Journal of Social Work and Disabilities Rehabilitation, 7*(1), 47–62.

U.S. Department of Health and Human Services. (2010). *Healthy People 2020: Understanding and improving health* (2nd ed.). Washington, DC: U.S. Government Printing Office. Retrieved March 26, 2011, from http://www.healthypeople.gov/2020/default.aspx.

U.S. Department of Labor. (2005). *Work activity of high school students: Data from the National Longitudinal Survey of Youth 1997* (USDL reports: 05-732). Retrieved June 16, 2005, from http://www.bls.gov/nls/nlsy97r6 .pdf

U.S. Department of Labor, Office of Disability Employment Policy. (2009). *Customized employment: Applying practical solutions for employment success, Vol. II.*, retrieved March 27, 2011 from http://www.dol.gov/odep/pubs/publicat.htm

U.S.Department of Labor, Employment and Training Administration. (2005). *Map of state One-Stop websites*. Retrieved June 16, 2005, from http://www.doleta.gov/ usworkforce/onestop/onestopmap.cfm

United States Social Security Administration Annual Statistical Supplement. (2009). *Table 7.E2—Percentage distribution of federally administered awards, by sex, age, and eligibility category, 2009*. Retrieved March 20, 2011, from http://www.ssa.gov/policy/docs/statcomps/supplement/2010/7e.html

Van Naarden Braun, K., Yeargin-Allsopp, M., & Lollar, D. (2009). Activity limitations among young adults with developmental disabilities: A population-based follow-up study. *Research in Developmental Disabilities, 30*(1), 179–91.

von Schrader, S., Erickson, W.A., & Lee, C.G. (March 17, 2010). *Disability Statistics from the Current Population Survey (CPS)*. Ithaca, NY: Cornell University Rehabilitation Research and Training Center on Disability Demographics and Statistics (StatsRRTC). Retrieved March 27, 2011, from www.disabilitystatistics.org

Wehman, P., & Kregel, J. (1985). A supported work approach to competitive employment of individuals with moderate and severe handicaps. *Journal of The Association for Persons with Severe Handicaps, 10*(3), 132–136

Wehmann, P., & Mullaney-Wittig, K. (2009). *Transition IEPs: A curriculum guide for teachers and transition practitioners*, (3rd ed.). Ann Arbor, MI: Academic Therapy Press.

Wetherow, D., & Wetherow, F. (2004). *Microboards and microboard association design, development and implementation*. Available on the Internet at Community Works.org (http://www.communityworks.info/articles/microboard.htm)

Wolf-Branigin, M., Schuyler, V., White, P.H. (2007). Improving quality of life and career attitudes of youth with disabilities: Experience from the Adolescent Employment Readiness Center. *Research in Social Work Practicum, 17*(3), 324–333

Workforce Investment Act (WIA) of 1998, PL 105-220, 29 U.S.C. §§ 2801 *et seq.*

World Health Organization. (2001). *International Classification of Functioning, Disability and Health (ICF)*. Geneva, Switzerland: Author.

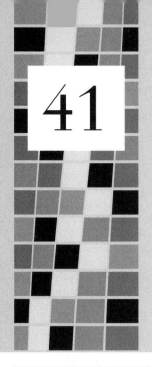

41

Health Care Delivery Systems and Financing Issues

Angelo P. Giardino and Renee M. Turchi

Upon completion of this chapter, the reader will

- Define the term *children and youth with special health care needs* and understand the impact of this diagnosis on health care delivery and financing issues

- Describe the complexity involved in developing a system that adequately coordinates various services and supports for these children

- Explain the importance of the medical home and care coordination in caring for children and youth with special health care needs

- Discuss trends in insurance coverage in the provision of health care to these children

- Describe how public health care programs and benefits contribute to these children and their families

The federal Maternal and Child Health Bureau (MCHB) defines children and youth with special health care needs (CYSHCN) as "those who have or are at increased risk for a chronic physical, developmental, behavioral or emotional condition and who also require health and related services of a type or amount beyond that required by children generally" (McPherson et al., 1998). Developing a clear definition of children and youth with special health care needs has fostered research investigating prevalence, quality of care, and health outcomes for this population. According to the nationally representative National Survey of Children with Special Health Care Needs (NS-CSHCN), conducted in 2005–2006, 14% of U.S. children and youth (birth through 17 years of age) have special

health care needs, and 22% of U.S. households with children include at least one child or youth with a special health care need (U.S. Department of Health and Human Services [USDHHS], 2007). The NS-CSHCN survey confirms that CYSHCN is a diverse group comprised of all races, ethnicities, ages, family incomes, and levels of functional abilities. Yet, not all children with developmental disabilities have special health care needs, and not all CYSHCN have developmental disabilities. For example, children with learning disabilities do not generally have special medical needs, and children with asthma, who do have special medical needs, do not generally have developmental disabilities. Therefore, the term CYSHCN includes both a subgroup of children with developmental disabilities (e.g., cerebral palsy, **meningomyelocele**) and a group of typically developing children with complex medical problems (e.g., hemophilia, diabetes, severe asthma; Davis et al., 2007). Understanding the similarities and differences between the groups informs clinical decision making, policy development, and resource allocation. However, each group shares similarities around health care structure, processes, policies, and outcomes. In addition, there is cohort of children that fall into both groups (having a developmental disability and complex medical problems). Table 41.1 lists the more common diagnoses found among the CYSHCN represented in the 2005–2006 NS-CHSCN.

Developing an effective health care system (which includes a medical home) for CYSHCN is the focus of this chapter. Optimal functioning of high performing, quality medical home and care coordination systems are paramount for CYSHCN. Several of the core features of this system, however, are important for all children. Yet, CYSHCN may require an array of services beyond the primary care doctor, including those provided by specialists, therapists, pharmacists,

educators, mental health providers, and home health providers (Wells et al., 2000). Table 41.2 lists specific health services utilized by the CYSHCN represented in the 2005–2006 NS-CSHCN.

An Institute of Medicine (IOM, 2001) report a decade ago suggested that the fragmentation of health care in the United States jeopardizes quality of care. In order to address this, all children, whether with a disability or typically developing, should be provided comprehensive health care that is coordinated and occurs within a "medical home" framework that is described more fully below. Recently, four medical organizations have issued a joint statement calling for the medical home principles to be extended to all primary care for children, youth, and adults throughout the United States. They refer to this care model as the patient-centered medical home (Joint Principles, 2007).

THE CONCEPT OF A MEDICAL HOME

To help families with care coordination and to improve care, the American Academy of Pediatrics (AAP; 1992) called for all children to have

Table 41.1. Percent of children with special health care needs with selected conditions

Health conditions	Percent
Allergies	53.0%
Asthma	38.8%
Attention deficit disorder/attention-deficit/hyperactivity disorder	29.8%
Depression, anxiety, or other emotional problems	21.1%
Migraine or frequent headaches	15.1%
Intellectual disability	11.4%
Autism or autism spectrum disorder	5.4%
Joint problems	4.3%
Seizure disorder	3.5%
Heart problems	3.5%
Blood problems	2.3%
Cerebral palsy	1.9%
Diabetes	1.6%
Down syndrome	1.0%
Muscular dystrophy	0.3%
Cystic fibrosis	0.3%

From U.S. Department of Health and Human Services, Health Resources and Services Administration, Maternal and Child Health Bureau. (2007). The National Survey of Children with Special Health Care Needs Chartbook 2005–2006 (p. 18). Rockville, MD: U.S. Department of Health and Human Services. p. 18. Retrieved from http://mchb.hrsa.gov/cshcn05/MI/NSCSHCN.pdf

Table 41.2. Percent of children with special health care needs needing specific health services

Specific health care needs	Percent
Prescription drugs	86.4%
Preventive dental care	81.1%
Routine preventive care	77.9%
Specialty care	51.8%
Eyeglasses/vision care	33.3%
Mental health care	25.0%
Other dental care	24.2%
Physical, occupational, or speech therapy	22.8%
Disposable medical supplies	18.6%
Durable medical equipment	11.4%
Hearing aids/hearing care	4.7%
Home health care	4.5%
Mobility aids/devices	4.4%
Substance abuse treatment	2.8%
Communication aids/devices	2.2%

From U.S. Department of Health and Human Services, Health Resources and Services Administration, Maternal and Child Health Bureau. (2007). The National Survey of Children with Special Health Care Needs Chartbook 2005–2006 (p. 25). Rockville, MD: U.S. Department of Health and Human Services. p. 25. Retrieved from http://mchb.hrsa.gov/cshcn05/MI/NSCSHCN.pdf

"a medical home that provides accessible, continuous, comprehensive, family-centered, coordinated, and compassionate health care in an atmosphere of mutual responsibility and trust among clinician, child, and caregiver(s)" (American Academy of Pediatrics Policy Statement, 2002; Johnson & Kastner, 2005). The AAP (2002) subsequently expanded the statement with a more comprehensive interpretation of the concept along with operational definitions of a medical home that would make recognizing care consistent with the medical home principles easier to identify. Table 41.3 describes the ideal medical home.

Effective primary care has long been recognized as a valuable component for all children

Table 41.3. Attributes of the ideal medical home

Attributes	Description
A medical home provides care that is accessible.	The family can obtain care in the community, and there are no barriers to receiving care based on race, ethnic, or cultural background; based on type of health insurance, including Medicaid and the Children's Health Insurance Program (CHIP); or based on lack of insurance coverage. When families are forced to change insurance because of employer decisions, the health care practice makes an effort to accommodate the change and maintain continuity of care.
The medical home is family centered.	Family members are recognized by the clinicians and staff as the principal caregivers and partners in caring for the child. Information is shared with parents in an unbiased, ongoing, and complete manner. All care plans reinforce the family as the center of support and decision makers for the child.
Care from a medical home is continuous.	Families and children value the ongoing relationship with primary care providers, subspecialty clinicians, and staff. The medical home provides continuity of care as the child and family make the transition from the hospital to the community and to child care, to school, or to home-based care. The continuity of care from infancy through young adulthood is the foundation of the medical home; it allows the clinician to know the family and patient and permits the family to trust the physician and his or her staff. This continuity shapes clinical judgment so that unnecessary tests are avoided and psychosocial factors can be weighed in decision making. The long-term relationship finally fosters the young adult and family to make a smooth transition to adult-based care with a new provider with support and information from the pediatrician or pediatric nurse practitioner.
Primary care medical homes provide care that is comprehensive.	Families can receive health care or advice 24 hours per day, 7 days per week. The child can receive preventive, acute, or chronic care within the scope and knowledge of the clinician. Because of the complexity of medical conditions today, many children require appropriate referral to subspecialists for management of acute and chronic conditions.
Medical homes coordinate care.	Not only are families assisted in contacting and utilizing appropriate support, educational services, and community-based services, but also the care provided in hospital, ambulatory, and community settings is planned and coordinated to the benefit of the family and child. Medical records, care plans, and other information are shared between providers and across systems avoiding duplication and fragmentation.
Medical homes are characterized by compassion.	The clinic- and office-based teams in the medical home demonstrate concern for the well-being of the child and family. This compassion is communicated by every member of the staff and felt by the family.
Care in the medical home also must be culturally competent.	The medical home must be able to deliver care in cross-cultural situations; therefore, the staff members must value diversity, be aware of how their own culture affects their thoughts and actions, understand the dynamics when cultures interact, and have a practicewide cultural education program that helps ensure culturally competent clinical care and service delivery.
Care delivered by the medical home is community-based.	Primary care is community-based. Although children and families with special health care needs often require care by subspecialists who may not be available in their own community, the medical home should be in the community where the family lives whenever possible. The staff and clinicians of the medical home coordinate and communicate with the subspecialists. In addition, other providers—including pediatric physical, occupational, speech, and feeding therapists; home nursing staff; and providers of other important services—should be available in the community or as close to home as possible.

Source: American Academy of Pediatrics (1992).

in the highly specialized, technology-dependent, tertiary care–based health care delivery system in the United States. Starfield (1992) defined primary care as health care that is first contact (involving an initial physician to whom the family goes to for routine and nonroutine care), community-based (accessible), longitudinal (continuous), coordinated, and comprehensive. In addition, primary care clinicians for children (e.g., community pediatricians, family physicians, nurse practitioners) provide preventive care such as well-child examinations; immunizations; and vision, hearing, developmental, and medical screenings. Primary care also includes personalized care that demonstrates the clinician's knowledge of the patient and family environment, including work, personal, emotional and, at times, financial concerns. For the child and family, often the primary care team's medical home coordinates care with the pediatric subspecialist(s), the school system, and community providers to ensure comprehensive care. In a few instances, the subspecialist assumes the majority of the responsibilities for the medical home. In some unusual cases, the specialist may also provide well-child care (e.g., for a child with cystic fibrosis who is receiving care at a comprehensive center run by a pulmonologist).

Looking across several measures, the NS-CSHN in 2005–2006 sought to characterize how many CYSHCN received care that could be characterized as consistent with medical home principles, namely "ongoing comprehensive, coordinated, family-centered care in the child's community" (USDHHS, 2007, 46). On average, 47% of CYSCHN received care that met all of the following criteria, defined as reflecting an effective medical home:

- The child/youth has a personal doctor or nurse as well as a usual source of sick and well-child care and has not had problems obtaining needed referrals.

- The family is satisfied with the doctors' communications with each other, the school, and other related systems and receives help coordinating the child's or youth's care when needed.

- The doctor spends enough time with the child/youth, listens carefully, and is sensitive to the family customs and provides enough information.

- The parents feel like a partner in the child's or youth's care and receive interpretation when needed.

IMPORTANCE OF COORDINATION OF CARE

Given the many services that may be needed and the number of providers and professionals potentially involved in coordinating the various health care services required by a CYSHCN, coordinating care is important for the child's family and health care providers. The child's needs are complex, and a great deal of time, energy, and skill are required to ensure that the different agencies, institutions, and professionals work effectively together in developing a comprehensive plan of care (AAP, 1998, 1999, 2005). Required services may include some that are not traditionally seen as health related such as education and housing. Care coordination can avoid both excessive services (e.g., unnecessary repeated imaging studies) and deficient services (e.g., failure to arrange for medications to be provided at school). When provided, care coordination services are readily accepted by families and minimize the burden of the child's medical condition (Palfry et al., 2004).

According to the NS-CSHCN in 2005–2006, 46% of parents of CYSCHN received coordinated care, 32% lacked one or more elements of coordinated care, and 22% felt they did not need coordinated care. In response to a question about their ability to get help in coordinating their child's care, 55% of parents did not report that they needed any help with care coordination, 30% reported that they needed help and usually got it, and 15% reported they needed help and did not get it (USDHHS, 2007). Care coordination can have a favorable impact on the family's experience. An analysis of the NS-CSHCN in 2005–2006 found that those children who received adequate care coordination had an increased chance of receiving family-centered care, experiencing partnerships with professionals and indicating satisfaction with services (Turchi et. al, 2009).

Care coordination can also result in cost savings and decreased hospital stays (Liptak et al., 1998; Palfrey et al., 2004). Despite this value in reducing health care costs, more than half of the time that a health care provider spends with CYSHCN may involve care coordination that is not reimbursed by insurance (Antonelli & Antonelli, 2004; Antonelli, Stille, & Antonelli, 2008). Even when care coordination is available, many services may not be located in convenient, community-based settings, thus further depleting the family's energy and resources.

In an attempt to deal with these issues, insurers, hospitals, and public and private agencies have developed case management programs. The purpose and scope of these programs, however, vary with agency type and often are not focused on the overall coordination of care. As an example, a hospital case management program generally deals with patients at one point in time (i.e., at discharge from a hospital stay) and does not address the patient's needs beyond that episode. Hospitals currently use case managers principally to provide information to payers and assist with discharge planning. In the era of health care reform, however, the case manager's job description may broaden in the context of an accountable care organization (ACO; Watson, 2011). Case managers working for insurers and managed care organizations (MCOs) typically focus more on benefits management and resource utilization and less on care coordination, although some Medicaid MCOs do organize and coordinate a broader package of benefits (Abt Associates, 2000). Many social agencies and public programs provide case management services as these are often mandated by public policy. Title V programs, which are state programs for CYSHCN that are funded via block grants from the MCHB, have a special mandate to monitor and provide care coordination, but programs vary from state to state (USDHHS, 2008).

Although Medicaid payment for case management may be allocated for a child, families may find that their case manager lacks necessary medical knowledge or does not communicate adequately with their child's clinicians. Many specialty programs in children's hospitals have nurse specialists who help coordinate the medical care. These specialty-based care coordinators may have comprehensive information about the particular disorder (e.g., diabetes) but may lack knowledge about community or primary care level resources and other aspects of comprehensive medical care. This points to the importance of providing care coordination at the community practice (medical home) level. One of the few estimates of the cost of providing care coordination services in a community-based practice suggested that although substantial, it is not cost prohibitive (Antonelli & Antonelli, 2004).

Does the increased cost of the coordinated care found in a medical home produce better outcomes? In one study, the answer appears to be "yes" (Cooley et al., 2009); it used a measure of determining the consistency between the medical home principles and the care delivered to CYSCHN, namely the Medical Home Index (MHI). The MHI is a quality improvement tool that captures 25 dimensions of being a medical home and organizes them into six domains: 1) organizational capacity, 2) chronic condition management, 3) care coordination, 4) community outreach, 5) data management, and 6) quality improvement that generates a standardized score. The higher the MHI score is, the more "medical home-like" is the care being delivered. In a study of MHI scores collected from 43 primary care practices from 7 health plans across 5 states, higher MHI scores and higher individual domain scores were associated with increased organizational capacity, care coordination, and chronic condition management, and with significantly fewer hospitalizations. Higher chronic condition management scores were also associated with fewer emergency department visits (Cooley et al., 2009).

CHANGES IN FINANCING HEALTH CARE FOR CYSHCN

There are several perspectives on what constitutes an optimal care system for CYSHCN. These are synthesized and listed in Table 41.4. For most of its history, the health care system in the United States utilized a fee-for-service model in which the health care provider received a payment for each unit of service rendered (MacLeod, 2001). The typical payment was based on a "usual and customary" charge for the service. This system was a **retrospective payment system**. Payment was made after the service was rendered; it typically focused on sick care; and there was little incentive to deliver preventive services. This approach was criticized because of its potential to encourage health care professionals to provide too many acute care services (i.e., overutilization). In response to skyrocketing costs, the U.S. health care system experienced a revolution in the later years of the 20th century, and it continues to evolve toward a **prospective**, or prepayment, approach. If structured correctly, the prospective approach would encourage "appropriate" utilization, be focused on well and preventive services, and avoid utilization of unnecessary services (Deal, Shiono, & Behrman, 1998; Wagner, 2001). This is a particular issue for CYSHCN, whose health care costs may be as high as three times that of children in the general population (Newacheck & Kim, 2005). Table 41.5 compares expenditures and utilization for health care services for CYSHCN with those for typically developing children.

Table 41.4. Components of an optimal care system for children with special health care needs

- Integration of primary and specialty care in a way that combines the expertise of the specialists with the breadth of perspective provided by a generalist
- Integration of medical care with home- and community-based services, effectively linking the person with visiting nurses, Meals on Wheels, transportation, respite care, housekeeping, educational, and housing services
- Integration of patient and family perspectives into the care process and planning, using patient-centered communication and a consumer-oriented focus to service delivery
- Emphasis on functional status and quality of life so systems are tracked to be accountable for their effectiveness
- Improved screening and risk assessment to identify children early, when specialized services developmentally have the most effect
- Individual and group health education targeted to improve self-care skills and appropriate use of health care services
- Flexible gatekeeping that allows children and families access to a variety of services on a limited basis without prior authorization
- Comprehensive case management moving beyond benefit management and achieving real case coordination
- Coordination with public health, education, and social services, including collaborative arrangements, to organize and provide services
- An understanding of the differences between adult and childhood disability and the need for managed care models to be flexible in meeting pediatric needs
- Access to a medical home
- Fair reimbursement that compensates physicians for the increased time and complexity associated with care coordination (sometimes referred to as risk-adjusted rates in capitated systems)
- Viable systems of monitoring the care delivered

Sources: American Academy of Pediatrics (1998); McManus and Fox (1996a, 1996b); Sandy and Gibson (1996).

One of the principal proposals of health care reform is the development of accountable care organizations (ACOs). An ACO is defined as "a group of physicians, other healthcare professionals hospitals, and other healthcare providers that accept a shared responsibility to deliver a broad set of medical services to a defined set of patients across the age spectrum and who are held accountable for the quality and cost of care provided through alignment of incentives" (Joint Principles Statement on ACOs, 2011). The ACO would be given annual funding on a per-capita basis for providing comprehensive care. In this shared-risk model, if the ACO does not need to expend all the money, it is permitted to keep a portion; however, if it spends more it must be responsible for the financial loss. The foundation of ACOs lies in the primary care medical home and if adopted, will drive the health care financial discussion in the next decade.

Insurance Coverage: Public and Private

Access and use of health care services is affected by insurance coverage, family income, and sociodemographic factors (Blumberg & Carle, 2009; Singh et al., 2009). Health insurance for all Americans younger than age 65 is primarily private or commercial insurance provided by employers. The number of workers receiving employer-provided insurance, however, continues to decline, with a resultant reduction in the number of children covered under such plans (Children's Defense Fund, 2004). Employer-sponsored health insurance coverage continues to decline in the present decade (Gould, 2011).

As employer-based insurance coverage for children declines, coverage from public forms of insurance tends to increase. If this increase occurs at a slower rate than the decrease in private insurance, it results in an expanding number of uninsured children.

To avoid the problem of uninsured children, the federal government has developed several publicly funded insurance programs that provide avenues for children to receive health care coverage. Table 41.6 lists each program. In 1965, Medicaid was launched. Medicaid is a jointly funded federal/state program that serves as a societal safety net for children who are inadequately covered by private insurance, who do not have private insurance, or who meet other eligibility criteria. It should be noted that coverage under Medicare, the other kind of public insurance, is uncommon in children except for those with end-stage kidney disease. In addition, Congress created the Children's Health Insurance Program (CHIP) in 1997 and reauthorized it in 2009. CHIP provides states with an incentive to extend health care coverage to uninsured children who do not qualify for traditional Medicaid (Deal & Shiono, 1998; Eskin & Ranji, 2009). Many states have CHIP programs (also called SCHIP) with coverage that deviates from that of Medicaid. One study concluded that CHIP coverage may not be sufficient to care for CYSHCN, suggesting that care coordination and reviewing of insurer's coverage decisions should be integrated into CHIP program design (Markus et al., 2006). Despite the availability of public coverage via Medicaid and CHIP, there are children who do not have adequate health insurance coverage

Table 41.5. Comparison of health care expenditures and utilization between children and youth with special health care needs and children without disabilities

Category	Children and youth with special health care needs	Children without disabilities	Comparison
Hospital days	464 days/1,000	55 days/1,000	8 times higher
Physician visits	4.6 visits/year	1.9 visits/year	2 times more visits
Nonphysician professional visits	3 visits/year	0.6 visits/year	5 times more visits
Prescriptions	6.2 medications/year	1.8 medications/year	3 times the number of prescriptions
Home health provider days	3.8 days/year	0.04 days/year	95 times more days
Health care expenditures	$2,669/year	$676/year	4 times the cost
Out-of-pocket expenditures	$297/year	$189/year	1.5 times the cost

Source: Newacheck, Inkelas, and Kim (2004).

Secondary data analysis of 1999 and 2000 Medical Expenditure Panel Survey, with total sample of 13,792 children younger than 18 years of age and overall response rate of 65.5%. All comparisons are statistically significant.

(Children's Defense Fund, 2004; Newacheck, Halfon, & Inkelas, 2000).

The federal and state governments provide several other avenues for CYSHCN and their families to gain access to a range of health care services and funding for these services. These include 1) the Social Security Administration's Supplemental Security Income (SSI) program, which provides income support and/or access to Medicaid; 2) the MCHB's Title V programs, which provide services (e.g., case management) beyond the covered Medicaid services; 3) and the Individuals with Disabilities Education Improvement Act of 2004 (IDEA 2004; PL 108-446), which links educational and health care needs with Medicaid funding. In practical terms, these programs may demonstrate considerable state-to-state variability in eligibility criteria, types of services covered or offered, and amount of care provided.

Private–public insurance coverage issues and programmatic variability further complicate the task of fashioning care plans for CYSHCN. Children and families experience this variability most acutely when navigating through and around a number of agencies, institutions, and providers, each with its own set of eligibility requirements, regulations, and service provisions that may or may not meet the child's needs. In addition, publicly funded programs are coming under increased scrutiny as legislative and budgetary debates focus on cost cutting efforts (Reichard, 2011; Smith, 2004; White et al., 2005).

The NS-CSHCN also assessed insurance coverage and found that during the 2005–2006 time period CYSCHN were more likely than children in the general population to have insurance coverage. Only 3.5% of CYSCHN were uninsured at the time of the survey, and only 8.8% had been uninsured at any time in the 12 months prior to the survey (USDHHS, 2007). This compares to a 2006 national overall estimate of 11.6% of children being uninsured in the United States (Children's Defense Fund, 2007).

The NS-CSHCN also assessed the type of insurance held by children with special needs and found that 59% had solely private insurance provided by an employer, union, or directly from an insurance company; 28% had solely public insurance; 7% had a combination of private and public insurance; 4% were uninsured; and 2% had various forms of comprehensive coverage (USDHHS, 2007). Comparing the 2005–2006 administration of the NS-CSHCN with a previous version done in 2001 demonstrates a decreasing trend for CYSHCN having private insurance. In fact, 65% had private insurance in 2001 versus 59% in 2006; and while 22% had public coverage in 2001, 28% had this coverage in 2006.

Additionally, while two thirds of parents of CYSHCN responded that their child's coverage was adequate, one third thought coverage was usually or always inadequate (USDHHS, 2007). The adequacy of insurance coverage varied as a function of the type of insurance. Parents of CYSCHN who had only public insurance were less likely to view the insurance as inadequate compared to parents who had both private and public insurance (USDHHS, 2007). In addition,

Table 41.6. Overview of assistance programs for children with special health care needs

Program	Description
Supplemental Security Income (SSI)	SSI provides benefits to low-income people who meet financial and other eligibility requirements. SSI qualifies children and adults (including those with disabilities) for Medicaid health care services in many states.
Medicaid	Medicaid provides low-income individuals access to health coverage. States are mandated to cover a core set of benefits (e.g., hospital; outpatient physician services; laboratory and x ray; basic home health services; and early and periodic screening, diagnosis, and treatment [EPSDT]). EPSDT requires states to cover all medically necessary services for children, even those optional for adults.
Children's Health Insurance Program (CHIP)	CHIP funds states to insure children from working families with incomes too high to qualify for Medicaid but too low to afford private health insurance.
Title V	Provides children with special health care needs and their families with family-centered, coordinated, and community-based services, such as case management or care coordination, transportation, home visiting, and health education. Also, Title V helps to provide wraparound services (individualized direct services designed to support a child in his or her home, school, and community) and provides rehabilitation services for individuals younger than 16 who are blind or who have disabilities and who receive SSI. Title V may also provide partial funding for categorical programs (e.g., for children with spina bifida, cerebral palsy, sickle-cell disease, hemophilia).
Individuals with Disabilities Education Improvement Act of 2004 (IDEA 2004; PL 108-446)	IDEA guarantees all students with disabilities ages 3–21 the right to a free appropriate public education in the least restrictive environment. It also provides federal funds to states and local school districts to help pay the costs of special education, including related services such as speech-language and physical therapy.

Sources: U.S. Department of Education, Office of Special Education Programs (2010); U.S. Department of Health and Human Services, Centers for Medicare & Medicaid Services (2010-a); U.S. Department of Health and Human Services, Centers for Medicare & Medicaid Services (2010-b); U.S. Department of Health and Human Services, Health Resources and Services Administration, Maternal and Child Health Bureau (2010); and U.S. Social Security Administration (n.d.).

the NS-CSHCN assessed the financial impact on families of having a child with CYSHCN. Eighteen percent of parents reported that their child's condition caused financial problems for the family. Twenty percent of parents reported more than $1,000 of out-of-pocket expenditures per year, and 24% percent of parents indicated that they had to cut back or quit work in order to provide care for the child or youth (USDHHS, 2007).

The findings in the literature regarding the impact of various health benefit design approaches on children in general and those with special health care needs in particular are equivocal (Mitchell & Gaskin, 2004; Szilagyi, 1998). While some plan designs can successfully reduce inpatient hospital bed days and emergency department usage, the impact on primary care in the outpatient setting and access to specialists is less clear. One persistent concern around serving CYSHCN is that managed care organizations (MCOs) may reduce access to specialty services, especially when they involve high-cost procedures (Szilagyi, 1998). In the 2005–2006 NS-CSHCN survey, 16% of

parents reported that their CYSHCN did not receive at least one needed specialty service in the previous year, and 6% responded that they did not receive two or more services. Of note, only 3% reported not receiving any specialty care (USDHHS, 2007).

Wagner (1998) has proposed a chronic care model, based on experience and existing literature focusing on patient–provider interactions; the model is believed to result in improved care to both adults with chronic illnesses and CYSHCN. The model underscores how favorable outcomes for patients, families, and practice teams ensue when the medical home works in partnership with community resources and policies. See Figure 41.1 for a graphic representation of Wagner's chronic care model. The characteristics of this care model include:

- Providing care in the context of a medical home

- Having processes and incentives to improve the care delivery system

- Having information technology and clinical decision support for clinicians

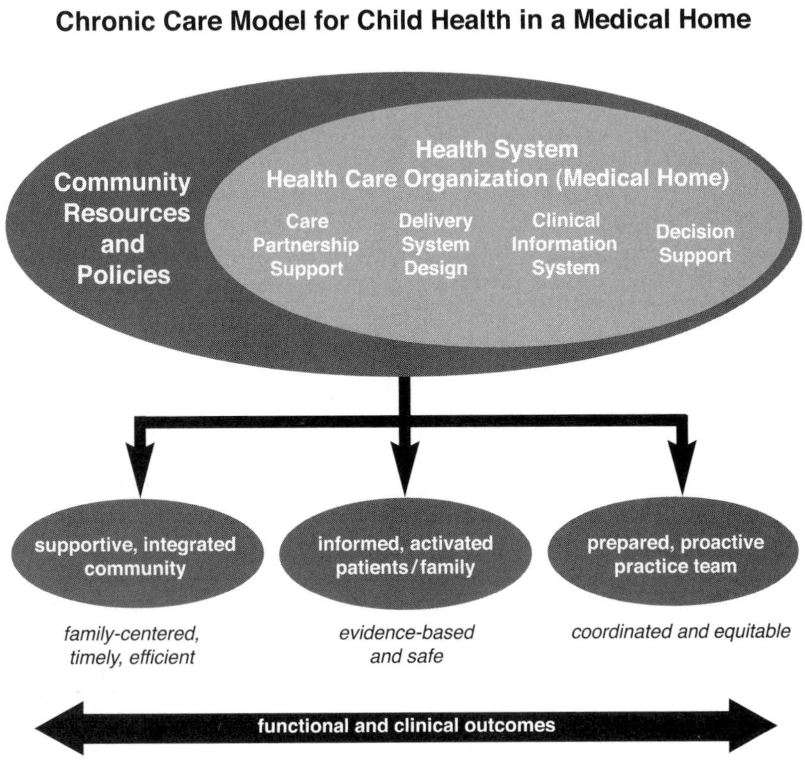

Chronic Care Model for Child Health in a Medical Home

Figure 41.1. A modification of the Wagner Chronic Care Model to reflect the unique aspects of of children with special health needs as defined by the National Initiative for Children's Healthcare Quality and to reflect the Institute of Medicine's quality of domain. (From Wagner, E.H. [1998], Chronic Disease Management: What Will It Take To Improve Care for Chronic Illness? *Effective Clinical Practice*, Aug/Sept 1998, Vol 1; adapted by permission.)

- Assuring a focus on effective self-management training and support
- Organizing team activities and practice systems around the unique needs of children, youth, and adults with chronic conditions
- Utilizing appropriate evidence-based guidelines in a measurable manner
- Fostering increased communication between primary care and specialty care providers
- Utilizing information systems in a way that produces disease registries, tracking systems and reminders about important care needs
- Providing care in the environment of a patient- and family-centered medical home

Beyond the chronic care model, additional innovations in health care delivery models have emerged over the last several years including ACOs, health insurances exchanges, and models for health care delivery. For example, Bodenheimer and Laing (2007) proposed the use of a "teamlet model" where the dyad of a practitioner and a medical assistant/health-care coach provides care collaboratively with patients to improve health-care delivery and quality.

The Centers for Medicare & Medicaid Services (CMS), which has federal oversight responsibility for Medicaid, has established a set of safeguards promoting attention to the unique aspects of caring for CYSHCN in a managed care environment. To deal with this issue, some states have conceived of "carveouts" for these children, in which the child is handled separately from the general population. CYSHCN also may be eligible for various Medicaid waivers, including 1) the Home and Community-Based Services Waiver (HCBS), sometimes referred to as a 1915(c) waiver, and 2) the Katie Beckett waiver (Peters, 2005). Both essentially waive (or permit exceptions to) certain federal requirements to provide home and community-based services as an alternative to institutionalization or continued hospitalization. Such waivers, for example, may permit a family with a CYSHCN to receive Medicaid in order to have health care services and support for keeping that child at home rather than in a hospital or chronic care facility. One advantage of the waivers is that family income may be exempted from consideration in determining eligibility for Medicaid. The waivers are state-run programs, however, so each state has different approaches to waivers with different eligibility requirements or services.

LOOKING TOWARD THE FUTURE

Measuring outcomes and demonstrating high quality results (e.g., pay-for-performance models) will become increasingly important in justifying the enhanced service delivery and higher costs for CYSHCN (Palfry et al., 2004). This will require rigorous collection of data on the health care services delivered and analysis of the data using increasingly sophisticated health services techniques.

The United States spent over $2.3 trillion dollars on health care in 2008 without improved outcomes compared to other countries that were spending fewer dollars for their population (CMS, 2011). Then, the year 2010 made history in the United States as The Patient Protection and Affordable Care Act (ACA) was signed by President Barack Obama. The recent health care debate and reform provides hope that health care transformation will continue for CYSHCN and will improve access and quality as well as reduce costs (Palfrey & Hall, 2010). States across the nation are operationalizing the Affordable Care Act in unique ways. Many models and ideas are being brought forth to ensure adequate coverage of children and adults, without compromising quality. Models such as ACOs, health insurance exchanges, and innovative infrastructure (e.g., teamlets, care

coordination) hold promise for the future of primary care. Innovations in how we deliver and measure health care quality are paramount to insure that all Americans have equal access to health care within a medical home.

Classically, the measurable dimensions of health care quality are the structure, the process, and the actual outcomes (Donabedian, 1980). Structure, from a quality and health services perspective, describes aspects of the health care system such as facilities, staffing patterns, and qualifications. Process in this context deals with the policies and procedures that govern aspects of care, such as technical and professional skills, documentation of care, safety practices, and the use of assessment tools. Finally, outcomes deal with the health status of the people served, their health-related knowledge and behavior, and their satisfaction with the care they receive (Monahan & Sykora, 1999). Table 41.7 lists the types of quality questions that can be answered when looking at structure, process, and outcomes, and Table 41.8 outlines potential problems with assessing outcomes. Related to quality improvement and outcomes measurement, the MHI, mentioned above, is a validated tool that offers a vehicle to measure six domains of a functioning medical home and provides a readily available framework from which to trend results (http://www.medicalhomeimprovement.org).

Table 41.7. Quality indicators in health care and the questions they address

Dimension	Indicators examined	Examples of questions
Structure	Facilities Equipment Conformance to standards Staffing patterns Personnel qualifications and experience Organizational structure descriptions Financing patterns	Are primary care and specialty care clinics and hospitals accessible? How is the service delivery system structured? Do clinicians providing care communicate with each other? Are the health care professionals well educated, well trained, and board certified? Are medical records well maintained?
Process	Technical and professional skill Documentation of care Safety practices Monitoring assessment tools	Was the blood test for lead done for a child at risk for lead poisoning? Was the child with asthma treated in the most up-to-date manner?
Outcome	Health status Health-related knowledge Health-related behavior Satisfaction with care	Did the patient get better? Was the impact of the disability reduced? Does a child with special health care needs have the highest level of functioning possible given what is known to be possible? If not, why not?

Source: Monahan & Sykora (1999).

Note: Not all outcomes are the result of purely clinical decision making. Clinicians need to acknowledge that parents of children with special health care needs and other consumers of health care also consider personal preferences and experience when making health care plan choices.

Table 41.8.   Potential problems with assessing outcomes

Self-limited conditions may improve or resolve on their own/even without therapy over time, so attributing the improvement to the treatment may be difficult.

Treatment of some chronic conditions is only partially effective and is not expected to be curative, so the presence of the condition cannot be used as a measure because the diagnosis does not change even though the treatment makes an improvement.

Lack of understanding of the natural history of some chronic conditions leads some authorities to disagree on what is expected and what the result of therapy should be.

External factors that may be involved in improvement, such as supportive family involvement and the responsiveness of community supports, are not easily measured but surely can have an impact on outcome.

Source: Monahan & Sykora (1999).

SUMMARY

Given the many services needed and the number of providers and professionals involved, coordinating health care services for CYSHCN presents a unique challenge to the child's family and health care providers. The complexity of the child's needs necessitate a great deal of time, energy, and skill to coordinate the efforts of different agencies, institutions, and professionals so that they work effectively together in a comprehensive plan of care. This coordination is particularly complex because of the labor-intensive nature of the comprehensive case management necessary and because the child's needs may span a range of services, including some that are not traditionally seen as health-related. Further complicating matters are the many federal and state agencies and programs involved in providing and funding services and the revolutionary changes currently occuring in the heath care marketplace. All of this points to the importance of each child having a medical home and effective case management to assist the family in navigating this system.

REFERENCES

Abt Associates, Inc. (2000, June). *Evaluation of the District of Columbia's demonstration program, "Managed Care System for Disabled and Special Needs Children": Final report summary.* Retrieved November 20, 2001, from http://aspe.hhs.gov/daltcp/reports/dc-frs.htm

American Academy of Family Physicians. (2011). *Joint Principles Statement of Accountable Care Organizations.* Retrieved July 7, 2011, from http://www.aafp. org/online/etc/medialib/aafp_org/documents/policy/private/healthplans/payment/acos/20101117. Par.0001.File.tmp/AAFP-ACO-Principles-2010.pdf.

American Academy of Pediatrics. (1992). American Academy of Pediatrics Ad Hoc Task Force on Definition of the Medical Home: The medical home (RE9262). *Pediatrics, 90,* 774.

American Academy of Pediatrics. (1998). Managed care and children with special health care needs: A subject review (RE9814). *Pediatrics, 102,* 657–660.

American Academy of Pediatrics. (1999). Care coordination: Integrating health and related systems of care for children with special health care needs (RE9902). *Pediatrics, 104,* 978–981.

American Academy of Pediatrics. (2002). Medical Home Initiatives for Children with Special Needs Project Advisory Committee: The medical home. *Pediatrics, 110,* 184–186.

American Academy of Pediatrics. (2005). Council on Children with Disabilities: Care coordination in the medical home: Integrating health and related systems of care for children with special health care needs. *Pediatrics, 116,* 1238–1244.

Antonelli, R.C., & Antonelli, D.M. (2004). Providing a medical home: The cost of care coordination services in a community-based general pediatric practice. *Pediatrics, 113*(5), 1522–1528.

Antonelli, R.C., Stille, C.J., & Antonelli, D.M. (2008). Care coordination for children and youth with special health care needs: A descriptive, multisite study of activities, personnel costs, and outcomes. *Pediatrics, 122,* e209–e216.

Bodenheimer, T., & Laing, B.Y. (2007). The teamlet model of primary care. *Annals of Family Medicine, 5,* 457–61,

Blumberg, S.J., & Carle, A.C. (2009). The well-being of the health care environment for CSHCN and their families: A latent variable approach. *Pediatrics, 124*(4), S361–7.

Center for Medical Home Improvement.CMHI. http://www.medicalhomeimprovement.org/index.html

Centers for Medicare and Medicaid Services, Office of the Actuary, National Health Statistics Group. (2011). *National Health Care expenditure Data.* Retrieved from www.cms.gov/NationalHealthExpendData.

Children's Defense Fund. (2004). *CDF calls on country to insure all children during "cover the uninsured week."* Washington, DC: Children's Defense Fund.

Children's Defense Fund. (2007). *In harm's way: True stories of uninsured texas children.* Available at http://www.childrensdefense.org/child-research-data-publications/data/in-harms-way-true-stories-of-uninsured-texas-children.pdf

Cooley, W.C., McAllister, J.W., Sherrieb, K., & Kuhlthau, K. (2009). Improved outcomes associated with medical home implementation in pediatric primary care. *Pediatrics 124*(1), 358–364. doi:10.1542/peds.2008–2600

Davis, M.M., & Brosco, J.P. (2007). Being specific about being special: Defining children's conditions and special health care needs. *Archives of Pediatrics and Adolescent Medicine, 161*(10), 1003–1005.

Deal, L.W., & Shiono, P.H. (1998). Medicaid managed care and children: An overview. *The Future of Children, 8*(2), 93–104.

Donabedian, A. (1980). *The definition of quality and approaches to its assessment.* Ann Arbor, MI: Health Administration Press.

Eskin, R., & Ranji, U. (2009). Children's Coverage and SCHIP Reauthorization. *The Henry J. Kaiser Family Foundation. Health Policy Explained*. Retrieved from http://www.kaiseredu.org/Issue-Modules/Childrens-Coverage-and-SCHIP-Reauthorization/Background-Brief.aspx

Gould, E. (2011). *2010 marks another year of decline for employer-sponsored health insurance coverage*. Retrieved from http://www.epi.org/publication/2010-marks-year-decline-employer-sponsored/

Individuals with Disabilities Education Act (IDEA) of 1990, PL 101-476, 20 U.S.C. §§ 1400 *et seq.*

Individuals with Disabilities Education Improvement Act of 2004, PL 108-446, 20 U.S.C. §§ 1400 *et seq.*

Institute of Medicine. (2001). *Crossing the quality chasm: A new health system for the 21st century*. Washington, DC: National Academies Press.

Johnson, C.P., & Kastner, T.A. (2005). Helping families raise children with special health care needs at home. *Pediatrics 115*(2), 507–511.

Joint Principles of the Patient-Centered Medical Home. (February, 2007). Retrieved from www.pcpcc.net/content/joint-principles-patient-centered-medical-home.

Liptak, G.S., Burns, C.M., & Davidson, P.W., & McAnarney, E.R. (1998). Effects of providing comprehensive ambulatory services to children with chronic conditions. *Archives Pediatrics and Adolescent Medicine, 152*, 1003–1008.

MacLeod, G.K. (2001). An overview of managed health care. In P.R. Kongstvedt (Ed.), *The managed health care handbook* (4th ed., pp. 3–16). Gaithersburg, MD: Aspen Publishers.

Markus, A., Rosenbaum, S., Stein, R.E., & Joseph, J. (2006). *From SCHIP benefit design to individual coverage decisions* (Policy brief #6). Washington, DC: The George Washington University Department of Health Policy.

McManus, M.A., & Fox, H.B. (1996a). Enhancing preventive and primary care. *Managed Care Quarterly, 4*(3), 19–29.

McManus, M.A., & Fox, H.B. (1996b). Enhancing preventive and primary care for children with chronic or disabling conditions served in health maintenance organizations. In P.D. Fox & T. Fama (Eds.), *Managed care and chronic illness: Challenges and opportunities* (pp. 197–112). Gaithersburg, MD: Aspen Publishers.

McPherson, M., Arango, P., Fox, H., Lauver, C., McManus, M., Newacheck, P.W., … Strickland, B. (1998). A new definition of children with special needs. *Pediatrics, 102*, 137–140.

Mitchell, J.M., & Gaskin, D.J. (2004). Do children receiving Supplemental Security Income who are enrolled in Medicaid fare better under fee-for-service or comprehensive capitation model? *Pediatrics, 114*(1), 196–204.

Monahan, C.A., & Sykora, J. (1999). *Developing and analyzing performance measures: A guide for assessing quality care for children with special health care needs*. Vienna, VA: National Maternal and Child Health Clearinghouse.

National Initiative for Children's Healthcare Quality (NICHQ). Medical Home Index. Chronic Care Model for Child Health in a Medical Home. http://www.nichq.org/resources/medical_home_toolkit.html

Newacheck, P.W., Halfon, N., & Inkelas, M. (2000). Commentary: Monitoring expanded health insurance for children: Challenges and opportunities. *Pediatrics, 105*, 1004–1005.

Newacheck, P.W., Inkelas, M., & Kim, S.E. (2004). Health services use and health care expenditures for children with disabilities. *Pediatrics, 114*(1), 79–85.

Newacheck, P.W., & Kim, S.E. (2005). A national profile of health care utilization and expenditures for children with special health care needs. *Pediatrics, 159*(1), 10–17.

Palfrey J.S., & Hall, R. (2010). Health care reform: The doorway to health care transformation. *Pediatrics, 126*(2), 374–5.

Palfry, J.S., Sofis, L.A., Davidson, E.J., Liu, J., Freeman, L., Ganz, M.L., & Pediatric Alliance for Coordinated Care. (2004). The pediatric alliance for coordinated care: Evaluation of a medical home model. *Pediatrics, 113*(5), 1507–1516.

Peters, C.P. (2005). *National Health Policy Forum, The George Washington University. Children with Special Care Needs: Minding the Gaps. Background Paper*. Retrieved from http://www.nhpf.org/library/background-papers/BP_CSHCN_06-27-05.pdf

Reichard, J. (2011). *Washington Health Policy Week in Review: Medicaid Discussions Heat Up as Funding Pressures Grow. The Commonwealth Fund*. Retrieved from http://www.commonwealthfund.org/Newsletters/Washington-Health-Policy-in-Review/2011/Jun/June-20-2011/Medicaid-Discussions-Heat-Up.aspx?view=print&page=all

Sandy, L.G., & Gibson, R. (1996). Managed care and chronic care: Challenges and opportunities. In P.D. Fox & T. Fama (Eds.), *Managed care and chronic illness: Challenges and opportunities* (pp. 8–17). Gaithersburg, MD: Aspen Publishers.

Smith, V. (2004, October). *The continuing Medicaid budget challenge: State Medicaid spending growth and cost containment in fiscal years 2004 and 2005*. Washington, DC: Kaiser Commission on Medicaid and the Uninsured.

Starfield, B. (1992). *Primary care: Concept, evaluation and policy*. New York, NY: Oxford University Press.

Singh, G.K., Strickland, B.B., Ghandour, R.M., & van Dyck, P.C. (2009). Geographic disparities in access to the medical home among U.S. CSHCN. *Pediatrics, 124*(4), S352-60.

Szilagyi, P.G. (1998). Managed care for children: Effect on access to care and utilization of health services. *The Future of Children 8*(2), 39–59.

U.S. Department of Education, Office of Special Education Programs. (2010). *IDEA*. Retrieved from http://idea.ed.gov/explore/home

U.S. Department of Health and Human Services. (2008). State MCH-Medicaid Coordination: A Review of Title V and Title XIX Interagency Agreements, (2nd ed). *Chapter One. Overview of Title V and Title XIX*. Retrieved from http://mchb.hrsa.gov/IAA/overview.htm

U.S. Department of Health and Human Services, Centers for Medicare & Medicaid Services. (2010a). *Children's Health Insurance Programs*. Retrieved from http://www.cms.gov/home/chip.asp

U.S. Department of Health and Human Services, Centers for Medicare & Medicaid Services. (2010b). *Medicaid*. Retrieved from http://www.cms.gov/home/medicaid.asp

U.S. Department of Health and Human Services, Health Resources and Services Administration, Maternal and Child Health Bureau. (2007). *The National Survey of Children with Special Health Care Needs Chartbook 2005–2006*. Rockville, Maryland: U.S. Department of Health and Human Services.

Retrieved from http://mchb.hrsa.gov/cshcn05/MI/NSCSHCN.pdf

U.S. Department of Health and Human Services, Health Resources and Services Administration, Maternal and Child Health Bureau. (2010). *Title V Block Grant to States.* Retrieved from http://mchb.hrsa.gov/programs/

U.S. Social Security Administration. (n.d.) *Supplemental Security Income (SSI).* Retrieved from http://www.ssa.gov/ssi

Turchi, R.M., Berhane, Z., Bethell, C., Pomponio, A., Antonelli, R., & Minkovitz, C.S. (2009). Care coordination for CSHCN: Associations with family-provider relations and family/child outcomes. *Pediatrics, 124*(4), S428–34.

Wagner, E.H. (1998). Chronic disease management: What will it take to improve care for chronic illness? *Effective Clinical Practice, 1,* 2–4.

Watson, A.C. (2011). Finding common ground in case management. *Professional Case Management,* March/April, 52–54.

Wagner, E.R. (2001). Types of managed care organizations. In P.R. Kongstvedt (Ed.), *The managed health care handbook* (4th ed., pp. 28–41). Gaithersburg, MD: Aspen Publishers.

Wells, N., Knauss, M.W., & Anderson, B. (2000). *What do families say about health care for children with special health care needs? Your voice counts!! The Family Partners Project report to families.* Unpublished manuscript, Family at the Federation for Children with Special Needs, Boston.

White, C., Fisher, C., Mendelson, D., & Schulman, K.A. (2005). *State Medicaid disease management: Lessons learned from Florida.* Lambertville, NJ: The Health Strategies Consultancy LLC, in collaboration with Duke University.

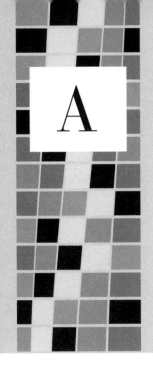

A Glossary

Arlene Gendron

AAC *See* augmentative and alternate communication.

ABA *See* applied behavior analysis.

abducens nerve The sixth nerve; controls the lateral resctus eye muscle.

abduction Moving part of the body away from one's mid-line.

ABR *See* auditory brainstem response.

abruptio placenta Premature detachment of a normally situated placenta; *also called* placental abruption.

abscesses Localized collections of pus in cavities caused by the disintegration of tissue, usually the result of bacterial infections.

accommodation 1) In special education, a change in how a student gains access to the curriculum or demonstrates his or her learning. This approach does not substantially alter the content or level of instruction (e.g., allowing a student additional time to take a test); 2) the change in the shape of the lens of the eye that allows it to focus on objects at varying distances.

acetabulum The cup-shaped cavity of the hip bone that holds the head of the femur in place, creating a joint.

acetylcholine A neurotransmitter for cholinergic neurons that innervate many tissues, including smooth muscle and skeletal muscle.

acid–base balance In metabolism, the ratio of acidic to basic compounds (or pH).

acidosis Abnormally high levels of acid in the bloodstream. The normal pH is 7.42; acidosis is generally less than pH 7.30.

acquired immunodeficiency syndrome (AIDS) Severe immune deficiency disease caused by human immunodeficiency virus (HIV).

actin Protein involved in muscle contraction.

acute inflammatory peripheral neuropathy The most common form is Guillain-Barre syndrome. It involves an ascending paralysis, with weakness beginning in the feet and hands and migrating towards the trunk. It can cause life-threatening complications, particularly if the breathing muscles are affected or if there is dysfunction of the autonomic nervous system. The disease is usually triggered by an acute infection.

adaptive technology Substitutes or makes up for the loss of function brought on by a disability (e.g., software that permits voice production through a computer for an individual who cannot speak).

adduction Moving a body part, usually a limb, toward the mid-line.

adenine One of the four nucleotides (chemicals) that comprise DNA.

adenoid Lymphatic tissue located behind the nasal passages.

adenoidectomy The surgical removal of the adenoids.

adenoma sebaceum Benign cutaneous growths, usually seen around the nose, that resemble acne; these occur in individuals with tuberous sclerosis (*see Appendix B*).

adenotonsillectomy Surgical removal of adenoids and tonsils.

adjustment disorders A group of psychiatric disorders, usually of childhood, associated with difficulty adjusting to life changes.

adrenaline A potent stimulant of the autonomic nervous system. It increases blood pressure and heart rate and stimulates other physiological changes needed for a "fight or flight" response.

advance directives In children with severe disabilities or diseases, the term is used to define the level of intervention a parent wants provided in the event of life-threatening emergency or illness in the child.

AED *See* automated external defibrillator.

afferent Pertaining to the neural signals sent from the peripheral nervous system to the central nervous system (CNS). Sensory fibers carry signals from muscles, skin, and joints back to the brain.

AFO *See* ankle-foot orthosis.

AFP *See* alpha-fetoprotein.

afterbirth *See* placenta.

agenesis of the corpus callosum Absence of the band of white matter that normally connects the two hemispheres of the brain.

agonist A muscle that works in concert with another muscle to produce movement.

agyria Absence of the normal convolutions on the surface of the brain.

AIDS *See* acquired immunodeficiency syndrome.

alcohol-related neurodevelopmental disorder (ARND) *Previously called* fetal alcohol effects (FAE); refers to the range of neurological and developmental impairments that can affect a child who has been exposed *in utero* to alcohol. The most severe of these effects is fetal alcohol syndrome.

alleles Alternate forms of a gene that may exist at the same site on the chromosome.

alopecia The partial or complete absence of hair from areas of the body where it normally grows.

alpha-fetoprotein (AFP) Fetal protein found in amniotic fluid and serum of pregnant women. Its measurement is used to test for meningomyelocele and Down syndrome in the fetus and is a chemical typically found in the fetal spinal fluid, brain, and spinal cord.

alternative technology *See* adaptive technology.

alveoli Small air sacs in the lungs. Carbon dioxide and oxygen are exchanged through their walls.

amalgam An alloy of mercury and silver used in dental fillings.

amaurosis Blindness.

amblyopia Partial loss of sight resulting from disuse atrophy of neural circuitry during a critical period of development, most often associated with untreated strabismus in children.

amino acid Building block of protein needed for normal growth.

amino acid disorders Inborn errors of metabolism resulting from an enzyme deficiency involving amino acids, the building blocks of protein.

amniocentesis A prenatal diagnostic procedure performed in the second trimester in which amniotic fluid is removed by a needle inserted through the abdominal wall and into the uterine cavity.

amniotic fluid Clear fluid that surrounds the fetus during pregnancy, acting as a physical buffer for fetal movements and physical development. It is formed by fetal urine production and lung fluid secretion during fetal respirations.

amygdala A part of the brain involved in sensory procession and emotions.

anaphase The stage in cell division (mitosis and meiosis) when the chromosomes move from the center of the nucleus toward the poles of the cell.

anaphylaxis A life-threatening hypersensitivity response to a medication or food, marked by breathing difficulty, hives, and shock.

anemia Disorder in which the blood has either too few red blood cells or too little hemoglobin.

anencephaly Neural tube defect (NTD) in which either the entire brain or all but the most primitive regions of the brain are missing.

ankle-foot orthosis (AFO) The AFO stabilizes the position of the foot and provides a consistent stretch to the Achilles tendon.

anophthalmia Congenital absence of the eye globes.

anorexia A severe loss of appetite.

anotia Congenital absence of the external ear (auricle).

antagonists Muscles that work at cross-purposes (e.g., the adductor and abductor muscles of the hip oppose each others' actions).

antecedents Events or contextual factors that precede the manifestation of a behavior.

anterior The front part of a structure.

anterior chamber The space between the cornea and lens of the eye.

anterior fontanelle The membrane-covered area on the top of the head; *also called* the "soft spot." It generally closes by 18 months of age.

anterior horn cells Cells in the spinal column that transmit impulses from the pyramidal tract to the peripheral nervous system.

anthropometrics Measurements of the body and its parts.

antibody A protein formed in the bloodstream to fight infection.

anticholingeric medications A group of medications that acts by antagonizing the effects of the neurotransmitter acetylcholine.

anticipation A term used in genetics to denote an expansion in triplet repeats from one generation to the next, leading to a more severe manifestation of the disease (e.g., in fragile X syndrome).

anticonvulsants Medications used for control of seizures.

antidepressants Medications used to control major depression.

antigen A substance that, when introduced into the body, triggers the production of an antibody by the immune system, which will then kill or neutralize the antigen that is recognized as a foreign and potentially harmful invader.

antihistamine A drug that counteracts the effects of histamines, substances involved in allergic reactions.

antipsychotic medications Medications used to treat psychosis; the atypical antipsychotics have also been found to be useful in treating aggression and self-injury in children with severe intellectual disability.

antipyretics Medications used to treat fever.

antiretroviral agents (ARVs) A category of medications used to treat retroviral infections (i.e., HIV/AIDS).

anuria In chronic renal (kidney) failure, the absence of urine production.

anxiety disorders Psychiatric disorders characterized by feelings of anxiety. The disorders include panic attacks, separation anxiety, obsessive-compulsive disorder (OCD), and posttraumatic stress disorder (PTSD).

aorta The major artery, originating in the left ventricle of the heart and supplying oxygenated blood to the body and brain.

Apgar scoring system Scoring system developed by Virginia Apgar to assess neurological status in the newborn infant. Scores range from 0 to 10.

aphasia A class of language disorder that ranges from having difficulty remembering words to being completely unable to speak, read, or write due to damage to the brain.

apical At the tip of a structure.

apnea A lack of spontaneous breathing effort; brief breathing arrests.

apneic Pertaining to an episodic arrest of breathing.

apoptosis Programmed cell death.

applied behavior analysis (ABA) A treatment method, commonly used in autism, that uses behavioral learning theory to change behavior.

apraxia The inability to perform coordinated movements or manipulate objects in the absence of a motor or sensory impairment.

aqueous humor The watery fluid in the eyeball that fills the anterior chamber (the space between the lens and the cornea).

architectonic dysplasias Developmental malformations affecting the neuronal architecture of the brain.

areflexia Lack of deep tendon reflexes.

ARND *See* alcohol-related neurodevelopmental disorder.

arterial blood gas A laboratory profile test of sampled arterial blood, including pH, PaO_2, and $PaCO_2$.

arterial-venous malformation (AVM) Birth defect of blood vessels, most commonly in the brain, that can be associated with a disastrous postthrombotic hemorrhage.

arthritis An inflammatory disease of joints.

articular Referring to the surface of a bone at a joint space.

articulation 1) The formulation of individual speech sounds; 2) the connection at a joint.

ARVs *See* antiretroviral agents.

ASDs *See* autism spectrum disorders.

asphyxia Interference with oxygenation of the blood that leads to loss of consciousness and possible brain damage.

aspiration Inhalation of a foreign body, usually a food particle, into the lungs.

aspiration pneumonia Inflammation of the lung(s) caused by inhaling a foreign body, such as food, into the lungs; an infection by the aspiration of food into the lung.

asplenia Nonfunctioning spleen.

assent Agreement to research or treatment, given by a child or minor who is too young to give legally valid informed consent.

assistive devices Any device used to assist in a body function (e.g., a wheelchair).

assistive technology Technology (often software) to improve communication, movement, independence, and so forth.

astigmatism A condition of unequal curvature of the cornea that leads to blurred vision.

astrocytes   Support cells in the central nervous system (CNS) that help form the white matter.

asymmetrical tonic neck reflex (ATNR)   A primitive reflex, *also called* the fencer's response, found in infants; usually is no longer evident by 3 months of age. When the neck is turned in one direction, the arm shoots out on the same side and flexes on the opposite side; similar changes occur in the legs.

ataxia   An unbalanced gait or movement of any part of the body caused by a disturbance of cerebellar control. Movements are jerky and uncoordinated, without the smooth flow of normal motion.

ataxic   Erratic and uncoordinated voluntary movement.

ataxic cerebral palsy   A form of dyskinetic cerebral palsy in which the prominent feature is ataxia; characterized by abnormalities of voluntary movement involving balance and position of the trunk and limbs in space (ataxia). Ataxic cerebral palsy may be associated with increased (spastic) or decreased (hypotonic) muscle tone.

athetoid cerebral palsy   A form of dyskinetic cerebral palsy associated with athetosis.

athetosis   Constant random, slow, writhing involuntary movements of the limbs.

atlantoaxial instability (AAI)   Excessive movement at the junction between the atlas (C1) and axis (C2) bones in the upper spine as a result of either a bony or ligamentous abnormality. This is a common finding in Down syndrome.

atlantoaxial subluxation   Partial dislocation of the upper spine, a particular risk in Down syndrome.

ATNR   *See* asymmetrical tonic neck reflex.

atonic   Pertaining to the absence of normal muscle tone.

atopic dermatitis   Eczema.

atresia   Congenital absence of a normal body opening; often occurs with microtia and refers to the absence of the opening to the external ear canal.

atria   The two upper chambers of the heart.

atrial septal defect   A congenital heart defect in which where there is lack of closure of the wall separating the two upper chambers of the heart.

attention-deficit/hyperactivity disorder (ADHD)   A developmental disorder characterized by impulsivity, hyperactivity, and inattention to a degree that leads to impairment in functioning.

audiometry   A hearing test using a device called an audiometer that yields results in the form of a graph showing hearing levels in sound intensity at various wavelengths of sound presented through earphones.

auditory agnosia   Inability to distinguish different sounds in the presence of normal hearing.

auditory brainstem response (ABR)   A test of central nervous system (CNS) hearing pathways.

augmentative and alternative communication (AAC)   Devices that assist individuals who lack the ability to speak (e.g., a microchip-powered voice output augmentative device for a person with dysarthria).

augmentative devices   Devices used to increase an area of functioning that is deficient, sometimes severely, but for which there are some residual abilities.

aura   A sensation, usually visual and/or olfactory, marking the onset of a seizure.

auricle   The outer ear.

autism spectrum disorders (ASDs)   A group of related developmental disabilities including autistic disorder (or autism), Asperger's Disorder, and pervasive developmental disorder-not otherwise specified.

autoimmune   Pertaining to a reaction in which one's immune system attacks other parts of the body.

automated external defibrillator (AED)   Portable electronic device that automatically diagnoses the potentially life-threatening cardiac arrhythmias of ventricular fibrillation and ventricular tachycardia in a patient and can provide an electrical impulse to correct the arrhythmia.

automatic movement reactions   *See* postural reactions.

automatic reinforcement   A behavior that produces internal consequences that can reinforce and thus produce functional relationships that maintain the problem behavior.

automatisms   Automatic fine motor movements (e.g., unbuttoning one's clothing) that are part of a seizure.

autonomic   Describing the part of the nervous system that regulates certain automatic functions of the body (i.e., heart rate, sweating, and bowel movement).

autonomic nervous system   Controls involuntary activities of the cardiovascular, digestive, endocrine, urinary, respiratory, and reproductive systems.

autonomy The ability and/or right to be self-determining, an important concept in participating in human trials research.

autosomal dominant Mendelian inheritance pattern in which a single copy of a gene (from either mother or father) leads to expression of the trait.

autosomal recessive Mendelian inheritance pattern in which identical copies of a gene from both mother and father are required to result in the expression of a trait.

autosomes The first 22 pairs of chromosomes. All chromosomes are autosomes except for the two sex chromosomes.

avascular necrosis Destruction of bone from microvascular occlusion.

aversive Pertaining to a stimulus, often unpleasant, that decreases the likelihood a particular response will subsequently occur.

AVM *See* arterial-venous malformation.

axon A long, slender projection of a nerve cell, or neuron, that conducts electrical impulses away from the neuron's cell body.

babinski sign Upgoing toe when the sole of the foot is stroked firmly.

backward chaining Method of teaching a task in which the instructor begins by teaching the last step in a sequence because this step is most likely to be associated with a potent positive reinforcer.

bacteremia Spread of a bacterial organism throughout the bloodstream.

banding In genetics, pertaining to a series of dark and light bars that appear on chromosomes after they are stained. Each chromosome has a distinct banding pattern.

barotrauma Injury related to excess pressure, especially to the lungs or ears.

basal 1) Near the base; 2) relating to a standard or reference point (e.g., basal metabolic rate).

basal ganglia Brain structure at the base of the cerebral hemispheres involved in motor control, cognition, emotions, and learning.

baseline In behavior management, the frequency, duration, and intensity of a behavior prior to intervention.

behavior Refers to any action that one person can perform and that another person can observe.

beriberi Disease caused by a deficiency of the vitamin B1 (thiamin) and manifested as edema, heart problems, and peripheral neuropathy.

beta-blockers Medications (e.g., propranolol) that were initially used to control high blood pressure and have subsequently been found also to be useful in treating tremor migraine headache.

binocular vision The focusing of both eyes on an object to provide a stereoscopic image.

biotin One of the B-complex vitamins needed to activate a number of important enzymatic reactions in the body.

bipolar disorder A psychiatric disorder manifested by cycles of mania and depression; *previously called* manic-depression.

blastocyst The embryonic group of cells that exists at the time of implantation.

blepharitis Inflammation of the eyelids.

blood PaO$_2$ A measurement of the partial pressure of arterial oxygen (i.e., the amount of oxygen in the blood).

blood pH Blood acidity normally around 7.40.

blood poisoning *See* sepsis.

body mass index (BMI) A measurement of the relative percentages of fat and muscle mass in the human body, in which weight in kilograms is divided by height in meters and the result used as an index of obesity.

bolus 1) A small rounded mass of food made ready by tongue and jaw movement for swallowing; 2) a single dose of a large amount of medication given to rapidly attain a therapeutic drug level.

botulinum toxin (Botox) The neurotoxin that produces botulism (food poisoning). Neurotoxin used in the treatment of neuromuscular disorders such as rigidity and spasticity.

botulism Poisoning by botulin toxin and manifested as muscle weakness or paralysis.

BPD *See* bronchopulmonary dysplasia.

brachial plexus Network of nerve fibers, running from the spine through the neck, the axilla (armpit region), and into the arm.

brachialis A muscle in the upper arm.

brachycephaly Tall head shape with flat back part of the skull.

bradycardia Abnormal slowing of the heart rate, usually to fewer than 60 beats per minute.

braille A system of writing and printing for people who are blind or severely visually impaired.

brainstem The primitive portion of the brain that lies between the cerebrum and the spinal cord.

branchial arches A series of arch-like thickenings of the body wall in the pharyngeal region of the embryo.

bronchopulmonary dysplasia (BPD) A chronic lung disorder that occurs in a minority of premature infants who previously had respiratory distress syndrome. It is associated with "stiff" lungs that do not permit adequate exchange of oxygen and carbon dioxide, frequently leads to dependence on ventilator assistance for extended periods, and markedly increases the risk for the child developing asthma in the future.

bronchospasm Acute constriction of the bronchial tube, most commonly associated with asthma.

bruxism Repetitive grinding of the teeth.

bulging fontanel Bulging soft spot on the crown of the head.

bulk Foodstuffs that increase the quantity of intestinal contents and stimulate regular bowel movements. Fruits, vegetables, and other foods containing fiber provide bulk in the diet.

caffeine A central nervous system (CNS) stimulant found in coffee, tea, and cola.

calcify To become hardened through the laying down of calcium salts.

calculus An abnormal collection of mineral salts on the tooth, predisposing it to decay; *also called* tartar; when plaque becomes calcified.

callus A disorganized network of bone tissue that forms around the edges of a fracture during the healing process.

camptodactyly Deformity of fingers or toes in which they are permanently flexed.

cancellous Referring to the lattice-like structure in long bones (e.g., the femur).

cardiomegaly Enlarged heart.

cardiopulmonary resuscitation (CPR) An emergency procedure involving manual pumping of the chest combined with rescue breathing which is performed in an effort to preserve intact brain function until further measures are taken to restore spontaneous blood circulation and breathing in a person in cardiac arrest.

cardiorespiratory arrest Slowing or stopping of breathing and/or heart rate.

cardiorespiratory monitor A device used to monitor heart and respiratory rate.

case control study An observational epidemiologic study of people with a specific disease (or other outcome) of interest and a suitable control (e.g., comparison, reference) group of people without the disease.

catalyze To stimulate a chemical reaction via a compound that is not used up.

cataracts Clouding of the lenses of the eyes.

catheterization Use of a tube to infuse or remove fluids.

caudal Posterior pole of the developing embryo.

caudal regression syndrome Defects that may occur during embryonic life that can result in major malformations of the lower vertebrae, pelvis, and spine.

caudate nucleus Located within the basal ganglia, it is an important part of the brain's learning and memory system.

CBF *See* cerebral blood flow.

cecostomy Surgical formation of a permanent artificial opening into the cecum, the end of the colon.

celiac disease Congenital malabsorption syndrome that leads to the inability to gain weight and the passage of loose, foul-smelling stools. It is caused by intolerance of cereal products that contain gluten (e.g., wheat). Affected individuals should avoid wheat and other grains.

central hypoventilation Shallow breathing leading to low oxygen level resulting from disordered cerebral control of respiration.

central nervous system (CNS) The portion of the nervous system that consists of the brain and spinal cord. It is primarily involved in voluntary movement and thought processes.

central venous line A catheter that is advanced through a peripheral vein to a position directly above the opening to the right atrium of the heart. It is used to infuse long-term medication and/or nutrition.

centrioles Tiny organelles that migrate to the opposite poles of a cell during cell division and align the spindles.

centromere The constricted area of the chromosome that usually marks the point of attachment of the sister chromatids to the spindle during cell division.

cephalocaudal From head to tail; refers to neurological development that proceeds from the head downward.

cephalohematoma A swelling of the head resulting from bleeding of scalp veins. Often found in newborn infants, it is usually not harmful.

cerebellum A cauliflower-shaped brain structure located just above the brainstem beneath the occipital lobes at the base of the skull that is principally involved in muscle tone and coordination of movement.

cerebral blood flow (CBF) Poorly autoregulated blood flow within the early developing brain, making the newborn particularly vulnerable to any changes in blood pressure.

cerebellar cognitive affective syndrome A syndrome associated with cerebellar injury that includes impairment of executive functions such as planning, set-shifting, verbal fluency, abstract reasoning and working memory; difficulties with spatial congnition including visual-spatial organization and memory; personality change with blunting of affect or disinhibited and inappropriate bahavior.

cerebral contusion A bruise on the cerebrum.

cerebral hemisphere Either of the two halves of brain substance.

cerebral palsy A disorder of movement and posture due to a nonprogressive defect of the immature brain.

cerebral vascular accident (CVA) A thrombotic (clot) or hemorrhagic (bleed) stroke that can damage large regions of the brain in the location of a particular blood vessel (artery or vein).

cerebrospinal fluid (CSF) Clear, watery fluid that fills the ventricular cavities within the brain and circulates around the brain and spinal cord.

cerumen Ear wax.

cervical Pertaining 1) to the cervix, or 2) to the neck.

cesarean section (C-section) A surgical operation for delivering a baby through incising the uterus.

CHARGE syndrome A syndrome defined by Colaboma of the eye, Heart defects, Atresia of the choanae, Retardation of growth and/or development, Genital and/or urinary abnormalities, and Ear abnormalities and deafness. These children may have significant vision and hearing impairments.

cheilitis An inflammation of the lips.

chelation therapy The use of an oral, intravenous, or topical medication to remove metal from the body, most commonly used in lead poisoning.

chemotaxis The phenomenon in which cells direct their movements according to certain chemicals in their environment. This is critical to early development (e.g., movement of sperm towards the egg during fertilization) and subsequent phases of development (e.g., migration of neurons or lymphocytes) as well as in normal function.

chemotherapy Drugs used to treat cancer.

chest physiotherapy (CPT) A general term referring to treatments generally performed by respiratory therapists to improve breathing by the indirect removal of mucus from the breathing passages.

Chiari type II malformation An abnormality, wherein the brain stem and part of the cerebellum are displaced downward toward the neck, rather than remaining within the skull.

cholelethiasis Gall stones.

CI *See* cochlear implant.

circle of support A group of volunteer advocates, such as family members, friends, and neighbors, who make sure that an individual with a developmental disability has a support system that meets all of his or her needs.

choanal atresia Congenital closure of the nasal passage; part of the CHARGE association.

cholelithiasis Gall stones.

cholesteatoma A complication of otitis media in which skin cells from the ear canal migrate through the perforated eardrum into the middle ear, or mastoid region, forming a mass that must be removed surgically.

chorea A disorder marked by involuntary jerky movements of the extremities.

choreoathetosis Movement disorder, characteristic of dyskinetic cerebral palsy, involving frequent involuntary spasms of the limbs; when chorea and athetosis are seen together.

chorioamnionitis An infection of the amniotic sac that surrounds and contains the fetus and amniotic fluid.

chorion The outermost covering of the membrane surrounding the fetus.

chorionic villi Tiny projections that sprout from the chorion to give a maximum area of contact with the maternal blood. Embryonic blood is carried to the villi by the branches of the umbilical arteries, and after circulating through the capillaries of the villi, is returned to the embryo by the umbilical veins. The villi are part of the border between maternal and fetal blood during pregnancy.

chorionic villus sampling (CVS) A prenatal diagnostic procedure done in the first trimester of pregnancy to obtain fetal cells for genetic analysis; minute biopsy of the chorion.

chorioretinitis An inflammation of the retina and choroid that produces severe visual loss.

choroid The middle layer of the eyeball between the sclera and the retina.

choroid plexus Cells that line the walls of the ventricles of the brain and produce cerebrospinal fluid.

chromatids Term given to chromosomes during cell division.

chromosomes Threadlike strands of DNA and associated proteins in the nucleus of cells that carry the genes transmitting hereditary information.

ciliary body Located behind the iris, this structure allows drainage out of the eye in the angle where the cornea meets the iris through a spongelike meshwork to Schlemm's canal.

ciliary muscles Small muscles that affect the shape of the lens of the eye, permitting accommodation.

CK *See* creatine kinase.

cleft Term used in reference to a congenital deformity of the lip or palette.

clonus Alternate muscle contraction and relaxation in rapid succession.

clubfoot A congenital foot deformity; *also called* talipes equinovarus.

CMV *See* cytomegalovirus.

CNS *See* central nervous system.

coagulation Blood clotting.

coarctation A congenital narrowing, such as of a blood vessel, most commonly of the aorta.

cochlea The snail-shaped structure in the inner ear containing the hearing organ.

cochlear implant (CI) A device surgically implanted in the cochlea of the ear that permits a form of hearing in individuals with deafness.

codons Triplets of nucleotides that form the DNA code for specific amino acids.

cognitive strategy instruction (CSI) CSI teaches metacognitive strategies (thinking about thinking) to improve learning and performance. It is beneficial when teaching more complex material involving problem solving and decision making.

cognitive-behavioral therapy (CBT) A type of psychotherapy that focuses on feelings about behavior.

cohort study An epidemiologic study of subgroups of a population identified with some common characteristic (e.g., an exposure, an ethnic background) that are followed or traced over a period of time for the occurrence of disease.

colic A condition in infancy marked by uncontrollable crying usually caused by abdominal discomfort and often the result of gastroesophageal reflux (GER).

coloboma Congenital cleft in the retina, iris, or other ocular structure.

comorbid A coexisting condition that worsens an underlying disorder.

competent Legally recognized to be able to make decisions for oneself. Minors are presumed to be incompetent, except under certain specified conditions that may vary from state to state.

competing stimuli Stimuli that displace the problem behavior, such as providing food or mouthing toys to children that display pica (eating of nonfood items).

competitive employment Individuals with disabilities must have the same skills requisite for any employee to succeed in the workplace: knowledge base for the job, appropriate social skills, effective communication skills, and motivation. Individuals with disabilities also must have appropriate independent living skills and the skills and abilities to manage their disability-related needs, such as hiring and managing personal care attendants and transportation services.

complete learning trials Refers to an opportunity to respond that is controlled by the trainer.

compliance training An important prerequisite to instructional training. The instructor orients the child to attend to the instructor and then issues a developmentally appropriate "do" request.

computed tomography (CT) An imaging technique in which x-ray "slices" of a structure are viewed and synthesized by a computer, forming an image. CT scans are less clear than magnetic resonance imaging (MRI) scans but are better at localizing certain tumors and areas of calcification.

concave Having a curved, indented surface.

concussion A clinical syndrome caused by a blow to the head, characterized by transient loss of consciousness.

conductive In reference to hearing the conduction and amplification of sound through the middle ear.

cones Photoreceptor cells of the eye associated with color vision.

congenital Originating prior to birth.

congenital myopathies A group of inherited muscle disorders often associated with mitochondrial dysfunction.

conjunctiva The mucous membrane that lines the inner surface of the eyelid and the exposed surface of the eyeball.

consanguinity Familial relationship, such as the marriage of first cousins.

conscience A personal sense, generally intuitive and urgent, of the way one should respond under specific circumstances.

consequences Events or contextual factors that occur subsequent to a behavior and may or may not be causally related to it.

conservatorship A circumstance in which the court declares an individual unable to take care of legal matters and appoints another individual (a conservator) to handle these matters on the individual's behalf.

contiguous gene syndrome A genetic syndrome resulting from defects in a number of adjacent genes.

contingent stimulation Applying punishment following the occurrence of a misbehavior.

contingent withdrawal The removal of access to positive reinforcement following a misbehavior.

continuous positive airway pressure (CPAP) Involves providing a mixture of oxygen and air under continuous pressure; this prevents the alveoli from collapsing between breaths.

continuum A spectrum.

contracture A shortening of muscle fibers and soft tissue around a joint that causes decreased mobility and is almost always irreversible.

contralateral Opposite side.

contusion (of brain) Structural damage limited to the surface layer of the brain caused by trauma.

convex Having a curved, elevated/protruding surface, such as a dome.

cooperative learning An instructional method that includes a range of team-based learning strategies.

copy number variability (CNV) When the number of copies of a particular gene varies from one individual to the next.

cordocentesis *See* percutaneous umbilical blood sampling (PUBS).

cornea The clear dome that covers and protects the iris of the eye.

corpus callosotomy Surgical procedure in which the corpus callosum is cut to prevent the generalized spread of seizures from one hemisphere to another.

corpus callosum The bridge of white matter connecting the two cerebral hemispheres and permitting the exchange of information between the two hemispheres.

cortex The surface of the cerebral hemisphere, composed principally of neurons and glia.

cortical Pertaining to the cortex or gray matter of the brain.

cortical visual impairemt Visual impairment caused by damage to the part of the brain related to vision. Although the eye is normal, the brain cannot properly process the information it receives. The degree of vision loss may be mild or severe and can vary greatly, even from day to day.

corticospinal pathways White matter pathways leading from the brain through the spinal corticospinal tract; *see* pyramidal tract.

cortisol A steroid.

CPR *See* cardiopulmonary resuscitation.

CPT *See* chest physiotherapy.

cranial sutures Fibrous material connecting skull bones.

craniofacial Relating to the skull and bones of the face.

craniosynostosis Premature closure of cranial bones.

creatinine Product produced by muscle tissue and normally filtered from the blood by the kidney.

creatine kinase (CK) An enzyme released by damaged muscle cells. Its level is elevated in muscular dystrophy.

crib death *See* sudden infant death syndrome (SIDS).

Crohn's disease An inflammatory bowel disorder.

crossover The exchange of genetic material between two closely aligned chromosomes during the first meiotic division.

cryotherapy The use of freezing temperatures to destroy tissue.

cryptorchidism Undescended testicles.

C-section *See* cesarean section.

CSF *See* cerebrospinal fluid.

CT *See* computed tomography.

customized employment A blend of services designed to increase employment options for individuals with significant disabilities such as self-employment, entrepreneurship, job carving and restructuring, personal agents, and customized training.

CVA *See* cerebral vascular accident.

CVS *See* chorionic villus sampling.

cystic fibrosis An autosomal recessively inherited disorder of the secretory glands leading to malabsorption and lung disease.

cystometrogram (urodynamics) A procedure in which fluid is injected into the bladder and pressure is measured.

cytomegalovirus (CMV) A virus that may be asymptomatic or cause symptoms in adults that may resemble mononucleosis. In the fetus, it can lead to severe malformations similar to congenital rubella.

cytoplasm The contents of the cell outside the nucleus.

cytosine One of the four nucleotides (chemicals) that comprise DNA.

DAI *See* diffuse axonal injury.

dB *See* decibel.

DDH *See* developmental dislocation of the hip.

debridement The removal of dead tissue (e.g., after a burn or an infection).

decibel (dB) A measure of loudness used in hearing testing.

decubitus ulcers Bed sores.

delay Refers simply to a slower than expected rate in the acquisition of skills, usually defined with reference to widely accepted developmental milestones.

deletion Loss of genetic material from a chromosome.

delirium An organically based psychosis characterized by impaired attention, disorganized thinking, altered and fluctuating levels of consciousness, and memory impairment. It may be caused by encephalitis, diabetes, or intoxication and is usually reversed by treating the underlying medical problem.

delusions False beliefs, often quite bizarre, that are symptoms of psychosis or drug intoxication.

dementia A progressive neurological disorder marked by the loss of memory, decreased speech, impairment in abstract thinking and judgment, other disturbances of higher cortical function, and personality change (e.g., Alzheimer's disease).

dental caries Tooth decay.

dental lamina A thickened band of tissue along the future dental arches in the human embryo.

dental organ The embryonic tissue that is the precursor of the tooth; *also called* tooth bud.

dental plaque Patches of bacteria, bacterial byproducts, and food particles on teeth that predispose them to decay.

dental sealant Plastic substance administered to teeth, most commonly the molars, to increase their resistance to decay; consists of a plastic coating that is bonded to the chewing surface of molars to prevent decay.

dentin The principal substance of the tooth surrounding the tooth pulp and covered by the enamel.

deoxyribonucleic acid (DNA) The fundamental component of living tissue. It contains an organism's genetic code.

depolarization The eliminating of the electrical charge of a cell.

depolarizing current An electrical current causing a change in cell membrane voltage.

depressed fracture Fracture of bone, usually the skull, that results in an inward displacement of the bone at the point of impact. It requires surgical intervention to prevent damage to underlying tissue.

deprivation In behavior management, denial of access to a reinforcing item or event.

dermal sinus A cavity lining extending from the skin surface to a deeper structure, most notably the spinal cord.

descriptive analysis Involves the quantitative, direct observation of the individual's behaviors as well as antecedent events and consequences under naturalistic conditions.

descriptive and functional analysis Observation period in behavior management that precedes treatment.

detoxification The conversion of a toxic compound to a nontoxic product.

developmental cerebeller cognitive affective syndrome A syndrome described in children who survive prematurity-related cerebellar injury and have deficits range from impaired executive function to serve behavioral disturbances that fall into the autism spectrum.

developmental delay Refers to a significant lag in the attainment of milestones in one or more areas of development.

developmental deviance Refers to nonsequential unevenness in the achievement of milestones within one or more streams of development.

developmental disabilities A group of chronic conditions that are attributable to an impairment in physical, cognitive, speech/language, psychological, or self-care areas and that are manifested during the developmental period (younger than 21 years of age).

developmental dislocation of the hip (DDH) A congenital hip dislocation, usually evident at birth, occurring more commonly in girls.

developmental dissociation Refers to a significant difference in developmental rates between two areas.

developmental regression Loss of previously attained milestones.

deviate *See* diverge.

dextrose A simple sugar similar to glucose and used to medically correct or prevent low blood sugar.

diagnostic test A test used to definitively confirm or exclude the presence of a disease or condition in a particular individual.

dialysis A detoxification procedure of the blood (i.e., hemodialysis) or across the peritoneum (i.e., peritoneal dialysis) used to treat kidney failure.

diaphysis The shaft of a long bone lying under the epiphysis.

diastematomyelia A congenital defect in which the spinal cord is divided into halves by a bony or cartilaginous divider, often seen in spina bifida.

diencephalon A part of the forebrain.

differential reinforcement A behavior management technique in which a preferred alternate behavior is positively reinforced while a less preferred behavior is ignored.

differential reinforcement of alternative behaviors (DRA) When the delivery of the reinforcer is contingent on the performance of alternative, more appropriate behaviors.

differential reinforcement of other behaviors (DRO) Consists of the delivery of reinforcers (e.g., attention) contingent on the absence of problem behaviors.

diffuse axonal injury (DAI) Diffuse injury to nerve cell components, usually resulting from shearing forces. This type of traumatic brain injury is commonly associated with motor vehicle accidents.

diffusion-weighted imaging (DWI) A new form of magnetic resonance imaging (MRI) scanning that can identify with great sensitivity areas of brain, especially white matter, that have suffered an acute injury.

diopters Units of refractive power of a lens.

diplegia A form of spastic cerebral palsy, most often found in former premature babies, in which the legs are predominantly affected.

diploid Having paired chromosomes in nondividing cells (i.e., 46 chromosomes in 23 pairs).

diplopia Double vision.

direct instruction (DI) A codified approach to teacher-led instruction that provides explicit instruction with teacher modeling, extensive practice through choral response, brisk pacing, and immediate corrective feedback. The DI technique is very successful for teaching fundamental reading skills, and building reading fluency and reading comprehension.

disability Refers to a decrement in the ability to perform some action, engage in some activity, or participate in some real-life situation or setting.

discrepancy model In education this is often called the "wait to fail" model. As the child ages, they will fall far enough behind to have a significant difference between their ability (IQ) and their achievement.

dislocation The displacement of a bone out of a joint space.

disorders of carbohydrate metabolism Inborn errors of metabolism involving enzyme deficiencies in the breakdown of sugars.

dissociation A child may demonstrate an uneven pattern of skills, such that in some areas progress is fairly typical, whereas in other areas the child demonstrates a significant departure (delay or deviation) from the expected course.

distal Involving muscles or body segments farther from the center of the body.

distension Constipation.

diuretics Medications used to reduce intercellular fluid buildup in the body (edema), especially in the lungs.

diverge A child demonstrates functional or behavioral characteristics that are not typical for any child at any age.

diving reflex Named for its presence in diving seals, this also occurs in infants during hypoxic ischemic encepolopathy (HIE) and results in the redistribution of blood away from "nonvital organs" (e.g., kidneys, liver, lungs, intestines, and skeletal muscles) to preserve the perfusion of the "vital organs" (i.e., heart, brain, and adrenal glands). This reflex, if prolonged, may result in insufficient blood supply and damage to the nonvital organs.

DMD *See* Duchenne muscular dystrophy.

DNA *See* deoxyribonucleic acid.

DNR *See* do not resuscitate.

do not resuscitate (DNR) Medical orders that state that, should a patient develop a cardiopulmonary arrest, no attempts at resuscitation would be undertaken; *also called* "No Code" orders.

dominant In genetics, referring to a trait that only requires one copy of a gene to be expressed phenotypically. For example, having brown eyes is a dominant trait, so a child receiving a gene for brown eyes from his or her mother or father (or from both parents) will have brown eyes.

dopamine A neurotransmitter involved in attention deficits (e.g., attention-deficit/hyperactivity disorder [ADHD]) and motor function (e.g., Parkinson's disease).

dorsal Back.

dorsal induction Describes the processes of primary and secondary neurulation during embryogenesis.

dorsiflexion Upward movement of the foot.

dorsolateral Involving both the back and side of a body part.

double effect Principle of a moral argument used to defend certain actions that can be anticipated to have both good and bad outcomes.

double helix The coiled structure of DNA; a structure that resembles a twisted ladder.

dual diagnosis Intellectual disability and psychiatric disorder.

dual discrepancy model The student *both* performs below the level evidenced by classroom peers as well as shows a learning rate substantially below that of classroom peers.

Duchenne muscular dystrophy (DMD) *See Appendix B.*

ductus arteriosus An arterial connection open during fetal life that diverts the blood flow from the pulmonary artery into the aorta, thereby bypassing the not-yet-functional lungs.

ductus venosus Open during fetal life, it is a shunt that allows oxygenated blood from the placenta to bypass the liver and return to the systemic circulation for distribution to the rest of the body.

duodenal atresia Congenital absence of a portion of the first section of the small intestine; often seen in individuals with Down syndrome.

duodenum The first part of the small intestine; the upper part of the small intestine.

DWI *See* diffusion-weighted imaging.

dynamic In the context of orthotics, capable of active movement.

dysarthria Difficulty with speech due to impairment of oral motor structures or musculature.

dyscalculia Learning disability affecting skills in mathematics.

dyscontrol syndrome Intermittent explosive disorder out of proportion to the event that provokes it.

dysgraphia Learning disability in areas of processing and reporting information in written form.

dyskinesia An impairment in the ability to control movements characterized by spasmodic or repetitive motions

dyskinetic cerebral palsy Type of "extrapyramidal" cerebral palsy often involving abnormalities of the basal ganglia and manifesting as rigidity, dystonia, or choreoathetosis.

dyslexia Learning disability affecting reading skills, which commonly causes the reader to see a word's letters in reverse order.

dysmorphic Unusual facial appearance as a result of a genetic disorder.

dysmotility Abnormal motility of the gut.

dysostosis An abnormal bony formation.

dysphagia Difficulty in swallowing.

dysphasia Impairment of speech consisting of a lack of coordination and failure to arrange words in proper order due to a central brain lesion.

dysplasia Abnormal tissue development.

dyspraxia Inability to perform coordinated movements despite normal function of the central and peripheral nervous systems and muscles.

dysthymia A mild form of depression characterized by a mood disturbance that is present most of the time and is associated with feelings of low self-esteem, hopelessness, poor concentration, low energy, and changes in sleep and appetite; seen most commonly in adolescents.

dystocia Structural abnormalities of the uterus that cause a difficult labor or childbirth.

dystonia A disorder of the basal ganglia associated with altered muscle tone leading to contorted body positioning.

dystonic cerebral palsy A form of dyskinetic cerebral palsy, the most prominent feature of which is dystonia.

E. coli *See Escherichia coli.*

Eagle Barrett syndrome Formerly "prune belly syndrome."

ECG *See* electrocardiogram.

echocardiography An ultrasonic method of imaging the heart. It can be used to detect congenital heart defects even prior to birth

echolalic Pertaining to immediate or delayed repetition of a word or phrase said by others; often evident in children with autism spectrum disorders.

ECMO *See* extracorporeal membrane oxygenation.

ecological systems model Can be used to understand the interactive nature of family existence within *microsystem, mesosystem, exosystem,* and *macrosystem.*

ectoderm Outer cell layer in the embryo.

ectodermal dysplasia Abnormal skin development.

ectopias Congenital displacement of a body organ or tissue.

ectopic pregnancy Embryo implanted outside of the uterus.

ectrodactyly Congenital absence of all or parts of digits.

eczema A common skin condition, often occurring in childhood, marked by an itchy inflammatory reaction manifested by tiny blisters with reddening, swelling, bumps, and crusting; *also called* atopic dermatitis.

EDC *See* estimated date of confinement.

EDD Estimated due date; *also called* estimated date of confinement.

edema An abnormal accumulation of fluid in the tissues of the body.

EEG *See* electroencephalogram.

efferent Pertaining to the impulses that go to a nerve or muscle from the central nervous system (CNS); for example motor fibers transmit impulses from the brain to initiate movement.

effusion   A middle-ear infection associated with fluid accumulation.

Ehlers Danlos syndrome   *See Appendix B.*

EKG   *See electrocardiogram.*

ELBW   *See extremely low birth weight.*

electrocardiogram (EKG, ECG)   The graphic record of an electronic recording of heart rate and rhythm.

electroencephalogram (EEG)   A recording of the electrical activity in the brain that is often used in the evaluation of seizures.

electrolytes   Minerals contained in the blood, such as sodium, potassium, chloride.

electromyography (EMG)   A technique for measuring muscle activity and function; recording of electric currents associated with muscle contractions are useful in the diagnosis of a variety of neuromuscular disorders, including anterior horn cell disease, neuropathies, neuromuscular junction disorders, and some myopathies.

electroretinogram (ERG)   A graphic record of the electrical activity of the retina.

elixir   Hydroalcoholic liquid intended for oral use.

eloquent cortex   The area of the cortex involved in the production of speech.

emancipated minor   A teenage minor who is legally free of parental control for giving informed consent to any medical treatment.

embryo   The earliest stage of conceptional development after fertilization and during the first 8 weeks of pregnancy. The placenta and most of the primitive organs are formed into the major systems during this time.

embryotic period   The first 8 weeks of pregnancy.

EMG   *See electromyography.*

enamel   The calcified outer layer of the tooth.

encephalitis   Inflammation of the brain, generally from a viral infection.

encephalocele   A malformation of the skull that allows a portion of the brain, which is usually malformed, to protrude; a neural tube defect characterized by a sac-like protrusion of the brain and the membranes that cover it through an opening in the skull. This defect is caused by failure of the neural tube to close completely during fetal development.

encephalopathy   Disorder or disease of the brain.

enclaves   Once considered a viable employment option for individuals with severe disabilities; it brings together groups of individuals with disabilities at one site with a common job coach engaged around a work task.

endocardial cushion defect   A congenital heart defect, found often in Down syndrome, where there is a lack of closure of the wall separating the two sides of the heart.

endocarditis   Inflammation of the inner lining of the heart.

endochondral ossification   Formation of bone from cartilage.

endoderm   The inner cell layer in the embryo.

enriched environments   A type of treatment that focuses on providing stimuli that compete with problem behaviors.

enteral nutrition   Feeding directly into the stomach through the nose or mouth to ensure that nutritional requirements are met.

enteric nervous system   The subdivision of the autonomic nervous system that controls the gastrointestinal system.

enterobacter   A rod-shaped bacteria that can cause gastrointestinal symptoms.

enuresis   Incontinence.

ependomomas   Tumors developing from cells that line both the hollow cavities-ventricles of the brain and the canal containing the spinal cord.

ephiphysis   Growth area in long bones.

epicanthal folds   Crescent-shaped fold of skin on either side of the nose, commonly associated with Down syndrome.

epidemiology   The study of the distribution and determinants of disease frequency in specific populations.

epidural anesthesia   Pain relief by infusing an anesthetic agent into the epidural space of the spine.

epidural hematoma   Localized collection of clotted blood lying between the skull and the outer (dural) membrane of the brain, resulting from the hemorrhage of a blood vessel resting in the dura. This most often results from traumatic head injury.

epigenetics   Changes in gene expression that do not permanently alter the DNA sequence.

epiglottis   A lid-like structure that hangs over the entrance to the windpipe and prevents aspiration of food or liquid into the lungs during swallowing.

epilepsy   A disorder of the brain characterized by repeated seizures and by the neurobiologic, cognitive, psychological, and social consequences of this condition.

epiphyses   The end plates of long bones where linear growth occurs.

epithelial Pertaining to cells that are found on exposed surfaces of the body, (e.g., skin, mucous membranes, intestinal walls).

equinus Involuntary extension (plantar flexion) of the foot (like a horse); this position is often found in spastic cerebral palsy. It leads to toe walking.

ERG *See* electroretinogram.

erythrocytosis An abnormal increase in the number of circulating red blood cells.

erythropoietin A protein that regulates red blood cell production.

Escherichia coli (E. coli) Bacteria that can cause infections ranging from diarrhea to urinary tract infection to sepsis.

esophageal atresia A congenital defect in which there is a stricture in the esophagus, preventing food from entering the stomach.

esophagus Tube through which food passes from the pharynx to the stomach.

esotropia A form of strabismus in which one or both eyes turn in; "cross-eyed."

estimated date of confinement (EDC) Expected date of delivery; *also called* estimated due date (EDD).

estrogen Female sex hormone.

etiology Refers to the cause of a medical condition.

eustachian tube Connection between oral cavity and middle ear, allowing equilibration of pressure and drainage of fluid.

everted Turned outward.

evidence-based research instruction Defined as "research that involves the application of rigorous, systematic, and objective procedures to obtain reliable and valid knowledge relevant to education activities and programs" (U.S. Department of Education, 2007).

excitotoxic Pertaining to excitotoxins, neurochemicals that can cause neuronal cell death and have been implicated in hypoxic brain damage and acquired immunodeficiency syndrome (AIDS) encephalopathy.

executive function The cognitive tasks related to taking in, organizing, processing and acting on information. Deficits are present in people with autism spectrum disorders (ASDs), learning differences, and attention-deficit/hyperactivity disorder (ADHD).

exotropia A form of strabismus in which one or both eyes turn out; "wall-eyed."

expressive language Communication by spoken language, gesture, signing, or body language.

extension Movement of a limb at a joint to bring the joint into a more straightened position.

extinction The process through which reinforcement is withheld for a previously reinforced response, resulting in a decrease in the future occurrence of that response; *see* planned ignoring.

extinction burst A transient increase in the frequency and intensity of a challenging behavior before a subsequent reduction occurs.

extracorporeal membrane oxygenation (ECMO) An extreme and invasive life support technique that involves putting a patient onto a heart–lung bypass machine.

extract In the context of medication, a concentrated preparation.

extrapyramidal cerebral palsy *See* dyskinetic cerebral palsy.

extrapyramidal system Areas of the brain involved in subconscious, automatic aspects of motor coordination.

extremely low birth weight (ELBW) Term often used to describe an infant with a birth weight less than 1,000 grams (2¼ pounds).

fading Behavioral instruction process by which prompts are withdrawn gradually.

FAE *See* fetal alcohol effects.

failure to thrive (FTT) Inadequate growth of both weight and height in infancy or early childhood caused by malnutrition, chronic disease, or a congenital anomaly.

family-centered care An approach to health care that is based on mutual respect which promotes optimal health outcomes and treatment adherence by encouraging shared decision making in daily patient interactions.

fatty acid oxidation disorders Inborn errors of metabolism involving enzyme deficiencies in the breakdown of fatty acids.

febrile Having an elevated body temperature. A child is considered febrile when registering a fever above 100.4 degrees Fahrenheit (38 degrees Celsius).

FEES Flexible endoscopic evaluation of swallowing.

Feingold diet This diet involves removing synthetic colors, flavors, artificial preservatives, salicylates, and sweeteners from the diet.

femur Long bone in the thigh connecting the hip to the knee.

fencer's response *See* asymmetrical tonic neck reflex (ATNR).

fertilization The entrance of a sperm into the egg resulting in a conception.

FES *See* functional electrical stimulators.

fetal alcohol effects (FAE) Former term for alcohol-related neurodevelopmental disorder (ARND; *see Chapter 3*).

fetal heart rate (FHR) Normally 120–140 beats per minute and routinely monitored by ultrasound throughout labor to indicate fetal well-being versus fetal distress (i.e., FHR < 100).

fetal heart rate monitoring Monitoring fetal heart rate with ultrasound.

fetus Refers to the stages of development during pregnancy after the first eight weeks.

FHR *See* fetal heart rate.

fibroma A benign fibrous tumor of connective tissue.

FISH *See* fluorescent *in situ* hybridization.

fissures On the brain, these are deeper than sulci, are first visible during fetal development, and separate each hemisphere into four functional areas or lobes.

flexion Movement of a limb to bend at a joint.

flexor A muscle with the primary function of flexion or bending at a joint.

flexor and extensor spasms Spasms of bending of a limb toward or away from the body.

flora In medicine, bacteria normally residing within a body organ and not causing disease, such as *E. coli* in the intestine.

fluency Aspect of speech, that is, producing speech in a fluid manner.

fluorescent *in situ* hybridization (FISH) Technology used to diagnose a number of microdeletion syndromes.

fMRI *See* functional magnetic resonance imaging.

focal Localized.

focal neurological changes Findings on neurological exams that are abnormal and indicative of a lesion in a particular part of the brain; *also called* focal neurological impairments.

folic acid A vitamin, a deficiency of which during early pregnancy has been linked to neural tube defects.

foramen ovale A tiny window between the right atrium and the left atrium.

forebrain The front portion of the brain during fetal development; *also called* the prosencephalon.

forward chaining A behavior management technique in which the first skill in a sequence is taught first and the last skill is taught last.

fovea centralis The small pit in the center of the macula; the area of clearest vision, containing only cones.

frame shift A type of gene mutation in which the insertion or deletion of a single nucleotide leads to the misreading of all subsequent codons as the three base pair reading frame is shifted.

free level In pharmacotherapy, the amount of active drug that is able to produce an effect on the body.

free radicals Chemical compounds, the abnormal accumulation of which has been linked to cancer and neurotoxicity.

frequency Cycles per second, or hertz (Hz), a measure of sound.

frontal lobe Controls both voluntary motor activity and important aspects of cognition (Brodal, 2010).

FTT *See* failure to thrive.

functional (experimental) analysis *See* applied behavioral analysis.

functional electrical stimulators (FES) Provide neural stimulation to increase mobility.

functional magnetic resonance imaging (fMRI) A neuroimaging procedure that permits evaluation of the effects of activities, such as reading, on brain function.

fundoplication An operation in which the top of the stomach is wrapped around the opening of the esophagus to correct gastroesophageal reflux (GER).

FXS Fragile X syndrome (*see Chapter 1*).

G tube *See* gastrostomy tube.

GABA *See* gamma-aminobutyric acid.

galactosemia An inborn error of metabolism involving an enzyme deficiency that prevents the breakdown of the sugar galactose, a component of many foods.

gamma-aminobutyric acid (GABA) An amino acid that acts as an inhibitory neurotransmitter.

ganglia Masses of nerve cell bodies.

gastrocolic reflex A trigger that results in an urge to defecate; it generally occurs 30–60 minutes after a meal.

gastroenteritis An acute illness marked by vomiting and diarrhea usually associated with a viral infection (e.g., rotavirus in infants) that generally lasts a few days; *also called* stomach flu.

gastroesophageal duodenoscopy Endoscopy in which a flexible instrument with a light source examines the esophagous, stomach, and small bowel.

gastroesophageal reflux disease (GER/GERD) The backward flow of food into the esophagus after it has entered the stomach; acid reflux.

gastrointestinal (GI) tract The stomach and small intestine.

gastrojejunal (G-J) tube A feeding tube that is inserted through a gastrostomy site and threaded through the stomach and duodenum into the jejunum (the second part of the small intestine).

gastrojejunostomy (G-J) Surgical procedure to prepare for gastrojejunostomy (G-J) tube.

gastroschisis Congenital malformation of the abdominal wall resulting in the protrusion of abdominal contents.

gastrostomy An operation in which an artificial opening is made into the stomach through the wall of the abdomen. This is usually done in order to place a feeding tube into the stomach.

gastrostomy tube (G tube) A permanent tube placed directly through the skin and into the stomach.

GBS *See* group B *Streptococcus*.

GDD *See* global developmental delay.

gene A molecular unit of heredity consisting of stretches of DNA and RNA that code for a type of protein or for an RNA chain that has a function in the organism.

genome The complete set of hereditary units (genes) in an organism.

genomic imprinting A condition manifested differently depending on whether the trait is inherited from the mother or father; *also called* uniparental disomy. An example is a deletion in chromosome 15q11–q13, which when inherited from the mother results in Angelman syndrome and when inherited from the father results in Prader-Willi syndrome.

genotype The genetic composition of an individual.

genu verum Bowed legs.

GERD *See* gastroesophageal reflux.

germ cells The cells involved in reproduction (i.e., sperm, eggs).

German measles *See* rubella.

GI *See* gastrointestinal tract.

G-J tube *See* gastrojejunal tube.

glaucoma Increased pressure within the anterior chamber of the eye which can cause blindness.

glia Cells that compose the white matter and provide a support function for neurons.

global developmental delay (GDD) Significant delays in two or more of the following domains: gross motor/fine motor, speech/language, cognition, social/personal, and activities of daily living (ADL).

globus pallidus A subcortical area of the brain that is a major component of the basal ganglia and is part of the extrapyramidal system.

glossoptosis Protruding tongue.

glucose A sugar; *also called* sucrose; contained in fruits and other carbohydrates.

glutaminergic neurons Brain cells that release the chemical glutamate, an exactatory neurotransmitter.

gluten-/casein-free diet Involves removing all wheat and milk products from the child's diet.

glycine An amino acid that can serve as an excitotoxin, causing seizures.

glycogen The chief carbohydrate stored in the body, primarily in the liver and muscles.

GMPCS *See* gross motor function classification system.

goiter Enlargement of the thyroid gland.

Golgi apparatus The intracellular organelle that packages proteins in a form that can be released through the cell membrane and carried throughout the body.

goniometry Use of a hinged measuring tool to determine joint range of motion.

graduated guidance A behavior management technique in which only the level of assistance (guidance) necessary for the child to complete the task is provided.

graft versus host disease A mechanism of the body's immune system that destroys foreign proteins. It can be life-threatening when it occurs in a child who has received a bone marrow or organ transplant and has a suppressed immune system. Symptoms include diarrhea, skin breakdown, and shock.

grammar The system of and rules for using units of meaning (morphemes) and syntax in language.

grapheme A unit, such as a letter, of a writing system.

gravida/para The number of times a woman has been pregnant (gravid) and has delivered (parous) a living infant.

grey matter The part of the brain rich in neurons. It comprises the cortex.

gross motor function classification system (GMFCS) An assessment of ambulatory ability for children with cerebral palsy.

group B *Streptococcus* (GBS) Bacteria, causing one of the most common and severe neonatal infections.

guanine One of the four nucleotides (chemicals) that comprises DNA.

guided compliance A behavior management technique involving the use of graduated guidance to teach functional tasks.

Guillain-Barré syndrome An acute inflammatory peripheral neuropathy (*see Appendix B*).

gynecomastia Excessive breast growth in males.

gyri Convolutions of the surface of the brain; *singular*: gyrus.

habilitation The teaching of new skills to children with developmental disabilities. It is called habilitation rather than rehabilitation because these children did not possess these skills previously.

haemophilus influenzae A bacteria that can cause serious infections in children including meningitis

hallucinations Sensory perceptions without a source in the external world. These most commonly occur as symptoms of psychosis, drug intoxication, or seizures.

hamartomas A benign (not cancer) growth made up of an abnormal mixture of cells and tissues normally found in the area of the body where the growth occurs

hand splints A form of low-tech assistive device to children with cerebral palsy or neuromuscular disorder.

haploid Having a single set of human chromosomes, 23, as in the sperm or egg.

hCG *See* human chorionic gonadotropin.

hearing loss A condition characterized by a decrease in the ability to hear based on decreased intensity, loudness as measured in decibels (dB), or frequency of sound.

hemangiomas Congenital abnormal masses of blood vessels, such as "birth marks."

hematocrit Percentage of red blood cells in whole blood, normally about 35%–40%.

hematologic Relating to the blood system.

hematopoietic Relating to the formation of red blood cells.

hematuria Blood in the urine.

hemihypertrophy Asymmetric overgrowth of the face or limbs.

hemiplegia Spasticity and weakness on one side of the body.

hemispherectomy Surgical removal of most of one cerebral hemisphere for treatment of intractable generalized seizures.

hemodialysis A detoxification procedure in which an individual's blood is gradually removed through an artery, passed through an artificial kidney machine, and then returned cleansed. It is used most commonly to treat chronic renal (kidney) failure.

hemoglobin Blood protein capable of carrying oxygen to body tissues.

hemolytic Excessive breakdown of red blood cells.

hemolytic anemia Anemia due to the destruction of red blood cells.

hemostat A small surgical clamp used to constrict a tube or blood vessel.

hepatomegaly Enlarged liver.

hepatosplenomegaly Enlargement of the liver and spleen.

herpes simplex virus (HSV) A virus that can lead to symptoms that range from cold sores to genital lesions to encephalitis; also a cause of fetal malformations and sepsis in early infancy.

hertz (Hz) Cycles per second; a measure of the frequency of sound.

heterotopia Migration and development of normal neural tissue in an abnormal location in the brain.

heterozygous Carrying two genes that are dissimilar for one trait.

hexosaminidase An enzyme, a deficiency of which leads to Tay-Sachs disease.

HIE *See* hypoxic ischemic encephalopathy.

high stakes testing One of the most controversial tenets of the No Child Left Behind (NCLB) Act of 2001. Under NCLB, all students, in all schools, in all districts must take standardized assessments to determine whether they are functioning on grade level in the areas of reading/language arts, math, and science, regardless of disability.

high-tech assistive technology Complicated and often expensive to own and maintain form of assistive technology.

hippocampus A region of the brain in the floor of each lateral ventricle that has a central role in the formation of memories, emotion and rapid learning of new information.

hippotherapy The therapeutic use of horseback riding.

Hirschsprung disease Congenitally enlarged colon.

HMD *See* Hyaline member disease.

holoprosencephaly A congenital defect manifest by impaired cleavage of the cerebral hemispheres.

homeobox (HOX) A group of genes involved in early embryonic development.

homeostasis Metabolic equilibrium of the body.

homozygous Carrying identical genes for any given trait.

HOX *See* homeobox.

HSV *See* herpes simplex virus.

human chorionic gonadotropin (hCG) The hormone secreted by the embryo that prevents its expulsion from the uterus. A pregnancy test measures the presence of this hormone in the blood or urine.

Hyaline membrane disease (HMD) A disorder characterized by respiratory distress in the newborn period, principally in premature infants. *Also called* RDS.

hybrid Offspring of parents of different species.

hydrocephalus A condition characterized by the abnormal accumulation of cerebrospinal fluid within the ventricles of the brain. In infants, this leads to enlargement of the head and compression of the brain.

hyperacusis Unusual sensitivity to certain sounds such as a vacuum cleaner, often found in children with autism.

hyperalimentation *See* parenteral feeding.

hyperbilirubinemia Excess accumulation of bilirubin in the blood, which can result in jaundice, a yellowing of the complexion and/or the whites of the eyes, or kernicterus, the yellow staining of certain central parts of the brain.

hypercholesterolemia Elevated cholesterol levels in blood.

hyperglycemia High blood sugar level as seen in diabetes.

hyperimmune globulin Blood that is especially rich in antibodies against a virus.

hyperkalemia Elevations in levels of potassium in the blood.

hyperopia Farsightedness.

hyperparathyroidism High level of blood parathyroid hormone, which causes abnormalities in calcium and phosphorous metabolism.

hyperphagia Pathological overeating.

hyperreflexia Increased deep tendon reflexes, such as the knee jerk.

hypersynchronous In the context of the central nervous system (CNS), pertaining to the discharge of many neurons at the same time that leads to a seizure.

hypertelorism Widely spaced eyes.

hypertension Elevated blood pressure.

hyperthyroidism Condition resulting from excessive production of thyroid hormone.

hypertonia Increased muscle tone as seen in spastic cerebral palsy.

hypertrichosis Excessive hair growth.

hypertrophy Overgrowth of a body part or organ.

hypocalcemia Low blood calcium level.

hypogenitalism Having small genitalia.

hypoglycemia Low blood sugar level, usually below a concentration of 40–50 milligrams of glucose per 100 milliliters of blood for a period of time.

hypogonadism Decreased function of sex glands with resultant retarded growth and sexual development.

hypomania Symptoms not severe enough to meet full mania criteria with being silly not

euphoric, talks fast or too much but not pressured, babbling incoherently.

hypopharynx The area at the back of the throat where the larynx sits next to the entrance to the esophagus.

hypoplasia Defective formation of a tissue or body organ leading it to be small and underdeveloped.

hypoplastic lungs Small lungs that are not fully developed.

hypospadias A congenital defect in which the opening of the urethra is on the underside, rather than at the end, of the penis.

hypotension Low blood pressure.

hypothalamus A portion of the brain that directs a number of important bodily functions including many autonomic functions of the peripheral nervous system. Connections with structures of the endocrine and nervous systems enable the hypothalamus to play a vital role in maintaining homeostasis. The hypothalamus also influences various emotional responses.

hypothermia Excessively low body temperature.

hypothyroidism Condition resulting from deficient production of thyroid hormone.

hypotonia Decreased muscle tone.

hypoxemia Seriously low blood oxygen supply to the entire body.

hypoxic Having reduced oxygen content in body tissues.

hypoxic ischemic encephalopathy (HIE) An acute brain malfunction often resulting in coma caused by acute reduction in the blood flow and the oxygen supply to the brain.

hypsarrhythmia Electroencephalographic (EEG) abnormality seen in infants with infantile spasms. It is marked by chaotic spike–wave activity.

hysterectomy The surgical removal of the uterus.

Hz *See* hertz.

ichthyosis Dry and scaly skin.

ictal Pertaining to a seizure event.

IDDM *See* insulin-dependent diabetes mellitus.

idiopathic Without an identifiable cause.

IEP *See* individualized education program.

IFSP *See* individualized family service plan.

IH *See* learning/instructional hierarchy.

ileostomy A surgically placed opening from the small intestine through the abdominal wall to divert bowel or bladder contents after an operation.

ileum Lower portion of the small intestine.

imitation training A behavior management technique in which the teacher demonstrates the desired behavior, asks the child to complete the action, and provides positive reinforcement when the task is completed.

immunoglobulin An antibody produced by the body after exposure to a foreign agent, such as a virus.

impact In reference to traumatic head injury, the forcible striking of the head against an object.

imperforate Lacking a normal opening in a body organ. The most common example in childhood is an absent or closed anus.

implantation The attachment and imbedding of the fertilized egg (blastocyst) into the mucous lining of the uterus.

in utero Occurring during fetal development.

in vitro fertilization Fertilization of harvested eggs and allowing them to develop in culture to the blastomere, or eight-cell stage, at which point they are implanted into the uterus of the recepient.

inborn error of metabolism An inherited enzyme deficiency leading to the disruption of normal bodily metabolism (e.g., phenylketonuria [PKU]).

incidence The rate of occurrence of new cases of a disorder in a population expressed as a function of time.

incidental teaching An ardent attempt to catch the child complying with commands or following instructions in his or her everyday life and to praise (reinforce) the performance.

incisors Front teeth used for cutting.

incus One of the three small bones in the middle ear that help amplify sound.

independent residential alternatives (IRA) Independent living centers; group homes designed for 1–3 individuals.

indirect assessment Simplest method of gathering information about behavioral function that consist of questionnaires and rating scales that are completed by caregivers

individualized education program (IEP) A written plan, mandated by federal law, that maps out the objectives and goals that a child receiving special education services is expected to achieve over the course of the school year.

individualized family service plan (IFSP) A written plan detailing early intervention and related services to be provided to an infant or toddler with disabilities in accordance with federal law.

inertial Pertaining to the tendency to keep moving in the same direction as the force that produced the movement.

infantile spasms A seizure type in infancy marked by brief flexor spasms, usually lasting 1–3 seconds.

inferior In anatomy, below.

inferior vena cava The main vein feeding into the baby's heart.

influenza An acute illness caused by a virus that attacks respiratory and gastrointestinal tracts.

informed consent The written consent of a person to undergo a procedure or treatment after its risks and benefits have been explained in easily understood language.

inhaled nitric oxide (iNO) A new therapeutic gas for treating persistent pulmony hypertension of the neonate (PPHN). It is mixed with the baby's oxygen supply in miniscule amounts and directly stimulates pulmonary function.

instructional training A behavior management technique in which the teacher describes the desired behavior, asks the child to perform it, and provides positive reinforcement upon completion of the task.

insulin-dependent diabetes mellitus (IDDM) A disorder in which blood sugar level is high enough to require treatment with insulin.

insult An attack on a body organ that causes damage to it. This may be physical, metabolic, immunological, or infectious.

integrative medicine Refers to a practice that combines conventional and types of complementary and alternative treatments for which there is evidence of safety and effectiveness.

intellectual disability Significantly subaverage general intellectual functioning accompanied by significant limitations in adaptive functioning; *previously called* mental retardation.

intensity Strength.

interictal In an individual with a seizure disorder, pertaining to the periods when seizures are not occurring.

internal capsule The area of white matter in the brain that separates the caudate nucleus and the thalamus from the lenticular nucleus. The internal capsule contains both ascending and descending axons so it can control distant movement.

interpersonal psychotherapy (IPT) A time-limited psychotherapy that focuses on building interpersonal skills

interphase The period in the cell life cycle when the cell is not dividing.

interval schedules Provision of reinforcement based on the passage of a certain amount of time relative to the child's performance of a behavior or task.

intrathecal The infusion of medication into the spinal space.

intrauterine growth restriction (IUGR) Restricted growth in the fetus, producing a small for gestational age at-birth baby, often resulting from abnormal placental development.

intravenous Infusion into a vein.

intraventricular hemorrhage (IVH) A hemorrhage into the cerebral ventricles.

intubation Insertion of a tube through the nose or mouth into the trachea to permit mechanical ventilation.

inversion In genetics, the result of two breaks on a chromosome followed by the reinsertion of the missing fragment at its original site but in the inverted order.

ionic Pertaining to mineral ions, a group of atoms carrying a charge of electricity.

iris The circular, colored membrane behind the cornea that surrounds the pupil.

ischemia A decreased blood flow to an area of the body that leads to tissue death.

isochromosome A chromosome with two copies of one arm and no copy of the other.

isometric contraction Muscular contraction against resistance in which the length of the muscle remains the same.

ITP *See* individualized transition plan.

IUGR *See* intrauterine growth restriction.

IVH *See* intraventricular hemorrhage.

J tube *See* jejunostomy tube.

Jacksonian seizure Spread of focal epileptiform activity to contiguous brain areas resulting in seizure which starts in one part of the body and involves adjacent body regions as seizure evolves.

jaundice A yellowing of the complexion and the whites of the eyes resulting from hyperbilirubinemia.

jejunostomy (J) tube A tube placed through the skin of the abdomen and directly into the jejunum to provide nutrition.

jejunum The second portion of the small intestine.

karyotyping Photographing the chromosomal makeup of a cell. In a human, there are 23 pairs of chromosomes in a normal karyotype.

ketogenic diet Special diet high in fat used to promote the use of ketones as an energy source; used in some children with intractable epilepsy.

ketosis The buildup of acid in the body, most often associated with starvation, inborn errors of metabolism, or diabetes.

Klebsiella pneumoniae A bacteria that can cause pneumonia, especially in immunocompromised individuals.

kyphoscoliosis A combination of humping and curvature of the spine.

kyphosis An excessive anterior (forward) curvature of the spine creating a hump.

labyrinth One of the major components of the inner ear, the other being the cochlea.

lactase Enzyme necessary to digest the milk sugar lactose.

lactic acid Chemical produced in muscles as a result of anaerobic glucose metabolism.

lacrimal gland Gland that produces tears.

lactose Milk sugar composed of glucose and galactose.

laminar Layered.

lanugo Fine body hair found in premature infants.

large for gestational age (LGA) Weighing more than 4 kilograms, about 9 or more pounds at birth. This typically occurs in infants of diabetic mothers.

lateral To the side; away from the mid-line.

lateral ventricles Cavities in the interior of the cerebral hemisphere containing cerebrospinal fluid. They are enlarged with hydrocephalus or with brain atrophy.

Law of Effect Functional relationship between behavior and its consequences.

LBW *See* low birth weight.

learned helplessness Occurs when families, teachers, and other well-intentioned people often protect youth with disabilities from making mistakes and avoid discussing the ramifications of a child's disability as they help them prepare for adulthood.

learning disability A developmental disability characterized by difficulty with certain academic skills such as reading or writing in individuals with normal intelligence.

learning/instructional hierarchy (IH) IH describes behaviors to be learned and mastered, not only by their form but by the level of proficiency with which they are performed.

left ventricular hypertrophy Enlargement of the left side of the heart.

lens The biconvex, translucent body that rests in front of the vitreous humor of the eye and precisely focuses the light rays on the retina.

lentiform nucleus A large, cone-shaped mass of gray matter just lateral to the internal capsule of the brain.

lesions Injuries or loss of function.

leukemias Blood cell cancers.

LGA *See* large for gestational age.

ligament A sheet or band of tough, fibrous tissue connecting bones or cartilage at a joint.

ligamentous laxity Double jointedness; hyperflexiblity.

linear fracture Break of a bone in a straight line; refers to a type of skull fracture or fracture of a long bone (arm or leg).

lipid metabolism The creation and/or breakdown of lipids including cholesterol and fat-soluble vitamins.

lipoma A benign, fatty tissue tumor.

lissencephaly A congenital abnormality marked by a "smooth" brain due to incomplete neuronal proliferation and migration and resultant lack of folds (gyri) and grooves (sulci).

listeria monocytogenes The causative agent of listeriosis.

locus Focus or location.

lordosis An excessive posterior (backward) curvature of the spine.

low birth weight (LBW) Term often used to describe an infant with a birth weight less than 2,500 grams (5½ pounds).

lower esophageal sphincter (LES) The muscular valve connecting the esophagus and stomach and normally preventing reflux.

low-tech assistive technology An assistive device that does not require batteries or other electric sources to operate.

lumbar Pertaining to the lower back.

lumbar puncture The tapping of the subarachnoid space to obtain cerebrospinal fluid from the lower back region. This procedure is used to diagnose meningitis and to measure chemicals in the spinal fluid; *also called* a spinal tap.

lymphadenopathy Enlargement of lymph nodes.

lymphocyte A type of white blood cell.

lymphoma A cancerous growth of lymphoid tissue.

lyonization The genetic principle discovered by Mary Lyon that there is X-chromosome inactivation in females.

lysosome Minute organelle in cells that contains enzymes used to digest potentially toxic material.

macrocephaly Large head size.

macroorchidism Having abnormally large testicles; found in fragile X syndrome.

macrosomia Large body size.

macrostomia Large mouth.

macula The area of the retina that contains the greatest concentration of cones and the fovea centralis, where central vision is processed.

magnetic resonance imaging (MRI) Imaging procedure that uses the magnetic resonance of atoms to provide clear images of interior parts of the body. It is particularly useful in diagnosing structural abnormalities of the brain.

magnetic resonance spectroscopy (MRS) A study that can be done as part of a regular MRI scan. Rather than provide a picture of the brain, it analyzes the presence and amount of certain metabolic components in various brain regions. It is particularly helpful in diagnosing certain inborn errors of metabolism, such as mitochondrial disorders (*see Appendix B*).

major depression A prolonged period of depressed mood.

malleus One of the three small bones in the middle ear that help amplify sound.

malnutrition Inadequate nutrition for typical growth and development to occur.

malocclusion The improper fitting together of the upper and lower teeth.

mandible Lower jaw bone.

mania A distinct period of abnormally and persistently elevated, expansive, or irritable mood. This mood disturbance is sufficiently severe to cause impairment in function.

manic depression *See* bipolar disorder.

Marfan syndrome Disorder of connective tissue the strengthens the body's structures. (*see Appendix B*).

mass spectrometry A technique used for identifying chemical, drug, or metabolic abnormalities in the blood or urine.

mastoiditis Infection of the mastoid air cells that rest in the temporal bone behind the ear. This is an infrequent complication of chronic middle-ear infection.

mature minor A teenage minor who may give consent because the physician judges that he or she understands the nature, purpose, and risks of the proposed treatment; generally limited to minors at least 15 years old where the treatment is for the patient's own benefit and is judged necessary by conservative medical opinion (compare with *emancipated minor*).

maxilla The bony region of the upper jaw.

maxillary hypoplasia Incomplete development of the upper jaw.

MBD *See* metabolic bone disease.

meconium The thick and tarry stool that is formed during fetal life consisting of swallowed amniotic fluid debris, gastrointestinal mucous and green bile secretions from the liver, and sloughed off gastrointestinal epithelial cells; is not normally passed until after birth.

medial Toward the center or mid-line.

median plane The mid-line plane of the body. It runs vertically and separates the left and right halves of the body.

medical assistive technology Subset of assistive technology that is used for primarily medical or life-sustaining reasons (e.g., ventilators, feeding pumps).

medical home Involves a trusting partnership between a child, a child's family, and the pediatric primary care team who oversees the child's health and well-being within a community-based system that provides uninterrupted care to support and sustain optimal health outcomes.

medication *See Appendix C.*

medium chain fatty acids Fatty acids that can bypass the normal uptake process and go directly to the liver.

medulloblastomas Cerebellar tumors.

megavitamin therapy The use of more than 10 times the average daily required amount of vitamins; *also called* orthomolecular therapy.

meiosis Reductive cell division occurring only in eggs and sperm in which the daughter cells receive half (23) the number of chromosomes of the parent cells (46).

melanocytes Pigment-forming skin cells.

melatonin A naturally occurring hormone available as an over-the-counter preparation for which there is evidence of efficacy in improving sleep onset in children with disabilities who have sleep problems.

Mendelian traits Dominant and recessive traits inherited according to the genetic principles put forward by Gregor Mendel.

meningeal Related to the meninges, the three membranes enveloping the brain and spinal cord.

meningitis Infection, often bacterial, of the meninges or sac that surround the brain.

meningocele Protrusion of the meninges through a defect in the skull or vertebral column, a neural tube defect.

meningoencephalitis A generalized and often devastating infection of the brain and central nervous system.

meningomyelocele Protrusion of meninges and malformed spinal cord through a defect in the vertebral column; *also called* myelomeningocele.

menses Menstrual flow.

mental retardation *See* intellectual disability.

mentation Thinking.

mesencephalon Midbrain region.

mesoderm Middle cell layer in the embryo.

messenger ribonucleic acid (mRNA) RNA, synthesized from a DNA template during transcription, that mediates the transfer of genetic information from the cell nucleus to ribosomes in the cytoplasm, where it serves as a template for protein synthesis.

metabolic bone disease (MBD) *Previously called* renal osteodystrophy, results from abnormalities in calcium, phosphorous, vitamin D, and parathyroid hormone.

metaphase The stage in cell division in which each chromosome doubles.

metaphyses The ends of the shaft of long bones connected to the epiphyses.

methionine An amino acid.

methylation The attachment of methyl groups to DNA at the cytosine base that turns gene function off.

microcephaly Abnormally small head.

microdeletion A microscopic deletion in a chromosome associated with a loss of a small number of contiguous genes; a chromosomal deletion spanning several genes that is too small to be detected under the microscope using conventional cytogenetic methods but can be detected using newer molecular genetic techniques such as FISH and microarrays.

microdeletion syndromes Genetic disorders caused by mutations in a small number of contiguous genes, an example being velocardiofacial syndrome; *see* contiguous gene syndrome.

micrognathia Receding chin.

microphthalmia Small eye.

micropreemie Term often used to describe an infant born weighing less than 800 grams (1.75 pounds).

microswitches Switches used to control computers, environmental control systems, or power wheelchairs that have been adapted so that less pressure than normal is required for activation.

microtia Small ear.

microtrauma Small injuries such as stress cracks or fractures that occur in the growth area or cartilage of growing bones as a result of high impact or overloading.

mid-tech assistive technology An assistive device that generally requires battery/ electrical power or is more complex in its use; for example, teletypewriter (TTY) devices for those who are deaf, home-infusion pumps, suction machines, and sophisticated manual wheelchairs.

MII *See* multiple intraluminal impedance.

milligram One thousandth of a gram.

milliliter One thousandth of a liter; equal to about 15 drops.

missense mutation Gene error (mutation) resulting from the replacement of a single nucleic acid for another, resulting in a misreading of the DNA code.

mitochondrial myopathy Congenital muscle disorder caused by a mutation in the mitochondrial DNA.

mitosis Cell division in which two daughter cells of identical chromosomal composition to the parent cell are formed. Each contains 46 chromosomes.

mixed cerebral palsy A form of cerebral palsy with spastic and dyskinetic components; this term is used when more than one type of motor pattern is present and when one pattern does not clearly predominate over another.

MOs *See* motivating operations.

modification In special education, a substantial change in the method or scoring scale used to assess a student's academic performance or knowledge (e.g., using a portfolio of work to demonstrate a student's learning).

molded ankle-foot orthoses A plastic insert for the shoe that is used to treat toe walking.

monosomy Chromosome disorder in which one chromosome is absent. The most common example is Turner syndrome, XO (*see Appendix B*).

monosomy X Turner syndrome (*see Appendix B*).

morbidity Medical complication of an illness, procedure, or operation.

moro reflex A primitive reflex elicited when a newborn infant experiences a sudden drop of the head and neck or a loud noise. The infant responds with sudden extension and then flexion of the neck, arms, and legs, and then cries irritably.

morphemes The smallest linguistic units of meaning.

morula The group of cells formed by the first divisions of a fertilized egg.

mosaic trisomy Type of Down syndrome in which the individual has two distinct populations of cells, one containing 46 chromosomes and the other containing 47 chromosomes.

mosaicism The presence of two genetically distinct types of cells in one individual.

MOSF *See* multi-organ system failure.

motivating operations (MOs) Play a central role in the operant learning conceptualization of motivation; produces two effects: 1) a change in the value of a consequence, and 2) a corresponding change in the strength of motivation.

motor point block The injection of a denaturing agent into the nerve supply of a spastic muscle. This effectively interrupts the nerve supply at the entry site to a spastic muscle without compromising sensation and results in the return of tone towards normal.

MRI *See* magnetic resonance imaging.

mRNA *See* messenger ribonucleic acid.

MRS *See* magnetic resonance spectroscopy.

MS/MS *See* tandem mass spectrometer.

mucopolysaccharides Product of metabolism that may accumulate in cells and cause a progressive neurological disorder (e.g., Hurler syndrome, *see Appendix B*).

multifactorial Describing an inheritance pattern in which environment and heredity interact.

multi-organ system failure (MOSF) This devastating condition can result from the diving reflex during severe hypoxic ischemic encephalopathy (HIE).

multiple intraluminal impedance (MII) A relatively new technology that measures the movement of fluids, solids, and air in the esophagus.

muscle spindles Muscle fibers that are part of the reflex arc that controls muscle contraction.

muscle and tendon structures Muscle and tendons associated with long bones such as the tibia, fibia, and femur that are more succeptable to injury during growth periods.

musculoskeletal Referring to the muscle and bone support system of the body.

mutation A change in the genomic sequence resulting in a variant form that may be transmitted to subsequent generations and may be associated with disease.

myasthenia gravis Neuromuscular disorder involving the muscles and the nerves that control them (*see Chapter 13*).

myelinated Insulating sheath around many nerve fibers in the white matter, increasing the speed at which impulses are conducted.

myelination The production of a coating called myelin around an axon, which quickens neurotransmission; a process that involves elaboration of supportive structures that improve transmission of electrical impulses from one part of the nervous system to another.

myelomeningocele   *See* meningomyelocele.

myoclonus   Irregular, involuntary contraction of a muscle.

myoglobinuria   The spillage of myoglobin, the oxygen-transporting protein of muscle, into the urine. This can occur with trauma, vascular problems, certain drugs and other situations that destroy or damage the muscle, releasing myoglobin into the circulation and thus to the kidneys.

myopathies   A muscular disease in which the muscle fibers do not function for any one of many reasons, resulting in muscular weakness. The most common example is muscular dystrophy.

myopia   Nearsightedness.

myosin   Protein necessary for muscle contraction.

myotonia   Abnormal rigidity of muscles when voluntary movement is attempted.

myringotomy   The surgical incision of the eardrum, usually accompanied by the placement of pressure-equalization tubes, to drain fluid from the middle ear.

nasal cannula   A plastic prong placed in the nose and connected to a tube that delivers an oxygen/air mixture.

nasal pillows   A prop attached to an oxygen line to permit the flow of oxygen directly into the nose.

nasogastric (NG) tube   A feeding tube placed in the nose and extended into the stomach.

nasojejunal tube   A feeding tube placed in the nose and extended through the stomach and into the jejunum.

nasopharynx   Posterior portion of the oral cavity above the palate.

NCS   *See* nerve conduction studies.

NDT   *See* neurodevelopmental therapy.

NEC   *See* necrotizing enterocolitis.

necrosis   Death of tissue.

necrotizing enterocolitis (NEC)   Severe inflammation of the small intestine and colon, most common in premature infants.

negative punishment   Involves the contingent removal of a consequence (i.e., positive reinforcer).

negative reinforcement   Behavioral phenomenon in which an individual's behavior permits an unpleasant event to be avoided or escaped, with a resultant increase in this behavior in the future.

neonatal intensive care unit (NICU)   Hospital unit specializing in providing newborn life support treatments.

neonatal seizure   Seizures in newborn infants appear different than in older children. The seizure may manifest as arm and/or leg tonic/clonic movements seeming like bicycling or rowing. Movements may also be more subtle including spasmodic lip smacking or tongue thrusting, ocular movements such as excessive blinking or prolonged eye opening/staring, or episodes of apnea and bradycardia.

nerve blocks   Direct injection of denaturing agents into motor nerves to decrease spasticity.

nerve conduction studies (NCS)   Involves placing needle electrodes at various points on the body to test motor and sensory function of the peripheral nerves.

nerve conduction velocity   Measure of nerve function.

neuropores   The rostral and caudal openings of the neural tube which close around six weeks gestational age.

neural fold   During embryonic life, the fold created when the neural plate expands and rises; later it becomes the spinal column.

neural network   A network involving many brain regions working in concert to store and use information obtained from the environment.

neural plate   Earliest fetal brain mass development derived from the ectodermal germ layer of the embryo in the first 7 weeks of gestation.

neural proliferation   A sustained period of vigorous cellular division which peaks between 6 and 22 weeks gestational age, giving rise to precursors of the future neuronal and glial populations of the brain.

neural tube   The stage of central nervous system (CNS) development that follows neural plate formation, which subsequently gives rise to the various parts of the brain (i.e., the forebrain folding into the cerebrum and the hindbrain into the cerebellum, brainstem, and spinal cord).

neural tube defects (NTDs)   Birth defects of the brain and spina cord (i.e., spina bifida and anencephaly).

neurodevelopmental treatment (NDT)   An intervention approach used with children with neurologically based motor disabilities such as cerebral palsy.

neurogenesis   The birth of neurons.

neurogenic   Originating in, starting from, or caused by the nervous system or nerve impulses.

neuroleptic malignant syndrome   A rare toxic reaction to a medication in which there is a potentially life-threatening high fever, most commonly a problem with anesthetic agents.

neuromuscular Affecting both muscles and nerves.

neuron Any of the impulse-conducting cells that constitute the brain, spinal column, and nerves, consisting of a nucleated cell body with one or more dendrites and a single axon; also called a nerve cell.

neurotoxicant A chemical compound that can damage neurons; *also called* neurotoxin.

neurotransmitter A chemical released at the synapse that permits transmission of an impulse from one nerve to another.

neurulation Sequential central nervous system (CNS) developmental processes of neuron cell proliferation and migration of nascent neurons outward from the center of the developing brain to the outer cortex.

neutropenia Low white blood cell count.

NG tube *See* nasogastric tube.

NICU *See* neonatal intensive care unit.

nondisjunction Failure of a pair of chromosomes to separate during mitosis or meiosis, resulting in an unequal number of chromosomes in the daughter cells.

nonsense mutation Gene defect in which a single base pair substitution results in the premature termination of a message and the resultant production of an incomplete and inactive protein; *see* missense mutation.

norepinephrine A neurotransmitter.

NTDs *See* neural tube defects (*see Chapter 25*).

nucleotide bases The nucleic acids that form DNA—adenine, guanine, cytosine, and thymine.

nutritive assistive devices Devices that assist in providing nutrition to an individual who cannot take oral feeding. These include nasogastric and gastrostomy feeding tubes.

nystagmus Involuntary rapid movements of the eyes (jiggling of the eyes) due to abnormalities in the cerebellum.

oblique muscles Eye muscles whose primary function is to rotate the eyes. Their secondary function is to handle moving the eyes horizontally and vertically.

obsessive-compulsive disorder (OCD) A psychiatric disorder in which recurrent and persistent thoughts and ideas that cannot be suppressed (obsessions) are associated with repetitive behaviors (compulsions), such as excessive handwashing.

obstructive uropathy Pathologic condition that blocks urine flow.

occipital lobe The posterior area of the brain where the visual receptive cortex is located.

OCD *See* obsessive-compulsive disorder.

ocular Pertaining to the eye.

oculomotor nerve The third cranial nerve controls the four eye muscles not controlled by the trochlear and abducens nerves.

oligodendrocytes A type of glial brain cell.

oligohydramnios The presence of too little amniotic fluid, which may result in fetal deformities, including clubfoot and hypoplastic lungs.

oliguria Decreased passage of urine.

omphalocele Congenital herniation of abdominal organs through the navel.

onychomycosis A fungal infection of the nails.

oophorectomy Surgical removal of the ovary or ovaries.

operant control Control established and maintained by operant contingencies (i.e., the relationships in effect between the behavior and its consequences).

ophthalmologist Physician specializing in treatment of diseases of the eye.

ophthalmoscope An instrument containing a mirror and a series of magnifying lenses used to examine the interior of the eye.

opiate antagonists A category of medications that block endorphin receptors of the brain.

opisthotonos Abnormal positioning of the body in which the back is arched while the head and feet touch the bed; holding the head arched backward.

optic chiasm Located just before the nerves enter the brain, it is where crossover of nerve fibers occurs.

optic nerve Transmits visual information from the retina to the brain.

optokinetic Pertaining to movement of the eyes.

oral pharyngeal musculature Muscles in the throat.

oral preparatory phase (Phase I) The step preceding swallowing in which food is formed into a bolus in the mouth.

oral transport (Phase II) The transport of a bolus of food to the back of the mouth so that it can be swallowed; primarily under volitional control.

organ of Corti A series of hair cells in the cochlea that form the beginning of the auditory nerve.

organic acidemias Inborn errors of metabolism involving enzyme deficiencies in the breakdown of organic acids (e.g., methylmalonic aciduria; *see Appendix B*); *also called* organic acid disorders and organic acidurias.

ornithine transcarbamylase An enzyme in the urea cycle. An inborn error of metabolism involving a deficiency of this enzyme leads to episodes of encephalopathy.

orocutaneous stimulation This stimulation therapy mimics the temporal organization of sucking and can enhance the premature infant's acquisition of a functional suckle pattern.

oropharynx The part of the pharynx between the soft palate and the upper edge of the epiglottis.

orthomolecular therapy *See* megavitamin therapy.

orthopedic Relating to bones or joints.

orthosis Orthopedic device (e.g., a splint or brace) used to support, align, or correct deformities or to improve the function of limbs; *plural*: orthoses; *also called* orthotic.

orthotic Device that supports or corrects the function of a limb or the torso; *also called* orthosis.

orthotist Professional trained in the fitting and construction of splints, braces, and artificial limbs.

osmolarity The concentration of dissolved particles in a liquid.

ossicles The three small bones in the middle ear—the stapes, incus, and malleus.

osteoarthritis Degenerative joint disease.

osteoblasts Cells that produce bony tissue.

osteoclast Cell that absorbs and removes bone.

osteoid The substrate of bone.

osteopenia The loss of bony tissue resulting in low bone density.

osteopetrosis A genetic disorder marked by deficient osteoclastic activity. A buildup of bone encroaches on the eye, brain, and other body organs, leading to early death; bone weakness.

osteotomies Surgical cuts through the bone to correct deformities.

ostomy An artificial opening in the abdominal region, for example, for discharge of stool or urine.

otitis media Middle-ear infection.

otoacoustic emissions Low-intensity sound energy emitted by the cochlea subsequent to sound stimulation as measured by a microphone coupled to the external ear canal.

ototoxic Toxic to the auditory nerve, leading to hearing impairment.

oval window Connects the middle to the inner ear.

overt strokes Involves a focal (localized) neurological deficit that lasts more than 24 hours and results from an occlusion of one of the large anterior cerebral circulation vessels.

oxidative phosphorylation A chemical reaction occurring in the mitochondrion, resulting in energy production.

oximeter An instrument that measures oxygen saturation in the bloodstream.

oxygenation The provision of sufficient oxygen for bodily needs.

pachygyria Abnormal convolutions on the surface of brain.

palatal Relating to the palate, the back portion of the roof of the mouth.

palate The roof of the mouth.

pancreatitis An inflammation of the pancreas.

panic disorder A psychiatric disorder in which the patient has episodes of sudden and irrational fears associated with hyperventilation and palpitations.

paraplegia Paralysis of the legs and lower body.

parapodium A reciprocal gait orthosis or a hip-knee-ankle-foot orthosis used in combination with crutches or a walker.

parasomnia Sleep disturbances (i.e., night terrors, sleep walking).

parenchymal Tissue within a body organ.

parenteral feeding Intravenous provision of high-quality nutrition (i.e., carbohydrates, protein, fat) used in children with malabsorption, malnutrition, and short bowel syndrome; *also called* hyperalimentation; parenteral feeding is usually administered in a hospital setting on a short-term basis.

parenting networks Parents who educate and support one another.

paresthesias Numbness with skin sensations such as burning, prickling, itching, or tingling.

parietal lobe The middle-upper part of the hemisphere of the brain; brain region involved in integrating sensory information and in visual-spatial processing.

Parkinson's disease A progressive neurological disease, usually occurring in older people, associated with tremor, slowed movements, and muscular rigidity.

parotid The salivary gland beside the ear.

paroxysmal Intermittent.

partial graduated guidance Instructor uses minimal physical contact but much praise in helping the child learn a desired task.

parvovirus A group of extremely small DNA viruses. Intrauterine infection with one type of parvovirus increases the risk of miscarriage but has not been shown to result in fetal malformations.

patella Kneecap.

patent ductus arteriosus (PDA) The persistence of a fetal passage permitting blood to bypass the lungs.

patent foramen ovale (PFO) A tiny open window in the atrial wall of the heart passing oxygenated blood from the right atrium into the left atrium, thus bypassing circulation to the fetal lungs *in utero*.

paternalism Imposing a decision on another person for that person's welfare (e.g., the theory that "doctor knows best").

PBIS *See* positive behavior interventions and supports.

PCB *See* polychlorinated biphenyl.

PDA *See* patent ductus arteriosus.

PDD pervasive developmental disorder (*see Chapter 21*).

PEEP *See* positive end expiratory pressure.

penetrance The percentage of people with a particular genetic mutation who express symptoms of the disorder. A disorder shows reduced penetrance when some people with the genetic defect are completely without symptoms.

percutaneous umbilical blood sampling (PUBS) A prenatal diagnostic procedure for obtaining fetal blood for genetic testing; *also called* cordocentesis.

percutaneously Through the skin.

perfusion The passage of blood through the arteries to an organ or tissue.

periodontal disease Disease of the gums and bony structures that surround the teeth.

periosteum Fibrous tissue covering and protecting all bones.

peripheral nervous system The parts of the nervous system other than the brain and spinal cord.

peripheral venous lines Catheters that are placed in a superficial vein of the arm or leg to provide medication.

peristalsis The voluntary constriction and relaxation of the muscles of the esophagus and intestine, creating wavelike movements that push food forward.

peritoneal Referring to the membrane surrounding the abdominal organs.

periventricular leukomalacia (PVL) Injury to part of the brain near the ventricles caused by lack of oxygen; occurs principally in premature infants.

periventricular region The area surrounding the ventricles.

peroxisome A cellular organelle involved in processing fatty acids.

persistent pulmonary hypertension of the newborn/persistent fetal circulation (PPHN/PFC) Persistent high pulmonary blood pressure in the newborn period due to vasoconstriction of the pulmonary arterial blood vessels and resulting in severe hypoxia.

pervasive developmental disorder (PDD) One of the autism spectrum disorders (*see Chapter 21*).

pes cavus High-arched foot.

pes planus Flat feet.

pesticide A chemical used to kill insects.

PET scan *See* positron emission tomography.

petechiae A small purplish spot, usually on the skin, caused by a minute hemorrhage.

PFO *See* patent foramen ovale.

PGD *See* preimplantation genetic diagnosis.

pH probe A small sensor, which detects the pH, or acidity, above the gastroesophageal junction.

phalanges Bones of the fingers and toes.

pharyngeal Pertaining to the pharynx or back of the throat.

pharyngeal transfer phase (Phase III) The transfer of a food bolus from the mouth to the pharynx on its way to being swallowed; begins when the bolus passes the faucial arches (near the tonsils) and triggers the start of the swallowing cascade.

pharynx The back of the throat.

phenothiazines Antipsychotic medications that affect neurochemicals in the brain and are used to control aggressive behavior and psychotic symptoms.

phenotype The physical appearance of a genetic trait.

phenylalanine An amino acid, the elevation of which causes phenylketonuria (PKU).

phenylketonuria (PKU) Birth defect in which a child is born without the ability to break down amino acids called phenylalanine.

philtrum Groove between nose and mouth.

phobias Irrational fears.

phocomelia Congenitally foreshortened limbs.

phoneme The smallest unit of sound in speech.

phonetic Pertaining to the sounding out of words.

phonological processing disorder A developmental disorder in which there is difficulty learning the rules about which sounds go together in specific positions within words when sounds are voiced or voiceless.

phonology The set of sounds in a language and the rules for using them.

photoreceptors Receptors for light stimuli; the rods and cones in the retina.

physes   Growth plates of a developing long bone.

physiotherapy   Physical therapy.

pica   The hunger for or ingestion of nonfood items.

pitch   The frequency of sounds, measured in cycles per second, or hertz (Hz). Low-pitched sounds have a frequency less than 500 Hz and a bass quality. High-pitched sounds have a frequency greater than 2,000 Hz and a tenor quality.

PKU   *See* phenylketonuria (*see Chapter 19 and Appendix B*).

placebo   An inactive substance used as a control in a study to determine the effectiveness of a drug.

placenta   The organ of nutritional exchange between the mother and the embryo. It has both maternal and embryonic portions, is disc-shaped, and is about 7 inches in diameter. The umbilical cord attaches in the center of the placenta. *Also called* the afterbirth; *adjective*: placental.

placenta accreta   Abnormal adherence of the chorionic villi to the uterus.

placenta previa   Condition in which the placenta is implanted in the lower segment of the uterus, extending over the cervical opening.

placental abruption   *See* abruptio placenta; early separation of the placenta from the uterine wall.

planned ignoring   A behavior management technique based on withholding positive reinforcement following the occurrence of a nondangerous, nondestructive challenging behavior; *also called* extinction.

plantarflexion   A toe-down motion of the foot at the ankle.

plantargrade   Flat on the floor.

plasma   The noncellular content of blood; *also called* serum.

plasmapheresis   The removal of blood followed by filtering the plasma and reinfusing the blood products. This procedure is done to remove toxins and antibodies as in Guillain-Barré syndrome.

plasticity   The ability of an organ or part of an organ to take over the function of another damaged organ; the ability of the nervous system to change or adapt.

pneumocystis carinii pneumonia   Lung infection often seen in immunocompromised individuals, such as those with acquired immunodeficiency syndrome (AIDS).

point mutation   A mutation in a single nucleotide (DNA) base leading to a genetic syndrome (e.g., sickle cell disease).

polar body testing   Polar bodies are the by-products of the egg's division during meiosis. The two polar bodies are essentially discarded by the egg. By analyzing the polar bodies, it is possible to infer the genetic status of the egg.

polio   Viral infection of the spinal cord causing an asymmetrical ascending paralysis, now prevented by vaccination.

polychlorinated biphenyl (PCB)   One of a group of organic compounds originally used in industry and now recognized as an environmental pollutant.

polydactyly   Extra fingers or toes.

polyhydramnios   The presence of excessive amniotic fluid; often associated with certain fetal anomalies such as esophageal atresia

polymicrogyria   A brain with too many convoluted gyri that are smaller than normal, due to abnormal neuronal migration during embryogenesis of the central nervous system.

polysomnogram   Procedure performed during sleep that involves monitoring the electroencephalogram (EEG), electrocardiogram (EKG), and respiratory efforts. It is used to investigate individuals with sleep disorders, including sleep apnea; also called a sleep study.

polyuria   Excessive passage of urine.

POR   *See* prevalence odds ratio.

positive behavioral interventions and supports (PBIS)   Positive reinforcement used to control undesired behaviors.

positive end expiratory pressure (PEEP)   Technique administered to a child who is on a mechanical ventilator in which positive pressure is administered between mechanical breaths.

positive pressure ventilation   Application of positive pressure to the inspiratory phase when the patient has an artificial airway in place and is connected to a ventilator.

positive punishment   Involves the contingent delivery of a consequence (*sometimes termed* an aversive stimulus).

positive reinforcement   A method of increasing desired behaviors by rewarding them; exists when the contingent delivery of an outcome produces an increase in the likelihood of the behavior(s) upon which it is contingent.

positive reinforcers   Any tangible (e.g., food, toy) or action (e.g., hug) that is reinforcing to an individual and will lead to a subsequent increase in the behavior that preceded it.

positive support reflex (PSR)   Primitive reflex present in an infant, in which the child reflexively accepts weight on the feet when bounced, appearing to stand briefly.

positron emission tomography (PET) Imaging study utilizing radioactive labeled chemical compounds to study the metabolism of an organ, most commonly the brain.

posterior In back of or the back part of a structure.

postictal Immediately following a seizure episode.

postterm birth Birth after the 42nd week of gestation.

posttraumatic stress disorder (PTSD) Psychiatric disorder in which a previously experienced stressful event is reexperienced psychologically many times and associated with anxiety and fear.

postural reactions Normal reflexlike protective responses of an infant to changes in position; *also called* automatic movement reactions.

PPHN/PFC *See* persistent pulmonary hypertension of the newborn/persistent fetal circulation.

PPV *See* positive pressure ventilation.

pragmatics The study of language as it is used in a social context (e.g., conversation).

precocious puberty A condition in which the changes associated with puberty begin at an unexpectedly early age.

preeclampsia Disorder of late pregnancy characterized by high blood pressure with swelling and/or protein in the mother's urine, seen especially in teenagers and women older than 35 years; *also called* toxemia of pregnancy; blood toxemia of pregnancy.

preference assessments Assessments to identify high-preference stimuli that may be potential reinforcers in a behavior management program.

preimplantation genetic diagnosis (PGD) Refers to procedures that are performed on embryos prior to implantation. PGD is considered another approach to prenatal diagnosis. When used to screen for a specific genetic disease, it avoids selective pregnancy termination as the method makes it highly likely that the baby will be free of the disease under consideration. PGD is an adjunct to assisted reproductive technology and requires in vitro fertilization (IVF) to obtain oocytes or embryos for evaluation.

premolar Teeth in the back of the mouth used for grinding.

prenatal screening Noninvasive (usually maternal blood) tests used to screen for genetic disorders in the fetus.

presbyopia A decrease in the accommodation of the lens of the eye that occurs with aging.

preterm birth Birth prior to the 37th week of gestation; prematurity.

prevalence odds ratio (POR) The burden or status of a disease in a defined population at a specified time, including all cases of disease in the population whether they are newly diagnosed or previously recognized.

priapism Painful and long-lasting penile erections.

primary neurulation The process by which the neural plate develops a midline groove the edges of which fold over, converge, and close to form the neural tube.

primitive reflexes Infantile reflexes that tend to fade in the first year of life (i.e., the suck, startle, and root) (*see Chapter 26*).

prompts Cues (e.g., verbal, visual) that direct the child to participate in a targeted activity.

prone Face down.

prophase The initial stage in cell division when the chromosomes thicken and shorten to look like separate strands.

prophylaxis Use of a preventive agent.

proprioception Ability to sense the position, location, orientation and movement of body parts.

proptosis Appearance of protruding eyes.

prosencephalon *See* forebrain. The forward-most bulge, gives rise to the left and right cerebral hemispheres.

prosocial Socially acceptable.

prosody The intonation and rhythm of speech.

proteinuria Protein in urine.

proximal Describing the part nearest the midline or trunk

proxy consent Consent for treatment or research given by a parent or guardian for a child or an incompetent adult.

pseudohypertrophy Enlarged but weak muscle, as found in muscular dystrophy.

pseudomonas A bacterial infection that most commonly causes pneumonia in immuno-compromised patients.

PSR *See* positive support reflex.

psychoeducational Pertaining to the testing of intelligence, academic achievement, and other types of psychological and educational processes.

psychological assessment Incorporates test scores into a broadly based assessment of a child's abilities and functioning; *also called* psychological testing.

psychosis A psychiatric disorder characterized by hallucinations, delusions, loss of contact with reality, and unclear thinking; *adjective*: psychotic.

psychotherapy Nonpharmacological treatment for an individual with an emotional disorder. Various types of psychotherapy range from supportive counseling to psychoanalysis with services usually provided by a psychologist, psychiatrist, or social worker.

ptosis Droopy eyelids.

PTSD *See* posttraumatic stress disorder.

PUBS *See* percutaneous umbilical blood sampling.

pulmonary Pertaining to the lungs.

pulmonary hypertension Increased back pressure in the pulmonary artery leading to decreased oxygenation and right heart failure.

pulmonary vascular obstructive disease This leads to increased back pressure in the arteries that connect the heart to the lungs and results in congestive heart failure.

pulmonary vascular resistance (PVR) Vasoconstriction of the pulmonary blood vessels normally high during fetal life, which should relax immediately upon birth with the first breaths of life.

pulmonary vasodilation Relaxation of the lung's blood vessels soon after birth to establish lung circulation and extinguish fetal circulation.

pulp The soft tissue under the dentin layer in teeth containing blood vessels, lymphatics (lymph vessels), connective tissue, and nerve fibers.

pulse oximeter A device that measures oxygen tension noninvasively.

punishment In behavior management, a procedure or consequence that decreases the frequency of a behavior through the use of a negative stimulus or withdrawal of a preferred activity/object.

pupil The aperture in the center of the iris.

purine A type of organic molecule found in RNA and DNA.

purpuric Bruising indicating bleeding into the skin.

purpuric skin lesions Bruising.

putamen A part of the lentiform nucleus that is lateral to the globus pallidus in the brain. It is associated with the corpus striatum and receives connections from the suppressor centers of the cortex.

PVL *See* periventricular leukomalacia.

PVR *See* pulmonary vascular resistance.

pyloric stenosis A congenital narrowing of the opening from the stomach to the small bowel.

pylorus The sphincter at the junction of the stomach and the duodenum.

pyramidal tract A nerve tract; *also called* the corticospinal tract, leading from the cortex into the spinal column and involved in the control of voluntary motor movement. Damage to this tract results in spasticity, commonly seen in cerebral palsy.

pyridoxine Vitamin B_6.

quadriplegia Paralysis of all four extremities.

quickening The first signs of life felt by the mother as a result of fetal movements in the fourth or fifth month of pregnancy.

rad A measure of radioactivity.

radiograph A medical x ray.

ratio schedules Provision of reinforcement following a set number of correct responses.

real-time ultrasonography The use of sound waves to provide a moving (real-time) image used in fetal monitoring.

rebound A phenomenon in which as a medication dose wears off, a person's behavior or symptoms become worse than when completely off medication.

receptive aphasia Impairment of receptive language due to a disorder of the central nervous system (CNS).

receptive language The cognitive processing involved in comprehending oral, symbolic, or written language.

recessive Pertaining to a trait that is expressed only if the child inherits two copies of the gene; from the Latin word for "hidden."

recti muscles Eye muscles that converge the eyes towards the nose for near activities and diverge the eyes for far ones.

red reflex The reddish-orange reflection from the eye's retina that is observed when using an opthalmoscope or retinoscope.

refracted Bent, toward a focal point.

reframing Reinterpreting a behavior by viewing it from a different lens-frame and focusing on the adaptive and positive aspects rather than negative one.

reinforcer A response to a behavior that increases the likelihood that the behavior will occur in the future.

related services Services (e.g., transportation, occupational and physical therapy) that supplement the special education services provided to a child with a developmental disability.

renal dysplasia Small, abnormal kidneys.

repetitive microtrauma Small injury of lesion that can become problematic if repetitive.

representative payee Often required by programs and services in order to disburse funds to an individual with developmental disabilities.

resonance In linguistics and speech-language pathology, the balance of air flow between the nose and the mouth.

resonance disorders Abnormal amounts of nasality, often caused by structural malformations such as enlarged adenoids and tonsils, or structural anomalies such as a deviated septum.

respiratory technology assistance Medical devices used to replace or augment a vital body function.

response to intervention (RTI) Represents a shift in thinking about students who have difficulty learning at the same rate as their peers. Students with learning difficulties are provided supplementary instruction within general education, with special education being the final rung on the ladder of support. RTI also concerns the diagnosis of students with specific learning disabilities (SLD). RTI was introduced by the Individuals with Disabilities Education Improvement Act of 2004 (IDEA 2004) as an alternate and preferred method for diagnosing children with SLD. It is likely that when IDEA is next reauthorized, RTI will be the only acceptable method for diagnosing SLD.

retina The photosensitive nerve layer that lines the back of the eye, senses light, and creates impulses that travel through the optic nerve to the brain.

retinopathy Disorder of the retina.

retinopathy of prematurity (ROP) A disorder involving abnormal blood vessel development in the retina of the eye in a premature infant. It has been linked to excessive provision of oxygen.

retinoscope An instrument used to detect errors of refraction in the eye.

retro-illumination In split-lamp examination of the eye, it is a method of illuminating a structure by using the light that is reflected by the iris or by a lens containing a cataract.

retrospective payment system Pertaining to a fee-for-service health care model in which payment occurs after services are rendered.

retrovirus The class of viruses that includes human immunodeficiency virus (HIV), the causative agent of acquired immunodeficiency syndrome (AIDS).

Rh incompatibility Condition occurring when an Rh+ baby is born to an Rh– mother. This leads to breakdown of red blood cells in the baby and the excessive release of bilirubin, predisposing the Rh+ baby to kernicterus.

rhabdomyolysis Breakdown of muscle tissue.

rhombencephalon The hindbrain region of the embryo.

ribonucleic acid (RNA) A nucleic acid that is an essential component of all cells, composed of a long, usually single-stranded chain of nucleotide units that contain the sugar ribose. It is essential for protein synthesis within the cell.

ribosome Intracellular structure involved in protein synthesis. It reads the genetic code delivered to it by mRNA.

rickets Bone disease resulting from nutritional deficiency of vitamin D.

rights Moral or legal claims by one party against another.

rigid Pertaining to increased tone marked by stiffness.

ring chromosome A ring-shaped chromosome formed when deletions occur at both tips of a normal chromosome with subsequent fusion of the tips, forming a ring.

RNA *See* ribonucleic acid.

rods Photoreceptor cells of the eye associated with low-light vision.

rolandic epilepsy An inherited benign form of epilepsy occurring in children and characterized by sudden episodes of arrested speech and muscular contractions of the side of the face.

rootlets Small branches of nerve roots.

ROP *See* retinopathy of prematurity.

rostral Anterior pole of the developing embryo.

RTI *See* response to intervention.

rubella A viral infection. Generally causes a mild elevation of temperature and skin rash and resolves in a few days. However, when it occurs in a pregnant woman during the first trimester, it can lead to intrauterine infection and severe birth defects; *also called* German measles.

SAH *See* subarachnoid hemorrhage.

salicylates Chemicals found in many food substances and in aspirin.

saline A salt solution.

sarcomeres The contractile units of the muscle fiber.

Sarnat neurological score The most popular system for grading the severity of hypoxic ischemic encephalopathy (HIE); it ranges from 1 (*mild*) to 3 (*severe*) in neonates.

satiation Having had enough or too much of something.

saturated fatty acid A type of fatty acid in the diet that has been linked to heart disease more frequently than unsaturated fatty acids have been.

scala media Fluid-filled cavity within the cochlea of the ear.

schizencephaly A severely malformed brain with clefts formed because of a neuronal migrational defect during early embryogenesis.

schizophrenia A psychiatric disorder with characteristic psychotic symptoms (i.e., prominent delusions, hallucinations, catatonic behavior, and/or flat affect).

Schlemm's canal The passageway in which the aqueous fluid leaves the eye.

sclera The thick, white nontransparent fibrous covering in the eye.

scoliosis Lateral curvature of the spine.

screening test A test designed to screen for, but not definitively diagnose, a particular condition.

SDH *See* subdural hemorrhage.

seborrheic dermatitis Dandruff.

secondary Occurring as a consequence of a primary disorder.

secondary neurulation A series of events at the lower edge of the neural tube in which the caudal eminence develops into the bottom most segments of the spine and elements of the lower intestine.

second-trimester ultrasonography An ultrasound conducted in the 13th–14th week to test for Down syndrome and other congenital anomalies.

secretin Hormone produced in the duodenum that stimulates secretion of pancreatic enzymes.

seizure threshold Tolerance level of the brain for electrical activity. If level of tolerance is exceeded, a seizure occurs.

selective serotonin reuptake inhibitors (SSRIs) Commonly used medications for treatment of depression and anxiety. They act by decreasing reuptake of serotonin from the synaptic cleft, resulting in more serotonin being available for neurotransmission.

selective vulnerability Refers to a susceptibility of specific regions and cells to injury.

self-injurious behavior (SIB) or aggressions The intentional, direct injuring of body tissue most often done without suicidal intentions.

semantics The study of and conventions governing meanings of words.

sensorineural Involving the cochlea or auditory nerve.

sensory integration (SI) therapy Therapy that uses controlled sensory stimulation combined with a meaningful adaptive response to achieve changes in learning and behavior. A common method used in occupational therapy.

separation anxiety Excessive concern about separation, usually of mother from child (e.g., school phobia).

sepsis Infection that has spread throughout the bloodstream and can be life threatening; *also called* blood poisoning.

sequential modification If desired changes in behavior are not observed to occur across settings and behaviors, concrete steps are taken to introduce the effective intervention (e.g., positive reinforcement) to each of the behaviors or settings to which transfer of effects is inadequate.

serotonin reuptake inhibitors A group of psychoactive drugs, an example being fluoxetine (Prozac) used to treat depression.

serum *See* plasma.

sex chromosomes The X and Y chromosomes that determine gender.

sex-linked trait *See* X-linked trait.

SGA *See* small for gestational age.

shadowing Technique in which the instructor keeps his or her hands within an inch of the child's hands as the child proceeds to complete the task.

shared decision making Patient or proxy and physician participate together in committing to a treatment decision.

SI therapy *See* sensory integration therapy.

SIB *See* self-injurious behavior or aggressions.

SIDS *See* sudden infant death syndrome.

silent stroke A stroke without any outward symptoms.

single nucleotide polymorphisms (SNPs) DNA sequence variations in the population.

single photon emission computed tomography (SPECT) An imaging technique that permits the study of the metabolism of a body organ, most commonly the brain.

single-gene defect A mutation or error in a single gene leads to disease. Examples include sickle-cell disease and phenylketonuria.

sleep apnea Brief periods of arrested breathing during sleep, most commonly found in premature infants and in older children and adults with morbid obesity.

sleep myoclonus Sudden jerking movements of the body associated with various sleep stages that may be confused with a seizure.

small for gestational age (SGA) Refers to a newborn whose weight is below the third percentile for gestational age; prematurely born infants.

SNPs *See* single nucleotide polymorphisms.

social-negative reinforcement The removal of some unwanted or aversive event contingent on a behavior may also result in strengthening of that behavior and may take the form of escape or avoidance from the unwanted event.

social-positive reinforcement Events or stimuli that follow the occurrence of a behavior may function to strengthen that behavior.

soft neurological signs A group of neurological findings that are normal in young children, but when found in older children suggest immaturities in central nervous system (CNS) development (i.e., difficulty performing sequential finger–thumb opposition, rapid alternating movements).

soft spot *See* anterior fontanelle.

somatic Relating to the body.

somatic nervous system (SNS) Part of the peripheral nervous system associated with the voluntary control of body movements via skeletal muscles and with sensory reception of touch, hearing, and sight.

spastic Pertaining to increased muscle tone in which muscles are stiff and movements are difficult; caused by damage to the pyramidal tract in the brain.

spastic diplegia A form of cerebral palsy primarily seen in former premature infants that is manifested as spasticity of both lower extremities with only mild involvement of upper extremities.

spastic hemiplegia A form of cerebral palsy in which one side of the body demonstrates spasticity and the other side is unaffected.

spastic hypertonicity Increased muscle tone and a positive Babinski response, two of the hallmark features of spastic cerebral palsy.

spastic quadriplegia A form of cerebral palsy in which all four limbs are affected. Increased muscle tone (i.e., spasticity) is caused by damage to the pyramidal tract in the brain.

spasticity Abnormally increased muscle tone.

speaking valve A valve that can be used by children who have tracheostomy tubes to permit vocalizations.

specific language impairment A significant deficit in linguistic functioning that does not appear to be accompanied by deficits in hearing, intelligence, or motor functioning.

specific learning disability Includes disorders that affect the ability to understand or use spoken or written language; it may manifest in difficulties with listening, thinking, speaking, reading, writing, spelling, and/or doing mathematical calculations.

SPECT *See* single photon emission computed tomography.

spectrum of developmental disabilities The various neurological disorders that result from abnormalities in cognitive, motor, and neurobehavioral function.

speech and language disorders Problems in communication and related areas such as oral-motor function.

splenomegaly Enlarged spleen.

spermatocytes Sperm.

spina bifida A developmental defect of the spine, a neural tube defect; *also called* spinal dysraphism.

spina bifida occulta Generally benign congenital defect of the spinal column not associated with protrusion of the spinal cord or meninges; the most common neural tube defect.

spinal braces A form of low-tech assistive device to children with cerebral palsy or neuromuscular disorder.

spinal cord The thick, whitish cord of nerve tissue that extends from the base of the brain down through the spinal column.

spinal dysraphism *See* spinal bifida.

spinal muscular atrophy Congenital neuromuscular disorder of childhood associated with progressive muscle weakness.

spinal tap *See* lumbar puncture.

spindle In mitosis and meiosis, a weblike figure along which the chromosomes are distributed.

spondyloepipheseal dysplasia Congenital structural abnormality of vertebral column caused by a lack of mineralization of bone.

spontaneous recovery In behavior management, the recurrence of an undesirable behavior after it has been extinguished.

sporadic In genetics, describing a disease that occurs by chance and carries little risk of recurrence.

SSRIs *See* selective serotonin reuptake inhibitors.

standardized rating scales Questionnaires concerning specific behaviors that have been completed for large samples of children so that norms and normal degrees of variation are known.

stapes One of the three small bones in the middle ear, collectively called the ossicles, that help amplify sound.

staphylococcus aureus The bacteria resulting in Staph infections such as cellulitis.

static encephalopathy Is characterized by significantly delayed development, with the acquisition of new skills at a slower rate than is typical.

static Unchanging.

status epilepticus A seizure lasting more than 30 minutes.

stenosis An abnormal narrowing.

stereotypic movement disorder Disorder characterized by recurring purposeless but voluntary movements (e.g., hand flapping in children with autism); *also called* stereotypies.

stereotypies *See* stereotypic movement disorder.

steroids 1) Medications used to treat severe inflammatory diseases and infantile spasms; 2) certain natural hormones in the body.

stimulant Medication used to treat attention-deficit/hyperactivity disorder (e.g., methylphenidate).

stomach flu *See* gastroenteritis.

strabismus Deviation of one or both eyes during forward gaze; the loss of this coordinated movement leads to misalignment of the eye; crossed eyes.

subacute progressive encephalopathy Characterized by a gradual and insidious loss of previously obtained cognitive and motor milestones.

subarachnoid Beneath the arachnoid membrane, or middle layer, of the meninges.

subarachnoid hemorrhage (SAH) Hemorrhage into the fluid-filled space between the arachnoid membrane and the underlying brain that can compress or contuse the underlying brain.

subdural Resting between the outer (dural) and middle (arachnoid) layers of the meninges.

subdural hematoma Localized collection of clotted blood lying in the space between the dural and arachnoid membranes that surround the brain. This results from bleeding of the cerebral blood vessels that rest between these two membranes.

subdural hemorrhage (SDH) Hemorrhage between the tough outer membrane (dura) and the meninges surrounding the brain and spinal cord that can compress or contuse the underlying brain.

subluxation Partial dislocation.

submucosal A supporting layer of loose connective tissue directly under a mucous membrane, (i.e., below the palate).

substrate A compound acted upon by an enzyme in a chemical reaction.

sucrose *See* glucose.

sudden infant death syndrome (SIDS) Diagnosis given to a previously well infant (often a former premature baby) who is found lifeless in bed without apparent cause; *also called* crib death.

sulci Furrows of the brain; *singular:* sulcus.

superior In anatomy, above.

supine Lying on the back, face upward.

supported employment Defined by the Rehabilitation Act Amendments of 1986 (PL 99-506) and 1992 (PL 102-569) as employment in an inclusive setting with ongoing support services for an individual with a disability.

suppository Small solid body shaped for ready introduction into one of the orifaces of the body other than the oral cavity such as the rectrum, urethra, or vagina.

surfactant A lipoprotein normally secreted into the alveoli with the first breaths of life that acts like a soap bubble and allows for a significant decrease in the alveolar membrane's surface tension, thus making breathing much easier and the lungs much more flexible immediately after birth.

surveillance The ongoing monitoring of disease in the population.

surveillance devices Devices such as cardiorespiratory monitors, and pulse oximeters.

sutures In anatomy, the fibrous joints between certain bones (e.g., skull bones).

synapses The minute spaces separating one neuron from another. Neurochemicals breach this gap.

syncopal episode Fainting spell.

syndactyly Webbed hands or feet.

synophrys Confluent eyebrows.

syntax Word order.

syphilis A sexually transmitted disease that can cause an intrauterine infection in pregnant women and result in severe birth defects.

syringomas Benign sweat glad tumors.

syringomyelia A chronic disease of the spinal cord characterized by the presence of fluid.

syrinx A pathological tube-shaped cavity in the spinal cord.

systemic Involving the body as a whole.

T cell lymphocyte population White blood cells responsible for recognizing and chemically encoding into immunologic memory any foreign bacterial substances.

tachycardia Rapid heart rate.

tachypnea Rapid breathing.

talipes equinovarus *See* clubfoot.

tandem mass spectrometer (MS/MS) A machine that separates and quantifies ions based on their mass-to-charge ratio. It is used in newborn screening to detect a number of inborn errors of metabolism.

tangential migration Cells migrate parallel to the surface of the brain and perpendicular to the radial glia.

tangibles Rewards given in positive reinforcement procedures (e.g., food, toys).

tardive dyskinesia A potentially severe movement disorder resulting from the long-term use of phenothiazines or other antipsychotic medication.

target behaviors Behaviors selected for assessment and management.

tartar *See* calculus.

TCD *See* transcranial Doppler.

telangiectasia Abnormal cluster of small blood vessels.

telehealth Electronic and video-based communication.

teletypewriter (TTY) An electronic device for text communication via a telephone line used when one or more of the parties has hearing or speech difficulties.

telophase The final phase in cell division in which the daughter chromosomes are at the opposite poles of the cell and new nuclear membranes form.

temporal lobe Brain region involved in visual and auditory processing. The area of the cortex primarily involved in communication and sensation.

tendons Fibrous cords by which muscles are attached to bone or to one another.

teratogens Agents that can cause malformations in a developing embryo.

testosterone Male sex hormone.

tethered Tied down.

tetraploid Having four copies of each chromosome (i.e., 92 chromosomes). This is incompatible with life.

thalamus Region of the brain situated in the posterior part of the forebrain that relays sensory impulses to the cerebral cortex.

thickening agents Can transform any thin liquid into a nectar, honey, or milkshake-like consistency.

thimerosal A mercury-containing organic compound that was used as a preservative in vaccines.

thoracolumbar kyphosis Curvature of the mid-lower spine in the front to back plane.

thrombocytopenia Low platelet count.

thrombophilia A genetic tendency for one's blood to clot more than normal.

thrush Monilial (fungal) yeast infection of the oral cavity sometimes seen in infants.

thymine One of the four nucleotides (chemicals) that comprise DNA.

thymus A gland in the chest which plays a key role in regulating immune responses.

thyrotoxicosis A form of hyperthyroidism leading to severe symptoms.

tics Brief repetitive movements or vocalizations that occur in a stereotyped manner and do not appear to be under voluntary control.

time-in A behavioral procedure which dramatically increases pleasant social and physical contact between the child and caregiver.

time-out A procedure whereby the possibility of positive reinforcement is withdrawn for a brief amount of time following the occurrence of a targeted challenging behavior.

TLR *See* tonic labyrinthine reflex.

tocolysis Use of medications to stop preterm labor.

Todd's paralysis Reversible weakness of one side of the body following a seizure.

tonic labyrinthine reflex (TLR) Primitive reflex in which the infant retracts the arms and extends the legs when the neck is tilted backwards, stimulating the labyrinth; *also called* tonic labyrinthine response.

tonic-clonic Spasmodic alteration of muscle contraction and relaxation.

tonotopically Arranged spatially by tone as found in the cochlea of the inner ear.

tooth bud *See* dental organ.

torticollis Wry neck in which the neck is painfully tilted to one side; a form of dystonia.

toxemia *See* preeclampsia.

toxoplasma gondii Microorganism causing toxoplasmosis.

toxoplasmosis An infectious disease caused by a microorganism, which may be asymptomatic in adults but can lead to severe fetal malformations.

trachea Windpipe.

tracheal intubation Introducing a tube into the airway to facilitate breathing.

tracheoesophageal fistula A congenital connection between the trachea and esophagus leading to aspiration of food and requiring surgical correction.

tracheomalacia Softening of the cartilage of the trachea.

tracheostomy The surgical creation of an opening into the trachea to permit insertion of a tube to facilitate mechanical ventilation.

tracheostomy tube A catheter that is inserted into the trachea for the purpose of supplying air to a blocked airway.

trachoma A bacterial infection causing blindness in developing countries.

transcranial Doppler (TCD) An instrument that emits ultrasonic beams to diagnose vascular disease in the head.

transcription The process in which mRNA is formed from a DNA template.

transition individualized education program (transition IEP) A written plan for an adolescent receiving special education services that maps out his or her postschool education, services, and employment and adult living goals. It is required by federal law (IDEA, 2004) to be part of the student's individualized education program (IEP) starting at age 16; *previously called* individualized transition plan (ITP).

transitional (fetal) circulation Circulatory changes occurring at birth in the lungs and around the heart, resulting from pulmonary vasodilation and closure of the ductus arteriosus and the foramen ovale (the two fetal bypasses around the lungs during fetal life).

translation A process where the mRNA moves out of the nucleus into the cytoplasm, where it provides instructions for the production of a protein.

translocation The transfer of a fragment of one chromosome to another chromosome.

tremor A trembling motion.

treponema pallium Microorganism causing syphilis.

trichotillomania Hair-pulling disorder.

triplet repeat expansion Abnormal number of copies of identical triplet nucleotides (as occurs in fragile X syndrome; *see Chapter 1*).

triploid Having three copies of each chromosome (i.e., 69 chromosomes), which is generally incompatible with life.

trisomy A condition is which there are three copies of one chromosome rather than two (e.g., trisomy 21, Down syndrome).

trochlear nerve The fourth cranial nerve controls the superior oblique eye muscle.

trophoblast The outermost layer of cells that attaches the fertilized egg to the uterine wall.

TTY *See* teletypewriter.

tubers Benign growths found in the brain of an individual with tuberous sclerosis.

twinning The production of twins.

tympanometry The measurement of flexibility of the tympanic membrane as an indicator of a middle-ear infection or fluid in the middle ear.

tympanostomy A small tube inserted through the tympanic membrane after myringotomy to aerate the middle ear; often used in the treatment of recurrent or persistent otitis media (middle ear infection).

tyrosine An amino acid.

UES *See* upper esophageal sphincter.

umbilical cord prolapse The umbilical cord being born before rather than after the baby, thereby becoming compressed by the fetus during the delivery process and interfering with oxygen flow to the fetus during labor; typically occurs with polyhydramnios.

undernutrition Inadequate nutrition to sustain normal growth.

uniparental disomy *See* genomic imprinting.

unsaturated fatty acid A type of dietary fat, certain kinds of which have been linked to heart disease.

upper esophageal sphincter (UES) A muscle at the entrance to the esophagus.

urea End product of protein metabolism.

uremia The abnormal accumulation of urinary waste products in the blood present in renal (kidney) failure.

ureterostomy Surgical procedure creating an outlet for the ureters through the abdominal wall.

urethra Canal through which urine passes from the bladder.

urodynamics A test that accesses how the bladder and urethra are performing their job of storing and releasing urine.

valgus Condition in which the distal body part is angled away from the mid-line.

varicella The virus that causes chickenpox and shingles.

varus Condition in which the distal body part is angled toward the mid-line.

vasoconstriction A decrease in the diameter of blood vessels.

vasodilation Relaxation and dilation of blood vessels.

vaso-occlusive episode In sickle-cell disease, the sudden restriction of blood flow due to sickle shaped cells blocking capillaries.

ventilator A machine that provides a mixture of air and oxygen to an individual in respiratory failure.

ventral Front.

ventral induction Describes development of the prosencephalon, its division into two sections, the telencephalon and diencephalon, and cleavage of the telencephalon into two cerebral hemispheres.

ventricles Fluid filled cavities, especially in the heart or brain.

ventricular septal defect A congenital heart defect in which the wall separating the two lower chambers of the heart does not close during embryonic development.

ventricular system Interconnecting cavities of the brain containing cerebrospinal fluid.

ventriculoperitoneal shunt (VP shunt) Tube connecting a cerebral ventricle with the abdominal cavity; used to treat hydrocephalus by draining cerebrospinal fluid into the child's abdominal cavity.

ventriculo-subgaleal shunt Implanted as a temporary measure for treatment of hydrocephalus, draining cerebrospinal fluid from the ventricles to the scalp.

vertebral arches The bony arches projecting from the body of the vertebra.

vertex presentation Downward position of infant's head during vaginal delivery.

vertical transmission Mother to child transmission of infection, especially in HIV.

very low birth weight (VLBW) Term often used to describe an infant with a birth weight less than 1,500 grams (3⅓ pounds).

vesicles Small bladder-like cavities containing specific chemicals (neurotransmitters) that are released from the axon of a neuron.

vesicostomy The surgical creation of an opening for the bladder to empty its contents through the abdominal wall.

vestibular system Three ring-shaped bodies located in the labyrinth of the ear that are involved in maintenance of balance and sensation of the body's movement through space.

villi Vascular projections, such as those coming from the embryo that become part of the placenta; *singular:* villus.

visceral Relating to the soft internal organs of the body, especially those contained within the abdominal and thoracic cavities.

vision impairment A condition characterized by a loss of visual acuity, where the eye does not see objects as clearly as usual, or a loss of visual field, where the eye cannot see as wide an area as usual without moving the eyes or turning the head.

vitiligo A skin disease marked by patches of lack of pigment.

vitreous humor The gelatinous content of the eye located between the lens and retina.

VLBW *See* very low birth weight.

volunteering An opportunity for adolescents to gain valuable insight into the world of work, to develop skills, and to build work-related experience.

VP shunt *See* ventriculoperitoneal shunt.

watershed area Area of tissue lying between two major arteries and thus poorly supplied by blood.

watershed infarct Injury to brain due to lack of blood flow in the brain tissues between interfacing blood vessels.

work-study employment Part-time work for students sanctioned by the school either on or off campus.

xerosis Dryness of eyes.

xerostomia Dry mouth.

X-linked trait A trait transmitted by a gene located on the X chromosome; *previously called* sex-linked.

zygote Fertilized egg.

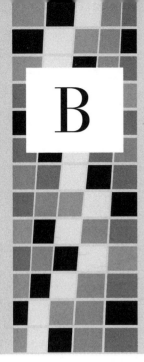

B Syndromes and Inborn Errors of Metabolism

Kara L. Simpson

The underlying cause of a developmental disability can be explained in some children by a single genetic or teratogenic mechanism. An understanding of the etiology can shed light on the reason for clinical features such as physical malformations, cognitive impairments, and behavior problems. Making a diagnosis in such cases may be important for physicians to implement appropriate medical management or to provide genetic or prenatal counseling. Other professionals may also find that a diagnosis assists them in the development of more global aspects of the child's care, including educational, physical, occupational, and speech-language therapy. The direct benefit to families includes the ability to gather information specific to their child's condition and to seek out support from other parents and/or affected individuals through support groups, conferences, and the Internet. Finally, attaining a specific diagnosis can lead patients, families, and health-care professionals to the appropriate disease-oriented organization, which is often a great source of information and support (not just medical, but emotional and sometimes financial as well). For all of these reasons, the search for an etiology of a child's developmental disability may focus on syndrome identification.

By definition, a *syndrome* is a recurring, recognizable pattern of structural defects and/or secondary effects that represents a single etiology. Syndromes may have a genetic basis (chromosomal, single gene defects; see Chapter 1), can be environmental (teratogens; see Chapter 3), or can be complex (caused by more than one genetic and/or environmental

factor). Genetic syndromes affect multiple organ systems because the genetic defect is usually contained in every cell of the body. This abnormality may interfere with typical development or cause abnormal differentiation of more than one tissue of the body. Most genetic and teratogenic syndromes are of prenatal onset and are evident at birth, usually because of an unusual appearance (i.e., dysmorphic features) or multiple congenital abnormalities. Syndromes are usually stable conditions, and neurological regression is uncommon. A *sequence* is a situation where a single event leads to a single anomaly which has a cascading effect of local and/or distant deformations and/or disruptions. An *association* is a nonrandom occurrence of anomalies with no consistent etiology.

Unlike most syndromes, *inborn errors of metabolism* are usually not evident at birth. During pregnancy, the mother's normal metabolism usually protects the fetus. After delivery, however, there may be an accumulation of toxic metabolites as a result of an enzyme deficiency. The presentation of inborn errors varies from metabolic crisis and death within days of birth to occasional episodes in response to external factors later in childhood. Some metabolic disorders are treatable, and many in this category of genetic conditions are detectable with newborn screening through biochemical or molecular testing (see Chapters 5 and 19). Others, despite early diagnosis and treatment, still lead to irreversible effects.

Although the clinical features associated with certain syndromes and inborn errors of metabolism have been known for centuries (e.g., Down syndrome, congenital hypothyroidism), the chromosomal and molecular basis of the disorders have only been characterized since the 1960s. An increasing number of genetic and biochemical tests can now be utilized to confirm a clinically suspected diagnosis. This is of particular importance because different therapeutic options (or the opportunity to participate in clinical research trials) may be available to individuals on the basis of a genetic diagnosis, particularly in the cases of molecularly based therapies. In addition, a genetic diagnosis allows for accurate recurrence risk estimates and appropriate genetic counseling for other family members.

Diagnostic testing in patients with developmental delay, intellectual disability, congenital anomalies, and dysmorphic features has evolved significantly in the last several years with the addition of the popular cytogenetic microarrays based on comparative genomic hybridization (CGH) and single nucleotide polymorphism (SNP) array analyses. With the array CGH, copy number variants (CNVs) are determined by comparing the hybridization pattern intensities between a patient's DNA and control DNA. Microarrays are generally limited by the length and spacing between probes but this resolution has continued to increase, allowing for the identification of chromosomal imbalances with greater precision and accuracy. The appeal of microarrays is especially great in those patients with no clear syndrome pattern. However, it should be noted that microarray reports are frequently not straightforward and often contain changes of unknown significance. It is recommended that the ordering of microarrays be done by geneticists as they have the appropriate resources to explain the results and consequences to patients. (See Manning, M., & Hudgins, L. [2010]. Array-based technology and recommendations for utilization in medical genetics practice for detection of chromosomal abnormalities. *Genetics in Medicine, 12*(11), 742–745.)

Research on the cognitive abilities of individuals with genetic syndromes is uncovering specific learning and behavior patterns for many syndromes. These are called behavioral phenotypes, and they can be used to establish rational and attainable educational goals to promote a child reaching his or her full cognitive and functional potential. (Behavioral phenotypes in neurogenetic syndromes. [2010]. *American Journal of Medical Genetics Part C: Seminars in Medical Genetics, 154C*(4), 387–485).

Insight into an individual's specific condition, the behavioral phenotype, cognitive abilities, and learning strengths and weakness can be of particular importance in the classroom. References addressing the cognitive and behavioral abilities of individuals with specific genetic conditions are included in this appendix.

Many excellent resources concerning genetic conditions exist for families and health care professionals caring for children with disabilities. Some useful ones include the following

- **The Genetic Alliance** is a nonprofit organization with a directory of support groups, foundations, research organizations, patient advocacy groups, and tissue registries. The Genetic Alliance is based in Washington, D.C. (202-966-5557; http://www.geneticalliance.org; e-mail: info@geneticalliance.org).

- **GeneTests** (http://ncbi.nlm.nih.gov/sites/GeneTests) GeneTests is administered by the University of Washington and funded by the National Institutes of Health (NIH), the Health Resources and Services Administration (HRSA), and the U.S. Department of Energy (DOE). GeneTests has a directory of clinics and laboratories that provide genetic testing. In addition, some educational tools for professionals are available. Also within GeneTests is GeneReviews, which provides peer-reviewed articles on genetic conditions that include information on diagnosis, management, and genetic counseling of individuals with specific inherited disorders and their families. It also provides relevant resources specific to each disease.

- **The National Organization for Rare Disorders** (NORD; 203-744-0100; toll free: 800-999-6673 [voicemail only]; http://www.rarediseases.org) is a nonprofit patient advocacy organization dedicated to orphan diseases (disorders occurring in less than 200,000 individuals in the United States). NORD provides information about diseases, referrals to patient organizations, research grants and fellowships, advocacy for the rare-disease community, and medication assistance programs.

- **The Online Mendelian Inheritance in Man** (OMIM; http://www.ncbi.nlm.nih.gov/omim) catalog describes all known Mendelian disorders and over 12,000 genes, providing clinical, biochemical, genetic, and therapeutic information. OMIM is authored and edited at the McKusick-Nathans Institute of Genetic Medicine, Johns Hopkins University School of Medicine.

- **The National Coalition for Health Professionals Education in Genetics** (NCHPEG; http://www.nchpeg.org) is committed to a national effort to promote health professional education and access to information about advances in human genetics. The NCHPEG web site offers targeted web-based educational programs for a variety of professionals including dieticians and nutritionists, physician assistants, genetic counselors, speech-language pathologists and audiologists, and dentists. They also have tools to aid in family history-taking and general core competencies in genetics.

- **The Genetics Home Reference**, sponsored by the U.S. National Library of Medicine (http://ghr.nlm.nih.gov/), is an excellent resource for health care professionals, teachers, and families, providing basic information about genetics and searchable disease-specific data.

HOW ENTRIES ARE ORGANIZED

This appendix lists a number of syndromes and inborn errors of metabolism that are often associated with developmental disabilities. Included in each listing are the disease category, principal characteristics, pattern of inheritance, frequency of occurrence (prevalence or incidence), treatment options when available, and recent references that further define the syndrome. Cognitive and behavioral changes are noted for disorders in which common developmental abnormalities are widely accepted as being part of the syndrome or inborn error. When known, the causative gene or chromosome location is listed. In describing the chromosomal location, the first number or letter indicates the chromosome on which there is a genetic change (mutation), and the subsequent letter (*p* or *q*) indicates the short or long arm of the chromosome, respectively. The term *ter* is used when the site is at the terminal end of one arm of the chromosome, and *cen* is used when the site is near the **centromere**. The numbers following the *p* or *q* specify the location on the chromosome. For example, Aarskog-Scott syndrome is located on the short arm of the X chromosome at position 11.21, designated as Xp11.21. The inheritance patterns of genetic traits are listed as autosomal recessive (AR), autosomal

dominant (AD), X-linked recessive (XLR), X-linked dominant (XLD), mitochondrial (M), new mutation (NM; i.e., diseases caused by new mutations that arise in the sperm or the egg), or sporadic (SP; i.e., noninherited). Each syndrome has been assigned to a disease category which is defined next. Although this appendix lists a number of the more commonly recognized syndromes associated with developmental disabilities, it is not intended to be all inclusive. Specific medical terminology is defined in the Glossary (see Appendix A).

DISEASE CATEGORIES

auditory disorders Diseases that affect hearing.

chromosome abnormality Disorder due to a duplication, loss, or rearrangement of chromosomal material.

chromosome breakage syndrome Syndromes associated with increased rates of chromosomal breakage or instability due to defects in DNA repair mechanisms or genomic instability which leads to chromosomal rearrangements.

connective tissue disorders Disorders that affect the connective tissue, the tissue that helps support, binds together, and protects organs.

contiguous gene defect A disorder due to deletion of multiple genes that are adjacent to one another.

endocrine disorder Disorders affecting the endocrine systems glands and secretions (hormones).

inborn error of metabolism Genetic disorders that disrupt metabolism. Most are due to defects of single genes that code for enzymes that break down substrates. Each inborn error of metabolism has been categorized based on the main type of metabolism affected (e.g., carbohydrate, amino acid, organic acid, lysosomal storage disease, copper).

imprinting defect Group of disorders where there is a defect in the process of genomic imprinting (where certain alleles are expressed based on the parent of origin).

malformation Birth defect that results from intrinsic defects in genes that control development.

multiple congenital anomalies Structural defects that are present at birth and affect multiple structures and organs.

neurological disorders Disorders mainly affecting the brain, spinal cord, and nerves.

neuromuscular disease Diseases that affect the muscles and/or the nerves that control them.

ophthalmologic disorders Diseases that affect the eye.

overgrowth syndromes Disorders in which there is an abnormal increase in the size of the body or of a specific body part.

peroxisomal disorders A group of disorders caused by a deficiency in enzymes within the peroxisome (an organelle involved in metabolism of very long chain fatty acids, biosynthesis of plasmalogens, and energy metabolism), or proteins encoded by genes for normal peroxisome assembly.

skeletal dysplasia A group of disorders characterized by abnormalities of bone and cartilage.

SYNDROMES AND DISORDERS

Aarskog-Scott syndrome (facio-digito-genital dysplasia) *Disease category:* Multiple congenital anomalies. *Clinical features:* Short stature, brachydactyly (short fingers and toes), widow's peak, broad nasal bridge with small nose, hypertelorism, shawl scrotum, cryptorchidism (undescended testes); learning disabilities and behavioral problems are present in a subset of patients. *Associated complications:* Ptosis, eye movement problems, strabismus, orthodontic problems, occasional cleft lip/ palate. *Cause:* Mutations in the *FGD1* gene at Xp11.21. *Inheritance:* XLR with partial expression in some females. *Prevalence:* Unknown, phenotypic overlap with other conditions.
References: Kaname, T., Yanagi, K., Okamoto, N., & Naritomi, K (2006). Neurobehavioral disorders in patients with Aarskog-Scott syndrome with novel *FGD1* mutations. *American Journal of Medical Genetics Part A, 140*(12), 1331–1332.
Orrico, A., Faivre L., Clayton-Smith, J., Azzarello-Burri, S.M., Hertz J.M ... Jacquemont, S. (2010). Aarskog–Scott syndrome: Clinical update and report of nine novel mutations of the *FGD1* gene. *American Journal of Medical Genetics Part A, 152A*, 313–318.
Taub, M., & Stanton, A. (2008). Aarskog syndrome: A case report and literature review. *Optometry, 79*(7), 371–377.

achondroplasia *Disease category:* Skeletal dysplasia. *Clinical features:* The most common form of short stature, associated with rhizomelic (proximal) shortening of the arms and legs, large head with typical facial features including frontal bossing and midface hypoplasia, genu varum (bow legs), and trident appearance of the hands. Hypotonia and motor delay is common. Cognitive development and life span are usually normal, although cervical spinal cord compression and upper airway obstruction increases risk of death in infancy. Children with achondroplasia should be monitored for changes in their neurological status, particularly if there are concerns about delayed motor development. *Prevalence:* Varied reports of 1:15,000 to 1:25,000 live births. *Cause:* 98% of affected individuals have a common point mutation in the gene coding for fibroblast growth factor receptor 3 (*FGFR3*). *Inheritance:* AD although 80% of cases are caused by NM.
References: Horton, W.A., Hall, J.G., & Hecht, J.T. (2007). Achondroplasia. *Lancet, 370*, 162–172.
Trotter, T.L., & Hall, J.G. (2005). Health supervision for children with achondroplasia. *Pediatrics, 116*, 771–783.
Wynn, J., King, T.M., Gambello, M.J., Waller, D.K., & Hecht, J.T. (2007). Mortality in achondroplasia study: A 42-year follow-up. *American Journal of Medical Genetics Part A, 143A*, 2502–2511.

acrocephalosyndactyly, type I *See* Apert syndrome.

acrocephalosyndactyly, type II *See* Carpenter syndrome.

acrocephalosyndactyly, type V *See* Pfeiffer syndrome.

acrofacial dysostosis (Nager syndrome) *Disease category:* Multiple congenital anomalies. *Clinical features:* Micrognathia (small jaw), malar hypoplasia (underdeveloped cheeks), downward slant of eyelids, high nasal bridge, external ear defects, occasional cleft lip/palate, asymmetric limb anomalies (hypoplastic thumb or radius [a bone in the lower arm]). *Associated complications:* Scoliosis, severe conductive hearing loss, occasional heart or kidney defects, intellectual disability present in 16%. *Cause:* Current candidate gene is ZFP37 linked to chromosome 9q32. *Inheritance:* Most cases NM with evidence of AD inheritance, rare reports of AR. *Prevalence:* Rare.
References: Dreyer, S.D., Zhou, L, Machado, M.A., Horton, W.A., Zabel, B., Winterpacht, A., & Lee, B. (1998). Cloning, characterization, and chromosomal assignment of the human ortholog of murine *Zfp-37*, a candidate gene for Nager syndrome. *Mammalian Genome, 9*, 458–462.

Hunt, J.A., & Hobar, P.C. (2002). Common craniofacial anomalies: The facial dysostoses. *Plastic and Reconstructive Surgery, 110,* 1714–1726.

Herrman, B., Karzon, R., & Molter, D.W. (2005). Otologic and audiologic features of Nager acrofacial dysostosis. *International Journal of Pediatric Otorhinolaryngology, 69,* 1053–1059.

McDonald, J.T., & Gorski, J.L. (1993). Nager acrofacial dysostosis. *Journal of Medical Genetics, 30,* 779–782.

adrenoleukodystrophy (X-linked ALD)

Disease category: Neuromuscular disease. (*For neonatal form, see* adrenoleukodystrophy, neonatal form.) *Clinical features:* Progressive neurological disorder of white matter resulting from accumulation of very long chain fatty acids; three main phenotypes are seen in affected males. Those with the childhood cerebral form develop normally until between the ages of 4 and 8. Symptoms initially resemble attention deficit disorder or hyperactivity. Impairment of cognition, behavior, vision, hearing, and motor function develop following initial symptoms and lead to total disability within 2 years. A second phenotype called adrenomyeloneuropathy (AMN) manifests most commonly in the late twenties as progressive paraparesis (paralysis), sphincter disturbances, sexual dysfunction, and often, impaired adrenocortical function. The third phenotype is known as "Addison disease only" and presents with primary adrenocortical insufficiency between age 2 and adulthood without evidence of neurologic abnormality (but can develop later). *Associated complications:* Progressive intellectual deterioration, seizures, endocrine abnormalities, conductive hearing loss. *Cause:* Mutations in *ABCD1* gene at Xq28. The ALD protein product is localized to the peroxisomal membrane. *Inheritance:* XLR, with intrafamilial variability ranging from classical childhood-onset ALD to adult-onset ALD to Addison disease. 93% of affected individuals inherit the *ABCD1* mutation from one parent; 7% from NM. Approximately 20% of females who are carriers develop neurologic manifestations that resemble AMN but have later onset and milder disease than affected males. *Prevalence:* 1:20,000–1:50,000. *Treatment:* Corticosteroid replacement therapy for adrenal insufficiency (will not alter neurologic symptoms). Bone marrow transplant can provide long-term stability and may reverse some neurologic complications in the early stages. Dietary modifications including "Lorenzo's oil" (oleic acid and erucic acid) have been shown to lower VLCFA levels but clinical effects are still under investigation.

References: Berger, J., Pujol, A., Aubourg, P., & Forss-Petter, S. (2010). Current and future pharmacological treatment strategies in x-linked adrenoleukodystrophy.

Cartier, N., & Aubourg, P. (2010). Hematopoietic stem cell transplantation and hematopoietic stem cell gene therapy in X-linked adrenoleukodystrophy. *Brain Pathology, 20*(4), 857–62.

Ferrer, I., Aubourg, P., & Pujol, A. (2010). General aspects and neuropathology of x-linked adrenoleukodystrophy. *Brain Pathology, 20*(4), 817–830.

Kaga, M., Furushima, W., Inagaki, M., & Nakamura, M. (2009). Early neuropsychological signs of childhood adrenoleukodystrophy (ALD). *Brain & Development, 31,* 558–561.

adrenoleukodystrophy, neonatal form (NALD)

Disease category: Peroxisomal disorder (*For childhood form, see* adrenoleukodystrophy [X-linked ALD].) *Clinical features:* A disorder of peroxisome biogenesis and an intermediate presentation of the Zellweger syndrome spectrum. Peroxisomes are minute organelles in certain cells that are involved in the processing of long chain fatty acids. NALD can present in the neonatal period but generally manifests later in childhood because of developmental delays, hearing loss, or visual impairment. The condition is slowly progressive, and hearing and vision worsen with time. Some individuals may develop progressive degeneration of myelin, a leukodystrophy, which may lead to loss of previously acquired skills and eventually death. *Associated complications:* Intellectual disability, cataracts, visual and auditory impairment, liver dysfunction, hypotonia, and hemorrhage/intracranial bleeding. *Cause:* Mutations in twelve different *PEX* genes resulting in absence of peroxisomes have been identified. *Inheritance:* AR. *Prevalence:* 1 in 50,000 with variation among populations.

References: Ebberink, M., Kofster, J., Wanders, R.J., & Waterham, H.R. (2010). Spectrum of *PWX6* mutations in Zellweger syndrome spectrum patients. *Human Mutation, 31,* E1058–E1070.

Wanders, R.J.A., & Waterham, H.R. (2005). Peroxisomal disorders I: Biochemistry and genetics of peroxisome biogenesis disorders. *Clinical Genetics, 67*(2), 107–133.

Aicardi syndrome *Disease category:* Neurologic. *Clinical features:* Infantile spasms, agenesis (absence) of the corpus callosum, and abnormalities of eyes (specifically chorioretinal lacunae. *Associated complications:* Poorly controlled seizures, visual impairment, cortical malformations, vertebral and rib abnormalities, vascular malformations or malignancy, micropthalmia, hypotonia, microcephaly, moderate to severe intellectual disability. Survival varies, but mean age of death is about 8.3 years and median age of death is about 18.5 years. *Cause:* No gene or candidate region on the X chromosome has been definitively identified. *Inheritance:* XLD/NM; previously it has been assumed that mutations are lethal in males as Aicardi syndrome has been seen almost exclusively in females or 47, XXY Klinefelter males. More recently there have been rare reports of 46, XY male patients. *Prevalence:* Between 1:105,000 and 1:167,000 in the United States. *References:* Aicardi, J. (2005). Aicardi syndrome. *Brain and Development, 27,* 164–171.

Anderson, S., Menten, B., Kogelenberg, M., Robertson, S., Waginger, M., Mentzel, H.J. ... Willems, P. (2009). Aicardi syndrome in a male patient. *Neuropediatrics, 40*(1), 39–42.

Aicardi-Goutières syndrome (AGS) *Disease category:* Neurologic. *Clinical features:* Early onset encephalopathy whose clinical features mimic those of acquired *in utero* viral infection. Normal pregnancy, delivery, and neonatal period in 80% of those affected. 20% present with brain calcifications *in utero* and present at birth with abnormal neurologic findings, hepatosplenomegaly, elevated liver enzymes, and thrombocytopenia. The rest of affected infants present at variable times, and it is usually after a period of normal development. They present with subacute onset of severe encephalopathy characterized by extreme irritability, intermittent sterile pyrexias, loss of skills, and slowing of head growth. *Associated complications:* Peripheral spasticity, dystonic posturing of upper limbs, truncal hypotonia, poor head control, and seizures. Almost all affected individuals have severe intellectual and physical impairment. *Cause:* Four causative genes have been found. A three prime repair exonuclease gene called *TREX1* (3p21.3-p21.2), and 3 different ribonuclease H2 subunits: *RNASEH2B* (13q14.1), *RNASEH2C* (11q13.2), and *RNASEH2A* (19p13.13). *Inheritance:* Majority of cases are AR although there are AD/NM mutations in *TREX1*. *Prevalence:* Unknown.

References: Crow, Y., & Rehwinkel, J. (2009). Aicardi-Goutieres syndrome and related phenotypes: Linking nucleic acid metabolism with autoimmunity. *Human Molecular Genetics, (R2),* R130–6.

Goutieres, F. (2005). Aicardi-Goutieres syndrome. *Brain and Development, 27,* 201–206.

Rice, G., Patrick, T., Parmar, R., Taylor, C.F., Aeby, A., Aicardi, J...Crow, Y.J. (2007). Clinical and molecular phenotype of Aicardi-Goutieres syndrome. *American Journal of Human Genetics, 81*(4), 713–725.

alcohol-related neurodevelopmental defects (ARND) Previously called fetal alcohol effects (FAE); *see Chapter 3.*

Alexander disease *Disease category:* Neurologic. *Clinical features:* Progressive cortical white matter neurological disorder that mostly affects infants and children and results in early death. General characteristics of the disease include seizures, intellectual disability, white matter abnormalities, and megalencephaly. The neonatal form usually ends in death within 2 years. The infantile form presents by age 2, and affected children survive up to several years. The juvenile form presents between ages 4 and 10 (and occasionally in the teens) and affected individuals survive until early teens to mid 20s and 30s. An adult form has been described although with variable presentation. *Associated complications:* Hydrocephalus, demyelination, progressive spasticity, visual impairment; bulbar signs are present in some patients. *Cause:* Mutations in the *GFAP* gene are known to be causative, (coding for glial fibrillary acidic protein at 17q21). *Inheritance:* Majority of cases caused by a NM with AD inheritance when passed from an affected individual; rare AD families have been reported. *Prevalence:* Rare.

References: Balbi P., Salvini, S., Fundarò, C., Frazzitta, G., Maestri, R., Mosah, D... Sechi, G (2010). The clinical spectrum of late-onset Alexander disease: A systematic literature review. *Journal of Neurology, 257*(12), 1955–1962.

Messing, A., Daniels, C.M., & Hagemann, T.L. (2010). Strategies for treatment in Alexander disease. *Neurotherapeutics, 7,* 507–515.

Rong, L., Johnson, A.B., & Salomons, G. (2005). Glial fibrillary acidic protein mutations in infantile, juvenile, and adult forms of Alexander disease. *Annals of Neurology, 57,* 310–326.

Sawaishi, Y. (2009). Review of Alexander disease: Beyond the classical concept of leukodystrophy. *Brain and Development, 31,* 493–498.

Angelman syndrome *Disease category:* Imprinting defect/multiple congenital defect/contiguous gene defect. *Clinical features:* Severe developmental delay or intellectual disability, severe speech impairment, gait ataxia, and unique behavior with an inappropriate happy demeanor that includes frequent laughing, smiling, and excitability. *Associated complications:* Seizures, microcephaly. Behavioral features include hyperactivity, short attention span, hand flapping, feeding problems, chewing/mouthing behaviors, fascination with water, abnormal food-related behaviors. *Cause:* Deletion of 15q11–q13 on the maternally inherited chromosome, paternal inheritance of both copies of chromosome 15 (uniparental disomy, or UPD), a point mutation in the maternal copy of the *UBE3A* gene or an imprinting defect (due to deletion or epigenetic effect). *Inheritance:* All three causes arise as a result of NM; mutations in the *UBE3A* gene may be passed in an AD fashion. *Prevalence:* 1:10,000–1:20,000.

References: Pelc, K., Cheron, G., & Dan, B. (2008). Behavior and neuropsychiatric manifestations in Angelman syndrome. *Neuropsychiatric Disease and Treatment, 4*(3), 577–584.

Van Buggenhout, G., & Fryns, J.P. (2009). *European Journal of Human Genetics, 17,* 1367–1373.

Williams, C.A. (2010). The behavioral phenotype of the Angelman syndrome. *American Journal of Medical Genetics Part C: Seminars in Medical Genetics, 154C,* 432–437.

Apert syndrome (acrocephalosyndactyly, type I) *Disease category:* Craniosynostosis. *Clinical features:* (Craniosynostosis) premature fusion of the cranial sutures with misshapen head (turribrachycephalic skull shape), high forehead, and flat occiput (back part of head); hypertelorism with downward slant; moderate-to-severe midface hypoplasia (flat mid-face) and nasal bridge; severe syndactyly (webbing of fingers or toes); limb anomalies; cleft palate, hypertelorism, and fused cervical vertebrae. *Associated complications:* Hydrocephalus, varying degrees of intellectual disability, hearing loss, teeth abnormalities, occasional heart and kidney anomalies. *Cause:* Mutations in the fibroblast growth factor receptor-2 (*FGFR2*) gene on chromosome 10q26. *Inheritance:* Majority of cases are caused by a NM, with AD inheritance when passed from

an affected individual. *Incidence:* 1:100,000. *Treatment:* Early neurosurgical correction of fused sutures improves appearance and may reduce risk of intellectual disability; plastic/orthopedic surgery for limb anomalies.

References: Carinci, F., Pezzetti, F., Locci, P., Becchetti, E., Carls, F., Avantaggiato, A. ... Bodo, M. (2005). Apert and crouzon syndromes: Clinical findings, genes and extracellular matrix. *The Journal of Craniofacial Surgery, 16*(3), 361–368.

Kreiborg, S., & Cohen, M. (2010). Ocular manifestations of Apert and Crouzon syndromes: qualitative and quantitative findings. *The Journal of Craniofacial Surgery, 21*(5), 1354–1357.

ARND Alcohol-related neurodevelopmental disorder; *see Chapter 3.*

arthrogryposis multiplex congenital *Disease category:* Neuromuscular disease. *Clinical features:* Nonprogressive joint contractures that begin prenatally; flexion contractures at the fingers, knees, and elbows, with muscle weakness around involved joints. *Associated complications:* Occasional kidney and eye anomalies, cleft palate, defects of abdominal wall, scoliosis. *Cause:* Multiple; most frequently related to an underlying neuropathy, myopathy (muscle weakness), or *in utero* crowding; may be associated with maternal myasthenia gravis; nerve conduction studies/electromyography (EMG) and muscle biopsy may be beneficial in determining the basis of the condition (myopathic versus neurogenic). Intelligence is usually normal. *Inheritance:* Usually SP and may be caused by teratogenic exposure; however both AD or AR inheritance also have been reported. *Incidence:* Ranges from 1:3,000– 1:12,000. *Treatment:* Casting of affected joints or surgery, if indicated.

References: Fassier, A., Wicart, P., Dubousset, J., & Seringe, R. (2009). Arthrogryposis multiplex congenital: Long-term follow-up from birth until skeletal maturity. *Journal of Child of Orthopaedics, 3,* 383–390.

Nordone, T., & Li, P. (2010). Arthrogryposis multiplex congenita in association with bilateral temporormandibular joint hypomobility: Report of a case and review of literature. *Journal of Oral and Maxillofacial Surgery, 68,* 1197–1204.

ataxia telangiectasia *Disease category:* Chromosome breakage syndrome. *Clinical features:* Slowly progressive ataxia, telangiectasias (dilation of capillaries, especially in the sclera [whites of eye] and behind the earlobe), immune defects, elevated alpha-fetoprotein in blood, small cerebellum. *Associated complications:* Dystonia or choreoathetosis, dysarthric speech (imperfect articulation due to decreased motor control), increased sensitivity to radiation, increased risk of malignancy (especially leukemia or lymphoma), eye movement abnormalities, finger contractures, increased risk of sinus and pulmonary infections; intelligence is typically unaffected but may decline with disease progression. Survival is typically past 25 years and some live into their fifties. *Cause:* Mutation in the *ATM* gene (*A*taia-*T*elangiectasia *M*utated) on chromosome 11q22.3. Involved in cellular responses to DNA damage and cell cycle control. *Inheritance:* AR. *Prevalence:* 1:40,000–1:100,000 live births in the United States. *Treatment:* IVIG (intravenous immunoglobulin) replacement therapy for those with frequent and severe infections and low IgG levels; aggressive pulmonary hygiene for those with chronic bronchiectasis; steroids temporarily improve neurologic function but symptoms reappear within days of discontinuation; avoidance of excessive ionizing radiation; treatments are under investigation aimed at improving neurological symptoms.

References: Crawford, T.O., Skolasky, R.L., Fernandez, R., Rosquist, K.J., & Lederman, H.M. (2006). Survival probability in ataxia telangiectasia. *Archives of Disease in Childhood, 91*(7), 610–611.

Lavin, M., Gueven, N., Bottle, S., & Gatti, R.A. (2007). Current and potential therapeutic strategies for the treatment of ataxia-telangiectasia. *British Medical Bulletin, 81–82,* 129–147.

McGrath-Morrow, S., Gower, W.A., Rothblum-Oviatt, C., Brody, A.S., Langston, C., Fan, L.L. … Lederman, H.M. (2010). Evaluation and management of pulmonary disease in ataxia-telangiectasia. *Pediatric Pulmonology, 45,* 847–859.

Bardet-Biedl syndrome (BBS) *Disease category:* Multiple congenital anomalies. *Clinical features:* Retinal dysfunction, polydactyly (extra fingers or toes), obesity, learning disabilities, genital abnormalities, renal anomalies. *Associated complications:* Speech delay/disorder, developmental delay, behavioral abnormalities, eye abnormalities, ataxia, diabetes, heart abnormalities, abnormal liver function, specific facial features, night blindness. *Cause:* Mutations have been found in 14 genes: *BBS1, BBS2, ARL6/BBS3, BBS4, BBS5, MKKS/BBS6, BBS7, TTC8/BBS8,* *B1/BBS9, BBS10, TRIM32/BBS11, BBS12, MKS1/BBS13,* and *CEP290/BBS14* linked to chromosomal loci: 17q23, 16q21, 15q22.3-q23, 14q32.1, 12q21.3, 12q21.2, 11q13, 9q31-q34.1, 8q21.13-q22.1, 7p14, 4q27, 4q27, 3p12-q13, 2q31, 20p12. *Inheritance:* Generally AR although in some families, mutations in more than one BBS locus may result in a clinical phenotype of BBS. *Prevalence:* 1:100,000.

References: Sapp, J.C., Nishimura, D., Johnston, J.J., Stone, E.M., Héon, E., Sheffield, V.C., & Biesecker, L.G. (2010). Recurrence risks for Bardet-Biedl syndrome: Implications of locus heterogeneity. *Genetics in Medicine, 12*(10), 623–627.

Batten disease (neuronal ceroid lipofuscinosis, juvenile) *Disease category:* Neurological disorder. *Clinical features:* Typical development until rapid vision loss begins between 4 and 10 years; children become completely blind within 2 to 4 years of the onset of vision loss. Gradual onset of ataxia, myoclonic, generalize tonic-clonic or focal seizures happens between ages 9 and 18. Early death usually occurs by late teens or early 20s, although some patients have lived into their 30s. *Associated complications:* Gradual intellectual decline, spasticity, psychosis, kyphoscoliosis, decline in speech, behavioral problems, sleep disturbance. *Cause:* The genes *CLN3, PPT1, TPP1,* and *CLN9* are associated with juvenile neuronal ceroid-lipofuscinosis. *Inheritance:* AR. *Incidence:* 1.3–7:100,000 live births. Many other forms of neuronal ceroid lipofuscinosis exist including infantile, late infantile, juvenile, and adult forms. Mutations in 8 CLN genes (plus 2 more that have not been identified) cause various forms of neuronal ceroid lipofuscinosis.

References: Adams, H., Kwon, J., Marshall, F.J., de Blieck, E.A., Pearce, D.A., & Mink, J.W. (2007). Neuropsychological symptoms of juvenile-onset Batten disease: Experiences from two studies. *Journal of Child Neurology, 22,* 621–627.

Adams, H., Beck, C.A., Levy, E., Jordan, R., Kwon, J.M., Marshall, F.J. … Mink J.W. (2010). Genotype does not predict severity of behavioural phenotype in juvenile neuronal ceriod lipofuscinosis (Batten disease). *Developmental Medicine and Child Neurology, 52*(7), 637–643.

Kohlschutter, A., & Shulz, A. (2009). Towards understanding the neuronal ceroid lipofuscinoses. *Brain and Development, 31,* 499–502.

Becker muscular dystrophy (BMD) *See* muscular dystrophy.

Beckwith-Wiedemann syndrome *Disease category:* Overgrowth syndrome/imprinting defect/ contiguous gene syndrome. *Clinical features:* Macrosomia (large body size); large organs, especially the tongue; neonatal hypoglycemia (low blood sugar), embryonal tumors (Wilms tumor, hepatoblastoma, neuroblastoma, rhabdomyosoarcoma), omphalocele (congenital defect in abdominal wall containing the intestine), ear creases/pits, renal abnormalities. *Associated complications:* Advanced growth for the first 6 years, with advanced bone age, occasional **hemihyperplasia** (abnormal cell proliferation leading to asymmetrical overgrowth), kidney or adrenal anomalies, occasional intellectual disability (may be due to untreated hypoglycemia). *Cause:* Abnormal transcription and regulation of genes in the imprinted domain on chromosome 11p15.5, two copies of paternal 11p15.5 (paternal uniparental disomy or UPD), methylation abnormalities of gene *KCNQ1OT1 (DMR2)* or *H19 (DMR1)*, mutations in *CDKN1C*, or maternal rearrangments involving 11p15.5. *Inheritance:* Majority of cases are caused by a NM with AD inheritance with variable penetrance when passed from an affected individual. *Incidence:* 1:13,700 live births. *Treatment:* Early treatment of hypoglycemia is critical; surgical repair of omphalocele.

References: Choufani, S., Shuman, C., & Weksberg, R. (2010). Beckwith-Wiedemann syndrome. *American Journal of Medical Genetics Part C, 154C,* 343–354.

Weksberg, R., Shuman, C., & Beckwith, J. (2010). Beckwith-Weidemann. *European Journal of Human Genetics, 18,* 8–14.

biotinidase deficiency *See* multiple carboxylase deficiency, late onset, juvenile form.

Bloom syndrome *Disease category:* Chromosome breakage syndrome. *Clinical features:* Pre- and postnatal growth retardation, sparse subcutaneous fat, red, sun-sensitive skin lesion appears on the nose and cheeks after sun exposure, high incidence of multiple cancers. *Associated complications:* Mild intellectual disability or learning disability, gastroesophageal reflux, common infections, infertility in males, reduced fertility in females, non–insulin dependant diabetes, immunoglobulin deficiency, chronic lung disease. *Cause:* Mutations in the *BLM* gene which encodes the *BLM* RecQ protein on chromosome 15q26.1. *Inheritance:* AR. *Prevalence:* Overall prevalence

is rare, although it is seen more commonly in the Ashkenazi Jewish population.

References: Diaz, A., Vogiatzi, M.G., Sanz, M.M., & German, J. (2006). Evaluation of short stature, carbohydrate metabolism and other endocrinopathies in Bloom's syndrome. *Hormone Research, 66,* 111–117.

Thomas, E.R., Shanley, S., Walker, L., & Eeles, R. (2008). Surveillance and treatment of malignancy in Bloom syndrome. *Clinical Oncology, 20*(5), 375–379.

BMD muscular dystrophy, Becker type *See* muscular dystrophy, Duchenne and Becker types.

Börjeson-Forssman-Lehmann syndrome *Disease category:* Multiple congenital anomalies. *Clinical features:* Obesity, short stature, postpubertal gynecomastia (breast enlargement in males), large ears, coarse facial appearance, small external genitalia, eye anomalies, tapering fingers, varying degree of intellectual disability. *Associated complications:* Seizures, abnormal head size ranging from microcephalic to macrocephalic, hypotonia. *Cause:* Causative gene *PHF6* linked to chromosome Xq26.3. *Inheritance:* XLR, with females less severely affected than males. *Prevalence:* Rare.

References: Carter, M.T., Picketts, D.J., Hunter, A.G., & Graham, G.E. (2009). Further clinical delineation of the Borjeson-Forssman-Lehmann syndrome in patients with *PHF6* mutations. *American Journal of Medical Genetics Part A, 149A,* 246–250.

De Winter, C.F., van Dijk, F., Stolker, J.J., & Hennekam, R.C. (2009). Behavioural phenotype in Borjeson-Forssman-Lehmann syndrome. *Journal of Intellectual Disability Research, 53*(4), 319–328.

Brachmann de Lange syndrome *See* de Lange syndrome.

Canavan disease (spongy degeneration of central nervous system) *Disease category:* Neurological disorder. *Clinical features:* Progressive neurological disorder consisting of macrocephaly, hypotonia progressing to spasticity with age, visual impairment, and early death. Symptoms begin at 3–6 months of age; children do not develop ability to sit, walk, or talk. Despite limitations, children are interactive. *Associated complications:* Feeding difficulties with progressive swallowing problems, gastroesophageal reflux, severe intellectual disability, head lag. *Cause:* Deficiency in the enzyme aspartoacylase caused by a mutation in the *ASPA* gene on chromosome 17pter–p13. *Inheritance:* AR. *Prevalence:* Rare in most populations; about 1:6,400–1:13,456 in Ashkenazi Jewish population.

References: Kumar, S., Mattan, N.S. & de Vellis, J. (2006). Canavan disease: A white matter disorder. *Mental Retardation and Developmental Disabilities Research Reviews, 12,* 157–165.

Namboodiri, A., Peethambaran, A., Mathew, R., Sambhu, P.A., Hershfield, J., Moffett, J.R., & Madhavarao, C.N. (2006). Canavan disease and the role of N-acetylaspartate in myelin synthesis. *Molecular and Cellular Endocrinology, 252,* 216–223.

Carpenter syndrome (acrocephalosyndactyly, type II) *Disease category:* Craniosynostosis. *Clinical features:* Craniosynostosis, flat nasal bridge, malformed and low-set ears, short digits, syndactyly and/or polydactyly, obesity, **hypogenitalism** and/or cryptorchidism. *Associated complications:* Congenital heart defects, hearing loss; 75% have mild intellectual disability. *Cause:* Causative gene RAS-Associated Protein *RAB23*, which encodes an essential negative regulator of Sonic hedgehog signaling pathway. *Inheritance:* AR. *Prevalence:* Rare.

References: Robinson, L.K., James, H.E., Mubarak, S.J., Allen, E.J., & Jones, K.L. (1985). Carpenter syndrome: Natural history and clinical spectrum. *American Journal of Medical Genetics, 20,* 461–469.

Jenkins, D., Seelow, D., Jehee, F.S., Perlyn, C.A., Alonso, L.G., Bueno, D.F. … Wilkie, A.O. (2007). *RAB23* mutations in Carpenter syndrome imply an unexpected role for hedgehog signaling in cranial-suture development and obesity. *American Journal of Human Genetics, 80*(6), 1162–1170.

cerebrohepatorenal syndrome *See* Zellweger syndrome.

CHARGE syndrome *Disease category:* Multiple congenital anomalies. *Clinical features:* CHARGE is an acronym that stands for: **C**oloboma (defect in iris or retina), **h**eart defect, choanal **a**tresia (congenital blockage of the nasal passages), **r**etarded growth and development, **g**enital anomalies, and **e**ar anomalies with or without hearing loss. *Associated complications:* Hypogenitalism, cryptorchidism, occasional cleft lip/palate, varying degrees of intellectual disability ranging from normal intelligence to profound intellectual disability, behavioral problems, potentially severe visual and hearing impairments. Survival ranges widely from 5 days to 46 years. *Cause:* Mutations in the chromodomain helicase DNA-binding protein-7 (*CHD7*)

and semaphorin-3E gene (*SEMA3E*) have been shown to cause CHARGE. *Inheritance:* Majority of cases are caused by a NM, with evidence of AD inheritance when passed from an affected individual; associated with increased paternal age. Usually SP; approximately 8% of cases are familial. *Prevalence:* 1:8,500 to 1:12,000; more common in females than males.

References: Wullfaert, J., Scholte, E.M., Dijkhoorn, Y.M., Bergman, J.E., van Ravenswaaij-Arts, C.M., & van Berckelaer-Onnes, I.A. (2009). Parenting stress in CHARGE syndrome and the relationship with child characteristics. *Journal of Developmental and Physical Disabilities, 21*(4), 301–313.

Zentner, G.E., Layman, W.S., Martin, D.M., & Scacheri, P.C. (2010). Molecular and phenotypic aspects of *CHD7* mutation in CHARGE syndrome. *American Journal of Medical Genetics Part A, 152A,* 674–686.

chondroectodermal dysplasia *See* Ellis-van Creveld syndrome.

chromosome 22q11 microdeletion syndromes (i.e., DiGeorge syndrome, velocardiofacial syndrome [VCFS], Shprintzen syndrome) *Disease category:* Multiple congenital anomalies/contiguous gene. *Clinical features:* Microdeletions within the long arm of chromosome 22 have varying presentations, including DiGeorge syndrome, VCFS, and isolated outflow tract defects of the heart. Characteristic facial appearance that includes a small, open mouth; short palpebral fissures (eyelid openings); flat nasal bridge; bulbous nasal tip; protuberant, low-set ears; varying degrees of palatal abnormalities ranging from cleft to velopharyngeal insufficiency; classic DiGeorge syndrome is associated with immune deficiency, hypoparathyroidism leading to hypocalcemia, hypotonia, and congenital heart defect (especially conotruncal defects). *Associated complications:* Feeding problems in infancy, rare seizures, hypernasal speech, psychiatric illness, developmental disabilities ranging from learning disability to more significant cognitive delays; gross and fine motor delays; expressive language is delayed more significantly than receptive language. *Cause:* 1.5- to 3.0-Mb hemizygous deletion of chromosome 22q11.2. Haploinsufficiency of the *TBX1* gene in particular is responsible for most of the physical malformations. There is evidence that point mutations in the *TBX1* gene can also cause the disorder. *Inheritance:* AD. 93% from NM, 7% received the deletion from an affected parent; one parent occasionally has a chromosomal rearrangement involving 22q, which increases the risk for recurrence; risk to offspring of affected individuals is 50%. *Prevalence:* A 2003 Centers for Disease Control (CDC) study found an overall prevalence of about 1:6,000 in Caucasians, African Americans, and Asians, and 1:3,800 in the Hispanic population in the United States.

References: Drew, L.J., Crabtree, G.W., Markx, S., Stark, K.L., Chaverneff, F., Xu, B. ... Karayiorgou, M. (2011). The 22q11.2 microdeletion: Fifteen years of insights into the genetic and neural complexity of psychiatric disorders. *International Journal of Developmental Neuroscience. 29*(3): 259–281.

Roizen, N.J., Higgins, A.M., Antshel, K.M., Fremont, W., Shprintzen, R., & Kates, W.R. (2010). 22q11.2 Deletion syndrome: Are motor deficits more than expected for IQ level? *Journal of Pediatrics, 157*(4), 658–661.

Cohen syndrome *Disease category:* Multiple congenital anomalies. *Clinical features:* Characteristic facial features including thick hair and eyebrows, long eyelashes, wave-shaped palpebral fissures, bulbous nasal tip, smooth or shortened philtrum; retinal dystrophy; progressive high myopia; acquired microcephaly; global developmental delay and variable intellectual disability; hypotonia; and joint hyperextensibility. *Associated complications:* Short stature, small or narrow hands and feet, truncal obesity appearing in teen years after initial poor weight gain, friendly disposition. *Cause:* Mutations in the *COH1* gene linked to chromosome 8q21–q22. *Inheritance:* AR. *Prevalence:* Unknown, although it is overrepresented in certain populations such as the Finnish population and the Amish.

References: Parri, V., Katzaki, E., Uliana, V., Scionti, F., Tita, R., Artuso, R... Ariani, F. (2010). High frequency of *COH1* intragenic deletions and duplications detected by MLPA in patients with Cohen syndrome. *European Journal of Human Genetics, 18,* 1133–1140.

Waite, A., Somer, M., O'Driscoll, M., Millen, K., Manson, F.D., & Chandler, K.E. (2010). Cerebellar hypoplasia and Cohen syndrome: A confirmed association. *American Journal of Medical Genetics Part A, 152A*(9), 2390–2393.

congenital facial diplegia *See* Moebius sequence.

Cornelia de Lange syndrome *See* de Lange syndrome.

craniofacial dysostosis *See* Crouzon syndrome.

cri-du-chat syndrome (chromosome 5p–syndrome) *Disease category:* Multiple congenital anomalies/Contiguous gene syndrome. *Clinical features:* Pre- and postnatal growth retardation, cat-like cry in infancy, hypertelorism with downward slant, microcephaly, low-set ears, micrognathia, single palmar crease, cognitive deficits ranging from learning difficulties in some patients to moderate or severe intellectual disability in others. Receptive language skills are better then expressive language. *Associated complications:* Severe respiratory and feeding difficulties in infancy, hypotonia, inguinal (groin) hernias, occasional congenital heart defects, sleep disturbance, hyperactivity. *Cause:* Partial deletion of chromosome 5p15.2-deletions can range from involving only the 5p15.2 band to the entire short arm. There is evidence that deletion of the telomerase reverse transcriptase gene (*TERT*) is specifically involved in the phenotypic changes. *Inheritance:* Usually NM; in 12% of cases, a parent carries a balanced translocation. *Prevalence:* 1:20,000–1:50,000.

References: Pituch, K., Green, V.A., Didden, R., Whittle, L., O'Reilly, M.F., Lancioni, G.E., & Sigafoos, J. (2010). Educational priorities for children with cri-du-chat syndrome. *Journal of Developmental and Physical Disabilities, 22*(1), 65–81.

South, S.T., Swensen, J.J., Maxwell, T., Rope, A., Brothman, A.R., & Chen, Z. (2006). A new genomic mechanism leading to cri-du-chat syndrome. *American Journal of Medical Genetics Part A, 140*(24), 2714–2720.

Crouzon syndrome (craniofacial dysostosis) *Disease category:* Craniosynostosis. *Clinical features:* Craniosynostosis, shallow orbits with proptosis (protuberant eyeballs), hypertelorism, strabismus, parrot-beaked nose, short upper lip, maxillary hypoplasia (small upper jaw), conductive hearing loss. *Associated complications:* Increased intracranial pressure, intellectual disability, seizures, visual impairment, agenesis of corpus callosum, occasional cleft lip or palate, obstructive airway problems. *Cause:* Mutations in fibroblast growth factor receptor-2 (*FGFR2*) gene on chromosome 10q25.3–q26. *Inheritance:* AD with variable expression; up to 25% may represent new mutations. *Prevalence:* Unknown.

References: Papagrigorakis, M., Vilos, G.A., Apostolidis, C., Daskalopoulou, E., & Vlachogiannis, M. (2011). Long-term surgical cure of severe obstructive sleep apnea in an adult patient with craniofacial dysostosis (Crouzon's syndrome): A case report and literature review. *Sleeping and Breathing, 15*(2), 239–248.

Goriely, A., Lord, H., Lim, J., Johnson, D., Lester, T., Firth, H.V., & Wilkie, A.O. (2010). Germline and somatic mosaicism for *FGFR2* mutation in the mother of a child with Crouzon syndrome: Implications for genetic testing in "paternal age-effect" syndromes. *American Journal of Medical Genetics Part A, 152A*, 2067–2073.

Perlyn, C.A., Morriss-Kay, G., Darvann, T., Tenenbaum, M., & Ornitz, D.M. (2006). A model for the pharmacological treatment of Crouzon syndrome. *Neurosurgery, 59*(1), 210–215.

de Lange syndrome (Brachmann de Lange syndrome, Cornelia de Lange syndrome) *Disease category:* Multiple congenital anomalies. *Clinical features:* Prenatal growth retardation, postnatal short stature, hypertrichosis (excessive body hair), synophrys (confluent eyebrows), anteverted nostrils, depressed nasal bridge, long philtrum, thin upper lip, microcephaly, low-set ears, limb and digital anomalies, eye problems (myopia, ptosis, or nystagmus). *Associated complications:* Severe intellectual disability, occasional heart defect, gastrointestinal problems, features of autism, self-injurious behavior, occasional hearing loss. *Cause:* Mutations in the Nipped-B-like gene (*NIPBL*), which is linked to chromosome 3q26.3 are found in 50% of cases. Mutations in *SMC1A* (formerly *SMC1L1*) linked to Xp11.22-p11.21 have been identified in a small percentage of individuals. A mild version of Cornelia de Lange has been associated with the *SMC3* gene. *Inheritance:* AD or XL, 99% NM. Those with *NIPBL* mutations have a 50% chance of passing it on. *Prevalence:* Published estimates range from 1:10,000 to 1:100,000.

References: Deardorff, M., Kaur, M., Yaeger, D., Rampuria, A., Korolev, S., Pie, J. … Krantz, I.D. (2007). Mutations in cohesion complex members *SMC3* and *SMC1A* cause a mild variant of Cornelia de Lange syndrome with predominant mental retardation. *American Journal of Human Genetics, 80* (3), 485–494.

Musio A., Selicorni, A., Focarelli, M.L., Gervasini, C., Milani, D., Russo, S. … Larizza, L. (2006). X-linked Cornelia de Lange syndrome owing to *SMC1L1* mutations. *Nature Genetics, 38*, 528–530.

DiGeorge syndrome *See* chromosome 22q11 microdeletion syndromes.

DMD muscular dystrophy, Duchenne type *See* muscular dystrophy, Duchenne and Becker types.

Down syndrome *Disease category:* Chromosome abnormality/multiple congenital anomalies. *Clinical features:* Hypotonia, flat facial profile, upward-slanting palpebral fissures, small ears, small nose with low nasal bridge, single palmar crease, short stature, intellectual disability, congenital heart disease. *Associated complications:* Atlantoaxial (upper cervical spine) instability; hyperextensible large joints; strabismus; thyroid dysfunction; predisposition toward immune disorders and leukemia; eye abnormalities, including strabismus, nystagmus, cataracts, or glaucoma; narrow ear canals and high incidence of middle-ear infections with potential hearing loss; neurological abnormalities include risk of seizures and early-onset Alzheimer's disease. *Cause:* Extra chromosome 21 caused by trisomy, mosaicism, or translocation. *Inheritance:* NM; usually nondisjunction chromosomal abnormality. Recurrence risk in the absence of translocation is 1%–2% in women younger than 35 years and the same as the typical maternal age-related risk in women over 35 years old at delivery. If translocation is present in parent, recurrence risk is higher and is dependent on sex of carrier parent. *Prevalence:* 1–1.5:100,000. *Incidence:* 1:800 births. *See also Chapter 18.*

References: Feeley, K.M., & Jones, E.A. (2008). Strategies to address challenging behaviour in young children with Down syndrome. *Down Syndrome Research and Practice, 12*(2), 153–163.

Rigoldi, C., Galli, M., & Albertini, G. (2010). Gait development during lifespan in subjects with Down syndrome. *Research in Developmental Disabilities, 32*(1), 158–163.

Van Duijin, G., Dijkxhoorn, Y., Scholte, E.M., & van Berckelaer-Onnes, I.A. (2010). The development of adaptive skills in young people with Down syndrome. *Journal of Intellectual Disability Research, 54*(11), 943–954.

Dubowitz syndrome *Disease category:* Multiple congenital anomalies. *Clinical features:* Prenatal onset of growth deficiency, postnatal short stature, eczema, sparse hair; mild microcephaly, cleft palate, dysmorphic facial features, including high forehead, broad nasal bridge, ptosis, epicanthal folds. *Associated complications:* Intellectual disability, behavioral disturbances, recurrent infections, increased frequency of malignancy, occasional hypospadias (abnormality in the location of the male urethra) or cryptorchidism, hypoparathyroidism. *Cause:* Unknown. *Inheritance:* AR. *Prevalence:* Rare.

References: Tsukahara, M., & Opitz, J.M. (1996). Dubowitz syndrome: Review of 141 cases, including 36 previously unreported patients. *American Journal of Medical Genetics, 63,* 277–289.

Yesilkaya, E., Karaer, K., Bideci, A., Camurdan, O., Perçin, E.F., & Cinaz, P. (2008). Dubowitz syndrome: A cholesterol metabolism disorder? *Genetic Counseling, 19,* 287–290.

Duchenne muscular dystrophy (DMD) *See* muscular dystrophy, Duchenne and Becker types.

ectrodactyly–ectodermal dysplasia–clefting (EEC) syndrome *Disease category:* Ectodermal dysplasia. *Clinical features:* Ectrodactyly (split hands or feet), ectodermal dysplasia (abnormal skin development), sparse hair, cleft lip and palate, lacrimal (tear) duct abnormalities; intelligence is not usually affected. *Associated complications:* Occasional renal (kidney) or genital anomalies, hearing impairment, hypodontia (underdeveloped teeth), lymphoma associated with *EEC3* only. *Cause:* Mutations in *p63* gene at 3q27 cause EEC type 3; EEC type 1 have been linked to chromosome 7q21–q22. *Inheritance:* AD with variable penetrance and expressivity. *Prevalence:* Unknown. *See also* Ehlers-Danlos syndrome.

References: Birgfeld, C., Glick, P., Singh, D., LaRossa, D., & Bartlett, S. (2007). Midface growth in patients with ectrodactyly-ectodermal dysplasia-clefting syndrome. *Plastic and Reconstructive Surgery, 120*(1), 144–150.

Clements, S.E., Techanukul, T., Coman, D., Mellerio, J.E., & McGrath, J.A. (2010). Molecular basis of EEC (ectrodactyly, ectodermal dysplasia, clefting) syndrome: Five new mutations in the DNA-binding domain of the *TP62* gene and genotype-phenotype correlation. *British Journal of Dermatology, 162*(1), 201–207.

Edwards syndrome *See* trisomy 18 syndrome.

EEC syndrome *See* ectrodactyly-ectodermal dysplasia-clefting syndrome.

Ehlers-Danlos syndrome (EDS) *Disease category:* Connective tissue disorder. *Clinical features:* At least 10 distinct forms have been described. All include aspects of skin fragility, easy bruisability, joint hyperextensibility, and hyperelastic skin. Classic (previously type I and II) and hypermobility (previously type III) forms are most commonly described and have similar clinical presentations with the previously mentioned features; the vascular form (previously type IV) is characterized by severe blood vessel involvement with risk of spontaneous arterial rupture; the progeroid (premature aging) form is characterized by wrinkled face, curly/fine hair, scanty eyebrows and eyelashes, and periodontitis in addition to the other usual signs of EDS; type V has been questioned as to whether it is a actually a distinct phenotype; the kyphoscoliotic (type VI) form is characterized by eye involvement, including corneal fragility and kyphoscoliosis (curvature of the spine); the arthrochalasia type (type VIIA &B) presents with congenital bilateral hip dislocation; the dermatosparaxis type (previously type VIIC) includes delayed closure of the fontanelles, characteristic facies, edema of the eyelids, blue sclerae, short stature and fingers; the periodontitis type (previously type VIII) includes periodontal disease; cardiac valvular form has the typical signs as well as cardiac valvular defects. *Associated complications:* Occasional intellectual disability, premature loss of teeth, mitral valve prolapse, intestinal hernias, premature delivery from premature rupture of membranes, scoliosis, abnormalities of thymus. *Cause:* Each form is associated with an abnormality in the formation of collagen. The classic form is caused by mutations in the *COL5A1* and *COL5A2* genes; hypermobility form is caused by mutations in the *COL3A1* gene as well as the tenascin XB gene (*TNXB*); the vascular type is caused by mutations in the *COL3A1* gene; the progeroid form is caused by mutations in *B4GALT7* gene; mutations in the lysyl hydroxylase gene (*PLOD*) cause some cases of kyphoscoliotic form; arthrochalasia type are caused by mutations in the *COL1A1* and *COL1A2* gene. Dermatosparaxis type is linked to the *ADAMTS2* gene; cardiac valvular type is linked to *COL1A2*. A possible new form of EDS was discovered in 2010 to be like the kyphoscoliotic form but without lysyl hydroxylase deficiency and has been linked to the gene *CHST14*. *Inheritance:* Classic, hypermobility, vascular, arthrochalasia and periodontitis types are all AD. Progeroid, kyphoscolotic, dermatospraxia and cardiac valvular are all AR. *Prevalence:* Classic type is 1:20,000; hypermobility type ranges from 1 in 5,000–1:20,000; kyphoscolotic form estimates around 1:100,000; vascular type 1:250,000; the rest unknown. *See also* ectrodactyl-ectodermal dysplasia-clefting syndrome.

References: Malfait, F., Wenstrup, R.J., & De Paepe, A. (2010). Clinical and genetic aspects of Ehlers-Danlos syndrome, classic type. *Genetics in Medicine, 12*(10), 597–605.

Miyake, N., Kosho, T., Mizumoto, S., Furuichi, T., Hatamochi, A., Nagashima, Y. … Matsumoto, N. (2010). Loss-of-function mutations of *CHST14* in a new type of Ehlers-Danlos syndrome. *Human Mutation, 31,* 966–974.

Savasta, S., Merli, P., Ruggieri, M., Bianchi, L., & Spartà, M.V. (2011). Ehlers-Danlos syndrome and neurological features: A review. *Child Neurology, 27*(3), 365–371.

Ellis-van Creveld syndrome (chondroectodermal dysplasia) *Disease category:* Ectodermal dysplasia. *Clinical features:* Short-limbed dwarfism (final height 43–60 inches or 109 to 152cm), polydactyly, nail abnormalities, neonatal teeth, underdeveloped and premature loss of teeth, congenital heart defect in 50%; intelligence is usually not affected. *Associated complications:* Severe cardiorespiratory problems in infancy specifically atrial septation (producing a common atrium in the heart), hydrocephalus, severe leg deformities. *Cause:* Mutations in the *EVC* and *EVC 2* genes located on chromosome 4p16. *Inheritance:* AR. *Prevalence:* Rare, more common in the Amish population.

References: Tompson, S.W., Ruiz-Perez, V.L., Blair, H.J., Barton, S., Navarro, V., Robson, J.L. … Goodship, J.A. (2007). Sequencing EVC and EVC2 identifies mutations in two-thirds of Ellis-van Creveld syndrome patients. *Human Genetics, 120*(4), 662–670.

Ulucan, H., Gül, D., Sapp, J.C., Cockerham, J., Johnston, J.J., & Biesecker, L.G. (2008). Extending the spectrum of Ellis van Creveld syndrome: a large family with a mild mutation in the EVC gene. *BMC Medical Genetics, 9*(92).

facio-auriculo-vertebral spectrum *See* oculoauriculovertebral spectrum.

faciodigitogenital dysplasia (FGDY) *See* Aarskog-Scott syndrome.

FAE *See* fetal alcohol effects.

familial dysautonomia (Riley-Day syndrome) *Disease category:* Neurological disorder. *Clinical features:* Absent or sparse tears, absence of fungiform papillae (knob-like projections) on tongue, diminished pain and temperature sensation, postural hypotension, abnormal sweating, episodic vomiting, swallowing disorder, ataxia, decreased reflexes. *Associated complications:* Feeding difficulties, scoliosis, joint abnormalities, hypertension, aseptic necrosis of bones (damage to bony tissue unassociated with infection or injury). Neuronal degeneration is progressive. *Cause:* Mutation of *IKBKAP* gene (stands for inhibitor of kappa light polypeptide gene enhancer in B-cells, kinase complex associated protein) localized to chromosome 9q31–q33. *Inheritance:* AR. *Prevalence:* Rare; 1:36 carrier frequency in Ashkenazi Jewish population.

References: Axelrod, F.B. (2006). A world without pain or tears. *Clinical Autonomic Research, 16,* 90–97.

Gold-von Simson, G., Goldberg, J.D., Rolnitzky, L.M., Mull, J., Leyne, M., Voustianiouk, A. … Axelrod, F.B. (2009). Kinetin in familial dysautonomia carriers: Implications for a new therapeutic strategy targeting mRNA splicing. *Pediatric Research, 65*(3), 341–346.

Sands, S.A., Giarraffa, P., Jacobson, C.M., & Axelrod, F.B. (2006). Familial dysautonomia's impact on quality of life in childhood, adolescence, and adulthood. *Acta Pædiatrica, 95,* 457–462.

FAS *See* fetal alcohol syndrome.

fetal alcohol effects (FAE) Former term for alcohol-related neurodevelopmental effects (ARND); *see Chapter 3.*

fetal alcohol syndrome (FAS) *See Chapter 3.*

fetal face syndrome *See* Robinow syndrome.

fetal hydantoin syndrome Phenytoin syndrome.

FGDY faciogenital dysplasia *See* Aarskog-Scott syndrome.

***FMR1*-related disorders (fragile X syndrome, fragile X-associated tremor/ataxia syndrome (FXTAS), and *FMR1*-related primary ovarian insufficiency)** *Disease category:* Neurological disorder/triplet repeat expansion. *Clinical features:* Males with full mutations typically have a large head, long face, prominent forehead and chin, protruding ears, behavioral problems such as hyperactivity, hand flapping, hand biting, temper tantrums, and sometimes autism. *Associated complications:* Abnormalities of connective tissue with finger joint hypermobility or joint instability, mitral valve prolapse, large testes. Females heterozygous for full-mutation alleles can have similar phenotypes as males but with lower frequency and generally milder involvement. Both males and females with permutations are known to develop FXTAS-late-onset progressive cerebellar ataxia and intention tremor. Twenty-one

percent of females who are carriers of permutation alleles develop primary ovarian insufficiency (cessation of menses before age 40). *Cause:* Mutation in *FMR1* gene on Xq27–q28; molecular analysis reveals an increase in cytosine-guanine-guanine (CGG) trinucleotide repeats in the coding sequence of the *FMR1* gene. Normal allele sizes vary from 6 to approximately 55 CGG repeats. Phenotypically unaffected individuals have premutations, with allele size ranging from 55 to 200 but are at risk for FXTAS and POI. Allele sizes of greater than 200 CGG repeats generally indicate a full mutation with phenotypic expression of the syndrome. *Inheritance:* X-linked with genetic imprinting (full mutations are not inherited from the father) and anticipation (number of repeats may increase in subsequent generations). *Prevalence:* 16–25:100,000 males; prevalence of females affected with fragile X is presumed to be half the male prevalence. *See also Chapter 11.*
References: Boyle, L., & Kaufmann, W.E. (2010). The behavioral phenotype of *FMR1* mutations. *American Journal of Medical Genetics Part C: Seminars in Medical Genetics, 154C*(4), 469–476.
Rodriguez-Revenga, L., Pagonabarraga, J., Gómez-Anson, B., López-Mourelo, O., Madrigal, I., Xunclà M. ... Milà, M. (2010). Motor and mental dysfunction in mother-daughter transmitted FXTAS. *Neurology, 75*(15), 1370–1376.
Symons, F.J., Byiers, B.J., Raspa, M., Bishop, E., & Bailey, D.B. (2010). Self-injurious behavior and fragile X syndrome: Findings from the national fragile X survey. *American Journal on Intellectual and Developmental Disabilities, 115*(6), 473–81.
5p– syndrome   *See* cri-du-chat syndrome.
45,X   *See* Turner syndrome.
47,X   *See* XXX, XXXX, and XXXXX syndromes.
fragile X syndrome   *See FMR1*-related disorders
Friedreich ataxia   *Disease category:* Neurological disorder/triplet repeat expansion. *Clinical features:* Slowly progressive neurological disorder characterized by limb and gait ataxia, dysarthria, nystagmus, pes cavus (high-arched feet), hearing loss, kyphoscoliosis (backward curve of the spine). In rare cases, progression is rapid. Onset is usually between age 10–15. *Associated complications:* Delayed motor milestones, cardiomyopathy (heart muscle weakness), and/or congestive heart failure; increased risk of insulin-dependent diabetes mellitus; impaired color vision.

Cause: Usually homozygous guanine-adenosine-adenosine (GAA) expansions in intron 1 of the frataxin (*FXN*) gene on chromosome 9q13; point mutations in the *FXN* have also been identified. Normal alleles are 5–33 GAA repeats; premutation alleles are 34–65 uninterrupted GAA repeats; full disease-causing alleles are 66-1700 GAA repeats. *Inheritance:* AR. *Prevalence:* Approximately 2–4:100,000. *Treatment:* Supportive care includes physical therapy, orthopedic surgery to correct progressive scoliosis, and close cardiology follow-up. Antioxidants such as Idebenone have been used with intial success. Additional studies must be done to confirm these results and monitor long-term effects.
References: Delatycki, M.B. (2009). Evaluating the progression of Friedreich ataxia and its treatment. *Journal of Neurology, 256*(1), 36–41.
Mancuso, M., Orsucci, D., Choub, A., & Siciliano, G. (2010). Current and emerging treatment options in the management of Friedreich ataxia. *Neuropsychiatric Disease and Treatment, 6,* 491–499.
G syndrome   *See* Opitz GBB syndrome.
GBS   *See* Guillain-Barre Syndrome.
galactosemia   *Disease category:* Inborn error of metabolism: carbohydrate. *Clinical features:* Jaundice, lethargy, hypotonia in the newborn period; poor weight gain with vomiting and diarrhea; bleeding diathesis; cataracts; liver dysfunction; varying degrees of intellectual impairment (severe if untreated); visual-perceptual impairments; verbal dyspraxia. *Associated complications:* Ovarian failure, hemolytic anemia, increased risk of sepsis (particularly *E. coli* in neonate), cerebellar ataxia, tremors, choreoathetosis. Some newborns have a mild variant galactosemia (Duarte galactosemia), which is not associated with developmental delays, cataracts, or hepatocellular damage. Nutritional intervention is not usually necessary or is restricted only to children under 1 year of age. *Cause:* Onset of clinical features is in part dependant on the ingestion of dietary galactose; individuals diagnosed by newborn screening in whom galactose has been withheld still experience some cognitive deficits, speech defects, cataracts and ovarian failure (females). *Cause:* A deficiency of the enzyme galactose-1-phosphate uridyltransferase or (GALT), less commonly, galactokinase (both are enzymes required for digestion of galactose, a natural sugar found in milk). The GALT gene is on chromosome

9p13. *Inheritance:* AR. *Prevalence:* 1:10,000–1:30,000 in the United States. *Treatment:* Galactose-free diet.

References: Cuthbert, C., Klapper, H., & Elsas, L. (2008). Diagnosis of inherited disorders of galactose metabolism. *Current Protocols in Human Genetics, 17,* Unit 17.5.

Panis, B., Gerver, W.J., & Rubio-Gozalbo, M.E. (2007). Growth in treated classical galactosemia patients. *European Journal of Pediatrics, 166,* 443–466.

Gaucher disease *Disease category:* Inborn error of metabolism: lysosomal storage disease. *Clinical features:* Three clinically distinct forms, the most common of which (type I) has onset in adulthood including enlarged spleen and liver, anemia, thrombocytopenia, and bone involvement; it is distinguished by the lack of neurological involvement. Most individuals with type I go undiagnosed. Type II presents in infancy with an enlarged spleen, hematological abnormalities, bony lesions, abnormalities of skin pigmentation, limited psychomotor development and rapidly progressive course. Most children will die within the first 2 to 4 years of life. Type III is more variable with ataxia, seizures, eye movement disorder, and dementia with onset before age 2 but with a more slowly progressive course. There is also a perinatal lethal form associated with ichthyosiform or collodion skin abnormalities and nonimmune hydrops fetalis (accumulation of fluid, or edema). *Associated complications:* Rare associated features such as cardiac valvular involvement and Parkinsonian features have been associated with specific genotypes. *Cause:* Accumulation of glucosylceramide due to deficiency of the enzyme beta-glucosidase from mutations in the *GBA* gene on chromosome 1q21. *Inheritance:* AR. *Prevalence:* Rare in general population; prevalence of type I estimated to be approximately 1:855 in the Ashkenazi Jewish population. *Treatment:* Enzyme replacement therapy improves rate of bone loss, reduces spleen size, and so forth but does not seem to affect neurological symptoms; thus it is generally used only in individuals with type 1 bone marrow transplantation.

References: Biegstraaten, M., Mengel, E., Maródi, L., Petakov, M., Niederau, C., Giraldo, P. ... van Schaik, I.N. (2010). Peripheral neuropathy in adult type 1 Gaucher disease: A 2-year prospective observational study. *Brain, 133*(10), 2909–2019.

Gupta, N., Oppenheim, I.M., Kauvar, E.F., Tayebi, N., & Sidransky, E. (2011). Type 2 Gaucher disease: Phenotypic variation and genotypic heterogeneity. *Blood Cells and Molecular Disease, 46*(1), 75–84.

globoid cell leukodystrophy *See* Krabbe disease.

glutaric acidemia, type I (a disorder of organic acid metabolism) *Disease category:* Inborn error of metabolism: organic acidemia. *Clinical features:* Macrocephaly, hypotonia, basal ganglia lesions causing a movement disorder (dystonia), and seizures present between 6 and 18 months, interrupting otherwise typical development. This disorder may mimic dyskinetic cerebral palsy. *Associated complications:* Episodic acidosis, vomiting, lethargy, and coma. Intellectual disability is usual, although intellectual functioning may remain intact. *Cause:* Mutations in the glutaryl-CoA dehydrogenase (*GCDH*) gene on chromosome 19p13.2 result in accumulation of glutaric acid and to a lesser degree of 3-hydroxyglutaric and glutaconic acids. *Inheritance:* AR. *Prevalence:* Overall frequency is 1:100,000; 1:30,000 in Sweden; and 1:50,000 in the United States. It is more common in certain ethnic groups such as in the Amish population. *Treatment:* Low protein diet and supplemental oral carnitine.

References: Bijamia, S., Wiley, V., Carpenter, K., Christodoulou, J., Ellaway, C.J., & Wilcken, B. (2008). Glutaric aciduria type I: Outcome following detection by newborn screening. *Journal of Inherited Disease, 31*(4), 503–507.

Hedlund, G., Longo, N., & Pasquali, M. (2006). Glutaric academia type 1. *American Journal of Medical Genetics Part C: Seminars in Medical Genetics, 142C*(2), 86–94.

glutaric acidemia, type II (multiple acyl-CoA dehydrogenase deficiency) *Disease category:* Inborn error of metabolism: organic acidemia. *Clinical features:* Severe metabolic acidosis, hypoglycemia, and cardiomyopathy, and urine with a characteristic odor of sweaty feet, similar to that present in isovaleric acidemia. Dysmorphic facial features (macrocephaly, large anterior fontanelle [soft spot], high forehead, flat nasal bridge, and malformed ears) are seen in one half of cases. This condition also can present later in life with episodic vomiting, acidosis, and hypoglycemia. *Associated complications:* Muscle weakness, liver disease, cataracts, respiratory distress, renal (kidney) cysts. *Cause:* Mutations in at least three different genes—*ETFA*, *ETFB*, and *ETFDH*—have been identified. No clinical differences with respect to causative gene have been identified. *Inheritance:* AR. *Prevalence:* Rare. *Treatment:* Diet with supplemental riboflavin and carnitine.

References: Angle, B., & Burton, B.K. (2008). Risk of sudden death and acute life-threatening events in patients with glutaric acidemia type II. *Molecular Genetics and Metabolism, 93*(1), 36–39.

Liang, W.C., Ohkuma, A., Hayashi, Y.K., López, L.C., Hirano, M., Nonaka, I. ... Nishino, I. (2009). ETFDH mutations, CoQ10 levels, and respiratory chain activities in patients with riboflavin-responsive multiple acyl-CoA dehydrogenase deficiency. *Neuromuscular Disorders, 19*(3), 212–216.

glycogen storage diseases (glycogenoses) *Disease category:* Inborn error of metabolism: carbohydrate. *Clinical features:* More than 12 forms of glycogen storage diseases are currently known, all caused by defects in the production or breakdown of glycogen and resulting in a wide spectrum of clinical features. They share varying degrees of liver and muscle abnormalities and can be broken down by whether they primarily affect the muscle (and therefore present with muscle cramps, easy fatigability, and progressive muscle weakness) or the liver (where an enlarged liver and decreased blood sugar are the initial symptoms). In all disease forms, patient organs have excessive glycogen accumulation. Types I (glucose-6-phosphate deficiency), II (Pompe disease, acid alpha-glucosidase deficiency), III (amylo-1, 6-glycosidase deficiency), and VI (hepatic phosphorylase deficiency) are the most common and represent almost 95% of cases. Common clinical features include hypoglycemia, short stature, enlarged spleen, and muscle weakness. *Associated complications:* Hypotonia, renal (kidney) abnormalities, gouty arthritis, bleeding abnormalities, hypertension, respiratory distress; type II disease characteristically has severe cardiac, muscle, and neurological involvement. *Cause:* Deficiencies in the various enzymes involved in the synthesis and degradation of glycogen. There are many genes and chromosome locations associated with glycogenoses. *Inheritance:* All except type IX (previously type VIII) are inherited as AR; type IX is XLR. *Prevalence:* Combined incidence of 1:20,000–1:25,000. *Treatment:* Increased protein intake and overnight tube feeding of starch to maintain normoglycemia have been shown to be useful for supportive care. This treatment also prevents growth and developmental problems, and can mollify the biochemical abnormalities. No more specific treatment, however, is yet available for any of the glycogenoses. Liver transplantation has been attempted in types I, III, and IV, with correction of the biochemical abnormalities but not all sequelae.

References: Lee, Y.C., Chang, C.J., Bali, D., Chen, Y.T., & Yan, Y.T. (2011). Glycogen-branching enzyme deficiency leads to abnormal cardiac development: Novel insights into glycogen storage disease IV. *Human Molecular Genetics, 20*(3), 455–465.

Ozen, H. (2007). Glycogen storage diseases: New perspectives. *World Journal of Gastroenterology, 13*(18), 2541–2553.

Shin, Y.S. (2006). Glycogen storage disease: Clinical, biochemical, and molecular heterogeneity. *Seminars in Pediatric Neurology, 13*(2), 115–120.

GM2 gangliosidosis, type I *See* Tay-Sachs disease.

Goldenhar syndrome *See* oculoauriculovertebral spectrum.

Guillain-Barré Syndrome (GBS) *Disease category:* Neuromuscular disease. *Clinical features:* GBS is an acute inflammatory demyelinating polyneuropathy. Pain and the development over one to several days of muscle weakness, with the inability to walk and a loss of deep tendon reflexes. The weakness affects both sides of the body symmetrically, usually starting in the lower extremities. The arms are involved later, with maximum weakness occurring by 3 weeks. Most children with GBS begin to recover 2–3 weeks after the symptoms began. About 85% of affected children are able to walk within 6 months; however, some have residual weakness. The mortality rate is 3%, and the chance of relapse has been reported as 7% in children. *Cause:* It can follow an upper respiratory or gastrointestinal (GI) viral infection. A specific type of GI infection produced by the bacteria *campylobacter jejuni* has been particularly associated with GBS. GBS is considered an autoimmune disease. Although rare familial cases have been reported, it is thought to be a multifactorial disease with both genetic and environmental factors contributing to its occurrence. *Incidence:* 0.4–1.7 cases per 100,000 people each year. Diagnosis: Spinal fluid analysis and electromyographic evaluation. *Treatment:* Treatment is mostly supportive. About 10%–20% need to be placed on a ventilator. Medical treatment includes the use of intravenous immune globulin (IVIG) and/or plasmapheresis.

References: Hughes, R.A., & Cornblath, D.R. (2005). Guillain-Barré syndrome. *The Lancet, 9497,* 1653–1666.

Van Doorn, P.A., Kuitwaard, K., Walgaard, C., van Koningsveld, R., Ruts, L., & Jacobs, B.C. (2010). IVIG treatment and prognosis in Guillain-Barre syndrome. *Journal of Clinical Immunology, 30*(1), S74–S78.

Van Doorn, P.A., Ruts, L., & Jacobs, B.C. (2008). Clinical features, pathogenesis, and treatment of Guillain-Barre syndrome. *Lancet Neurology, 7*(10), 939–950.

Hallermann-Streiff syndrome (oculomandibulodyscephaly with hypotrichosis) *Disease category:* Skeletal dysplasia. *Clinical features:* Proportionate short stature; characteristic facial appearance, including small eyes, small, pinched nose, and small mouth; sparse, thin hair; frontal bossing (prominent central forehead). *Associated complications:* Various eye abnormalities, including nystagmus, strabismus, cataracts, and/or decreased visual acuity; neonatal teeth and other dental abnormalities; narrow upper airway or tracheomalacia (softening of the tracheal cartilages), with related respiratory difficulty; frequent respiratory infections, snoring, and feeding difficulties; clinical overlap with oculodentodigital dysplasia (ODDD) has been suggested; intellectual disability has been reported in some cases. *Cause:* Unknown, believed to be genetic; one patient has been identified with a homozygous mutation in the *GJA1* gene known to be causative in ODDD. *Inheritance:* Most reported cases are not inherited from an affected parent and are assumed to be caused by a NM. *Prevalence:* 150 cases known to exist. *References:* Morice-Picard, Marlin, S., Rooryck, C., Fayon, M., Thambo, J.B., Demarquez, J.L. ... Lacombe, D. (2009). Hallerman-Streiff-like syndrome presenting with laterality and cardiac defects. *Clinical Dysmorphology, 18,* 116–119.

Pizzuti, A., Flex, E., Mingarelli, R., Salpietro, C., Zelante, L., & Dallapiccola, B. (2004). A homozygous *GJA1* gene mutation causes a Hallermann-Streiff/ODDD spectrum phenotype. *Human Mutation, 23,* 286.

hemifacial microsomia *See* oculoauriculovertebral spectrum.

hereditary progressive arthroophthalmopathy *See* Stickler syndrome.

holocarboxylase synthetase deficiency *See* multiple carboxylase deficiency, infantile or early form.

holoprosencephaly *Disease category:* Malformation. *Clinical features:* This classification encompasses a spectrum of midline defects of the brain and face, which occur after failed or abbreviated midline cleavage of the developing brain during the third to fourth weeks gestation. The most severe are incompatible with life. Individuals who survive have varying degrees of disability ranging from typical development with hypotelorism (widely spaced eyes) to alobar holoprosencephaly (brain without segmentation into hemispheres) and cyclopia (single central eye). *Associated complications:* Seizures, endocrine abnormalities, micropenis and other genital anomalies, cleft of retinae, and intellectual disability. Facial anomalies are seen in 80% of cases. *Cause:* Genetically heterogeneous; sonic hedgehog (*SHH*) gene on chromosome 7q36 implicated in some cases; many cases have involved mutations in different genes, such as those located at 2p21 (*SIX3* gene), 13q32 (*ZIC2* gene), 18p11.3 (*TGIF* gene), 22q22.3 (*HPE1* gene), 2q37.1, 9q22.3 (*PTCH1*), 14q13, 2q14 (*GLI2* gene), and to 1q41-q42; cases may be caused by a single gene or a larger chromosomal abnormality. *Inheritance:* May be part of a syndrome or caused by teratogenic exposure; as an isolated birth defect may be AD or AR. *Prevalence:* 1:250 gestations but 1:8,000 live births.

References: Hahn, J.S., Barkovich, A.J., Stashinko, E.E., Kinsman, S.L., Delgado, M.R., & Clegg, N.J. (2006). Factor analysis of neuroanatomical and clinical characteristics of holoprosencephaly. *Brain and Development, 28*(7), 413–9.

Lacbbawan, F., Solomon, B.D., Roessler, E., El-Jaick, K., Domené, S., Vélez, J.I. ... Muenke, M (2009). Clinical spectrum of *SIX3*-associated mutation sin holoprosencephaly: Correlation between genotype, phenotype, and function. *Journal of Medical Genetics, 46*(6), 389–98.

Holt-Oram syndrome *Disease category:* Multiple congenital anomalies. *Clinical features:* Upper-limb defect ranging from hypoplastic (incompletely formed), abnormally placed or absent thumbs to hypoplasia of radius, ulna, or humerus (arm bones) to complete phocomelia (foreshortened limbs); 85%–95% of affected individuals also have congenital heart defect (atrial septal defect and ventricular septal defect are most common). *Associated complications:* Occasional abnormalities of chest muscles and vertebral anomalies. *Cause:* Mutations in the *TBX5* gene on chromosome 12q2. *Inheritance:* AD with variable expression; may increase in severity with each generation. *Prevalence:* Approximately 1:100,000.

References: Basson, C.T., Cowley, G.S., Solomon, S.D., Weissman, B., Poznanski, A.K., Traill, T.A. ... Seidman, C.E. (1994). The clinical and genetic spectrum of Holt-Oram syndrome (heart–hand syndrome). *The New England Journal of Medicine, 330,* 885–891.

Boogerd, C.J., Dooijes, D., Ilgun, A., Mathijssen, I.B., Hordijk, R., van de Laar, I.M. ... Postma, A.V. (2010). Functional analysis of novel TBX5 T-box mutations associated with Holt-Oram syndrome. *Cardiovascular Research, 88*(1), 130–139.

McDermott, D., Bressan, M.C., He, J., Lee, J.S., Aftimos, S., Brueckner, M. ... Basson, C.T. (2005). TBX5 Genetic testing validates strict clinical criteria for Holt-Oram syndrome. *Pediatric Research, 58*(5), 981–986.

homocystinuria *Disease category:* Inborn error of metabolism: amino acid. *Clinical features:* Downward dislocation of lens of the eye (with myopia); tall, slim physique; hypopigmentation (fair skin); and sparse, thin hair. Two forms have been described, differing in their responsiveness to pyridoxine (vitamin B_6). *Associated complications:* Mild to moderate intellectual disability in one half to three fourths of untreated individuals; a vascular event such as myocardial infarction and stroke occurs in 50% of affected individuals by age 30 due to increased risk for blood clots; behavioral disorders, cataracts, or glaucoma; scoliosis; osteoporosis. *Cause:* Inherited defect in the enzyme cystathionine beta-synthetase caused by mutations in the *CBS* gene on chromosome 21q22. *Inheritance:* AR with variable expressivity. *Incidence:* Ranges from 1:65,000 in Ireland to 1:344,000 worldwide. *Treatment:* Folic acid supplementation, use of betaine, and dietary restriction of methionine have shown promise; pyridoxine is used in the rare individuals who have the pyridoxine-responsive form of the disease. Early treatment with pyridoxine in responsive cases may allow typical intelligence. Treatment with above agents significantly reduces risk of vascular events.

References: Elsaid, M.F., Bener, A., Lindner, M., Alzyoud,M., Shahbek, N., Abdelrahman, M.O. ... Hoffmann G.F. (2007). Are heterozygotes for classical homocystinuria at risk of vitamin B_{12} and folic acid deficiency? *Molecular Genetics and Metabolism, 92*(1–2), 100–103.

Skovby, F., Gaustadnes, M., & Mudd, S.H. (2010). A revisit to the natural history of homocystinuria due to cystathionine B-synthase deficiency. *Molecular Genetics and Metabolism, 99,* 1–3.

Yap, S. (2003). Classical homocystinuria: Vascular risk and its prevention. *Journal of Inherited Metabolic Disorders, 26,* 259–265.

Hunter syndrome (MPS II) *See* mucopolysaccharidoses (MPS).

Huntington disease (HD; previously called Huntington chorea), juvenile *Disease category:* Neurologic/triplet repeat expansion. *Clinical features:* Juvenile onset progressive neurological disorder. For cases to be considered juvenile HD onset must occur by 20 years of age. Children present with dysarthria, clumsiness, hyperreflexia, rigidity, and oculomotor disturbances. *Associated complications:* Joint contractures, swallowing dysfunction, seizures. *Cause:* Expansion of CAG (cytosine-adenineguanine) trinucleotide repeat in *Huntington* gene on chromosome 4p16.3 (normal number of CAG repeats is 11–34; individuals affected with juvenile HD have greater than 60 CAG repeats). *Inheritance:* AD with anticipation (earlier onset with each generation, especially when paternally inherited). Progression in children with paternally inherited disease is more rapid than in children with maternally inherited disease. *Prevalence:* 3:100,000–7:100,000; juvenile onset disease accounts for 5%–10% of all cases of HD.

References: Toufexis, M., & Gieron-Korthals, M. (2010). Early testing for Huntington disease in children: Pros and cons. *Journal of Child Neurology, 25*(4), 482–484.

Ribai, P., Nguyen, K., Hahn-Barma, V., Gourfinkel-An, I., Vidailhet, M., Legout, A. ... Dürr, A. (2007). Psychiatric and cognitive difficulties as indicators of juvenile Huntington disease onset in 29 patients. *Archives of Neurology, 64*(6), 813–9.

Hurler syndrome (MPS IH) *See* mucopolysaccharidoses (MPS).

hypophosphatasia *Disease category:* Skeletal dysplasia. *Clinical features:* A disorder of calcium and phosphate metabolism with symptoms ranging from a severe infantile form (which can be rapidly fatal) to a relatively mild childhood form. A total of 6 forms of the disease have been described (perinatal lethal, perinatal benign, infantile, childhood, adult, and odontohypophosphatasia [dental only]). Features include short stature, bowed long bones, craniosynostosis, hypocalcemia. *Associated complications:* Seizures, multiple fractures, premature loss of teeth. The perinatal lethal form presents as short limbs and poor ossification of the skeleton, and affected infants usually die from pulmonary insufficiency. The benign perinatal form is usually identified by prenatal ultrasound but the skeletal manifestations slowly resolve with an eventual phenotype similar to the childhood or adult types. The childhood form presents with an early loss of secondary teeth, short stature, and delayed walking with a waddling gait. Joint pain and nonprogressive muscle weakness may also be present and the features resemble rickets. *Cause:* Mutations in the "tissue nonspecific" alkaline phosphatase gene (*ALPL*) on chromosome 1p36. *Inheritance:* AR (severe forms), AR/AD (milder forms). *Incidence:* 1:100,000; incidence of severe infantile form is 1:250 in Mennonite families from Manitoba, Canada.

References: Fauvert, D., Brun-Heath, I., Lia-Baldini, A.S., Bellazi, L., Taillandier, A., Serre, J.L. … Mornet, E. (2009). Mild forms of hypophosphatasia mostly result from dominant negative effect of severe alleles or from compound heterozygosity for severe and moderate alleles. *BMC Medical Genetics, 10,* 51.

Mornet, E. (2008). Hypophosphatasia. *Best Practice and Research: Clinical Rheumatology, 22*(1), 113–27.

Zanki, A., Mornet, E., & Wong, S. (2008). Specific ultrasonographic features of perinatal lethal hypophophatasia. *American Journal of Medical Genetics A, 146A*(9), 1200–4.

incontinentia pigmenti *Disease category:* Dermatologic disorder. *Clinical features:* Swirling patterns of hyperpigmented skin lesions; tooth abnormalities; microcephaly; ocular abnormalities; thin, wiry hair; hairless lesions, intellectual disability in approximately one third of cases. *Associated complications:* Spasticity, seizures, vertebral or rib abnormalities; strabismus, hydrocephalus, history of male miscarriages. *Cause:* Mutations in *IKBKG* (previously *NEMO*) gene on chromosome Xq28, skewed X-inactivation. A deletion of exons 4-10 is present in about 80% of affected individuals. *Inheritance:* XLD with lethality in males. Living affected males have been found with 47, XXY karyotype or somatic mosaicism. *Prevalence:* Rare.

References: Fusco, F., Pescatore, A., Bal, E., Ghoul, A., Paciolla, M., Lioi, M.B. … Ursini, M.V. (2008). Alterations of the IKBKG locus and diseases: An update and a report of 13 novel mutations. *Human Mutation, 29*(5), 595–604.

Jessup, C.J., Morgan, S.C., Cohen, L.M., & Viders, D.E. (2009). Incontinentia pigmenti: Treatment of IP with topical tacrolimus. *Journal of Drugs in Dermatology, 8*(10), 944–946.

O'Doherty, M., Mc Creery, K., Green, A.J., Tuwir, I., & Brosnahan, D. (2011). Incontinentia pigmenti—opthalmological observation of a series of cases and review of the literature. *British Journal of Ophthalmology, 95*(1), 11–16.

infantile Refsum disease *See* Refsum disease, infantile.

isovaleric acidemia *Disease category:* Inborn error of metabolism: organic acidemia. *Clinical features:* A disorder of organic acid metabolism; an acute, often fatal neonatal form is characterized by acidosis and coma; a chronic form presents with recurrent attacks of ataxia, vomiting, lethargy, and ketoacidosis. Attacks are generally triggered by infection or increased protein load. Urine smell of sweaty feet is characteristic. *Associated complications:* Seizures, intellectual disability if untreated, enlarged liver, vomiting, hematologic abnormalities. *Cause:* Deficiency of the enzyme isovaleryl-CoA dehydrogenase; gene linked to chromosome 15q14–q15. *Inheritance:* AR. *Prevalence:* Rare. *Treatment:* Treatment consisting of a low-protein diet with supplemental oral glycine and carnitine has resulted in a relatively good cognitive outcome.

References: Berry, G.T., Yudkoff, M., & Segal, S. (1988). Isovaleric acidemia: Medical and neurodevelopmental effects of long-term therapy. *Journal of Pediatrics, 113,* 58–64.

Loots, D.T., Mienie, L.J., & Erasmus, E. (2007). Amino acid depletion induced by abnormal amino-acid conjugation and protein restriction in isovaleric academia. *European Journal of Clinical Nutrition, 61*(11), 1323–1327.

Vockley, J., & Ensenauer, R. (2006). Isovaleric academia: New aspect of genetic and phenotypic heterogeneity. *American Journal of Medical Genetics C: Seminars in Medical Genetics, 142C*(2), 95–103.

Joubert syndrome *Disease category:* Multiple congenital anomalies. *Clinical features:* Structural cerebellar abnormalities ("molar tooth sign" on MRI), hypotonia in infancy which develops into ataxia, abnormal eye movements, retinal dysplasia or coloboma, abnormal breathing pattern, developmental delay/intellectual disability and behavioral problems; characteristic facial appearance including large head, prominent forehead, ptosis, epicanthal folds, upturned nose, tongue protrusion. *Associated complications:* Retinal dystrophy, renal disease, ocular colobomas, occipital encephalocele, hepatic fibrosis, polydactyly, oral hamartomas, and endocrine abnormalities. Cognitive abilities range from moderate to severe intellectual disability. *Cause:* Joubert syndrome has been linked to multiple different genes: *INPP5E* gene on chromosome 9q34.3, *TMEM216* gene on chromosome 11q13, *AHI1* gene on chromosome 6q23, *NPHP1* gene on chromosome 2q13, *CEP290* gene, also called *NPHP6* on chromosome 12q21.32, *TMEM67* gene on chromosome 8q21, *RPGRIP1L* gene on chromosome 16q12.2, *ARL13B* on chromosome 3q11.2, *CC2D2A* gene on chromosome 4p15.3, and *CXORF5* gene on chromosome Xp22.3 *Inheritance:* AR or XLR. *Prevalence:* Rare.

References: Coene, K.L. (2009). OFD1 is mutated in X-linked Joubert syndrome and interacts with LCA5-encoded lebercilin. *American Journal of Human Genetics, 85*(4), 465–81.

Edvardson, S., Shaag, A., Zenvirt, S., Erlich, Y., Hannon, G.J., Shanske, A.L. … Elpeleg, O. (2010). Joubert syndrome 2 (JBTS2) in Ashkenazi Jews is associated with a TMEM216 mutation. *American Journal of Human Genetics, 86*(1), 93–97.

juvenile neuronal ceroid lipofuscinosis *See* Batten disease.

Kabuki syndrome *Disease category:* Multiple congenital anomalies. *Clinical features:* Microcephaly, trapezoid philtrum (area between base of nose and upper lip), prominent posteriorly rotated ears, preauricular pit (small hole/indentation on the ear), long palpebral fissures, thick eyelashes, ptosis, sparse broad arched eyebrows, congenital heart defect, hirsutism (excessive hair), café au lait spots, cryptorchidism, small penis, hypotonia, joint hyperextensibility. *Associated complications:* Cleft palate, recurrent ear infections, hearing loss, aspiration pneumonia, feeding difficulties, malabsorption, anal stenosis, imperforate anus, scoliosis, congenital hip dislocation, increased susceptibility to infections, seizures, intellectual disability, premature thearche (breast development), hemolytic anemia, congenital hypothyroidism. *Cause:* Mutations in the *MLL2* gene on chromosome 12q12-q14 (78% pick-up rate). *Inheritance:* NM with AD inheritance when passed on from an affected individual. *Prevalence:* Rare.

References: Armstrong, L., Abd El Moneim, A., Aleck, K., Aughton, D.J., Baumann, C., Braddock, S.R. … Allanson, J.E. (2005). Further delineation of Kabuki syndrome in 48 well defined new individuals. *American Journal of Medical Genetics, 132*, 265–272.

Ng, S., Bigham, A.W., Buckingham, K.J., Hannibal, M.C., McMillin, M.J., Gildersleeve, H.I. … Shendure, J. (2010). Exome sequencing identifies MLL2 mutations as a cause of Kabuki syndrome. *Nature Genetics, 9*, 790–793.

Sanz, J.H., Lipkin, P., Rosenbaum, K., & Mahone, E.M. (2010). Developmental profile and trajectory of neuropsychological skills in a child with Kabuki syndrome: Implications for assessment of syndromes associated with intellectual disability. *Clinical Neuropsychology, 24*(7), 1181–1192.

Kearns-Sayre syndrome *Clinical features:* Short stature, progressive external ophthalmoplegia, retinitis pigmentosa, heart block, cerebellar ataxia. *Associated complications:* Visual impairment, hearing loss, myopathy, endocrine abnormalities, diabetes mellitus, dementia. *Cause:* Deletions in mtDNA (90% have a 2–10kb mtDNA deletion) *Inheritance:* Maternal, through mtDNA.

kinky hair syndrome *See* Menkes syndrome.

Klinefelter syndrome (XXY syndrome) *Disease category:* Chromosomal abnormality. *Clinical features:* Occurring only in males; tall, slim stature; long limbs; relatively small penis and testes; gynecomastia (breast enlargement) in 40%. *Associated complications:* Intention tremor (involuntary trembling arising when attempting a voluntary, coordinated movement) in 20%–50%, low to average intelligence, infertility, behavioral disorders, scoliosis, osteoporosis and reduced muscle strength, vascular problems; 8% have diabetes mellitus as adults, risk of extragonadal mid-line germ cell tumors. Patients may appear to have no physical changes prior to puberty with the exception of long legs. *Cause:* Chromosomal nondisjunction resulting in 47, XXY karyotype. *Inheritance:* NM caused by the presence of an additional X chromosome; about 50% of cases caused by maternal non-disjunction (error in the separation of chromosomes), while 50% are caused by paternal nondisjunction. *Prevalence:* 1:500 males. *Treatment:* Hormone treatment is needed in adolescence for the development of secondary sex characteristics.

References: Geschwind, D.H., Boone, K.B., Miller, B.L., & Swerdloff, R.S. (2000). Neurobehavioral phenotype of Klinefelter syndrome. *Mental Retardation and Developmental Disabilities Research Reviews, 6*, 107–116.

Giltay, J.C., & Maiburg, M.C. (2010). Kline-felter syndrome: Clinical and molecular aspects. *Expert Review in Molecular Diagnosis*, *10*(6), 765–76.

Klippel-Feil syndrome *Disease category:* Multiple congenital anomalies. *Clinical features:* Cervical vertebral fusion, hemivertebrae (incomplete development of one side of one or more vertebrae). *Associated complications:* Congenital scoliosis, torticollis (wry neck), low hairline; sacral agenesis (absence of tailbone), hearing loss, occasional congenital heart defect, extra, fused, or missing ribs, middle-ear abnormalities, genitourinary abnormalities, pain. *Cause:* Subgroup has been linked to the *GDF6* gene on chromosome 8q22.2. *Inheritance:* AD with variable expressivity and reduced penetrance most common; AR and nongenetic causes have been reported. *Incidence:* Approximately 1:40,000, with a slight female predominance.

References: Tassabehji, M., Fang, Z.M., Hilton, E.N., McGaughran, J., Zhao, Z., de Bock, C.E. ... Clarke, R.A. (2008). Mutation sin *GDF6* are associated with vertebral segmentation defects in Klippe-Feil syndrome. *Human Mutations*, *29*(8), 1017–1027.

Tracy, M.R., Dormans, J.P., & Kusumi, K. (2004). Klippel-Feil syndrome: Clinical features and current understanding of etiology. *Clinical Orthopaedics and Related Research*, *424*, 183–190.

Klippel-Trenauny-Weber syndrome *Disease category:* Multiple congenital anomalies. *Clinical features:* Asymmetric hypertrophy of limb, face (lips, cheeks, tongue, teeth) or other body parts, hemangiomas (benign congenital tumors made up of newly formed blood vessels), arteriovenous fistulas. *Associated complications:* Dependent on the area of hypertrophy; complications may affect any organ/body part including spinal cord (resulting in weakness or paralysis), kidneys (renal obstruction), brain (intracranial hypertension). *Cause:* Linked to the *VG5Q* (*AGGF1*) gene at 5q13.3. *Inheritance:* Believed to pass as an AD trait, where individuals are not affected unless a second, somatic (mutation arising after fertilization) occurs. *Prevalence:* Unknown.

References: Ceballos-Quintal, J.M., Pinto-Escalante, D., & Castillo-Zapata, I. (1996). A new case of Klippel-Trenaunay-Weber (KTW) syndrome: Evidence of autosomal dominant inheritance. *American Journal of Medical Genetics*, *63*, 426–427.

Hu, Y., Li, L., Seidelmann, S.B., Timur, A.A., Shen, P.H., Driscoll, D.J., & Wang, Q.K. (2008). Identification of association of common *AGGF1* variants with susceptibility for Klippel-Trenanunay syndrome using the Structure Association Program. *Annals of Human Genetics*, *72*(5), 636–643.

Tian, X.L., Kadaba, R., You, S.A., Liu, M., Timur, A.A., Yang, L. ... Wang, Q. (2004). Identification of an angiogenic factor that when mutated causes susceptibility to Klippel-Trenaunay syndrome. *Nature*, *427*, 640–644.

Krabbe disease (globoid cell leukodystrophy) *Disease category:* Progressive neurologic disorder. *Clinical features:* In the classic form, symptoms begin at 4–6 months of age with irritability, progressive stiffness, optic atrophy, cognitive deterioration, and early death, often before age 2. Approximately 10%–15% of cases have onset of symptoms between 6 months and 17 years of age, and have slower disease progression. *Associated complications:* Hypertonicity, opisthotonos (back arching), visual and hearing impairment, episodic unexplained fevers, seizures; peripheral neuropathy. *Cause:* Deficiency of the galactocerebrosidase enzyme resulting from a mutation in the *GALC* gene on chromosome 14q24.3–q32.1. *Inheritance:* AR. *Incidence:* 1:100,000; may be increased in specific populations such as the Druze kindred in Israel (carrier frequency of 1:6). *Treatment:* Hematopoietic stem cell transplantation has been performed in a small number of patients, but success is unclear.

References: Kemper, A., Knapp, A.A., Green, N.S., Comeau, A.M., Metterville, D.R., & Perrin, J.M. (2010). Weighing the evidence for newborn screening for early-infantile Krabbe disease. *Genetics in Medicine*, *12*(9), 539–543.

Sakai, N. (2009). Pathogenesis of leukodystrophy of Krabbe disease: Molecular mechanism and clinical treatment. *Brain and Development*, *31*, 485–487.

Siddiqi, Z.A., Sanders, D.B., & Massey, J.M. (2006). Peripheral neuropathy in Krabbe disease: Effect of hematopoietic stem cell transplantation. *Neurology*, *67*, 268–272.

Landau-Kleffner syndrome (LKS) *Disease category:* Neurologic. *Clinical features:* Selective aphasia (loss of speech), regression in receptive and/or expressive language ability, with some recovery in older children, seizures (80% of patients), paroxysmal electroencephalogram, electrical status epilepticus in slow-wave sleep with or without clinical seizures. *Associated complications:* Behavioral disturbances similar to those in autism. Males more frequently affected than females. The younger the age of onset, the worse the prognosis for possibility of recovery. *Cause:* Unknown. *Inheritance:* Possibly AR. *Prevalence:* Unknown; at least 170 children have been reported in the medical literature with approximately 1:440 children with epilepsy being diagnosed with LKS; predominance of affected males. *Treatment:* Treatment of seizures with antiepileptic medications. *See also* Chapter 27.

References: Billard, C., Fluss, J., & Pinton, F. (2009). Specific language impairment versus Landau-Kleffner syndrome. *Epilepsia,* *50*(7), 21–24.

Duran, M.H., Guimarães, C.A., Medeiros, L.L., & Guerreiro, M.M. (2009). Landau-Kleffner syndrome: Long-term follow-up. *Brain and Development, 31*(1), 58–63.

McVicar, K.A., & Shinnar, S. (2004). Landau-Kleffner syndrome, electrical status epilepticus in slow wave sleep, and language regression in children. *Mental Retardation and Developmental Disabilities Research Reviews, 10,* 144–149.

Laurence-Moon-Bardet-Biedl syndrome *See* Bardet-Biedl syndrome.

Leber hereditary optic neuropathy (Leber's congenital amaurosis, LHON) *Clinical features:* Bilateral central vision loss. *Associated complications:* Occasionally seen with multiple sclerosis, dystonia, or movement disorder. *Cause:* Primarily associated with point mutations in mtDNA. *Inheritance:* Maternal, through mtDNA. Males are more commonly affected.

Leber's congenital amaurosis *See* mitochondrial disorders.

Leigh syndrome (subacute necrotizing encephalomyopathy) *Clinical features:* Encephalopathy, ophthalmoplegia, optic atrophy, myopathy. *Associated complications:* Developmental delay and regression, ataxia, spasticity, hypertrophic cardiomyopathy, early death. Onset usually between 3 and 12 months of age, often after a viral infection. *Cause:* Mutations in many different nuclear and mitochondrial genes involved in energy metabolism including respiratory chain complexes I, II, III, IV, and V as well as tRNA proteins, and pyruvate deydrogenase complex. *Inheritance:* Maternal, AR, XLR.

Lennox-Gastaut syndrome *See Chapter 27.*

Lesch-Nyhan syndrome *Disease category:* Inborn error of metabolism: nucleic acid.

Clinical features: An inborn error of purine metabolism associated with elevated levels of uric acid in blood and urine. Affected males appear symptom free at birth but then present with hypotonia and developmental delay during the first year. Dystonia (abnormal movements) and spasticity develop, accompanied by severe involuntary self-injurious behavior, including biting of fingers, arms, and lips. *Associated complications:* Cognitive impairment, seizures in 50%, hematuria (blood in urine), kidney stones, and ultimate kidney failure without treatment. *Cause:* Defect in enzyme hypoxanthine-guanine phosphoribosyl transferase caused by a mutation in the *HPRT* gene on Xq26–q27.2. *Inheritance:* XLR. Affected females with skewed X-inactivation have been reported. Carrier females are typically unaffected although some have increased uric acid excretion. *Prevalence:* 1:380,000. *Treatment:* Allopurinol is useful in preventing kidney and joint deposition of uric acid. Spasticity is treated with Baclofen or benzodiazepines. Numerous medications have been used in management of self-injurious behavior without much success.

References: Ceballos-Picot, I., Mockel, L., Potier, M.C., Dauphinot, L., Shirley, T.L., Torero-Ibad, R. ... Jinnah, H.A. (2009). Hypoxanthine-guanine phosphoribosyl transferase regulates early developmental programming of dopamine neurons: Implications for Lesch-Nyhan disease pathogenesis. *Human Molecular Genetics, 18*(13), 2317–2327.

Schretlen, D.J., Ward, J., Meyer, S.M., Yun, J., Puig, J.G., Nyhan, W.L. ... Harris, J.C. (2005). Behavioral aspects of Lesch-Nyhan disease and its variants. *Developmental Medicine and Child Neurology, 47*(10), 673–677.

lissencephaly syndromes (e.g., Miller-Dieker syndrome) *Disease category:* Malformation. *Clinical features:* A group of disorders characterized by lissencephaly (smooth brain) in which Miller-Dieker syndrome is the prototype; lissencephaly syndromes can be divided into subgroups based on features. Classical lissencephaly (formerly lissencephaly type I), the most common form, is defined by the presence of a very thick cortex and subcortical band heterotopia, whereas other types of lissencephaly present with other brain malformations, including agenesis of the corpus callosum and severe cerebellar hypoplasia. Features include agyria or **pachygyria** (absent or decreased cerebral convolutions, respectively), progressive spasticity, microcephaly; characteristic facial appearance with short nose, broad nasal bridge, upturned nose, hypertelorism, prominent upper lip, malformed or malpositioned ears. *Associated complications:* Intellectual disability, infantile spasms, late tooth eruption, poor weight gain, **dysphagia** (swallowing difficulty), congenital heart defect, intestinal atresia (congenital closure). *Cause:* Six genes have been defined to date that cause lissencephaly: *LIS1* (on chromosome 17p13.3), *14-3-3* epsilon (on chromosome 17p13.3), *DCX* (on chromosome Xq22.3), *RELN* (on chromosome 7q22), and *ARX* (on chromosome Xp22.13), *TUBA1A* (on chromosome 12q12-q14); a deletion of one copy (haploinsufficiency) of any of the above genes is sufficient to cause one of the lissencephaly syndromes. *Inheritance:* NM with AD inheritance when passed from an affected individual, or XLR (males are typically affected while females have milder phenotype); possibly increased recurrence risk if one parent has a balanced chromosomal translocation of chromosome 17p. *Prevalence:* Rare.

References: Haverfield, E, Whited, A.J., Petras, K.S., Dobyns, W.B., Das, S. (2009). Intragenic deletions and duplications of the *LIS1* and *DCX* genes: A major disease-causing mechanism in lissencephaly and subcortical band heterotopia. *European Journal of Human Genetics, 17,* 911–918.

Wynshaw-Boris, A. (2007). Lissencephaly and *LIS1*: Insights into the molecular mechanisms of neuronal migration and development. *Clinical Genetics, 72*(4), 296–304.

Lowe syndrome (oculocerebrorenal syndrome) *Disease category:* Multiple congenital anomalies. *Clinical features:* Bilateral cataracts at birth, hypotonia, absent deep tendon reflexes, kidney dysfunction (proximal renal tubular dysfunction), dysmorphic facies. *Associated complications:* Poor weight gain, short stature, vitamin D-resistant rickets, seizures, visual impairment (corrected acuity is usually 20/100), glaucoma, intellectual disability in 75%, behavioral problems, intention tremor, craniosynostosis, peripheral neuropathy (damage to nerves). Female carriers have characteristic findings in the lens (opacities) of each eye. *Cause:* Abnormal inositol phosphate metabolism caused by mutations in the *OCRL1* gene on chromosome Xq26.1. *Inheritance:* XLR with one third of cases being NM. *Prevalence:* 1:100,000.

References: Addis, M., Meloni, C., Congiu, R., Santaniello, S., Emma, F., Zuffardi, O. ...

Cau, M. (2007). A novel interstitial deletion in Xq25, identified by array-CGH in a patient with Lowe syndrome. *European Journal of Medical Genetics, 50*(1), 79–84.

Bockenhauer, D., Bokenkamp, A., van't Hoff, W., Levtchenko, E., Kist-van Holthe, J.E., Tasic, V., & Ludwig, M. (2008). Renal phenotype in Lowe syndrome: A selective proximal tubular dysfunction. *Clinical Journal of the American Society of Nephrology, 3*(5), 1430–1436.

mandibulofacial dysostosis *See* Treacher Collins syndrome.

maple syrup urine disease (MSUD) *Disease category:* Inborn error of metabolism: amino acid. *Clinical features:* A disorder of branched chain amino acid metabolism with four identified clinical variants (classic, intermittent, intermediate, and thiamine-responsive); the classic form comprises 75% of cases and is characterized by a maple syrup odor in the cerumen and urine from birth to 7 days of age, severe opisthotonos (spasm with body in a bowed position and head and heels bent backward), hypertonia, hypoglycemia, lethargy, and respiratory difficulties. Symptoms appear within the first 48 hours of life; if untreated, it is most often fatal within 1 month. Untreated survivors have severe intellectual disability and spasticity. The intermittent form presents with periods of ataxia, behavior disturbances, drowsiness, and seizures. Attacks are triggered by infections, excessive protein intake, or other physiological stresses. Individuals with the intermediate form usually demonstrate mild to moderate intellectual disability. *Associated complications:* Acidosis, hypoglycemia, growth retardation, feeding problems; acute episodes are characterized by muscle fatigue, vomiting, impaired cognitive ability, hyperactivity, sleep disturbance, hallucinations, dystonia, and ataxia. *Cause:* Deficiency in branched chain alpha-ketoacid dehydrogenase caused by mutations in the genes (at chromosomal locations 1p31, 6p22–p21, and 19q13.1–q13.2) making up this enzyme complex: BCKDHA, BCKDHB and DBT. *Prevalence:* 1:185,000; increased prevalence in Mennonite population with an incidence of 1:380. *Inheritance:* AR. *Treatment:* High-calorie diet with restriction of leucine, supplementation with isoleucine and valine. If instituted early (within 2 weeks of birth), the prognosis is good for typical intelligence. Thiamine is used in the thiamine-responsive form. Orthotopic liver transplantation is effective for classic MSUD.

References: Puckett, R.L., Lorey, F., Rinaldo, P., Lipson, M.H., Matern, D., Sowa, M.E. … Abdenur, J.E. (2010). Maple syrup urine disease: Further evidence that newborn screening may fail to identify variant forms. *Molecular Genetics and Metabolism, 100*(2), 136–142.

Shellmer, D.A., et al. (2011). Cognitive and adaptive functioning after liver transplantation for maple syrup urine disease: A case series. *Pediatric Transplantation, 15*(1), 58–64.

Zinnanti, W.J., Lazovic, J., Griffin, K., Skvorak, K.J., Paul, H.S., Homanics, G.E. … Flanagan, J.M. (2009). Dual mechanism of brain injury and novel treatment strategy in maple syrup urine disease. *Brain, 132*(4), 903–918.

Marfan syndrome *Disease category:* Connective tissue disorder. *Clinical features:* Tall, thin body, upward dislocation of ocular lens, myopia, spiderlike limbs, hypermobile joints. Average intelligence expected, although learning disabilities have been reported in up to 50% of children. *Associated complications:* Aortic dilatation or dissection, congestive heart failure, mitral valve prolapse, emphysema, sleep apnea, and scoliosis. *Cause:* Mutation in the fibrillin (*FBN-1*) gene located on chromosome 15q15–q21.3. *Inheritance:* AD with wide clinical variability. *Prevalence:* Estimated to be about 1:5,000. *Treatment:* Use of Losartan, an angiotensin II type 1 receptor blocker has been shown to prevent aortic aneurysm through the inhibition of transforming growth factor beta in mice. Doxycycline has also been shown to normalize aortic vasomotor function and suppress aneurysm growth. Trials continue with both of these medications.

References: Dean, J.C. (2007). Marfan syndrome: Clinical diagnosis and management. *European Journal of Human Genetics, 15*(7), 724–733.

Hilhorst-Hofstee, Y., Hamel, B.C., Verheij, J.B., Rijlaarsdam, M.E., Mancini, G.M., Cobben, J.M. … Pals, G. (2011). The clinical spectrum of complete *FBN1* allele deletions. *European Journal of Human Genetics, 19*(3), 247–252.

Maroteaux-Lamy syndrome (MPS VI) *See* mucopolysaccharidoses.

McCune-Albright syndrome (polyostotic fibrous dysplasia) *Disease category:* Endocrine disorder. *Clinical features:* Large café-au-lait spots with irregular borders; fibrous dysplasia of bones (thinning of the bone with replacement of bone marrow with fibrous tissue, producing pain and increasing deformity), bowing of long bones, premature onset of puberty; advanced bone age. *Associated complications:* Hearing or visual impairment, hyperthyroidism, hyperparathyroidism (increased activity of the parathyroid gland, which controls calcium metabolism), abnormal adrenal function, increased risk of malignancy, occasional spinal cord anomalies. *Cause:* Postmitotic mutation in the *GNAS1* gene (causing a defect in the enzyme adenyl cyclase) localized to 20q13. *Inheritance:* NM arising after fertilization (somatic mosaic) will be passed in an AD fashion if reproductive organs involved; theoretically lethal unless present in the mosaic form. *Testing:* Mutations in the *GNAS1* gene were only present in 46% of patients presenting with the classic triad. Other tissue types may need to be tested to confirm the presence of the common mutation. *Prevalence:* Unknown.

References: Chapurlat, R.D., & Orcel, P. (2008). Fibrous dysplasia of bone and McCune-Albright syndrome. *Best Practice and Research: Clinical Rheumatology, 22*(1), 55–69.

Lietman, S.A., Schwindinger, W.F., & Levine, M.A. (2007). Genetic and molecular aspects of McCune-Albright syndrome. *Pediatric Endocrinology Reviews, 4*(4), 380–385.

MELAS (*m*itochondrial myopathy, *e*ncephalopathy, *l*actic *a*cidosis, and *s*troke-like episodes) *See* mitochondrial disorders.

Menkes syndrome (kinky hair syndrome) *Disease category:* Inborn error of metabolism: copper. *Clinical features:* An inborn error of copper metabolism presenting at age 1–2 months with "steely" texture of hair and characteristic face with pudgy cheeks. *Associated complications:* Seizures, feeding difficulties, severe intellectual disability, recurrent infections, visual loss, bony abnormalities with tendency toward easy fracture, thrombosis, early death. *Cause:* Copper deficiency from decreased absorption and/or missing enzymes caused by mutations in the adenosine triphosphatase *ATP7A* gene at Xq13. *Inheritance:* XLR. *Prevalence:* 1:100,000. *Treatment:* Treatment with copper-histidine has been found to prevent neurological deterioration when provided before the age of 2 months. Treatment provided after 2 months of age cannot prevent neurologic, connective tissue, or bone complications.

References: Kaler, S.G., Holmes, C.S., Goldstein, D.S., Tang, J., Godwin, S.C., Donsante,

A. ... Patronas, N. (2008). Neonatal diagnosis and treatment of Menkes disease. *New England Journal of Medicine, 358*, 605–614.

Kaler, S.G., Liew, C.J., Donsante, A., Hicks, J.D., Sato, S., & Greenfield, J.C. (2010). Molecular correlates of epilepsy in early diagnosed and treated Menkes disease. *Journal of Inherited Metabolic Disease, 33*(5), 583–589.

MERRF (myoclonic epilepsy with ragged red fibers) *See* mitochondrial disorders.

metachromatic leukodystrophy (Arylsulfatase A deficiency) *Disease category:* Inborn error of metabolism: lysosomal storage disorder. *Clinical features:* One of a group of lysosomal storage disorders in which lysosomes, the cell structures that digest toxic materials, are missing a necessary enzyme; the resulting accumulation of toxins leads to varying degrees of progressive neurological impairment, ranging from unsteady gait to severe rigidity and choreoathetosis. Muscle weakness and ataxia are common. Onset of the infantile form is by age 2 years and usually results in death by age 5 (50%–60% of cases). The juvenile form generally begins between 4 and 10 years of age, is rarer (20%–30% of cases), and progresses more slowly. Two distinct adult onset forms exist, one presenting with neurologic/motor involvement and the other with behavioral abnormalities. *Associated complications:* Seizures, abdominal distension, mental deterioration. *Cause:* Mutations in the arylsulfatase A (*ASA*) gene on chromosome 22q cause ASA enzyme deficiency and result in the accumulation of sphingolipid sulfatide. *Inheritance:* AR. *Prevalence:* 1:40,000 in Sweden; rarer elsewhere. *Treatment:* Bone marrow transplantation may have beneficial effects on some tissues types but does not affect lipid storage in the brain.

References: Gieselmann, V., & Krageloh-Mann, I., & Krägeloh-Mann, I. (2010). Metachromatic leukodystrophy—an update. *Neuropediatricsm 41*(1), 1–6.

Mahmood, A., Berry, J., Wenger, D.A., Escolar, M., Sobeih, M., Raymond, G., & Eichler, F.S. (2010). Metachromatic leukodystrophy: A case of triplets with the late infantile variant and a systematic review of the literature. *Journal of Child Neurology, 25*(5), 572–580.

Smith, N.J., Marcus, R.E., Sahakian, B.J., Kapur, N., & Cox, T.M. (2010). Haematopoietic stem cell transplantation does not retard disease progression in the psycho-cognitive variant of late-onset metachromatic leukodystrophy. *Journal of Inherited Metabolic Disease,* doi: 10.1007/s10545-010-9240-1

methylmalonic aciduria *Disease category:* Inborn error of metabolism: organic acidemia. *Clinical features:* An organic acidemia with multiple subtypes. In the infantile/non-B_{12} responsive phenotype (most common form), infants are normal at birth but then develop lethargy, vomiting, dehydration, hepatomegaly, hypotonia and encephalopathy. There is a rarer intermediate B_{12}-responsive type, which presents in the first few months to years with anorexia, poor weight gain, hypotonia and developmental delay. The atypical/benign adult subtype is associated with increased urinary excretion of methylmalonic acid but they may remain asymptomatic. *Associated complications:* Variable developmental delay, renal failure, metabolic stroke affecting the basal ganglia, movement disorder with choreoathetosis, dystonia, para/quadriparesis, pancreatitis, growth failure, immune dysfunction, and optic nerve atrophy. *Cause:* Isolated methylmalonic aciduria is found in patients with mutations in the MUT gene (*6p21*) causing partial, mut(-), or complete, mut(0), enzyme deficiency. This form is unresponsive to B_{12} therapy. Various forms of isolated methylmalonic aciduria also occur in a subset of patients with defects in the synthesis of the MUT coenzyme adenosylcobalamin (AdoCbl) and are classified according to complementation group: cblA, caused by mutation in the *MMAA* gene (4q31.1-q31.2), and cblB, caused by mutation in the *MMAB* gene (12q24). Combined methylmalonic aciduria and homocystinuria may be seen in complementation groups cblC, cblD, and cblF. *Inheritance:* AR. *Prevalence:* 1:50,000–1:100,000. *Treatment:* Treatment consists of a low-protein, high calorie diet and supplemental hydroxycobalamin (B_{12}) injections in those who have a B_{12}-responsive form; carnitine is also given. Liver and liver/kidney transplant has been performed to avoid continual damage to the kidneys, and some success has been reported.

References: Hauser, N.S., Manoli, I., Graf, J.C., Sloan, J,. & Venditti, C.P. (2011). Variable dietary management of methylmalonic acidemia: Metabolic and energetic correlations. *American Journal of Clinical Nutrition, 93*(1), 47–56.

Lee, N.C., Chien, Y.H., Peng, S.F., Huang, A.C., Liu, T.T., Wu, A.S. ... Hwu, W.L. (2008). Brain damage by mild metabolic derangements in methylmalonic acidemia. *Pediatric Neurology, 39*(5), 325–329.

Morioka, D., Kasahara, M., Horikawa, R., Yokoyama, S., Fukuda, A., & Nakagawa, A. (2007). Efficacy of living donor liver transplantation for patients with methylmalonic acidemia. *American Journal of Transplantation*, 7(12), 2782–2787.

Miller-Dieker syndrome   *See* lissencephaly syndromes.

mitochondrial disorders (mitochondrial encephalopathies and myopathies)   *Disease category:* Inborn error of metabolism/mitochondrial disorders. *Clinical features:* This diverse group of disorders is linked by a common etiology: abnormal function of the mitochondria (energy-producing intracellular structures) or mitochondrial metabolism. Mitochondrial disorders can affect every organ system. Common features include ptosis, external ophthalmoplegia (paralysis of the external eye muscles), myopathy, cardiomyopathy, short stature, and hypoparathyroidism. *Associated complications:* Seizures, sensorineural hearing loss, optic atrophy, retinitis pigmentosa (pigmentary changes in retina causing loss of peripheral vision and clumping of pigment), cataracts, diabetes, migraine, intestinal pseudo-obstruction, reflux, renal problems, exercise intolerance. *Cause:* Genes encoding nuclear DNA and mitochondrial DNA (mtDNA) are known to cause mitochondrial disorders. Mutations in different genes may cause the same symptoms. *Inheritance:* AR, AD, NM, or may be inherited from the mother through mtDNA. *Prevalence:* 1:8,500 for all mitochondrial disorders combined. *Treatment:* Early diagnosis and treatment of diabetes, eye abnormalities, and cardiac disease. Coenzyme Q10 and riboflavin have been used with some reported benefit. Six mitochondrial disorders are discussed next.

References: Chinnery P.F., Majamaa, K., Turnbull, D., & Thorburn, D. (2006). Treatment for mitochondrial disorders. *Cochrane Database of Systematic Reviews*, 1(CD004426). doi: 10.1002/14651858.CD004426.pub2.

DiMauro, S. (2004). Mitochondrial diseases. *Biochemica et Biophysica Acta*, *1658*, 80–88.

Falk, M., & Sondheimer, N. (2010). Mitochondrial genetic diseases. *Current Opinion in Pediatrics*, *22*(6), 711–716.

Thornburn, D.R. (2004). Mitochondrial disorders: Prevalence, myths, and advances. *Journal of Inherited Metabolic Disease*, *27*, 349–362.

MELAS (*m*itochondrial myopathy, *e*ncephalopathy, *l*actic *a*cidosis, and *s*troke-like episodes)   *Clinical features:* Migraine headaches, seizures, stroke-like episodes, encephalopathy (degenerative disease of the brain), myopathy. *Associated complications:* Progressive hearing loss, cortical blindness, ataxia, dementia, and lactic acidosis, recurrent vomiting, hemiparesis. *Cause:* A mutation in mtDNA encoding transfer RNA causes reduced mitochondrial protein synthesis. *Inheritance:* Maternal, through mtDNA.

MERRF (*m*yoclonic *e*pilepsy with *r*agged *r*ed *f*ibers)   *Clinical features:* Myoclonic epilepsy, ataxia, spasticity, myopathy. *Associated complications:* Optic atrophy, sensorineural hearing loss, peripheral neuropathy, diabetes, cardiomyopathy, dementia, lipomas (fatty tumors); characteristic ragged red muscle fibers are seen on muscle biopsy examination. *Cause:* Mutations in mtDNA encoding transfer RNA. *Inheritance:* Maternal, through mtDNA.

Moebius sequence (congenital facial diplegia)   *Disease category:* Multiple congenital anomalies. *Clinical features:* Expressionless face and facial weakness (bilateral in 92% of cases and unilateral in 8%) due to palsies of the 6th, 7th, and occasionally 12th cranial nerves; occasional abnormalities of fingers and legs; micrognathia; eye abnormalities including esotropia ("cross-eyed") and vision problems including myopia, astigmatism, and amblyopia; craniofacial malformations. *Associated complications:* Feeding difficulties, oral motor dysfunction, articulation disorder, occasional tracheal or laryngeal anomalies, gross and fine motor delay and dysfunction. Intellectual disability in 10%–50%. *Cause:* Linked to chromosomes 13q12–q13 and 1p34. *Inheritance:* Not well characterized, most reported cases are SP, possibly due to a NM; rare reports of AR, AD and X linked cases with variable expressivity. *Prevalence:* 1:50,000.

References: Briegel, W. (2006). Neuropsychiatric findings of Möbius sequence-a review. *Clinical Genetics*, *70*(2), 97–97.

Cattaneo, L., Chierici, E., Bianchi, B., Sesenna, E., & Pavesi, G. (2006). The localization of facial motor impairment in sporadic Möbius syndrome. *Neurology*, *66*(12), 1907–1912.

Grazidadio, C., Lorenzen, M.B., Rosa, R.F., Pinto, L.L., Zen, P.R., Travi, G.M. ... Paskulin, G.A. (2010). New report of a familial case of Moebius syndrome presenting skeletal findings. *American Journal of Medical Genetics Part A*, *152A*(8), 2134–2138.

monosomy X *See* Turner syndrome.

Morquio syndrome (MPS IV) *See* mucopolysaccharidoses.

MSUD *See* maple syrup urine disease.

mucopolysaccharidoses (MPS) *Disease category:* Inborn error of metabolism: lysosomal storage disorder. *Clinical features:* Glycosaminoglycans accumulate within the lysosomes in these seven distinguishable forms of the disorder, each with two or more subgroups. Features shared by most include coarse facial features, thick skin, hirsutism (excessive hair), corneal clouding, and organomegaly (enlargement of spleen and liver). Growth deficiency, intellectual disability, cardiomyopathy, and skeletal dysplasia are also seen. Intelligence is normal in MPS type IV (Morquio syndrome) and MPS type VI (Marataux-Lamy). *Inheritance:* All are AR except MPSII, Hunter syndrome which is XLR. The various MPS disorders are differentiated by their clinical features, enzymatic defects, genetic transmission, and urinary mucopolysaccharide pattern. *Prevalence:* Overall estimated to be 1: 22,500. MPS I (Hurler, Scheie, & Hurler-Scheie), MPS II (Hunter), and MPS III (Sanfilippo) syndromes are discussed next. Others include MPS IV (Morquio), MPS VI (Maroteaux-Lamy), and MPS VII (Sly) syndromes.
References: Muenzer, J. (2004). The mucopolysaccharidoses: A heterogeneous group of disorders with variable pediatric presentations. *Journal of Pediatrics, 144,* S27–S34.
Neufeld, E.F., & Muenzer, J. (2001). The mucopolysaccharidoses. In C.R. Scriver, A.L. Beaudet, W.S. Sly, et al. (Eds.), *The metabolic and molecular bases of inherited disease* (pp. 3421–3452). New York, NY: McGraw-Hill.

MPS I (Hurler syndrome, Scheie syndrome, Hurler-Scheie syndrome) Due to the wide spectrum of clinical variability seen in patients with MPS I, patients with the mild form were originally thought to have a distinct disorder from those with severe symptoms. The mild condition was called Scheie syndrome (previously called MPS V), and the severe form of the disorder was previously called Hurler syndrome. Determination of a common enzyme deficiency in both conditions led to the realization that these conditions represented the variable presentation of a single disease. They are now denoted as having severe MPS I or attenuated MPS I. *Clinical features:* Patients with the severe MPS I are

normal at birth but then gradual coarsening of facial features in early childhood becomes apparent; they also have hypertrichosis (excessive hair); large skull; organomegaly; prominent lips; corneal clouding; dysostosis (malformed bones); stiffening of joints. There is progressive intellectual deterioration and spasticity and by age 3, growth typically stops. Death typically occurs by age 10. The attenuated form is characterized by hearing loss, cardiac valvular disease, progressive restriction in range of motion with typical stature, typical intelligence (although some may have learning disabilities), and survival into adulthood. *Associated complications:* Chronic ear infections, hearing loss, occasional hernia and cardiac valve changes, visual impairment, brain cysts, airway obstruction. *Cause:* Deficiency of enzyme alpha-L-iduronidase caused by mutations in the iduronidase gene on chromosome 4p16.3. *Inheritance:* AR. *Incidence:* 1:100,000 for the severe form and 1:500,000 for the attenuated form. *Treatment:* Hematopoietic stem cell transplantation (HSCT) in some severe MPS I patients can increase survival, improve facial coarseness and hepatosplenomegaly, improve hearing and maintain normal heart function (but does not improve skeletal manifestations or corneal clouding). HSCT may slow the course of cognitive decline in those with mild impairment. Enzyme replacement therapy with Aldurazyme is licensed for treatment of non-CNS manifestations of MPS I.

MPS II (Hunter syndrome) *Clinical features:* Features include short stature; enlarged liver and spleen; coarsening of facial features, with hypertrichosis beginning in early childhood; hoarse voice. Intellectual disability is mild or absent in the attenuated form of the disease; this subtype is compatible with survival to adulthood. The severe form is highlighted by progressive intellectual deterioration first noted between 2 and 3 years of age; death occurs before age 15 in most cases and is similar to severe MPS I, but with clear corneas. *Associated complications:* Sensorineural hearing loss, retinitis pigmentosa with visual loss, macrocephaly, stiffening of joints, particularly those in the hands, cardiac valve disease, hernia; respiratory insufficiency; chronic diarrhea, seizures. *Cause:* Deficiency of enzyme iduronate-2-sulfatase caused by mutations in this gene on chromosome Xq28. *Inheritance:* XLR. *Incidence:* 1:100,000–1:170,000 male births. *Treatment:* Minimal success has been reported with bone marrow transplantation. Enzyme replacement therapy for MPS II is now available (Idursulfase/Elaprase). No information is yet available on the outcome of using the drug for patients under age 5 or who have severe pulmonary compromise or severe central nervous system disease. Elaprase does not cross the blood-brain barrier and thus it is not expected that there would be any effect on CNS disease.

MPS III (Sanfilippo syndrome) *Clinical features:* Four distinct types representing four different enzyme defects with similar clinical features; clinical features present between 2 and 6 years in children who otherwise appear typical. There is mild coarsening of facial features, coarse hair and hirsutism, absence of corneal clouding, mild enlargement of liver, joint stiffness, sleep disorders, and progressive mental deterioration. Deterioration is most rapid in type IIIA; death occurs by 10–20 years in most cases. *Associated complications:* Severe behavioral disturbances by age 4–6 years, dysostosis, diarrhea in 50%, progressive spasticity and ataxia, precocious puberty, central breathing problems with advancing disease. *Cause:* Type IIIA: Deficiency of enzyme heparan sulfatase caused by mutations in sulfamidase gene on 17q25.3. Type IIIB: Deficiency of enzyme alpha-N-acetylglucosaminidase caused by mutations in the *NAGLU* gene on 17q21. Type IIIC: Deficiency of enzyme acetyl-CoA: alpha-glucosaminide N-acetyltransferase caused by mutations in a gene linked to chromosome 14. Type IIID: Deficiency of enzyme N-acetyl-alpha-glucosaminine-6sulfatase caused by mutations in the G6S gene linked to chromosome 12q14. *Inheritance:* AR. *Incidence:* 1:73,000–1:280,000. *Treatment:* Treatment is supportive only. Bone marrow transplantation has not been successful.

multiple acyl-CoA dehydrogenase deficiency *See* glutaric acidemia, type II.

multiple carboxylase deficiency, infantile or early form (holocarboxylase synthetase deficiency) *Disease category:* Inborn error of metabolism: cofactor deficiency. *Clinical features:* Disorder of biotin metabolism characterized by seizures, hypotonia, lethargy, coma, skin rash, alopecia (loss of hair from skin areas where it is normally present), and acidosis. Often, the presenting feature

is feeding difficulty or respiratory distress. *Associated complications:* Intellectual disability, hearing impairment, optic atrophy with visual impairment, recurrent infections, vomiting. *Cause:* Mutations in *HCLS* causing enzyme deficiencies of holocarboxylase synthetase, or 3-methylcrotonyl-CoA carboxylase. *Inheritance:* AR. *Prevalence:* Rare. *Treatment:* Oral biotin supplementation. Prenatal treatment with oral biotin corrects lethargy, hypotonia, and vomiting.

References: Tammachote, R., Janklat, S., Tongkobpetch, S., Suphapeetiporn, K., & Shotelersuk, V. (2010). Holocarboxylase synthetase deficiency: Novel clinical and molecular findings. *Clinical Genetics, 78*(1), 88–93.

Van Hove, J.L., Josefsberg, S., Freehauf, C., Thomas, J.A., Thuy le, P., Barshop, B.A. ... León-Del-Río, A. (2008). Management of a patient with holocarboxylase synthetase deficiency. *Molecular Genetics and Metabolism, 95*(4), 201–205.

multiple carboxylase deficiency, late onset, juvenile form (biotinidase deficiency) *Disease category:* Inborn error of metabolism: cofactor deficiency. *Clinical features:* A disorder characterized by varying degrees of intellectual disability, hypotonia, seizures (often infantile spasms), alopecia, skin rash, delayed myelination and lactic acidosis; the onset of symptoms usually occurs between 2 weeks and 2 years of age. *Associated complications:* Hearing and visual impairment, respiratory difficulties and apnea, recurrent infections. *Cause:* Defects in various enzymes for biotin transport or metabolism; genetic mutations have been identified in the biotinidase gene on chromosome 3p25 and the holocarboxylase synthetase gene on chromosome 21q22.1. *Inheritance:* AR. *Incidence:* 1:60,000–1:140,000. *Treatment:* Supplementation with oral biotin; response is better if used early in the course of the disease.

References: Cowan, T.M., Blitzer, M.G., Wolf, B. & Working Group of the American College of Medical Genetics Laboratory Quality Assurance Committee. (2010). Technical standards and guidelines for the diagnosis of biotinidase deficiency. *Genetics in Medicine, 12*(7), 464–470.

Pindolia, K., Jordan, M., & Wolf, B. (2010). Analysis of mutations causing biotinidase deficiency. *Human Mutation, 31*(9), 983–991.

muscular dystrophy, Duchenne (DMD) and Becker (BMD) types *Disease category:*

Neuromuscular disease. *Clinical features:* Progressive proximal muscular degeneration, muscle wasting, hypertrophy (enlargement) of calves, cardiomyopathy; onset of symptoms in DMD occurs before 3 years. Loss of ability to walk independently occurs by adolescence in DMD. The onset in BMD is later, and the progression is slower. *Associated complications:* Congestive heart failure, scoliosis, flexion contractures, respiratory compromise, and intestinal motility dysfunction (causing constipation); approximately one third of boys with DMD have learning or intellectual disabilities. *Cause:* Mutations in the gene that encodes dystrophin localized to Xp21.1. *Inheritance:* XLR with one third of cases due to a NM. *Incidence:* DMD 1:3,500 male births; BMD 1:20,000 males. There are reports of females with clinical features of DMD as the result of X-chromosome rearrangements involving the *DMD* locus because they have Turner syndrome (i.e., complete or partial absence of an X chromosome) or nonrandom X-chromosome inactivation. *Treatment:* Glucocorticosteroids have been shown to prolong ambulation; prednisone has been shown to improve strength and function. *See also Chapter 13.*

References: Wingeier, K., Giger, E., Strozzi, S., Kreis, R., Joncourt, F., Conrad, B. ... Steinlin, M. (2010). Neuropsychological impairments and the impact of dystrophin mutations on general cognitive functioning of patients with Duchenne muscular dystrophy. *Journal of Clinical Neuroscience, 18*(1), 90–95.

myasthenia gravis *Disease category:* Neuromuscular disease. *Clinical features:* Proximal muscle weakness, facial muscle weakness, difficulty chewing, ptosis, dysarthria, dysphagia, ventilatory insufficiency *Cause:* Failure of chemical transmission at the neuromuscular junction. It is an autoimmune disorder in which antibodies interfere with neuromuscular transmission. Although in rare instances genetic in origin, it is most often acquired as an autoimmune disorder. *Incidence:* 1:30,000. *Treatment:* Directed at removing the offending antibody and increasing the level of acetylcholine in the synaptic cleft; the immunological approach has employed corticosteroid medication, immunoglobulin, plasmapheresis, and the surgical removal of the thymus gland. Transient symptom improvement due to increased neurotransmitter levels in the synaptic cleft is achieved with pyridostigmine (Mestinon). Using these various treatment approaches, individuals with myasthenia can lead quite typical lives.

References: Mandawat, A. (2010). Comparative analysis of therapeutic options used for myasthenia gravis. *Annals of Neurology. 68*(6), 797–805.

Jani-Acsadi, A., & Lisak, R.P., (2010). *Myasthenia gravis. Current Treatment Options in Neurology, 12*(3), 231–243.

myotonic dystrophy (Steinert's disease) *Disease category:* Neuromuscular disease. *Clinical features:* The most prominent feature is myotonia, a form of dystonia involving increased muscular contractility combined with decreased power to release (e.g., a strong handshake with the inability to release it). Other features include myopathy, dysarthria, ptosis, and frontal balding. The age of onset varies from childhood to adulthood. The congenital form is severe, with neonatal hypotonia, motor delay, intellectual disability, and facial muscle palsy. In the congenital form, feeding difficulties and severe respiratory problems are common. Classic myotonia does not begin until around 10 years of age. *Associated complications:* Cataracts, cardiac conduction abnormalities, diabetes, and hypogonadism. *Cause:* Cytosine-thymine-guanine (CTG) expansion mutations in the muscle protein kinase gene on chromosome 19q13. Severity varies with the number of CTG repeats. Unaffected people have 5–30 repeat copies. Those with the classical adult form have more than 100 copies, and individuals with the congenital form usually have more than 2,000 copies. The correlation between the number of repeats, severity, and age of onset, however, is not always consistent. Myotonic dystrophy has also been associated with CCTG repeat expansion in the *CNBP(ZNF9)* gene (3q13.3-q24). Normal alleles have up to 30 repeats; those affected have 75–11,000 repeats with an average of 5,000. *Inheritance:* AD with genetic anticipation (repeat expands in subsequent generations and the onset of symptoms becomes earlier); with rare exception, it is the mother who transmits mutations, causing the congenital form. *Prevalence:* 1:8,000; increased prevalence in certain areas of Quebec.

References: Douniol, M., Jacquette, A., Guilé, J.M., Tanguy, M.L., Angeard, N., Héron, D. ... Cohen, D. (2009). Psychiatric and cognitive phenotype in children and adolescents with myotonic dystrophy. *European Child and Adolescent Psychiatry, 18*(12), 705–715.

Lopez, C., Nakamori, M., Tomé, S., Chitayat, D., Gourdon, G., Thornton, C.A., & Pearson, C.E. (2010). Expanded CTG repeat demarcates a boundary for abnormal CpG methylation in myotonic dystrophy patient tissues. *Human Molecular Genetics, 20*(1), 1–15.

Raheem, O., Olufemi, S.E., Bachinski, L.L., Vihola, A., Sirito, M., Holmlund-Hampf, J. ... Krahe, R. (2010). Mutant (CCTG) expansion causes abnormal expression of zinc finger protein 9 (ZNF9) in myotonic dystrophy type 2. *American Journal of Pathology, 177*(6), 3025–3036.

Nager syndrome *See* acrofacial dysostosis.

NARP (*n*europathy, *a*taxia, *r*etinitis *p*igmentosa) *Clinical features:* Retinitis pigmentosa, sensory neuropathy. *Associated complications:* Seizures, dementia, ataxia, proximal weakness. *Cause:* Mutation in the ATP synthase 6 gene. *Inheritance:* Maternal, through mtDNA.

neonatal adrenoleukodystrophy *See* adrenoleukodystrophy, neonatal form.

neurofibromatosis, type I (von Recklinghausen disease) *Disease category:* Neurological disorder. *Clinical features:* Multiple café-au-lait spots, axillary (armpit) and inguinal (groin) freckling, nerve tumors (fibromas) in body and on skin, Lisch nodules (brown bumps on the iris of the eye). *Associated complications:* Glaucoma, scoliosis, hypertension, attention-deficit/hyperactivity disorder (ADHD), macrocephaly or hydrocephalus, visual impairments (secondary to optic gliomas), increased risk of numerous malignant and benign tumors in the nervous system (malignant peripheral nerve sheath tumors in 8%–13% of patients), verbal and nonverbal learning disabilities occur in 30%–65% of patients. *Cause:* Mutation in NF1 gene, which codes for neurofibromin protein, on chromosome 17q11.2. *Inheritance:* AD with variable expression. Approximately 50% represent NM. *Prevalence:* 1:3,000.

References: Huijbregts, S. (2010). Cognitive and motor control in neurofibromatosis type I: Influence of maturation and hyperactivity-inattention. *Developmental Neuropsychology, 35*(6), 737–751.

Lorenzo, J., Barton, B., Acosta, M.T., & North, K. (2011). Mental, motor, and language development of toddlers with neurofibromatosis type 1. *Journal of Pediatrics, 158*(4), 660–665.

neurofibromatosis, type II *Disease category:* Neurological disorder. *Clinical features:* Bilateral vestibular schwannomas (benign tumors of auditory nerve), cranial and spinal tumors, neuropathy, café-au-lait spots (usually fewer than six); in contrast to type I, no Lisch nodules or axillary freckling are seen. *Associated complications:* Deafness (average age of onset is 20 years), cataracts or other ocular abnormalities, meningiomas (tumor of the meninges); tumor growth rates are variable within the same patients and between patients. *Cause:* Mutation in tumor-suppressor (*NF2*) gene encoding merlin protein on chromosome 22q12.2; genotype/phenotype studies show that nonsense mutations (mutations that create a stop codon) are associated with more severe disease presentation than other types of genetic mutations. *Inheritance:* AD with significant variability between patients; up to 50% may represent NM. *Prevalence:* 1:60,000. *Incidence:* 1:25,000. *Treatment:* Mortality is lower for patients treated in specialty centers. Microsurgery and radiation therapy are both commonly used.

References: Asthagiri, A.R., Parry, D.M., Butman, J.A., Kim, H.J., Tsilou, E.T., Zhuang, Z., & Lonser, R.R. (2009). Neurofibromatosis type 2. *Lancet, 373*(9679), 1974–1986.

Evans, D.G., Kalamarides, M., Hunter-Schaedle, K., Blakeley, J., Allen, J., Babovic-Vuskanovic, D. ... Giovannini, M. (2009). Consensus recommendations to accelerate clinical trials for neurofibromatosis type 2. *Clinical Cancer Research, 15*(16), 5032–5039.

neuronal ceroid lipofuscinosis, juvenile *See* Batten disease.

Niemann-Pick disease, types A and B *Disease category:* Inborn error of metabolism: lysosomal storage disorder. *Clinical features:* Lysosomal storage disorder; type A presents in infancy with poor weight gain, enlarged liver and spleen, rapidly progressive neurological decline. Death occurs by age 2–3 years. *Associated complications:* Intellectual disability, ataxia, myoclonus, eye abnormalities, coronary artery disease, lung disease; type B is variable but compatible with survival to adulthood and may cause few or no neurological abnormalities. Main clinical features of type B are enlargement of the spleen and liver resulting in liver dysfunction, as well as cardiac disease, lipid abnormalities, pulmonary involvement, and growth retardation. *Cause:* Sphingomyelinase enzyme deficiency caused by mutations in the sphingomyelinase (*SMPD*) gene on chromosome 11p15.4. *Inheritance:* AR. *Prevalence:* Rare; incidence of type A is increased in Ashkenazi Jewish population, type B is seen equally in all ethnic groups.

References: McGovern, M.M., Aron, A., Bro-die, S.E., Desnick, R.J., & Wasserstein, M.P. (2006). Natural history of Type A Nie-mann-Pick disease: Possible endpoints for therapeutic trials. *Neurology, 66,* 228–232.

McGovern M.M., Wasserstein, M.P., Giugli-ani, R., Bembi, B., Vanier, M.T., Mengel, E. ... Cox, G.F. (2008). A prospective, cross-sectional survey study of the natural history of Niemann-Pick disease type B. *Pediatrics, 122,* e341–e349.

Noonan syndrome *Disease category:* Multiple congenital anomalies. *Clinical features:* Short stature, characteristic facial features, includ-ing triangular shape, deep philtrum, down-slanting palpebral fissures, ptosis, low-set ears, low posterior hairline, short or webbed neck, congenital heart defects (usually pulmonary valve stenosis, or hypertrophic cardiomy-opathy), shield-shaped chest; one third have mild intellectual disability *Associated complica-tions:* Sensorineural deafness, malocclusion of teeth, learning disabilities with deficits in ver-bal learning, attention-deficit/hyperactivity disorder, poor motor coordination, bleeding, and lymphatic abnormalities. *Cause:* 4 genes are linked to Noonan Syndrome: *PTPN11* (50%), *SOS1* (10%–13%), *RAF1* (3%–17%), and *KRAS* (<5%). *Inheritance:* AD, 25%–50% NM. *Prevalence:* 1:1,000–1:2,500. *Treatment:* Human growth hormone has been used to treat short stature in some patients with Noonan syndrome.

References: Allanson, J.E., Bohring, A., Dörr, H.G., Dufke, A., Gillessen-Kaesbach, G., Horn, D. ... Zenker, M. (2010). The face of Noonan syndrome: Does phenotype pre-dict genotype. *American Journal of Medical Genetics A, 152A*(8), 1960–1966.

Lee, D.A., Portnoy, S., Hill, P., Gillberg. C., & Patton, M.A. (2005). Psychological pro-file of children with Noonan syndrome. *Developmental Medicine and Child Neurology, 47,* 35–38.

Romano, A.A., Allanson, J.E., Dahlgren, J., Gelb, B.D., Hall, B., Pierpont, M.E. ... Noonan, J.A. (2010). Noonan syndrome: Clinical features, diagnosis, and manage-ment guidelines. *Pediatrics, 126*(4), 746–759.

oculoauriculovertebral spectrum (facio-auriculo-vertebral spectrum; Goldenhar syndrome; hemifacial microsomia) *Dis-ease category:* Multiple congenital anoma-lies. *Clinical features:* Unilateral external ear deformity ranging from absence of an ear to microtia (tiny ear), preauricular (earlobe) tags or pits, middle-ear abnormality with vari-able hearing loss, facial asymmetry with small size unilaterally, macrostomia (large mouth), occasional cleft palate, microphthalmia or eyelid coloboma. *Associated complications:* Ver-tebral anomalies, occasional heart and renal (kidney) defects, intellectual disability in 10%. *Cause:* Unknown. Recent array-CGH studies on a cohort of patients were unable to identify a recurrent chromosomal abnormal-ity. *Inheritance:* Genetically heterogeneous; may be SP in some cases resulting from ges-tational maternal diabetes; additionally cases with clear AR and AD inheritance have been reported. *Prevalence:* 1:45,000 in Northern Ireland, presumably less common in other populations. *Incidence:* 1:3,000–1:5,000.

References: Rooryck, C., Souakri, N., Cailley, D., Bouron, J., Goizet, C., Delrue, M.A. ... Arveiler, B. (2010). Array-CGH analy-sis of a cohort of 86 patients with oculoau-riculovertebral spectrum. *American Journal of Medical Genetics Part A, 152A*(8), 1984–1989.

Vendramini-Pittoli, S., & Kokitsu-Nakata, N.M. (2009). Oculoauriculovertebral spec-trum: Report of nine familial cases with evi-dence of autosomal dominant inheritance and review of the literature. *Clinical Dys-morphology, 18*(2), 67–77.

oculocerebrorenal syndrome *See* Lowe syndrome.

oculomandibulodyscephaly with hypotri-chosis *See* Hallermann-Streiff syndrome.

Optiz GBB syndrome (Opitz-Frias syndrome; Opitz oculogenitolaryngeal syndrome; previously separate and called G syndrome and BBB syndrome; [G refers to surname of original patient described.]) *Disease cat-egory:* Multiple congenital anomalies. *Clinical features:* Hypertelorism (wide-spaced eyes), hypospadias, imperforate (without an opening) anus, dysphagia, bifurcated (divided) nasal tip, broad nasal bridge, widow's peak, occasional cleft lip/palate, mild to moderate intellectual disability in two thirds of affected individu-als. *Associated complications:* Gastroesophageal reflux, esophageal dysmotility (poor move-ment of food through the esophagus), hoarse cry, occasional congenital heart defect, agen-esis of corpus callosum, platelet abnormali-ties, structural cerebellar anomalies, including Dandy-Walker malformation. *Cause: MID1* gene on Xp22.3 is known to cause the X linked form. The gene believed to cause the AD form has been linked to deletion of 22q11.2. *Inheri-tance:* AD and XLR. In both the AD and XLR forms symptoms are more severe in males than in females. *Prevalence:* Unknown.

References: Erickson, R.P., Díaz de Ståhl, T., Bruder, C.E. ... Dumanski, J.P. (2007). A patient with 22q11.2 deletion and Opitz syndrome-like phenotype has the same deletion as velocardiofacial patients. *American Journal of Medical Genetics Part A,143A*(24), 3302–3308.

Hsieh, E.W., Vargervik, K., & Slavotinek, A.M. (2008). Clinical and molecular studies of patients with characteristics of Opitz G/BBB syndrome shows a novel MID1 mutation. *American Journal of Medical Genetics, 146A*(18), 2337–2345.

osteogenesis imperfecta *Disease category:* Connective tissue disorder. *Clinical features:* Seven clinically distinct forms of this metabolic disease of bone have been described. Type I is characterized by typical height or mild short stature, bone fragility, and blue sclera. Type II usually presents with severe bone deformity and death in the newborn period. Type III is characterized by progressive bone deformity, short stature, triangular face, severe scoliosis, and dental abnormalities. Type IV is clinically similar to type I, but presents with normal sclerae, milder bone deformity, variable short stature, and dental abnormalities. Type V is similar to type IV but with hyperplastic callus formation at fracture sites, calcification of the interosseous membrane between the radius and ulna and the presence of a radioopaque metaphyseal band adjacent to the growth plates. Type VI is characterized by severe bone deformity with moderate short stature and a fish scale pattern of bone deposition. Type VII causes moderate bone deformations, mild short stature, with a shortening of the long bones (humerus and femur). *Associated complications:* Increased prevalence of fractures (may be confused with physical abuse) that decreases after puberty; scoliosis; mitral valve prolapse; occasionally progressive adolescent-onset hearing loss. *Cause:* Mutations in one of the genes regulating collagen formation. Type I maps to 17q21–q22 (*COLA1*). Types IIA, II and IV map to both the *COLA1* gene and 7q21–q22 (*COLA2*). Type IIB has been linked to *CRTAP* on 3p22, 3p24.1-p22. Type VI is caused by mutation in the *FKBP10* gene on 17q21. Type VII is also caused by mutations in the *CRTAP* gene on 3p22, 3p24.1-p22 (allelic to Type IIB). The genetic cause of type V has yet to be determined. *Inheritance:* Type I, IV, V: AD; type IIA: AD (all type IIA cases are NM; recurrence risk is 6% due to gonadal

mosaicism); type IIB: AR. Type III is occasionally AR, types VI and VII are AR (type VII is only seen in indigenous peoples in northern Quebec and some South African families). *Prevalence:* 1:30,000. *Treatment:* Cyclic intravenous pamidronate therapy to increase bone mineral density. (*See Chapter 13.*)

References: Alanay, Y., Avaygan, H., Camacho, N., Utine, G.E., Boduroglu, K., Aktas, D. ... Krakow, D. (2010). Mutations in the gene encoding the RER protein FKBP65 cause autosomal recessive osteogenesis imperfecta. *American Journal of Human Genetics, 86*(4), 551–559.

Shapiro, J.R., & Sponsellor, P.D. (2009). Osteogenesis imperfecta: Questions and answers. *Current Opinion in Pediatrics, 21*(6), 709–716.

pentasomy X *See* XXXXX syndrome.

Pfeiffer syndrome (acrocephalosyndactyly, type V) *Disease category:* Craniosynostosis. Three subtypes of Pfeiffer syndrome have been described with a range of clinical severity. *Clinical features:* Mild craniosynostosis with brachycephaly, flat mid-face, broad thumbs and toes, hypertelorism, and partial syndactyly. *Associated complications:* Hydrocephalus, airway obstruction due to mid-face hypoplasia, hearing impairment, seizures, occasional intellectual disability. *Cause:* Mutations in the genes that code for fibroblast growth factor receptors 1 and 2 (*FGFR1* and *FGFR2*) on chromosomes 8p11.2–p11.1 and 10q26, respectively. *Inheritance:* AD with many cases due to NM. *Prevalence:* 1:100,000.

References: Fearon, J.A., & Rhodes, J. (2009). Pfeiffer syndrome: A treatment evaluation. *Plastic and Reconstructive Surgery, 123*(5), 1560–1569.

Vogels, A., & Fryns, J.P. (2006). Pfeiffer syndrome. *Orphanet Journal of Rare Diseases, 1*, 19.

phenylketonuria (PKU) *Disease category:* Inborn error of metabolism: amino acid. *Clinical features:* Inborn error of amino acid metabolism without acute clinical symptoms; intellectual disability, microcephaly, abnormal gait, and seizures may develop in untreated individuals. Treated individuals have still been found to have mild cognitive deficits, especially in executive function. Pale skin and blond hair are common features. *Associated complications:* Behavioral disturbances, cataracts, skin disorders, movement disorders. *Cause:* Classically caused by a deficiency of the enzyme phenylalanine hydroxylase, which is associated with a mutation in the *PAH* gene on chromosome

12q24.1. *Inheritance:* AR. *Prevalence:* 1:10,000 among Caucasians in the United States. *Treatment:* Early identification is available through newborn screening. A phenylalanine-restricted, low-protein diet should be continued at least until adulthood and in females during childbearing years. Returning to a regular diet even in adulthood may cause reduction of IQ. Specialized formulas are available for individuals who need to be on the restricted diet. Sapropterin dihydrochloride (Kuvan), a synthetic formulation of the cofactor tetrahydrobiopterin (BH4) is approved to reduce blood phenylalanine levels in patients with hyperphenylalaninemia due to tetrahydrobiopterin-responsive PKU. *See also Chapter 19.*

References: Harding, C.O., & Blau, N. (2010). Advances and challenges in phenylketonuria. *Journal of Inherited Metabolic Disease,* 33(6), 645–648.

Trefz, F.K., Scheible, D., & Frauendienst-Egger, G. (2010). Long-term follow-up of patients with phenylketonuria receiving tetrahydrobiopterin treatment. *Journal of Inherited Metabolic Disease.* doi: 10.1007/s10545-010-9058-x.

White, D.A., Waisbren, S., & van Spronsen, F.J. (2010). The psychology and neuropathology of phenylketonuria. *Molecular Genetics and Metabolism,* 99(1), 1–2.

phenytoin syndrome (fetal hydantoin syndrome) *Disease category:* Malformation. *Clinical features:* Intrauterine growth restriction with microcephaly and minor dysmorphic craniofacial features and limb defects including hypoplastic nails and distal phalanges. *Associated complications:* Growth problems and developmental delay, or intellectual disability. *Cause:* Maternal ingestion of phenytoin (Dilantin) during pregnancy. *Prevalence:* About one third of children whose mothers are taking this drug during pregnancy have features of phenytoin syndrome. *Treatment:* Surgical correction of cranial facial and limb defects when required and feasible.

Reference: Nicolai, J., Vles, J.S., & Aldenkamp, A.P. (2008). Neurodevelopmental delay in children exposed to antiepileptic drugs *in utero*: A critical review directed at structural study-bias. *Journal of Neurological Science,* 271(1–2), 1–14.

Pierre-Robin sequence *Disease category:* Malformation. *Clinical features:* Micrognathia, cleft palate, glossoptosis (downward displacement of tongue). *Associated complications:* Neonatal feeding problems, apnea or respiratory distress, upper airway obstruction, GI reflux.

Cause: Impaired closure of the posterior palatal shelves early in development; this defect can be an isolated finding or can be associated with trisomy 18, Stickler syndrome, or other syndromes. *Inheritance:* AR; a rare X-linked form also exists. *Prevalence:* Unknown. *Treatment:* Surgical procedure (mandibular distraction osteogenesis) can be used to correct micrognathia, which alleviates many of the feeding and respiratory problems.

References: Al-Samkari, H.T., Kane, A.A., Molter, D.W., & Vachharajani, A. (2010). Neonatal outcomes of Pierre Robin sequence: An institutional experience. *Clinical Pediatrics,* 49(12), 1117–1122.

Drescher, F.D., Jotzo, M., Goelz, R., Meyer, T.D., Bacher, M., & Poets, C.F. (2008). Cognitive and psychosocial development of children with Pierre Robin sequence. *Acta Paediatrica,* 97(5), 653–656.

PKU *See* phenylketonuria.

polyostotic fibrous dysplasia *See* McCune-Albright syndrome.

Prader-Willi syndrome *Disease category:* Multiple congenital anomalies/imprinting defect/contiguous gene. *Clinical features:* Short stature, poor weight gain in infancy, hyperphagia (abnormally increased appetite), almond-shaped eyes, viscous (thick) saliva, hypotonia, particularly in neck region, hypogonadism with cryptorchidism, small hands and feet, hypopigmentation. *Associated complications:* Mild to moderate intellectual disability, behavior problems (tantrums, obsessive compulsive disorder, rigidity, food stealing, skin picking), obstructive sleep apnea, high pain threshold, osteoporosis, neonatal temperature instability, type 2 diabetes. *Cause:* Approximately 75% have a microdeletion on the long arm of the paternally inherited chromosome 15 (15q11–q13); 25% have maternal uniparental disomy. *Inheritance:* NM with AD inheritance when passed from an affected individual. *Incidence:* 1:10,000–1:30,000. *Prevalence:* 1:50,000.

References: Benson, L.A., Maski, K.P., Kothare, S.V., & Bourgeois, B.F. (2010). New onset epilepsy in Prader-Wili syndrome: Seminology and literature review. *Pediatric Neurology,* 43(4), 297–299.

Buiting, K. (2010). Prader-Willi syndrome and Angelman syndrome. *American Journal of Medical Genetics Part C,* 154C(3), 365–376.

Whittington, J. & Holland, A. (2010). Neurobehavioral phenotype in Prader-Willi Syndrome. *American Journal of Medical Genetics Part C,* 154C(4), 438–447.

propionic acidemia *Disease category:* Inborn error of metabolism: organic acidemia. *Clinical features:* A disorder of organic acid metabolism characterized by episodes of vomiting, lethargy, and coma; hypotonia, bone marrow suppression, enlarged liver (hepatomegaly), characteristic facies with puffy cheeks and exaggerated Cupid's bow upper lip. *Associated complications:* Impaired antibody production, intellectual disability, seizures in half, abnormalities of muscle tone, lack of appetite, prolonged drowsiness, rapid difficult breathing; a late-onset form of propionic acidemia has been described with average onset at 16 months. *Cause:* Deficiency of enzyme propionyl-CoA carboxylase (PCC) caused by mutations in the *PCCA* gene on chromosome 13q32 and the *PCCB* gene on chromosome 3q21–q22. *Inheritance:* AR. *Prevalence:* 1:2,000–1:5,000 in Saudi Arabia; rare elsewhere. *Treatment:* Treatment consists of a diet low in valine, isoleucine, threonine, and methionine with supplement of carnitine. A commercial formula is available. Hemofiltration and peritoneal dialysis have been used with some success in patients in metabolic crisis. Some success has been documented in treating hyperammonemia in propionic acidemia patients with N-carbamylglutamate (Carbaglu). Liver transplantation has been used in some cases and is considered an option for patients who continue to experience episodes of hyperammonemia in spite of maximal medical treatment.

References: Ah Mew, N., McCarter, R., Daikhin, Y., Nissim, I., Yudkoff, M., & Tuchman, M. (2010). N-carbamylglutamate augments ureagenesis and reduces ammonia and glutamine in propionic acidemia. *Pediatrics, 126*(1), e208–e214.

Barshes, N.R., Vanatta, J.M., Patel, A.J., Carter, B.A., O'Mahony, C.A., Karpen, S.J., & Goss, J.A. (2006). Evaluation and management of patients with propionic acidemia undergoing liver transplantation: A comprehensive review. *Pediatric Transplant, 10*(7), 773–781.

Johnson, J.A., Le, K.L., & Palacios, E. (2009). Propionic acidemia: Case report and review of neurologic sequelae. *Pediatric Neurology, 40*(4), 317–320.

Refsum disease, infantile *Disease category:* Neurologic/peroxisomal disorder. *Clinical features:* Poor weight gain, absent or tiny ear lobes, high forehead, single palmar crease, flat facial profile and nasal bridge, retinal degeneration/retinitis pigmentosa, hypotonia, liver enlargement and dysfunction. *Associated complications:* Sensorineural hearing impairment, intellectual disability, peripheral neuropathy, hypercholesterolemia (elevated blood cholesterol level), anosomia (inability to smell); there is also a late-onset form of this disease. *Cause:* Accumulation of phytanic acid, very long chain fatty acids, di- and trihydroxy-cholestanoic acids, and pipecolic acid due to defect in peroxisomal function. Mutations in *PEX1* (7q21-q22), *PEX2* (8q21.2), and *PEX26* (22q11.21) genes have been linked to infantile Refsum disease. *Inheritance:* AR. *Prevalence:* Rare. *Treatment:* Restriction of dietary intake of phytanic acid or eliminating phytanic acid by plasmapheresis or lipid apheresis has been shown to reduce phytanic acid concentrations in plasma by 50%–70% leading to improvement of ichthyosis, sensory neuropathy and ataxia.

References: Wanders, R.J., & Waterham, H.R. (2005). Peroxisomal disorders I: Biochemistry and genetics of peroxisome biogenesis disorders. *Clinical Genetics, 67*(2), 107–133.

Van Maldergem, L., Moser, A.B., Vincent, M.F., Roland, D., Reding, R., Otte, J.B. ... Sokal, E. (2005). Orthotopic liver transplantation from a living-related donor in an infant with a peroxisome biogenesis defect of the infantile Refsum disease type. *Journal of Inherited Metabolic Disease, 28*(4), 593–600.

retinitis pigmentosa *Disease category:* Ophthalmalogic. *Clinical features:* A group of diseases associated with retinal degeneration, constricted visual fields, and progressive blindness; initial symptom is night blindness occurring in adolescence or adult life and loss of peripheral vision. *Associated complications:* May occur as an isolated condition or as part of over 30 syndromes (e.g., Usher syndrome, mitochondrial disorders). *Cause:* More than 35 different genes have been identified to date. Additional causative genes are anticipated. *Inheritance:* AD in 15%–25% of cases, AR in 5%–20%, and XLR in 5%–15%. A genetic cause is yet to be identified in the remaining 40%–50%. A rare digenic form where individuals are heterozygous for mutations in two genes also exists. Recurrence risk depends on cause and family history. *Incidence:* 1:3,500–1:4,000 in the United States and Europe.

References: Simpson, D.A., Clark, G.R., Alexander, S., Silvestri, G., & Willoughby, C.E. (2011). Molecular diagnosis for heterogenous genetic disease with targeted high-throughput DNA sequencing applied to retinitis pigmentosa. *Journal of Medical Genetics.* 48(3), 145–151.

Musarella, M., & MacDonald, I. (2010). Current concepts in the treatment of retinitis pigmentosa. *Journal of Ophthalmology.* doi: 10.1155/2011/753547.

Rett syndrome (Rett's disorder) *Disease category:* Progressive neurologic disorder. *Clinical features:* Typical development for 6–9 months, followed by progressive encephalopathy. Features of autism, loss of purposeful hand use with characteristic wringing of hands, hyperventilation, ataxia, spasticity. *Associated complications:* Postnatal onset of microcephaly, seizures. *Cause:* Mutations in the methyl-CpG binding protein 2 (*MeCP2*) gene at Xq28. Mutations in *CDKL5* (Xp22) have been found in individuals with what has been characterized as the early-seizure onset variant of Rett. *Inheritance:* XLD with severe, neonatal encephalopathy or lethality in males. *Prevalence:* 1:10,000 among females.

References: Didden, R., Korzilius, H., Smeets, E., Green, V.A., Lang, R., Lancioni, G.E., & Curfs, L.M. (2010). Communication in individuals with Rett syndrome: An assessment of forms and functions. *Journal of Developmental and Physical Disabilities, 22*(2), 105–118.

Neul, J.L., Kaufmann, W.E., Glaze, D.G., Christodoulou, J., Clarke, A.J., Bahi-Buisson, N. … RettSearch Consortium. (2010). Rett syndrome: Revised diagnostic criteria and nomenclature. *Annals of Neurology.* 68(6), 944–50.

Riley-Day syndrome *See* familial dysautonomia.

Robinow syndrome (fetal face syndrome) *Disease category:* Skeletal dysplasia. *Clinical features:* Slight to moderate short stature, short forearms, macrocephaly with frontal bossing (prominent central forehead), flat facial profile with apparent hypertelorism, small, upturned nose, hypogenitalism, micrognathia, small face, tented upper lip with occasional clefting of the lower lip, hypertrophy of the gums, deficiency of the lower eyelid giving the appearance of protruding eyes (exophthalmos), congenital heart defects. *Associated complications:* Vertebral or rib anomalies, dental malocclusion, genital hypoplasia, inguinal (groin) hernia, enlarged liver and spleen, developmental delay in 15% of cases. *Cause:* Mutations in the *ROR2* gene on 9q22. AD form has been linked to deletions of 1q41q42.1 *Inheritance:* Rarely AD; AR form is most common, is clinically more severe, and is often accompanied by rib anomalies. *Prevalence:* Rare.

References: Mazzeu, J.F., Pardono, E., Vianna-Morgante, A.M., Richieri-Costa, A., Ae Kim, C., Brunoni, D. … Otto, P.A. (2007). Clinical characterization of autosomal dominant and recessive variants of Robinow syndrome. *American Journal of Medical Genetics Part A, 143*(4), 320–325.

Mazzeu, J.F., Vianna-Morgante, A.M., Krepischi, A.C., Oudakker, A., Rosenberg, C., Szuhai, K. … Brunner, H.G. (2010). Deletions encompassing 1q41q42.1 and clinical features of autosomal dominant Robinow syndrome. *Clinical Genetics,* 77, 404–407.

Rubinstein-Taybi syndrome *Disease category:* Multiple congenital anomalies. *Clinical features:* Growth retardation, broad thumbs and toes, maxillary hypoplasia (small upper jaw), high-arched palate, down-slanted palpebral fissures, prominent nose, pouting lower lip, short upper lip, occasional agenesis of corpus callosum. *Associated complications:* Apnea, constipation, reflux, feeding difficulties, hypotonia, cardiac defects, renal anomalies, ophthalmologic problems, keloid (scar) formation, glaucoma, cryptorchidism, moderate to severe intellectual disability (IQ scores range from 25–79 and average 36–51), and behavior problems. *Cause:* Mutations of the CREB binding protein (*CBP*) gene on chromosome 16p13.3, most often an interstitial microdeletion of this chromosome locus, as well as mutations of the EP300 gene (22q13). *Inheritance:* Most cases are due to a NM with AD inheritance when passed from an affected individual. *Prevalence:* 1:125,000.

References: Bartsch, O., Kress, W., Kempf, O., Lechno, S., Haaf, T., & Zechner, U. (2010). Inheritance and variable expression in Rubinstein-Taybi syndrome. *American Journal of Medical Genetics Part A, 152A*(9), 2254–2261.

Verhoeven, W., Tuinier, S., Kuijpers, H.J., Egger, J.I., & Brunner, H.G. (2010). Psychiatric profile in rubinstein-taybi syndrome. A review and case report. *Psychopathology, 42*(1), 63–68.

Russell-Silver syndrome (Silver-Russell syndrome) *Disease category:* Imprinting defect/multiple congenital anomalies. *Clinical features:* Short stature (beginning with intrauterine growth retardation), skeletal asymmetry with hemihypertrophy (enlargement of one side of the body) in 60%;

triangular facies, beaked nose, thin upper lip, narrow, high-arched palate, blue sclerae, occasional café-au-lait spots, fifth finger clinodactyly, genital anomalies in males; motor and cognitive developmental delay and learning disabilities. *Associated complications:* Delayed fontanelle (soft spot) closure, hypocalcemia in neonatal period with sweating and rapid breathing, increased risk of fasting hypoglycemia as toddler, feeding difficulties, precocious sexual development, vertebral anomalies. *Cause:* 44% of patients have a hypomethylation of the imprinting control region 1 (ICR1) in 11p15.5 affecting the expression of H19 and IGF2. 4%–10% of the patients carry a maternal UPD of chromosome 7. Chromosomal rearrangements have also been reported. *Inheritance:* NM with AD inheritance when passed from an affected individual; maternal uniparental disomy; AR in rare cases. Recurrence risk is generally low but can be increased in cases of familial epimutations or chromosomal rearrangements. *Prevalence:* Unknown.

References: Eggermann, T. (2010). Russell-Silver syndrome. *American Journal of Medical Genetics Part C, 154C*(3), 355–364.

Wakeling, E.L., Amero, S.A., Alders, M., Bliek, J., Forsythe, E., Kumar, S. ... Cobben, J.M. (2010). Epigenotype-phenotype correlations in Silver-Russell syndrome. *Journal of Medical Genetics, 47*(11), 760–768.

Saethre-Chotzen syndrome *Disease category:* Craniosynostosis. *Clinical features:* Short stature, brachycephaly (forshortened skull), acrocephaly, radioulnar synostosis (fusion of lower arm bones), syndactyly of the second and third fingers, and third and fourth toes, fifth finger clinodactyly, craniosynostosis, small ears, flat facies with long pointed nose and low hairline and facial asymmetry, shallow asymmetric eye orbits with hypertelorism. *Associated complications:* Late closing fontanelles (soft spot of forehead), deafness, strabismus, proptosis, lacrimal (tear) duct abnormalities. *Cause:* Mutations in the *TWIST* transcription factor gene on chromosome 7p21. *Inheritance:* AD. *Prevalence:* 1:25,00–1:50,000.

References: Foo, R., Guo, Y., McDonald-McGinn, D.M., Zackai, E.H., Whitaker, L.A., & Bartlett, S.P. (2009). The natural history of patients treated for TWIST1-confirmed Saethre-Chotzen syndrome. *Plastic and Reconstructive Surgery, 124*(6), 2085–2095.

Woods, R.H., Ul-Haq, E., Wilkie, A.O., Jayamohan, J., Richards, P.G., Johnson, D. ... Wall, S.A. (2009). Reoperation for intracranial hypertension in TWIST1-confirmed Saethre-Chotzen syndrome: A 15-year-review. *Plastic and Reconstructive Surgery, 123*(6), 1801–1810.

Sanfilippo syndrome (MPS III) *See* mucopolysaccharidoses.

Scheie syndrome (MPS V) *See* mucopolysaccharidoses.

Silver-Russell syndrome *See* Russell-Silver syndrome.

Sly syndrome (MPS VII) *See* mucopolysaccharidoses.

Smith-Lemli-Opitz syndrome *Disease category:* Inborn error of metabolism-cholesterol synthesis. *Clinical features:* Microcephaly, short nose with upturned nostrils, low serum cholesterol, syndactyly of second and third toes, genitourinary abnormalities, renal anomalies, and lung malformations. *Associated complications:* Intrauterine growth restriction, postnatal growth retardation, hypotonia, moderate to severe intellectual disability, motor and language delay, seizures, feeding difficulties and vomiting, photosensitivity, occasional heart defect. Specific behavioral features include: irritability, sleep disturbance, self-injurious behavior. *Cause:* Defect in cholesterol metabolism (conversion of 7-DHC to cholesterol) caused by mutations in the sterol delta-7-reductase gene (*DHCR7*) on chromosome 11q12–q13. Clinical features result from deficiency of cholesterol as well as toxic accumulation of 7-DHC. *Inheritance:* AR. *Prevalence:* 1:20,000–1:40,000. *Treatment:* Dietary modifications, including cholesterol supplementation.

References: Chan, Y.M., Merkens, L.S., Connor, W.E., Roullet, J.B., Penfield, J.A., Jordan, J.M. ... Jones, P.J. (2009). Effects of dietary cholesterol and simvastatin on cholesterol synthesis in Smith-Lemli-Opitz syndrome. *Pediatric Research, 65*(6), 681–685.

Porter, F.D. (2008). Smith-Lemli-Opitz syndrome: Pathogenesis, diagnosis and management. *European Journal of Human Genetics, 16*(5), 535–541.

Tierney, E., Conley, S.K., Goodwin, H., & Porter, F.D. (2010). Analysis of short-term behavioral effects of dietary cholesterol supplementation in Smith-Lemli-Opitz syndrome. *American Journal of Medical Genetics Part A, 152A*(1), 91–95.

Smith-Magenis syndrome (SMS) *Disease category:* Multiple congenital anomalies/

Contiguous gene syndrome. *Clinical features:* Feeding difficulties, poor weight gain, hypotonia, hyporeflexia, lethargy, distinctive facial features, developmental delay, cognitive impairment and significant behavioral abnormalities including sleep disturbance, sterotypies (such as a "self-hug" and "lick and flip"), self-injurious behavior including self-hitting, self-biting. *Associated complications:* skeletal anomalies, short stature, brachydactyly, ophthalmologic abnormalities, otolaryngologic abnormalities, peripheral neuropathy, cardiac and renal anomalies. *Cause:* Microdeletion at chromosome 17p11.2 or mutations including the gene *RAI1*. *Inheritance:* Most cases represent new mutations with AD inheritance when passed from an affected individual. *Prevalence:* 1:25,000.

References: Laje, G., Morse, R., Richter, W., Ball, J., Pao, M., & Smith, A.C. (2010). Autism spectrum features in Smith-Magenis syndrome. *American Journal of Medical Genetics Part C, 154C*(4), 456–462.

Wolters, P.L., Gropman, A.L., Martin, S.C., Smith, M.R., Hildenbrand, H.L., Brewer, C.C., & Smith, A.C. (2009). Neurodevelopment of children under 3 years of age with Smith-Magenis syndrome. *Pediatric Neurology, 41*(4), 250–258.

Sotos syndrome *Disease category:* Overgrowth syndrome. *Clinical features:* An overgrowth syndrome characterized by a distinctive head shape, macrocephaly, downslanting eyes, flat nasal bridge, accelerated growth with advanced bone age, high forehead, hypertelorism, and prominent jaw. *Associated complications:* Increased risk of abdominal tumors, hypotonia, marked speech delay, congenital heart defects, varying degrees of cognitive impairment. *Cause:* Mutations in the *NSD1* gene have been found to be causative; in addition, submicroscopic deletions have been identified at chromosome 5q35. *Inheritance:* AD with the majority of cases due to a NM. *Prevalence:* 1:14,000.

References: de Boer, L., Röder, I., & Wit, J.M. (2006). Psychosocial, cognitive, and motor functioning in patients with suspected Sotos syndrome: A comparison between patients with and without *NSD1* gene alterations. *Developmental Medicine and Child Neurology, 48*(7), 582–588.

Leventopoulos, G., Kitsiou-Tzeli, S., Kritikos, K., Psoni, S., Mavrou, A., Kanavakis, E., & Fryssira, H. (2009). A clinical study of Sotos syndrome patients with review of the literature. *Pediatric Neurology, 40*(5), 357–364.

spongy degeneration of central nervous system *See* Canavan disease.

Stickler syndrome (hereditary progressive arthroophthalmopathy) *Disease category:* Connective tissue disorder. *Clinical features:* Flat facies, myopia, cleft of hard or soft palate, spondyloepiphyseal dysplasia (lag of mineralization of bone). *Associated complications:* Hypotonia, hyperextensible joints, occasional scoliosis, risk of retinal detachment, cataracts, arthropathy in late childhood or adulthood, occasional hearing loss or cognitive impairment. *Cause:* Mutations in type 2, type 9 and type 11 procollagen genes (*COL2A1, COL9A1, COL11A1, COL11A2*), which have been linked to chromosomes 12q13.11–q13.2, 6q13, 1p21, and 6p21.3, respectively. *Inheritance:* AD with variable expression, AR (*COL9A1* mutations). *Prevalence:* 1:7,500–1:9,000.

References: Hoornaert, K.P., Vereecke, I., Dewinter, C., Rosenberg, T., Beemer, F.A., & Leroy, J.G. (2010). Stickler syndrome caused by *COL2A1* mutations: Genotype-phenotype correlation in a series of 100 patients. *European Journal of Human Genetics, 18*(8), 872–880.

Richards, A.J., McNinch, A., Martin, H., Oakhill, K., Rai, H., Waller, S. ... Snead, M.P. (2010). Stickler syndrome and the vitreous phenotype: Mutation in *COL2A1* and *COL11A1*. *Human Mutation, 31*(6), E1461–E1471.

Van Camp, G., Snoeckx, R.L., Hilgert, N., van den Ende, J., Fukuoka, H., Wagatsuma, M. ... Usami, S. (2006). A new autosomal recessive form of Stickler syndrome is caused by a mutation in the *COL9A1* gene. *American Journal of Human Genetics, 79*(3), 449–457.

Sturge-Weber syndrome *Disease category:* Multiple congenital anomalies. *Clinical features:* Flat facial "port wine stains," seizures, glaucoma, intracranial vascular abnormality. *Associated complications:* Hemangiomas (benign congenital tumors made up of newly formed blood vessels) of meninges; may be progressive in some cases, with gradual visual or cognitive impairment and recurrent stroke-like episodes, hemiparesis, hemiatrophy, and hemianopia (decreased vision in one eye). *Cause:* Unknown. *Inheritance:* Usually SP, possibly due to somatic mosaicism; AD in a few reported cases. *Incidence:* 1:50,000. *Treatment:* Pharmacologic therapies can be used to treat seizures, surgical intervention can be used for glaucoma, and laser therapy can be used to remove vascular facial features.

References: Alkonyi, B., Govindan, R.M., Chugani, H.T., Behen, M.E., Jeong, J.W., & Juhász, C. (2011). Focal white matter abnormalities related to neurocognitive dysfunction: An objective diffusion tensor imaging study of children with Sturge-Weber syndrome. *Pediatric Research, 69*(1), 74–79.

Turin, E., Grados, M.A., Tierney, E., Ferenc, L.M., Zabel, A., & Comi, A.M. (2010). Behavioral and psychiatric features of Sturge-Weber syndrome. *Journal of Nervous and Mental Disease, 198*(12), 905–913.

subacute necrotizing encephalomyopathy Leigh syndrome; *See* mitochondrial disorders.

sulfatide lipidosis *See* metachromatic leukodystrophy.

TAR syndrome *See* thrombocytopenia-absent radius syndrome.

Tay-Sachs disease (GM2 gangliosidosis, type I) *Disease category:* Inborn error of metabolism: lysosomal storage disease. *Clinical features:* A lysosomal storage disorder leading to a progressive neurological condition characterized by deafness, blindness, and seizures; development is typical for the first several months of life. Subsequently, there is an increased startle response, hypotonia followed by hypertonia, cherry-red spot in maculae, optic nerve atrophy. There is rapid decline and fatality by age 5 years. An adult form of this enzyme deficiency presents with ataxia. *Associated complications:* Feeding abnormalities, aspiration. *Cause:* Deficiency of the enzyme hexosaminidase A caused by mutation in the *HEXA* gene at chromosome 15q23–q24. *Inheritance:* AR. *Prevalence:* 1:112,000; 1:3,600 in Ashkenazi Jewish population (although extensive genetic counseling of carriers identified through carrier screening programs the incidence in the Ashkenazi Jewish population of North America has been reduced by more than 90%); increased frequency in the Cajun and French Canadian populations.

References: Elstein, D., Doniger, G.M., Simon, E., Korn-Lubetzki, I., Navon, R., & Zimran, A. (2008). Neurocognitive testing in late-onset Tay-Sachs disease: A pilot study. *Journal of Inherited Metabolic Diseases, 31*(4), 518–523.

Schneider, A., Nakagawa, S., Keep, R., Dorsainville, D., Charrow, J., Aleck, K. … Gross, S. (2009). Population-based Tay-Sachs screening among Ashkenazi Jewish young adults in the 21st century: Hexosaminidase A enzyme assay is essential for accurate testing. *American Journal of Medical Genetics Part A, 149A*(11), 2444–2447.

tetrasomy X *See* XXXX syndrome.

Tourette syndrome *Disease category:* Neurological disorder. *Clinical features:* Chronic vocal or motor tics (irrepressible, repetitive, non-rhythmic movements and vocalizations) present for at least 1 year, obsessive-compulsive disorder (OCD), attention-deficit/hyperactivity disorder (ADHD). Age of onset is typically between age 3 and 8 years with onset of motor tics most often preceding vocal tics. The course of the tics is waxing and waning and peak symptom intensity is usually in late childhood (mean age 10 years) Fluctuation occurs in adolescence and by early adulthood there is often significant improvement. *Associated complications:* Learning difficulties, language-based learning problems, habit disorders such as trichotillomania (chronic hair pulling), pathologic nail biting and skin picking, mood disorders such as bipolar disorder and major depressive disorder, anxiety. *Cause:* Unknown although *SLITRK1* has been implicated as a candidate gene but studies have not been conclusive. Environmental factors are thought to be involved as well since concordance rate is not 100% between monozygotic twins. *Inheritance:* Unknown. *Prevalence:* 0.3%–1%. Males are affected more often than females with an approximate 4:1 ratio. *Treatment:* Typical and atypical neuroleptics such as haloperidol and pimozide, alpha adrenergic agonist such as clonidine, habit reversal therapy, surgical intervention for a small subset with intractable Tourettes disorder, repetitive transcranial magnetic stimulation.

References: Bloch, M., State, M., & Pittenger, C. (2011). Recent advances in Tourette syndrome. *Current Opinion in Neurology, 24*(2), 119–125.

Jankovic, J., & Kurlan, R. (2011). Tourette syndrome: Evolving concepts. *Movement Disorders, 26*(6), 1149–1156.

State, M. (2011). The genetics of Tourette disorder. *Current Opinion in Genetics & Development, 21*(3), 302–309.

thrombocytopenia-absent radius syndrome (TAR syndrome) *Disease category:* Multiple congenital anomalies. *Clinical features:* Radial aplasia (absence of one of the lower arm bones) with normal thumbs; thrombocytopenia (platelet deficiency) is present in all cases and symptomatic in 90% of cases; 50% of patients have dysmorphic features including micrognathia (small jaw) and low posteriorly rotated ears. *Associated complications:* Knee joint abnormalities, neonatal foot swelling, occasional congenital heart or renal (kidney) defect, gastrointestinal bleeding, and occasional intracerebral bleeding. *Cause:* Unknown. Presence of the minimally deleted 200-kb region at chromosome band 1q21.1 is necessary but not sufficient to cause TAR. A modifier is likely present. *Inheritance:* AR. *Prevalence:* 0.5–1:100,000. *Treatment:* Platelet infusions.

References: Klopocki, E., Schulze, H., Strauss, G., Ott, C.E., Hall, J., Trotier, F. … Mundlos, S. (2007). Complex inheritance pattern resembling autosomal recessive inheritance involving a microdeletion in thrombocytopenia-absent radius syndrome. *American Journal of Human Genetics, 80*(2), 232–240.

Oishi, S., Carter, P., Bidwell, T., Mills, J., & Ezaki, M. (2009). Thrombocytopenia absent radius syndrome: Presence of brachiocarpalis muscle and its importance. *Journal of Hand Surgery, 34*(9), 1696.

Treacher Collins syndrome (mandibulofacial dysostosis) *Disease category:* Multiple congenital anomalies. *Clinical features:* Characteristic facial appearance with malformation of external ears, small chin, flattened midface, cleft palate. *Associated complications:* Conductive or mixed (conductive and sensorineural) hearing loss; defects of middle and inner ear; respiratory and feeding problems, apnea; intelligence is average in 95% of cases. *Cause:* 93% of patients have mutations in *TCOF1* gene on chromosome 5q32–q33. *POLR1D*, which encodes a subunit present in RNA polymerase I (PolI) and RNA polymerase III (PolIII), has recently also been linked to Treacher Collins. *Inheritance:* AD. 60% NM. *Incidence:* 1:10,000–1:50,000. *Treatment:* Surgical repair of most malformations.

References: Dauwerse, J., Dixon, J., Seland, S., Ruivenkamp, C.A., van Haeringen, A., Hoefsloot, L.H. … Wieczorek, D. (2011). Mutations in genes encoding subunits of RNA polymerases I and III cause Treacher Collins syndrome. *Nature Genetics. 43*(1), 20–22.

Thompson, J.T., Anderson, P.J., & David, D.J. (2009). Treacher Collins syndrome: Protocol management from birth to maturity. *Journal of Craniofacial Surgery, 20*(6), 2028–2035.

trisomy 13 syndrome (Patau syndrome) *Disease category:* Chromosome abnormality/ multiple congenital anomalies. *Clinical features:* Microphthalmia, coloboma, corneal opacity, cleft lip and palate, polydactyly, scalp defects, dysmorphic features, low-set ears,

flexion deformity of fingers. *Associated complications:* Cardiac defects, kidney and gastrointestinal tract anomalies, eye abnormalities, visual impairment, sensorineural hearing loss, profound intellectual disability, cerebral palsy. 50% die within the first month of life. *Cause:* Nondisjunction (usually in maternal meiosis I) resulting in extra chromosome 13; rarely parental translocation. *Inheritance:* NM; usually nondisjunction chromosomal abnormality; may recur in families in presence of parental translocation. *Incidence:* 1:15,000–1:20,000 births.

References: Crider, K.S., Olney, R.S., & Cragan, J.D. (2008). Trisomies 13 and 18: Population prevalences, characteristics, and prenatal diagnosis, metropolitan Atlanta, 1994–2003. *American Journal of Medical Genetics Part A, 146*(7), 820–826.

De Souza, E., Halliday, J., Chan, A., Bower, C., & Morris, J.K. (2009). Recurrence risks for trisomies 13, 18, and 21. *American Journal of Medical Genetics Part A, 149A*(12), 2716–2722.

trisomy 18 syndrome (Edwards syndrome) *Disease category:* Chromosome abnormality/ Multiple congenital anomalies. *Clinical features:* Prenatal onset of growth retardation, low-set ears, clenched fists, "rocker-bottom" feet, congenital heart defects, microphthalmia, coloboma, corneal opacity; 30% die within first month of life, 50% by second month, and only 10% survive their first year. *Associated complications:* Feeding problems, aspiration, conductive hearing loss, profound intellectual disability. *Cause:* Nondisjunction resulting in extra chromosome 18. *Inheritance:* NM; usually nondisjunction chromosomal abnormality, may recur in families in presence of parental translocation. *Incidence:* 1:7,500 births.

References: Crider, K.S., Olney, R.S., & Cragan, J.D. (2008). Trisomies 13 and 18: Population prevalences, characteristics, and prenatal diagnosis, metropolitan Atlanta, 1994–2003. *American Journal of Medical Genetics Part A, 146*(7), 820–826.

De Souza, E., Halliday, J., Chan, A., Bower, C., & Morris, J.K. (2009). Recurrence risks for trisomies 13, 18, and 21. *American Journal of Medical Genetics Part A, 149A*(12), 2716–2722.

trisomy 21 *See* Down syndrome; *see also* Chapter 18.

trisomy X *See* XXX syndrome.

tuberous sclerosis complex *Disease category:* Neurologic. *Clinical features:* Hypo-pigmented

areas on skin, adenoma sebaceum (acne-like facial lesions), infantile spasms, iris depigmentation, retinal defects, calcium deposits in brain, benign tumor of the kidneys, pulmonary lesions. *Associated complications:* Seizures, mild to moderate intellectual disability, tumors of the heart, increased risk of malignancy, hypoplastic tooth enamel and dental pits, renal (kidney) cysts, hypertension. *Cause:* Mutations in the *TSC1* and *TSC2* genes on chromosomes 16p13 and 9q34, respectively. *Inheritance:* AD with variable expressivity. ²/₃ NM. *Incidence:* 1:5,800.
References: D'Agati, E., Moavero R, Cerminara C, & Curatolo P. (2009). Attention-deficit/hyperactivity disorder (ADHD) and tuberous sclerosis complex. *Journal of Child Neurology, 24*(10), 1282–1287.
de Vries, P.J. (2010). Targeted treatments for cognitive and neurodevelopmental disorders in tuberous sclerosis complex. *Neurotherapeutics, 7*(3), 275–282.
Salerno, A.E., Marsenic, O., Meyers, K.E., Kaplan, B.S., & Hellinger, J.C. (2010). Vascular involvement in tuberous sclerosis. *Pediatric Nephrology, 25*(8), 1555–1561.

Turner syndrome (45,X; monosomy X) *Disease category:* Chromosome abnormality. *Clinical features:* Affecting females only, the physical features include short stature, broad chest with widely spaced nipples, short neck with low hairline and extra skin at nape ("webbed" appearance), "puffy" hands and feet. *Associated complications:* "Streak" ovaries causing infertility and delayed puberty, congenital heart defect (often coarctation of aorta), small ear canals, eye involvement (strabismus, ptosis, nystagmus, cataracts), chronic otitis media in 90% with frequent hearing loss, hypothyroidism, renal (kidney) disease; intelligence is usually average, but prevalence of learning disabilities is high. *Cause:* Nondisjunction chromosome abnormality resulting in one copy of sex chromosome. *Inheritance:* NM; usually nondisjunction chromosomal abnormality. *Prevalence:* 1:4,000. *Incidence:* 1:2,000 *Treatment:* Growth hormone has been used successfully to increase eventual adult height. Hormone replacement therapy is needed to initiate puberty (*see also Chapter 1*).
References: Burnett, A.C., Reutens, D.C., & Wood, A.G. (2010). Social cognition in Turner's Syndrome. J*ournal of Clinical Neuroscience, 17*(3), 283–286.
Hong, D., Scaletta Kent, J., & Kesler, S. (2009). Cognitie profile of Turner syndrome.

Developmental Disabilities Research Reviews, 15(4), 270–278.
Thomas, J., & Yetman, A.T. (2009). *Expert Review of Cardiovascular Therapy, 7*(12), 1631–1641.

urea cycle disorders *Disease category:* Inborn error of metabolism: amino acid. *Clinical features:* this group of disorders results from defects in any of the first five enzymes (CPSI, OTC, ASS, ASL, ARG) in the urea cycle or the cofactor producer (NAGS) which break down the excess nitrogen from protein degradation. Severe deficiencies or complete absence of the first four enzymes results in the accumulation of ammonia and other precursor metabolites during the first few days of life. Infants often appear normal initially but rapidly develop lethargy, vomiting, anorexia, hyperventilation or hypoventilation, hypothermia, seizures, neurologic posturing, cerebral edema/encephalopathy and coma. Partial urea cycle enzyme deficiencies are milder, and ammonia accumulation may be triggered by illnesses or stress at almost any time of life thus delaying diagnosis by months to years. Deficiency of the fifth enzyme in the pathway causes arginase deficiency, which does not typically have the same frequency of hyperammonemic episodes but results in seizures, intellectual disability and severe spasticity. Citrin deficiency and hyperornithinemia, hyperammonemia, homocitrullinuria (HHH) syndrome also occur due to defects in two transporters. *Associated complications:* Loss of appetite, cyclical vomiting, lethargy, behavioral abnormalities, delusions, hallucinations and psychosis can occur during hyperammonemic episodes. Developmental delay, attention-deficit/hyperactivity disorder, and intellectual disability are common, especially in those patients who have had significantly elevated ammonia levels. Liver failure occurs in some patients. *Cause:* mutations or deletions involving the genes encoding the enzymes, cofactor and transporter proteins of the urea cycle. *Inheritance:* AR, except OTC which is X-linked. *Prevalence:* 1:30,000 although undiagnosed partial defects may make the number much higher. *Treatment:* Hemodialysis for rapidly lowering ammonia levels, ammonia scavenging medications (IV for acute hypermmonemia and oral for daily use), restricted protein diet to reduce excess nitrogen, and amino acid supplementation, liver transplantation in some infants with complete defects.
References: Krivitzky, L., Babikian, T., Lee, H.S., Thomas, N.H., Burk-Paull, K.L., &

Batshaw M.L. (2009). Intellectual, adaptive, and behavioral functioning in children with urea cycle disorders. *Pediatric Research, 66*(1), 96–101.

Scaglia, F. (2010). New insights in nutritional management and amino acid supplementation in urea cycle disorders. *Molecular Genetics and Metabolism, 100*(1), S72–S76.

Seminara, J., Tuchman, M., Krivitzky, L., Krischer, J., Lee, H.S., Lemons, C. ... Batshaw, M.L. (2010). Establishing a consortium for the study of rare diseases: The urea cycle disorders consortium. *Molecular Genetics and Metabolism, 100*(1), S97–S105.

Usher syndromes *Disease category:* Auditory/ophthalmologic. *Clinical features:* Approximately 10 subtypes exist; all have progressive sensorineural deafness, nystagmus, retinitis pigmentosa, central nervous system defects (e.g., loss of sense of smell, vertigo, epilepsy). Type 1 is characterized by profound hearing loss, absent vestibular function, and retinitis pigmentosa in childhood. Individuals with type 2 have normal vestibular function and less severe hearing loss with onset of retinitis pigmentosa in the second decade. Type 3 can be differentiated by the presence of a progressive loss of hearing. *Associated complications:* Ataxia, psychosis, cataracts, occasional cognitive impairment; more than 50% of adults with a combination of congenital blindness and deafness have Usher syndrome. *Cause:* Seven chromosome loci (5 genes) have been identified for type 1 alone (*MYO7A, USH1C, CDH23, PCDH15, SANS*). Three loci have been identified for type 2, although only two genes have been identified: *USH2A* and *GPR98(VLGR1)*. A fourth loci has been postulated but is unknown. One loci and gene has been identified for type 3: *CLRN1*. *Inheritance:* AR. *Prevalence:* 4.4:100,000. *Treatment:* Cochlear implants may be beneficial for some individuals with type 1, while hearing aids are effective for individuals with type 2.

References: Kimberling, W.J., Hildebrand, M.S., Shearer, A.E., Jensen, M.L., Halder, J.A., Trzupek, K. ... Smith R.J. (2010). Frequency of Usher syndrome in two pediatric populations: Implications for genetic screening of deaf and hard of hearing children. *Genetics in Medicine, 12*(8), 512–516.

Yan, D., & Liu, X.Z. (2010). Genetics and pathological mechanisms of Usher syndrome. *Journal of Human Genetics, 55*(6), 327–335.

VATER/VACTERL association *Disease category:* Multiple congenital anomalies. *Clinical features:* Vertebral defects, anal atresia (imperforate anus), genitourinary anomalies, tracheoesophageal fistula (problem with connection between trachea and esophagus), radial (lower arm) and other limb defects, renal (kidney) anomalies. VACTERL is an expanded definition including cardiac malformations and limb anomalies. Diagnosis is made if 3 of 7 defects are present. *Associated complications:* Poor weight gain, ear anomalies, facial clefting; respiratory, cardiac, and renal (kidney) abnormalities that can be severe. Intelligence is usually not affected. *Cause:* Unknown. Mutation in the *HOXD13* gene on 2q31-q32 was identified in 1 patient with VACTERL association. *Inheritance:* Usually SP, no recognized genetic or teratogenic cause; rare families with AR pattern. *Prevalence:* 1.6:10,000.

References: Solomon, B.D., Pineda-Alvarez, D.E., Raam, M.S., & Cummings, D.A. (2010). Evidence for inheritance in patients with VACTERL association. *Human Genetics, 127*(6), 731–736.

Wheeler, P.G., & Weaver, D.D. (2005). Adults with VATER association: Long-term prognosis. *American Journal of Medical Genetics Part A, 128A*(3), 212–217.

velocardiofacial syndrome (VCFS) *See* chromosome 22q11 microdeletion syndromes.

von Recklinghausen disease *See* neurofibromatosis, type I.

Waardenburg syndrome *Disease category:* Auditory/pigmentary. Four clinical subtypes exist with types I and II accounting for the majority of cases. *Clinical features:* Widely spaced eyes (type I), heterochromia (irises of different colors), white hair forelock, nonprogressive sensorineural hearing loss, musculoskeletal abnormalities (type III). Types I and II have virtually identical clinical features with the only distinguishing characteristic being telecanthus (abnormally long distance from the inside corner of the eye to the nose) which is found in type I, but not in type II. Type III has telecanthus and upper limb abnormalities. Type IV (also known as Waardenburg-Shah syndrome) has the additional feature of Hirschsprung disease. *Associated complications:* Impaired vestibular function leading to ataxia, premature graying, vitiligo (patches of skin depigmentation), occasional glaucoma. *Cause:* Types I and III: Mutations in *PAX3* gene on chromosome 2q35; type II: Mutations in various genes, including the microphthalmia-associated transcription factor (*MITF*) gene on chromosome 3p14.1–p12.3. Type IV is caused by mutations in the *EDNRB* gene on 13q22, the *EDN3* gene on 20q13, and *SOX10* on 22q13. *Inheritance:* AD, AR. *Prevalence:* 1:20,000–1:40,000.

References: Pau, H., Gibson, W.P., Gardner-Berry, K., & Sanli, H. (2006). Cochlear implantations in children with Waardenburg syndrome: An electrophysiological and psychophysical review. *Cochlear Implants International,* 7(4), 202–206.

Pingault, V., Ente, D., Dastot-Le Moal, F., Goossens, M., Marlin, S., & Bondurand, N. (2010). Review and update of mutations causing Waardenburg syndrome. *Human Mutation,* 31(4), 391–406.

Weaver syndrome *Disease category:* Multiple congenital anomalies. *Clinical features:* Micrognathia; distinctive chin with dimple; hypertelorism; macrocephaly; downslanting palpebral fissures; long philtrum; depressed nasal bridge; hoarse, low-pitched cry; deep set nails. *Associated complications:* Accelerated growth with advanced bone age, hypertonia, camptodactyly (permanently flexed fingers), intellectual disability. *Cause:* Mutations have been identified in the *NSD1* gene on chromosome 5q35. *Inheritance:* Select case reports suggest AD inheritance, but most cases are isolated, suggesting NM. *Prevalence:* Unknown.

References: Basel-Vanagaite, L. (2010). Acute lymphoblastic leukemia in Weaver syndrome. *American Journal of Medical Genetics Part A,* 152A(2), 383–386.

Rio, M., Clech, L., Amiel, J., Faivre, L., Lyonnet, S., Le Merrer, M. … Cormier-Daire, V. (2003). Spectrum of *NSD1* mutations in Sotos and Weaver syndromes. *Journal of Medical Genetics,* 40, 436–440.

Williams syndrome *Disease category:* Multiple congenital anomalies/contiguous gene. *Clinical features:* Characteristic "elfin" facies (full lips and cheeks, fullness of area around the eyes), short stature, starlike pattern to iris; hoarse voice, communication delay in early childhood, followed by increasing verbal abilities later in life, characteristic friendly, talkative, extroverted personality, congenital heart defect, often supravalvular aortic stenosis. *Associated complications:* Hypercalcemia (increased blood calcium level), stenosis (stricture) of blood vessels, kidney anomalies, hypertension, joint contractures, mild to moderate intellectual disability (but with characteristic strength in verbal abilities). *Cause:* Microdeletion of a segment of chromosome 7q11.23 consisting of approximately 28 genes. *Inheritance:* AD; all cases are the result of NM (sporadic deletions). *Prevalence:* 1:7,500–1:8,000.

References: Mervis, C.B., & John, A.E. (2010). Cognitive and behavioral characteristics of children with Williams syndrome: Implications for intervention approaches. *American Journal Medical Genetics Part C,* 154C(2), 229–248.

Morris, C.A. (2010). The behavioral phenotype of Williams syndrome: A recognizable pattern of neurodevelopment. *American Journal Medical Genetics Part C,* 154C(4), 427–431.

Wilson disease *Disease category:* Inborn error of metabolism: copper. *Clinical features:* Liver dysfunction, jaundice, Kayser-Fleischer ring in cornea, low serum ceruloplasmin (enzyme important in regulation of copper in body). *Associated complications:* Movement disorders, dysphagia (difficulty swallowing) or other oral-motor dysfunction, behavioral disturbances; if left untreated, death from liver failure within 1–3 years of onset. *Cause:* Mutations in the copper metabolism gene, *ATP7B*, on chromosome 13q14.3–q21.1 lead to intracellular accumulation of copper in liver. *Inheritance:* AR. *Prevalence:* 1:30,000. As high as 1:10,000 in China, Japan, and Sardinia. *Treatment:* Administration of copper-chelating agents in conjunction with a low copper diet. Liver transplant is used in those that fail to respond to medical therapy.

References: Bruha, R., Marecek, Z., Pospisilova, L., Nevsimalova, S., Vitek, L., Martasek, P. … Ferenci, P. (2011). Long-term follow-up of Wilson Disease: Natural history, treatment, mutations analysis and phenotypic correlation. *Liver International,* 31(1), 83–91.

Takeyama, Y., Yokoyama, K., Takata, K., Tanaka, T., Sakurai, K., Matsumoto, T. … Sakisaka, S. (2010). Clinical features of Wilson disease: Analysis of 10 cases. *Hepatology Research,* 40(12), 1204–1211.

Wolf-Hirschhorn syndrome *Disease category:* Multiple congenital anomalies/contiguous gene. *Clinical features:* Hypertelorism; characteristic broad, beaked nose ("Greek warrior helmet appearance"), downturned mouth, short philtrum, microcephaly, marked intrauterine growth retardation and premature birth, ear anomalies, severe intellectual disability with reductions in receptive and expressive language. *Associated complications:* Hypotonia, psychomotor delays, growth delay, renal anomalies, hypodontia (decreased number of teeth) resulting in feeding problems, seizures, occasional heart defect or cleft palate. *Cause:* Partial deletion of 4p16.3; some research shows that the *LEMT1* gene may be responsible as well as the Wolf-Hirschhorn syndrome candidate-1 gene (*WHSC1*). *Inheritance:* Occurs as a result of a NM; recurrence risk is greater if parent has a balanced translocation. *Prevalence:* 1:50,000.

References: Battaglia, A., Filippi, T., & Carey, J.C. (2008). Update on the clinical features and natural history of Wolf-Hirschhorn (4p-) syndrome: Experience with 87 patients and recommendations for routine health supervision. *American Journal of Medical Genetics Part C, 154C*(4), 246–251.

Fisch, G.S., Grossfeld, P., Falk, R., Battaglia, A., Youngblom, J., & Simensen, R. (2010). Cognitive-behavioral features of Wolf-Hirschhorn syndrome and other subtelomeric microdeletions. *American Journal of Medical Genetics Part C, 154C*(4), 417–426.

X-linked ALD *See* adrenoleukodystrophy.

XXX (trisomy X; 47,XXX); XXXX (tetrasomy X); and XXXXX (pentasomy X) syndromes *Disease category:* Chromosome abnormality. *Clinical features:* Females with XXX syndrome generally have above-average stature but otherwise typical physical appearance; 70% have significant learning disabilities; language delay/problems are also present in some girls. Significant malformations have been described in some patients including gonadal dysgenesis (nonfunctional ovaries), dysmorphic facial appearance, atrophic or dysplastic (absent or shrunken) kidneys, and vaginal and uterine malformations. XXXX syndrome is associated with a mildly unusual facial appearance, behavioral problems, and moderate intellectual disability. XXXXX syndrome presents with severe intellectual disability and multiple physical defects. *Associated complications:* Infertility, delayed pubertal development. *Cause:* Nondisjunction during meiosis. *Inheritance:* NM; usually nondisjunction chromosomal abnormality, may recur in families in presence of parental translocation. *Incidence:* 1:800 liveborn females.

References: Ottesen, A.M., Aksglaede, L., Garn, I., Tartaglia, N., Tassone, F., Gravholt, C.H. ... Juul, A. (2010). Increased number of sex chromosomes affects height in a nonlinear fashion: A study of 305 patients with sex chromosome aneuploidy. *American Journal of Medical Genetics Part A, 152*(A), 1206–1212.

Stochholm, K., Stochholm, K., Juul, S., & Gravholt, C.H. (2010). Mortality and incidence in women with 47, XXX and variants. *American Journal of Medical Genetics Part A, 152*(A), 367–372.

XXY syndrome *See* Klinefelter syndrome.

XYY syndrome *Disease category:* Chromosome abnormality. *Clinical features:* Subtle findings, including tall stature, severe acne, large teeth. *Associated complications:* Poor fine-motor coordination; learning disabilities; language delay; varying degrees of behavioral disturbances, including tantrums and aggression; increased risk for autism. *Cause:* Extra Y chromosome resulting from nondisjunction. *Inheritance:* NM; usually nondisjunction chromosomal abnormality, may recur in families in presence of parental translocation. *Prevalence:* 1:1,000.

References: Leggett, V., Jacobs, P., Nation, K., Scerif, G., & Bishop, D.V. (2010). Neurocognitive outcomes of individuals with a sex chromosome trisomy: XXX, XYY, or XXY: A systematic review. *Developmental Medicine and Child Neurology, 52*(2),119–129.

Ross, J.L., Zeger, M.P., Kushner, H., Zinn, A.R., & Roeltgen, D.P. (2009). An extra X or Y chromosome: Contrasting the cognitive and motor phenotypes in childhood in boys with 47, XYY syndrome or 47, XXY Klinefelter syndrome. *Developmental Disabilities Research Reviews, 15*(4), 309–317.

Zellweger syndrome (cerebrohepatorenal syndrome) *Disease category:* Multiple congenital anomalies/Peroxisomal disorder. *Clinical features:* The most severe of the known peroxisomal disorders; affected infants have intrauterine growth retardation, characteristic facies (high forehead, upslanting palpebral fissures, hypoplastic supraorbital ridges, and epicanthal folds), hypotonia, eye abnormalities (cataracts, glaucoma, corneal clouding, retinitis pigmentosa), early onset of seizures. Death occurs by 1 year of age in most cases. *Associated complications:* Severe feeding difficulties with poor weight gain, liver disease, occasional cardiac disease, extremity contractures, kidney cysts. *Cause:* Impaired peroxisome synthesis caused by mutations in a number of genes, including peroxin-1 (*PEX1*) at chromosome 7q21–q22, pereoxin-3 (*PEX3*) at chromosome 6, peroxin-5 (*PEX5*) at chromosome 12, peroxin-2 (*PEX2*) at chromosome 8, peroxin-6 (*PEX6*) at chromosome 6, peroxin-12 (*PEX12*), peroxin-26 (*PEX26*) at chromosome 22 (The peroxisome is a cellular organelle involved in processing fatty acids). *Inheritance:* AR. *Prevalence:* 1:50,000.

References: Ebberink, M.S., Mooijer, P.A., Gootjes, J., Koster, J., Wanders, R.J., & Waterham, H.R. (2011). Genetic classification and mutational spectrum of more than 600 patients with a Zellweger syndrome spectrum disorder. *Human Mutation, 32*(1), 59–69.

Krause, C., Rosewich, H., & Gärtner, J. (2009). Rational diagnostic strategy for Zellweger syndrome spectrum patients. *European Journal of Human Genetics, 17*(6), 741–748.

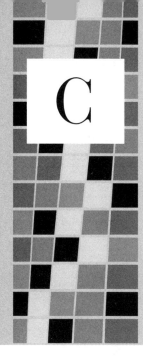

C

Commonly Used Medications

Michelle L. Bestic

This appendix contains information about commonly used medications but is not meant to be used to prescribe medication. The generic name of each drug is in capital letters. The trade name is in parentheses; not all preparations are included. The drug categories, uses, standard applications, and common side effects are listed. Please note that uses and standard applications may change during the life of this edition and that additional side effects may be discovered. Drug interactions and contraindications such as hepatic or renal insufficiency are not included; use of any medication should be discussed with a health care provider familiar with the individual's medical background.

REFERENCES

Children's National Medical Center. (2006). *CNMC Hospital Formulary (Intranet version)*. Washington, DC: Author.

MICROMEDEX Thomson Healthcare. (1974–2006). *MICROMEDEX Healthcare Series: Vol. 125*. Greenwood Village, Co: Author.

Taketomo, C.K., Hodding, J.H., & Kraus, D. M. (Eds). (2011–2012). *Pediatric dosage handbook* (18th ed.). Cleveland, OH: Lexicomp.

Medication	Category	Use(s)	Standard applications	Side effects
ACYCLOVIR (Zovirax)	Antiviral agent	Used primarily to treat or prevent infections caused by herpes simplex viruses or varicella	**C, L, O, T, and injection:** varies with clinical situation	Renal impairment, malaise, headache, gastrointestinal irritation, rash/hives, elevated liver function tests, adverse hematologic effects
ALPRAZOLAM (Xanax, Xanax XR)	Benzodiazepine	Anxiety, panic attacks	**T, L:** Titrate starting at minimal doses of 0.125 mg three times daily; safety and efficacy in children <18 is not known	Drowsiness, fatigue, depression, decreased salivation, dysarthria, ataxia, addictive potential; avoid abrupt withdrawal
AMITRIPTYLINE (Elavil)	Tricyclic antidepressant	Depression, migraine prophylaxis, neuropathic pain, anxiety	**T, injection:** 1–1.5 mg/kg/day, given in three doses; not recommended for children <12 years	Sedation, dry mouth, blurred vision, dizziness, urinary retention, confusion; cardiac arrhythmia (rarely)
AMOXICILLIN (Amoxil)	Antibiotic	Treatment of susceptible infections most commonly acute otitis media, upper respiratory or respiratory tract, and so forth.	**C, T, L, chewables:** 20–90 mg/kg/day, given in two to three doses	Diarrhea, rash, nausea, allergic reactions
AMOXICILLIN AND CLAVULANIC ACID (Augmentin, Augmentin ES, XR)	Antibiotic, penicillin	Treatment of susceptible infections, including otitis media, sinusitis, pneumonia, and so forth.	**T, L, chewables:** 50 mg/kg/day, given in two doses	Diarrhea (worse than with amoxicillin alone), rash, nausea
AMPHETAMINE salts (Amphetamine, Dextroamphetamine, Lisdexamfetamine; Adderall and Adderall XR, Dexedrine, Vyvanse)	Stimulant	Attention-deficit/hyperactivity disorder, narcolepsy	**C, T:** One to three doses daily; not recommended for children younger than 3 years; 3-to-5-year-old: 2.5 mg/day initially, with an increase of 2.5 mg/week until optimal response; children older than 6 years: 5 mg once or twice daily initially, with an increase of 5 mg/week until optimal response; extended release is dosed once daily	Insomnia, loss of appetite, emotional lability, addictive potential, arrhythmia, visual disturbances; not recommended for children younger than 3 years of age; caution in seizure and cardiac patients
ARIPIPRAZOLE (Abilify)	Antipsychotic, atypical	Bipolar disorder, agitation, psychosis, Tourette syndrome, autism spectrum disorder	**T, L:** Initial 2 mg daily titrate after one week to 5 mg then titrate (if needed) weekly by 5 mg increments to max 30 mg/day	Nausea, weight gain, akathisia, somnolence, extrapyramidal effects, fatigue, blurred vision; rarely blood dyscrasias

Drug	Class	Indications	Dosage	Side Effects
ATOMOXETINE (Strattera)	Norepinephrine reuptake inhibitor, selective	Attention-deficit/hyperactivity disorder	**C:** Initial: 0.5 mg/kg/day, increase after minimum of 3 days to ~1.2 mg/kg/day; may administer as either a single daily dose or 2 evenly divided doses in morning and late afternoon/early evening; maximum daily dosage: 1.4 mg/kg or 100 mg, whichever is less	Headache, palpitations, decreased appetite, abdominal pain, nausea, vomiting, weight loss; FDA warning letter cautions about severe liver injury
BACLOFEN	Skeletal muscle relaxant	Spasticity of cerebral or spinal origin	**T:** 5 mg, two or three times daily initially; increase by 5 mg every 4–7 days to a maximum of 30–80 mg/day; *Intrathecal:* 50–600 mcg/day delivered by implantable pump	Drowsiness, muscle weakness, constipation, rarely nausea, dizziness, paresthesia (numbness and tingling); abrupt withdrawal can cause severe sequelae
BENZTROPINE (Cogentin)	Anticholinergic	Movement disorders associated with antipsychotics such as haloperidol	**T, injection:** Initiate therapy 0.02–05 mg/kg/dose; gradually increase in increments of 0.5 mg twice daily; maximum dosage: 6 mg/day	Gastrointestinal upset, drowsiness, dizziness or blurred vision, dry mouth, difficult urination, constipation, tachycardia
BOTULINUM TOXIN A (Botox)	Antispasticity agent	Spasticity in cerebral palsy and spinal cord injury, strabismus, migraines	Injections are administered by a qualified practitioner; the total dosage (usually 4 units/kg) is divided between affected limbs every 2–3 months	Diffuse skin rash, paralysis with overdose, muscle weakness
BUDESONIDE (Pulmicort, Rhinocort)	Corticosteroid, inhaled, nasal, systemic	Maintenance and prophylactic treatment of asthma, rhinitis, nasal polyps, Crohn's disease	*Nebulized:* 0.25–1 mg/day *Inhaled:* 180–1200 mcg/day as single dose or twice daily *Nasal:* 1–2 sprays in each nostril daily	Nausea, cough, oral candidiasis, hoarseness, dry mouth, epistaxis (bloody nose)
BUPROPION (Wellbutrin, SR, XL, Budeprion SR, XL, Zyban)	Antidepressant (dopamine reuptake inhibitor)	Depression, attention-deficit/hyperactivity disorder, smoking cessation	**T:** Safety and efficacy in children <18 years has not been established; adult dosage range 150–450 mg/day	Decreased seizure threshold, nausea, agitation, anxiety, insomnia, decreased appetite, tachycardia, headache, dry mouth; FDA warns of possible increased suicidal risks in children and adolescents
BUSPIRONE (BuSpar)	Antianxiety agent	Anxiety, aggression, depression, attention-deficit/hyperactivity disorder	**T:** Safety and efficacy in children <18 years has not been established	Chest pain, ringing in the ears, dizziness, drowsiness, restlessness, dyskinesia (rare)

(continued)

Key: C, capsule; IM, intramuscularly; L, liquid suspension or elixir; O, ointment; P, powder; S, suppository; T, tablet.

Medication	Category	Use(s)	Standard applications	Side effects
CALCIUM UNDECYLENATE (10%; Caldesene powder)	Skin agent	Diaper rash	**O, P:** Apply three or four times daily after bath or changing	Irritation, allergic reaction
CARBAMAZEPINE (Carbatrol; Tegretol, Tegretol XR)	Antiepileptic	Epilepsy–partial, generalized or mixed seizures; bipolar disorder, neuralgia, agitation	**C, T, L: chewable:** 5–20 mg/kg/day; blood level should be maintained at 4–14 mcg/ml	Unsteady gait, double vision, drowsiness, slurred speech, dizziness, tremor, headache, nausea, abnormalities in liver function, hypersensitivity reactions with very bad rashes especially in people of Asian descent; FDA warning of reported aplastic anemia and agranulocytosis
CARNITINE (also called L-CARNITINE; Carnitor)	Nutritional supplement	Primary and secondary carnitine deficiency, especially in inborn errors of metabolism; valproic acid–induced deficiency	**T, L, injection:** 50–100 mg/kg/ day divided into doses given every 6 hours; titrate slowly to therapeutic response. Maximum 399 mg/kg or 3g.	Nausea, vomiting, abdominal cramps, diarrhea, body odor, chest pain, headaches, hypertension with IV
CEPHALEXIN (Keflex, Biocef)	Antibiotic	Used to treat susceptible infections of the respiratory tract, skin, and urinary tract; prophylaxis against infective endocarditis	**C, T, L:** 25–100 mg/kg/day divided every 6–8 hours; maximum dosage: 4,000 mg/day	Headache, rash, nausea, vomiting, diarrhea, hypersensitivity
CETIRIZINE (Zyrtec)	Antihistamine, alpha/ beta agonist decongestant	Allergies, itching	**T, C, L:** 6–12 months 2.5 mg daily; 12 months–2 years 2.5 mg daily or twice daily; 2–5 years 5 mg daily or divided twice daily; >6 years 5–10 mg daily	Dry mouth, headache, nausea, somnolence
CHLORAL HYDRATE (Aquachloral, Noctec)	Hypnotic, nonbenzodiazepine	Sedation	**C, S, syrup:** 5–15 mg/kg every 8 hours to a maximum dosage of 2 g/day	Gastrointestinal irritation, dizziness, unsteady gait, hangover effect, paradoxical excitement, hypotension, myocardial/respiratory depression, hallucinations (rare)
CHLORPROMAZINE (Thorazine)	Antipsychotic, typical	Psychosis, anxiety, aggression, severe hyperactivity in individuals with intellectual disability (rarely used now because of newer drugs with fewer side effects), intractable hiccups, nausea/vomiting	**T, S, C, injection, syrup, L:** 2.5–6 mg/kg/day to a maximum of 40 mg in children younger than 5 years or 75 mg in children 5–12 years old	Drowsiness, tardive dyskinesia (involuntary movements of face and tongue), hypotensive, weight gain, lower seizure threshold, electrocardiogram changes, agranulocytosis (depletion of white blood cells), rash, hyperpigmentation of skin

CIMETIDINE (Tagamet)	Histamine (H2) antagonist	Gastroesophageal reflux, gastric/duodenal ulcers, mast cell disease	**T, L:** 20–40 mg/kg/day, given 4 times daily	Rarely diarrhea, headache, decreased white blood count, liver toxicity
CITALOPRAM (Celexa)	Antidepressant (selective serotonin reuptake inhibitors)	Depression, panic disorder, obsessive-compulsive disorder	**T, L:** Adult dosage 20–40 mg daily	Somnolence, insomnia, nausea, dry mouth, increased sweating, agitation, restlessness; FDA warns of possible increased suicidal risks in children and adolescents
CLARITHROMYCIN (Biaxin, XL)	Antibiotic	Wide-spectrum drug used against staph infection, strep throat, and mycoplasma ("walking pneumonia") infections	**T, L:** 15 mg/kg/day, given twice daily for 7–14 days	Stomach upset, diarrhea, nausea, cardiac arrhythmias, but tolerated better than erythromycin
CLOMIPRAMINE (Anafranil)	Tricyclic antidepressant	Obsessive-compulsive disorder, trichotillomania (hair-pulling disorder)	**C:** Initiate at 25 mg/day; gradually increase during the first 2 weeks, as tolerated, to a daily maximum of 3 mg/kg or 100–200 mg, whichever is smaller	Drowsiness, dry mouth, blurred vision, flushing, constipation, central nervous system depression
CLONAZEPAM (Klonopin)	Benzodiazepine	Seizures; infantile spasms; anxiety, panic disorders	**T:** 0.01–0.2 mg/kg/day (usual maintenance dosage is 0.5–2 mg/day, given twice daily)	Sedation, hyperactivity, confusion, depression; do not stop abruptly—tolerance to the drug can develop
CLONIDINE (Catapres; Nexiclon XR)	Alpha-2 adrenergic agonist	Hypertension, attention-deficit/hyperactivity disorder, Tourette syndrome, pain management	**T:** 0.005–0.025 mg/kg/day, increase every 5–7 days as needed; sustained-release patch. Oral suspension and tablets also available	Dry mouth, sedation, hypotension, drowsiness, dermatologic reactions with patch. Do not discontinue abruptly.
CLORAZEPATE (Tranxene)	Benzodiazepine	Adjunctive therapy for partial seizures, anxiety	**T:** 3.75–7.5 mg/dose twice daily; increase dosage by 3.75 mg at weekly intervals, not to exceed 60 mg/day in two to three divided doses	Hypotension, drowsiness, dizziness (see also side effects of DIAZEPAM)
CLOTRIMAZOLE (Lotrimin, Mycelex)	Antifungal, topical, oral	Antifungal, Candida albicans (yeast) infections	**Cream:** Apply twice daily for 2–4 weeks; **Troche (oral)** 10 mg dissolved 3–5 times/day	Skin irritation, peeling, nausea and vomiting with oral
CLOZAPINE (Clozaril, Foxaclo)	Atypical antipsychotic	Schizophrenia in which standard antipsychotic drug treatment has not worked	**T:** 12.5–25 mg once or twice daily, increase slowly to target response. Usual range 25–400 mg/day (**Note:** All patients must be registered in Novartis' distribution system prior to starting the medication)	Hypotension, seizure, weight gain, sedation, extrapyramidal effects; FDA warning for seizures, agranulocytosis, myocarditis, and other cardiovascular and respiratory effects

(continued)

Key: C, capsule; IM, intramuscularly; L, liquid suspension or elixir; O, ointment; P, powder; S, suppository; T, tablet.

Medication	Category	Use(s)	Standard applications	Side effects
COLLOIDAL OATMEAL (e.g., Aveeno)	Skin treatment	Dry skin, itching	**Oil, cleansing bar, cream, lotion:** Add to bath or apply as needed	Allergic reaction
CORTICOTROPIN (Acthar, ACTH)	Corticosteroid, systemic	Infantile spasms and Lennox-Gastaut syndrome, many off-label uses	**Injection, IM, SC:** 75 units/m²/dose given twice daily; many regimens exist, but ACTH is generally used for weeks-months and then tapered off slowly	Glucose in urine, hypertension, cataracts, brittle bones, altered behavior, Cushing's syndrome, immunosuppression
CYPROHEPTADINE (Periactin)	Histamine (H1) antagonist	Allergies, migraines, appetite stimulation, spasticity, urticaria	**T, L:** 0.25 mg/kg/day divided 2–3 times/day or 2–4 mg given 2–3 times/day; Maximum 12–16 mg	Weight gain, nausea, gastrointestinal irritation, dry mouth, somnolence
DANTROLENE SODIUM (Dantrium)	Skeletal muscle relaxant	Spasticity in cerebral palsy or spinal cord injury, malignant hyperthermia prevention	**C:** 0.5 mg/kg twice daily initially; increase by 0.5 mg/kg every 4–7 days to a maximum of 2 mg/kg/dose, given 2–4 times daily; injection for malignant hyperthermia	Weakness, drowsiness, lethargy, dizziness, tingling sensation, nausea, diarrhea; FDA warning for hepatotoxicity (liver function should be monitored); long-term side effects in children are not known
DESIPRAMINE (Norpramin)	Tricyclic antidepressant	Depression, anxiety, attention-deficit/hyperactivity disorder, neuropathic pain	**T:** Not recommended in children younger than 12 years; 1–5 mg/kg/day in divided doses; maximum 150 mg/day	Hypotension, dizziness, constipation, somnolence, dry mouth, blurred vision, sudden death from cardiac arrhythmia (rarely); FDA warning of possible increased risk of suicidal thinking and behavior
DEXTROAMPHETAMINE (Dexedrine, Dexedrine-Spansules, DextroStat, Procentra)	Stimulant	Attention-deficit/hyperactivity disorder, narcolepsy	**C, L, T (5 mg):** 2.5–5 mg once daily titrate weekly to response; Maximum 40 mg/day; sustained release available	Insomnia, restlessness, decreased appetite, irritability, headache, abdominal cramps, decreased appetite; FDA warning for potential for abuse, cardiac events; not recommended for children under 3 years of age
DIAZEPAM (Valium, Diastat)	Benzodiazepine	Sedation, aggression, anxiety, spasticity, seizures, status epilepticus	**C, T, L:** 0.12–0.8 mg/kg/day given three to four times daily; **Rectal gel (Diastat):** Not recommended for infants younger than 6 months; safety and efficacy not established in children younger than 2 years; 2–5 years, 0.5 mg/kg; 6–11 years, 0.3 mg/kg; older than 11 years, 0.2 mg/kg; not to exceed 20 mg/dose; injection is available	Sedation, weakness, depression, ataxia, memory disturbance, difficulty handling secretions and chewing/swallowing foods, anxiety, paradoxical reactions (e.g., anxiety, agitation), respiratory and cardiac depression, rash, low white blood cell count; drug dependence can occur

DIPHENHYDRAMINE (Benadryl, various brands)	Antihistamine	Sedation, allergies, hives, extrapyramidal symptoms, motion sickness	**C, T, O, L:** 5 mg/kg/day given at 6–8 hour intervals to a maximum dosage of 300 mg/day; injection is available	Sedation, insomnia, dry mouth, dizziness, euphoria, gastrointestinal upset, paradoxical excitation
DULOXETINE (Cymbalta)	Antidepressant (norepinephrine serotonin reuptake inhibitor)	Depression, neuropathy, fibromyalgia, anxiety	**C:** Adult dose: 20–60 mg/day; safety and efficacy not established in children <18 years	Dry mouth, nausea, diaphoresis, headache, insomnia, fatigue, FDA warning of possible increased risk of suicidal thinking and behavior; dizziness
DUODERM	Skin treatment	Skin ulcers/sores, second-degree burns, and minor abrasions	Sterile occlusive dressing with hydroactive or gel formula	Allergic reaction to tape or gel formula
ERYTHROMYCIN (various brands)	Antibiotic, prokinetic agent	Used against staph infection, strep throat, and mycoplasma ("walking pneumonia") infections;	**C, O, T, L:** 30–50 mg/kg/day, given four times daily; injection is available	Nausea, vomiting, diarrhea, cardiac dysrhythmias; interactions with other drugs
ERYTHROMYCIN (2%) (T-STAT)	Antibiotic, topical	Acne	**Solution on pads:** Apply to clean area twice daily	Skin dryness, peeling, skin irritation
ESCITALOPRAM (Lexapro)	Antidepressant (selective serotonin reuptake inhibitors)	Depression, anxiety, obsessive compulsive disorder, panic disorder	**T, L:** Children >12 years, initial 10 mg once daily increase to 20 mg after 3 weeks	FDA warning of possible increased risk of suicidal thinking and behavior
ETHOSUXIMIDE (Zarontin)	Antiepileptic	Absence seizures	**C, L:** 15–40 mg/kg/day, given twice daily to a maximum of 1.5 g/day; blood level: 40–80 mcg/l	Sedation, unsteady gait, anorexia, rash, stomach distress, blood dyscrasias
FAMOTIDINE (Pepcid)	H2 antagonist	Gastrosophageal reflux; ulcers, decreases stomach acidity	**C, T, L:** 1 mg/kg/day, given twice daily with meals; maximum dosage: 80 mg/day; injection is available	Headache, dizziness, constipation, diarrhea
FELBAMATE (Felbatol)	Antiepileptic	Lennox-Gastaut syndrome; also effective in generalized and secondary generalized seizures, partial seizures	**T, L:** 15–45 mg/kg/day divided 3–4 times/day	Anorexia, vomiting, insomnia, headache, rash, risk of life-threatening hepatitis and aplastic anemia; FDA recommends close monitoring
FLUCONAZOLE (Fluconazole, Diflucan)	Antifungal	Treatment or prophylaxis of susceptible fungal infections, including oral and vaginal Candida albicans (yeast) infections	**T, L:** 6 mg/kg once on first day of therapy, then 3 mg/kg/ dose daily for 14–21 days; for vaginal candidiasis: a single 150 mg dose may be given, injection is available	Dizziness, headache, rash, increased liver enzymes nausea; inhibits the metabolism of many drugs so screen for possible drug interactions

(continued)

Key: C, capsule; IM, intramuscularly; L, liquid suspension or elixir; O, ointment; P, powder; S, suppository; T, tablet.

Medication	Category	Use(s)	Standard applications	Side effects
FLUOXETINE (Prozac)	Antidepressant (selective serotonin reuptake inhibitors)	Depression, self-injurious behavior, Tourette syndrome, obsessive-compulsive disorder, anxiety, bulimia, panic disorder	**T, C, L:** Safety and efficacy in children has not been established; adults should initially receive 20 mg/day in morning to a maximum dosage of 80 mg/day	Anxiety, agitation, sleep disruption, decreased appetite, seizures; FDA warns of possible increased suicidal risks in children and adolescents
FOSPHENYTOIN (Cerebyx)	See PHENYTOIN; intravenous substitute for phenytoin	See PHENYTOIN	See PHENYTOIN	See PHENYTOIN
FUROSEMIDE (Lasix)	Diuretic	Diuresis	**T, L, injection:** 1 mg/kg/dose given 1–4 times daily; Maximum 6 mg/kg/dose	Electrolyte abnormalities
GABAPENTIN (Neurontin)	Antiepileptic	Adjunctive therapy in partial and secondarily generalized seizures, neuropathic pain	**C, T, L:** 10–15 mg/kg/day titrated up to 40–50 mg/kg/day in divided doses	Sedation, dizziness, unsteady gait, emotional lability; do not withdraw abruptly
GLYCOPYRROLATE (Robinul)	Anticholinergic	Decrease drooling in cerebral palsy	**T:** 40–100 mcg/kg/dose every 3–4 hours as needed for secretions; injection is available	Rapid heart rate, orthostatic hypotension, drowsiness, blurred vision, dry mouth, constipation
GUANFACINE (Tenex, Intuniv extended release)	Alpha-2 agonist	Hypertension, attention-deficit/hyperactivity disorder, Tourette syndrome	**T:** Initial 1 mg/day may increase 1 mg/week to maximum dosage of 4 mg/day	Dry mouth, sedation, hypotension, headache, nausea; do not discontinue abruptly
HALOPERIDOL (Haldol)	Antipsychotic, typical	Self-injurious behavior, Tourette syndrome, severe agitation, psychosis	**T, L:** 0.01–0.03 mg/kg/day for agitation; 0.05–0.15 mg/kg/ day, in two or three daily doses, for psychosis; and 0.05–0.075 mg/kg/day, in two or three daily doses, for Tourette syndrome, IM	Extrapyramidal effects, hypotension, nausea, vomiting, electrocardiogram changes, neuroleptic malignant syndrome, lower seizure threshold in epilepsy, anticholinergic effects
HYDROCORTISONE (e.g., Caldecort, Cort-Dome, Hytone)	Corticosteroid, topical	Eczema, dermatitis	**O, cream, gel, liquid:** Apply thin film 2–4 times daily	Skin irritation, dryness, rash
HYDROCORTISONE, POLYMYXIN-B, NEOMYCIN (Cortisporin)	Corticosteroid + antibiotic, topical	Steroid-responsive skin conditions with secondary infection	**O, cream:** Apply sparingly and massage into skin two or three times daily.	Local irritation

IBUPROFEN (Advil, Motrin)	Nonsteroidal anti-inflammatory (NSAID)	Inflammatory diseases and rheumatoid disorders, including juvenile rheumatoid arthritis (JRA); mild to moderate pain; fever; dysmenorrhea; migraines	*C, T, L:* 5–10 mg/kg/dose given every 6–8 hours; maximum dose: 40 mg/kg/day; *JRA:* 30–50 mg/kg/day in 3–4 divided doses; start at lower end of dosing range and titrate; maximum: 2.4 g/day; *Pain:* 4–10 mg/kg/dose every 6–8 hours	Gastrointestinal irritation, rash, dizziness, increased bleeding risk, renal effects (higher doses; elderly); caution in ulcer and renal patients; FDA warning of possible increased risk of cardiovascular thrombotic events and serious gastrointestinal events
IMIPRAMINE (Tofranil, Janimine)	Tricyclic antidepressant	Depression, enuresis, neuropathy	*C, T:* 1.5 mg/kg/day, given in three daily doses to a maximum dosage of 5 mg/kg/day; enuresis 25 mg at bedtime, increase to 50 mg if no response	Dry mouth, drowsiness, constipation, electrocardiogram abnormalities, increased blood pressure, urinary retention, FDA warning of possible increased risk of suicidal thinking and behavior
ISOTRETINOIN (Accutane, Claravis)	Skin treatment	Severe acne	*C:* 0.5–2 mg/kg/day, given in two divided doses for 15–20 weeks	Drying of mucous membranes, photosensitivity, dry skin, cheilitis, itching, retinoid dermatitis; known teratogen: must be part of iPledge program to receive to eliminate fetal exposure
LAMOTRIGINE (Lamictal)	Antiepileptic	Adjunct or monotherapy for a variety of seizures; bipolar disorder	*T, L:* Initial 0.3 mg/kg/day in 1–2 doses titrated slowly (every 2 weeks) to usual maintenance dose of 4.5–7.5 mg/kg/day (lower dose if coadministered with valproic acid)	Sedation, dizziness, ataxia, headaches, nausea, vomiting, severe and potentially life-threatening skin reactions
LANOLIN, PETROLATUM, VITAMINS A and D, MINERAL OILS (A & D Ointment)	Skin treatment	Diaper rash	*O:* Apply thin film at each diaper change	Allergic reaction
LANSOPRAZOLE (Prevacid)	Proton pump inhibitor	Treatment or relief of ulcers, gastroesophageal reflux disease; adjuvant therapy in the treatment of *Helicobacter pylori* associated gastritis	*C, L, T:* 15–30 mg given once or twice daily depending on age and condition treated; maximum dosage: 60 mg/day; injection (IV) is available	Abdominal pain, nausea, flatulence, increased appetite, headache, fatigue, rash
LEVETIRACETAM (Keppra)	Antiepileptic	Adjunctive therapy in a variety of seizure types, migraine prophylaxis	*T, L:* Initially, 20 mg/kg/day divided twice daily. Dosage is increased to 40–60 mg/kg/day as tolerated; Maximum daily dosage: 3,000 mg/day; injection is available	Somnolence, nausea, anorexia, dizziness, behavior changes, irritability

Key: C, capsule; IM, intramuscularly; L, liquid suspension or elixir; O, ointment; P, powder; S, suppository; T, tablet.

(continued)

Medication	Category	Use(s)	Standard applications	Side effects
LEVOTHYROXINE (Syn-throid, Levothroid, Levoxyl)	Thyroid product	Hypothyroidism	*T:* <1 year 6–15 mcg/kg/day; 1–5 years, 5–6 mcg/kg/ day; 6–12 years, 4–5 mcg/ kg/day; older than 12 years, 2–3 mcg/kg/day; injection is available	Heart palpitations, nervousness, tremor, excessive sweating, diarrhea, weight loss
LINDANE (Kwell)	Antiparasitic, topical	Scabies and lice	*Cream, lotion:* Apply thin layer and massage into body from neck down; wash off after 8–12 hours; *Shampoo:* apply to dry hair, massage thoroughly into hair, and leave on for 4 minutes; then form lather and rinse well	None with prescribed use; FDA warning of risk of seizures with overuse in small children; should be reserved for patients who do not respond to other treatments
LITHIUM CARBONATE (Eska-lith, Lithobid)	Antipsychotic	Mood stabilizer, bipolar disorder, depression	*C, T, L:* 15–60 mg/kg/day divided in three to four doses; do not exceed 1,800 mg/day. Therapeutic range: mania, 0.6–1.5 mEq/l; bipolar disorder, 0.8–1 mEq/l	Sedation, confusion, seizures, rash, hypothyroidism, diarrhea, muscle weakness, gastrointestinal irritation, renal dysfunction, tremor
LORATADINE (Claritin, Alavert)	Antihistamine H1 antagonist	Allergies, urticaria	*C,T,L:* 2–5 years 5 mg daily; >6 years 10 mg daily	Sedation, dry mouth, headache
LORAZEPAM (Ativan)	Benzodiazepine	Anxiety, status epilepticus, agitation, sedation, antiemetic	*T, L, injection:* 0.05 mg/kg/dose every 4–8 hours as needed; do not exceed 4 mg/dose, IM	Sedation, weakness, depression, unstable gait, memory disturbance, difficulty handling secretions and chewing/swallowing foods
MAGNESIUM HYDROX-IDE AND ALUMINUM HYDROXIDE (Alamag)	Antacid, laxative	Antacid for reflux; also helps treat constipation	*T, L:* 2–4 teaspoons with meals and at bedtime	Minimal; may accumulate in renal dysfunction patients
METHYLPHENIDATE/ DEXMETHYLPHENIDATE (e.g., Concerta, Daytrana, Metadate, Metadate CD, Metadate ER, Methylin, Methylin ER, Ritalin, Daytrana; Focalin, Focalin XR)	Stimulant	Attention-deficit/hyperactivity disorder	*C,L,T, patch:* Dose varies with each product. Generally do not exceed 60 mg/day	Appetite suppression, insomnia, arrhythmia, anxiety, headache, irritability
METHYLPREDNISOLONE (Solu-Medrol, Medrol)	Corticosteroid	Reduction of airway inflammation during acute asthma attacks, inflammatory conditions, many others	*Injection:* 1–2 mg/kg/dose; *Orally:* 1–2 mg/kg/dose, twice daily for 3–5 days	Side effects usually mild with short-term use

Medication	Classification	Indication	Forms/Dosage	Side effects
METOCLOPRAMIDE (Reglan)	Prokinetic agent	Antireflux, increases gastric emptying	**T, L:** 0.1–0.5 mg/kg/day, given four times daily	Acute movement disorder (dystonia), drowsiness, sedation, anxiety, leukopenia
MICONAZOLE (2%; e.g., Monistat)	Antifungal, topical	Antifungal, *Candida albicans* (yeast) infections	**S, O, cream:** Apply twice daily for 2–4 weeks	Skin irritation, peeling, pruritis
MINERAL OIL (e.g., AlphaKeri, Fleet enema)	Skin treatment, laxative	Emollient for dry skin	**Soap, oil, spray:** Add to bath or rub into wet skin as needed; rinse; **Oral:** 1–3 ml/kg/day	Allergic reaction (topical) nausea and diarrhea (oral)
MINERAL OIL, PETROLATUM, LANOLIN (Nivea, Lubriderm)	Skin treatment	Emollient for dry skin, constipation	**Cream, lotion, bath oil:** Apply as needed	Allergic reaction
MONTELUKAST (Singulair)	Leukotriene receptor antagonist	Asthma, allergies	**T, granules, sprinkles:** 6 months–5 years 4 mg daily; 6–14 years 5mg daily; >15 10 mg daily	Headache, altered behavior, eosinophilia (rare)
MUPIROCIN (2%; Bactroban)	Antibiotic, topical	Antibiotic for impetigo, secondary infections of skin ulcers, burns	**O:** Apply sparingly three times daily; may cover with gauze	Burning, itching, pain at site of application
NALTREXONE (ReVia)	Opioid antagonist	Opiate antagonist for treatment of self-injurious behavior	**T:** 50 mg/day in adults; safety and efficacy in children <18 years has not been established	None in opioid-free individuals
NORTRIPTYLINE (Pamelor, Aventyl)	Tricyclic antidepressant	Depression, neuropathic pain, nocturnal enuresis, attention-deficit/hyperactivity disorder	**C, T, L:** Not recommended for children <12 years; Usual dosage 10–60 mg/day	Dry mouth, drowsiness, constipation, electrocardiogram abnormalities, mania, sedation; FDA warning of possible increased risk of suicidal thinking and behavior
NYSTATIN (Mycostatin)	Antifungal	Treatment of yeast and thrush infections in the mouth and gastrointestinal tract	**O, T P, cream:** Apply twice daily; **Oral suspension:** Swish and swallow 400,000–600,000 units 4 times/day	Diarrhea (reported with oral form), redness, skin irritation, gastrointestinal upset
OLANZAPINE (Zyprexa)	Antipsychotic, atypical	Treatment of the manifestations of psychotic disorders, Tourette syndrome, anorexia nervosa, autism spectrum disorder	**T, C, injection (IM):** Start at 2.5 mg once daily; titrate dose weekly as required, up to a maximum dosage of 20 mg/day	Edema, weight gain, hyperglycemia, somnolence, orthostatic hypotension, increase in lipids, akathisia, asthenia, dizziness, tremor, FDA warning of possible increased risk of suicidal thinking and behavior

(continued)

Key: C, capsule; IM, intramuscularly; L, liquid suspension or elixir; O, ointment; P, powder; S, suppository; T, tablet.

Medication	Category	Use(s)	Standard applications	Side effects
OMEPRAZOLE (Prilosec)	Proton pump inhibitor	Treatment or relief of ulcers, gastroesophageal reflux disease; adjuvant therapy in the treatment of *Helicobacter pylori* associated gastritis	**L, C, T:** Dose varies with age from 5–20 mg daily or given in divided doses twice daily; maximum dosage: 40 mg/day	Abdominal pain, diarrhea, nausea, flatulence, increased appetite, taste changes, headache
OXCARBAZEPINE (Trileptal)	Antiepileptic	Generalized tonic-clonic, complex partial, and simple partial seizures as both adjunctive and monotherapy	**T, L:** 8–10 mg/kg in two divided doses, usually not to exceed 600 mg/day; do not exceed the maximum adult dosage of 2,400 mg/day	Ataxia, dizziness, gastrointestinal irritation, headache, somnolence, tremor, vision disturbances, hyponatremia
OXYBUTYNIN (Ditropan)	Antispasmodic agent, urinary	Antispasmodic for neurogenic bladder	**T, L:** 0.2 mg/kg/dose 2–4 times/day or 5 mg twice daily, up to 5 mg 3 times/day, maximum: 15 mg/day, patch; topical gel one packet/day	Palpitations, drowsiness, dizziness, insomnia, dry mouth, nausea, vomiting, constipation, urinary hesitancy or retention, blurred vision, decreased tears, decreased sweating
PAROXETINE (Paxil)	Antidepressant (selective serotonin reuptake inhibitor)	Depression, obsessive-compulsive disorder, anxiety disorders, self-injurious behavior	**T, L:** 10–20 mg/day to start; increase dosage as needed by 10 mg/day weekly. Maximum dosage is 60 mg/day	Somnolence, headache, insomnia, nausea, constipation, decreased appetite, palpitations, asthenia, sexual dysfunction; FDA warns of possible increased suicidal risks in children and adolescents
PENICILLIN (e.g., Pen V K)	Antibiotic	Drug of choice for strep throat, which in severe cases can be treated by a single intramuscular injection of Bicillin	**T, L:** 25–50 mg/kg/day, given 3–4 times daily for 7–14 days; injection is available	Allergic reactions, diarrhea, nausea
PERMETHRIN (Nix, Elimite)	Antiparasitic, topical	Scabies and lice	**Cream, lotion:** Apply thin layer and massage into body from neck down; wash off after 8–14 hours; **Shampoo:** Apply to towel-dried hair, massage thoroughly into hair, and leave on for 10 minutes; then rinse well. May repeat in 1 week if live mites reappear.	Pruritis, hypersensitivity, burning, stinging, rash
PETROLATUM, MINERAL OIL AND WAX, ALCOHOL (Eucerin)	Skin treatment	Emollient for dry skin, itching	**Cream, lotion, facial lotion with sunscreen, cleansing bar:** Apply as needed	Allergic reaction

PHENOBARBITAL (Luminal)	Antiepileptic	Generalized tonic-clonic, simple partial, and secondarily generalized seizures	**C, T, L:** 2–5 mg/kg/day for children; 1–2 mg/kg/day for adolescents; therapeutic blood level: 15–40 mcg/ml; injection is available	Paradoxical hyperactivity, sedation, learning difficulties in older children, behavioral difficulties in 50% of children younger than 10 years, irritability, unsteady gait, respiratory depression
PHENYTOIN (Dilantin)	Antiepileptic	Generalized tonic-clonic and complex partial seizures	**C, T, injectable, suspension:** Maintenance dosage: 4–10 mg/kg/day; blood level:10–20 mcg/ml; free level: 1–2 mcg/ml, chewable	Swelling of gums, excessive hairiness, rash, coarsening of facial features, possible adverse effects on learning and behavior; risk of birth defects if taken during pregnancy; nystagmus and unsteady gait with toxic levels; blood dyscrasias; decreased bone density
PREDNISOLONE (Prelone)	Corticosteroid, systemic	Reduction of airway inflammation during acute asthma attacks, inflammatory conditions (many), nephrotic syndrome	**T, L:** 1 mg/kg/dose, twice daily for 3–5 days; injection; doses vary depending on condition treated	Side effects usually mild with short-term use but may result in headache, mood changes, hypertension or edema; long-term use may result in congestive heart failure, osteoporosis, weight gain, increased risk of infection, Cushing's syndrome, glaucoma, and thinning skin
PREDNISONE (Deltasone)	Corticosteroid, systemic	Reduction of airway inflammation during acute asthma attacks, inflammatory conditions (many)	**T, L:** 1 mg/kg/dose, twice daily for 3–5 days; doses vary depending on condition treated	Side effects usually mild with short-term use but may result in headache, mood changes, hypertension or edema; long-term use may result in congestive heart failure, osteoporosis, weight gain, increased risk of infection, Cushing's syndrome, glaucoma and thinning skin
PRIMIDONE (Mysoline)	Antiepileptic	Generalized tonic-clonic and complex partial seizures	**T, L:** 10–25 mg/kg/day for children; 125–250 mg three times daily for adolescents; therapeutic blood level: 5–12 mcg/ml, also metabolized to phenobarbital (of which therapeutic blood level is 15–40 mcg/ml)	Drowsiness, dizziness, nausea, vomiting, leucopenia (low white blood cell count), systemic lupuslike syndrome, nystagmus (jerky eye movements), personality change (see also side effects of PHENOBARBITAL)

(continued)

Key: C, capsule; IM, intramuscularly; L, liquid suspension or elixir; O, ointment; P, powder; S, suppository; T, tablet.

Medication	Category	Use(s)	Standard applications	Side effects
QUETIAPINE (Seroquel)	Antipsychotic, atypical	Bipolar disorder, psychosis, depression, autism spectrum disorder	**T:** Children >10 years: 50 mg divided twice daily titrated up to lowest effective dose. Maximum dosage: 600 mg/day	Hyper or hypotension, elevated lipids, weight gain, gastrointestinal irritation, somnolence, tremor, extrapyramidal effects, dizziness, asthenia, FDA warning of possible increased risk of suicidal thinking and behavior
RANITIDINE (Zantac)	Histamine H2 antagonist	Gastroesophageal reflux (decreases stomach acidity), ulcers	**C, T, L:** 2–8 mg/kg/day, given twice daily; injection	Headache, gastrointestinal upset, rarely liver toxicity
RISPERIDONE (Risperdal)	Antipsychotic, atypical	Self-injurious behavior, psychosis, Tourette syndrome, aggression, pervasive developmental disorders	**T, L:** Pediatric patients may start with 0.25–0.5 mg twice daily; slowly increase as needed; dosages greater than 10 mg/day should be avoided.	Hypotension, sedation, dizziness, movement disorder, headache, constipation, weight gain, urinary retention, agranulocytosis
SELENIUM SULFIDE (2.5%; Selsun Blue)	Skin treatment	Scalp conditions (dandruff or seborrhea)	**Lotion, shampoo:** Apply to wet scalp, wait 3 minutes, rinse, repeat; use twice a week for 2 weeks, and then as needed	Skin irritation, dry or oily scalp, hair loss and discoloration
SERTRALINE (Zoloft)	Antidepressant (selective serotonin reuptake inhibitors)	Depression, anxiety, obsessive-compulsive disorder, posttraumatic stress syndrome	**T, L:** 50 mg/day initially to a maximum of 200 mg/day in adults; safety and efficacy not established in children	Somnolence, headache, agitation, sleep disruption, decreased appetite, nausea, diarrhea, tremors, sweating, seizures; FDA warns of possible increased suicidal risks in children and adolescents
THEOPHYLLINE (Aerolate Slo-Bid, Theo-Dur, Uniphyl)	Respiratory agent	Bronchodilator; may be used in conjunction with other treatments for acute or chronic asthma	**C, T, L:** Ages 6 weeks to 6 months: 10 mg/kg/day; children ages 6 months to 1 year: 12–18 mg/kg/day; children ages 1–9 years: 20–24 mg/kg/day; children ages 9–12 years: 20 mg/kg/day; children ages 12–16 years: 18 mg/kg/day; maximum adult dosage: 900 mg/day; injection (IV) is available, IM	Nausea, vomiting, stomach pain (especially common at high blood levels), gastroesophageal reflux, anorexia, nervousness, tachypnea

Drug	Classification	Indication	Dosing	Side Effects/Warnings
THIORIDAZINE (Mellaril)	Antipsychotic, typical	Self-injurious behavior, psychosis	**T, L:** Not recommended for children <2 years; children ages 2–12 years: 0.5–3 mg/kg/day; children >12 years with mild disorders: 10 mg, two or three times daily; children >12 years with severe disorders: 25 mg, two or three times daily	Drowsiness, hypotension, movement disorder, electrocardiogram abnormalities, retinal abnormalities; FDA warning for QT prolongation on electrocardiogram
THIOTHIXENE (Navane)	Antipsychotic, typical	Self-injurious behavior, psychosis	**C, L:** 2 mg, three times daily, increase to 20–30 mg/day if needed; not recommended for children <12 years	Movement disorder (tardive dyskinesia), neuroleptic malignant syndrome, rapid heart rate, hypotension, drowsiness, bone marrow suppression
TIAGABINE (Gabitril)	Antiepileptic	Adjunct for partial seizures	**T:** 12–18 years: initially 4 mg once daily for 1 week; then 8 mg/day in two divided doses for 1 week; then increase weekly by 4–8 mg/day; increase weekly by 2–4 mg/day in two to four divided doses daily; titrate dosage to response; maximum dosage: 32 mg/day	Dizziness, headache, sleepiness, central nervous system depression, memory disturbance, unsteady gait, emotionality, tremors, abdominal pain
TOLNAFTATE (Tinactin)	Antifungal, topical	Antifungal, ringworm	**Cream, P:** Apply small amount of cream or powder to affected area 2–3 times a day for 2–4 weeks	Nontoxic, skin irritation
TOPIRAMATE (Topamax)	Antiepileptic	Refractory partial seizures, Lennox-Gastaut syndrome	**T, sprinkles:** Initially 1–3 mg/kg/day in two divided doses for 1 week, then increase by 1–3 mg/kg/day each week; titrate dosage to response; usual dose range: 6–9 mg/kg/day in two divided doses; some children may require more than 15 mg/kg/day	Edema (swelling), language problems, abnormal coordination, depression, difficulty concentrating, fatigue, dizziness, unsteady gait, sleepiness, weight loss, somnolence, weakness, nystagmus; seek immediate medical attention if blurry vision occurs
TRIAMCINOLONE (Kenalog, Aristocort [skin]; Azmacort [respiratory])	Corticosteroid, inhaled, systemic, topical	Eczema, dermatitis	**T, L, O, P, cream, lotion:** Apply thin film two to four times daily	Skin irritation, rash, dryness,
TRIMETHOPRIM AND SULFAMETHOXAZOLE (TMP/SMZ) (Bactrim, Septra)	Antibiotic	Treatment or prophylaxis of susceptible infections, including urinary tract infections, otitis media, sinusitis, and so forth.	**T, L:** 8–20 mg/kg of TMP/day, given twice daily; injection is available	Bone marrow suppression (rare), allergic reactions, photosensitivity, gastrointestinal irritation, rash

Key: C, capsule; IM, intramuscularly; L, liquid suspension or elixir; O, ointment; P, powder; S, suppository; T, tablet.

(continued)

Medication	Category	Use(s)	Standard applications	Side effects
VALPROIC ACID (Depakene, Depacon, Depakote)	Antiepileptic, mood stabilizer	Myoclonic, simple absence, and generalized tonic-clonic seizures; Lennox-Gastaut syndrome; infantile spasms; also used to treat aggression and mood disorders, bipolar disorder, impulsive aggression, intermittent explosive disorder, migraine prophylaxis	**C, syrup, sprinkle, injection:** 15–60 mg/kg/day; therapeutic blood level: 50–100 mcg/ml; Depakote ER may be dosed less frequently than the other preparations	Hair loss, weight loss or gain, abdominal distress, tremor, agranulocytosis, low platelet count; risk of birth defects if taken during pregnancy; FDA warning for potentially fatal liver damage (risk is 1/800 in children with developmental disabilities <2 years who are taking more than one antiepileptic drug) and pancreatitis
VENLAFAXINE (Effexor, XR)	Antidepressant (norepinephrine-selective reuptake inhibitors)	Depression, anxiety, attention-deficit/hyperactivity disorder, panic disorder	**T,C:** Initial 12.5 mg/day increase weekly by 12.5–25 mg of 75 mg daily	Hypertension, diaphoresis, weight loss, gastrointestinal irritation, asthenia, insomnia, tremor, dizziness, somnolence, headache; FDA warns of possible increased suicidal risks in children and adolescents
ZINC OXIDE, COD LIVER OIL, LANOLIN, PETROLATUM (Caldesene ointment)	Skin treatment	Diaper rash	**O:** Apply three or four times daily after diaper change or bath	Allergic reaction
ZIPRASIDONE (Geodon)	Antipsychotic, atypical	Bipolar disorder, psychosis, agitation, Tourette's syndrome	**C:** Doses of 5–40 mg/day have been reported; injection is available, IM	Orthostatic hypotension, gastrointestinal irritation, hyperglycemia, weight gain, extrapyramidal effects, insomnia, somnolence, QTc prolongation, FDA warnings of blood dyscrasias
ZONISAMIDE (Zonegran)	Antiepileptic	Adjunctive therapy in partial seizures, infantile spasms, and Lennox-Gastaut syndrome	**C:** Not approved < 16 years; adult dosing: 100 mg/day titrated every 2 weeks by 100 mg to max of 400 mg/day	Somnolence, dizziness, ataxia, loss of appetite, gastrointestinal discomfort, headache, agitation/irritability, confusion, rash, visual disturbances

Key: C, capsule; IM, intramuscularly; L, liquid suspension or elixir; O, ointment; P, powder; S, suppository; T, tablet.

818

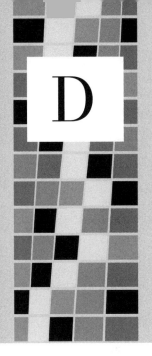

D Childhood Disabilities Resources, Services, and Organizations

This appendix lists a number of organizations, Internet sources, and other resources that provide services and assist in research in the area of childhood developmental disabilities. The resources cited are a representative sample and are not intended to be all inclusive. A brief description follows each listing.

GENERAL

Federal Agencies

Administration on Developmental Disabilities (ADD)
http://www.acf.hhs.gov/programs/add/
Program within the U.S. Department of Health and Human Services promoting the independence and economic and social well-being of individuals with developmental disabilities and their families by ensuring that needed services and assistance for community life are available and that families participate in the design of such services.

Eunice Kennedy Shriver National Institute of Child Health and Human Development (NICHD)
http://www.nichd.nih.gov/
Established in 1962 as part of the National Institutes of Health. Funds research and offers information related to human development, health, and developmental disabilities.

Maternal and Child Health Bureau (MCHB)
http://mchb.hrsa.gov

Established in 1912 as part of the Health Resources and Services Administration (HRSA). Provides funding and governs programs designed to ensure equal access for all to quality health care in a supportive, culturally competent, family, and community setting.

Office of Disability Employment Policy
http://www.dol.gov/odep
One of the oldest presidential committees in the United States. Promotes acceptance of people with physical and intellectual disabilities in the world of work, in both the public and the private sectors. Promotes the elimination of barriers, both physical and attitudinal, to the employment of people with disabilities.

Office of Special Education and Rehabilitative Services (OSERS)
http://www.ed.gov/about/offices/list/osers
Part of the U.S. Department of Education. Responds to inquiries, and researches and documents information on operations serving the field of disabilities. Specializes in providing information on federal funding for programs serving people with disabilities, federal legislation affecting individuals with disabilities, and federal programs benefiting people with disabilities.

Social Security Administration
http://www.ssa.gov
Mission is to advance the economic security of the nation's people through compassionate and vigilant leadership in shaping and managing America's Social Security programs. Provides

information to the U.S. population on policy; programs and services; and, more specifically, resources for people with disabilities.

Finances

Children's Defense Fund (CFD)

http://www.childrensdefense.org

Private nonprofit organization dedicated to educating about, advocating for, and studying the needs of children, especially low-income children, minority children, and children with disabilities. Mission focuses on giving children a head start (child care), a healthy start (child health), a fair start (family income), a safe start (violence prevention, child welfare, and mental health), and a moral start (ethics, morality, and self-discipline).

Libraries and Clearinghouses

Cochrane Library

http://www.thecochranelibrary.com

Searchable, online database of systematic reviews of the effects of health care interventions related to pregnancy and neonatal outcomes. Also available on DVD-ROM.

Early Childhood Research & Practice (ECRP)

http://www.ecrp.uiuc.edu

Web site of a peer-reviewed, bilingual electronic journal sponsored by the ERIC Clearinghouse on Elementary and Early Childhood Education (ERIC/EECE) at the University of Illinois at Urbana–Champaign. Covers topics related to the development, care, and education of children from birth to approximately age 8. Also includes articles and essays that present opinions and reflections, as well as letters to the editor.

Medline Plus Health Information

http://www.medlineplus.gov

Web site presents health information from NLM and contains extensive information for professionals and the public on diseases/conditions and medicines, lists of hospitals, a medical encyclopedia/dictionary, information in Spanish, and links to current clinical trials.

National Dissemination Center for Children with Disabilities (NICHCY)

http://www.nichcy.org

Web site contains information about specific disabilities, early intervention services for infants and toddlers, special education and related services for children in school, resources and connections in every state, individualized education programs, parent materials, disability organizations, professional associations, education rights and law requirements, and the transition to adult life. Publishes *Research Connections in Special Education* and *OSEP Digests*.

National Library of Medicine (NLM)

http://www.nlm.nih.gov

Part of the National Institutes of Health. Is the world's largest medical library and is a national resource for all U.S. health sciences libraries. Collects materials in areas of biomedicine; health care; biomedical aspects of technology; humanities; and the physical, life, and social sciences.

PubMed

http://www.ncbi.nlm.nih.gov/entrez/query.fcgi

Search engine allows users to research and obtain peer-reviewed articles and abstracts published by major journals of medical research.

Professional Societies

American Academy of Pediatrics (AAP)

http://aap.org

The professional association of pediatricians. Committed to the optimal, physical, mental, and social health and well-being of infants, children, adolescents, and young adults. Publishes a major pediatric medical journal, *Pediatrics*.

American Academy of Pediatrics (AAP) Policies

http://aappolicy.aappublications.org

Web site includes policy statements and guidelines developed by the AAP. Also offers links to printable handouts for parents that provide important health messages based on these statements.

American College of Obstetricians and Gynecologists (ACOG)

http://www.acog.org

Professional organization of obstetrician-gynecologists, dedicated to the advancement of women's health through education, advocacy, practice, and research. Provides online physician directory. Bookstore offers patient information pamphlets, professional resources, and multimedia resources.

American Medical Association (AMA)

http://www.ama-assn.org

Develops and promotes standards in medical practice, research, and education; advocates for patients and physicians. Publishes a leading medical journal, *JAMA: The Journal of the American Medical Association*.

Association of University Centers on Disabilities (AUCD)

http://www.aucd.org

Represents the professional interests of the national network of 61 university centers for excellence in developmental disabilities education, research, and service (UCEs; formerly called university affiliated programs, or UAPs) that serve people with developmental disabilities.

National Association of Developmental Disabilities Councils

http://www.nacdd.org

Organization of developmental disability councils that exist in each state to provide information on and advocate for resources and services for people with developmental disabilities and their families.

Society for Disability Studies

http://www.uic.edu/orgs/sds

Works to explore issues of disability and chronic illness from scholarly perspectives. Publishes *Disability Studies Quarterly*; holds an annual conference that brings together scholars from a broad spectrum of fields as well as artists and community-based activists.

CHILD DEVELOPMENT AND DIAGNOSIS OF DISABILITIES

Birth Defects

Genetics Home Reference

http://ghr.nlm.nih.gov

Genetics Home Reference provides consumer-friendly information about the effects of genetic variations on human health.

March of Dimes

http://www.marchofdimes.com

Awards grants to institutions and organizations for development of genetic services, perinatal care in high-risk pregnancies, prevention of premature delivery, parent support groups, and other community programs. Campaign for Healthier Babies distributes information about birth defects and related newborn health problems. Spanish-language materials available.

National Society of Genetic Counselors

http://www.nsgc.org

Includes a searchable database of counselors.

Child Development

Ages and Stages: Birth to 12 months

http://www.extension.iastate.edu/Publications/PM1530A.pdf

Web site features a publication from the Iowa State University Extension program that presents information about the physical, mental, emotional, and social development of children between birth and 12 months of age. Provides

ideas and tips for parents to facilitate these milestones.

Child Development Institute

http://www.childdevelopmentinfo.com

Web site for parents on child development, parenting, child psychology, teenagers, health, safety, and learning disabilities.

East Tennessee Children's Hospital: Developmental Milestones

http://www.etch.com/healthdevms.cfm

Web site presents a brief overview of typical and atypical developmental milestones from birth to 15 months. Site also provides links to information about feeding and swallowing, physical therapy and occupational therapy, and language development.

KidsHealth

http://kidshealth.org

Sponsored by the Nemours Foundations Center for Children's Health. Web site offers a wide variety of information pertaining to child health issues. Contains helpful explanations of basic medical terminology and articles and resources for parents and professionals. Available in Spanish.

National Center for Education in Maternal and Child Health

http://www.ncemch.org

Disseminates publications and fact sheets to the public and professionals in the field and develops and maintains database of topics, agencies, and organizations related to maternal and child health.

Pediatric Development and Behavior

http://www.dbpeds.org

Independent web site created to promote better care and outcomes for children and families affected by developmental, learning, and behavioral problems by providing access to clinically relevant information and educational material for medical providers, other service delivery professionals, and parents.

WebMD Health

http://my.webmd.com

Provides a variety of useful information on mainstream health topics. Offers reliable information about identifying symptoms of illness and reports on highlighted topics.

ZERO TO THREE

http://www.zerotothree.org

National, nonprofit organization whose mission is to promote the healthy development of infants and toddlers by supporting and strengthening families, communities, and those who work on their behalf. Web site includes various policies, research reports, and technical assistance resources for parents and professionals.

Environmental Toxicants

American Association on Intellectual and Developmental Disabilities (AAIDD) Environmental Health Initiative
http://www.aaidd.org/ehi/index.cfm
AAIDD's goals are to raise awareness about the complex links between exposure to neurotoxic chemicals and developmental disabilities, and to raise awareness that those living with intellectual disabilities and related developmental disabilities may be at greater risk of secondary health effects from toxic exposures than individuals without disabilities.

National Library of Medicine, Environmental Health and Toxicology Webpages
http://sis.nlm.nih.gov/enviro.html
The NLM has aggregated a large number of resources at a single web portal.

Pediatric Environmental Health Specialty Units (PEHSU)
www.pehsu.net
There are 10 PEHSUs in the United States. Any health professional, parent, school teacher or other person can contact their regional PEHSU for information about children's health and the environment.

Genetics

GeneTests
http://www.ncbi.nlm.nih.gov/sites/GeneTests/
Free medical genetics information resource developed for physicians, other health care providers, researchers, and the public. Provides *GeneReviews*, peer-reviewed articles describing the application of genetic testing to the diagnosis, management, and genetic counseling of patients; international directories for genetic testing laboratories and genetic and prenatal diagnosis clinics; and various educational materials.

Genetic Alliance
http://www.geneticalliance.org
International organization of families, health professionals, and genetic organizations dedicated to enhancing the lives of individuals living with genetic conditions through the provision of education, policy, and information services. Staff is available to address questions about

genetics and to connect callers with support groups and informational resources. An annual conference is held in Washington, D.C.

Genetics Society of America
http://www.genetics-gsa.org
Professional organization that aims to bring together genetic investigators and provide a forum for sharing research findings. Cooperates in the organization of an international congress held every 5 years under the auspices of the International Genetics Federation. Publishes the journal *GENETICS* and other resources.

Online Mendelian Inheritance in Man (OMIM)
http://www.ncbi.nlm.nih.gov/omim
Web site database of human genes and genetic disorders with textual information, pictures, and reference information.

Neurocognitive Assessment

American Psychological Association
http://www.apa.org/topics/testing/index.aspx
Web site addresses major considerations and issues in psychological testing.

National Council on Measurement in Education
http://www.ncme.org
Organization working to advance the science and practice of measurement in education.

The Standards for Educational and Psychological Testing
http://www.apa.org/science/programs/testing/standards.aspx
A key reference for test developers and professionals, developed jointly by the American Educational Research Association (AERA), the American Psychological Association (APA), and the National Council on Measurement in Education (NCME).

Prematurity

BLISS
http://www.bliss.org.uk
Site created by parents for parents that provides information about causes of prematurity and levels of neonatal care.

Emory Pediatrics Developmental Progress Clinic
http://med.emory.edu/PEDIATRICS/NEONATOLOGY/DPC/index.htm
Information regarding medical complications with implications for development focusing on prematurity and other neonatal medical

complications associated with developmental problems, developmental care in the neonatal intensive care unit, neurodevelopmental implications of neonatal trauma, developmental milestones specifically for children born prematurely, information regarding issues beyond infancy, Georgia state resources, frequently asked questions and answers, and web links.

Family Practice Notebook
http://www.fpnotebook.com/NICCH16.htm
Information on the outcomes of infants born prematurely. Also gives neurological outcomes for 24–26 weeks' gestation and links to the references that support these outcomes.

March of Dimes PeriStats Database
http://www.marchofdimes.com/peristats/
PeriStats provides free access to maternal and infant health-related data at the United States, state, county, and city level.

Mayo Clinic: Premature Birth
http://www.mayoclinic.com/health/premature-birth/DS00137
Provides information related to prematurity, such as causes of premature delivery, signs and symptoms during pregnancy, and when to seek medical help. Also includes information on the difficulties a child born prematurely may have, the course of care he or she will receive in the neonatal intensive care unit, and what to expect upon discharge.

Medline Plus: Premature Babies
http://www.nlm.nih.gov/medlineplus/prematurebabies.html
Resource for health care professionals. Sections include drug information, an encyclopedia, a dictionary, news pages, and other resources. Provides links to information (e.g., car-seat safety for premature infants) that can be printed out and shared with parents.

Parents of Premature Babies
http://www.preemie-l.org
Supports families and caregivers of premature infants. Offers a discussion forum and an e-mail list, as well as a unique mentoring program for new parents of premature infants who are matched with parents of an older premature infant.

Premature Babies: Caring for Your Baby
http://familydoctor.org/handouts/283.html
Web site maintained by the American Academy of Family Physicians as an all-encompassing resource to address typical parent concerns. Includes discussions about the special care

needed by premature babies, growth and development, feeding issues, sleep patterns, vision and hearing, immunizations, and travel concerns such as car seat placement.

Premature Babies
Guide at Keep Kids Healthy
http://www.keepkidshealthy.com/newborn/premature_babies.html
General resource for parents. It defines the risk factors for having a premature baby; describes neonates at various gestational ages; defines common medical problems that premature babies often face; and answers common parent questions related to feeding, going home, and possible long-term problems.

Premature Baby–Premature Child
http://prematurity.org
Web site developed by parents of children who were born prematurely and who went on to have developmental issues.

Premature-infant.com
http://premature-infant.com
Web site has touching stories and supportive information for parents, along with insights for medical personnel. Contains resource links to related problems/concerns. Also provides information regarding gastroesophageal reflux disease, infant massage, kangaroo care, positioning, pain, respiratory syncytial virus (RSV), and feeding issues.

The Vermont Oxford
http://www.vtoxford.org
Web site provides information for the institutions that participate in its database. Database tracks the progress of high-risk infants within certain criteria and provides good statistical analysis and research options to those who participate.

DEVELOPMENTAL DISABILITIES AND DISABLING ILLNESSES

Acquired Immunodeficiency Syndrome (AIDS)

Centers for Disease
Control and Prevention (CDC)
National Sexually Transmitted Diseases (STD) and AIDS Hotline (English: 800-342-2437; Spanish: 800-344-7432; TTY: 800-243-7889; http://www.cdc.gov). Weekday hotline that provides confidential information on transmission and prevention of human immunodeficiency

virus (HIV)/AIDS and other STDs, testing, local referrals, and educational materials to the public.

Office of National AIDS Policy
http://www.whitehouse.gov/onap/aids.html
Provides broad direction for federal AIDS policy and fosters interdepartmental communication on HIV and AIDS. Works closely with the AIDS community in the United States and around the world.

Attention-Deficit/
Hyperactivity Disorder (ADHD)

A.D.D. WareHouse
http://www.addwarehouse.com
Mail-order resource for ADHD-related books, games, videotapes, and other materials for clinicians, parents, teachers, adults, and students.

Attention Deficit Disorder Association
http://www.add.org
National organization that provides education, research, and public advocacy. Especially focused on the needs of adults and young adults with ADHD.

CHADD (Children and Adults with Attention-Deficit/Hyperactivity Disorder)
http://www.chadd.org
Support group for parents of children with attention disorders. Provides continuing education for both parents and professionals, serves as a community resource for information, and advocates for appropriate educational programs.

Autism Spectrum Disorders (ASDs)

American Academy of Pediatrics
http://www.aap.org/healthtopics/autism.cfm
Web site provides professional and family/community resources and information about autism spectrum disorders. Includes links for audiotaped interviews of experts for families and professionals about pertinent topics, to the *AAP Toolkit: AUTISM: Caring for Children with Autism Spectrum Disorders Resource Toolkit for Clinicians*, as well as policy statements pertinent to ASDs.

Autism Society of America
http://www.autism-society.org
Provides information about autism, including options, approaches, methods, and systems available to parents and family members of children with autism and the professionals who work with them. Advocates for the rights and needs of individuals with autism and their families.

Autism Speaks
http://www.autismspeaks.org
Dedicated to helping families find answers, through funding research and education efforts and, most significantly, by spearheading the development of a national registry of individuals with autism.

International Rett Syndrome Association
http://www.rettsyndrome.org
Provides information, referral, and support to families and acts as a liaison with professionals.

National Center on Birth Defects and Developmental Disabilities (NCBDDD): Autism Information Center
http://www.cdc.gov/ncbddd/autism/index.htm
Web site has unique feature: link to the Autism Spectrum Disorders Kids' Quest, a series of informative sites provided by the NCBDDD for the purpose of educating children about developmental disabilities. Site also provides information about current research on autism spectrum disorders (ASDs) by the Centers for Disease Control and Prevention (CDC) and other federal agencies. Serves as a link for information regarding various state funding programs for ASDs.

Blindness

American Association for Pediatric Ophthalmology and Strabismus (AAPOS)
http://aapos.org
Provides resources for patients and families regarding frequently asked questions of ocular conditions. Resource for locating a pediatric ophthalmologist in your area.

American Foundation for the Blind (AFB)
http://www.afb.org
Works in cooperation with other agencies, organizations, and schools to offer services to individuals who are blind or who have visual impairments; provides consultation, public education, referrals, and information; produces and distributes talking books; publishes and sells materials for professionals in the blindness field.

American Printing House for the Blind (APH)
http://www.aph.org
Nonprofit publishing house for people with visual impairments. Has books in braille and large type and on audiotape and computer disk, as well as a range of aids, tools, and supplies for education and daily living.

Learning Ally (Previously Recording for the Blind & Dyslexic)

http://www.learningally.org

Produces and distributes textbooks on audiotape, computer disk, and CD-ROM; individuals or institutions who have memberships may borrow these materials. Also provides reference librarian services for individual members.

Lighthouse International (previously National Association for Visually Handicapped)

www.lighthouse.org

Provides informational literature, guidance, and counseling in the use of visual aids, emotional support, and referral services for parents of partially sighted children and for people who work with these children. Publishes free large-print newsletter.

National Braille Association

http://www.nationalbraille.org

Produces and distributes braille reading materials for people with visual impairment. Collection consists of college-level textbooks, materials of general interest, standard technical tables, and music.

National Federation of the Blind

http://www.nfb.org

Strives for complete inclusion of people who are blind into society on the basis of equality. Offers advocacy services for these individuals in such areas as discrimination in housing and insurance. Operates a job referral and listing system for individuals to find competitive employment. Runs an aids and appliances department, a scholarship program for college students, and a loan program for people who are going into business for themselves. Publishes monthly and quarterly publications.

National Library Service for the Blind and Physically Handicapped

http://www.loc.gov/nls

Administers a national library service through a network of participating public libraries to provide braille and recorded books and magazines on free loan to anyone who cannot read standard print because of visual or physical disabilities.

Prevent Blindness America

http://www.preventblindness.org

Committed to the reduction of preventable blindness. Provides information to people who are blind, professionals working with these individuals, and the public.

United States Association of Blind Athletes (USABA)

http://www.usaba.org

Aims to ensure that legally blind individuals have the same opportunities as their sighted peers in recreation and sports programs at all levels, from developmental to elite. Works to change negative stereotypes related to the abilities of individuals who are blind and other people with disabilities. Publishes a newsletter. Web site has links to related sites and event calendars with sport descriptions.

Cerebral Palsy

American Academy for Cerebral Palsy and Developmental Medicine (AACPDM)

http://www.aacpdm.org/

Multidisciplinary scientific society that fosters professional education, research, and interest in the problems associated with cerebral palsy.

Cerebral Palsy, Erbs Palsy, All Types of Cerebral Palsy

http://www.cerebralpalsy.org

Web site provides information about causes, risk factors, and types of cerebral palsy. Includes links and resources about types of help available and how to find help. Also discusses treatment interventions and special education issues.

Cerebral Palsy: Hope Through Research

http://www.ninds.nih.gov/disorders/cerebral_palsy/detail_cerebral_palsy.htm

Web site discusses diagnostic questions related to cerebral palsy. Includes questions related to causes and treatments available. Also provides information about current research projects being conducted concerning cerebral palsy. Available in Spanish.

Cerebral Palsy—Neurology Channel

http://www.neurologychannel.com/cerebral palsy

Web site includes information about cerebral palsy, including types, causes, treatments, risk factors, complications, and prognosis. Also provides information about orthopedic and neurological surgeries for cerebral palsy.

Children's Disabilities and Special Needs

http://www.comeunity.com/disability/cerebral_palsy

Web site contains general articles related to cerebral palsy and articles about research concerning cerebral palsy in children born prematurely. Provides links to books and resources.

CP Resource Center

http://www.cpparent.org
Web site provides general information about cerebral palsy, its causes, and some treatments. Contains a dictionary to help parents understand medical terms they may hear. Also lists books for further reading.

United Cerebral Palsy

http://www.ucp.org
Provides direct services to children and adults with cerebral palsy that include medical diagnosis, evaluation and treatment, special education, career development, counseling, social and recreational programs, and adapted housing.

Deafness and Speech Disorders

ADARA (formerly Professional Workers with the Adult Deaf [PRWAD] and the American Deafness and Rehabilitation Association)

http://www.adara.org
Serves professionals who work with deaf individuals and people interested in learning about deafness. Publishes a journal and newsletter by subscription; offers memberships.

Alexander Graham Bell Association for the Deaf

http://nc.agbell.org
A free membership organization that provides general information and information on resources related to hearing loss. They publish materials and books on these subjects and provide information about scholarships and financial aid for individuals who are deaf and hard of hearing.

American Society for Deaf Children

http://www.deafchildren.org
Provides information and support to parents and families with children who are deaf or hard of hearing.

American Speech-Language-Hearing Association (ASHA)

http://www.asha.org
Professional and scientific organization and certifying body for professionals providing speech-language and hearing services. Conducts research in communication disorders, publishes several journals, and provides consumer information and professional referral.

Apraxia—KIDS

http://www.apraxia-kids.org
Web site maintained by Childhood Apraxia of Speech Association of North America (CASANA). Provides comprehensive information and resources, including a free online newsletter, related to diagnosis and treatment, educational programs, and the medical and insurance aspects of childhood apraxia. Spanish-language materials are available.

Augmentative and Alternative Communication–Rehabilitative Engineering Research Center (AAC-RERC)

http://aac-rerc.psu.edu/
Collaborative research programs that develop and disseminate information and activities that seek to advance and promote augmentative and alternative communication (AAC) technologies for individuals with disabilities who use them, as well as for professionals who manufacture, recommend, and distribute them.

Boys Town National Research Hospital

http://www.boystownhospital.org/home.asp; http://www.babyhearing.org/
Two web sites that provide a variety of resources relating to children with hearing, language, and learning disabilities and the research currently underway at Boys Town National Research Hospital. The site titled "Baby Hearing" is offered in a Spanish-language version.

Centers for Disease Control and Prevention

http://www.cdc.gov/hearingloss
Web site provides comprehensive information about hearing loss. It is sponsored by the National Center on Birth Defects and Developmental Disabilities of the U.S. federal government's Centers for Disease Control and Prevention. This web site and its Hearing Loss Team provides free brochures, fact sheets, and other educational materials.

Collaborative Early Intervention National Training e-Resource

http://center.uncg.edu
Target audience for web site is professionals who serve families with infants and toddlers who are deaf or hard of hearing. Provides graduate-level, web-based training for service providers. Site also offers an extensive list of resources for professionals and families.

Deafness Research Foundation

http://www.drf.org
Solicits funds for the support of research into the causes, treatment, and prevention of deafness and other hearing disorders.

Described and Captioned Media Program
http://www.dcmp.org/
Government-sponsored distribution of open-captioned materials to eligible institutions, individuals, and families. Program promotes and provides equal access to communication and learning for students who are blind, visually impaired, deaf, hard of hearing, or deaf-blind.

Hands and Voices
http://www.handsandvoices.org
A nationwide nonprofit organization that is a parent-driven, parent/professional collaborative group dedicated to supporting families and their children who are deaf or hard of hearing, as well as the professionals who serve them. Web site offers a wealth of information and resources related to hearing loss, technology, communication and educational methodologies, and advocacy.

Hearing Loss
Association of America (HLAA)
http://www.shhh.org
Educational organization that provides assistance to individuals who are deaf or hard of hearing to participate fully in society. Publishes a journal, newsletter, and other materials; provides advocacy and outreach programs and an extensive network of local chapters and self-help groups; and hosts an annual convention.

Helen Keller National Center
for Deaf-Blind Youths and Adults
http://www.hknc.org/
The center offers a residential training facility for deaf-blind individuals and has representatives in 10 regional offices across the nation who can assist with information, training, and support. Also maintains a national registry of people who are deaf-blind.

International Hearing Society
http://ihsinfo.org/IhsV2/Home/Index.cfm
Provides information on how to proceed when hearing loss is suspected. Also offers free consumer kit, facts about hearing aids, and a variety of literature on hearing-related subjects.

Laurent Clerc National
Deaf Education Center
http://clerccenter.gallaudet.edu/infotogo
Web site provides a comprehensive resource related to the educational, linguistic, social, and emotional development of deaf or hard of hearing children. Information is included about assistive devices and hearing aids, learning sign language or speech reading, and classroom issues related to education of children with deafness.

National Center for Stuttering
http://www.stuttering.com/homepag.htm
Provides free information for parents of young children just starting to show symptoms of stuttering; runs training programs in current therapeutic approaches for speech-language professionals; provides treatment for people older than 7 years of age who stutter.

National Consortium on Deaf-Blindness
http://www.nationaldb.org/
A national technical assistance and dissemination center for children and youth who are deaf-blind. Web site provides information about deaf-blindness, disability, education and technical assistance, technology, and medical and health resources.

National Institute on
Deafness and Other Communication
Disorders/National Institutes of Health
http://www.nidcd.nih.gov/
A web site, sponsored by the U.S. federal government, that provides health information about all hearing-related topics including ear infections, deafness and hearing aids, as well as balance, smell, taste, voice, and speech and language disorders. The institute offers free publications, information about clinical trial participation, and links to organizations related to deafness and communication disorders.

Speech and Language
Development in Young Children
http://members.tripod.com/Caroline_Bowen/devel1.htm
Web site presents information about the acquisition of language in early childhood. Provides information about how language is learned and the role of the parent in facilitating these skills. Language and communication milestones are presented along with a section on when to seek professional help.

Speech Therapy Activities
http://www.speechtx.com
Web site provides free, printable speech-language activities for speech-language pathologists and parents.

Down Syndrome

The Association for
Children with Down Syndrome
http://www.acds.org
Offers information and referral services, including a free list of publications.

Down Syndrome: Health Issues

http://www.ds-health.com

For parents and professionals. Web site includes articles concerning specific health issues related to Down syndrome, such as gastroesophageal reflux, blood disorders, and thyroid function. Information also provided about health guidelines and controversies in the care of children and adults with Down syndrome.

National Down
Syndrome Congress (NDSC)

http://ndsccenter.org

Provides information, advocacy, and support. Has annual convention for families in the summer and publishes a newsletter, *Down Syndrome News*.

National Down Syndrome Society (NDSS)

http://www.ndss.org

National advocate for the values, acceptance, and inclusion of people with Down syndrome. Works with affiliate groups to advance research, increase public awareness, and improve education opportunities.

Epilepsy

American Epilepsy Society

http://www.aesnet.org

Promotes research and education for professionals dedicated to the prevention, treatment, and cure of epilepsy.

Epilepsy Foundation

http://www.efa.org

Provides programs of information and education, advocacy, support of research, and the delivery of needed services to people with epilepsy and their families.

International League Against Epilepsy

http://www.ilae-epilepsy.org

Global nonprofit organization that disseminates knowledge about epilepsy and fosters research, education, training, and improved services and care. Has official working relationship with the World Health Organization.

Fetal Alcohol Spectrum Disorder

Family Empowerment Network (FEN)

http://www.fammed.wisc.edu/fen

National nonprofit organization that exists to empower families affected by fetal alcohol syndrome and other drug-related birth defects, through education and support; also publishes a newsletter, *The FEN Pen*.

National Organization on
Fetal Alcohol Syndrome (NOFAS)

http://www.nofas.org

Nonprofit organization founded in 1990; dedicated to eliminating birth defects caused by alcohol consumption during pregnancy and to improving the quality of life for those individuals and families affected.

PREVLINE: Prevention
Online (National Clearinghouse
for Alcohol and Drug Information)

http://ncadi.samhsa.gov

The world's largest resource for current information and materials concerning substance abuse. Distributes brochures, offers resources for parents and teachers on prevention, and has English- and Spanish-speaking information service staff available to answer questions.

Genetic Syndromes and
Inborn Errors of Metabolism

There are many support organizations and networks for children with various syndromes and inborn errors of metabolism and their families. Resources for more common syndromes (e.g., Down syndrome) appear in their own sections in this appendix, but a representative sample of others is listed here. For a more complete listing, contact the National Organization for Rare Disorders (NORD [see later listing]).

5p Minus Society

http://www.fivepminus.org

Family support and information group for parents, grandparents, and guardians of individuals with 5p- (cri-du-chat) syndrome. Publishes a newsletter and sponsors an annual meeting.

Angelman Syndrome Foundation, Inc.

http://www.angelman.org

Organization that sponsors research, and provides information to families and providers. Sponsors a biennial conference and has a mentorship program for newly diagnosed families.

The American Society of Human Genetics

http://www.ashg.org

Professional organization for human genetics specialists. Publishes *The American Journal of Human Genetics* and other resources.

Arthrogryposis Multiplex
Congenita Support, Inc.

http://www.amcsupport.org

Group that aims to provide more information and support for families of children with arthrogryposis multiplex congenital. Provides resources for physical therapists and other providers to families.

Association for Glycogen Storage Disease
http://www.agsdus.org
Association that aims to create public awareness, provide family support, and stimulate research. A quarterly newsletter, *The Ray*, is published, and a conference is held annually.

Avenues
http://www.avenuesforamc.com
Publishes a semiannual newsletter that provides lists of parents, physicians, and experienced medical centers concerned with people with arthrogryposis multiplex congenita.

Children's Craniofacial Association
http://www.ccakids.com
Supports families and children with craniofacial patients, encourages public awareness and education, and publishes a quarterly newsletter, and educational brooklets.

Children's Tumor Foundation: Ending Neurofibromatosis through Research
http://www.ctf.org
Foundation dedicated to improving the health and well-being of individuals and families affected by neurofibromatosis by supporting research, providing information for families, assisting in developmental clinical centers and expanding public awareness.

Cornelia de Lange Syndrome Foundation
http://www.cdlsusa.org
Supports parents and children affected by de Lange syndrome, encourages research, and disseminates information to increase public awareness through a newsletter and informational pamphlet.

Ehlers Danlos National Foundation
http://www.ednf.org
Funds research and provides information and support to families and medical providers. Sponsors annual conference.

FRAXA Research Foundation
http://www.fraxa.org
Supports scientific research aimed at finding a treatment and a cure for fragile X syndrome. Funds grants and fellowships at universities worldwide. Runs an e-mail list on which individuals may post strategies and questions. Publishes *FRAXA Newsletter*, *Medication Guide for Fragile X Syndrome* (by Michael Tranfaglia) and *Fragile X A to Z: A Guide for Families* (edited by Wendy Dillworth; downloadable from the web site free of charge).

Little People of America, Inc.
http://www.lpaonline.org
Nationwide organization dedicated to helping people of short stature. Provides fellowship, moral support, and information to people who are shorter than typical, or individuals with dwarfism. The toll-free helpline provides information on organizations, products and services, and doctors in the caller's area.

The National Fragile X Foundation
http://www.FragileX.org
Provides information, medical and genetic referrals, sponsors research grants, and provides educational resources.

National Gaucher Foundation
http://www.gaucherdisease.org
Publishes quarterly newsletter, operates support groups and chapters, provides referrals to organizations for appropriate services, and funds research on Gaucher disease.

National MPS Society
http://www.mpssociety.org
Raises money to provide student fellowships and fund research for mucopolysacchoride disorder, collaborates with other lysosomal storage diseases, patient support groups, supports families by providing resource guides, publish a newsletter, *Courage*, and hold a yearly conference.

The National Organization for Rare Disorders (NORD)
http://www.rarediseases.org
A nonprofit patient advocacy organization dedicated to orphan diseases (disorders occurring in fewer than 200,000 individuals in the United States). NORD provides information about diseases, referrals to patient organizations, research grants and fellowships, advocacy for the rare-disease community, and medication assistance programs.

National PKU Alliance
http://www.npkua.org
Raises money to fund research, supports local phenylketonuria (PKU) organizations, educates communities about issues faced by individuals and families affected with PKU.

National Tay-Sachs and Allied Diseases Association
http://www.NTSAD.org
Promotes genetic screening programs nationally, has updated listing of Tay-Sachs disease–prevention centers in a number of countries, provides educational literature to general public and professionals, and coordinates peer group support for parents.

National Urea Cycle Disorders Foundation
http://www.nucdf.org
Provides information and support for families. Supports and stimulates medical research and increased awareness by the public and the legislators of issues related to urea cycle disorders.

Organic Acidemia Association
http://www.oaanews.org
A volunteer nonprofit organization whose mission is to empower families and health care professionals with knowledge in organic acidemia metabolic disorders.

Osteogenesis Imperfecta Foundation
http://www.oif.org
Supports research on osteogenesis imperfecta and provides information to those with this disorder, to their families, and to other interested people.

Prader-Willi Syndrome Association
http://www.pwsausa.org
National organization that provides information education and support services on Prader-Willi syndrome to parents, professionals, and other interested people. Provides research funding, bimonthly newsletter, and an annual national conference for families and professionals.

Rare Diseases Clinical Research Network
http://rarediseasesnetwork.epi.usf.edu
National network made up of 19 distinctive consortia that are working together to improve availability of rare disease information, treatment, clinical studies, and general awareness for both patients and the medical community. The RDCRN also aims to provide up-to-date information for patients and to assist in connecting patients with advocacy groups, expert doctors, and clinical research opportunities.

**Support Organization for Trisomy
18, 13, and Related Disorders (SOFT)**
http://www.trisomy.org
Chapters in most states provide support and family packages with a newsletter and appropriate literature underscoring the common problems for children with trisomy 13 or trisomy 18 during pregnancy, life and after passing. Holds a yearly conference for families and professionals.

Tourette Syndrome Association
http://www.tsa-usa.org
Offers information, referral, advocacy, education, research, and self-help groups for those affected by Tourette syndrome.

Tuberous Sclerosis Alliance
http://www.tsalliance.org
Offers public information about manifestations of the disease to newly diagnosed individuals, their families, and interested professionals. Referrals are made to support groups located in most states. Funds research through membership fees and donations.

United Leukodystrophy Foundation
http://www.ulf.org
Maintains 24-hour hotline to provide family support, provides educational resources, supports research, puts out a quarterly newsletter, and runs an annual conference.

**The United Mitochondrial
Disease Foundation**
http://www.umdf.org
Promotes research and education for the diagnosis, treatment, and cure of mitochondrial disorders and provides support to affected individuals and families.

Intellectual Disability

**American Association on Intellectual
and Developmental Disabilities (AAIDD)**
http://www.aaidd.org
Professional organization that promotes cooperation among those involved in services, training, and research in intellectual disabilities. Encourages research, dissemination of information, development of appropriate community-based services, and the promotion of preventive measures designed to further reduce the incidence of intellectual disability.

The Arc of the United States
http://thearc.org
National advocacy organization working on behalf of individuals with intellectual disabilities and their families; has more than 1,000 state and local chapters.

**President's Committee for People
with Intellectual Disabilities (PCPID)**
http://www.acf.hhs.gov/programs/pcpid/index.html
Advises the President and the Secretary of Health and Human Services on all matters pertaining to intellectual disabilities; publishes annual reports and information on the rights of people with intellectual disabilities.

Learning Disorders

Dyslexia Research Institute
http://www.dyslexia-add.org
Provides training, workshops, and seminars for professionals.

International Dyslexia Association (IDA)
http://www.interdys.org
Devoted to the study and treatment of dyslexia; provides information and referrals; sponsors conferences, seminars, and support groups; and has two regular publications and more than 40 branches in the United States and abroad.

LD Online
http://www.ldonline.org
Resources on learning disabilities for parents, students, teachers, and other professionals. Interactive web site provides basic information on learning disabilities and the latest research and news; also offers e-mail consultation by experts on learning disabilities, resource lists, personal stories, bulletin boards, and materials/resources for purchase.

Learning Disabilities Association of America (LDA)
http://www.ldanatl.org
Encourages research and the development of early detection programs, disseminates information, serves as an advocate, and works to improve education for individuals with learning disabilities.

National Center for Learning Disabilities (NCLD)
http://www.ld.org
Promotes public awareness of learning disabilities and provides computerized information and referral services to consumers and professionals on learning disabilities. Publishes *Their World*, an annual magazine for parents and professionals.

Schwablearning.org
http://www.schwablearning.org
An online parent's guide to helping children with learning disabilities and attention-deficit/hyperactivity disorder (ADHD), including information on identifying disabilities and on managing home, school, and learning. Site also has resources and publications for families.

Neural Tube Defects

Spina Bifida Association of America
http://www.sbaa.org
Provides information and referral for new parents and literature on spina bifida; supports a public awareness program; advocates for individuals with spina bifida and their families; supports research; and conducts conferences for parents and professionals.

Neuromuscular and Musculoskeletal Disorders

Cure CMD
http://curecmd.org/
Support group for families affected by congenital muscular dystrophy, also provides research funding.

Families of SMA
http://www.fsma.org/
Support group for families affected by spinal muscular atrophy.

Guillain-Barré Syndrome Foundation International
http://www.gbsfi.com
Provides emotional support to individuals with Guillain-Barré syndrome and their families; fosters research; educates the public about the disorder; develops nationwide support groups; and directs people with this syndrome to resources, meetings, newsletters, and symposia.

Harvard Neuromuscular Disease Project
http://www.childrenshospital.org/cfapps/research/data_admin/Site2549/mainpageS2549P0.html
Conducts research in the genetics of neuromuscular diseases, especially muscular dystrophy.

Manton Center for Orphan Disease Research
http://www.childrenshospital.org/cfapps/research/data_admin/Site2673/mainpageS2673P0.html
Research center devoted to the study of rare diseases, including inherited neuromuscular conditions.

Muscular Dystrophy Association
http://www.mdausa.org
Health care agency that fosters research and provides direct services to individuals with muscular dystrophy; is concerned with conquering muscular dystrophy and other neuromuscular diseases.

Myasthenia Gravis Foundation of America
http://www.myasthenia.org/
Support group for myasthenia gravis.

National Scoliosis Foundation
http://www.scoliosis.org
Nonprofit organization with state chapters; dedicated to informing the public about scoliosis and promoting early detection and treatment of scoliosis. Publishes *Spinal Connection Newsletter*.

Scoliosis Research Society
http://www.srs.org
Sponsors and promotes research on the etiology
and treatment of scoliosis and spinal disorders.

**Spinal Muscular Atrophy
Foundation (SMA Foundation)**
http://www.smafoundation.org/
Provides support for research into potential
therapies for SMA.

Traumatic Brain Injury (TBI)

Brain Injury Association of America
http://www.biausa.org
Provides information to educate the public, poli-
ticians, businesses, and educators about brain
injury, including effects, causes, and prevention.

Traumatic Brain Injury Resource Guide
http://www.neuroskills.com
Web site includes educational information,
books, local support groups, and research.

INTERVENTIONS, SERVICES, AND OUTCOMES

Assistive Technology

ABLEDATA
http://www.abledata.com
National database of information on assistive
technology and rehabilitation equipment.

Alliance for Technology Access
http://www.ataccess.org
A resource and demonstration center open
to people with disabilities, their families, and
professionals and others interested in adaptive
technology.

**Assistive Technology Outcomes
Measurement System (ATOMS)**
http://www.atoms.uwm.edu
A center which has done research and developed publications on outcomes of the use of
assistive technology.

**Center for Applied Special Technology
(CAST)**
http://www.cast.org
CAST is a nonprofit research and development organization that works to expand learning opportunities for all individuals, especially
those with disabilities, through Universal
Design for Learning.

Independent Living Aids
http://www.independentliving.com
Sells aids that make daily tasks easier for those
with physical disabilities; also carries clocks,
calculators, magnifying lamps, and easy-to-see
low-vision and talking watches for individuals
with visual impairments.

Michigan's Assistive Technology Resource
http://www.copower.org/At/atlinks.htm
Provides free information on low-tech devices
and equipment available for individuals with
disabilities.

**National Center for
Technology Innovation (NCTI)**
http://www.nationaltechcenter.org
NCTI assists researchers, developers, and
entrepreneurs in creating innovative learning
tools for all students, with special focus on students with disabilities.

**Rehabilitation Engineering
and Assistive Technology
Society of North America (RESNA)**
http://www.resna.org
Multidisciplinary organization of professionals
interested in the identification, development,
and delivery of technology to people with disabilities. Offers numerous publications.

Behavior and Mental Health

**American Academy of Child
and Adolescent Psychiatry (AACAP)**
http://www.aacap.org
National nonprofit organization comprised
of child and adolescent psychiatrists. Provides information for professionals and families to aid in the understanding and treatment
of childhood and adolescent developmental,
behavioral, and mental health disorders. Parent
and caregiver fact sheets and information on
research, practice, and membership are available on the web site.

American Psychiatric Association (APA)
http://www.psych.org
International organization for physicians, dedicated to the diagnosis and treatment of mental
health and substance-use disorders.

American Psychological Association (APA)
http://www.apa.org
National scientific and professional organization that develops and promotes standards in
psychological practice, research, and education.
Dedicated to the dissemination of psychological knowledge to professionals, students, and
the general public through meetings, reports,
and publications.

Association for Behavior Analysis International (ABA International)
http://www.abainternational.org
International organization that promotes the experimental, theoretical, and applied analysis of behavior. Disseminates professional and public information. Also publishes two scholarly journals, *The Behavior Analyst* and *The Analysis of Verbal Behavior*.

Behaviour Change Consultancy
http://www.behaviourchange.com
Provides advice, support, project management, policy development, and training to schools, local educational authorities, and parents on the subjects of disaffection. Also gives advice on social, emotional, and behavioral difficulties, as well as behavior management.

Bright Futures at Georgetown University
http://www.brightfutures.org/mentalhealth
Web site explains the Bright Futures materials that help providers operationalize the guidelines for mental health promotion in children. Site also contains materials to download, including a mental health fact sheet, a listing of supporting organizations, and training tools.

Head Start/Administration on Children and Families
http://www.headstartinfo.org
Web site contains a wealth of information on the Head Start and Early Head Start programs. A special feature is The Mental Health Toolkit, an annotated bibliography of a variety of articles, books, and federal programs, services, and publications.

Journal of Applied Behavior Analysis
http://seab.envmed.rochester.edu/jaba
Psychology journal that publishes research about applications of the experimental analysis of behavior to social problems. Published by The Society for the Experimental Analysis of Behavior.

Research and Training Center (RTC) on Family Support and Children's Mental Health
http://www.rtc.pdx.edu
This federally funded RTC is dedicated to promoting effective community-based, culturally competent, family-centered services for families and their children who are or may be affected by mental health, emotional, or behavioral disorders.

Early Intervention

Child and Family Studies Research Programs
http://jeffline.tju.edu/cfsrp/
Conducts research and offers resources and training for professionals working with infants, toddlers, and young children with disabilities and their families.

Child Development Web
http://www.childdevelopmentweb.com/Information/EIprograms.asp
Web site offers information on early intervention for parents and families of children who might be eligible for services. Early Intervention Programs section is part of the Information Link on The Child Development web's home page. Site contains information on obtaining services in the United States, an explanation of early intervention programs and processes, and a breakdown of the services that are available through early intervention. Provides contact information for early intervention in each state.

Contemporary Practices in Early Intervention
http://www.teachingei.org
A distance-learning program to train early interventionists to provide evidence-based, culturally competent, family-centered early childhood practices to infants, toddlers, and young children with disabilities and their families.

Early Childhood Outcomes Center
http://www.fpg.unc.edu/~eco
Offers information and resources for state and local early childhood administrators, technical assistance providers, teachers, other direct service providers, and families.

Kid Source
http://www.kidsource.com
Web site defines early intervention and provides support for intervening as early as a disability or developmental difficulty has been identified. Site also contains a basic, although limited, reference list.

The National Early Childhood Technical Assistance Center (NECTAC)
http://www.nectac.org/
Offers tools and information on a vast range of topics for early childhood professionals.

National Scientific Council on the Developing Child at Harvard University

http://www.developingchild.net

Presents scientific research on early childhood and early brain development to guide public policy.

Education

American Educational Research Association (AERA)

http://www.aera.net

International professional organization with the goal of advancing educational research and its practical education. Members are educators, counselors, evaluators, graduate students, behavioral scientists, and directors or administrators of research, testing, or evaluation.

Association on Higher Education and Disability (AHEAD)

http://www.ahead.org

Professional organization committed to full participation in higher education for people with disabilities.

Association for Supervision and Curriculum Development (ASCD)

http://www.ascd.org

Professional membership organization for educators with interest in instruction, curriculum, and supervision. Publishes the journal *Educational Leadership*.

Building the Legacy: IDEA 2004—Part C

http://idea.ed.gov and http://idea.ed.gov/explore/view/p/,root,statute,I,C

Comprehensive information about IDEA 2004 Part C, which funds and regulates early intervention services for infants and toddlers with disabilities and their families.

Council for Exceptional Children (CEC)

http://www.cec.sped.org

Provides information to teachers, administrators, and others concerned with the education of gifted children and children with disabilities. Maintains a library and database (ERIC Clearinghouse on Disabilities and Gifted Education; http://www.ericec.org) on research in special and gifted education; provides information and assistance on legislation. Publishes the journals *Exceptional Children* and *Teaching Exceptional Children*.

Federal Resource Center for Special Education (FRC)

http://www.rrfcnetwork.org

Supports a nationwide technical assistance network to respond to the needs of students with disabilities, especially those from underrepresented populations. Web site provides information and links from a variety of federally funded projects.

National Association of Private Special Education Centers (NAPSEC) (formerly National Association of Private Schools for Exceptional Children)

http://www.napsec.org

A nonprofit association that represents more than 200 schools nationally and more than 600 at the state level through its Council of Affiliated State Associations. Provides special education and therapeutic services for children in public or private educational placements. Also provides a free referral service to parents and professionals seeking appropriate placement for children with disabilities and publishes a directory of member schools.

National Dissemination Center for Children with Disabilities

http://nichcy.org/laws/idea/legacy

This web site presents a training curriculum on IDEA 2004, the federal law governing special education and early intervention for children with disabilities.

National Information Center for Educational Media (NICEM)

http://www.nicem.com

Provides database of educational audiovisual materials, including videotapes, motion pictures, filmstrips, audiotapes, and slides.

Tots 'n Tech Research Institute

http://tnt.asu.edu/

Provides information on assistive technology and other adaptation options for infants and toddlers.

What Works Clearinghouse (WWC)

http://ies.ed.gov/ncee/wwc

The WWC was established in 2002 by the Institute of Education Sciences at the U.S. Department of Education to provide educators, policymakers, researchers, and the public with a central and trusted source of scientific evidence about "what works" in education.

Family and Sibling Supports

Beach Center on Disability

http://www.beachcenter.org

Research and training center that disseminates information about families with members who have developmental disabilities. Publishes a newsletter, and offers many other publications.

Bureau of Primary Health Care
http://bphc.hrsa.gov/quality/Cultural.htm
Web site uses a variety of stories to illustrate values and principles one needs to appreciate and understand when providing culturally competent care to individuals with disabilities or special health care needs.

The Center for Universal Design
http://www.ncsu.edu/project/design-projects/udi/
Provides publications and information to parents and professionals concerning accessible housing design and financing issues; makes referrals to local organizations.

Center on Human Policy
http://thechp.syr.edu/
Involved in a range of local, state, national, and international activities, including policy studies, research, information, and referral.

Children's Disabilities Information
http://www.childrensdisabilities.info/prematurity/followup.html
Support site for parents that contains articles, lists of books, and web links on premature infants and prematurity. Has several links for parents of children with disabilities, including parenting children with special needs, articles on several disorders, and support network links. Contains general information that is written in easily understandable terms.

The Compassionate Friends
http://www.compassionatefriends.org
National and worldwide organization that supports and aids parents in the positive resolution of the grief experienced upon the death of a child; fosters the physical and emotional health of bereaved parents and siblings.

Easter Seals
http://www.easter-seals.org
Nonprofit, community-based health agency dedicated to increasing the independence of people with disabilities, especially those with autism. Offers a range of quality services, research, and programs.

Exceptional Parent
http://www.eparent.com
Magazine published since 1971 that provides straightforward, practical information for families and professionals involved in the care of children and young adults with disabilities; many articles are written by parents.

Family Village: A Global Community of Disability-Related Resources
http://www.familyvillage.wisc.edu
Global community that integrates information, resources, and communication opportunities on the Internet for people with cognitive and other disabilities, for their families, and for people who provide services and support to these individuals.

Family Voices
http://www.familyvoices.org
Web site for a national, grassroots clearinghouse for information and education concerning the health care of children with special health needs. Contains links to all state chapters and the various projects the organization conducts.

Federation for Children with Special Needs
http://www.fcsn.org
Offers parent-to-parent training and information; projects include Technical Assistance for Parent Programs (TAPP), Collaboration Among Parents and Health Professionals (CAPP), and Parents Engaged in Educational Reform (PEER). Part of the National Early Childhood Technical Assistance System (NEC*TAS) consortium.

National Organization on Disability
http://www.nod.org
Promotes the acceptance and understanding of the needs of citizens with disabilities, through a national network of communities and organizations; facilitates exchange of information regarding resources available to people with disabilities.

PACER Center (Parent Advocacy Coalition for Educational Rights)
http://www.pacer.org
Provides education and training to help parents understand special education laws and to obtain appropriate school programs for their children. Workshops and program topics include early intervention, emotional disabilities, and health/medical services. Also provides a disability-awareness puppet program for schools, child abuse—prevention program services, newsletters, booklets, extensive written materials, and videotapes.

Parent Educational Advocacy Training Center (PEATC)
http://www.peatc.org
Professionally staffed organization that helps parents to become effective advocates for their

children with school personnel and the educational system.

Parent to Parent

http://www.p2pusa.org

State and local chapters provide one-to-one, parent-to-parent support by matching trained parents with newly referred parents on the basis of their children's disabilities and/or family issues they are encountering or have encountered.

The Sibling Support Project

http://www.siblingsupport.org

National program dedicated to the interests of brothers and sisters of people with special health and developmental needs. Primary goal is to increase the availability of peer support and education programs for such siblings.

Special Child

http://www.specialchild.com

Sponsored by the Resource Foundation for Children with Challenges (RFCC). Web site provides parent testimonials, diagnosis-related information, parent support, and a wide variety of information regarding educational and early intervention services.

TASH

http://www.tash.org

Advocates inclusive education and community opportunities for people with disabilities, disseminates research findings and practical applications for education and community living, and encourages sharing of experience and expertise. Publishes a newsletter and a journal.

Team Advocates for Special Kids (TASK)

http://www.taskca.org

Offers training, education, support, information, resources, and community awareness programs to families of children with disabilities and the professionals who serve them. Conducts an advocacy training course and other workshops, and publishes a bimonthly newsletter. TASK's Tech Center (a member of the Alliance for Technology Access) conducts one-to-one guided exploration of technology to determine appropriate adapted hardware and software for people with disabilities.

Tools for Coping with Life's Stressors

http://www.coping.org

Web site contains many links to help parents in coping with issues related to raising a child with special health care needs, such as tools for communication and tools for a balanced lifestyle. Also provides information about early identification and intervention.

Feeding, Growth, and Nutrition

American Dietetic Association

http://www.eatright.org

World's largest association of food and nutrition professionals. Web site offers healthy lifestyle and nutrition tips and referrals to registered dieticians. Publishes the *Journal of the American Dietetic Association*.

ComeUnity's Resources for Feeding and Growth of Children

http://www.comeunity.com/premature/child/growth/resources.html

Web site contains links to recommended parent discussion lists, articles, and hospitals/institutions that offer feeding therapy.

Dysphagia Resource Center

http://www.dysphagia.com

Web site contains links to resources on swallowing and swallowing disorders.

Food and Drug Administration (FDA)

http://www.fda.gov

Part of the U.S. Department of Health and Human Services. Provides the latest federal warnings and updates about foods, drugs, medical devices, vaccines, animal feed, cosmetics, and radiation-emitting products. Has links for children, consumers, patients, and health care professionals.

Formula Manufacturers

The following web sites contain information about special formulas required by some infants and children with developmental disabilities:

- http://www.meadjohnson.com
  (Enfamil Premium Infant, Pregestimil, metabolic formulas)

- http://www.abbottnutrition.com
  (Similac Advance, Similac Soy Isomil, metabolic formulas)

- http://www.shsna.com
  (metabolic, ketogenic, and hypoallergenic formulas)

- http://www.gerber.com
  (Gerber Good Start)

New Visions

http://www.new-vis.com

Provides education and therapy services to professionals and parents working with children with feeding, swallowing, oral-motor, and pre-speech problems. Mealtimes catalog offers therapy materials, tapes, and books.

Health Care

AAP Medical Home Information
http://www.medicalhomeinfo.org/how/care_delivery/
This site features several tools and protocols that can assist with coordination of care for children with chronic conditions.

Guide to the Health Care Reform and Affordable Care Act
http://www.whitehouse.gov/healthreform/healthcare-overview#healthcare-menu
White House guide to Health Care Reform and the Affordable Care Act of 2010.

Institute for Child Health Policy
http://www.ichp.edu
Mission is to research, evaluate, formulate, and advance health policies, programs, and systems that promote the health and well-being of children and youth through applied knowledge to health-related–systems and outcomes for children and youth.

Maternal and Child Health Bureau/CDC National Survey of CYSHCN (2005–2006)
http://nschdata.org/viewdocument.aspx?item=256
http://mchb.hrsa.gov/cshcn05/NF/intro.htm
These sites offer searchable statistics on child and adolescent health in the United States.

State-level Data from the National Survey of CYSHCN 2005–2006
http://cshcndata.org/Content/Default.aspx
Allows searching of state-level data about child and adolescent health.

Supporting the Health Care Transition from Adolescence to Adulthood in the Medical Home
http://aappolicy.aappublications.org/cgi/content/abstract/pediatrics;128/1/182?rss=1
Publication jointly authored by the AAP, the American Academy of Family Physicians, and the American College of Physicians, published in July 2011, that provides an overview of the role and components of transition with an algorithm for providers.

20th Anniversary of Americans with Disabilities Act
http://www.census.gov/newsroom/releases/archives/facts_for_features_special_editions/cb10-ff13.html
This is a link provided by the U.S. Census Bureau detailing the American with Disabilities Act.

Legal Issues

Administration for Children and Families (ACF)
http://www.acf.dhhs.gov
Web site is from the federal agency that provides assistance to the various entities that provide family assistance, child support, child care, Head Start, child welfare, and other programs related to helping families and children.

American Bar Association Center on Children and the Law
http://www.abanet.org/child
Offers information and advocacy to professionals and parents of children and adolescents with disabilities.

American Civil Liberties Union (ACLU)
http://www.aclu.org
Nonprofit organization that is the largest public-interest law firm in the United States. Offers links to disability rights topics.

Center for the Child Care Workforce
http://www.ccw.org
Web site is maintained by a division of the American Federation of Teachers Educational Foundation that was set up to support the education of children, advocacy of early child care and education, and compensation of professionals who work with children. Site provides many resources available for teachers about educating children and a newsletter to help professionals keep current on issues of interest.

Disabilities Rights Education and Defense Fund (DREDF)
http://www.dredf.org
Law and policy center to protect the rights of people with disabilities. Offers referral and information regarding the rights of people with disabilities. Educates legislators and policy makers about issues affecting the rights of people with disabilities; also educates the public about the Americans with Disabilities Act (ADA) of 1990 (PL 101-336).

Do2Learn
http://www.do2learn.com
Web site discusses the legal rights of children with special health care needs and their parents in regard to creating the individual family service plan (IFSP). Includes parent-friendly links to sites that provide information about amendments to the Individuals with Disabilities Education Act (IDEA) and other legal concerns.

Early Child Development

http://www.worldbank.org/children

Web site is a knowledge source designed to assist policy makers, program managers, and practitioners in their efforts to promote the healthy growth and integral development of young children. Site is in Spanish, Portuguese, French, and Arabic.

Illinois Department of Human Services

http://www.dhs.state.il.us/ei

Web site provides a library of information services to parents, providers, educators, policy makers, students, and others interested in early intervention issues. Resource library contains books, periodicals, audiovisual, and other reference materials that can be issued for use on loan. Information is for multiple audiences, but the site also offers *Early Intervention*, a quarterly newsletter directed specifically toward parents.

Indiana First Steps Early Intervention

http://www.infirststeps.com/matrix/default.asp

Target audience includes therapists, parents, service coordinators, and other service providers for children from birth to age 3. Provides information pertaining to therapists; mainly on administrative issues, enrollment, reimbursement, and training. Parent information available for choosing a provider; also provides other early childhood links.

National Association of Protection and Advocacy Systems (NAPAS)

http://www.icdri.org/legal/natpai.htm

Web site provides links to protection and advocacy agencies, located across the United States, mandated by federal law to serve and protect the rights of people with disabilities.

National Early Childhood Technical Assistance Center

http://www.nectac.org

Program that provides responsive technical assistance to the programs supported under the Individuals with Disabilities Education Act (IDEA) for infants and toddlers with disabilities (Part C of IDEA) and for preschoolers with disabilities (Section 619-Part B of IDEA) in all states and participating jurisdictions, as well as to the projects funded by the Office of Special Education Programs under the Early Education Program for Children with Disabilities. Offers informational links to IDEA, publications, and other resources.

Office of Special Education Programs (OSEP)

http://www.ed.gov/about/offices/list/osers/osep/index.html

Web site is from the division of the Department of Education that oversees IDEA. Provides information regarding IDEA and other special education initiatives.

Parents Helping Parents (PHP)

http://www.php.com

Web site is sponsored by a California-based not-for-profit organization for parents of children with disabilities. An international consulting organization for family resources. Site provides valuable information for parents regarding laws concerning the rights of children with disability, and health care issues. Provides regional and state-specific information about support groups for parents and siblings, as well as information on topics such as special education, IDEA, the No Child Left Behind Act of 2001 (PL 107-110), and other special education initiatives.

Medications

Drug InfoNet

http://www.druginfonet.com

Web site that provides information about drugs, diseases, and pharmaceutical manufacturing, as well as links to related sites.

Occupational and Physical Therapy

American Occupational Therapy Association (AOTA)

http://www.aota.org

Professional organization of occupational therapists; provides such services as accreditation of educational programs, professional publications, public education, and continuing education for practitioners.

American Physical Therapy Association (APTA)

http://www.apta.org

Professional membership association of physical therapists, physical therapist assistants, and physical therapy students. Operates clearinghouse for questions on physical therapy and disabilities. Publishes bibliographies on a range of topics.

Oral Health Care

American Academy of Pediatric Dentistry

http://www.aapd.org

National organization representing the specialty of pediatric dentistry. Dedicated to improving and maintaining the oral health of children, adolescents, and people with special health care needs. Publishes the journal *Pediatric Dentistry*.

American Society of Dentistry for Children

http://www.ucsf.edu/ads/asdc.html

Professional organization for specialists in pediatric dentistry. Dedicated to improving the dental health of children through the dissemination of knowledge to professionals and the general public through educational programs, public service efforts, and research. Publishes the *Journal of Dentistry for Children*.

National Institute of Dental and Craniofacial Research

http://www.nidr.nih.gov

Institute dedicated to the promotion of oral, dental, and craniofacial health through study of ways to promote health, prevent diseases and conditions, and develop new diagnostics and therapeutics.

Special Care Dentistry

http://www.SCDonline.org

National organization of dentists, dental hygienists, dental assistants, nondental health care providers, health program administrators, hospitals, agencies that serve people with special needs, and other advocacy and health care organizations. Publishes the journal *Special Care in Dentistry*.

Recreation and Sports

American Alliance for Health, Physical Education, Recreation and Dance (AAHPERD)

http://www.aahperd.org

National organization supporting and assisting individuals involved in physical education, recreation, dance, as well as health, leisure, fitness, and education. An alliance of six national associations. Offers numerous publications.

American Association of Adapted Sports Programs

http://www.aaasp.org

Mission is to enhance the health, independence, and future economic self-sufficiency of youth with physical disabilities by facilitating a national sports movement and assisting communities in creating the best member programs possible for youth with disabilities who wish to compete.

Disabled Sports USA (DS/USA)

http://www.dsusa.org

Offers summer programs and competitions, fitness programs, "fitness is for everyone" videos, and winter ski programs. Local chapters offer activities (e.g., camping, hiking, biking, horseback riding, 10K runs, water skiing, whitewater rafting, rope courses, mountain climbing, sailing, yachting, canoeing, kayaking, aerobic fitness, skiing). Provides year-round sports and recreational opportunities to people with orthopedic, spinal cord, neuromuscular, and visual impairments, through a national network of local chapters.

Girl Scouts of the USA

http://www.girlscouts.org

Open to all girls ages 5–17 (or kindergarten through grade 12). Runs camping programs, sports and recreational activities, and service programs. Incorporates children with disabilities into general Girl Scout troop activities. Published the book *Focus on Ability: Serving Girls with Special Needs*.

International Committee of Sports for the Deaf

http://www.deaflympics.com

Gives a history of accomplishments of deaf athletes. Links to regional confederations and technical delegates throughout the world.

Little League Baseball, Challenger Division

http://www.littleleague.org/divisions/challenger.asp

Online resource provides information and opportunities for boys and girls with disabilities to experience the emotional development and the fun of playing Little League baseball.

National Center on Physical Activity and Disability

http://www.ncpad.org

Encourages and supports people with disabilities who wish to increase their overall level of activity and participate in some form of regular physical activity. Offers searchable directories of organizations, programs, and facilities that provide opportunities for accessible physical activity; adaptive equipment vendors; conferences and meetings; and references to journal articles, books, videos, and more. Provides fact sheets on a variety of physical activities for people with disabilities.

The National Sports Center for the Disabled

http://www.nscd.org

Provides therapeutic recreation programs designed for individuals with disabilities who require adaptive equipment and/or special instruction. Offers summer and winter programs; has some scholarships.

Special Olympics International
http://www.specialolympics.org
Largest organization to provide year-round sports training and athletic competition for children and adults with intellectual disabilities and certain other significant cognitive impairments. Local, state, and national games are held throughout the United States and in more than 150 countries; world games held every 4 years.

Wheelchair Sports, USA
http://www.wsusa.org
Governing body of various sports of wheelchair athletics, including swimming, archery, weightlifting, track and field, table tennis, and air weapons. Publishes a newsletter.

Yoga for the Special Child
http://www.specialyoga.com
A comprehensive program of yoga techniques designed to enhance the natural development of children with special needs.

Transition to Adulthood

Fedcap Rehabilitation Services
http://www.fedcap.org
Services include vocational training and job placement for adults with severe disabilities and/or other disadvantages.

Going to College
http://www.going-to-college.org/
Information for teenagers with disabilities about what college entails and how to plan for it.

Healthy and Ready to Work Information Center
http://www.hrtw.org
Network that works with local agencies to ensure that all youth with special health care needs receive the services necessary to make the transition to all aspects of adulthood, including adult health care, employment, and independence.

I'm Determined.org
http://www.imdetermined.org/
Lesson plans, brochures, and information about teaching self-determinations skills to adolescents with disabilities, with material for parents, youth, and educators.

Institute for Child Health Policy
http://www.ichp.edu
Mission is to research, evaluate, formulate, and advance health policies, programs, and systems that promote the health and well-being of children and youth through applied knowledge to health-related–systems and outcomes for children and youth.

Job Accommodation Network (JAN)
http://askjan.org/
Information and resources to make workplaces accessible to those with disabilities.

National Center on Accessibility
http://www.ncaonline.org
Works with departments of parks, recreation, and tourism throughout the United States to improve accessibility. Sponsors several training sessions each year throughout the United States to educate employers on making their workplaces accessible.

National Center on Physical Activity and Disability
http://www.ncpad.org
Mission of the National Center on Physical Activity and Disability (NCPAD) is to promote substantial health benefits that can be gained from participating in regular physical activity.

National Council on Independent Living
http://www.ncil.org
A national membership association of nonprofit corporations that advances the full inclusion of people with disabilities in society and the development of centers for independent living. Provides members with technical assistance and training, publishes a quarterly newsletter, and sponsors a national conference.

National Gateway to Self Determination
http://www.aucd.org/ngsd/template/index.cfm
Federally funded initiative that has established a model for promoting self-determination and compiled a comprehensive searchable database on interventions.

National Health Care Transition Center
http://www.gottransition.org
Information and tools for health care professionals, state policy makers, families, and youth to assist youth as they transition to adult health care.

National Home of Your Own Alliance
http://alliance.unh.edu/nhoyo.html
This program is dedicated to helping people with disabilities become homeowners and in controlling their homes.

**National Institute on Disability
and Rehabilitation Research (NIDRR)**
http://www.ed.gov/about/offices/list/osers/nidrr
Provides leadership and support for a comprehensive program of research related to the rehabilitation of individuals with disabilities.

**National Rehabilitation
Information Center (NARIC)**
http://www.naric.com
Rehabilitation information service and research library; provides quick-reference and referral information, bibliographic searches, and photocopies of documents. Publishes several directories and resource guides.

Think College!
http://www.thinkcollege.net
Information, activities, and tools for teachers, students, and parents about postsecondary education options for youth with intellectual disabilities.

Index

Tables and figures are indicated by *t* and *f*, respectively.